Primary
Nursing Practice

Primary
Nursing Practice

GLORIA CALIANDRO, R.N., Ed.D.
Associate Professor
Seton Hall University
South Orange, New Jersey

BARBARA L. JUDKINS, R.N., Ed.D.
Associate Professor
Department of Nursing
College of Health
University of Central Florida
Orlando, Florida

Scott, Foresman/Little, Brown College Division
SCOTT, FORESMAN AND COMPANY
Glenview, Illinois Boston London

Library of Congress Cataloging-in-Publication Data

Primary nursing practice.

  Includes bibliographies and index.
  1. Nursing.   2. Medicine, Clinical.   3. Nurse and
patient.   I. Caliandro, Gloria.   II. Judkins, Barbara L.
[DNLM: 1. Primary Nursing Care. WY 101 P9523]
RT41.P852   1988   610.73   87-17072
ISBN 0-673-39731-9

1   2   3   4   5   6   7   8   9   10 – RRC – 94   93   92   91   90   89   88

Printed in the United States of America

Acknowledgments

Pages 209–211: The relaxation exercises are adapted from Patricia A.
Flynn, *Holistic Health: The Art and Science of Care.* Bowie, MD:
Robert J. Brady, Co., 1980. Reprinted by permission.

Photographs by Lori Bennett

This book is dedicated to Dr. Jean Campbell,
former Chairman of the Department of Nursing,
Skidmore College, our friend and mentor

PREFACE

This textbook, *Primary Nursing Practice,* derives from a philosophy of nursing care which departs from that found in most settings today. As described in chapter 1, primary nursing care is comprehensive, client-centered care given by a nurse who acts autonomously and assumes full accountability for the quality of care given. It emphasizes a one-to-one relationship between the client and nurse and continuity of care as long as the client needs it. This is achieved in part through planning and coordinating the efforts of other nurses, health care personnel, family, and other caregivers. Primary nursing, being a philosophy of care, does not depend upon a setting. It may be practiced anywhere at any time.

This textbook focuses on issues and health problems encountered in advanced clinical practice at an undergraduate level and by beginning students at the graduate level. Since this textbook bridges the gap between undergraduate and graduate education, practicing nurses will also find the content useful to their nursing care. The textbook assumes background knowledge of the behavioral, physical, and biological sciences, and also of nursing process. Students and graduates who have mastered first-level nursing skills will find this book valuable in helping them define their role as professional nurses providing primary nursing care to clients and families in a variety of settings. Although the content does not relate to nursing care rendered in intensive, acute-care situations, it does provide the reader with information needed to see these situations in perspective and begin to plan for the long-term care of clients who have little ability to care for themselves.

Unique to this textbook is an approach that provides a framework for primary nursing practice and examines the nurse's role as primary care planner and provider in wellness and illness in various settings. The text explains how to use nursing concepts in practice and covers selected health problems of various age groups from beginning families through old age.

In developing the theme of primary nursing, the editors chose to divide the book into six units. Unit One provides the framework for primary nursing. In chapter 1 the reader is introduced to the philosophy of primary nursing in the context in which it evolved and is continuing to evolve. Chapter 2 presents two concepts foundational to primary nursing—caring and self-care. Nursing is a caring profession that aims to enable others to achieve a higher level of self-care. In order to do this, the nurse must not only have a solid base of knowledge and skills in nursing, but be able to communicate effectively, the subject of chapter 3. Unit One continues with discussions of accountability and quality assurance, legal and ethical issues that the nurse encounters in primary nursing practice, and research. In chapter 8, the reader is reminded of reality as the author discusses nursing in the context of systems. Although primary nursing emphasizes autonomy, the nurse quickly learns that knowing how to function effectively within a system contributes greatly to personal and professional satisfaction and success.

In Unit Two, the reader is exposed to the concept of supporting wellness in communities. One of the major foci of primary nursing practice is to foster wellness and self-care regardless of the setting. The unit begins with assessment of a community and continues with two subjects that illustrate the impact of a community upon the individual—health belief systems and social welfare. In the chapter on nutrition and self-care, the reader is introduced to the role of the nurse in meeting a basic need essential to wellness—food—in the context of self-care. The two chapters on school health and occupational health represent primary nursing practice in distinct types of communities—the school and the workplace. The unit concludes with a chapter on home care, one of the fastest growing segments of health care.

Unit Three develops the idea that primary nursing involves dealing with people under stress and in crisis. The reader is introduced to concepts of stress and methods of stress reduction and to crisis theory and intervention. The unit continues by focusing on one common response to stress and crisis—grief. The following chapters discuss two other situations in which the levels of stress and crisis can be significant—substance abuse and abusive families. The unit concludes with a discussion of cancer nursing, a clinical situation in which the nurse commonly encounters stress and crisis; the authors explore this subject from the standpoint of barriers to care and how to overcome them.

Primary Nursing Practice is based on the belief that nursing is a caring profession that works with clients and families throughout the life span. Units Four through Six deal with content related to the growing family, young adults and middle-aged adults, and the older person. These units aim to illustrate the scope of problems and situations the primary nurse may encounter. Because of the necessary limitations of textbook size, topics are selective.

Subjects such as family planning, working mothers, special families, and the chronically ill child were chosen for Unit Four to illustrate common problems and situations in the growing family. In Units Five and Six, major health problems of adults are discussed with emphasis upon application of the concepts of primary nursing. For example, the first chapter in Unit Six helps the reader acquire a perspective on aging and its problems,

and these problems are then explored in subsequent chapters dealing with diseases that occur primarily in the older person.

Themes developed throughout the book include the nursing process, ethical and legal issues related to nursing practice, and the value of research. Primary nursing practice can provide many fruitful opportunities for nursing research. Likewise, it is an area where application of research findings is necessary for the maintenance and improvement of quality of care. In the development of their chapters, all the authors have based their work upon current research in nursing and related fields.

Finally, this textbook attempts to present an integrated approach to nursing. Content from the major fields of nursing—medical-surgical, obstetrical, pediatric, psychiatric, and community nursing—is brought together within a common framework, that of primary nursing practice. Both students and practicing nurses should gain valuable insights into their own role as health care planners and providers.

G.C.
B.L.J.

CONTENTS

.

UNIT ONE
A Framework for Primary Nursing Practice   3

1. *Introduction to Primary Nursing Practice* by Gloria Caliandro   5

2. *Caring and Self-Care* by Josephine Disparti   17

3. *Communication and Self-Care* by Gloria Caliandro   36

4. *Accountability and Quality Assurance* by Nadine Johnson   47

5. *Legal Responsibilities* by Kathleen M. Nokes   64

6. *Ethical Issues* by Kathleen M. Nokes   80

7. *Research and Nursing Practice* by Jean C. Kijek   90

8. *Negotiating the System* by Barbara J. Stevens Barnum   97

UNIT TWO
Supporting Wellness in Communities   109

9.   *Nursing Assessment of a Community* by Sylviagene Meneshian   111

10. *Health Beliefs in Sociocultural Perspective* by Judith M. Treistman   119

11. *Nutrition and Self-Care* by Josephine Disparti   133

12. *School Health* by Josephine Disparti   151

13. *Occupational Health* by Patricia Moccia   168

14. *Home Care* by Marilyn D. Harris   183

UNIT THREE

Primary Practice in Stress and Crisis   201

15. *Stress and Stress Management* by Alene Harrison   203

16. *Crisis Theory and Intervention for the Nurse
    in General Practice* by Lynn Miller-Seidman   215

17. *Grief and Grieving* by Pamella Hay Hosang   225

18. *Substance Abuse* by Alicia Georges   236

19. *Abuse in Families* by Marjory J. Martin   249

20. *Overcoming Barriers to Primary Cancer Nursing Care*
    by Constance H. Engelking and Nancy E. Steele   266

UNIT FOUR

Primary Nursing with Parents and Growing Families   309

21. *Family Planning* by Linda K. Huxall   311

22. *Breast-feeding* by Nancy Jackson   327

23. *Working Mothers* by Nancy Jackson   349

24. *Older Parents* by Nancy Jackson   362

25. *Special Families* by Nancy Jackson   374

26. *The Chronically Ill Child* by Helen Lerner   380

27. *Sudden Infant Death Syndrome* by Theresa McCoy Clifford   398

UNIT FIVE

Primary Practice with Young Adults and Adults
in Middle Years   411

28. *Caring for Adults with Sexually Transmitted Diseases*
    by Claudette Mobley   413

29. *Adults with Tuberculosis* by Sonya Appel   429

30. *Adults with Hypertension* by Rosemary Collins   447

31. *Adults with Chronic Renal Failure and End-Stage Renal Disease*
    by Marjatta Herranen   470

32. *Adults with Coronary Artery Disease* by Gloria Caliandro   486

33. *Adults with Diabetes* by Carolyn Auerhahn   504

34. *Adults with Human Immunodeficiency Virus Infection
    and Acquired Immunodeficiency Syndrome* by Jo Anne Bennett   522

UNIT SIX
Primary Practice with Older Adults   541

35. *The Older Adult* by Terry T. Fulmer   543

36. *Chronic Obstructive Pulmonary Disease* by Gloria Caliandro   558

37. *Older Adults with Cerebral Vascular Disease* by Joanne Damon   575

38. *Caring for the Person with Arthritis* by Mila Amorin-Nodelman
    and Daisy Cruz-Richman   594

39. *Older Adults with Degenerative Neuromuscular Disease*
    by Joanna Hoffman   615

Index   637

CONTRIBUTING AUTHORS

·

Mila Amorin-Nodelman, R.N., M.S., M.Ed.
Formerly Assistant Professor
College of Nursing
Skidmore College
New York, New York

Sonya Appel, R.N., M.S.
Infection Control Practitioner
Northern Westchester Hospital Center
Mt. Kisco, New York

Carolyn Auerhahn, R.N.C., M.S.
Instructor in Clinical Nursing
School of Nursing
Columbia University
New York, New York

Barbara J. Stevens Barnum, R.N., Ph.D.
Director
Division of Health Services, Sciences, and Education
Teachers College
Columbia University
New York, New York

Jo Anne Bennett, R.N., M.A., C.N.A.
Nursing Consultant and Team Nurse
Departments of Clinical Services and Education
Gay Men's Health Crisis, Inc.
New York, New York

Gloria Caliandro, R.N., Ed.D.
Associate Professor
Seton Hall University
South Orange, New Jersey

Theresa McCoy Clifford, R.N., M.S.
Consultant
Nanvet, New York

Rosemary Collins, R.N., M.Ed.
Nursing Staff Development Educator
Andrus Pavilion, St. John's Riverside Hospital
Yonkers, New York

Daisy Cruz-Richman, R.N., M.S., M.Ed.
Assistant Professor
College of Nursing
State University of New York
Health Science Center at Brooklyn
Brooklyn, New York

Joanne Damon, R.N.C., M.Ed.
Clinical Assistant Professor
School of Nursing
University of North Carolina at Chapel Hill
Chapel Hill, North Carolina

Josephine Disparti, B.N.S., M.P.H.
Manager of Student Programs
National Center for Homecare Education and
    Research
New York, New York

Constance H. Engelking, R.N., M.S., O.C.N.
Adjunct Instructor of Medicine
New York Medical College
Valhalla, New York

Terry T. Fulmer, R.N., Ph.D.
Associate Professor of Nursing
School of Nursing
Columbia University
New York, New York

Alicia Georges, R.N.C., M.A.
Lecturer, Department of Nursing
Lehman College
Bronx, New York

Marilyn D. Harris, R.N., M.S.N., C.N.A.A.
Executive Director
Visiting Nurse Association of Eastern Montgomery
    County
Abington, Pennsylvania

Alene Harrison, R.N., M.S.
Associate Professor of Nursing
Wilkes College
Wilkes-Barre, Pennsylvania

Marjatta Herranen, R.N., M.A.
Formerly Nurse Clinician
Renal Treatment Center
Mt. Sinai Medical Center
New York, New York

Joanna Hoffman, R.N., M.S.N., M.Ed.
Instructor
School of Nursing
Hunter College
New York, New York

Pamella Hay Hosang, R.N., Ed.D.
Associate Professor of Nursing
Department of Nursing
Medgar Evers College
Brooklyn, New York

Linda K. Huxall, R.N., M.N.
Instructor
Nursing Services Division
Tulsa Junior College
Tulsa, Oklahoma

Nancy Jackson, R.N., M.A.
Instructor
School of Nursing
The City College of New York
New York, New York

Nadine Johnson, R.N., M.S.N., C.P.Q.A.
Nursing Quality Assurance Coordinator
North Central Bronx Hospital
Bronx, New York

Barbara L. Judkins, R.N., Ed.D.
Associate Professor
Department of Nursing
College of Health
University of Central Florida
Orlando, Florida

Jean C. Kijek, R.N., Ph.D.
Chair and Associate Professor
Department of Nursing
College of Health
University of Central Florida
Orlando, Florida

Helen Lerner, R.N., Ed.D.
Assistant Professor
Parent Child Nursing
Department of Nursing
Lehman College
Bronx, New York

Marjory J. Martin, R.N., Ed.D.
Assistant Professor
School of Nursing
Fairfield University
Fairfield, Connecticut

Sylviagene Meneshian, R.N., B.S., M.A.
Community Health Staff Nurse
Westchester County Health Department
White Plains, New York

Lynn Miller-Seidman, R.N., B.S., M.S.
Associate Director of Nursing
Hillcrest Hospital
Flushing, New York

Claudette Mobley, R.N., M.A.
Assistant Director of Nursing
Visiting Nurse Services in Westchester
White Plains, New York

Patricia Moccia, R.N., Ph.D.
Associate Professor and Chair
Department of Nursing Education
Teachers College
Columbia University
New York, New York

Kathleen M. Nokes, R.N., Ph.D.
Consultant
New York, New York

Nancy E. Steele, R.N., M.S.N.
Oncology Clinical Nurse Specialist
Northern Westchester Hospital Center
Mt. Kisco, New York

Judith M. Treistman, R.N., Ph.D.
Chair
Department of Parent-Child Health
School of Nursing
Health Sciences Center
State University of New York at Stony Brook
Stony Brook, New York

The support and contribution of Alice Akan
and Christina Gomboschi Wasserman
are gratefully acknowledged

Primary
Nursing Practice

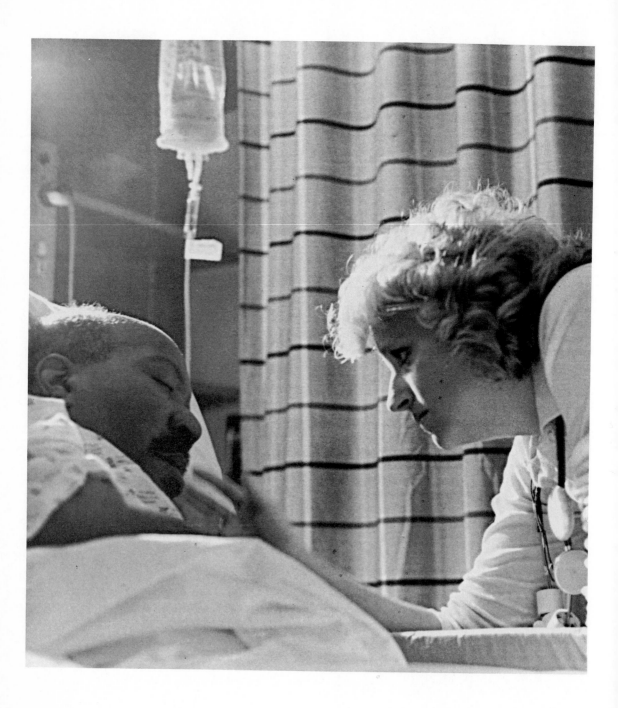

UNIT ONE

A Framework for Primary Nursing Practice

■

In chapter 1 the reader is introduced to the concept of primary nursing practice and, through a discussion of the social and historical evolution of this philosophy of care, is shown how it arrived at its current stage and how it differs from other forms of nursing practice. In chapter 2 the concept of caring and self-care helps to convey the message that nursing is a caring profession that aims to assist others to better care for themselves. Chapter 3 presents an overview of communication as it relates to primary nursing practice. Accountability, one of the criteria for primary nursing practice, is covered in chapter 4. Chapters 5 and 6 deal with legal and ethical issues, respectively.

The subject of chapter 7 is research. The type and quality of care connoted by the philosophy of primary nursing in this textbook require the application of current research findings from nursing and related fields to practice. Primary nursing is also viewed as a source rich in questions suitable for research.

Any evolving form of practice necessarily must deal with the realities of the present. For nursing, this is learning to exist and evolve within systems, the subject of chapter 8, the concluding chapter of this unit.

Introduction to Primary Nursing Practice

GLORIA CALIANDRO

■

OBJECTIVES

After completing this chapter, the reader will be able to:

- Explain the concept of primary nursing.
- Identify characteristics of primary nursing.
- Explain the historical and social context in which primary nursing emerged.
- Explain the relationship between educational preparation and practice environments and primary nursing.
- Describe the responsibilities of individual nurses choosing primary nursing.

Primary nursing is a philosophy of nursing in which comprehensive, client-centered care is given by a nurse who acts autonomously and assumes full accountability for the quality of care given. At the heart of this philosophy of nursing is a one-to-one relationship between client and nurse that promotes continuity of care as long as the client needs care. In order to provide continuity of care, the nurse works with the client, the client's family, and other health care professionals by setting health care goals, either independently or cooperatively, by providing direct care, and by coordinating the efforts of others.

Characteristics of Primary Nursing

Primary nursing is *holistic* care. It begins with the premise that a person is a psychological, physical, spiritual, social, and cultural unity. Consequently problems of one dimension of the person affect other dimensions, and care that focuses on only one dimension will not only be incomplete, but probably also have limited effectiveness. An example that illustrates this point is the case of a woman in her midfifties who was admitted to the hospital for pneumonia. It was winter, and when she arrived at the clinic, she was not only quite dirty but also insufficiently clothed for the weather. After spending a week in the hospital she was discharged. But three weeks later she was back. None of the staff was surprised to see her return. They knew it was highly probable, for the woman lived on the streets. She slept in doorways and ate what few substantial meals she could afford to buy in a local coffee shop. But there were many days when she lived on rolls and coffee. The staff also knew that the woman would return to the hospital several more times before the winter was over because she simply did not have the emotional and financial resources to care for herself. For the previous three years she had been in a mental hospital, but when health care costs soared and budget cuts came, she was discharged to the community to live as best she could with public assistance. The prospect of this woman attaining an acceptable level of physical health is poor until members of the helping professions assist her to deal with her basic problems—poverty, mental illness, and inability to care for herself.

Primary nursing is *individualized* care. It emphasizes the uniqueness of each human being and the need of each human being to be viewed as one of a kind. As William James, psychologist and philosopher, wrote: "There is little difference between one man and another; but what little there is, is very important" (9). It is true that we have a lot in common. Some problems each of us have simply because we are human. And there are solutions to problems that we all use because we have collectively learned that they work. But the fact remains that the way I experience my problems is different from the way you experience yours by virtue of the fact that you are you and I am me. My world is as contained in my perception of my world as is yours. Therefore, when helping a person to solve health problems, it is important for the nurse to remember how differently each of us responds to what we share in common.

Primary nursing is *goal-directed* care that emphasizes the use of the nursing process to help solve client health problems. Recently, while teaching a class on the nursing process to a group of registered nurses pursuing baccalaureate degrees, I stressed the importance of giving nursing care that focuses on solving nursing problems. A member of the class remarked, "But we can't just concentrate on nursing problems. What are we going to do about all the other care the patients need—all the doctors' orders and so forth?"

Although primary nursing emphasizes the solution of nursing problems using the nursing process, it is not limited to that. Comprehensive nursing care can be divided into two broad categories: independent care, which centers on the solution of nursing problems, and interdependent care, in which nurses cooperate with other health care professionals and assist them with the solution of problems outside the scope of nursing. Both categories of care are important, but unfortunately many nurses spend most of their time assisting others while neglecting their independent contributions to client care. Why do they do this? One reason is that others expect them to and assign enough tasks to fill the nurses' time. Another reason is that nurses expect to help others, especially physicians, whose orders give immediate structure to care. But most important is the fact that nurses are only beginning to understand and value what they can do for the client that no other member of the health care team can do—give holistic, client-centered, comprehensive nursing care. We will not be respected as autonomous professionals until we demonstrate to others how important the independent component of nursing is by developing it into an accepted body of knowledge and skills that we use consistently wherever we are. The vehicle by which nurses express the independent component of nursing is the nursing process.

The Nursing Process

The nursing process is systematic problem solving that involves four generally accepted steps. The first is *assessment* of the client's health status. Data are collected from a variety of sources—clients, their families, other health care personnel, and the findings of laboratory and diagnostic tests. The nursing history, which focuses on data related to areas of nursing concern, and the comprehensive assessment of the client, the client's family, and environment are important parts of data collection. But data are meaningless until they are interpreted. Tentative nursing problems or diagnoses are identified and the adequacy of the data for either accepting or rejecting the validity of these nursing diagnoses is determined. If the data are inadequate but diagnoses seem likely, then more data are collected before reaching a conclusion. The assessment step ends with the statement of nursing diagnoses, defined as client health needs and problems that require nursing intervention.

Planning is the second step in the nursing process. For each of the nursing diagnoses identified in the preceding step, the nurse specifies the desired resolution or goal. This is determined collaboratively between the nurse and the client. What do the client and the nurse want to accomplish as a result of nursing care? What do they want the client to be and do today, next week, or several months from now? Collaboration in this step of the nursing process is important because the nurse and the client bring different perspectives to the situation. The nurse sees the situation from the perspective of a professional, whereas the client sees it from the perspective of a person who, at this time, is a recipient of nursing care. Both are valid perspectives, yet the success of

nursing intervention depends on how much they agree on goals.

Immediate, intermediate, or long-range goals may be set for a nursing diagnosis. Whether a goal is labeled one of these depends on the nature of the problem, how quickly it can be solved, the client's abilities and resources, and the client's level of commitment to reaching it. Some diagnoses require only brief, intense intervention, whereas others cannot possibly be solved except with prolonged care. It is important to identify time frames for goal achievement. This helps to sharpen the focus of what nurses do daily and keep down health care costs. It also helps to motivate clients and boost their morale.

Once the goals of nursing care are determined, then strategies for meeting them are selected. This may involve such activities as teaching, counseling, referral, physical care, and therapeutic use of self. The planning step ends with the delineation of care needed to meet nursing goals. The delineation of nursing care, commonly called nursing orders, should be specific enough to communicate to others precisely what is to be done, when it should be done, and by whom it should be done.

Implementation of the nursing care plan is the third step in the nursing process. The nurse may implement the plan of care alone or delegate parts of it to others—for example, the client, another health care provider, or a member of the client's family. When care is delegated, the primary nurse still assumes responsibility for the care and is accountable for its quality. Therefore, it is important to determine in advance whether the caregiver has the knowledge and skills necessary to provide quality care.

The fourth and final step is *evaluation*. Logically, goals should be evaluated, but goals are usually broad and do not easily lend themselves to objective measurement. Thus a first step in evaluation is to translate goals into measurable objectives or outcome criteria. These are usually stated as observable client behaviors, but they may also be other client characteristics, such as decreased redness of the skin. Whatever they are, outcome criteria must be directly related to the goals and should be stated as specifically as possible.

Outcome criteria are evaluated consistently. In an acute care setting, such as a hospital, this may be every shift or every day. In long-term care and community settings this may be every week. Nursing diagnoses and strategies for achieving nursing goals are modified, and the overall quality of nursing care is judged on the basis of outcome criteria evaluation. This evaluation forms an important part of the nurse's progress notes, as it communicates to others the progress that has been made in the independent component of nursing care.

Thinking and the Nursing Process

The type of thinking used most often in the nursing process is vertical thinking. This is defined as analytical thinking in which a person looks at a problem, selects what appears to be the best solution, and then implements that solution. It is an expedient way to deal with problems because the number of possible solutions is limited.

An alternative way of thinking is lateral thinking (5). Instead of looking at a problem and deciding that there is a right or wrong or best way to deal with it, one suspends judgment and thinks of as many alternative solutions as possible. What commonly happens is that one begins to see the problem differently. This can open up a whole array of ideas that would never have been considered if one had moved as expediently as possible toward solving the problem as it was originally defined.

If we accept each person as someone who responds uniquely to the world, then it seems plausible that the way a problem is defined for one person may not be the way that problem should be defined for another. And the solutions that are best for one person may not be best for another. Lateral thinking allows us to consider these possibilities. In an effort to consistently do what is right for clients, nurses may actually do less than they could to meet the individual needs of clients.

There is a place for lateral thinking in the nursing process. It can be invaluable at the steps of problem identification and strategy planning. Although a promising way to solve what seems to be the correct problem is found, it can be profitable to continue thinking and perhaps come up with an even better way of understanding the problem and its solution. Through lateral thinking new and exciting approaches to nursing care can evolve.

Primary Nursing and Client Rights

Primary nursing recognizes the need and the right of the client to participate in care, and thus involves the client in all phases of the nursing process. The importance of this should not be minimized, for clients have a perspective about themselves that no one else can have. Clients can help validate nursing problems, choose strategies for intervention as appropriate, assist in implementing the strategies, and evaluate the effectiveness of care.

Clients' participation in their own care derives from the principle of autonomy. According to this principle, a person has the right to self-determination; to make decisions and to take action based on those decisions (1). There are, however, legal boundaries to this right. A person may not make a decision that, according to the law, infringes on the rights of others. Also, a person may be deemed legally incompetent, and the power to decide may be transferred to another person. For a more detailed discussion of the legal and ethical basis of primary nursing practice, see chapters 5 and 6.

Settings for Primary Nursing

Primary nursing may begin in primary, secondary, or tertiary health care settings. Perhaps some day the American public will have a primary nurse just as it has a family physician, someone who is the principal source of care over an extended period. Ideally the relationship would begin with a healthy, young family and continue as the family matures. But we are a long way from that kind of nursing care. Most primary nursing care today will be initiated in either a secondary health care setting (e.g., a hospital) or a tertiary care setting (e.g., a nursing home). The question then arises, how can we adapt the philosophy of primary nursing care to the realities of the settings in which nurses work? A nurse in a hospital does not follow the client into the community, except in rare instances. Nor does the community nurse care for the hospitalized client. Nurses provide care for specified periods within the context of the setting in which they work. But they can coordinate their efforts to provide continuity of care.

Primary nursing is a viable philosophy of nursing care as long as there is good communication and coordination between nurses caring for a client, regardless of the setting in which the care is given. Care may be initiated by a hospital nurse, with the bulk of care being given in the community by another nurse. Likewise, a community nurse may initiate a plan of care that a hospital nurse modifies during an acute episode of illness. Then when the client is discharged to the community again, the community nurse resumes care. The major difference between this approach to nursing care and that seen most often today is the continuity made possible by communication and by coordination of the efforts of all nurses involved in a client's care.

Early experiments with primary nursing were performed in hospital settings. At that time emphasis was placed on twenty-four-hour responsibility for the care of a group of patients. This certainly did not mean that a nurse gave care for twenty-four hours, but a nurse was responsible for planning and coordinating the care so that quality was assured. To some extent, primary nursing has been stymied because of the confusion about what twenty-four-hour responsibility means. When a physician or social worker cares for a client, he or she assumes twenty-four-hour responsibility but does not provide round-the-clock care. The physician or social worker remains apprised of the client's condition and needs and modifies his or her care as necessary, the emphasis being on continuity of care and working with others to provide this continuity.

Historically, nurses have tended to think in terms of blocks of care, the blocks being the time they are assigned to work. Responsibility ended with the nursing shift, except perhaps for the head nurses and nursing administrators. That is an entirely different perspective in terms of relationship with the client and is incompatible with primary nursing.

Primary Nursing in Perspective

To fully appreciate what primary nursing is and why it is important today, it must be considered from historical and social perspectives. It must be put in the context of where we have been and where we are going in health care.

Florence Nightingale's Contribution

The introduction of modern nursing is credited to Florence Nightingale, who developed her ideas about nurses and nursing on the battlefields of Turkey during the Crimean War (1854–56). It was a difficult time for the British government. The death rate among British soldiers was extraordinarily high, not so much from their wounds as from the care they received once they reached the military hospitals. Journalists, eager to keep the public informed, aroused reformers with their stories of needless suffering owing to substandard care, and the reformers in turn pressured the government into action. Conditions in the hospitals had to be improved.

The British government turned to Florence Nightingale for help, not only because she was a trained nurse in a country where trained nurses were almost nonexistent but also because she was an extraordinary woman. A member of a prominent English family, Miss Nightingale was well educated, well traveled, and well connected in society. She was also a highly capable administrator. Miss Nightingale agreed to go with a small group of nurses to the Crimea. The government gave her its orders, but that is where her problems began. She was to make major changes in the way the army cared for its sick, yet she had no authority to do anything. Every move she made, with the exception of the assignment of her nurses, had to be approved by the military physician in charge. The military did not want Miss Nightingale. She was a woman in a man's world at a time when women, especially those of the privileged class, stayed home and took care of their families. She was an intelligent, capable, determined intruder who rankled medical officers as much as she endeared herself to the enlisted men.

Miss Nightingale accomplished her objectives despite the army. When the army blocked her way, she simply went around it, going to her supporters in England— and she had many there. They backed her with their influence as well as with their money, over which she retained control. Even the chef of a well-known London club joined her at his own expense and completely reorganized the military kitchens so that the food would be edible. The work she did was amazing. It ranged from the most basic services—housekeeping and laundry—to an impressive system of keeping records to yield statistics. Between managing all of these services, she and her nurses gave comprehensive nursing care.

When the war was over and she returned to England, Miss Nightingale established her own school of nursing, although she never actually directed it herself. She had learned a valuable lesson in the Crimea: in order to do what you want to do, you must have authority and control your own money. The Nightingale school was established with funds given to her by supporters and was not controlled by the hospital to which it was attached. Its primary purpose was educating nursing students, not providing staff for the hospital. Teachers either presented classes voluntarily and without remuneration or were paid by the school's own funds. Although Miss Nightingale believed in nurses obeying physicians in medical matters, she firmly believed that no one, including physicians, should have authority over nurses except nurses (10, 11, 16, 19).

Visiting Nurses

One of the earliest practice models resembling primary nursing as we know it today in the United States was developed by Lillian Wald and her colleagues at the Henry Street Settlement on the Lower East Side, New York City, in 1893. In some ways Lillian Wald's biographical profile resembled that of Florence Nightingale. She was intelligent, well educated, and a member of an affluent family. At the time she decided to move to the Lower East Side and establish her nursing service she was a student in the Woman's Medical College of New York. With her friend Mary Brewster, Wald moved into an apartment on the top floor of a tenement on Jefferson Street. She believed that they would have to become part of the community if they were going to be accessible to their clients and provide the kind of care needed—comprehensive, individualized care that encouraged people to help themselves. Teaching, counseling, and management were as much a part of the care the nurses gave as physical care.

One of the remarkable characteristics of Wald's nursing service, which in later years became the Visiting Nurse Service of New York, was that it was developed and controlled by nurses. Although Wald insisted on clients having a physician while receiving nursing care, the care she and her nurses gave was not limited to assisting with or performing those duties delegated by the physician. Their primary objective was to give nursing care. These visiting nurses had a great deal of autonomy and authority (2).

Development of Nursing Education in Hospitals

The single greatest force that shaped nursing throughout the modern era, however, was not nurses, but hospitals. Nursing education began in the United States during the latter part of the nineteenth century in response to the needs of hospitals for a labor force to care for a growing number of clients. The first school, modeled after the Nightingale school in England, was established at Bellevue Hospital in New York City in 1873. Unlike its English counterpart, it was not financially independent and was controlled by the hospital. Providing care was priority and education of nurses, what little there was, was secondary (10).

The nursing staff on a typical unit in a metropolitan hospital in the latter part of the nineteenth and early part of the twentieth centuries consisted of a trained nurse, who functioned as a supervisor and, as time permitted, as a teacher of nursing students, who did most of the work on the unit. Few nurses remained in hospitals after completing their training, as the work was grueling, the pay and status were low, and the nurses had little time for themselves. As one writer described the situation, nurses were little more than cogs in a vast authoritarian labor system (10). Efficiency, economy, obedience, and silent endurance characterized the nurses who succeeded in the system. Consequently nurses left the hospitals as soon as they could and became private duty nurses in the homes of clients who could afford their services.

Team Nursing

During World War II, team nursing emerged in response to an acute shortage of professional nurses, many of whom had gone into military service, and the proliferation of untrained personnel providing care in civilian hospitals. The major responsibility of the professional nurse (often the only one on the team) was to supervise and coordinate the activities of team members—practical nurses, aides, and volunteers.

Team nursing, with its emphasis on division of labor in order to economically and efficiently perform a variety of tasks, exists today. It is not uncommon to find a group of nurses caring for a group of clients where one nurse is designated the medication nurse and another, the treatment nurse. Although efficiency and economy may be accomplished, this model of nursing practice has limitations, the most significant being the relationship between a nurse and a client. No one nurse assumes a primary relationship; therefore no one nurse can be held accountable for the quality of care the client receives. Also, no one nurse can experience the satisfaction of knowing that his or her care made the major difference in the client's well-being.

Modern Primary Nursing Practice Models

The evolution of primary nursing is, in large measure, a reaction of nurses to the limitations of task-oriented, functional nursing, including team nursing, and an expression of their desire to practice nursing in a manner more consistent with current ideas about what professional nursing is.

In 1963 Lydia Hall established a model of nursing practice at the Loeb Center for Nursing and Rehabilitation of the Montefiore Hospital and Medical Center in

New York. That model aimed to address the limitations of existing practice models. Her model emphasized a one-to-one relationship between nurse and client, with the nurse autonomously making decisions about nursing care and assuming responsibility and accountability for the quality of care given over a twenty-four-hour period. This one-to-one relationship began on admission to the Center and ended when the client was discharged (7).

Several years later the University of Minnesota Hospitals in Minneapolis adopted a similar model of nursing called primary nursing. It emphasized assigning a client to a nurse (the primary nurse) from the day of admission to the day of discharge or transfer, twenty-four-hour responsibility of the primary nurse for planning and evaluating care regardless of who gave it, client involvement in care, discharge planning, and communication between care givers (3, 15).

Today's Nurses

Today there are more well-educated nurses than at any point in our history and the number is growing. Whereas in 1977 there were 203,700 nurses with baccalaureate degrees employed in nursing, by 1983 there were 347,100. The number with advanced degrees is even more impressive. Before 1950 there were only fourteen registered nurses with doctorates in the United States. By 1983 there were 3,648 with doctorates and 79,900 with master's and higher degrees employed in nursing (6). These nurses are capable of functioning at a much higher level than in the past, and if a lesson is to be learned from the study of reality shock, it is this: nurses want a practice model more consistent with what they are taught in school—comprehensive, individualized care rendered autonomously.

Health Care Costs

In 1965 Congress legislated Medicare and Medicaid, both of which went into effect in July 1966. Since then the cost of health care to the American public from these two laws has soared, as shown in Table 1.1.

Medicare and Medicaid costs are only part of the problem. In 1970 personal health expenditures in the United States reimbursed by third-party payment were $65.4 billion. By 1983 these costs were $313.3 billion.

In an effort to cope with these soaring health care costs, Congress mandated in 1972 the establishment of

Table 1.1
Medicare and Medicaid Costs* 1970, 1983

Source	1970	1983
Medicare	$7.1	$62.6
Medicaid	$4.8	$32.3

*In billions of dollars

Source: U.S. Bureau of the Census, Statistical Abstract of the United States: 1985, 105th ed. Washington, D.C., 1984.

professional standard review organizations in all states to improve the quality of care and make it more effective. Then, in 1983, the Social Security Law was amended to provide for prospective payment of health care costs through diagnostic-related groups (DRGs). Under this system hospitals receive prospective reimbursement for Medicare patients on the basis of projected costs, including specified lengths of hospitalization, for a number of medical diagnoses. If the client's care can be given at less cost, the hospital may keep the profit. Likewise, if the client's care exceeds allowable costs, the hospital bears the additional expense (17, 18). For additional information about DRGs, see chapter 4.

Cost containment is having far-reaching effects on health care. Clients are being discharged from hospitals earlier and sicker than in the past. The average length of hospital stay in nongovernmental, not-for-profit, short-term general and other special hospitals in 1970 was 8.2 days; in 1983 it was 7.7 days (8). This means that clients are being discharged earlier and with greater needs for nursing care that will prepare them to care for themselves than in the past. The distinction between the acuity and complexity of care given in the hospital and that given in the community is becoming increasingly blurred. Nurses in the community are giving care that in the past was seen almost exclusively in hospitals. And nurses working in hospitals increasingly are being forced to consider the long-term implications of the care they initiate, particularly as it relates to self-management. Never before have nurses in hospitals needed to comprehend the nature and scope of community nursing, and vice versa, and how nurses can work together to deliver comprehensive, long-term care that will achieve a high degree of client compliance as they do now. We have reached the stage in the development of nursing where we can appreciate that nursing is nursing wherever it is practiced.

Consumerism and the Self-Help Movement

Consumerism and the self-help movement reflect public reaction to changes in American society that occurred after the Great Depression of the 1930s. The Social Security Act, passed in 1935, was one of the first pieces of federal legislation that would, in succeeding years, reach into many aspects of Americans' lives, such as housing, nutrition, income support, and health care. As government involvement in areas traditionally reserved for individuals and families grew and industry more strongly affected the quality of goods and services and the environment, Americans responded by reasserting their rights and reviving the spirit of self-reliance. In the area of health care, Americans realized that they could no longer afford to abrogate their personal responsibility for their own health to institutions and groups whose primary focus was care of the sick and injured. The diseases we get and our level of health are determined by the way we live. The women's health movement, hospices, birthing centers, and the patient's bill of rights of the American Hospital Association exemplify some of the directions consumerism and self-help have taken.

From Industrial Power to Information Power

The self-help movement in health care was spurred on by the dissemination of information that people needed to care for themselves. Since the mid-1950s, when satellite communications began, we have been rapidly transforming ourselves from an industrial society to an information society (13). In the past, power resulted from control of industry. Now power is in the hands of those who have information. Medical research has made tremendous progress in the twentieth century. The scope of information available about the cause and treatment of diseases has expanded exponentially. But information is not knowledge until it is presented in such a way that people can understand it. A growing cadre of science reporters is doing that for the American public. Whereas in the past members of the medical establishment were almost the sole possessors of knowledge about diseases, this is no longer true. Americans are becoming increasingly knowledgeable and, as a result, are demanding better care that meets their needs as human beings.

One has only to observe the number of people who are changing their life-styles to appreciate the impact of the self-help movement. More people are exercising regularly, eating better diets, smoking less, and trying to control the level of harmful stress in their environments.

Industries are instituting health maintenance and disease prevention programs for employees, such as physical fitness centers, health screening programs, and self-help groups for those who want to break habits such as smoking. Not only is a healthy employee more productive, but the cost to industry from employee time lost because of illness, as well as from medical and hospital expenses, is reduced.

Changes in Health Care Delivery

Along with the growth in self-care have come changes in how health care is delivered. For centuries, women have had their babies at home with the assistance of midwives. The delivery of babies in hospitals is a twentieth-century phenomenon. Now, with the growing popularity of birthing centers and natural childbirth methods, the delivery of babies is again becoming the natural family experience it used to be, with the family present and midwives in attendance. In death we are seeing a similar pattern. People are increasingly vocal about not wanting to die in the dehumanizing atmosphere of hospitals, surrounded by complex equipment they do not understand and that, in many instances, unnecessarily prolongs life. As a result there has been a marked increase in the number of hospices that offer care to the terminally ill and allow them to die in dignity, surrounded by loved ones, either at home or in hospice facilities.

Women's Rights Movement

Nursing has traditionally been a female occupation in a bureaucratic system dominated by men. With this position have come a number of problems—discrimination in terms of status and income, self-image problems such as low self-esteem and self-confidence, insecurity, inability to be assertive, and a lack of power and autonomy. All this is beginning to change, partially because of the effects of the women's rights movement. In 1966 the National Organization for Women (NOW) was founded for the purpose of achieving full equality for women. Activities of NOW and other women's rights groups include such projects as promoting legislation to stop discrimination against women and to protect their rights, and consciousness-raising sessions to help women become more aware of their potential and how to achieve it.

Women entering nursing today are different not only in terms of how they view themselves but in terms of how they view nursing and what they expect in the work situation. Kelly has observed that "women nurses entering the field are generally more comfortable with the tenets of feminism and see no need to take an inferior role in a profession they have chosen to make a career" (11). They are less willing to enter a bureaucracy in which the decisions are made at the top, without their participation, and in which priorities revolve around getting the work done to meet the institution's needs, instead of around how nurses can provide the kind of care that both satisfies the client's needs and gives the nurses a sense of professional accomplishment.

Primary nursing offers an alternative to the task-oriented care given by nurses with little authority and autonomy in bureaucratic institutions. With its emphasis on holistic, individualized care given on a continuing basis to a client who participates in the care to the extent of his or her abilities, primary nursing should meet some of the goals of society and nurses discussed earlier. But in order to be a significant alternative, it must be implemented on a much wider scale than it currently is.

Zander, observing second-generation primary nursing, wrote that for almost twenty years, primary nursing has been adapting to changes in economy, acuity, case types, personnel, and a developing profession, yet its enormous potential remains relatively untapped nationally. The reason she cites is confusion about how to render operative the central concepts of primary nursing. But she is optimistic for the future. Zander sees primary nursing as an opportunity to redefine and revitalize nursing practice (20).

Practice Model for Primary Nursing

Certain basic assumptions underlying primary nursing differ from other models of nursing practice. These are a collegial relationship between nurses; lateral lines of communication; individual responsibility, accountability, and authority; and decentralized decision making.

In a traditional model of nursing such as team nursing (see Figure 1.1), the relationship between nurses is hierarchical, implying superior and subordinate positions. Communication is basically vertical, especially as it relates to decision making and implementation. Decisions are made and transmitted down the hierarchy from top to bottom. Although responsibility is delegated as decisions move down the lines of the hierarchy, authority and accountability reside with those at the top of the hierarchy.

In the primary nursing model shown in Figure 1.2,

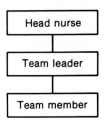

Figure 1.1. Team Nursing Model

the relationship between nurses is lateral. Although one nurse is designated a nurse manager, because there are managerial tasks inherent in any situation where a group of people work together (e.g., staffing schedules and client assignments), the relationship between all of the primary nurses is collegial, which implies relating and communicating across with one another rather than up and down. The primary nurse manager continues to have a client assignment, but it is less than that of the other nurses, to permit time for managerial tasks.

Decision making is decentralized in primary nursing. Primary nurses have the authority to autonomously make decisions related to the care of individual clients. The nurse manager, as well as any other nurse, may help the primary nurse make decisions, but the ultimate decision belongs to the primary nurse.

Determination of client assignments is a collaborative process between the primary nurses. Factors that influence the assignment of clients include the scope and complexity of care required by the client, the primary nurse's expertise in relation to the client's needs, and the probability that the nurse and the client (as well as the client's family) will be able to establish a relationship that will foster comprehensive care. The nurse manager assumes ultimate responsibility for deciding which primary nurse will work with a particular client.

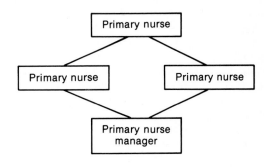

Figure 1.2. Primary Nursing Model

Maintaining a collegial relationship is important to successful primary nursing. With the emphasis on autonomy, one may assume that primary nurses work alone, separate from other nurses. This assumption is inaccurate. A primary nurse, by virtue of the kind of care given—holistic, comprehensive care—is a generalist. In many instances primary nurses will need the help of others to make and implement decisions. This is most often accomplished informally, by sitting down and talking about what is happening. A more formal approach is the client-centered nursing care conference, where primary nurses present and discuss their clients' problems and care. Primary nurses also need a collegial relationship for peer review. Although each nurse is accountable for the quality of care given, as professionals we are expected to assist one another to improve the quality of care by continual peer evaluation. Finally, primary nurses need a collegial relationship for mutual support.

Primary nursing will not emerge as a generally accepted philosophy of nursing that can be translated into a viable model of practice unless it receives support from nursing educators, employers, and nurses. Of the three, educators are probably the most important, for it is through education that a nurse is molded. If the formative period inculcates the essential ingredients for primary nursing, the nurse will be prepared not only to practice it but also to change the health care system to include it.

Socialization Process

Becoming a primary nurse is a process of socialization that begins when the student enters the nursing program. According to Cohen (4), socialization has four goals. Students must (a) learn the technology of the profession—the theory, facts, and skills; (b) learn to internalize the professional culture; (c) find a professionally and personally acceptable version of the role; and (d) integrate this professional role into other life roles. The first goal is primarily reached by exposure to the curriculum. The second goal may be reached in part by the curriculum, in which content related to the values, attitudes, and modes of behaving are presented; however, the most significant influence comes from interpersonal relationships—student-teacher, student-student, and student-nurse. To acquire a culture, one must live a culture. This means being exposed to other people who exemplify the culture on a continuing basis and assist

the student, who is, in essence, leaving one culture behind (the preprofessional culture) and acquiring a new one. The third and fourth goals relate to acquiring a self-identity, both intellectually and emotionally. The attainment of goals one and two contributes to this, but self-identity is accomplished when students internalize all the experiences they have been exposed to and find the meaning of these experiences for them. This interior process transcends what anyone else can do for them.

Leddy and Pepper, in their discussion of the development of the professional self-concept, relate the stages of development to Erikson's stages of the life cycle (12). Erikson identified eight stages that span from infancy to old age. Each stage has a primary task, the accomplishment of which affects development at each succeeding stage. Autonomy, a key concept in primary nursing, is the task to be accomplished at stage two (equivalent to early childhood). If students fail to acquire some degree of autonomy early in their educational experience, all other stages of professional development will be negatively affected. Likewise, if students are in an environment where autonomy is fostered, the mature nurse will be a very different person.

The usual relationship between teacher and student is one of authority figure and dependent learner. This is expected to some extent, yet if it is emphasized too much, students begin to internalize a dependent self-concept. Perhaps the relationship between faculty and students should be redefined as colleagues with differing levels of expertise working together on common problems. In a collegial relationship the contributions of each are valued and respected for their differences as well as for their similarities.

Impact of Primary Nursing
on Institutions

The implementation of primary nursing will have profound implications for the institutions in which nurses work, the most important being a shift from a bureaucracy to a decentralized system of care. This implies a shift in control from administration to the primary nurse and requires an entirely different perception of nurses by administration, one that may be difficult to achieve. As has been reiterated throughout this chapter, administrators generally do not think of nurses as autonomous, accountable practitioners, but tend to think of them as part of the labor force required to meet the institution's priorities.

Staffing patterns will change. Because primary nursing necessitates a well-educated, highly capable generalist in nursing, the nursing staff will be almost exclusively composed of professional nurses, preferably with a minimum of a baccalaureate education. Cost becomes an important factor to consider. Research has shown, however, that primary nursing can be less costly for an institution than team nursing (13).

Role relationships between health team members will change. The head nurse will no longer be the source of information and authority regarding client status and care, for there will be no head nurse. When other health team members want to know something about their clients or request care, they will have to relate directly to the primary nurse who is responsible for those clients.

The nature and scope of nursing practice will change as primary nursing is implemented. The degree to which health care administrations will be willing to accept holistic, comprehensive, client-centered care that fosters self-care and continuity depends on the demands for such care and whether or not it favorably affects total client care costs. This will be an area for negotiation between nurses and administrators. Cost containment is already decreasing the length of hospital stays. The question will be whether or not this type of care can be given in the period of time covered by third-party payment and whether or not it will reduce readmissions for relapses and complications. These areas are fruitful for nursing research.

Primary Nursing Today

Research has shown that nurses respond positively to primary nursing. Not only do they express greater satisfaction when assigned to settings in which primary nursing is practiced, but they also have fewer sick days than do nurses in team nursing settings (13).

As satisfying as primary nursing is, it can also be demanding. Assuming responsibility for comprehensive, holistic care means that nurses will have to keep up-to-date on changes in health care. This requires a commitment to professional and personal development through continuing education, which includes the latest in developments in nursing, medical, and health-related research. Although primary nurses are expected to help one another through a collegial relationship, the burden of preparation for responsibilities assumed resides with the primary nurse. Assuming responsibility for care means that the primary nurse will be a risk taker. No

longer will specified care be delegated; instead the nurse will be responsible for determining the nature and scope of care. Not all care will meet the expectations of clients and peers, exposing the nurse to criticism. Nurses will be able to support primary nursing to the extent that they are personally well grounded and professionally secure, and give mutual support through a collegial relationship.

Primary nursing has the potential for being the nursing system of the future. This philosophy of care is consistent with the aspirations and capabilities of better-educated nurses. Primary nursing is also in tune with the public's needs and desires. People who are increasingly dissatisfied with highly specialized, technological medicine are seeking an alternative that focuses on them as holistic individuals. Primary nursing does this. In a market where there will be increasing competition for clients, this can be one of the most potent factors in its promotion. But implementing primary nursing will require significant changes on the part of educators, employers, and nurses.

REFERENCES

1. Beauchamp, T. L., and J. F. Childress. *Principles of Biomedical Ethics.* New York: Oxford University Press, 1979. Chapter 3.
2. Caliandro, G. "The Visiting Nurse Movement in the Borough of Manhattan, New York City, 1877–1917." Ed.D. diss., Teachers College, Columbia University, 1970.
3. Ciske, K. L. "Primary Nursing: An Organization That Promotes Professional Practice." In *Primary Nursing,* ed. K. L. Ciske and G. G. Mayer. Wakefield, Mass.: Contemporary Publishing, 1977.
4. Cohen, H. A. *The Nurse's Quest for a Professional Identity.* Menlo Park, Calif.: Addison-Wesley, 1981.
5. deBono, E. *Lateral Thinking.* New York: Harper & Row, 1970.
6. *Facts About Nursing 84–85.* Kansas City, Mo.: American Nurses Association, 1985.
7. Hegyvary, S. T. *The Change to Primary Nursing.* St. Louis: C. V. Mosby, 1982.
8. *Hospital Statistics.* Chicago: American Hospital Association, 1984.
9. James, William. "The Will to Believe." In *Bartlett's Familiar Quotations.* 14th ed., ed. John Bartlett. Boston: Little, Brown, 1968.
10. Kalisch, P. A., and B. J. Kalisch. *The Advance of American Nursing.* 2nd ed. Boston: Little, Brown, 1986.
11. Kelly, L. *Dimensions of Professional Nursing.* 5th ed. New York: Macmillan, 1985.

12. Leddy, S., and S. M. Pepper. *Conceptual Bases of Professional Nursing.* Philadelphia: J. B. Lippincott, 1985.
13. Marram, G. "The Comparative Costs of Operating a Team and Primary Nursing Unit." In *Primary Nursing,* ed. K. L. Ciske and G. G. Mayer. Wakefield, Mass.: Contemporary Publishing, 1977.
14. Naisbitt, J. *Megatrends.* New York: Warner Books, 1984.
15. Nehls, D., et al. "Planned Change: A Quest for Nursing Autonomy." In *Primary Nursing,* ed. K. L. Ciske and G. G. Mayer. Wakefield, Mass.: Contemporary Publishing, 1977.

16. Nightingale, F. *Notes on Nursing.* New York: D. Appleton, 1861.
17. Shaffer, F. A. *DRGs: History and Overview.* New York: National League for Nursing, 1983.
18. Shaffer, F. A. "A Nursing Perspective of the DRG World," pt. 1. *Nursing and Health Care* 5:48, 1984.
19. Woodham–Smith, C. *Florence Nightingale.* New York: McGraw-Hill, 1951.
20. Zander, K. "Second Generation Primary Nursing: A New Agenda." *Journal of Nursing Administration* 15:18, 1985.

CHAPTER 2

Caring and Self-Care

JOSEPHINE DISPARTI

•

OBJECTIVES

After completing this chapter, the reader will be able to:

- Analyze the concept of caring.
- List the essential elements of caring according to Mayerhoff, Leininger, and Watson.
- Describe the relationship between caring, self-care, and nursing.
- List the factors that affect a health professional's capacity for caring.
- State some explanations for the therapeutic affect of caring on clients.
- Identify self-care as a basis for the nursing theories of Nightingale, Henderson, and Orem.
- Describe Orem's self-care theoretical framework for nursing.
- Compare the self-care model of nursing with more traditional models and with primary nursing practice.
- Identify significant areas of assessment and intervention that specifically relate to a self-care nursing framework.
- Identify three difficulties, realities, or controversies associated with the concept of self-care.

This chapter considers caring and self-care, two concepts that have particular significance for nurses in primary practice. These concepts are recognized as crucial and timely for both health providers and consumers. The stresses of contemporary life, the current state of the health care system, and the importance of behavioral change in the treatment and prevention of major health problems all point to the need for health professionals to maintain a caring approach and promote self-care on the part of their clients. At the same time there are factors operating that threaten this caring, self-care approach. These factors include an increasing emphasis on technological care, the maintenance of an authoritarian framework for provision of health and illness care, and economic competition with the associated imperatives for cost-effective, quantitative approaches.

Within nursing, the attention and recognition of the importance of the concepts of caring and self-care is, in part, an outgrowth of the attempt of the profession to conceptualize nursing and make nursing's contributions more visible and distinct. Some theorists argue that caring is the essence of nursing; others believe that it is the promotion of self-care abilities in clients that gives nursing its focus and content. These concepts are examined using the work of the major nurse theorists.

The two concepts are considered together because of their congruence and interrelatedness. Indeed, I faced a "chicken-and-the-egg" dilemma in deciding where to begin. Consider, for example, the following syllogism:

Nursing is a caring profession.
Self-care is the basis for caring for others.
Therefore, nurses are self-caring.

Consider further the proposition that self-care is not only the condition of caring but also the object or goal of the caring process. Underlying both concepts is the importance of nursing in helping people develop so that they live more complete, healthier lives and become as self-sufficient as possible.

The Meaning of Caring

There is a long tradition of nursing as a care-giving role. The public has come to expect sympathetic care from nurses; physicians have, at least in the past, written nursing orders for TLC (tender, loving care) and nurses have described themselves as care givers. Until recently, however, nurses have not fully appreciated the importance of this concept. Leininger points out that although nurses have long made claims to the concepts of care and nursing care, we have given the subject little attention.

> Concepts and theories related to caring appear essential to know and to link with ideas related to nursing care. Thus, it is time to focus on caring in research, teaching and practice in order to bring credence and legitimacy to a major implied and claimed concept that has been used in nursing for more than 100 years. (19, p. 7)

Many diverse ideas about caring are reflected in the nursing literature: concern, love, tenderness, compassion, empathy, helping, protecting, and comforting are all examples. In considering various definitions of caring some common themes arise that have to do with the components, purposes, and nature of caring. Three pertinent definitions are:

> Caring is helping another grow and actualize himself, is a process, a way of relating to someone that involves development, in the same way a friendship can only emerge through mutual trust and a deepening and qualitative transformation of the relationship. (25, p. 1)

> Caring is a feeling mandating relationship and because of the nature of the relationship, the feeling compels the caring person to do certain things, complete tasks, and move through given stages. (3, p. 59)

. . . those assistive, supportive, or facilitative acts toward or for another individual or group with evident or anticipated needs to ameliorate or improve a human condition or lifeway. (19, p. 9)

Some key points in these definitions are as follows:

- Caring is a process.
- Caring is commitment to action.
- Caring requires feeling, relationship between people.
- Caring has a purpose, which is the growth, development, or improvement of one or both persons in the caring relationship.

Essential Ingredients of Caring

Leininger (19), Mayerhoff (25), and Watson (36) further analyze caring by identifying the essential elements or ingredients encompassed by the concept. Table 2.1

shows their formulations. Mayerhoff, a philosopher, analyzes the caring process by describing some qualities or abilities that are essential for true caring to occur (25, p. 9).

Leininger studies caring from a nursing and anthropological perspective. By studying the caring phenomena from different cultural viewpoints, she is obtaining knowledge that nurses can use in providing both cultural-specific and cultural universal nursing care. She has identified certain ideas, or "constructs," of caring that are found in approximately thirty cultures (19, p. 13). Leininger points out that there are cultural differences in the perceptions of the care and that different constructs are preferred in different cultures.

Watson believes that the science of caring needs to approach human problems from two directions—the humanities and science—and that the base of the science of caring is formed by the interaction of those two domains. She identifies ten carative factors that she views

Table 2.1
Essential Elements of Caring

Mayerhoff's Major Ingredients of Caring (25, p. 9)	Leininger's Caring Constructs (19, p. 13)		Watson's Carative Factors (36, pp. 9–10)
Knowing	Comfort	Nurturance	Formation of humanistic-altruistic value system
Patience	Compassion Concern	Presence Protective behaviors	Instillation of faith and hope
Honesty	Coping behaviors	Restorative behaviors	Cultivation of sensitivity to self and others
Trust	Empathy Enabling	Sharing Stimulating behaviors	Development of helping-trust relationship
Humility	Facilitating Interest Involvement	Stress alleviation Succorance Support	Promotion and acceptance of positive and negative expression of feeling
Hope	Health consultative acts Health instruction acts	Surveillance	Utilization of scientific problem-solving methods for decision making
Courage	Health maintenance acts	Tenderness Touching	Promotion of interpersonal teaching and learning
Alternating rhythms	Helping behaviors Love	Trust Others	Provision for supportive, protective, and/or corrective mental, physical, sociocultural, and spiritual environment Assistance with human need gratification Allowance for existential-phenomenological forces

as primary and relevant to the science of caring (7, pp. 9–10). Watson points out that the carative factors are developed from a humanistic philosophy and are founded on a growing scientific base.

Although each writer approaches caring from a different perspective, there are remarkable similarities in what they present as basic to the caring process.

All three formulations present *knowledge* of self and others as basic—also, *feeling* for self and others. Each list of essential caring components includes qualities or behaviors that have to do with supporting, trusting, and encouraging another.

The works of Watson, Leininger, and Mayerhoff are strongly recommended for a better in-depth understanding of the caring process. Other sources important to review are from the writings of philosophers, humanistic psychologists, and other health professionals, such as Marcel (22), Teilhard de Chardin (34), Buber (6), Maslow (23), and Rogers (32).

Relationship of Caring to Nursing

How do we currently understand the caring process in nursing? Is the caring process really an essential component of nursing? Leininger has long held the position that "caring is the essence of nursing and the unique and unifying focus of the profession." She maintains that caring provides a "central focus for nursing decisions, practices and goals (18, p. 135)." Watson supports this in her differentiation between nursing's "core" and "trim." "Core" refers to those aspects of nursing that are intrinsic to the actual nurse-client process that produces therapeutic results in the person being served; "trim" refers to the "practice setting, the procedures, the specialized clinical focus, and the techniques and specific terminology surrounding the diverse orientations and preoccupations of nursing (36, p. xvi). Watson points out that although the trim is important, nursing is incomplete when there is an overemphasis on the "trim" to the neglect of the "core." '

Caring, therefore, is put forward as being essential to nursing—the thing without which there cannot be quality, professional, or effective nursing practice. It is useful to consider how closely the key points drawn from the definitions of caring relate to the practice of nursing.

Nursing as Process. Clearly there is agreement in many definitions of nursing that, like caring, nursing is a process that we readily describe as being creative, interactive, open, interpersonal, helping, therapeutic, deliberate, and problem solving.

The similarity between the caring process and the ideal nurse-client relationship can be seen in Figure 2.1. The interlocking circles and the two-directional arrow indicate a reciprocal process occurring, that is, the potential for a "working relationship" within an open, dynamic system. Between the nurse and client there occurs a mutual exploration (action and reaction) in which knowledge, responsibility, and decision making are shared and in which goals and means to those goals are negotiated. The nurse and client are viewed as two separate systems, both with their own unique personalities, abilities, life experiences, and beliefs, engaged in a mutually supportive exchange. The realization that both the nurse and the client have their own values, priorities, and definition of the problem to be solved is especially crucial for nurses practicing within a self-care framework.

The process—this giving and receiving of help—promotes the growth of both persons even though the original purpose of the relationship is the assistance of the client, and the capability for helping is generally greater in the nurse. As Mayerhoff points out, by his use of the term "primacy of the process," it is within the process itself that the growth occurs (25, pp. 1, 31). He indicates that it is the process that is crucial or primary in caring. The growth or development occurs in the present, during the process of caring, and the problem is always how to respond to the person or idea at the moment of interaction. Even in emergencies, or in isolated or rushed encounters with a client, the interaction can be growth producing if it is honest (not manipulative), shows respect for the client's need and ability to participate, and communicates an interest in helping the client.

In caring, the means to an end takes precedence. This

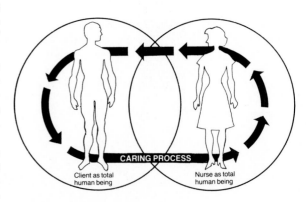

Figure 2.1. The Caring Process

is an important awareness of nurses. It indicates the significance of each encounter with our clients and helps us to explore the ability of nurses to care even when there is no known means to a cure or apparent solution to a problem.

If we contrast this ideal nurse-client process with another situation in which there is limited development or interaction, we discover something similar to the representation in Figure 2.2. The reciprocal, interactive nature of the relationship is replaced by a model that is more authoritarian, one-sided, and disease-centered and that tends to compartmentalize the client's problem and the nurse's helping role. The human dimension is diminished for both the nurse and the client. The only choice the client has is whether or not to comply.

In this model, nursing is a function, not a process, and the nurse is a technical or informational expert, as opposed to a helper, willing guide, and collaborator.

Nursing as Commitment to Action. The commitment to getting something done is fundamental to the profession of nursing. Nursing is conceptualized as action, as assisting the client to cope with or change a situation even when the direction in which to move is not apparent. The practical nature of the art of nursing—the giving of direct care (although usually perceived as physical care), the helping of people to cope with circumstances, and the overcoming of obstacles to care—are well known to the public.

Other health professionals are also concerned with assuring beneficial results in clients, but nursing has traditionally been in the best position by role preparation and philosophy to assume the job of helping the client whatever that helping takes. The current emphasis in nursing education on preparing nurses to be effective change agents and client advocates is a good example of commitment to action.

It is the nurse's knowledge of the client and her or his ability to empathize and enter into relationships that ensure or empower the commitment to action. The possession of a humanistic philosophy and knowledge of human needs, apparent or potential, leads the nurse into a position of involvement and dedication. Caring is the source and, ultimately, the practice of that commitment. "In care, one must by involvement with the objective fact, do something about the situation; one must make some decisions. This is where care brings love and will together" (24).

Watson points out that "primary preventive care occurs when nurses are committed to high-level health and wellness for themselves and others" (36, p. 18).

Nursing as Interpersonal Relationship. In many of our current definitions of nursing, the distinguishing characteristic of nursing is the nurse-client relationship. Interpersonal theory is an integral part of the present-day nursing curriculum. As the relationship deepens (develops by going through different stages), the potential for significant change or therapeutic effect increases (31). The nurse facilitates the development of the relationship by communicating caring through her or his openness, interest in understanding the client, warmth, and honesty. The client learns to trust the nurse and feels secure enough within the relationship to risk change and attempt an alteration in behavior. The interpersonal process is essentially the skill of communication.

The relationship, ideally, provides stimulation, inspires commitment, and gives satisfaction to both client and nurse.

Purpose of Nursing. It may be in this area that we can discern, at last, some separation between caring and nursing. How are the purposes of caring and the purposes of nursing similar to or different from each other? Nursing can be viewed as health caring or caring about another's health; however, we need, then, to consider

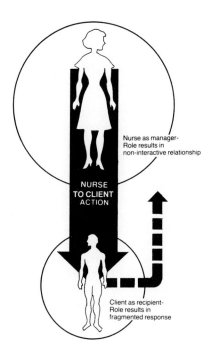

Nurse as manager-
Role results in
non-interactive relationship

NURSE
TO CLIENT
ACTION

Client as recipient-
Role results in
fragmented response

Figure 2.2. Non-interactive Model

what is meant by health. The purpose (goals) of nursing has evolved as we have gone from a clinical definition of health—the return to a homeostatic or asymptomatic condition, adequate role performance, cure of disease—to a broader definition of health—high-level wellness, realization of one's innate potential, coping with stress and change, and dying a peaceful death. We can see that nursing has gone from a physical-comforting, healing art to something that is more holistic, involves the client in different ways, and requires more autonomy and different strengths, abilities, and techniques.

Nursing practice is becoming geared more toward promoting growth, encouraging self-care, and teaching attitudes toward life and health and not exclusively toward physical and skilled technical care or health teaching and supervision. We still help people with their human needs, but we include higher-order needs, such as self-actualization, self-responsibility, and affiliation needs. Our understanding of the wholeness of human functioning has increased, and we are not dichotomizing between levels of need or seeing, for example, the physical aspects of people as separate from their social aspects. Our efforts are directed more at integration, and quality in the nursing (caring) process with clients.

When we define (understand) caring as a philosophy and as a science, it is difficult to distinguish between caring and nursing.

Certainly we can see that for nursing practice to be distinguished as holistic, primary, therapeutic, or high standard, the caring dimension is essential.

Caring, no longer just an inferred process in nursing, is being systematically studied and included in the newly developing conceptual nursing models. One conceptual model for nursing has been developed by Blattner in her book *Holistic Nursing*. The model is built on the work of E. O. Bevis (3), who provided six (of Blattner's nine) life processes that she thought were essential in nursing to help clients achieve optimal wellness. Blattner states that

> the goal of nursing is to use preventive, nurturative, and generative activities to assist clients towards achieving their own high level wellness. This is done by purposefully utilizing the nine life processes of self-responsibility, caring, stress, lifestyling, human development, problem solving, communication, teaching/learning, and leadership and change with self, client, and community. (4, p. 22)

The three life processes added by Blattner are caring, life-styling, and self-responsibility.

Factors That Affect the Capacity for Caring

It is important for health professionals to identify the factors that affect the capacity of human beings to care for others.

The following is a brief consideration of five significant areas:

1. one's personal philosophy,
2. predisposition of humans to be caring,
3. general growth and development of the person,
4. deliberate effort and study, and
5. setting in which care is given.

The Importance of Examining One's Philosophy. "In harmony with our own core of deepest values, we reach out to care for each other and our world" (16, p. 2).

If the practice of nursing depends on a caring ideology, it is evident that care givers need to examine their personal beliefs and values to determine if they are compatible with a caring and self-care philosophy. Two major points can be made.

Human actions are affected by our beliefs. Nursing actions are guided by nurses' philosophies about the human condition, the nature of human beings, and their capabilities. It follows, therefore, that if we wish to choose our actions rationally, so that they will be therapeutic, or have a positive affect on others, we need to be aware of our views and values. Failure to recognize our values could result in our practicing inappropriate caring (meeting our own needs rather than the client's) or our succumbing under pressure to dehumanizing practices.

A clear understanding of our philosophy helps us by guiding our practice according to personal and professional standards. It helps us make the moral and ethical decisions required in our clinical practice with clients. We can better recognize and respect the values of our clients when we are clear about our own values and beliefs. (Some hospitals have found it necessary to employ philosophers to help health professionals clarify the moral and ethical issues that arise in practice.)

An awareness of our philosophy gives us direction, a sense of security and acceptance that our interventions (or our doing nothing) have meaning and purpose for ourselves and our clients. We are better able to accept the decisions that clients make about themselves because we recognize that they may be based on values that are different from our own and because we know that the right to make those decisions belongs to the client. For many clients the quality of life may be a greater value than life or health in itself. Self-determination or body integrity may be a more significant moral consideration than prolongation of life (9). Acceptance of these differences of values between people enables a nurse to help clients make their own decisions and to uphold their rights even when they refuse needed treatment.

The following beliefs are compatible with a caring and self-care philosophy:

- The individuality of human beings is respected: the diversity of human beings is appreciated.
- The dignity and worth of the person is recognized: human actions are aimed at preserving and nourishing that worth.
- Human beings are whole beings with the components of mind, body, and spirit: holistic care is deserved and indicated.
- Life is precious: there is meaning and purpose to human existence.
- Human beings have a basic need to strive toward the realization of their full potential: there is considerable strength and potential for growth in each of us, despite negative conditioning.
- Human beings are rational: we have the ability and desire to act on our own behalf.
- Human beings are more similar than different: we are capable of understanding and helping one another.
- To care for others and to be cared for are basic human needs: people want to care for themselves and others.
- People have the right to make decisions about their bodies, their health, and even their lives: we assume the responsibility for those decisions.

Our Genetic Predisposition to Be Caring. There is a good deal of controversy about the relationship of genes to caring. According to Willard Gaylin, caring is a biologically programmed impulse essential for the survival of the human species. He says, "In all probability, the capacity for caring is part of the innate directive in our genes—the nurturing environment will simply allow it to emerge" (13, p. 98). We recognize this as the "nature versus nurture" debate, with a vote for nature. One anthropologist points out the significance of the choices we make in our attempt to understand humankind's ultimate nature:

We can opt for a number of perspectives drawn from theology, economics, philosophy, politics, biology, anthropology, sociology, psychology and

the harder sciences. It is these choices, made within a multiplicity of cosmological systems, which serve to elucidate the nature of man generally and human caring specifically. Man's morality was created by reason. Human genes have surrendered their primacy in human evolution to culture, and, to paraphrase Morley, while our genes may predispose us to speak, they do not tell us what to say. (26, p. 156)

General Growth and Developmental Experiences. The capacity for caring is primarily developed by experiences in childhood, within the nurturing environment of the family. At various stages and through changing forms of attachment and identification with caring adults, the growing child learns caring and gradually reduces his or her dependence on the caring "models" to become a person capable of caring for others.

Many of the abilities essential in the caring process are learned as we develop—our capacity to trust, to share, to achieve intimacy with others. Our moral development, social and cognitive achievements are all crucial for the understanding, commitment, and interpersonal skill required in caring for (helping) others. Nurses who have achieved a high degree of personal development will have the psychological maturity, the personal resources and sense of competency within their profession to enable them to help others develop.

Mayerhoff speaks to the need for care givers to have certain behavioral experiences. He suggests that caring begins with self-growth. "Only the man who understands and appreciates what it is to grow, who understands and tries to satisfy his own needs for growth, can properly understand and appreciate growth in another" (25).

A good example of how society affects our evolution into caring roles can be seen when we look at our sex-related roles. In the United States neither men nor women have learned to "care" properly; one sex has learned to give care and the other has learned to expect or receive care. It is good that this is changing. (Leininger notes in her studies how frequently the majority of cultures prescribed caring roles to women.)

We know all too well that the capacity for caring can be damaged or limited because of negative societal, cultural, and interpersonal experiences. In our clients we see much evidence of how the inability to care or be self-caring leads to abusive and violent actions against self and others.

Deliberate Effort and Study. Health professionals could improve their capacity for caring by deliberate effort to gain knowledge, skills, and experiences relevant to caring.

What areas are important to study? to analyze? The works of Mayerhoff, Leininger, and Watson suggest three areas: philosophy, anthropology, and the humanities.

Using Mayerhoff's ingredients of caring, one could analyze one's abilities in each of the eight areas to determine one's strengths and weaknesses. One might decide to work on an area of weakness, for example, patience. (Another author, Burnside, suggests that care givers analyze their philosophy of caring in three areas taken from existential philosophy: commitment, responsibility, and I-thou relationships [7, p. 10].)

Leininger points out the relevance of the study of culture to caring. She notes that care givers need to be in touch with their own preferred ways of expressing and receiving caring so that they can compare these ways with those of their clients. Cultures differ in understanding and expressing caring, and health professionals need to know this aspect of themselves and their clients in order to give appropriate, acceptable care (18, p. 138).

Watson stresses the importance of study of the humanities in the humanizing of one's values.

> Studying the humanities encourages the freeing of one's thoughts about and perceptions of people from different cultures. A foundation for empathy is laid as one becomes aware and appreciative of different ideas, tastes and divergent views of life, death, and the world in general. (36, p. 20)

Humanistic values and altruistic behavior can be developed through consciousness raising and a close examination of one's views, beliefs, and values. They can be further developed through, for example, experiences with different cultures, early experiences that have aroused compassion and other emotions, study of the humanities, literary and artistic experiences, value clarification exercises, and personal growth experiences (e.g., meditation and therapy).

A useful exercise for nurses who want to critique their individual caring behavior is to determine which clients they care about (in the sense of being committed to helping them and promoting their growth) and which clients they have difficulty caring for or helping. The underlying issues, once understood, would be more amenable to resolution. The nurses could examine their beliefs, behaviors, and feelings to determine how they promote or inhibit caring. Recognition of one's negative reac-

tions—such as dislike, confusion, fear, anger, repulsion, inadequacy—would be a first step in understanding the feelings that inhibit caring. It helps to objectively (scientifically) understand the person's behavior as (a) having developed and (b) serving some purpose for the person. Then what is ultimately done in a situation would be based on a less biased value system and on "objective" knowledge. At times the would-be care giver needs to admit his or her inability to help in a particular situation. Then caring might take the form of sending a client elsewhere.

Such self-knowledge would help a person choose the area of work that will give him or her the most satisfaction.

The Setting in Which Care Is Given. Setting can be viewed as anything ranging from the employing institution all the way to the societal environment. A setting can encourage or discourage caring. There may be pressures on nurses to conform in certain ways, and institutional sanctions against caring practices may be operating. Even good, caring people do noncaring things in noncaring settings. Nurses are just beginning to expect employing institutions to provide a supportive working environment that will permit the nurses to provide humane care. Nursing administrators are increasing their efforts to encourage, support, and "operationalize" the philosophy of caring. For example, one agency established the following criteria in their institution's statement of standards:

- Subscribe to a philosophy of service to whole persons.
- Have a statement of rights that is shared with patients and families.
- Maintain an administrative style that promotes communication, collaboration, innovation, and flexibility.
- Maintain a staff-patient ratio that promotes optimal patient/family care.
- Maintain an ongoing program for evaluation of care that includes input from both consumers and providers.
- Respect the physical and emotional needs of staff members.
- Foster the professional development of staff.
- Maintain a physical environment that is conducive to well-being. (30, p. 20)

The health care system itself can be viewed as a setting that affects one's capacity to be caring. Our institutions, professional practices, treatment modalities all influence the possibilities for producing growth in our clients. We recognize that much of our conventional health care is (a) not growth producing and (b) not supportive of care givers.

Often nurses do not receive support from other professionals when they adopt a caring approach toward clients. Support from co-workers is especially important because of the demanding, risk-taking nature of caring. It involves opening oneself to another; therefore, the emotional risks can only be attempted in a supportive environment. Unfortunately many health care settings are extremely stressful. There are staffing shortages and organization of care by tasks (fragmented care), and often practices are more technical than humanistic. Sufficient provisions for nurses to relax, become regenerated need to be made by health care employers.

How Does Caring Produce Beneficial Results in Clients?

How does caring help people? Studies in the fields of science and the humanities are attempting to provide explanations.

There are many sources in the literature about methods that nurses use to help their clients. These usually include teaching, counseling, direct services, providing emotional and social support, effecting environmental changes, and advocacy functions. The following ideas are an attempt to reflect on the caring dimension within those basic helping methods.

A Truly Caring Relationship, by Its Very Nature, Increases the Chances of Success. Because the nurse is open to real information and is sensitive to the client, she has the benefit of the client's honest contribution of information about a situation and how to remedy it. With more knowledge of her client (better data base), the nurse is more likely, with the help of the client, to make a correct assessment of needs and effective solutions. Furthermore, the relationship provides the energy to work at a problem, and it is resilient enough to withstand difficulties that necessarily arise. Anything attempted within that relationship will be more effective, more authentic. It is a relationship that maximizes the contribution of each partner. It has strength, energy, and flexibility. It is based on honesty and cooperation.

Caring Affirms the Other's Potential. When a nurse demonstrates caring in such ways as careful listening, acknowledging individual qualities, putting forth effort on behalf of the client, focusing on strengths, and indi-

cating appreciation of the client, one of two reactions occurs in the client. The positive information and feeling are received and incorporated into the client's feeling about himself—that is, the client's feeling is affirmed or strengthened—or the caring is perceived as being undeserved and not in keeping with the client's own belief or feeling about himself. In an attempt to reconcile this difference an "emotional dissonance" may result whereby the client searches for qualities within himself, and in so doing learns to recognize and accept the potential within himself.

The client who is a recipient of genuine caring may act in her own behalf out of a sense of obligation and gratitude for the nurse's effort—even out of lethargy—and may, in the process, learn a new behavior or discover new information that results in a real change or increased motivation. In this way the nurse creates a learning experience in caring that may help that client to care for herself and for others.

The nurse's belief and confidence in the client helps the client to have confidence in himself or herself. People often lack self-confidence and underestimate their capacity for change; they don't recognize their own resources.

Clients, like everyone else, need someone to give them encouragement, to acknowledge their effort, and to share (lend meaning to) their accomplishment.

We get our sense of self-worth partly from others' perceptions of us. If clients are treated as capable, trustworthy, and valuable, they often begin to feel that way about themselves. The positive reflection of a person's worth and potential may be especially needed to counterbalance negative feedback from the person's environment.

Caring Provides Essential Social and Emotional Support. Evidence from the social sciences is mounting regarding the importance of social relatedness to a person's physical health state. Health services are geared almost entirely to people as physical beings, not whole social beings. Increasingly, attempts are being made to understand the interrelationship between the physical and the behavioral sciences. Some of the findings in this emerging trend indicate that interpersonal interactions can influence physiologic responses and that social supports can modify disease susceptibility.

We have always known that emotional and psychological support is needed to sustain people in times of crisis, life tragedy, and acute and chronic illness. The emotional support sustains a person by compensating for some temporary lack of strength or coping ability.

A supportive, caring environment allows the person's own capacities to emerge and permits the client time for recuperation. Without such support the person is less able to take necessary action and may cease to function in her or his own behalf.

Many people are without a single, caring person to break their isolation and keep them in touch with reality. Having a caring nurse may provide the only relationship, the only supportive network to help a person cope with stressful life events and decrease susceptibility to illness. A goal of nursing intervention may be to help the client develop attachments and achieve better relationships with others.

In the area of primary prevention, people may need support to give up some satisfying but harmful health habits or to attempt some new behaviors intended to increase their level of wellness. This is the area of challenge for the future—how, through a caring nursing practice, to promote high-level health and self-care practices. We need to learn how to motivate people to change habits, to better understand how long it takes for people to succeed in changing their behavior, and to recognize factors that affect susceptibility to change and that determine health behavior.

Caring Promotes Mental States That Have a Healing or Therapeutic Effect.   Caring attempts to promote positive attitudes and is based on a belief system that positive things are possible. Nurses know how important it is to promote a sense of well-being in their clients. Clients prefer care givers who use humor or in some other way make them feel good. Recreational and other programs that encourage creativity and pleasure are desirable for people of all ages. A positive mental state makes people more likely to view themselves favorably and disposes them to take positive action.

There is considerable study and application of the proposition that mental states have substantial influence on our health. It is believed that, in the relationship between emotions and biochemistry, if negative emotions have negative effects (constriction of blood vessels, flooding of the endocrine system), then positive emotions, such as hope and optimism, should have a positive effect. (Norman Cousins has written about his success at self-healing using positive emotions [8].) Research is currently being conducted on brain sciences as they relate to healing, on therapeutic benefits of laughter, on the use of sound therapy, and on the intrinsic analgesic systems of the body (endorphins). We know people can learn conscious control over biological processes (biofeedback technology), and we have long

recognized the positive effects of placebos and hypnosis. There will probably be much study and experimentation in this area in the future. Much attention, for example, is being given to such healing methods as therapeutic touch and holistic approaches to care.

Looking back at the ingredients of caring as set down by Mayerhoff, Leininger, and Watson, one can see how many of the elements of caring are positive and meant to promote positive emotions in others—trust, hope, and faith, for example.

Caring may result in positive effects that are indirect. For example, a person who feels cared for may relax enough to gain benefits from other activities, such as taking nourishment or resting. Medication and specific treatments may be more effective as well if a person is in a state of mental and physical relaxation.

Caring Results in Finding Concrete Resources and Tangible Solutions.   In the process of caring, some real opportunities for change may be discovered. Options may be found through a counseling approach or an investigation of community resources. People may be directed to such growth activities as classes, self-help groups, and job-training programs. Helping someone to improve his or her housing conditions or to meet eligibility requirements for health insurance or income maintenance and food allowance is another way of demonstrating caring. When concrete help is pivotal to the welfare of the client, a caring person can be an essential, crucial resource. This requires patient and persistent effort by both nurse and client to successfully find and use community resources.

A negative spiraling of events can often be prevented. Intervention in crisis is a particularly important time of need and opportunity for the care giver. The care giver must have enough knowledge, however, to be able to anticipate the need for intervention and enough concern to try to change circumstances.

One major goal or purpose of the caring process is the promotion of self-care in clients.

The Concept of Self-Care

There can be little doubt that power is of overriding concern to human beings. It may be man's most central concern. What he is able to make happen by his own will and his own action determines the quality of his life, indeed his very existence. His belief in his own ability to stay alive, to meet his basic needs, to make real at least some of his hopes, to nourish and raise his children—these are a direct reflection of his perceptions of his own power in the world.

And the absence of power is terribly destructive. (12)

The self-care conceptual model has much appeal to nursing as we move away from a medical model perspective. It is closer to a nurse-directed nursing practice, makes explicit the purpose and value of nursing actions, and is extremely relevant to current health care needs. Whether it is in the area of health promotion or care in illness, people increasingly need to recognize the relationship of their actions and life-style to their health. The opportunity for nursing to be helpful is clear. People are becoming more knowledgeable about risk factors, more concerned about noxious agents in the environment, and increasingly dissatisfied with a highly technical, impersonal, and disease-oriented care system. Many are looking for alternative (and more health-enhancing) ways of caring for themselves. Many others, who are not aware that better states of health are possible, could be taught and encouraged to live in a more healthful way. The self-care model offers an opportunity to fully consider primary prevention. Nursing has a philosophy, knowledge base, and clinical approach that makes it well suited for the challenge of promoting healthful practices and self-care ability in people. Much is being written about self-care—as a concept, a theoretical nursing framework, and a consumer movement.

Levin and Katz define self-care as a "process whereby a layperson functions on his/her own behalf in health promotion and prevention and in disease detection and treatment at the level of the primary health resource in the health care system" (21, p. 44).

Nursing Theorists and Self-Care

The Concept of Self-Care Within Nursing. The concept of self-care, like that of caring, has traditionally been inferred and practiced by nurses since the beginning of organized nursing in the United States. Florence Nightingale's major focus was on the client's environment. She also stressed disease prevention and health promotion and described nurses as health teachers. She believed in the principle that people are responsible for their own health and, with the proper information and conditions, would care for themselves. Also inherent in her writings is the position that it is nature, not medicine, that is curative or promotive of health. In her famous *Notes on Nursing* she defined nursing as "that care that puts a person in the best condition for nature to restore or to preserve health and to cure illness" (28). She believed that nurses should focus on two things: educating the client and providing an environment conducive to health. In this way nature, in conjunction with the person's healthful practices, would act on behalf of that person.

Public health nursing is sometimes credited with originating the practice of promoting self-care. In that area of nursing the emphasis has been on helping the patient and the family to care for themselves by teaching, demonstrating the care, and helping people find and use community resources that would increase their self-sufficiency. Community health nursing is currently a field of nursing that is especially qualified to promote self-sufficiency, independence, and health.

Of the many nursing theorists who have defined the basic nature and practice of nursing, a few have presented the self-care dimension as essential. Two such theorists are Virginia Henderson and Dorothea Orem. Both see nursing as assistance with human needs and the promotion of self-care capacity. Henderson, in her definition/concept of nursing (Figure 2.3), stated that:

the unique function of the nurse is to assist the individual, sick or well, in the performance of those activities contributing to health or its recovery (or to peaceful death) that he would perform unaided if he had the necessary strength, will or knowledge. And to do this in such a way as to help him gain independence as rapidly as possible. (15, pp. 15–17)

She identified the following fourteen components of nursing care that the nurse either helped the client perform herself or himself or provided conditions under which the activities could be successfully performed:

1. Breathe normally.
2. Eat and drink adequately.
3. Eliminate body wastes.
4. Move, and maintain desirable postures.
5. Sleep and rest.
6. Select suitable clothing—dress and undress.
7. Maintain body temperature within normal range by adjusting clothing and modifying the environment.
8. Keep the body clean and well groomed, and protect the integument.
9. Avoid dangers in the environment and avoid injuring others.

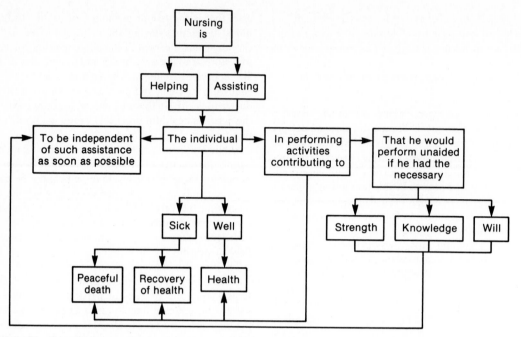

Figure 2.3. Dominant Themes in Henderson's Concept of Nursing; Formalization of Patient Agency Theme and Subsumption of Health Themes

Source: Dorothea Orem, ed., *Concept Formalization in Nursing: Process and Product.* The Nursing Development Conference Group. 2nd ed. (Boston: Little, Brown, 1979), p. 89.

10. Communicate with others in expressing emotions, needs, fears, or opinions.
11. Worship according to one's faith.
12. Work in such a way that there is a sense of accomplishment.
13. Play or participate in various forms of recreation.
14. Learn, discover, or satisfy the curiosity that leads to normal development and health and the use of the available health facilities (15, pp. 15–17).

The orientation of some of these components is clearly holistic and growth producing.

Dorothea Orem's Concept of Self-Care. Orem's framework emphasizes the self-care dimension of human functioning (Figure 2.4). She believes that human beings have the innate ability to care for themselves and that therefore, self-care should be the focal point of the nurse's thinking and behavior. According to Orem, "nursing has as its special concern the individual's need for self-care action and the provision and management

of it on a continuous basis in order to sustain life and health, recover from disease or injury, and cope with their effects" (29, p. 6).

Self-care is defined by Orem as the practice of activities that people initiate and perform on their own behalf in maintaining life, health, and well-being.

Three types of self-care requirements ("requisites") are described by Orem: universal, developmental, and health deviation (29, p. 41).

Universal self-care requisites are common to all human beings during all stages of the life cycle, adjusted to age, developmental state, and environmental and other factors. They are associated with life processes and with the maintenance of the integrity of human structure and functions.

The *universal self-care requisites* common to all human beings are as follows:

· Maintenance of sufficient intake of air
· Maintenance of sufficient intake of water
· Maintenance of sufficient intake of food
· Provision of care associated with elimination processes and excrements

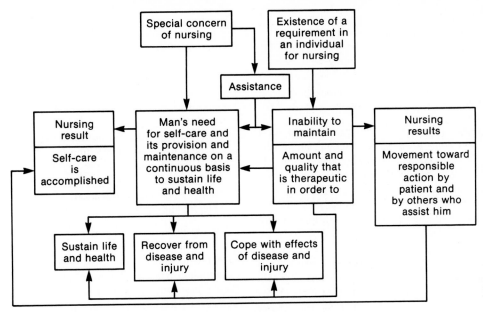

Figure 2.4. Dominant Themes in Orem's Concept of Nursing; Formalization of Term *Self-Care*

Source: Dorothea Orem, ed., *Concept Formalization in Nursing: Process and Product.* The Nursing Development Conference Group. 2nd ed. (Boston: Little, Brown, 1979), p. 90.

- Maintenance of a balance between activity and rest
- Maintenance of a balance between solitude and social interaction
- Prevention of hazards to human life, human functioning, and human well-being
- Promotion of human functioning and development within social groups in accord with human potential, known human limitations, and the human desire to be normal (29, p. 42)

Developmental self-care requisites are associated with human developmental processes, and with conditions and events occurring during various stages of the life cycle (e.g., prematurity, pregnancy) and events that can adversely affect development.

Health deviation self-care requisites are associated with genetic and constitutional defects and human structural and functional deviations, and with their effects, medical diagnosis, and treatment.

In each of these three areas (universal, developmental, and health deviation) self-care practices, actions, and abilities are examined to determine the degree to which the client is self-caring. Health deviation and therapies are examined in order to list the additional "therapeutic" demands placed on the client owing to the disease

process, disability, diagnosis, and treatment. The client's ability or potential for meeting these additional demands are also assessed. Any inability of the client to perform any of the types of demands is called a *self-care deficit*. It is the presence or absence of self-care deficits that determines if and what kind of nursing care is required. Nursing, then, is a "mediating" system that complements or overcomes self-care incapacities. After the deficits in universal, developmental, and therapeutic self-care abilities are identified, specific nursing systems are designed and implemented.

Three types of nursing systems are described by Orem. They reflect the varying roles assumed by the nurse and the client in the performance of health care activities.

1. *Wholly compensatory*—in this system the client has no active role and the nurse acts completely for the client. An example would be a client who is in a coma or otherwise incapacitated physically and/or mentally.
2. *Partly compensatory*—both the client and the nurse perform care measures but the distribution of responsibility varies with the patient's actual limitations, the client's readiness to learn or

perform certain activities, and the degree of knowledge and skill required for the activity.

3. *Supportive-Educative*—the client is capable of performing self-care or of learning how to but needs some assistance such as guidance and support, teaching, periodic consultation or attention to environmental factors. (29, p. 96)

The nursing systems use five basic methods of assistance: acting or doing for, guiding, teaching, supporting, and providing a developmental environment (29, p. 61). A given client may require different nursing systems as her or his condition or situation changes. Several articles have been written by nurses that apply Orem's theories to client care in different settings, with different conditions, stages of illness, diagnosis, and developmental periods.

For example, Barbara Bromley applies Orem's theory in her work as a hospital enterostomal therapist. She traces her care of one client, John, from preoperative counseling to discharge, showing how she revised Orem's three nursing systems (wholly compensatory, partly compensatory, and supportive-educative) based on the patient's changing needs, abilities, and readiness to engage in self-care.

A few days after the patient's surgery for cancer, in which a colostomy was prepared, Bromley discusses a period in which a partly compensatory nursing system was indicated: "John and I performed care together. As he grew stronger, I introduced new information and the necessary skills. Even though he didn't participate while I irrigated his colostomy, he was beginning to absorb what he would later need for self-care" (5).

Importance of Assessment

The process of assessment in self-care is essentially the same as that which most nurses use in the problem-solving (nursing process) method. The data base (client profile) is gathered by history taking; physical, mental, and emotional examinations; and consideration of laboratory results, known health problems, and so on. What is different is the deliberate, conscious focus on the client's self-care abilities and needs. The data base is examined to determine the client's physical, mental, emotional, and motivational capacities.

The data are analyzed to determine how the client's mental, physical, psychomotor, and psychological states affect his ability to decide and act in his own behalf.

Evaluate the client in the following specific areas:

- Self-concept
- Cognitive abilities
- Sensory function
- Learned skills
- Dexterity, coordination, and motor function
- Coping patterns
- Self-discipline and problem-solving ability
- Definition of health and knowledge of factors necessary to maintain health
- Type and availability of support systems
- Readiness to participate in health planning and care—degree of insight, recognition of need, or desire to change (motivation)
- Health and life goals

For example, a mental status examination will yield information about the person's self-concept and ability to make judgments and solve problems. A physical examination will give the nurse information about the client's psychomotor abilities and physical limitations. The client's diagnosis and life stage give pertinent information of special therapeutic or developmental needs.

Application of Orem's Treatment of the Person. A given client would be assessed for needs and abilities in each of Orem's areas of self-care requirements. An older adult with chronic obstructive pulmonary disease (COPD) would have, for example:

(area of universal self-care) deficit in sufficient air intake because of physiological changes in the pulmonary system with COPD
(developmental) needs owing to age and life cycle stage
(therapeutic self-care) client will have responsibilities related to diet, medication, and activity

Self-Care Concept Applied to Family and Community. Nurses can, and do, use self-care theory in working with families and communities. The underlying philosophy, principles, and methods are similar to those used with individual clients. Within the self-care philosophy the family (or community) is viewed, similarly, as having the capacity, desire, and responsibility for maintaining itself and developing in beneficial directions. The role and goal of the nurse would again be similar: to increase the self-competence of that family or community by a facilitative, assistive process dependent on the participation and collaboration of the family (community).

Assessment of the family and community could follow the method outlined by Orem. Viewed as units of service, the family (or community) can be assessed as to its structure, dynamics, stage of development, the presence of special needs, and the degree to which it functions successfully. With adequate conceptualizations of what constitutes a "healthy" family (community) and appropriate assessment tools, the nurse could assess capabilities and needs of the family (or community) in areas corresponding to Orem's universal, developmental, and therapeutic self-care.

Using standard family and community assessment tools, focus would be placed on the self-care dimension of the data base. For example, is the communication system in a family (or community) conducive to self-care action?

Comparison of Self-Care Model with a More Traditional, Medical Model

Significant differences exist between nursing practice in the two models. One major difference is the role of the nurse.

Lucille Kinlein, an independent nurse practitioner, defines nursing as assisting persons in self-care practices according to their states of health (17). She views the nurse as an extension of the client, not the physician, and sees self-care as providing the goal of the relationship between the client and the nurse. For Kinlein, nursing judgments are largely determined by the client's needs, practices, and desires. She sees the object of nursing as the entire person and the purpose of nursing as the promotion of his or her health (not disease) state. She adds that nursing can and should be independent as well as interdependent in all settings. Major areas of difference are identified and a comparison made in Table 2.2. (A similar comparison of practical models in an acute medical surgical setting has been done by Mullen [27].)

How to Promote Self-Care

What explains the failure of people to be self-caring? If we consider some of the explanations for this, the corresponding actions that nurses can take become clearer. People may not know how to act in their best interests, or for one or many reasons they choose not to; that is, they may act in ways that are not beneficial to them and that are against the advice of health professionals. Other considerations are environmental, societal, and peer pressure factors that may work against a person's efforts

to be self-caring. Table 2.3 gives some explanations and appropriate nursing actions to promote self-care.

Realities, Difficulties, Controversy Related to Nursing Self-Care Framework

Although it is true that the self-care nursing model provides an excellent opportunity for nurses to practice primary care, there are also difficulties with the practice of this model. Following are some ideas that are reflected in the literature and that have arisen in classroom discussions.

Resistance from Clients. Not all clients are enthusiastic about assuming more responsibility for themselves or for their health care. There may be a discrepancy between what the nurse and the client expect in each other's roles. (The tradition of self-responsibility is not clearly rooted in all cultures.) Many clients present with the expectation of the health professional being in charge, of being the "agent" of the cure, either by advice, diagnosis, or prescription of a pill. Alternatives to traditional medical treatment may seem unfamiliar, may postpone the time when relief or results are obtained, and may seem inappropriate to clients. (Why should a client learn relaxation when a pill will lower her blood pressure or change her mood?) Nurses, therefore, need to clarify with clients what their position and priorities are and to maintain the expectation that clients can learn to value and practice self-care. There are times when decision making about one's health or illness seems too great a responsibility, and people defer to the expert. Then health care providers have the dilemma of how much decision making to accept for the client, or how aggressively to inform him about his health options or prognosis.

Clients may be unable to change some of their behaviors easily because of society's values and overall influence on their lives. Much destructive behavior is encouraged in our contemporary society; consider, for example, the problems of overeating, substance abuse, smoking, auto accidents, environmental pollution, lack of exercise. Often in such cases, the client needs to be highly motivated, extremely resourceful, and psychologically strong to withstand or avoid negative societal influences.

Resistance from Other Professionals. Health professionals have differing beliefs about the desirability of promoting self-care in clients. Some believe that people will fail to seek professional care when they need it, or

Table 2.2
Major Areas of Difference in Nursing Models

	Traditional Nursing Model	Self-Care Nursing Model
Basic philosophy	The client is best helped by compliance, by following the prescription or advice of the "expert."	Client has the inherent right, responsibility, and capacity to act for self. Respect for person's free choice and ability to contribute to care plan
Objective of nursing action	To comply with predetermined priority or to give some care that is required by physical need of client or by physician order	To promote the self-care ability of the client To increase independence and promote development of the client
Locus of authority and decision making	Authority lies with the physician for medical, moral, nursing decisions. Limited judgment exercised by nurse or client	Nurse and client have a direct, legitimate relationship. Both contribute information, share in power to decide, assume responsibilities as appropriate. Physician is colleague or consultant.
Nursing actions	Direct care, doing something (teaching, doing procedure, monitoring vital signs, etc.) Carrying out orders to facilitate diagnosis and treatment of disease Management of other health workers, institutional representative	Direct care, teaching, counseling, guiding, supporting, all toward the goal of facilitating and promoting self-care capacity of client More attention to stimulation, motivation, creative teaching—learning efforts, improving problem-solving ability in client, involving client in all steps of nursing process, communication
Therapeutic orientation	Dependence on chemical or surgical cures, behavior modification Use of methods that are cost-effective and produce clearly measurable effects Stress alleviation through technological aids, medicines Emphasis on cure	Sees client as possessing considerable control over the therapeutic potential, and ability to prevent illness by self-responsibility, stress management, environmental adjustment, and life-style change More long-term, process-oriented goals necessitating an open-ended, continuous relationship with the client Emphasis on prevention

that there will be abuses in such areas as self-medication. There are also political power issues that arise because the self-care model opposes the present medical model, and therefore threatens the traditional client-professional interaction. There is the fear, by some, of the economic impact of reduced visits to physicians in favor of those who can help with common health maintenance issues or who are oriented toward health counseling and holistic care. Still others point out the danger of placing too much responsibility (blame) for health or illness on the person to the neglect of efforts to reform the health care system and improve environmental conditions. This could lead to government relinquishment of responsibility for the public's health and to penalties for those who do not give up harmful health-related activities.

Resistance from Employers, Health and Institution Administration. Self-care often depends on changing behaviors that have been learned over a lifetime. The current organization of health care does not offer the continuous access to the client that would allow the continuity and time necessary to fully understand and establish a working relationship with the client. Administrators, with their fiscal and survival concerns, are interested in promoting efficiency and productivity, which is often measured by the number of persons seen and the volume of reimbursable services rendered. Care

Table 2.3
Nursing Actions to Promote Self-Care

Why People Are Not Self-Caring	What Can Be Done
Poor or distorted self-image	Motivate them to learn about themselves, to like and value themselves. Help them accept and be proud of their uniqueness. Treat clients positively. Communicate your interest in, belief in, and liking for them.
Never learned how to take care of themselves	Help them gain the knowledge and skills they need. Direct them to sources of information and experiences in life skills, social relations, health maintenance. Show by role modeling and support and reinforce their efforts and intentions.
Lack awareness or in a state of unreadiness for self-care	Encourage them to get in touch with their own reality. Help them decide their priorities, to see future directions and possibilities for action. Encourage honesty and work toward reducing illusions. Work on supporting strengths and motivation.
Incapable of self-care because of mental or physical illness/disability	Offer assistance as needed; care here depends on treatment appropriate to the problem.
Act out of different values, norms, philosophies, priorities in ways that may not be health promoting	Help them to examine the reasons for their actions, to explore the effect of their actions, alternative practices that will be both health promoting and in keeping with the client's goals. Discover what is important to the person. Respect the client's values and choices—from the client's situation and point of view the behavior may be logical and necessary. Continue to offer support and information.
Possibly in a life situation where self-care cannot be easily practiced. Lack of resources, environmental pressures	Analyze the situation to determine factors—internal and external—that are preventing self-caring. Attempt to lessen environmental restraints, find needed concrete services (for example, child care, senior center, self-help group, legal aid, additional income). Help them find educational alternatives. Help groups to support, encourage consumer participation, political action, organize for change.

is fragmented and the work broken into tasks, with many types of workers working with the same client. Costs are based on the diagnosis and treatment services of physicians, so the difficulty becomes how to build in the time and how to receive reimbursement for efforts to promote caring and self-care.

Barbara Stevens points out the dilemma that nursing will face when nurses who have been educated in different nursing theories try to use various theoretical approaches on the same unit. A decision must be made or a consensus arrived at concerning the theory selected for use in particular service settings. Whatever model is chosen, that theory needs to be implemented and ac-

commodated in records, patterns of care, and so on (33).

Feasibility in All Settings. It may be that a self-care framework is not equally appropriate or possible in all settings. It may be easier within nonacute settings and in places where nurses are in independent roles, such as in community health nursing, where it is the mandate of the agency to promote self-sufficiency and independence. In acute settings—emergency areas, intensive care units—certain routines and controls necessary for client safety, along with the condition of the client, limit the choice and active involvement a client can have in determining his or her health care. The phase of the illness is an important factor; for example, in rehabilitation, when client independence is the goal, a self-care nursing framework is very relevant. Some writers have even pointed out that a self-care approach is crucial in situations where clients have already experienced a loss of control over their lives and need to regain some capacity to influence their lives (20). This is the case with clients who have been diagnosed as having incurable diseases; or who are in end-stage renal failure and are dependent on a machine for life; or who, because of advanced age, are cared for in a nursing home; or who have too few resources to be independent. In other words, those with the greatest need to be self-caring may be those least able to be, and care may be given to them in settings that least lend themselves to the respect for and promotion of self-care ability.

DISCUSSION QUESTIONS

1. Consider whether or not caring and self-care are essential processes within nursing. If they are not, what are the essential components?
2. Analyze your own capacity for caring and for promoting self-care in others.
   a. Explore your personal beliefs and philosophy.
   b. Trace the development of your caring capacity.
   c. Critique your ability in each of the areas of Mayerhoff's ingredients of caring.
3. Consider which clients you find it satisfying to work with and which you have difficulty working with. Identify the underlying issues and consider the implications for your future nursing practice.
4. Do you agree with the proposition that nurses cannot be effective in promoting growth or self-care ability in others unless they value and practice growth and healthful behavior in their own lives? What are the implications of such statements for individual nurses? for the nursing profession?
5. Consider for which clients a caring/self-care approach is most relevant. Consider the factors involved whenever this approach is not successful.
6. Evaluate the services provided by a health care agency you are familiar with as they relate to the concepts of care and self-care. (Evaluate the agency's philosophy and practices in such areas as client teaching, advocacy, client participation, contracting, clarifying client rights and responsibilities.)
7. Using Orem's self-care framework, assess the probable needs of clients you see in your clinical settings.

REFERENCES

1. Anna, D., D. Christensen, Ord Hoban, and Wells. "Implementing Orem's Conceptual Framework." *Journal of Nursing Administration*, November 1978, 8–11.
2. Backsheider, Joan E. "Self Care Requirements, Self Care Capabilities, and Nursing Systems in the Diabetic Nurse Management Clinic." *American Journal of Public Health,* December 1971, 1138–45.
3. Bevis, Em Olivia. "Caring: A Life Force." In *Caring: An Essential Human Need.* Proceedings of the Three National Caring Conferences. Thorofare, N.J.: Charles B. Slack, 1981, 49–60.
4. Blattner, Barbara. *Holistic Nursing.* Englewood Cliffs, N.J.: Prentice-Hall, 1981.
5. Bromley, Barbara. "Applying Orem's Self-Care Theory in Enterostomy Therapy." *American Journal of Nursing,* February 1980, 245–49.
6. Buber, Martin. *I and Thou.* 2nd ed. New York: Charles Scribner's Sons, 1958.
7. Burnside, I., P. Ebersole, and H. Monea. *Psychological Caring Throughout the Life Span.* New York: McGraw-Hill, 1979.
8. Cousins, Norman. *Anatomy of an Illness.* New York: W. W. Norton, 1979.
9. Curtin, Leah. "The Nurse-Patient Relationship: Foundations, Purposes, Responsibilities and Rights." In *Nursing Ethics: Theories and Pragmatics.* Bowie, Md.: Robert J. Brady, 1982.
10. Facteau, Lorna M. "Self-Care Concepts and the Care of the Hospitalized Child." *NCNO,* March 1980, 145–55.
11. Fromm, Eric. *The Art of Loving.* New York: Harper & Row, 1956.
12. Gans, Herbert. "Youth in the Ghetto," in *More Equality.* New York: Pantheon, 1973.
13. Gaylin, Willard. *Caring.* New York: Avon Books, 1976.
14. Harris, Judith K. "Self-Care Is Possible After Cesarean Delivery." *NCNO,* March 1980, 191–204.
15. Henderson, Virginia. *The Nature of Nursing.* New York: Macmillan, 1966.
16. Hyde, Ann. "The Phenomena of Caring," pt. 2. *Nursing Research Reports,* February 1976, 2.
17. Kinlein, M. Lucille. *Independent Nursing Practice with Clients.* Philadelphia: J. B. Lippincott, 1977.
18. Leininger, Madeleine. "Caring: A Central Focus of Nursing and Health Care Services." *Nursing and Health Care,* October 1980.
19. Leininger, Madeleine. "The Phenomenon of Caring: Importance, Research Questions, and Theoretical Considerations." In *Caring: An Essential Human Need.* Proceedings of the Three National Caring Conferences. Thorofare, N.J.: Charles B. Slack, 1981, 3–16.
20. Leinweber, Barbara. "The Hemodialysis Client: Nursing Focus on Self-Care." *Nephrology Nurse,* March–April 1981, 8–10.
21. Levin, L., and H. Katz. *Self-Care: Lay Initiatives in Health.* New York: Prodist, 1976.

22. Marcel, Gabriel. *Presence and Immortality*. Pittsburgh, Duquesne University Press, 1967.

23. Maslow, Abraham. *Toward a Psychology of Being*. 2nd ed. Princeton, N.J.: Van Nostrand Co., 1968.

24. May, Rollo. *Love and Will*. New York: W. W. Norton, 1969.

25. Mayerhoff, Milton. *On Caring*. New York: Harper & Row, 1971.

26. Morley, Peter. "Reflections in the Biopolitics of Human Nature and Altruism." In *Caring: An Essential Human Need*. Proceedings of the Three National Caring Conferences. Thorofare, N.J.: Charles B. Slack, 1981, 145–157.

27. Mullen, Virginia. "Implementing the Self-Care Concept in the Acute Care Setting." *NCNO*, March 1980, 189.

28. Nightingale, Florence. *Notes on Nursing*. New York: Dover Publications, 1969.

29. Orem, Dorothea. *Nursing: Concepts of Practice*. 2nd ed. New York: McGraw-Hill, 1980.

30. Paulen, Ann, and Catherine Rapp. "Person-Centered Caring." *Nursing Management,* September 1981, 20.

31. Peplou, Hildegard. *Interpersonal Relations in Nursing*. New York: G. P. Putnam's Sons, 1952.

32. Rogers, Carl. *On Becoming a Person*. Boston: Houghton Mifflin, 1972.

33. Stevens, Barbara. Address to the 6th Conference of Nurse Educators, Philadelphia, 1981.

34. Teilhard de Chardin, Pierre. *On Love*. New York: Harper & Row, 1967.

35. Walborn, Karen Ann. "A Nursing Model for the Hospice: Primary and Self-Care Nursing." *NCNO,* March 1980, 205–17.

36. Watson, Jean. *Nursing: The Philosophy and Science of Caring*. Boston: Little, Brown, 1979.

CHAPTER 3

Communication and Self-Care

GLORIA CALIANDRO

•

OBJECTIVES

After completing this chapter, the reader will be able to:

- Explain the importance of communication in the nursing process.

- Explain how self-concept, knowledge, attitudes and values, feelings, personality type, needs, and sociocultural factors influence communication and self-care.

- Discuss strategies for identifying and coping with selected factors that influence communication.

- Discuss communication techniques used to sustain the nurse-client relationship—active listening, collaborating, and negotiating.

- Analyze nurse-client communication and relationships in the context of self-care.

- Discuss factors that promote and inhibit communication between the primary nurse and health team members.

Communication is a vast subject that may be approached in a number of ways, each of which would be valid within the context of primary nursing and self-care. The discussion in this chapter is limited to two aspects of communication and self-care: communication between nurse and client and communication between members of the health team.

Communication Between Nurse and Client

A philosophy of primary nursing, introduced in chapter 1, briefly states that the one-on-one relationship between nurse and client that promotes continuity of care as long as the client needs it is at the heart of primary nursing.

From this philosophy the following premises about the nature of the relationship and communication that occurs in primary nursing care derive:

- The nurse-client relationship is central to primary nursing.
- A relationship is established, maintained, and terminated by communication between two persons. One cannot have a relationship without communication.
- One cannot refrain from communicating. Even the conscious attempt not to communicate communicates a message.
- The quality of a relationship depends on the quality of communication between two persons.
- The quality of nursing care primarily depends on the quality of the relationship between the nurse and the client and, consequently, on the quality of their communication.
- The nurse-client relationship arises out of mutual recognition of the client's need for nursing care; therefore, it differs in purpose and nature from other kinds of relationships. It is goal-directed, and in this instance the goal is self-care.
- The purpose and nature of a relationship

influence the communication that occurs between two persons.

Communication Model

A model of communication that incorporates the premises above and that elaborates on the scope and process of communication that facilitates self-care within the context of primary nursing is shown in Figure 3.1.

The reason for establishing the nurse-client relationship and the goal of the interaction is self-care. In order to achieve that goal, the nurse and the client enter into a problem-solving relationship, the quality and effectiveness of which depends on the ability of the nurse and the client to communicate.

Problem solving begins with the collection of data, a communication process in which the client shares what he or she knows and feels about the reason for seeking care and other background information that will enable the nurse to understand the client as well as the problem. The nurse uses various communication techniques—questioning, listening, observing, and touching—to collect information. The quality of assessment will depend not only on knowing what to assess, but also on the nurse's expertise in using communication techniques.

The assessment phase is also the beginning of the relationship between nurse and client. The nurse forms impressions of the client as a person by his or her behavior—how clearly ideas are articulated, how open and genuine the responses appear to be, and how receptive the client is to the nurse. The client, likewise, forms first impressions of the nurse—how competent, warm, and caring; how receptive to the client's expressed feelings and needs the nurse is; and his or her willingness to spend time with the client.

These first impressions are important to the kind of relationship that will be established and, consequently, to the progress the client makes toward achieving self-care. Negative first impressions usually require substantial time and energy to overcome, and in some

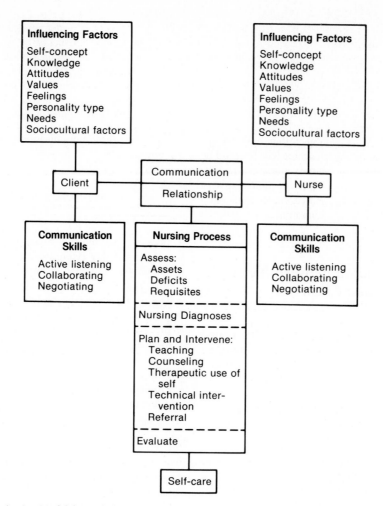

Figure 3.1. Communication Model for Self-Care in Primary Nursing

instances they may be permanent. Preplanning for assessment should include deciding not only what information needs to be collected in order to determine the client's assets, deficits, and requisites for nursing and how best to collect it, but also what impressions one wants to communicate and how to communicate them effectively so as to create a therapeutic relationship with the client. This requires insight into oneself, one's behavior, and one's communication skills.

Although nurses may assume that clients know what nursing care involves, experience indicates that clients have limited knowledge in most instances. It is important in the first encounters with the client to explain the

nature of the relationship they will be establishing, its focus and boundaries. It is also important to explain to the client what he or she can expect from the primary nurse, including such essentials as the client's rights to autonomy and privacy. In order to adequately convey the nature and scope of primary nursing to the client, the nurse first must understand it.

Of the five nursing skills used to implement the plan of nursing care, the model indicates that ·four—teaching, counseling, therapeutic use of self, and referral—are communication skills and the fifth—technical intervention—requires some degree of communication. Although it is beyond the scope of this chapter to elaborate on each of these skills, it is important to recognize that comprehensive nursing intervention, contrary to what many people presume, is predominantly communication.

The final step in the nursing process is also communication. In order to evaluate the effectiveness of care, data relevant to short- and long-range goals are collected and evaluated. This, ideally, is a collaborative process between the client and the nurse, with both contributing ideas and judgments from their individual perspectives.

In order to establish a therapeutic relationship that fosters self-care, both client and nurse use various communication skills. Three of the more important ones are active listening, collaborating, and negotiating. Each of these skills is discussed later in the chapter.

Both client and nurse bring to the relationship a background composed of personal and sociocultural factors that influence communication. These factors operate at both the conscious and the unconscious level. One of the nurse's responsibilities is to be alert to the possibility of unconscious influences both within herself or himself and the client, and to seek to validate and clarify them. The importance of these factors should not be underestimated.

Factors Influencing Communication and Self-Care

Selected factors that influence communication and self-care are shown in Figure 3.1. These are self-concept, knowledge, attitudes, values, feelings, needs, personality type, and sociocultural characteristics.

Self-Concept

The self-concept is what one believes oneself to be. It is "the composite of beliefs and feelings that one holds about oneself at a given point in time" (2, p. 174). It is formed from one's perceptions, particularly of the reactions of others, and directs one's behavior. The self-concept is not static, but evolves through interaction with others. It largely determines what we communicate about ourselves to others and the feedback we receive. One of the most important aspects of primary nursing care is to be able to identify how a person's self-concept affects the person, the nurse, and their relationship, and how the nurse can use communication skills to help the person change and achieve an optimum level of self-care.

The self-concept is a complex set of interacting aspects of the person. Nursing care that fails to appreciate the complexity of the self-concept and how it influences communication and self-care is not likely to be effective.

Illness has the ability to substantially alter one's self-concept. Changes caused by illness include physical changes resulting from altered physiology, trauma and surgery, loss of control as one assumes a dependent state, role changes, and reassessment of the meaning and purpose of life.

One of the goals of nursing is to help the client develop a more positive self-concept. Or, as Rogers wrote of the helping relationship, it is to enable the client not only to accept himself, but to actually like himself as well, and thus develop a quiet pleasure in being himself (24). The need to foster a positive self-concept assumes added importance when one considers the phenomenon of self-fulfilling prophecy. Watzlawick and colleagues state that a person elicits behavior in others consistent with the way the person thinks about herself. For instance, a person who believes that she is dependent, unable to learn, and incapable of caring for herself communicates this to others. They may respond by treating the person as if she were dependent and incompetent, thus bearing out the truth of the person's beliefs (27). A cycle of behavior may continue until the nurse, client, or someone insightful into the situation perceives what is happening, intervenes, and seeks to change the communication pattern.

It is important to explore the client's self-concept as it relates to self-care. Clients can be helped to become more self-reliant by acknowledging the reality of their self-concept for them, by encouraging them to express and explore positive as well as negative ideas and feelings about the ability to engage in self-care, and by giving honest, realistic feedback about their accomplishments as well as their problems. For some clients the greatest challenge will be not to acknowledge and explore problems, but to recognize and internalize their accomplishments. Some clients find it difficult to be successful; they are much more comfortable being not so.

Knowledge

Although studies have shown that knowledge about self-care does not necessarily lead to optimum self-care (14), a client's level of knowledge does affect the ability to effectively communicate about self-care. Assessment of clients includes their knowledge of their problems, themselves, and their care and their ability to comprehend what is being communicated. Assuming that a client comprehends, or is capable of comprehending, something usually leads to problems. Throughout the assessment the client's comprehension should be clarified in order to establish a valid base on which to build through teaching and counseling.

Equally important to communication is the nurse's ability to correctly perceive his or her own intellectual ability and to think of himself or herself as a source of knowledge. Aside from thoroughly knowing what one wishes to communicate, characteristics such as directness, clarity, honesty, and self-confidence help one to effectively communicate knowledge.

Attitudes and Values

It is important early in the nurse-client relationship to identify attitudes and values of both persons. As Hein wrote, "nothing is communicated as quickly or as surely as our attitudes. They affect how and what we communicate; they affect the transmission of our knowledge and they clearly imply the influence of our cultural heritage" (10, p. 67).

In order to appreciate the impact of attitudes on communication and self-care, attitudes need to be defined. Attitudes are "composed of an individual's beliefs, values, response sets, and perceptions about an object, person or process" (25). Together with motives, attitudes are principal determinants of behavior.

Because of their high correlation with behavior, it is important to be aware of the attitudes we have and do not have. This requires serious introspection and involves knowing rather than knowing about, especially oneself. In the context of building a helping relationship, Rogers wrote that whatever attitudes or feelings the helper experiences should be matched by an awareness of them. When this happens the helper becomes an integrated or unified person in that moment (24). In existential terms, this is achieving authenticity, a quality necessary for being perceived as trustworthy, consistent, and dependable. Rogers goes on to say that most of the failures to achieve a helping relationship can be traced to being unaware of attitudes, and thereby sending contradictory messages in communication.

Attitudes and values can either facilitate or inhibit communication. Attitudes that can facilitate communication and build relationships include investment (a willingness to put oneself into the relationship), warmth, acceptance, and objectivity. These attitudes not only help to build rapport, but also complement the client's identity as a unique human being. Attitudes that inhibit communication and serve as barriers to relationships include condescension, cautiousness (lack of spontaneity), inauthenticity (inability to be oneself), rejection, and authoritarianism.

Feelings

Emotions play a central role in the relationship established between client and nurse. Watson views the promotion and acceptance of the expression of positive and negative feelings as integral parts of the caring relationship and as important factors in the quality of care (26). Being able to explore and express feelings without the fear of judgment and with feedback that helps to place these feelings more solidly in the context of reality is essential to the development of trust. Without trust there cannot be a therapeutic relationship. These ideas are so basic to the nurse-client relationship that they may be taken for granted, minimized, or overlooked unless nurses consciously incorporate them into nursing care plans.

The relationship between nurse and client in primary nursing is long term and has the potential for greater depth than that found in other models of nursing practice. For this reason it is particularly important for primary nurses to explore not only their clients' feelings about the illness experience and self-care, but also their clients' and their own feelings about the relationship. Anger, disappointment, rejection, sadness, pleasure, and happiness are all bound to occur in any long-term relationship. Unless these feelings are recognized and appropriately expressed, they may be misinterpreted and block communication, thus impeding the client's progress toward self-care and health.

The degree to which feelings affect behavior varies from person to person and may vary within a person at different points in time, depending on the level of insight into oneself. Measures the nurse can use to help clients gain insight into how feelings affect communication and relationships include the following:

- Planning nurse-client contacts that focus on the exploration of feelings. The purpose and goals of these contacts and how they relate to self-care and health should be clarified so that clients better understand their value.
- Helping clients to distinguish between what they think about something or someone and what they feel. Listening to what the client says gives clues about whether the message deals with ideas or feelings. Calling it to the client's attention frequently helps refocus on feelings.

- Maintaining an accepting attitude. Acceptance does not mean agreement; it means that the validity of feelings as personal experience is recognized.
- Assisting the client to clarify feelings. What are the feelings? What evoked them? This is particularly important when dealing with people who have unresolved conflicts and displace feelings.

Nurses, too, need to explore how they feel about their relationships with their clients. Having a network of colleagues with whom one can talk, a support group, or a counselor can be an invaluable asset for the primary nurse, especially when the nurse perceives that relationships are becoming stressful and when personal feelings are beginning to adversely affect the client.

Personality Type

Based on Jungian psychology, the work of the late Isabel Briggs Myers and her colleagues gives considerable insight into personality types and how they influence personal preferences, interests, values, needs, habits of the mind, behavior, and communication. According to Myers, "much seemingly chance variation in human behavior is not due to chance; it is in fact the logical result of a few basic, observable differences in mental functioning" (20, p. 1). These differences can be organized into four categories: ways of perceiving, ways of arriving at judgments, relative interest in the outer versus the inner worlds, and attitudes toward dealing with the outer world.

There are two basic styles of perception, which Myers labels sensing and intuition. Sensing-type persons are very much aware of the external environment and much more interested in actualities, or what truly exists, than in possibilities. They depend on their five senses for defining their world and prefer living in the present to enjoyment of future pleasures. Intuitive-type persons rely much more on imagination and tend to suppress many of the impressions received through the senses. They may have little awareness of their surroundings unless they relate to a current interest or pursuit.

People differ in the way they arrive at judgments. For thinking-type people arriving at a conclusion is a logical process aimed at an impersonal finding. Such people collect the facts, organize them, and arrive at a conclusion based on them. They seem to be much more interested in things than in human relationships, and to suppress and undervalue feelings. Feeling-type people are

the opposite. Conclusions are reached subjectively. They value sentiment more than logic and are more interested in other people than in things. To them a decision is right if it feels right.

Individual persons may be classified according to their relative interest in the outer versus the inner world; they are either extraverts or introverts. For extraverts the real world is the outer world of people and things that must be experienced before they can understand it. They are very sociable and not particularly interested in ideas. The introverts' world is the opposite, one that is lived interiorly, a world of ideas that does not always take into account the external world around them.

The fourth classification relates to a person's attitude toward dealing with the outer world. A person is predominantly either perceptive or judging. Perceptive people are often viewed by others as indecisive because of a persistent feeling that they do not know quite enough about a situation to decide. They are curious, live in the present, and enjoy starting new projects, although they may not finish them. Their opposites, judging people, live according to plans and like to see matters settled as quickly as possible. They do not have difficulty making decisions and are prone to think that they know what others ought to do.

Given the fact that a person's personality type may be any combination of these characteristics, it is easy to appreciate the problems that may arise when trying to communicate with the person and establish a relationship that focuses on problem solving as it relates to health and self-care. Building productive relationships requires that both the client and the nurse recognize their personality types and respect the differences in the other. It is also important to remember that although a person has certain preferences, the auxiliary process (e.g., perception when the person is a judging type) can be developed through use (20).

Needs

Every person comes to a relationship with needs. In the context of this discussion the client's primary need is self-care. In order to achieve this, other needs—physical, emotional, social, cultural, and spiritual—must be considered.

The nurse also initiates a relationship because of needs that are as varied as the client's. Although the nurse's primary need may be defined as being a helper, what being a helper means to the nurse is highly personal and complex. It is both desirable and acceptable to enter a relationship because of needs; it is doubtful that a relationship could be established where there are none. But the quality of the relationship depends on the level of awareness of needs and their importance to the person, and the willingness of client and nurse to explore them.

Historically, nurses have been educated to value altruism, which is defined as "the unselfish concern for or devotion to the welfare of others" (25). This is certainly a necessary ingredient of a helping relationship, but in many instances it has been misconstrued to mean that the nurse should deny or ignore needs when entering into a helping relationship. Certainly the client's needs are a priority, but the needs of the nurse cannot be ignored, for they influence behavior and communication with others. This requires continuing self-examination in the context of the relationship, honesty and openness to areas in which change is needed. The inability to do these may result in a nontherapeutic relationship.

Having a professional support group of peers or other health team members can be invaluable to the primary nurse who maintains long-term, caring relationships with clients. Such a group provides an acceptable means for discussing needs and interactions and for coping with change.

Sociocultural Factors

Every person is a product of the social group and culture into which he or she was born and in which he or she was reared. Our sociocultural background is like a "lens through which experiences are perceived and behavioral choices made" (11). A person's sociocultural heritage determines, to a great extent, the language a person uses, the patterns of communication—with whom and how a person communicates—and the meaning attributed to communications. Culture also largely determines a person's concept of health, illness, care, and self-care and the behaviors associated with these. According to the idea of cultural relativism, a person can be understood only in the context of his or her cultural heritage.

Nursing is a transcultural interaction between a client who represents one culture and a nurse who represents at least two: the culture of origin and the subculture of nursing. As indicated in Figure 3.1, the outcome of their interaction is self-care. The ability of the nurse to foster self-care, and for the client to accept the nurse's assistance, will depend on their ability to clearly communicate their cultural perspectives and expectations and reach compatible understanding. This requires that the nurse, in particular, be open to learning about the cli-

ent's culture and refrain from judging until the client's perspective is understood.

Ethnonursing, an approach to nursing in which caretakers base their care on knowledge of the beliefs, values, perceptions, and behaviors of a particular cultural group, can help bridge the gap between the cultures of the nurse and the client. Leininger identifies three major types of ethnonursing care: (a) cultural accommodation, (b) cultural repatterning, and (c) cultural preservation (19). Each type of care has its place, depending on the effectiveness of the cultural practices to achieve mutually determined self-care outcomes.

The following cultural beliefs and practices illustrate differences that should be considered when planning and implementing nursing care. The first relates to the concept of social support. For the Mexican-American, illness is a family affair. When a person becomes ill the family rallies around the person, often in large numbers, and becomes involved in some way in the person's care (9). For the urban Latino who may be residing in a large city in the northeastern United States, the *compadrazgo* is an important support system to provide care in times of need. Dugan describes this as a fictive kin tie, a social bonding, that is not biologically or legally ascribed, and that includes men (compadres) and women (comadres) (6).

An area of cultural beliefs and practices that may lead to conflict is reliance on folk medicine. Naturopathy (9) and the use of sobadors to treat musculoskeletal disorders among Mexicans (1) may be difficult for the nurse schooled in traditional Western thought to appreciate. Yet, to the client, these may be quite acceptable. Self-care may also include seeking out several sources of care for a problem, depending on the client's beliefs about the causes of the problem. For example, if evil spirits are believed to be a cause, the client may consult a curandero (witchdoctor) while simultaneously seeking care from a nurse.

Cultural expectations for self-care also influence the way a client responds to care. For example, helping a disabled person to achieve an optimum level of functioning in activities of daily living and role fulfillment is a common nursing goal. If the client is from a village in Barbados, both family and client may have specific ideas about what a disabled person is expected to do. Village Barbadians do not expect disabled people to fulfill normative adult roles, although some do (8).

Finally, cultures that value independence are more likely to incorporate self-care values and practices into daily life than are cultures that do not (18). Studies of locus of control have demonstrated this. Nursing care that will most effectively assist the client toward self-care will recognize and provide for this cultural trait.

Communication Techniques for Sustaining Nurse-Client Relationships

Although a number of communication techniques can be used to sustain relationships between nurses and clients, three are considered essential: active listening, collaborating, and negotiating.

Listening

According to Rogers, real communication occurs when we listen with understanding. In order to do this a person must be able to "see the idea and attitude from the [other] person's point of view, to sense how it feels to him, to achieve his frame of reference in regard to the thing he is talking about" (24, pp. 331–32). What is required of the listener in order to achieve this level of understanding, which Rogers calls empathic understanding, or understanding with, not about, a person?

The first thing is courage. In order to enter another person's private world openly and nonjudgmentally we must be willing to take a risk, and for that courage is required. What is the risk? That as we begin to understand from another person's point of view, we are opening ourselves up to change. Nurses expect to facilitate change in clients; that is a common goal of nursing care. But for many of us, personal change as a result of interacting with the client can be frightening, and that takes courage.

Listening that enables the nurse to enter the client's private world is attentive listening. It requires concentration and undivided attention to both the content and the affect of the message, and sufficient feedback so the client knows that you are with him or her. It is particularly important to explore in depth the client's experiences related to self-care. What are some of the client's personal goals, and how does self-care fit into the overall plan for these goals? What is the client's self-image, and how does the ability to care for oneself impact on it? What is the quality of the relationships that the client has with people close to him or her? How will being able to care for oneself affect those relationships? How clearly does the client understand and express personal needs? How does the client feel about the issue of dependency? As these questions are explored, judgment should be suspended as the nurse clarifies and validates impressions with the client until both feel comfortable that the impressions do represent the client's experience. As Rogers wrote, "the tendency to react to any emotionally meaningful statement by forming an evaluation of it from our own point of view is . . . the major barrier to interpersonal communication" (24, p. 331). Effective and lasting change begins where the client is and builds on strengths while recognizing and overcoming limitations in meeting needs. And where the client is can be determined only when the nurse is willing to enter into, as much as possible, the client's world as he or she experiences it.

Collaborating

To collaborate means to willingly cooperate in some endeavor. Underlying this definition are certain assumptions. First, that there is commitment by the nurse and the client to the establishment and maintenance of a relationship and to fostering health and self-care in the client. The second assumption is that both client and nurse have something valuable to contribute to the endeavor. There is respect for the differences as well as for the similarities in what each brings to the relationship. The third assumption is that whatever transpires does so through joint planning and implementation. Although parts of an endeavor may be done individually by either nurse or client, they are done within the context of goals and plans that are jointly determined.

The collaborative process is divided into phases, the first being the initiation of the relationship. In this phase both client and nurse define who they are, what they have to offer, and what can and cannot be expected of them. This is equivalent to setting boundaries within which collaboration may occur. Having clearly defined boundaries fosters understanding between client and nurse and helps reduce misunderstanding that leads to tension and stress.

In the second phase, the working phase, the nursing process is implemented. As indicated in chapter 1, this involves assessment, identification of problems, specification of strategies for managing problems, statement of short- and long-range goals, and identification of client behaviors and characteristics that indicate goal achievement. This phase is a joint effort by nurse and client.

The third phase is the resolution phase, in which nurse and client agree that the client's problems have been resolved to their satisfaction, or at least to a reasonable level of expectation, and the need for nursing intervention ceases. Another important part of this phase is termination of the nurse-client relationship, either temporarily or permanently. Time is allotted in the final contacts for the client to discuss how he or she will feel about not having regular contacts with the nurse and for both to discuss the client's next phase of care—self-care without a nurse's assistance. It is important to spread the termination phase over several contacts so that feelings and questions that arise may be discussed.

As nurse and client collaborate, it is important to remember that the goals of collaboration are to foster self-care and promote compliance with a plan of care mutually determined by client and nurse. Research indicates that a number of factors influence compliance—demographic features of clients, characteristics of the disease (e.g., severity and duration), characteristics of the therapeutic regimen, characteristics of the source of care (e.g., clinic convenience, clinic waiting time), and sociobehavioral characteristics of the client (e.g., value system, level of motivation) (28). But two factors particularly relevant to this chapter that recur in the literature are the nurse-client relationship (3, 5, 13, 21) and the kind of communication that occurs between nurse and client (7, 13).

Kasch and Knutson suggest that the quality of the nurse-client relationship depends in part on whether or not the nurse uses either position-centered or person-centered speech. "Position-centered speech is grounded in the assumption that effective communication depends on everyone following the script, playing their role and following the rules and norms which implicitly govern nurse-patient interaction" (14, p. 153). Nurses who rely on this kind of speech tend to tell clients what to do and to rely on control strategies rather than on collaborative decision making. The nurse who uses person-centered speech is more likely to consider each client's subjective experience, attitudes, values, and personal beliefs about health care as the basis for intervention and to primarily rely on persuasion rather than control. The authors suggest that compliance is increased when nurses use person-centered speech.

Negotiating

In any long-term relationship there are bound to be conflicts, especially when the relationship exists to resolve problems. One approach to conflict resolution is authoritarian, with one person exerting power and control over another by determining the resolution. The other approach is the cooperative model, or negotiation,

which is defined as the mutual discussion and arrangement of terms of an agreement (25).

Not all conflicts can be negotiated. For instance, suppose a diabetic client being maintained on daily doses of insulin decides not to take insulin. The nurse caring for the client knows that insulin is necessary for the client's health and that it is part of the medical plan of care. A conflict ensues, but it is not one that can be resolved by negotiation. Whether or not the client takes insulin is not negotiable, and attempting to negotiate it makes the nurse liable to legal actions. Instead, the client is clearly informed about why the insulin is necessary and what will happen if it is not taken. Then the client is allowed to decide what he or she will do. Legally and ethically the power to make a decision about care resides with the client, assuming that the client is capable of deciding. Legally and ethically the nurse is obliged to behave in a responsible manner. In this instance it involves informing the client and the physician and not negotiating.

Many conflicts between nurse and client can be negotiated. For instance, a client is supposed to exercise for twenty minutes daily. A plan is worked out for the exercise, the client tries it, and it does not work to his or her satisfaction. A conflict ensues, but this conflict is appropriate for negotiation. There may be numerous exercise plans that fit better into the client's life-style than the original one. To insist on the client's following the original plan takes away the client's right to participate in decision making and blocks communication. A more satisfactory approach is to keep the goal in mind—twenty minutes of exercise daily—while exploring alternative ways of accomplishing it.

As indicated in chapter 8, some of the qualities of an effective negotiator are (a) being able to focus on the problem to be resolved while discussing alternatives, (b) being flexible concerning alternative solutions, (c) being able to listen while suspending judgment and analyzing suggestions dispassionately, (d) being able to get the facts and distinguish between them and opinions, and (e) understanding trade-offs. The latter is important. In negotiations, both parties give up something in order to get something else. Before entering into negotiation it is wise to prethink which trade-offs are acceptable and which are not. This helps to define the limits of negotiation.

The outcome of negotiation is an agreement or contract. Important elements of the nurse-client contract are specific goals, strategies for meeting them, a time frame, evaluation criteria, and a system of reward or reinforcement.

Communication with Other Members of the Team

Primary nursing is not practiced in isolation, but as part of a team that varies in composition, depending on the client's needs and resources. The most basic elements of a team, for most clients, are a physician, a nurse, family members, and, of course, the client. Their ability to collaborate as a team—the desired mode of functioning—depends on role clarification, commitment to working together as a team, and communication.

The need to clarify the roles of team members cannot be overemphasized. Each team member has a perception of his or her role that may or may not be consistent with that of other team members. For instance, physicians usually view themselves as captains of the ship, leaders, decision makers who are responsible for total care, including the prescription of nursing care, which they may or may not understand (23).

Primary nurses whose extended contacts with the client enable a long-term perspective of care similar to that of the physician may also see themselves as decision makers with significant contributions to make to the care of clients. Unless the role of each member is clarified by that member, conflict is inevitable. Primary nurses cannot assume that other team members understand them as professionals; it is part of their responsibility to clarify their role in the context of the team purpose. Although certain aspects of roles remain constant, how the roles will be expressed in a certain situation changes as the situation changes. Several team members may be qualified and able to fulfill a responsibility. The important thing is to decide who will do what and when and to clearly communicate this to all team members. Clarifying roles is a continuing process in a collaborative relationship.

Collaboration requires commitment to working together as a team. Identification of goals, developing and implementing plans for achieving them, and evaluating progress toward goals is a joint effort based on mutual respect for and support of other team members. Respect and support are not automatic endowments when one joins a team. They must be earned. Personal characteristics that foster respect and support are openness to suggestions by others, courtesy, positive self-image, assertiveness, maintenance of professional expertise, and flexibility in relating to others.

Collaboration also requires that team members continuously examine their ability to work together. What are their strengths? What are their weaknesses? What precipitates conflicts? How are individual members dealing with competition, power, and splitting? Do individual members make major decisions that affect other team members without consulting them first? How supportive are they of one another? How effective and efficient are team efforts in promoting self-care in clients? These are some of the more important questions that must be addressed if collaboration is to be maintained.

Of all the qualities essential for collaboration, none is more important than communication. Ideally, planned conferences would be scheduled regularly for the purpose of planning and evaluating the team's goals and activities. In reality this does not occur often for many reasons, for example, time, expense, and failure to appreciate the potential value of team conferences. More commonly communication is informal, with team members exchanging ideas and information when they happen to meet. Informal communication usually has serious limitations, two of them being the absence of some team members and the tendency to focus on current problems instead of a much broader picture.

Maintaining accurate, complete, well-written records of care is vital in terms of collaboration and legality. Ideally, goals for client care, with the contributions of each team member, would be clearly identified in the written record. This is particularly important when one considers that health care professionals are as liable for omission of needed care as they are for commission of careless acts (4). Maintaining joint progress notes can help ensure that each team member will read what the others write and have a clearer understanding of their care. For additional information about written records, the reader is referred to chapters 5 and 14.

REFERENCES

1. Anderson, R. "The Treatment of Musculoskeletal Disorders by a Mexican Bonesetter (Sobador)." *Social Science and Medicine* 24:43, 1987.
2. Bonham, P. A., and A. M. Cheney. "Concept of Self: A Framework for Nursing Assessment." In *Advances in Nursing Theory Development,* ed. P. L. Chinn. Rockville, Md.: Aspen Systems Corp., 1983, 173–90.
3. Brodish, M. S. "Nursing Practice Conceptualized: An Interaction Model." *Image* 14:5, 1982.
4. Creighton, H. "Legal Implications of Home Health Care." *Nursing Management* 18:14, 1987.
5. Dracup, K. A., and A. I. Meleis. "Compliance: An Interactionist Approach." *Nursing Research* 31:31, 1982.
6. Dugan, A. B. "Compadrazgo: A Caring Phenomenon Among Urban Latinos and Its Relationship to Health." In

Care: The Essence of Nursing and Health, ed. M. Leininger. Thorofare, N.J.: Charles B. Slack, 1984, 183–94.

7. Engel, N. S. "Confirmation and Validation: The Caring That Is Professional Nursing." *Image* 12:53, 1980.

8. Goerdt, A. "Social Integration of the Physically Disabled in Barbados." *Social Science and Medicine* 22:459, 1986.

9. Gonzalez, H. H. "Health Care Needs of the Mexican-American." In *Ethnicity and Health Care.* New York: National League for Nursing, 1976, 21–28.

10. Hein, E. C. *Communication in Nursing Practice.* 2nd ed. Boston: Little, Brown, 1980.

11. Horn, B. M. "Cultural and Religious Considerations." In *Medical-Surgical Nursing: Pathophysiological Concepts,* ed. M. Patrick et al. Philadelphia: J. B. Lippincott, 1986, 27–29.

12. Kanfer, F. H., and A. P. Goldstein. *Helping People Change.* 3rd ed. New York: Pergamon Press, 1986.

13. Kasch, C. R. "Toward a Theory of Nursing Action: Skills and Competency in Nurse-Patient Interaction." *Nursing Research* 35:226, 1986.

14. Kasch, C. R., and K. Knutson. "Patient Compliance and Interpersonal Style: Implications for Practice and Research." *Nurse Practitioner* 10:52, 1985.

15. Keirsey, D., and M. Bates. *Please Understand Me: Character and Temperament Types.* Del Mar, Calif.: Prometheus Nemesis Books, 1978.

16. Kobasa, S. C., and S. R. Maddi. "Existential Personality Theory." In *Current Personality Theories,* ed. R. Corsini. Ithaca, N.Y.: F. E. Peacock, 1977.

17. LaMonica, E. L. *The Humanistic Nursing Process.* Monterey, Calif.: Wadsworth, 1985.

18. Leininger, M. "Care: The Essence of Nursing and Health."

In *Care: The Essence of Nursing and Health,* ed. M. Leininger. Thorofare, N.J.: Charles B. Slack, 1984, 3–16.

19. Leininger, M. "Southern Rural Black and White American Lifeways with Focus on Care and Health Phenomena." In *Care: The Essence of Nursing and Health,* ed. M. Leininger. Thorofare, N.J.: Charles B. Slack, 1984, 133–60.

20. Myers, I. B., and P. B. Myers. *Gifts Differing.* Palo Alto, Calif.: Consulting Psychologists Press, 1980.

21. Patterson, G. R., and M. S. Forgatch. "Therapist Behavior as a Determinant for Client Noncompliance: A Paradox for the Behavior Modifier." *Journal of Consulting and Clinical Psychology.* 53:846, 1985.

22. Petosa, R. "Using Behavioral Contracts to Promote Health Behavior Change." *Health Educator* 15:22, 1984.

23. Richardson, A. T. "Nurses Interfacing with Other Team Members." In *Collaboration in Nursing,* ed. D. A. England. Rockville, Md.: Aspen Systems Corp., 1986, 163–86.

24. Rogers, C. *On Becoming a Person.* Boston: Houghton Mifflin, 1961.

25. *The Random House Dictionary of the English Language,* ed. J. Stein. Unabridged ed. New York: Random House, 1973.

26. Watson, J. *Nursing: The Philosophy and Science of Caring.* Boston: Little, Brown, 1979.

27. Watzlawick, P., J. B. Bavelas, and D. D. Jackson. *Pragmatics of Human Communication.* New York: W. W. Norton, 1967.

28. Yoos, L. "Compliance: Philosophical and Ethical Considerations." *Nurse Practitioner* 6:27, 1981.

29. Yura, H., and M. B. Walsh. *The Nursing Process.* 3rd ed. New York: Appleton-Century-Crofts, 1978.

CHAPTER 4

Accountability and Quality Assurance

NADINE JOHNSON

■

OBJECTIVES

After completing this chapter, the reader will be able to:

- Discuss the contributions of Florence Nightingale, industry, and federal legislation in the development of quality assurance activities.
- Discuss the nursing profession's responsibility to society in relation to health care.
- Define and discuss the concept of accountability.
- Describe how the concept of quality is related to standards.
- List three reasons why it is important to set and maintain standards.
- Identify how criteria are related to standards.
- Describe American Nurses' Association Standards of Practice.
- Choose one indicator of quality care that could be measured to improve the quality of care delivered within the students' own clinical setting by using the three selection criteria (i.e., benchmark of quality, known

or suspected problem, or areas of frequent nursing involvement/input).
- Define how *focused review* is related to the overall monitoring program.
- Define the concept of peer review.
- Discuss the concept of review and evaluation versus formal research.
- List three sources of data that can be used for monitoring activities.
- Define retrospective and concurrent time frames for data collection.
- Discuss the problem-solving process in relation to the American Nurses' Association Model for Quality Assurance.
- Identify at least two barriers to institutional change.
- Discuss the impact of prospective payment on health care and its potential impact on quality of care.

Nurses have long had a vital interest in the quality of nursing care being delivered to clients. There are myriad references in the nursing literature that address approaches and interventions that are said to represent quality care. Descriptions and definitions regarding what constitutes "quality" abound. Some nurses believe that quality care refers to meeting all the needs of a specific client. Others believe that it is adherence to the nursing process and subsequent documentation in the client care record.

In the American Academy of Nursing, Magnet Hospital Study, it was found that nurses in the magnet hospitals take enormous pride in the belief that they are providing high-quality nursing care to their patients (1). Quality assurance programs are viewed by these nurses as being constructive and, as one nurse stated, "the best thing that has happened to help nurses provide quality care" (1).

This chapter focuses on the concepts of accountability and quality nursing practice. These concepts may be viewed as *mechanisms* through which professional nurses implement change. This change has as its goal the improvement of the quality of nursing care planned and delivered by the professional nursing practitioner.

Historical Perspective

Florence Nightingale wrote about the assessment and assurance of the quality of nursing care back in 1858 during the Crimean War. She was able to bring public attention to the appalling conditions and mortality of British military personnel by using a set of standards to assess the care. Her report was instrumental in effecting change in the living conditions and health services provided for the military (20). Nightingale developed a multitude of standards for nursing care that are "precepts for every good nurse," whether the care is provided by a family member or a hired nurse. These standards relate to food service, bed type, mattress and linens, noise control, room ventilation, cleanliness, and personal hygiene (21). The death rate at one military

hospital fell from 42 percent to 2 percent six months after Nightingale was placed in charge. Nightingale implemented a quality assurance mechanism by setting standards, comparing actual care provided with the standards, and implementing change based on the findings (9).

Industry was the first to develop the quality control model. A product is inspected and tested according to governmental or industrial standards for the product. The quality control inspection might take place at any stage of production or after product completion. The concept and process were subsequently adapted by the health care industry. Clearly in health care, however, an inferior "product" cannot be recycled or discarded as an "irregular."

In the 1960s, in the era of the Great Society, legislation was enacted that provided health care for the aged and poor under Medicare, Medicaid, and Maternal and Child Health programs. In the years immediately after this legislation was passed, the quantity and cost of health care escalated. In response, Congress amended the Social Security Act (Public Law 92-602), which mandated that federally funded programs and providers were required to participate in quality and appropriateness of care review activities that were designed to cut costs through assuring appropriate utilization of health care resources while maintaining or assuring a level of quality. That was the beginning of widespread quality assurance activities in American health care.

Development of Quality Assurance Activities

By the middle of the 1970s common definitions and approaches to quality assurance activities had been developed. This was largely the result of the emergence of similar requirements for quality of care studies (then called audits) by governmental health regulatory agencies, professional standards review organizations (PSROs), and the voluntary accrediting agency, Joint Commission on Accreditation of Healthcare Organizations (JCAHO). This was the era in which *nursing audit* was the buzzword in nursing literature. It was usually a *retrospective* study of the medical record to audit a group of randomly selected patients with a similar problem or diagnosis. Most often these studies had a patient outcome focus—to validate whether or not the client achieved the defined elements of quality care. The problem with this approach was that measurement was only as good as the written record. It was impossible to ascertain whether appropriate care had been provided when documentation was poor. The most frequent recommendation resulting from these studies was to improve the quality of the written record (17, 18).

It was also in the 1970s that multidisciplinary client care audits were designed to foster better interdisciplinary approaches to improving quality care. There were also common approaches to criteria development using the *structure, process,* and *outcome* format for the first time. Again, these studies were also most often retrospective outcome audits, based on a medical diagnosis, that even used similar study design formats and tools provided by the JCAHO.

Also during this period, risk management programs developed that were often closely linked to quality assurance activities. Risk management was an outgrowth of the rise in malpractice lawsuits in health care. A risk manager's main functions were to track serious falls, medication errors, and other untoward occurrences, as well as to promote better systems to correct potentially hazardous practices and written documentation.

In the early 1980s the focus of quality assurance activities shifted somewhat when JCAHO changed its requirements. No longer was it sufficient to simply complete a certain number of required audits based on a chosen diagnosis, but a facility now had to have a written *plan* or *quality assurance mechanism* in place to integrate the quality assurance activities into the overall organizational structure of the facility on an ongoing basis. Further, the proposed studies were to be based on a problem in client care that had been identified by the facility or practitioners. The ultimate goal and emphasis of these studies was problem resolution—documented proof that the problem had been corrected or improved. Frequently the study (or limited aspects of it) was repeated numerous times until problem resolution was achieved. The emphasis was no longer on audit committees and completing a required number of studies, but on *assurance* of quality by solving priority problems of the facility in an integrated program approach.

In the late 1980s JCAHO again changed its requirements for quality assurance. (JCAHO requirements have, up to this point, largely shaped the approach and emphasis of quality assurance activities of hospitals and other accredited health care facilities; health care practitioners are free to conduct quality of care reviews using any other approach or methodology of preference within the constraints of the individual agency or facility structure.) The new requirement is that within the overall facility quality assurance program, each client care provider department or service (including the nursing service) must monitor and evaluate the quality and appropriateness of the care provided and resolve all identified problems. The difference is that the monitoring and evaluation are part of an ongoing, planned, systematic review and evaluation process, not necessarily the one-time, limited-sample studies, as were done previously. Another difference in this new approach is that problem identification became the result of the ongoing monitoring activities that had been the beginning point of the earlier problem-focused studies.

In this new approach, ongoing monitoring of important selected aspects, or *indicators,* of quality care will point to a possible problem. It is at this point that *focused review* of the problem area can be done until there is evidence of problem resolution. In the meantime the monitoring is continuing and the indicator that originally pointed to the problem can be continually assessed for evidence of progress toward the ultimate goal of problem resolution. The focused review (or smaller problem-focused substudy) helps to bring attention to the problem or better define it so that the appropriate actions for resolution can be undertaken. It is not always necessary to do a focused review of a problem that is indicated by the ongoing monitoring activity. Sometimes the actions that need to be taken are obvious and can be easily implemented. In such cases the next report of the ongoing monitoring activity will indicate the effectiveness of the actions taken. An example of this methodology as used in one hospital nursing department quality assurance program is as follows:

- Selected data from every medication error is collected, tabulated, and reported quarterly (i.e., ongoing, planned systematic monitoring of a selected indicator of quality).
- *Patterns* of problems are analyzed in committee to determine which common problems frequently recur.
- A pattern of frequent administration of medication by the incorrect route was related to administration of pre–cardiac catheterization medications (given intramuscularly instead of orally).

- The committee was unsure how big the problem really was and uncertain how many additional errors of this type either were not reported or were undetected. A focused review of this problem was recommended.
- A focused review of this specific problem was conducted for one month by nurses in the cardiac catheterization laboratory, who verified the route of premedication with the client on arrival to the procedure room.
- It was found that most, if not all, errors of this type were being detected and reported in the ongoing monitoring of errors program (no further problem was found in the focused review).
- Corrective actions to eliminate the problem were undertaken on the units that had been shown to have had errors.
- The quarterly ongoing reports on medication errors showed no further incidents related to pre–cardiac catheterization medications given by the incorrect route.

Management of data that is repetitive and ongoing lends itself well to computerized reporting systems. The development of personal computers has made it possible for facilities of any size to manage some of these large, ongoing data bases.

Another development of the late 1980s is that much more commonly the client care record is part of a computerized information management system. With such a system, indicators of quality care can be systematically retrieved to measure quality.

The introduction of the prospective payment system for Medicare by the federal government in the mid-1980s using diagnostic-related groups (DRGs) also had a tremendous impact on measuring the quality and appropriateness of care. The new system has hastened the use of computers for information management and, generally, has improved efficiency. It has also made possible some national standards and norms for each DRG as well as other quality indicators. Table 4.1 summarizes the development of quality assurance activities during the seventies and eighties.

Professionals and Quality Care

Society has long expected the professions to regulate themselves by the setting and monitoring of standards for professional practice. Phaneuf gives the explanation

Table 4.1
Development of Quality Assurance Activities

Period	The Definition of Quality
1970s	• Retrospective audit • Concurrent review • Outcome, process, structure • Nursing audit • Patient care audit, multidisciplinary audit • Risk Management
	The Organization for Quality
Early 1980s	• Quality Assurance • Problem focused • Problem identification and resolution • Quality assurance plan • Quality assurance program
	The Management of Quality Data
Late 1980s	• Ongoing systematic review and evaluation • Computers • Information management systems • Diagnostic related groups (DRGs) • National Standards and Data

Source: From Janet McBride, unpublished, 1982.

of the relationship between societal expectations and the professions:

> There is a social contract between society and the professions. Under its terms, society grants the professions authority over functions vital to themselves, and permits them considerable autonomy in the conduct of their own affairs. In return, the professions are expected to act responsibly; always mindful of the public trust. Self-regulation is at the heart of that relationship. It is the authentic hallmark of the mature professional. (22)

The appraisal of the quality of nursing services is an integral part of nursing's responsibility to the public trust. It is incumbent on the nursing profession to control and monitor its own practice in order to make the public feel secure about the appropriateness of the quality, quantity, and cost of nursing services. Nursing, as a profession, must not lose the public's trust.

There has, however, been a general erosion of that trust, and professionals have been required to show evidence that standards of professional practice are being met. Regulation in health care delivery systems has dramatically increased in the past decade. This clearly focuses on and specifically mandates accountability in the use of health resources.

Accountability

Accountability is a relatively new term in health care. It came to wide usage in the early 1970s, paralleling the rise of consumerism. Consumerism, and concomitant political and social changes of the Great Society (1963–68), had a significant impact on expectations about health care. Before this time Americans generally considered health care a privilege, not a right.

Even in the absence of health regulation, nurses would be professionally accountable for satisfying the public's trust, for validating that standards for care are being formulated and met. The concept of accountability for practice was weakly defined under "functional" and "team" nursing systems. It was impossible to focus responsibility for the quality of care delivered on any specific nurse. One could only ascertain whether the nursing *group* was meeting standards of care. Primary nursing, both as philosophy of practice and as a method of staffing, has provided the means for a professional nurse to be identified as responsible, liable, or answerable for exceeding, meeting, or failing to meet clearly established standards of practice (5).

Peer Review

Peer review is the process by which nurses who are actively engaged in the practice of nursing appraise the quality of nursing care in a given situation in accordance with established standards of practice (4). It is the appraisal of nursing care by *nurses;* it is *not* a review of nursing care conducted by a profession other than nursing. Peer review can be accomplished by (a) appraising the care rendered to clients and (b) appraising nurse performance, with primary focus on the nurse. The purposes of peer review are to:

- evaluate the quality and quantity of nursing care;
- identify the strengths and weaknesses of nursing care;
- provide evidence to be used as the basis of recommendations for new or altered policies and procedures to improve nursing care; and
- identify those areas of practice in which patterns

indicate more knowledge is needed by the practitioners (4).

Quality: The Concept

What does *quality* in nursing care mean? It validates the fact that nursing care meets, or compares favorably with, a norm or standard. This norm or *standard* is valued as representing excellence, or some characteristic or "goodness."

Quality Assurance Defined

The following compilation of some common interpretations of quality assurance has been adapted from an article by Schmadl (24).

American Nurses' Association: Estimation of the degree of excellence in (1) the alteration of the health status of consumers attained through providers' performance of (2) diagnostic, therapeutic, prognostic, and other health care activities. (3)

Quality assurance is a relatively new term conveying the broad idea that superiority or excellence in care is made secure or certain.

A program executed to make secure or certain the excellence of health care; the term is applied to programs as limited as that of an administrative unit of a health care agency or as broad as that of a community, a region, a state, or a nation. The program must have two major components: (1) the securing of measurements and ascertaining of the degree to which stated standards are met; (2) the introduction of changes based on information supplied by the measurements, with the view to improvement of the total effort and product of the unit or agency.

Quality assurance is an ongoing program in the nursing profession constructed and executed to secure and implement the excellence of health care. (4)

Brown: Quality assurance, when used in reference to health care, refers to the accountability of health personnel for the quality of care they provide.

Lang: Activities done to determine the extent to which a phenomenon fulfills certain values and activities done to assure changes in practices which will fulfill the highest levels of values.

Nichols: The term quality assurance is used to describe a process in which standards are set and action is taken to ensure achievement of standards. . . . It involves the description of the level of quality desired and feasible, and a system for ensuring its achievement.

Schmadl: Quality assurance involves assuring the consumer of a specified degree of excellence through continuous measurement and evaluation of structural components, goal-directed nursing process, and/or consumer outcome, using pre-established criteria and standards and available norms, and followed by appropriate alteration with the purpose of improvement. (24)

Zimmer: Quality assurance is estimation of the degree of excellence in patient health outcomes and in activity and other resource cost outcomes. (27)

As the variety of definitions indicates, the standard of "quality" may vary within a group of nurses and among consumers of the health care product. It is important to remember that it is the consumer of nursing services to whom we must assure the quality of the care. The changing societal values have reinterpreted and recast it as a "right." (The American Nurses' Association [ANA] has long affirmed this perception [4].) People have become consumers, buyers of goods and services. Dissatisfaction with the product, service, or provider has led to a dramatic increase in malpractice suits. This was to be expected as the public increasingly shows its concern for participation, information, and redress not only in the buying of goods, but also in the provision of services (5).

Standards of Nursing Practice

Standards for nursing describe a systematic approach to nursing practice. They are the objective measure of the level of appropriate care, the "goodness" of the level of care delivered by an accountable and responsible professional practitioner.

The standards of nursing practice reflect the beliefs and values of the profession, professionals, and consumers, as well as those of society at large, and model and guide the provision of nursing care.

Setting and Maintaining Standards—Why?

Quality cannot be assessed or described without standards against which to measure. In this era of cost containment in health care, it also is critical to define the role and practice of nursing so that actual costs of care can be established for further potential reduction and for reimbursement purposes.

In the Marker Model (26), standards are seen as the *means* to an end (quality care), not as an end in themselves. Quality must be defined through standards; thus compliance to standards is the definition of the concept "quality care." Likewise, noncompliance to a standard reveals a problem that must be pursued to resolution in a quality assurance program.

The setting of standards and the assurance of compliance to them guarantee the consumer a defined level of care.

In addition, setting and maintaining standards for care are:

- a professional obligation to define its scope of function;
- a consumer right;
- mandated by regulatory/accrediting agencies;
- a basis for evaluation of nursing staff, patient care, systems management;
- a basis for costing out nursing services;
- integral to effecting change in a system; and
- a basis for cost containment (26).

Types of Standards

There are three major categories of standards that may be written: structure, process, and outcome.

Structure Standards.   Structure standards often take a policy format. They define what conditions, systems, and equipment are needed to facilitate quality care. Structure standards may relate to anything in the care delivery process that is not associated with care giving. Often these standards are regulatory and legal requirements for a facility. Structure standards provide the basis for supporting the actual delivery of care. Such standards may relate to the following (26):

Physical plant and environment—room size, temperature, layout, maintenance, etc.
Patient population—adult or children, specialty (psychiatric, orthopedic, etc.)

Resources required
Staff credentialing
Quantity/Qualifications of staff
Equipment/Supplies

Process Standards. Process standards can be set in numerous formats, such as clinical nursing procedures, job descriptions, performance appraisals, clinical protocols, and standards of care. These standards may be directed at either the patient or the nurse. They define the actions or procedure to be carried out, as well as what constitutes care expectations. Nursing procedures give the nurse a step-by-step "recipe" to follow to accomplish a task, for example, colostomy irrigation. Process standards may also be a plan of care developed for a group of clients with similar problems or characteristics (e.g., preoperative client care). (These standard care plans may be preprinted.) Nursing procedures and standards of care are perhaps the most common examples of process standards.

Outcome Standards. The usual format for outcome standards is a goal statement. The standards are written to define the end result of the care to be given. They often describe elements of patient education or staff inservice education to be mastered. Goal statements that nurses write in nursing care plans are also examples of outcome standards that the nurse plans to assist the client to achieve. There are a number of established standards in three major realms of professional nursing practice: legal, professional, and regulatory. Examples of the standards to which nurses are accountable include state practice acts, state health codes, patient's bill of rights, ANA Code of Ethics, agency/institution policies and procedures, ANA Standards of Practice, clinical specialty standards, and JCAHO standards (if the facility seeks voluntary accreditation). The same generally accepted standards that define quality care are the standards that may be used in a malpractice suit to determine whether negligence is involved.

A number of client care standards developed by nurses have been published. In addition, guidebooks are available for nurses who want to create their own standards for clinical practice.

Although some professional and health care organizations have formulated standards for nurses or standards affecting nursing practice (e.g., ANA and JCAHO), these standards and the nursing process are still intertwined. Joint Commission on Accreditation of Healthcare Organizations standards also require that nursing written documentation reflect the use of the nursing process (14).

American Nurses' Association Standards

The development and implementation of standards of nursing practice, as a means to improve nursing practice, has long been a priority of the ANA. Between 1973 and 1975 the ANA approved its generic and specialty standards (Table 4.2).

The generic standards of practice are designed so that nursing care may be delivered in *any* setting—home, hospital, school, or community. They are global in nature and enable the nurse who is a generalist to practice in compliance with the highest expectations of professionalism. The specialty standards, on the other hand, although following the same general format as the generic, include *subject-specific items* for data collection, diagnosis, plan formulation, and outcome evaluation. The following is a noninclusive list of ANA Specialty Standards:

Table 4.2
American Nurses' Association Standards of Nursing Practice

Standard 1	The collection of data about the health status of the client/patient is systematic and continuous. The data are accessible, communicated, and recorded.
Standard 2	Nursing diagnoses are derived from health status data.
Standard 3	The plan of nursing care includes goals derived from the nursing diagnoses.
Standard 4	The plan of nursing care includes priorities and the prescribed nursing approaches or measures to achieve the goals derived from the nursing diagnoses.
Standard 5	Nursing actions provide for client/patient participation in health promotion, maintenance and restoration.
Standard 6	Nursing actions assist the client/patient to maximize his health capabilities.
Standard 7	The client's/patient's progress or lack of progress toward goal achievement is determined by the client/patient and the nurse.
Standard 8	The client's/patient's progress or lack of progress toward goal achievement directs reassessment, reordering of priorities, new goal setting and revision of the plan of nursing care.

Source: American Nurses' Association, *A Plan for Implementation of the Standards of Nursing Practice* (Kansas City, MO: The Association, 1975), p. 15.

Gerontological Nursing Practice
Maternal and Child Health Nursing Practice
Psychiatric and Mental Health Nursing Practice
Community Health Nursing Practice
Medical-Surgical Nursing Practice
Cardiovascular Nursing Practice
Orthopedic Nursing Practice
Nursing Practice: Operating Room
Emergency Nursing Practice
Rehabilitation Nursing Practice
Urologic Nursing Practice
Pediatric Oncology Nursing Practice
Nursing Staff Requirements for In-Patient Health
    Care Services
Continuing Education in Nursing
Outcome Standards for Cancer Nursing Practice

Nursing practice based on the implementation of the ANA standards is the responsibility of every nursing practitioner and is characterized by close communication between the client and the nurse, and the development and interpretation of health care plans and their effects on the client and family (11).

Joint Commission on Accreditation of Healthcare Organizations Standards

The JCAHO is a voluntary accreditation program for hospitals, long-term care institutions, and other health care institutions. These institutions pay the JCAHO a fee to schedule a visit by a survey team. The survey is conducted according to a manual of JCAHO standards for the major service departments in a facility, such as dietary, social service, infection control, nursing, special care units, and emergency services. Before the survey visit the hospital is required to post a notice of the forthcoming survey and solicit input from the hospital community at large of perceived problems or complaints. The survey team, which includes a nurse, may then focus on these problems in addition to completing the routine survey for compliance to its minimum standards for accreditation.

The JCAHO standards for nursing services describe how a nursing service in an agency should be administered, as well as some aspects of nursing practice. Nursing process and client education are emphasized, along with standards for the orientation, preparation, and credentialing of nurses. Because these standards have been developed in accordance with input from nursing leaders, they represent an excellent description of professional nursing practice in hospital and long-term care settings. Table 4.3 presents the requirements for quality assurance activities for nursing in a hospital setting.

Table 4.3
Joint Commission for Accreditation
of Healthcare Organizations
Standards for Nursing Services

Standard I	The nursing department/service shall be directed by a qualified nurse administrator and shall be appropriately integrated with the medical staff and with other hospital staffs that provide and contribute to patient care.
Standard II	The nursing department/service shall be organized to meet the nursing care needs of patients and to maintain established standards of nursing practice.
Standard III	Nursing department/service assignments in the provision of nursing care shall be commensurate with the qualifications of nursing personnel and shall be designed to meet the nursing care needs of patients.
Standard IV	Individualized, goal-directed nursing care shall be provided to patients through the use of the nursing process.
Standard V	Nursing department/service personnel shall be prepared through appropriate education and training programs for their responsibilities in the provision of nursing care.
Standard VI	Written policies and procedures that reflect optimal standards of nursing practice shall guide the provision of nursing care.
Standard VII	As part of the hospital's quality assurance program, the quality and appropriateness of the patient care provided by the nursing department/service are monitored and evaluated, and identified problems are resolved.

Source: American Nurses' Association, *A Plan for Implementation of the Standards of Nursing Practice* (Kansas City, MO: The Association, 1975), p. 15.

Many other agencies and nursing groups have published standards for nursing care for specific clients, diagnoses, settings, and procedures. Among these are the Duke University Nursing Services (7), which has written standards for many common medical and surgical client care problems; the American Association of Critical Care Nurses, which has formulated standards for the critically ill (2); and Johansen and co-workers, who have written standards for critical care nursing (13). Nurses who wish to write their own standards for practice can refer to several texts on writing standards (19, 26).

Indicators of Quality Care

Because it is not possible to measure every standard that exists or every facet of practice, it is necessary to determine what aspects of care are *indicators* of quality care. Indicators should be chosen that represent (a) known or suspected problems, (b) areas of frequent nursing involvement, and (c) benchmarks of quality care.

One cannot omit known problem areas from review and still expect to improve on or deliver quality care. Areas of frequent involvement for nurses include medication administration, client education, client assessment, counseling, and discharge planning. Benchmarks of quality care are those aspects of care that, in their absence, raise serious doubts that good care is being provided (e.g., high rates of facility-acquired decubiti, nosocomial infections, complications, and preventable accidents/incidents). The benchmarks of quality for each facility and discipline should be identified and included in the review and evaluation activities.

Review and Evaluation

As discussed earlier, a quality assurance program should have ongoing, planned, systematic review and evaluation of the quality and appropriateness of care, with the focus on resolution of identified problems. It is important to understand what is meant by review and evaluation. First of all, most quality assurance studies are not formal, controlled research and should not be considered as such. Their use is usually limited to a single setting; they are a pragmatic approach to problem solving that may or may not be replicated or applicable elsewhere. Table 4.4 shows the relationships between research and evaluation studies.

- *Not* formal studies
- *Is* focused on clinical aspects of patient care
- Results in *problem identification*
- Done on a *regular* basis
- Uses *multiple* data sources
- Reflected in baseline status reports:
  —Data reviewed
  —Problems identified
  —Status of problems (resolution and follow-up)

Figure 4.1. Review and Evaluation
Source: From Janet McBride, unpublished, 1982.

In addition, review and evaluation of quality should be focused on *clinical* aspects of care. The study should be done on a regular basis, either intermittently or continuously. It may use multiple data sources for measurement instead of using only the medical record. The results should be reflected in regular baseline status reports from which data can be readily reviewed, problems identified, or the status of problems previously identified may be assessed for resolution or further follow-up (see Figure 4.1).

Measuring Compliance with Standards

Criteria Selection and Development

Once standards have been developed (or recognized) and indicators or aspects of care that represent quality have been identified, there is a basis on which to begin the measurement process (see Figure 4.2). From the more general *standard* statements, any number of *criteria* statements can be developed. In effect, these cri-

Table 4.4
Differences Between Research and Evaluation

Activity	Research	Evaluation
Problem selection and definition	Responsibility of investigator	Determined by situation and constituents
Hypothesis testing	Formal statistical testing	Generally not done
Value judgment	Limited to selection of problem	Present in all phases of project
Replication of results	High likelihood	Low likelihood
Data collection	Dictated by problem	Heavily influenced by feasibility
Control of relevant variables	High	Low
Generalization of results	Can be high	Usually low

Source: Adapted from John K. Hemphill, in *Educational Evaluation: New Rules, New Means,* ed. Ralph W. Tyler, Sixty-eighth Yearbook of the National Society for the Study of Education, part 2 (Chicago: University of Chicago Press, 1969), pp. 190–91.

- Develop criteria that reflect the intent of the standards.
  - —Process
  - —Outcome
  - —Structure
- Select appropriate data source
  - —Written record (patient record)
  - —Observation
  - —Interview (patient questionnaires)
- Determine time frame
  - —Retrospective
  - —Concurrent
  - —Prospective

Figure 4.2. Measurement of Compliance with Standards
Source: From Janet McBride, unpublished, 1982.

teria *measure* the intent of the standard. By writing measurable criteria from established standards, one can compare actual practice with standards of practice expected. Because the standards are the representation of quality, or the "goodness" of care, nurses who meet the criteria are validating or "assuring" the quality of client care. Criteria that are written, developed, or adopted must be, first and foremost, clinically valid. They must be consistent with policies and procedures, rules and regulations, and standards of practice/protocols that exist. They should reflect the current scientific and professional literature and the very best in clinical knowledge and experience. They should help to identify or assess problems. Any type or combination (structure, process, or outcome) may be chosen, and any number of criteria may be developed, although the realities of time, expense, and ability to measure and manage the amount of resultant data must be considered (see Figure 4.3).

After criteria have been written or modified for a situation or facility, they should be shared with and agreed on by the staff. The staff members need to know exactly what they will be held accountable for and to have input if they are in disagreement.

- Best in knowledge and experience
- Literature
- Standards of care/practice
- Policies/procedures, rules and regulations
- Any type/any number
- Agreed on by staff
- Identify or assess problems

Figure 4.3. Requirements for Clinically Valid Criteria
Source: From Janet McBride, unpublished, 1982.

Data Source Selection

Selection of an appropriate approach to identify problems in the review and evaluation process must be made based on such factors as feasibility, cost, efficiency, and, especially, where the data resides. The source of data may be only the medical record for some reviews, but it may also include client questionnaires, client interviews, staff observations or interviews, administrative forms, logs, charts, algorithms or criteria maps, incident reports, or even combined approaches to these sources.

Time Frame

There may be little choice in the time frame selection if, for example, it is decided that the data is available only from client interview and the only appropriate access to the client for interview is during the current entry into the health care system. This would mandate that the review and evaluation activities be done in a *concurrent* time frame, that is, while client care and treatment are in progress. Review and evaluation activities are commonly performed concurrently. However, if the data are relevant only to the final outcome of care provided, it may be necessary, or most efficient, to review records after discharge from the health care facility or after receipt of care. This is *retrospective* review of care. It is also possible to review care prospectively, that is, before the receipt of care, although this type of review is less common and often not feasible.

Quality Appraisal Process

Appraisal of quality is not an end in itself, but rather a means of instituting appropriate change with the purpose of improvement. In client care studies it is frequently a temptation to consider data gathering the ultimate objective. It is easy to omit the most important, and hardest, part of the process—initiating changes based on the results of the evaluation studies.

There are several underlying assumptions in the quality appraisal and assurance process:

- Nursing care affects the outcome of the client's illness and influences his or her future health status.
- Identifiable outcomes exist that are primarily attributable to nursing care, even though nursing shares responsibility for client care with many health disciplines (10).
- Quality assurance accompanies the acceptance of

responsibility and accountability for professional practice.

- Quality of nursing care is a tangible and is therefore subject to measurement.
- When specific criteria or standards are applied, competency in the planning and execution of nursing care, of which recording and reporting are an integral part, can be evaluated through directly observable entities (8).

Up to this point the process of measuring quality has been discussed. Once the data have been gathered, one must begin the problem-solving process in order to resolve problems that are reflected by the data or to find opportunities to improve care. The ANA believes that it is possible to implement standards as well as solve problems by means of a quality assurance program and has proposed a model to assist implementation of such a program (Figure 4.4).

American Nurses' Association Model and Problem Solving

The first three steps in the model were discussed previously in the sections on standards, criteria, and measuring compliance to standards. Problem solving begins after data have been gathered and measurement is completed in step four.

The ANA model is flexible and can be used in different practice settings. The focus may be on the performance of an individual nurse or on that of a group of nurses; on an individual client or on a group of clients and the care provided; or on the institutional setting. The problem-solving process is easily integrated into this circular model. This circularity indicates the dynamic and constant process of care evaluation. The model is designed so that data can be fed into the process at any one of eight points.

1. Identify values. The major sources of values are societal, professional, and scientific (4). Keep in mind that each of these sources of values is subject to changes that may redefine quality, and thus our standards of practice.

The values of the care community may vary somewhat from those of society at large. The values of society may reflect its ethnicity or its predominant cultural or religious group. Each nurse also approaches a client and nursing care with his or her own value system.

The philosophy of the nurse, the institution, the nursing service, and the client, and the community expectations should be considered in this component of the model.

2. Identify structure, process, and outcome standards, and criteria. This process was described earlier. The following are examples of the three types of criteria statements:

The operating room had all the required equipment and staff. (Structure)
The operation was a success. (Process)
But the patient died. (Outcome)

3. Secure measurements needed to determine degree of attainment of standards and criteria. This topic was

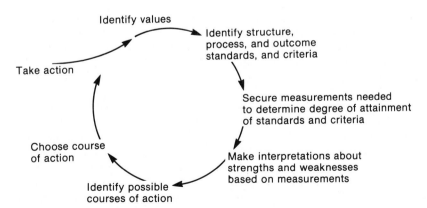

Figure 4.4. American Nurses' Association Model for Quality Assurance

Source: American Nurses' Association, *A Plan for Implementation of the Standards of Nursing Practice* (Kansas City, MO: The Association, 1975), p. 15.

also discussed earlier in relation to measuring compliance to standards. Methods to secure measurements include, but are not limited to, the following: direct client observation, external and internal peer review, concurrent monitoring programs/systems, retrospective audits, utilization review, self-assessment, client questionnaires, supervisor evaluation performance observation, and data from other sources, such as incidence rates for medications errors, nosocomial infections, falls, lost property, and client complaints. The method chosen for measurement will depend on the purpose of the measure, the tools available, and the human and fiscal resources of the institution (4).

At this point the measurement is completed and the problem-solving process begins.

4. *Make interpretations about strengths and weaknesses based on measurements.* In this step the degree of agreement between identified standards and criteria and the level of nursing practice is measured. Both strengths and weaknesses may be identified. It is important to document both. Strengths may later serve as a baseline for future studies to determine whether practice has maintained high compliance to standards. They may also be used as areas to encourage or commend the nursing staff. Professionals certainly need positive feedback from time to time!

5. *Identify possible courses of action.* Actions chosen should reinforce strengths and change the weaknesses of the nursing practice. Among the more commonly proposed actions are continuing education, in-service education, peer pressure, administrative changes, environmental changes, research, punitive or reward action, and self-initiated change (4). The actions chosen are based on the probable causes of strengths and weaknesses. The next step of the model could be based on wrong assumptions unless probable causes are interpreted. The need to determine the cause of weaknesses is demonstrated by the experience of one quality assurance committee. The committee found low compliance with documentation of daily weights in clients with congestive heart failure. The nurses could have assumed that the clients were being weighed but their weights were not being documented on the record. They could have then gone to next step in the model and proposed actions to encourage nurses to be more vigilant about documentation of weights. That would have proved a wasted effort because on further analysis of possible causes, they determined that it was largely bedfast clients, who require bedscales, who were not being weighed daily. The committee was aware of several problems with bedscale equipment on the unit and made *written* recommendation to administration that new

bedscales be purchased. Written documentation of lower attainment of standards owing to equipment problems resulted in the acquisition of equipment needed for quality care.

6. *Choose the best course of action.* From the possible alternatives, the action(s) most appropriate to the need should be chosen. It may be a continuing education program, in-service education, communication with other departments, rewards or recognition, punitive action, or counseling of individual practitioners.

7. *Take action.* Accountability for quality practice necessitates the implementation of action and subsequent documentation. The findings of the study and actions taken need to be formally reported through the existing accountability mechanism. In the example of the bedscales, once the nursing committee formally reported the deficiency and the need for the equipment through the quality assurance mechanism, the accountability for quality practice shifted to the level of organizational administration, which had the authority to grant or deny the needed resource.

8. *Follow-up to assure that the actions chosen were effective.* The ANA Model for Quality Assurance does not have an explicit step for follow-up. The follow-up step requires that weaknesses in practice be remeasured at a later interval, usually by the same method. The results of the restudy determine the effectiveness, or ineffectiveness, of the actions taken. It is possible that either the wrong cause or the wrong actions were chosen, and that a new course of action(s) should be determined. In the ANA model one would simply return to step three as a follow-up and proceed from that point.

Using the ANA Quality Assurance Model to Measure ANA Standards

Figure 4.5 shows an example of how the ANA quality assurance model might be used for nurses in private practice.

Establishing Quality Assurance Programs

Institutions or agencies that provide health care and are reimbursed by third-party payers are required to have an ongoing program to appraise care and services, to assure quality. The program must focus on both the cost and the quality of the services provided. The reasons for the existence of this systematic appraisal mechanism are statutory, regulatory, and professional. A quality assurance program may be for problem solving, for implementing standards, or for monitoring management effectiveness. The data gathered from the quality

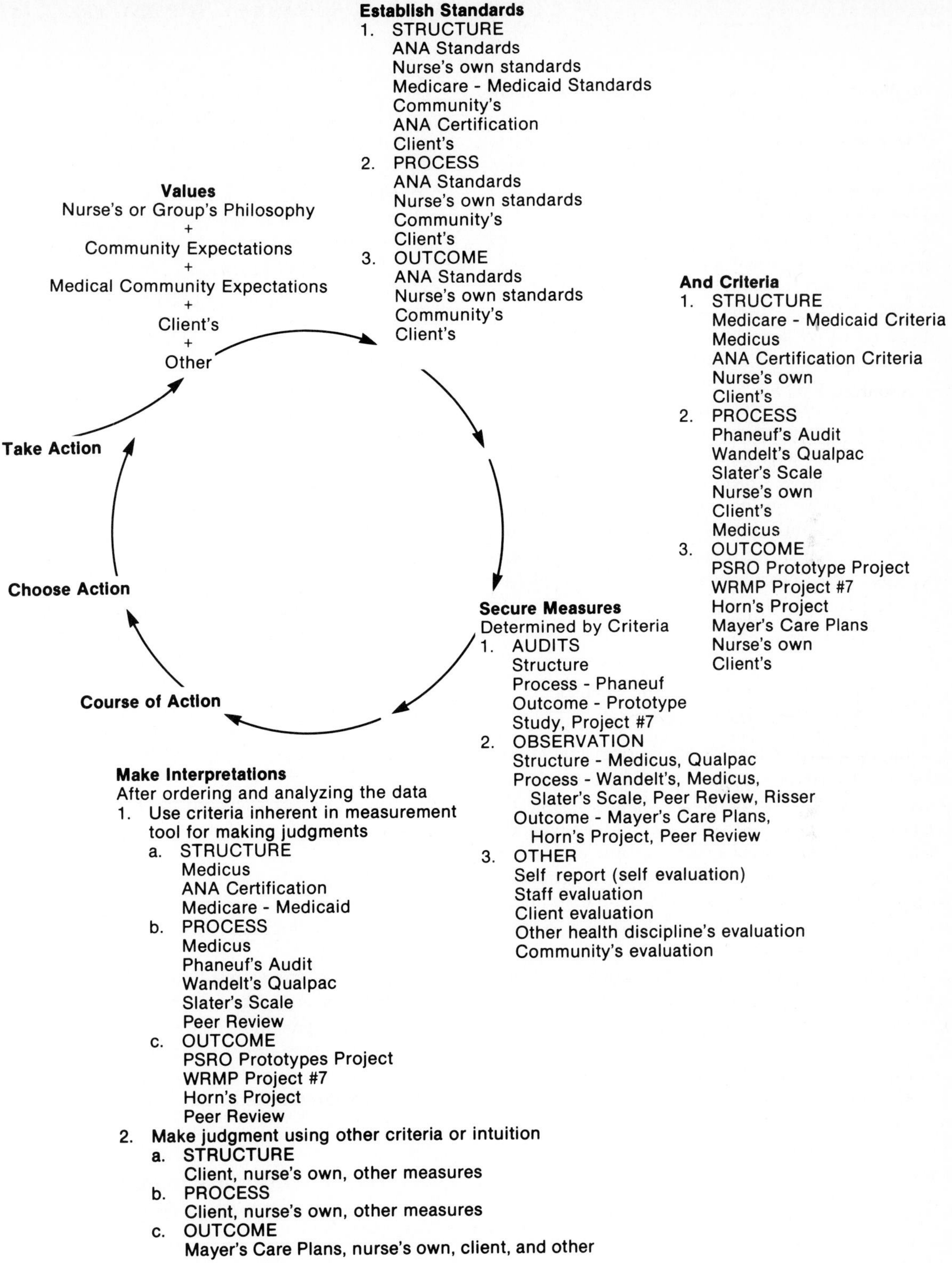

Establish Standards

1. STRUCTURE
   ANA Standards
   Nurse's own standards
   Medicare - Medicaid Standards
   Community's
   ANA Certification
   Client's
2. PROCESS
   ANA Standards
   Nurse's own standards
   Community's
   Client's
3. OUTCOME
   ANA Standards
   Nurse's own standards
   Community's
   Client's

Values

Nurse's or Group's Philosophy
+
Community Expectations
+
Medical Community Expectations
+
Client's
+
Other

Take Action

Choose Action

Course of Action

And Criteria

1. STRUCTURE
   Medicare - Medicaid Criteria
   Medicus
   ANA Certification Criteria
   Nurse's own
   Client's
2. PROCESS
   Phaneuf's Audit
   Wandelt's Qualpac
   Slater's Scale
   Nurse's own
   Client's
   Medicus
3. OUTCOME
   PSRO Prototype Project
   WRMP Project #7
   Horn's Project
   Mayer's Care Plans
   Nurse's own
   Client's

Secure Measures

Determined by Criteria

1. AUDITS
   Structure
   Process - Phaneuf
   Outcome - Prototype
   Study, Project #7
2. OBSERVATION
   Structure - Medicus, Qualpac
   Process - Wandelt's, Medicus,
   Slater's Scale, Peer Review, Risser
   Outcome - Mayer's Care Plans,
   Horn's Project, Peer Review
3. OTHER
   Self report (self evaluation)
   Staff evaluation
   Client evaluation
   Other health discipline's evaluation
   Community's evaluation

Make Interpretations

After ordering and analyzing the data

1. Use criteria inherent in measurement
   tool for making judgments
   a. STRUCTURE
      Medicus
      ANA Certification
      Medicare - Medicaid
   b. PROCESS
      Medicus
      Phaneuf's Audit
      Wandelt's Qualpac
      Slater's Scale
      Peer Review
   c. OUTCOME
      PSRO Prototypes Project
      WRMP Project #7
      Horn's Project
      Peer Review
2. Make judgment using other criteria or intuition
   a. STRUCTURE
      Client, nurse's own, other measures
   b. PROCESS
      Client, nurse's own, other measures
   c. OUTCOME
      Mayer's Care Plans, nurse's own, client, and other

Figure 4.5. Use of ANA Quality Assurance Model in Private Practice.

Source: American Nurses' Association, *A Plan for Implementation of the Standards of Nursing Practice.* (Kansas City, Mo.: The Association, 1975), p. 22.

assurance activities of a facility may be used by the managers to improve orientation of staff, to provide focus for in-service and continuing education programs, to budget staff and equipment, to assign staff, to modify or add policies or procedures, and to appraise staff performance (see Figure 4.6).

Quality assurance programs are generally conducted through evaluation of the *patterns* of problems or successes in the care of *groups* of clients, rather than by focusing on specific clients. Although problem solving for specific clients is a natural outcome of the process, a more global approach is usually taken. This approach is not inappropriate, since an individual client is likely to receive the same level of care as that shown by evaluation data for groups of clients with a similar problem.

Usually quality assurance activities are accomplished through a committee structure. The organization of the committee and the quality assurance program itself are at the discretion of the facility. Some factors to consider in developing a quality assurance program and organizing a committee to carry out the mission are delineated in Table 4.5.

Information Systems in the Quality Assurance Program

Facilities that have standards monitoring systems and other data systems may require tiered information systems (sometimes computerized) to make sure that the "right information is available to the right person at the right time," for data management. Unit-level nurses need more specific feedback to choose appropriate actions for change based on the results than does upper-level management. Also, there needs to be a channel, or accountability feedback mechanism, for nurses who provide the client care to report the actions that were taken to improve care as accountable professionals. Discussion of the need for incoming and outgoing flow of

---

- Improve clinical orientation
- Focus in-service and continuing education
- Budget staff and equipment
- Assign personnel
- Modify/add policies and procedures
- Performance appraisals
- Assess effectiveness of patient teaching/health promotion programs
- Planning clinical programs/projects

Figure 4.6. Uses for Quality Assurance Program Findings

Table 4.5
Factors Affecting the Organization
of a Quality Assurance Program/Committee

I. Purpose
  A. Assure quality patient care.
  B. Meet regulatory/accrediting requirements.
II. Objectives/Approach
  A. Identify and resolve problems.
  B. Develop/Monitor standards of care.
  C. Generate data for management.
III. Committee Composition
  A. All levels of staff
  B. Only management levels
  C. Only staff (nurses)
  D. Interdisciplinary participation
IV. Committee Functions
  A. Determine problems to be studied.
  B. Develop criteria/standards as basis for review.
  C. Retrieve data.
  D. Review data from multiple sources.
  E. Recommend or implement corrective action.
  F. Follow-up for problem resolution.
  G. Disseminate reports to appropriate levels.
  H. Perform secretarial functions—minutes, collate and display data, prepare reports, etc.
V. Reporting Mechanisms—"The Right Information to the Right Person at the Right Time"
  A. Tiered reporting systems
  B. Maintaining confidentiality of data

Source: From Janet McBride, unpublished, 1982.

information seems obvious and somewhat trivial; however, the reporting of data and then the actions taken can be a difficult challenge. It is, in effect, the essence of accountability.

Perhaps the overriding justification for a quality assurance program is professional accountability. As professional nursing practitioners, we have a desire and responsibility to assure, if not guarantee, our clients that care is accessible, acceptable, adequate, affordable, appropriate, comprehensive, effective, and efficient (27).

Introduction of Change and Improvement in Practice

The critical issue in quality assurance is whether or not the provision of data to people and organizations will result in changed behaviors.

The real barriers to quality assurance are not the problems in data retrieval and analysis, but the resistance to change among practitioners and health care institutions. In order to effectively plan change strategies it is important to understand the reasons for resistance. Luke and Boss identify the following ten barriers to change (16):

1. Autonomy expectations of health professionals
2. Collective benefits of stability
3. Calculated opposition to change (due to)
   a. Loss of prevailing advantage
   b. Protection of (current) quality
   c. Psychic cost of change
4. Programmed behavior (prevents innovation)
5. Tunnel vision (loss of perspective on a problem)
6. Limitation of resources
7. Sunk costs (any investment that is not convertible)
8. Accumulations of official constraints on behavior (statutes, regulations, and internal policies)
9. Unofficial and unplanned constraints on behavior (internal opposition)
10. Interorganizational agreements

Nurses who are interested in improving client care and who desire involvement in positive, planned change may be able to become involved in the quality assurance program in their practice setting. If such a program does not yet exist, or is in its infant stage, nurses may be able to advocate for beginning or improving the appraisal program. There are informal groups of nurses who are interested in quality assurance. These groups serve as resource colleagues for those nurses who are interested in initiating a quality assurance program. There are also numerous workshops designed to educate nurses about quality assurance strategies.

The Future: Quality Assurance and Prospective Payment Plans

Before the mid-1980s hospitals in the United States were reimbursed by third-party payers (i.e., Medicare) on the basis of clients' length of stay or the number of individual services that were provided. In essence, this fee-for-service system paid hospitals for doing as much as they could for clients. The cost of health care was escalating more rapidly than almost any other economic indicator,

and it was predicted that the federal Medicare fund would be depleted by the end of the decade. Congress decided that it was no longer willing to pay for so much of the nation's health care. The new plan enacted by Congress required that by 1986, hospitals in most states would be reimbursed by a prospective payment plan that was devised to save $20.4 billion in federal health costs by 1988. Although the prospective payment plan is a *federal* program for federally funded health care programs, such as Medicare, many other third-party payers, such as Blue Cross, have traditionally followed the lead of the government by instituting similar programs.

Prospective Payment—What Is It?

Under prospective payment plans, payment limits are established in advance. The rates are not the same for all hospitals. Adjustments to the payment rates are based on hospital location (i.e., urban or rural), the presence of teaching programs, and the case mix of clients. For example, a community hospital in a rural area may receive $2,000 to care for a client with pneumonia, whereas a teaching hospital in an urban area might receive $2,500. A hospital would receive a flat rate per diagnosis and would be paid for doing as much as possible for a client as long as the hospital did not exceed the prospective payment rate. Quality care will no longer be the most that can be offered to clients, but rather the most that can be provided at a reasonable cost. Prospective payment offers an incentive to hospitals to become cost-efficient. If a hospital spends less than the flat prospective payment rate, it can keep a percentage of the difference. If it spends more, it must absorb the expense (23).

Clearly this method of reimbursement contrasts dramatically with the traditional method by which hospitals have been reimbursed. Some observers claim that prospective payment is the health care revolution of the 1980s. Prospective payment has already had profound effects on health care delivery in the United States. The average length of stay in hospitals has already been dramatically reduced, as well as unnecessary admissions and hospital days. The result has been faster turnover of clients in hospitals, as well as clients who are much sicker on arrival and discharge than in the past. Much more ambulatory surgery is being done, and there is increased reliance on home and community care after the acute illness phase. Costs also are being reduced by eliminating superfluous tests and treatments. The challenge for the future for establishing and maintaining quality care is to make sure that the appropriate hospital resources are used, no more and no less, and that the quality of care is not sacrificed for cost containment.

Diagnostic-Related Groups

Currently, there is a list of 470 diagnostic-related groups (DRGs) that groups patients according to variables that influence the consumption of resources. Some of the variables are principal diagnoses, operating room procedures, the presence or absence of complications and comorbidity, age, and length of stay. When a client enters a hospital the proper DRG category for that client will be assigned by computer after the pertinent medical record information has been entered into the system. Once the proper DRG is assigned, the hospital will receive the flat rate for that DRG whether the client stays the standard number of days or not.

Effect of DRGs on Nursing Practice

Expert nursing care is crucial to a hospital's financial well-being. Although it is less costly to employ personnel with lesser qualifications than the registered nurse, it is critical that nothing prolong a client's stay or consume unnecessary resources. The registered nurse who is aware of a client's assigned DRG category will know the standard length of stay for that DRG and can plan ahead to accomplish the client education and discharge planning by that deadline.

Because clients are in the hospital for shorter periods and are leaving "sicker" than in the past, teaching clients and their families self-care is more important than ever, and anticipating what resources they will need at home is critical. In general, hospital readmission for the same problem or for complications resulting from the admission is at the hospital's expense. Third-party payers also are not willing to pay for preventable complications, such as decubiti, nosocomial infections, and injuries related to falls. Each of these can result in additional consumption of supplies and resources and may increase the length of stay, which in turn may drive up the cost beyond the reimbursed rate. Nursing intervention decreases the risk of complications that prolong hospitalization.

The new reimbursement system necessitates maximum productivity and cost-effectiveness in all hospital services, including nursing, which is the largest labor and financial component of any hospital. More will be expected of nurses who work in hospitals, public health departments, and visiting nurse associations. It will become even more important that nurses be freed from

nonnursing duties that may be performed more cost-effectively by other employees. Accurate and timely documentation of nursing assessments can decrease the need for costly diagnostic tests (6).

Nurses need to become aware of the cost of supplies and time, and even of their own value. Nurses who believe that managing money and resources is not their function are doing a disservice to themselves, their peers, and the consumers for whom they are supposed to be advocates (6).

REFERENCES

1. American Academy of Nursing Task Force. *Magnet Hospitals: Attraction and Retention of Professional Nurses.* Kansas City, Mo.: American Nurses' Association, 1983.
2. American Association of Critical Care Nurses. *Standards for Nursing Care of the Critically Ill.* Reston, Va.: Reston Publishing Co., 1980.
3. American Nurses' Association. *Guidelines for Review of Nursing Care at the Local Level.* Publ. No. NP-54. Kansas City, Mo.: American Nurses' Association, 1976, A-2.
4. American Nurses' Association. *A Plan for Implementation of the Standards of Nursing Practice.* Publ. No. NP-51. Kansas City, Mo.: American Nurses' Association, 1975, 22.
5. Betz, M. "From Whence Accountability?" *Nursing and Health Care,* November 1981, 482.
6. Byrnes, M. A. "DRGs: A New Era in Health Care." *New York State Nurses' Association. ENGW-State-Wide,* December–February 1984–85.
7. Duke University Nursing Services. *Quality Assurance: Guidelines for Nursing Care.* Philadelphia: J. B. Lippincott, 1980, 105–8, 437–44.
8. Felton, G., E. Frevert, K. Galligan, et al. "Pathway to Accountability: Implementation of a Quality Assurance Program." *Journal of Nursing Administration,* January 1976, 20.
9. Flanagan, L. *One Strong Voice.* Kansas City, Mo.: American Nurses' Association, 1976, 13.
10. Hegyvary, S. T., and R. K. D. Haussman. "The Relationships of Nursing Process and Patient Outcomes." *Journal of Nursing Administration,* 6 (9): 18, 1976.
11. Hegyvary, S. T., and R. K. D. Haussman. "Correlations of the Quality of Nursing Care." *Journal of Nursing Administration,* 6 (9): 22, 1976.
12. Hemphill, J. K. In *Educational Evaluation: New Roles, New Means,* ed. Ralph W. Tyler. Sixty-eighth Yearbook of the National Society for the Study of Education, part 2. Chicago: University of Chicago Press, 1969.
13. Johansen, B. C., C. V. Dungea, D. Hoffmeister, et al. *Standards for Critical Care.* St. Louis: C. V. Mosby Co., 1981.

14. Joint Commission on Accreditation of Hospitals. *Accreditation Manual for Hospitals.* Chicago: JCAH, 1987, 147–48.
15. Lang, N. A. "Quality Care: Individual and Collective Responsibility." *American Nurse,* September 1974.
16. Luke, R. D., and R. W. Boss. "Barriers Limiting the Implementation of Quality Assurance Programs." *Health Services Research,* Fall 1981, 306.
17. McBride, J. "What Has Audit Done for Nursing Practice?" *Quality Review Bulletin,* September 24, 1976, 24–26.
18. McGinnis, S. "History of Nursing Audit." *Quality Review Bulletin,* May–July 1975, 10–12.
19. Mason, E. J. *How to Write Meaningful Nursing Standards.* New York: John Wiley & Sons, 1978.
20. Nightingale, F. *Notes on Matters Affecting the Health, Efficiency and Hospital Administration of the British Army.* London: Harrison & Sons, 1858.
21. Nightingale, F. *Notes on Nursing: What It Is and What It Is Not.* New York: Dover Publications, 1969, 18.
22. Phaneuf, M. C. *The Nursing Audit: Self-Regulation in Nursing Practice.* 2nd ed. New York: Appleton-Century-Crofts, 1976, 5.
23. Sandrick, K. M. *What Doctors Should Know About DRGs.* Chicago: Care Communications, 1983.
24. Schmadl, J. C. "Quality Assurance: Examination of the Concept." *Nursing Outlook,* July 1979, 462.
25. Schroeder, P. S., and R. M. Maibusch. *Nursing Quality Assurance: A Unit-Based Approach.* Rockville, Md.: Aspen Publications, 1984.
26. Smith–Marker, C. G. *Setting Standards of Patient Care.* Handout. Resource Applications, October 1984.
27. Zimmer, M. J. *Quality Assurance for Nursing Care.* Proceedings of an institute jointly sponsored by the American Nurses' Association and the American Hospital Association. October 29–31, 1973, 4.

CHAPTER 5

Legal Responsibilities

KATHLEEN M. NOKES

.

OBJECTIVES

After completing this chapter, the reader will be able to:

- Identify how the model for legal decision making can be applied when faced with legal dilemmas.
- Apply principles of professional negligence to primary care situations.
- Identify informed consent issues in primary care.

Case law in health care has been established from conflicts arising in institutional settings, usually hospitals and, more recently, nursing homes. Relatively few lawsuits that involve nursing care given in primary care settings have gone to jury trial. Although the past gives little evidence of actual suits against nurses, it does point out the two areas of highest risk—client teaching and communication with other health care providers. This chapter first examines a model of legal decision making and then focuses on professional negligence and informed consent. Examples from law that involve primary care situations are integrated. A basic knowledge of the law-nursing interface is presumed.

Model of Legal Decision Making

When confronted with a legal dilemma, the nurse should look to the model of legal decision making for the answer. If the answer cannot be found through the model, the system has a gap that needs to be filled. The model, shown in Table 5.1, is hierarchical in that law assumes importance over rules and regulations, but rules are more binding than written policy. Common practice is least binding but is often where answers are found. The model is also hierarchical in that a lower level, such as a written policy, cannot be in conflict with the highest level, existing law. For example, in New York State a health care provider cannot tell the parents of a minor that their daughter plans to have an abor-

Table 5.1
Model of Legal Decision Making

Level 1:	Law; for example, Nurse Practice acts
Level 2:	Rules and Regulations; for example, unprofessional conduct standards
Level 3:	Written Policy; for example, protocols and standing orders
Level 4:	Common Practice: A. Community standards B. Professional standards

tion. A health care clinic, deciding that the parents have a right to know, cannot, in New York State, establish a notification policy. The model of legal decision making assumes that the health care providers are knowledgeable and holds the practitioner to the level of a reasonable, prudent person acting in a similar situation.

Level 1: The Law

Law is created in two ways: through legislation and through the court system or the judiciary. Legislation is said to establish policy, although it does reflect what the majority of people, represented by their elected officials, believe to be appropriate practice. If a current behavior is outdated, efforts are directed toward creating new legislation to change the practice. Politics, power, and chance have great influence on how our laws are shaped. The court system approach to creating law is more studied and usually more conservative. Civil law is built on past cases, and change in policy is avoided. The goal is to determine how the current dispute is similar to precedents. If there are similarities, the decision in the current case will be consistent with past decisions. Informed consent, or the right of a competent person to make decisions about himself or herself, has been a legal standard for more than eighty years. The basic principle—right to self-determination—has gone unchanged over the years. Technology has created new questions, especially in the care of the terminally ill. These new questions have generated litigation, but the basic principle underlying informed consent has remained unchanged.

Legislation. The most important legislation that all nurses must be knowledgeable about is the nurse practice act that is operative in the state in which they are practicing. Because health care is not specifically guaranteed as a right in the U.S. Constitution, each state can establish its own laws and regulations. The nurse practice acts vary from state to state and can differ widely. Nursing practice that is permissible in California can be grounds for charges of practicing medicine without a license in New Jersey. Nurses may hold licenses in as many states as they want and need to be aware of the regulations for reregistration in each state. A major difference is in continuing education requirements; in some states a specific number of hours are required, whereas in other states continuing education remains voluntary.

In the 1970s most states amended their practice acts to allow for more autonomous nursing practice. The changes created by these new acts are now being fought in the courts. A decision rendered in Missouri in 1983 is a particularly important one. In *Sermcheif v. Gonzales* the State Board for the Healing Arts, which is the regulatory agency for physicians in Missouri, charged that two nurse practitioners were "exceeding their scope of practice, that they often worked without immediate physician supervision, and that they dispensed controlled drugs under standing orders" (26, p. 132). Missouri had amended the nurse practice act, but the new legislation had stated that services in the care of the sick, prevention of disease, or conservation of health be performed in consultation with a physician. The two nurse practitioners were giving routine gynecological care to between three thousand and five thousand clients yearly in rural areas. The interventions included taking history; providing breast and pelvic examinations, Pap smears, gonorrhea cultures, and blood serology; providing and giving of information about oral contraceptives, condoms, and intrauterine devices; and other services. All actions were performed according to written standing orders and protocols signed by the agency physicians (40), who were also charged in the lawsuit.

The lower court in Missouri decided for the medical board. The case was appealed to the state supreme court, and the lower court decision was overturned; there was nothing in the law to prohibit the nurses' actions. The decision stressed that changes in the practice act revealed a desire on the part of the legislature to expand the scope of authorized nursing practice and to "avoid statutory constraints on the evolution of new functions for nurses" (26). The outcome of this case should be perceived as a victory for all primary nurse practitioners. After the final Missouri decision the Ohio Medical Board withdrew legal action that it had initiated. If the two nurses in Missouri had lost, independent nursing practice would have been severely threatened in many other states.

Some nurse practice acts have been revised to allow nurses to write prescriptions for drugs (17). However, in states where this function is not clearly permitted, the state boards are suspending the licenses of nurses who order prescription medications (17). The process of pre-scribing drugs varies greatly from state to state and is strictly regulated by rules and regulations, standing orders, and protocols. It is essential that all nurses know the status of this controversial issue in their state. Nurses who write prescriptions in states where the nurse practice act does not allow it are exceeding their legal function, and other nurses who are implementing those orders are acting unwisely. The state board of nursing can answer any questions about the legal status of prescription writing in the state and should be contacted if there is any uncertainty regarding this matter.

There is a fine difference between prescribing a medication and recommending that a person take an over-the-counter drug. Prescription writing is considered a medical act, whereas recommending that a competent adult go to a drugstore and buy vitamins or some other over-the-counter drug is considered part of the health teaching function of the registered nurse. This distinction is important. If the relationship between nurse and client is such that there is little medical input, for example, in an occupational health setting, the nurse could advise the client to let his doctor know if he decides to use the recommended over-the-counter drug. On the other hand, if the situation is such that a physician is responsible for the health team plan, as in a home care setting, the nurse should consult with the physician before recommending any over-the-counter drug. If the client is on a federally funded program, such as Medicaid, over-the-counter drugs can be prescribed and the client will not have to pay for them out of pocket.

Court Decisions.   Nurses need to be knowledgeable about two kinds of common law: criminal and civil. Driving while intoxicated is an example of criminal law violation, and professional negligence is an example of breach of civil law. Arrest is often a penalty for conviction in criminal law, whereas payment of monetary damages is usually the goal of punishment when a person is found guilty of violating a civil law.

Despite all the publicity about malpractice and the impact of the law on health care practice, few cases are ever brought before the court. The court process is lengthy and involves many appeals. Usually a number of years pass before an ultimate decision is reached. A case might even be brought before the U.S. Supreme Court if that body determines that the issues are of national interest. Most health care cases, however, are decided by the courts in the state where the conflict arose. Because the process is expensive and time-consuming, the interested parties often agree to a compromise solution before the court system is exhausted.

Most health care cases resulting in litigation arise from conflicts in care administered while the person is hospitalized. Until recently nurses have not often been named specifically in the suit because the hospital, under the principle of *respondeat superior,* has been held liable for the nurses' behavior. A compelling reason for this pattern is economics. Klein observes that for every malpractice claim that is paid, "another 24 go uncompensated" (22). The penalty for violation of civil law is payment of damages, but if that amount is insignificant, the expenses involved in preparation and defense of the case can exceed the amount of damages that may be awarded. Because the payment that lawyers usually receive is based on a percentage of the award—up to 30 percent—there can be little motivation for a lawyer to take a case in which damages are small or the possibility of payment remote.

Level 2: Rules and Regulations

Nurse practice acts are broad statements declaring what is permissible practice within a particular state. Court decisions establish principles that can be applied as new situations arise. Rules and regulations are usually more specific, especially when the state has defined unprofessional conduct and given examples of such behaviors. Unfortunately most states have not taken that important step and have general statements addressing such personal qualities as "good moral character."

The governor has the obligation to ensure that the state laws are upheld. The chief executive charges the state board of nursing to ensure that the nurses in that state practice safely. A license, because it is granted on condition, is not a permanent right, and the state may revoke it if the licensee does not continue to meet the standards set forth at licensure (2). Grounds for revocation of license are set forth in state statutes. Abuse of drugs and nursing while intoxicated are clear examples of reason to question whether or not the nurse should continue to practice. The development of peer assistance programs should help impaired nurses without compromising client safety. Unprofessional conduct is more difficult to operationalize, and most states use vague or general terms to describe unsafe conduct (2).

New York State, in 1977, revised its standards of unprofessional conduct for all groups licensed or certified by the Board of Education. These groups are as diverse as land surveyors, social workers, physicians, and nurses. There are general provisions related to such issues as advertising for all groups. Those for health professionals are specific definitions of unprofessional con-

duct and include behaviors such as abandonment, client abuse, inappropriate delegation and supervision of unlicensed and licensed personnel, insufficient documentation, dispensing drugs, and not wearing an identification badge. These rules and regulations hold the weight of law, and violation of one of these provisions affects the continuation of licensure in New York. Each health professional group monitors the conduct of its members through its state board, and the nursing board has been hearing an increasing number of unprofessional conduct charges since the institution of these new definitions.

Vagueness in rules and regulations can lead to different interpretation and litigation when one thinks that one has been unjustly accused. Clarity in expectations improves practice in that all professions are held to the same standards and the penalties for failure to conform are also uniform. The decision of the state board can always be appealed to the courts, but the temptation to pursue the matter lessens when there is universal agreement on inappropriate or unprofessional behaviors.

Level 3: Written Policies

Because of the vagueness of unprofessional conduct behaviors and the broad, sweeping intent of the law, written policies assume great importance. It is essential that these policies be written and that they be both specific and general. They must be specific in that they must speak to areas in practice where there is possible confusion, but they must also be general so that they do not restrict the practitioner's ability to use judgment. For example, a written policy would be needed concerning giving chemotherapy in a noninstitutional setting because this is a relatively new practice with potential hazards. The policy should specify who can administer the drug, how it should be given, and actions to take in the event of an anticipated emergency, such as extravasation with Adriamycin use. The policy should be general in that it should offer guidelines about how to choose a suitable vein, but it should not say that the drug should never be administered in the hand. The site of administration is a nursing judgment. If the policy specifies site and only a hand vein is available, and the nurse uses it and administers the drug safely, litigation is still possible because the nurse violated the written policy. It is essential that every nurse be thoroughly familiar with the written policies of the employing agency.

In *Utter v. United Hospital Center* (West Virginia, 1977) the jury found against the hospital, as employer, because nurses failed to notify the department chairperson about ineffective medical care. In this case a client developed signs of infection on the arm on the third day of hospitalization. The nurses notified the attending physician, who treated the arm. However, the arm continued to deteriorate, and after the family changed doctors it was necessary to amputate the arm. The hospital had a written policy stating that any nurse who believed that a client's medical care was inadequate must notify the department chairperson if, after discussing it with the attending physician, the situation was not resolved (5). Although the nurses testified that they thought the attending physician's treatment was appropriate, and therefore saw no need to notify the department chairperson, the jury found otherwise. Perhaps in the absence of the written policy, the hospital would not have been involved in the suit.

Written policies include job descriptions, procedure manuals, protocols, standing orders, and any other written material promulgated by the employing agency. Policies must reflect current practice and need to be reviewed and adapted frequently. Policies interfacing with medical practice must be accepted by the physicians associated with the agency. This approval should be in writing. If the nurses experience difficulty getting this approval or any action that indicates that the physicians are aware of the situation, the nursing department can write a memo stating, in essence, that "it is our understanding that the enclosed policy on cardiac arrest is acceptable to the medical department. It will be implemented starting January 16, 1986. If there is any disagreement with this action, please contact _____ before that date." A copy of the memo should go to all appropriate departments.

Although, ideally, nursing and medicine should collaborate in creating health care policies, occasionally people are of the thought that the less that is written down, the easier it will be to avoid responsibility. Nurses, being on the front lines, are often forced into action by the client's needs. In nebulous situations nurses find themselves taking unnecessary legal risks. If a recalcitrant medical department refuses to take clear stands, the nursing department is not powerless. Nurses can delineate what they believe to be appropriate policies and pressure administration to support those positions.

Level 4: Common Practice

Common practice is *not* established by the statement "we always do it this way." In fact, that explanation should create suspicions that the questionable act needs

a thorough examination. Common practice is established by community and professional standards.

Community Standards. Historically, the courts have recognized differences between rural and urban settings in identifying the level of care expected of a reasonable and prudent practitioner. More recently the courts have adopted a national standard that is expected of all providers. In the Alabama case *Lamont v. Brookwood Health Services, Inc.* (37), a client with prior nursing education alleged that the standard of nursing care she received as a client was below the acceptable level. The court concluded that the phrase "that degree of care, skill and diligence used by hospitals generally in the community refers to the national hospital community" (37). With the advent of mass communication and standardized educational programs, geographical differences have blurred and the standard of care required of any nurse is the same regardless of the specific area of the country in which she or he is practicing.

Another aspect of community standard refers to the kind of setting in which the nurse is practicing. If the setting is part of a statewide or citywide system, then there should be consistency between the institutions. For example, a nurse who works in a state-supported prison system must know the policies and expectations required throughout the system. If prisoners in one part of the state have twenty-four-hour access to nursing services but those in another part of the same state have nursing services only on a part-time basis, the latter group of prisoners could charge that their facility was not meeting the community standard of care in that they do not have twenty-four-hour access to nursing care.

Community standards change slowly but continually in the direction of increasing services. There is a critical mass theory that helps to determine when an agency is negligent. I will use an example to explain. All occupational health nurses, regardless of the specific setting, administer basic life support services when an employee has a cardiac arrest. One agency decides to offer advanced life support and then another agency follows and offers this service. When a certain undetermined number of settings offer advanced life support, those agencies that continue to offer only basic life support become negligent. The services that are offered can exceed the community standard, but if they fall below it, the service agencies expose themselves to charges of negligence. To use another example, if state laws require written doctor orders for physical restraint within twenty-four hours, an agency can choose to require that written order within four hours. It cannot choose to have the order written within thirty-six hours because the thirty-six-hour requirement falls below the legal standard.

Nurses who work in similar settings should be familiar with one another's activities. Specialty nursing organizations, such as the Occupational Health Nurses or the special interest groups within the American Nurses' Association (ANA), can provide such a forum. Networking and exchange of ideas are facilitated when communication channels are open.

Professional Standards. The ANA has promulgated nursing standards, and every nurse may be judged against those behaviors. National specialty organizations have also published standards against which the alleged negligence of nurse specialists is measured (32). These professional standards can be used by nurses to create policies, and they offer support when dealing with a reluctant administration. The standards of accrediting bodies will also be important in deciding what is reasonable and prudent practice (41, p. 33). In Pennsylvania a specific regulation states that guidelines promulgated by the professional associations and accrediting bodies will be the criteria for effective and safe nursing practice (41, p. 33). The importance of knowing the standard against which your actions will be judged was highlighted in the California case *Fein v. Permanente Medical Group* (1981).

Fein, a thirty-four-year-old attorney, was experiencing chest pains over a few days while he exercised. He went to Permanente and was examined by a nurse practitioner. The nurse practitioner consulted with a physician, and they both agreed that Fein had muscle spasms. Valium was prescribed. Fein returned to the emergency room at 1:30 the next morning and was seen by another physician, who ordered a chest x-ray. That physician agreed with the medical diagnosis of muscle spasm and gave Fein an injection of Demerol. At twelve noon the same day Fein returned to the emergency room and saw a third physician, who also agreed with the diagnosis of muscle spasm. That physician ordered an EKG, which showed changes consistent with an acute myocardial infarction, and then admitted Fein to the cardiac care unit. Later Fein sued. The trial judge, in instructing the jury, advised that the standard of care against which the nurse practitioner should be judged was "that of a physician or surgeon . . . when the nurse practitioner is examining a patient or making a diagnosis" (3).

The Permanente Medical Group appealed the $1 million decision against it, citing, among other things, that a nurse practitioner should not be judged against the standard required of a physician. The California supreme court, which heard the appeal and made the final decision, agreed that the jury should have been instructed that the standard of care to be applied "was that of another nurse practitioner, not physicians and surgeons" (18). The decision of negligence against Permanente stood because an EKG was not ordered until the third visit, but at least this important case clarified the reasonable and prudent standard against which nurse practitioners will be judged.

In summary, the hierarchical model of legal decision making can be used in every situation of legal confusion. It is a framework for making decisions and providing direction. Implicit in using this model is the need for knowledgeability of the nurse practice act in the state in which you are nursing; an understanding of the existing statewide rules and regulations; thorough familiarity with agency policies; and participation in continuing education workshops, journal reading, and communication within the professional nursing association. The adage is "ignorance of the law is never an excuse," and nurses in this day of accelerating change must keep abreast of the developments within the health care system at large and the nursing profession in particular.

Professional Negligence/Malpractice

In some respects there is an interchange of the meaning of the terms malpractice and professional negligence. One author proposes that either term means "the failure of a professional person to act in accordance with the prevalent professional standards or failure to foresee possibilities and consequences that a professional person, having the necessary skill and training to act professional, should foresee" (27). Some states, however, say that only physicians, because of the nature of the medical education necessary to perform the action in question, can be charged with malpractice. Other health care providers are charged with professional negligence. This distinction, which on the surface appears minor, has serious implications for nurses. In every state there is a *statute of limitations,* which is the period of time in which a lawsuit can be initiated after an alleged negligent act occurred. In most states the statute of limitations for an act of alleged malpractice is two years. The courts in a number of states have found that this statute of limitations does not apply to nurses and is in fact longer for nurses because they are not a group against which malpractice can be charged. *Bleiler v. Bodnar* (New York, 1980) illustrates this point.

In 1980 James Bleiler was struck in the eye by a small piece of metal. The next day he went to the emergency room of Tioga General Hospital, where he was interviewed by the nurse and treated by Dr. Bodnar, the emergency room physician. Dr. Bodnar failed to detect the metal fragment and ordered ointment and a follow-up appointment. Bleiler sought another opinion and had surgery the next day to remove the metal. He ultimately lost his eye.

Bleiler began proceedings against the emergency room physician for medical malpractice, against the nurse for the negligent taking or recording of his medical history, and against Tioga General Hospital for vicarious liability because of the alleged negligence of the doctor and the nurse (35). The suit was initiated after the two-and-a-half-year statute of limitations for malpractice in that state, but before the three-year statute of limitations for personal injury. The court dismissed the charges against the doctor because the statute of limitations had been exceeded but decided that the case against the nurse and the hospital could proceed because "medical malpractice does not apply to the malpractice of a hospital or nurse" (35). This decision was appealed, and the higher court found that:

> Obviously, not every negligent act of a nurse would be medical malpractice, but a negligent act or omission by a nurse that constitutes medical treatment by a licensed physician constitutes malpractice.

The higher court found that the statute of limitations was the same for nurses and physicians if the alleged action was similar (*Bleiler v. Bodnar* [65 NY 2d 65]).

In *Penkava v. Kasbohn* (4-75 NE 2d, 975, ILL) an Illinois court came to the same conclusion as the lower New York court. In this case the charges were dismissed against the doctor and the hospital because the statute of limitations for malpractice had been exceeded, but it allowed the suit to proceed against the nurse. The court noted that "the nurses are neither physicians nor a hospital and consequently the claim against the nurses is not covered by the limitations period set forth under the Medical Practices Act" (13). Nurses need to identify which statute of limitations will apply in negligence charges against them and to work with the legislature in making the length of time consistent with the statute for physicians.

In most cases, in order for professional negligence to be found, the plaintiff's attorney must prove four things:

1. that a standard of care existed in the given situation,
2. that the standard of care was breached or broken,
3. the proximate causation, and
4. damage (41).

Existence of Standard of Care

In order for a standard of care to exist, there must be a contractual relationship between the nurse and the client. Most nurses work under verbal contracts, which are as binding as written ones. The job description of the nurse can help describe the agency's expectations, and any areas of confusion should be clarified with the supervisor or with administration. The nurse cannot terminate care except in the following situations: (a) if the client agrees that the nursing services are no longer needed; (b) if the physician requests that the care be ended; and (c) if the nurse informs the patient and carefully documents that services are no longer indicated (11).

Before a primary nurse in a home care agency goes on vacation, she is often expected to set up the visiting schedule for the clients in her case load. In setting up this plan she turns the responsibility for the care of these clients to the nursing supervisor, who then delegates it to other nurses. If the primary nurse advised the supervisor that a visit was not indicated until the end of the next week, and it is later found that this period was excessive, the primary nurse would retain responsibility and may be found negligent. Horsley suggests that if, in good faith but nonetheless unwisely, the primary nurse visits the homebound client too infrequently and injury occurs as a result, the nurse could be charged with abandonment (11).

Once a contract between the nurse and the client is established, it cannot be broken without mutual agreement. One of the purposes of the phone call to the client before an initial home visit is to obtain the client's consent to accept services. Occasionally clients will refuse to be seen, and this refusal must be communicated to the referral source and be documented. If the visiting nurse visits the home and finds the environment dirty, cluttered, and unsafe, the nurse must explain to the client that services cannot be offered until the environment is improved. The nurse must be clear that services are available as soon as the environment is such that they can be offered safely. Often the name of a cleaning service is also suggested.

At the initial visit the nurse should also be clear that

the nursing services are being offered for a limited period of time, and that after that period the client may have to locate his or her own resources. If this is not specified, the client, who feels that he or she is being discharged prematurely, could charge the nurse with abandonment. In situations where care is perceived by the client as necessary longer than the home care agency will be reimbursed for providing it, referrals to other sources must be given to the client and initial contact with these referrals initiated. In a case where a client's needs have grown and the agency can no longer provide the extent of services necessary, the initial agency cannot discharge the person until the other agency has initiated services or the client is admitted to a hospital or a nursing home.

Nurses, when they accept employment by an agency, have contracted to provide nursing care to the people who are clients of the agency. The first principle of the ANA Code for Nurses specifies that nurses "provide services with respect for human dignity and the uniqueness of the client, unrestricted by considerations of social or economic status, personal attributes, or the nature of health problems." Nurses cannot refuse to care for clients of different ethnic backgrounds or with frightening health problems, such as acquired immunodeficiency syndrome. Clients, on the other hand, cannot require the agency to discriminate against its employees. Requests for the "white" nurse or the "young" nurse violate federal laws against discrimination and cannot be honored. It is usually best to explain to the client that the nurse assigned to that geographical area is the person who will be visiting, and if that is not satisfactory, the client should be offered referral to another agency.

When a client's condition has deteriorated quickly and hospitalization is indicated, the nurse's contract extends to the point at which the client is transferred into equally competent hands. The nurse should stay with the client until the ambulance personnel arrive. Even if the client is stable and other clients are awaiting the nurse's visit, one could argue that if the situation necessitates the use of an ambulance, a nurse would be acting unwisely to turn the health care of the person over to a family member until the ambulance arrives. For example, a community health nurse assesses that a client with a history of myocardial infarction is experiencing chest pain radiating down the left arm. She calls the emergency number and requests an ambulance but then decides that since the client's condition has not worsened, she will proceed to her next client. Between the time the nurse leaves and the ambulance arrives, the client suffers a cardiac arrest and cannot be resuscitated. It is easy to see how the nurse breached her contract with the client by not ensuring continuity of care.

When the ambulance arrives the nurse should make sure that the drivers are medically trained, although a 1985 decision, *Agoff v. Town, Village, or City of Jean Lafitte,* found that "failure of an ambulance attendant to have been trained in emergency medical aid was negligent per se" (9). The good Samaritan law does not apply in situations where there are preexisting contracts, and even in those emergencies where it does apply, the nurse's duty "to the injured party is not fulfilled until another of equal or higher skill assumes responsibility for that duty of care" (20).

It has been said that a nurse has a legal obligation to provide reasonable and prudent nursing care to a client. In community settings sometimes it is difficult to identify the client. This seems to be a difficulty particularly in occupational health settings. Although the health service is established for employees, other people, such as visitors or messengers, may drop in. The occupational health nurse needs to clarify with administration exactly what services are to be provided and to whom. If a messenger cuts himself and the nurse administers first aid, is the agency going to perceive this intervention as appropriate, or will it disclaim any responsibility for the nurse's behavior in treating the nonemployee? In an emergency situation, such as a cardiac arrest, the course of action is clear—the nurse would initiate cardiopulmonary resuscitation because nonintervention would result in brain death. It is the everyday situations that need clarification. Such clarification should be found in the written policies and common practice standards.

Breach or Break in Standard of Care

The second requirement that must be proved by the plaintiff's attorney in a professional negligence suit is that the standard of care was breached or broken. Expert witnesses testify as to the standard of care. Until recently suits alleging nursing professional negligence relied on physician expert witnesses to establish the standard of care owed by the nurse to the client (5). Now an increasing number of nurses are being called to testify as expert witnesses, both in disputes over nursing care and occasionally in areas commonly thought of as the exclusive domain of medicine.

The purpose of the expert witness is to identify for the jury what behaviors would be expected of reasonable and prudent practitioners in similar situations. In *Belmon v. St. Francis Cabrini Hospital* (427S2D541 LA, 1983) an appeals court upheld the expert testimony of a nurse who testified that the nurse's responsibility for a client increased when the client's partial thromboplastin time lengthened (5). The nurse's attorney had argued that interpretation of laboratory work was a medical function. In *Carter v. St. Vincent Infirmary* (690 SW 2d741, June 12, 1985, Arkansas) an appeals court also ruled that a nurse who had practiced for three years as an infection control practitioner was "qualified to testify on the effects of the herpes simplex virus and competent to conclude that the authorities cited by the defendant hospital were obsolete" (14). The trend of using nurses as expert witnesses is likely to continue. Nurses are often willing to testify and are proving to be excellent sources of reliable information.

Proximate Causation

The third condition necessary to prove malpractice is proximate causation. Written documentation is analyzed to demonstrate that either omission, not doing something, or commission, doing something incorrectly, led directly to the problem. There are four tests of direct causation. In two situations the burden of proof lies with the plaintiff, and in the other two situations the defendant needs to show that the action wasn't appropriate. One instance in which the *plaintiff* must prove negligence is called the "but for" situation. But for the action or nonaction of the *defendant,* the plaintiff's injury would not have occurred or would have occurred to a lesser degree (19). The other situation in which the burden of proof is with the plaintiff is when multiple causation is charged, when it is being alleged that the behavior of many people led to the negligent act.

The burden of proving innocence lies with the defendant in the substantial factor test, when "action or inaction of the defendants contributed a great deal to the plaintiff's injury," and in the case of *res ipsa loquitur.* In the latter case the injury speaks for itself, and there is no evidence of contributory negligence on the plaintiff's part. Examples of cases of *res ipsa loquitur* are when an instrument is left in an operative wound or when the injury is obvious, as for instance in a case where maggots had infested the nose and mouth of a comatose woman in a New York hospital (1985).

The client's record is examined minutely to identify if either action or nonaction led to the injury. The plaintiff's attorney will try to find inconsistencies, gaps in blocks of time, and descriptions that raise questions about the client's care. In a community setting the nurse is often the only health care provider seeing the client regularly. What is or is not in those notes is crucial. The

initial assessment is a gold mine of evidence if a lawyer is trying to prove that a client has been discharged prematurely or without needed follow-up. In one case when a client with a progressive neurological disease was discharged from the hospital, neither the sacral nor the heel decubitus was noted on her referral report. These decubiti needed medical attention and the primary nurse in the community health agency contacted the physician making the referral for orders. The decubiti continued to worsen despite treatment and the client had to be readmitted to the hospital. The client sued the hospital, the physicians in the hospital, the community health nurse, and the community health agency. One attorney advised that when trouble surfaces, a plaintiff's attorney may "sue everyone in sight" and name a nurse as defendant simply to make it easier to get a pretrial statement from the nurse (39).

Nurses working in any setting must document thoroughly. A good rule is to imagine defending what you have written five years later in a courtroom. Regan advises that judges and juries tend to place as much weight on what a nurse says about a client in distress as they do on what the attending or other physician recorded in medical progress notes regarding the same clinical incident (31). It is not necessary to write voluminously, but rather to document objectively. Chart vital signs, measure ankle edema and abdominal girth, and weigh clients, so that when the client is readmitted three days after your visit, you can safely say that there was no evidence of congestive heart failure during the time you assessed the client. When you report chest pain, also note whether it was relieved by rest and nitroglycerin, specify how many nitroglycerin tablets were given, how many attacks of chest pain the client experienced. Document all phone calls and record every caller's name on the chart. If the message was left with the physician's answering service, document that that was done. Document instructions that were given in case of an emergency. A thorough record will be your best defense in a lawsuit.

Avoid inconsistencies. If on Monday the client has a superficial burn on his arm from coffee, follow up on the condition of the burn at the next visit. Is it healing? What is the evidence for this judgment? Read the prior record immediately before the visit and make sure that the recommended plan is being implemented. This is important not only in litigation, but also if the agency wants to be reimbursed by a third-party payer. Gaps in time are red flags to the plaintiff's attorney. If the nurse planned to visit the next week, why is the next visit dated eight days later? Perhaps the client requested a deferred visit for personal reasons, but if that phone call is not documented, it will appear as if the nurse were negligent. Records should never be altered or rewritten because that destroys the documents' credibility. Alteration of medical documents is proved in court on the average of once a month, and the results are often catastrophic for the physician defendants. An alteration not only destroys the validity of the chart, but can also expose the defendant to punitive damages, which may include making public an accounting of all of his or her assets and income (1).

There is controversy about what documents must be produced by the defendant in a lawsuit. An increasing number of judges are deciding that routine reports and documents are not privileged communication (6). In *Villers v. Puritan–Bennett Corporation* (MA Appeals Court, No84-0076-CV Suffolk, February 2, 1984) a Massachusetts appeals court declared that a nurse must disclose the incident report, personal notes, and recorded statements to the hospital's insurance representatives (6). The case involved the malfunctioning of a respirator in the hospital's recovery room. With technology moving into the home, home health care providers should be alert to signs of equipment malfunctioning and know that reports associated with any problems will be used in future litigation.

Although Dunn advised that "giving telephone advice is hazardous to your professional health" (8), the telephone is often the vital link in community care. There must be a system of documenting every call. If the call relates to a client, use a nursing narrative sheet to document the call and any action taken. Keep the sheet with the rest of the client's record. If a staff nurse is calling the supervisor for clinical advice, the supervisor should document the call in a log and describe the advice given. The staff nurse should also document the call in the client's record. Logbooks should be kept between seven and ten years, according to Dunn, depending on the state's statute of limitations. This defensiveness may seem like a nuisance, but it is essential; the law presumes that information logged is true because it was written in the course of business. It may be the only way to show that you acted reasonably and prudently.

Damages

Damages are awarded for injury-related hospital and medical expenses, compensation for economic loss as a result of injury, and pain and suffering compensation (19). The highest amounts are awarded in the cases of young people who will need care for the remainder of their lives. Some state legislatures, for example, Maryland, have enacted laws to try to put an upper limit on the amount of damages that can be awarded, but such legislation is highly controversial. The major areas of dispute are over the percentage of the award that can go toward the lawyer's fees, and the amount that can be awarded for noneconomic damages. Maryland put a $250,000 ceiling on the amount that can be awarded for pain and suffering (24), but the Ohio court of appeals has struck down a $200,000 cap as being unconstitutional (45).

Lawyers point to studies that indicate that only one in six incidences of malpractice results in a lawsuit (39). Doctors complain that between 3 percent and 10 percent of their income is spent on malpractice insurance (42). Nurses are being brought into the professional negligence situation, but it is virtually impossible to get the exact number of nurses currently named in litigation. St. Paul Companies, the nation's largest medical malpractice carrier, reported that 2,487 claims, or 36 percent of the total claims, in the 1983–84 year fell in the nursing/client care category (45). The highest average cost of claims paid ($49,989) during the same period was in the labor/delivery nursing category, in which an additional 10 percent of the claims were filed. About 95 percent of all malpractice cases are settled out of court, and therefore never become public knowledge. As health care consumers view nurses as being more autonomous and separate from the hospital and the physician, more nurses will be sued individually. The best defense against malpractice charges has been and continues to be a good nurse-client relationship (39).

Professional Negligence

Inadequate Client Teaching

Although the function of client teaching is specified in most nurse practice acts, it is an essential responsibility of primary nurses. The nurse must teach the client, significant others, and unlicensed health care providers such as home health aides and personal care workers. A 1982 Joint Commission on the Accreditation of Hospitals survey revealed that 32 percent of all recommendations received by hospitals were because of deficiencies in client education and in client and family knowledge of self-care (23). The primary nurse often assumes responsibility for initial health teaching, along with reinforcement of the learning that was started by other health care providers. The areas that must be taught involve prevention of illness, for example, measures to stop smoking; health promotion, for example, anticipatory guidance for the new mother; and activities-of-daily-living adaptations secondary to illness. These adaptations would include care of any wounds, knowledge of the medical regimen, especially drugs, and prevention of further complications, for example, foot ulcers in the diabetic.

The physician or prescribing nurse practitioner is obliged to inform the client of any risks associated with the medical plan, especially when the client is taking medications (7). Some courts are finding that the physician must reveal even remote risks if they are severe (14). The nurse's responsibility in drug administration is to clarify and reinforce this teaching. Verbal teaching is important, but the client should also receive written material, especially if the instructions are complex or the client is having difficulty learning. The use of uniformly developed written instructions will help to substantiate a claim that teaching was done (7). At least two courts (in Texas and in California) have found physicians negligent for not warning a client that the prescribed drug may cause drowsiness while driving (7). The precise description of what has been taught and any written instructions given must be documented as part of the nursing intervention. This documentation saved the defendant nurses in the lawsuit *Christopher v. Dow Chemical Company* (428 S2d 1358LA, 1983).

In this Louisiana case an employee sued the company's physician and two occupational health nurses for negligence. The plaintiff had an eye injury, for which he was treated, and was instructed to return for follow-up the subsequent two days. The nurse's log indicated that he returned the second day but failed to return the third day. The employee disputed this, alleging that he had returned but was never treated. The court ruled against the employee because of the "nurse's documentation of the instructions and the employee's failure to comply with them" (7).

The opposite decision was reached in *Bass v. Barksdale* (671 SW 2d 476-TN), a case that aptly demonstrates the need to warn the client about every risk, however remote. Bass had tuberculosis and cataracts and was seen by Barksdale, who was the registered nurse in charge of the tuberculosis clinic. The physician had called the nurse, asking her about the drugs being used for tuberculosis. The physician prescribed ethambutal and isoniazid and Barksdale delivered these medications to the Bass home in April. At that time she informed the client and her sister that ethambutal could

affect Mrs. Bass's kidneys and to check the urine and observe whether it was a reddish color. Barksdale also warned Mrs. Bass that the drug could affect her vision, but the nurse never tested the client's eyes with an eye chart. By July, Bass's vision was deteriorating and a suit was brought against Barksdale. The court focused on whether appropriate warnings were given and whether adequate steps were taken to monitor the client, since no one ever checked her eyes. The court decided that Barksdale did not act reasonably and prudently in meeting the standard of care and so found against her (46).

In some states, such as Maryland, legislation has been passed that requires health care providers, including nurses, to inform parents in writing of certain information before administering the pertussis vaccine to their children. The information must include frequency, severity, and potential effects of the pertussis vaccine; symptoms and early warning signs; measures to reduce the risk; and whom to contact if symptoms appear (30). It is probably wise practice to convey such information to parents who are being asked to consent to any vaccination of their child.

The public perceives nurses as doers and is often confused when the nurse's primary intervention is teaching. Nurses should help consumers to understand that the purpose of nursing care is to help people help themselves. When this is unclear the consumer may perceive the nursing care as substandard.

The nurse is also responsible for teaching unlicensed health care providers and ensuring that a particular action is being performed correctly. Not only should the home health aide or personal care worker be able to return the demonstration, but the nurse should frequently observe the procedure being done. Agency insurance coverage often dictates what can be taught to unlicensed providers. Although the community health nurse can teach a significant other any procedure, the duties and responsibilities of unlicensed, paid providers can be quite restricted. The conflict between agency regulations, client needs, and unlicensed provider willingness can cause a real ethical dilemma.

Failure to Communicate

In a hospital setting a nurse can communicate with any number of doctors, pharmacists, supervisors, and administrators. In an emergency a team of practitioners are trained to respond immediately. In contrast, the nurse working in a community setting often works alone. The telephone is the vital link with outside resources, and at times it is inadequate. At such times the nurse must exercise flexibility, creativity, and excellent clinical judgment.

In a traditional community setting the physician authorizes the actions of the other health care team providers. Physician endorsement is necessary in home care settings, and physician review and support of standing orders and protocols is essential in many outpatient settings. Nurses in private practice can independently establish a nursing care plan, but they are expected to consult with other providers as the client's needs arise. Nurses must recognize this dependence on physician input and define it as a collaborate relationship. They must be able to clearly identify their unique contributions to the client's well-being and at the same time recognize when consultation is needed. For years nurses have been held negligent for failure to communicate. The Darling case, decided in 1965, held a nurse negligent for failure to notify administration when the physician, whom she had notified, gave her inappropriate medical advice. The law expects nurses to know that certain symptoms require medical input, but at the same time it refuses to recognize the nurse's ability to make a medical diagnosis. However, the law is upholding the responsibility of nurses to make a nursing diagnosis.

In *Cooper v. National Motor Bearing Company, Inc.* (288 P 2d581 Cal Dist Ct, App 1955) an employee was struck with a small piece of metal while he was working. He went to the occupational health nurse, who dressed the wound but did not probe for a foreign object. She treated the wound for ten months. At the end of that time, although the wound was essentially healed, a small red area remained, which spread and swelled. The employee eventually asked to see a physician, who did a biopsy. The results indicated that a malignant growth was present. The employee sued the nurse and the company for damages, and the court found both liable. In the decision the court said, "The nurse should be able to diagnose . . . sufficiently to know whether it is a condition within her authority to treat as a first aid case or whether it bears danger signs that should warn her to send the patient to a physician" (4).

The validity of a nursing diagnosis was identified in the court's opinion in *Cignetti v. Camel* (692 SW 2d239-MO). In this Missouri case, which involved a woman in labor, the court observed that "a registered nurse is authorized to make an assessment of persons who are ill and to render a nursing diagnosis, in her capacity as a professional adjunct to the treating physician" (47). As the court continues to recognize the nurse's responsibility to make assessments and take effective action, the potential of liability for failure to identify and act grows. Notification must be timely and the urgency with which the problem must be communicated depends on the condition. A pulse below sixty in a person who is taking digoxin must be brought to the physician's attention before the next dose is due. A nurse assessing a client in acute distress must notify the client's private physician if he or she is available. If the physician cannot be reached, the nurse should call for emergency care. The physician can be notified that a client is using Colace as needed rather than regularly, as prescribed, when it is convenient. It is the nurse's judgment that will be tested against the reasonable and prudent standard. It is probably better to overnotify than fail to communicate. However, this is to be tempered with allowing the nurse freedom to make judgments. Of course, all attempts at communication should be carefully documented.

All nurses must carry their own insurance against professional negligence. Even though the employing agency may have insured the nurse, this coverage may not be adequate. The employer may charge that the nurse is not covered by the policy because her behavior was inconsistent with agency protocols. The nurse should carry her own insurance because the amount of damages awarded against her may exceed the coverage bought by the hospital. The nurse should also carry personal negligence insurance in the event that the employer, in the face of a large loss, chooses to countersue him or her. The ANA offers its members professional negligence insurance at an additional cost, but nurse midwives and nurse anesthetists are not covered. In 1985 nurse midwives found it difficult to get insurance coverage, and this may portend a trend for nurses who work in more independent roles. Nursing is facing the professional negligence insurance challenge that many other professional groups have been coping with. The old answers to the questions of professional negligence seem to be less than satisfactory and new solutions are yet to be found.

Informed Consent

The issue of receiving permission before touching another person has long been settled by the U.S. judiciary system. The courts have determined that a truly informed consent is given only after the person understands the nature of the proposed procedure, its risks and benefits, and any alternative treatments that are available. The courts have also held that it is the responsibility of the person performing the procedure to convey this information. The instructions are given verbally, although written material is helpful to reinforce the information, especially in cases of high-risk procedures. Often a written consent is required, but the purpose of this form is only to substantiate that the proposed action was discussed with the client. Although any person can witness the client signing the consent form, a nurse is expected to assess that the client has fully given informed consent. In a proposed medical or surgical procedure, if the nurse determines that the client is deficient in essential knowledge, she or he must stop preparing the client for the procedure and ask the physician to clarify or expand on the procedure in question. It is the person performing the procedure who must divulge the information about it.

In the 1980s the major area of litigation in the informed consent issue is not whether the proposed procedure was discussed with the client, but how much information was shared. The courts have decided on an objective test to determine whether the client had enough material in order to make an informed decision. This objective test is "whether or not a reasonably prudent patient, fully advised of the material known risks, would have consented to the suggested treatment" (25). In most states the objective standard has replaced the subjective standard, based on what information the plaintiff would have needed to consent to the proposed procedure.

In the community setting the client has more control over how he will cooperate with the treatment plan. This is in contrast to a hospital situation, in which the client often feels intimidated by the environment and pressured by the providers to act in a certain way. The central issue in a community setting in informed consent is information not about the procedure per se, but about the behavior required of the client in order to cooperate most fully with the treatment. Giving information about medications and their side effects is probably the key potential risk area in community care. The person prescribing the medication must give the information necessary to ensure informed consent, while the other nurses who are involved with the client must frequently clarify and reinforce this material. The importance of client teaching is again highlighted.

Although the courts are clear in upholding the responsibility of the treating person to divulge common risks, there have been different opinions on the need to discuss low-probability risks. A Texas court in *Barclay v. Campbell* (683,SW2d, 498, 1985) found that because there was only a one in two hundred chance of the client

developing tardive dyskinesia from drug therapy, this risk did not have to be discussed with the client (28). Other courts have held that the client has the "right to be told of even an extremely rare complication if it is severe" (1). But a Pennsylvania court ruled, in *Bayer v. Smith* (497 A 2d646, August 23, 1985), that medical malpractice, rather than lack of informed consent, charges should be brought against a physician who failed to warn a client of the possibly life-threatening consequences of using Butazolidin (36). The distinction in the Pennsylvania case is not whether the physician should have disclosed the information, but under what set of rules he should be charged with failure to act reasonably and prudently.

The person prescribing the medication must convey the information. Indiana found that the pharmacist is not required to warn the client of potential side effects of drugs that he dispenses on prescription (*Ingram v. Hook's Drugs Inc.,* 476 NE 2d 881, April 16, 1985) (12). Nurses, under their health teaching responsibility, do have the obligation to expand and clarify when they are also caring for the client. The need to inform the client of potential risks and subsequent charges of negligence in the event of failure to inform may extend not only to the client, but also to the general public. The particular area of litigation with respect to the need to inform the public has been expanded when a medication impairs the person's ability to drive safely.

In *Kirk v. Michael Reese Hospital,* an Illinois case (483, NE 2d 906, IL App 1 District, 1985, August 28, 1985), physicians ordered both Prolixin and Thorazine to be administered, after which the client was discharged from the hospital. On leaving the hospital the client drank alcohol and drove his car, with the plaintiff as a passenger. The client lost control of the automobile and hit a tree, and the plaintiff sustained severe and permanent injuries. The plaintiff alleged that the hospital, as the party responsible for the providers administering the drug, the physician, and the drug company were negligent in failing to notify the plaintiff not to drive. The appeals court determined that the physician and the hospital had a duty to forewarn the client of adverse side effects and of the effect the drug would have on his ability to drive safely (24).

The competent person must be a knowledgeable participant in his or her care in every circumstance. This includes health care choices during the last period of life. To uphold this right, thirty-four states and the District of Columbia have enacted legislation known as living will laws. Among the requirements underlying the validity of a living will is the essential one that the per-

LIVING WILL DECLARATION

To My Family, Doctors, and All Those Concerned with My Care

I, _____ , being of sound mind, make this statement as a directive to be followed if for any reason I become unable to participate in decisions regarding my medical care.

I direct that life-sustaining procedures should be withheld or withdrawn if I have an illness, disease or injury, or experience extreme mental deterioration, such that there is no reasonable expectation of recovering or regaining a meaningful quality of life.

These life-sustaining procedures that may be withheld or withdrawn include, but are not limited to:

SURGERY   ANTIBIOTICS   CARDIAC RESUSCITATION
RESPIRATORY SUPPORT   ARTIFICIALLY ADMINISTERED FEEDING AND FLUIDS

I further direct that treatment be limited to comfort measures only, even if they shorten my life.

You may delete any provision above by drawing a line through it and adding your initials.

Other personal instructions:

These directions express my legal right to refuse treatment. Therefore, I expect my family, doctors, and all those concerned with my care to regard themselves as legally and morally bound to act in accord with my wishes, and in so doing to be free from any liability for having followed my directions.

Signed _____ Date _____

Witness _____ Witness _____

PROXY DESIGNATION CLAUSE

If you wish, you may use this section to designate someone to make treatment decisions if you are unable to do so. Your Living Will Declaration will be in effect even if you have not designated a proxy.

I authorize the following person to implement my Living Will Declaration by accepting, refusing and/or making decisions about treatment and hospitalization:

Name _____

Address _____

If the person I have named above is unable to act on my behalf, I authorize the following person to do so:

Name _____

Address _____

I have discussed my wishes with these persons and trust their judgment on my behalf.

Signed _____ Date _____

Witness _____ Witness _____

Figure 5.1. Living Will

Source: Courtesy of the Society for the Right to Die.

son be terminally ill before the living will can be executed (10). Figure 5.1 (on page 77) shows a copy of the living will disseminated by the Society for the Right to Die, an organization that believes that education is essential if people are to be able to knowledgeably decide on their health care. The major role of the primary nurse in this area is to educate the public about the need for one to be clear about one's wishes. Unfortunately most people seem reluctant to take the necessary steps to formally declare what they want done, so the decision is left to the health care provider, who must rely on input from family members. Because the opinion of a significant other may be biased, it is far better for a competent person to clearly make her or his own decisions while she or he is able to do so.

Once a person reaches eighteen, the age at which legal competency is achieved, only a court can declare that the person is no longer competent. Before age eighteen, the minor's parents or legal guardian must consent to treatment. After the age of competency only the person can make decisions for himself or herself, regardless of what other people think about the decision. Most states have a two-part definition of incompetence. First, the person must fall into a certain category, such as old age, mental illness, or mental retardation. Then it must be found that the person is unable to appropriately care for herself or himself or for her or his property (16). The impairment to appropriately care for oneself need not be life-threatening for incompetency to be determined by the court. The proceedings to initiate incompetency can be started by any interested party, and medical certification is not a prerequisite to the beginnings of proceedings. If, after hearing the evidence, the court determines that the person is incompetent, a legal guardian is named. The guardian then makes decisions for the incompetent person. These decisions include where the person will live and what treatments the person will receive. It is a tremendous responsibility and cannot be taken lightly.

Nurses often interact with elderly people who stubbornly hold on to their own homes. They refuse most medical interventions and will not consider nursing home placement. The son or daughter has no legal say in the decisions of the elderly person until the courts have determined if the older person is competent to make decisions. The nurse can find herself in the middle of a situation in which the son wants his mother in a nursing home but the mother refuses to go. If the mother falls or is harmed while staying at home, the agency can find itself sued by the son for negligence in the care of his mother, who may have subsequently died. The wisest action is for the agency to initiate legal proceedings. Many administrators still cling to the mistaken belief that action cannot be taken until a psychiatrist has given an opinion. It is the court's decision, not the opinion of the psychiatrist, that is legally binding.

DISCUSSION QUESTIONS

1. The written policy of the clinic calls for parental notification when a minor child is pregnant and desires an abortion. The nurse has just learned that state law prohibits notification and that if she follows the policy, she can be charged by the minor with breach of confidentiality. How should she proceed?
2. The employer assures the occupational health nurse that logs are internal records and can be discarded. Should the nurse dispose of this information?

REFERENCES

1. "Alterations of Medical Records." *Medical Liability Advisory Service* 10 (9): 3, 1985.
2. Cohn, S. "Revocation of Nurses' Licenses: How Does It Happen." *Law, Medicine & Health Care* 11 (1): 22, 1983.
3. Creighton, H. "Nurse Practitioner: New Decisions." *Nursing Management* 16 (8): 15, 1985.
4. Creighton, H. "Occupational Health Nurse's Liability." *Nursing Management* 16 (8): 49, 1985.
5. Cushing, M. "Legal Lessons on Patient Teaching." *American Journal of Nursing* 84:721, 1984.
6. Cushing, M. "Incident Reports: For Your Eyes Only?" *American Journal of Nursing* 85:873, 1985.
7. Cushing, M. "Lessons from History: The Picket Guard Nurse." *American Journal of Nursing* 85:1073, 1985.
8. Dunn, J. "Warning: Giving Telephone Advice Is Hazardous to Your Professional Health." *Nursing* 15 (8): 40, 1985.
9. "Failure to Train Ambulance Attendant Is Negligence; But Causation Not Found." *Medical Liability Advisory Service* 10 (5): 11, 1985.
10. Helm, A. "Final Arrangements, What You Should Know About Living Wills." *Nursing* 15:39, 1985.
11. Horsley, J. "Caution: Home Visits Can Be Hazardous to Your License." *RN* 45:89, 1982.
12. "Hospital Awards: Peltier v. Frankin Foundation Hospital." *Medical Liability Advisory Service* 10 (6): 6, 1985.
13. IL:RN's MD's and Limitations: Double Standard, Penkava v. Kasbohm (475 NE 2D, 975-ILL)." *Regan Report on Nursing Law* 25:3, 1985.
14. "Informed Consent for Prescriptions." *Medical Liability Advisory Service* 10 (9): 3, 1985.

15. "Informed Consent Not Required for Therapeutic Drugs: Boyer v. Smith." *Medical Liability Advisory Service* 10 (11): 5, 1985.

16. Kapp, M. "Legal Guardianship." *Geriatric Nursing* 2:366, 1981.

17. Kjervik, D. "Legal Parameters of Drug Prescriptions by NPs." *Nurse Practitioner* 10 (7): 44, 1985.

18. Klein, C. "Examination of Fein v. Permanente Medical Group." *Nurse Practitioner* 10 (8): 39, 1985.

19. Klein, C. "Malpractice." *Nurse Practitioner* 9 (2): 74, 1984.

20. Klein, C. "Good Samaritan Acts." *Nurse Practitioner* 9 (4): 66, 1984.

21. "Legal Questions: Whose Liability—Home Health Care Agency Setting Up IV at Home?" *Nursing Life* 5:14, 1985.

22. "Limits on Collateral Sources, Attorney's Fees, Dominate State Legislation in 1985." *Medical Liability Advisory Service* 10 (7): 1, 1985.

23. Longo, D., R. Laubenthal, and R. Redman. "Hospital Compliance with JCAH Nursing Standards: Findings from 1982 Surveys." *QRB* 10 (8): 243, 1984.

24. "Maryland Task Force Recommends Cap on Non-Economic Damages." *Medical Liability Advisory Service* 10 (12): 4, 1985.

25. "Mississippi Adopts Objective Test for Informed Consent." *Medical Liability Advisory Service* 10 (8): 9, 1985.

26. "Missouri NP Win Appeal in Medical Practice Suit." *American Journal of Nursing* 84:11, 1984.

27. Murchison, I., T. Nichols, and R. Hanson. *Legal Accountability in the Nursing Process.* St Louis: C. V. Mosby, 1982.

28. "No Consent Needed for 1 in 200 Risk." *Medical Liability Advisory Service* 10:3, 1985.

29. Northrop, C. "Legal Responsibilities of PHN." *Nursing Outlook* 33:316, 1985.

30. Northrop, C. "Government and Legal Influences on the Practice of Community Health Nursing." In *Community Health Nursing Process and Practice for Promoting Health,* ed. M. Stanhope and J. Lancaster. St. Louis: C. V. Mosby, 1984.

31. "Nurse's Notes: Valuable Legal Evidence." *Regan Report on Nursing Law* 23 (10): 1, 1983.

32. "Nurse Specialists: Prime Legal Targets." *Regan Report on Nursing Law* 23 (11):1, 1983.

33. "Nursing Homes Face Growing Malpractice Risk: Contract Liability Could Be Worse Than Tort." *Medical Liability Advisory Service* 10:1, 1985.

34. "Ohio Appeals Court Strikes Down Cap on Malpractice Damages." *Medical Liability Advisory Service* 10:10, 1985.

35. "Patient Loses Eye—Nurse Sued: History Issue." *Regan Report on Nursing Law* 25 (6): 1, 1984.

36. "Patient Communication." *Medical Liability Advisory Service* 10:3, 1985.

37. "Patient Alleges Substandard Nursing Care: Liability (Lamont v Brookwood Health Services Inc. [466 SO 20 1018-AL])." *Regan Report on Nursing Law* 25:2, 1984.

38. "Physician's Duty to Warn of Adverse Drug Effects Goes Beyond Patient to Public." *Medical Liability Advisory Service* 10:5, 1985.

39. Prigoff, M. "Straight Talk from a Hospital Attorney." *RN* 59:61, 1985.

40. "Proper Nursing Practice: Not Illegal Practice of Medicine (Sermcheif v. Gonzales [660 SW 683 MO])." *Regan Report on Nursing Law* 25:1, 1984.

41. Rocereto, L., and C. Maleski. *The Legal Dimensions of Nursing Practice.* New York: Springer, 1982.

42. "Ten Percent of NY Physicians Go for Malpractice Insurance, Study Says." *Medical Liability Advisory Service* 10:1, 1985.

43. Thomas, C. "State Report Missouri Lower Court Decision Overturned." *Nurse Practitioner* 9:2, 1984.

44. Thobaben, M., and L. Anderson. "Reporting Elder Abuse: It's the Law." *American Journal of Nursing* 85:371, 1985.

45. "Top 10 Hospital Malpractice Claims: St. Paul Insurance." *Medical Liability Advisory Service* 10:2, 1985.

46. "TB Patient Blinded by Treatment: Nurse Sued (Bass v. Barksdale [671 SW 20 476-TN])." *Regan Report on Nursing Law* 25 (4): 1, 1985.

47. "When RN's Assessment and MD's Diagnosis Differ (Cignetti v. Camel [692 SW 20 239-MO])." *Regan Report on Nursing Law* 25 (4): 1, 1985.

CHAPTER 6

Ethical Issues

KATHLEEN M. NOKES

.

OBJECTIVES

After completing this chapter, the reader will be able to:

☐ Identify differences between law and ethics.

☐ Identify differences in philosophical orientation between the individualistic and utilitarian perspectives.

☐ Examine how personal ethical beliefs impact on decision making.

The purpose of this chapter is to differentiate law from ethics; to explore the differences in philosophical perspective between focusing on the health of the person versus the public health orientation; to examine the major ethical issues in American society today; and to analyze how individual beliefs and environmental directives interact to influence a person's ethical decision making. Three case studies are presented that explore the issues of elder abuse, prisoner health care, and the person with acquired immunodeficiency syndrome (AIDS) returning to work. These cases illustrate the principles of different ethical schools and highlight the ethical dilemmas faced daily by nurses as they practice their profession. Some statements in this chapter are included as an attempt to challenge the nurse to reexamine his or her underlying belief systems so that these values can be confirmed, modified, or rejected.

Differences Between Law and Ethics

There are many differences between law and ethics. Law reflects societal values, whereas ethics is more the person's perception of what is right and wrong. Law reflects the consensus, whereas ethics is more individualistic. Law is written down, whereas a person's ethical beliefs can be more difficult to discern and may vary from situation to situation. Laws theoretically apply equally to all people, whereas ethical considerations may be influenced by a person's prior beliefs about the value of the people involved. Although law reflects the majority view, it can be in conflict with a person's ethical beliefs.

In South Africa the law encourages discrimination based on skin color, a position that many people find unethical. In the United States the law permits discrimination against a person who is living a gay or lesbian life-style, but some people find these laws ethically problematic. The federal budget is voted on by elected officials and establishes national priorities, but some find the focus on defense at the expense of social programs, like feeding children and the poor, ethically diffi-

cult. The law sets a clear direction; ethicists argue that they do not offer answers but frame the questions. Law is concrete, whereas ethics is fluid. In decision making, however, ethical beliefs can assume greater importance than the existing laws.

Individualistic Ethics

It has been argued that the conflict between the orientation of the individualistic focus of professional nursing and medicine and the goal of public health, which is care of aggregates, results in ethical dilemmas for the practitioners involved in community health (11). Both nursing and medicine focus on the one-on-one interaction between the practitioner and client. The client, whether identified as the individual, the family, or the community, is defined as the system. The practitioner focuses her or his attention on that system and seldom looks to how other systems impact on the client or how the client is impacting on other systems. This orientation may result from a need to achieve realistic goals and to not be overwhelmed by the magnitude of the specific problems. For example, students working with a chronically mentally ill population living in a single-room occupancy in New York City become overwhelmed when they focus on the total system and express feelings of powerlessness. They don't believe that they can make any impact on the clients' lives. They verbalize anger at the school for exposing them to such a hopeless situation and refuse to accept that they are making any difference. In reality, the staff repeatedly remark on the positive changes in client behavior that have been noted since the students have been visiting the facility. The faculty member, in group discussion, tries to focus the students in the single-room occupancy system on the changes that are possible and redirects the discussion when the students bring up their feelings of hopelessness. The faculty member is using an individualistic ethic, rather than a public health ethic that focuses on aggregates or groups of individuals.

Public Health Ethic

Utilitarianism is the school of ethical thought that underlies the public health ethic. This position, initially posed by John Stuart Mill, focuses on the consequences of actions. The important consideration is that the greatest number of people benefit so that they experience either the greatest amount of happiness or the least amount of harm. The public health ethic, to use the single-room occupancy example, would be concerned with how the total community is influenced by the hotel in its neighborhood. Influential factors would include health hazards posed by the clients' inability to manage their personal hygiene. These clients are having a lice epidemic and could be perceived as endangering the community when they use neighborhood facilities such as grocery stores, launderettes, and restaurants. Health professionals working in community health settings must balance the ethical dilemmas posed by the behaviors of their individual clients when these behaviors can harm the greater community. The traditional illustration of this dilemma is when a person refuses to be vaccinated against a communicable disease.

The public health ethic, which has influenced the passage of many of our health care laws, argues that a person's right to refuse to participate can be denied when society is at risk. Laws influenced by this public health ethic are firmly established in the American legal tradition. For example, a child cannot attend school without proper immunization. The parents' right to make decisions about their children is recognized in the need for the parents to consent to the vaccination. However, except in extreme medical situations or lengthy legal procedures, the parents must give their consent to the vaccination. If parental consent is absent, children are barred from school and the parents can be charged with child abuse because they are neglecting their children's education. The law gives an illusion of choice, but in reality, the parents must comply with what society has identified as being reasonable behavior. The health care professional who examines this situation can identify an ethical dilemma.

Ethical Dilemma

An ethical dilemma involves a choice between equally unsatisfactory alternatives, or a difficult problem that seems to have no satisfactory solution (3). It would seem possible that an ethical dilemma could also result when there is a conflict between two satisfactory solutions, but most discussions focus on ethical dilemmas resulting when the solutions available are less than optimum. Ethical dilemmas usually involve interrelationships in which there are conflicts and tensions (3). It is hard, and probably impossible, to conceive of a situation that is not interpersonal, since people are open systems interacting with the environment. The ethical dilemmas faced by health professionals result from their relationships with other professionals and with clients and from system demands. The major ethical conflicts faced by health professionals in the 1980s are questions of self-determination and allocation of scarce resources.

Self-Determination

The underlying question in the self-determination issue is whether a person is truly free to decide what actions are in his or her best interests. Self-determination recognizes that people are autonomous, which implies that they are independent, self-reliant, competent to make decisions, and able to exercise freedom of choice (10). Nursing students are often advised that their patients are autonomous and have a right to make their own decisions. This advice is given so frequently that it has become a truism. To give some illustrations, mentally ill patients can choose not to take psychotropic drugs, terminally ill patients can refuse food, and pregnant women can decide to have an abortion. But is the principle of self-determination realistic? Do people exist in a vacuum? Can a person ever make a decision considering only his or her best interest? Don't prior obligations, such as the responsibility of mother to child, impact on a person's ability to make decisions? What is the influence of poverty on the ability to make choices? Can a high-functioning mentally retarded person make decisions about who should be his friends?

Belief in self-determination as the overriding ethical principle has many limitations. It presumes that the person is an open system with control over the influences that impact on it. As an alternative, Rogers (25) argues that people interact with the environment with neither the person nor the environment having control. She says that the interaction between the person and the environment is mutual and simultaneous. Health professionals, especially nurses, must recognize the limitations of the premise of self-determination. Holding on to it as an ideal results in many ethical dilemmas for practitioners.

The intensity of the dilemma arising from this faulty belief can cause nurses to abandon any ethical consideration because they know the ideal can never be achieved.

Allocation of Scarce Resources

The ethical principle involved in the allocation of scarce resources is justice. Justice involves rights or claims that must be balanced and weighed against one another (10). Justice is often equated with fairness. Rawls's (10) theory of justice advocates that benefits and burdens should be distributed, keeping in mind the point of view of the least advantaged in society. He also suggests that ethical principles are valid if they are universal, public, and final. Universality is an important ethical consideration. It presumes that the principle will be applied equally to everyone. Universal principles are difficult to identify, but the right to live is usually accepted by all cultures and societies. By saying that the principle must be public, Rawls is suggesting that everyone in society is knowledgeable about the principle. The need for informed consent before touching another person is publicly known and so could be perceived as an ethical principle. By proposing that the ethical principle is final, Rawls is claiming that it assumes greater importance than legal considerations and customs.

Rawls's proposal that the position of the least advantaged must be considered in the allocation of benefits and burdens makes assumptions about the place of the poor in a society that Rawls would identify as just. In this society those who have would be obligated to assist those who have not. Great Society programs such as Medicaid and Medicare were created with this vision of society. But the public view has changed, and people are saying that resources are limited and choices must be made. Income is taxed to finance social programs, and some argue that taxes are growing excessive. The argument usually continues by posing that each person has an obligation to help herself or himself and that the obligation to help others should be voluntary and not regulated by the government.

Until the 1980s the health care industry proliferated and absorbed increasing amounts of the federal budget. This illusion of unlimited resources permitted decision making based on process considerations rather than on the bottom line. The orientation has changed, and now it is widely claimed that resources are limited. Some would argue that resources are decreased only because moneys are being shifted into other programs. Now that resources are perceived to be limited, justice in distributing the existing services becomes a primary factor and often poses ethical dilemmas for the health care professional. Primary prevention is not valued, and so funding for such programs is cut. Health teaching is considered a luxury, and people are told that they are responsible for their own behavior. The primary nurse in community services is forced to tell clients that services are limited and will be discontinued when preexisting regulations cite that recovery should have occurred, rather than when the client is again self-sufficient. The nurse, being on the front line, hears the client's outrage when services are cut and, in the face of the client's obvious need, has an ethical dilemma. Nurses are caught between employers and their need for reimbursement and the client's need for continuation of services. This ethical dilemma can cause severe conflict for the practitioner.

An Alternate Approach: Respect

Adoption of either the self-determination ethic or the majority benefit view is unsatisfactory. Both perspectives have limitations that result in either/or decisions. These approaches force a right or wrong answer, and in reality most ethical conflicts are more complex. Aroskar suggests that we should view others and ourselves as interconnected members of a system or community. The client is seen as part of a total system, and the client's decisions impact not only on the client, but also on his or her family and the health care providers. Respect for people requires that each person be treated in consideration of his or her uniqueness, as equal to every other, and that special justification be required for interference with a person's purposes, privacy, or behavior (6).

Using a principle of respect, the primary nurse would perceive each person as an individual but not as being isolated from other people. The nurse would identify that the client will impact on the nurse and influence the nurse's emotions, perceptions, and knowledge. The client would be respected for uniqueness, but this respect would be balanced by the needs of others in the community. An elderly woman living at home would be supported to stay there until she forgets to turn off her stove and endangers others in the building. A person with diabetes who refuses to comply with diet restrictions would be taught but then discharged when enough opportunities for learning had passed and the client still cheated. When admitting a person with multiple needs to a short-term program, the nurse would make clear that the services are limited in duration and that other options must be explored. The client can be discharged in good conscience when adequate time has passed. The occupational health nurse counsels the client with an alcohol problem and remains supportive when the employee is forced to resign but recognizes that the employee's behavior is endangering other workers. The nurse working with a client with rheumatoid arthritis respects the client's right to refuse to exercise only after the client understands the consequences; the nurse does not experience feelings of failure or guilt about the client's decision. Respect as the overriding value frees the nurse from guilt because the nurse is seen as part of the system, not as a controlling force. Respect also recognizes that there are times when the rights of the individual can be interfered with. Such circumstances would be when there is a threat to others or provision for common need.

A person's unique right to make a decision can be overturned if others in the community will be harmed by that decision. But it is essential that there be clear evidence that the community will be directly harmed by the decision. It is obvious that the paranoid person cannot shoot down someone he delusionally thinks is after him. On the other hand, there is no direct evidence that casual contact between a person with AIDS and others in the community will result in spread of the disease. The other reason for overturning a client's decision is if what is best for the community is different from what the person wants.

Elizabeth Bouvia, a twenty-six-year-old, severely handicapped person with cerebral palsy, went to court in California to ask that the court mandate the cooperation of Riverside County Hospital in her plan to starve herself to death (17). Bouvia argued that she had the right to determine the outcome of her life, but because of physical limitations, she needed assistance to die. The court found that such assistance was not within Bouvia's legal rights as a citizen. In this case, society's need was to refuse to grant Bouvia's wish because her request was perceived as unreasonable. In respecting one another it is assumed that one doesn't ask for too much. Bouvia's decision about continuation of her life was an essentially personal one until she asked society to help. The action she requested was too much. Bouvia was not terminally ill or brain dead; she was handicapped. If society, in the person of the court, had decided to help her die, this would have sent a clear message to other disabled people, one that is not consistent with the philosophy of the American culture. Such an action may be permissible in another society, especially one that is supposedly more primitive, in which disabled newborns are left to die, but it is out of character for our culture.

The issue of feeding may arise again in the case of prisoners who refuse to eat as a political statement. The executive director of the International Council of Nurses says that nurses should not participate in forced feedings; the prisoners should understand the consequences of their action, but the nurse should not intervene against the prisoners' wishes (15). This ethical directive may give some nurses difficulty.

Ethical Decision Making

Ethical decisions result from an interaction between a person's internal environment and the external environment. The person's internal environment is called mind-set. The external environment includes the mind-sets of other individual systems, such as providers and clients, and the structure of the larger social systems (4).

Internal Environments: Moral Reasoning

Lawrence Kohlberg (19) posited that there are six moral stages and that these can be grouped into three major levels: preconventional level (stages 1 and 2), conventional level (stages 3 and 4), and postconventional level (stages 5 and 6). He identified that people in stage 1 were usually under nine years of age. Children initially obey those in authority in order to avoid punishment. Then, as moral development continues, the person's selfish needs become primary and the person is said to be using a stage 2 orientation. Those who reason at these first two stages of moral development are identified as being at the preconventional level. Most adults develop into the conventional level of moral reasoning.

The major difference in the two stages in the conventional, or middle, level is the importance assigned to the overall needs of the system. People in stage 3 need to see themselves as good in their own estimation and in the perspective of others, but they lack a total system focus. In contrast, an orientation toward the importance of law, order, and duties is the organizing consideration for people reasoning with a stage 4 conventional orientation.

The highest, or postconventional, level is characterized by principled thinking (19), and only about 10 percent of the population develops to this level. On the principled level, stage 5, moral decision making focuses on the ability to freely adhere to contractual agreements. People in stage 6 are the most integrated, in that they recognize that people must be treated as ends in themselves. People seem to use more than one stage in their thinking about different situations (24). Research assessing the moral reasoning of nurses using this theory has consistently found that most nurses use a conventional level of moral reasoning.

Kohlberg claims that his theory is universal and therefore unaffected by culture or sex. Nokes (21) suggested that the theory is culturally biased in favor of values inherent in the United States, and Gilligan (13) offered a reinterpretation of moral reasoning from a feminist perspective. Because most nurses are women, Gilligan's work is of particular interest.

Gilligan says that responsibility and relationships, rather than rights, are the primary considerations. She identified three moral perspectives and how people in each stage view responsibility and relationships differently. There is an initial focus on caring for the self in order to ensure survival. The need to preserve oneself is the major determinant in an ethical dilemma situation. If a nurse perceives that she will lose her job if she acts ethically, that nurse, using a stage 1 perspective, would choose to do whatever is necessary to keep her position. As the person moves into the second perspective, this initial view is perceived as being selfish.

Using the second-stage perspective, good is equated with caring for others. Nursing is often equated with caring, and nurses are told that the clients' needs come first. We are made to feel virtuous and ethical when we care for others rather than for ourselves. The third perspective focuses on the dynamics of relationships and dissipates the tension between selfishness and responsibility through a new understanding of the interconnections between other and self. It is similar to Aroskar's concept of respect, in that interconnectedness is recognized. Nurses, using the third perspective, can see two points of view simultaneously and tolerate these conflicts. They can choose actions and make decisions considering both their own needs and the rights of others in the circumstances. They recognize that in most situations there is no absolute right or wrong decision, but a series of possibilities. Nurses who view ethical dilemmas using Gilligan's third perspective respect the rights of their clients and expect respect in return from clients and from other health care providers.

External Environments

A number of environmental factors impact on ethical decision making. These include client behaviors, professional standards, rules and regulations of the employing agency, and requirements of third-party payers, including Medicare and Medicaid.

Client Behaviors

In the ideal world the nurse teaches, the client learns and integrates information into behavior, the doctor is accessible and cooperative, and the family members are supportive. But the reality is often different. The client retains ultimate control over her or his behavior. The diabetic client cheats on cake, the hypertensive client omits medication, the wife doesn't position her husband. These noncompliant behaviors can cause ethical problems for the nurse. The nurse recognizes the consequences of failure to follow the care plan and, being a helping professional, would like to prevent them. The nurse must recognize that competent adults have the right to make their own choices, but that the nurse also has the right to terminate care as long as the client has had the option to learn (9). The legal implications of this rather frustrating situation have been discussed in chapter 5.

Professional Standards

The major ethical standard for registered professional nurses is the Code for Nurses (Figure 6.1). The code was first established in 1950 and has periodically been revised since that time. A code is a profession's framework for making ethical decisions and establishing professional expectations (29). Although some may claim that the Code for Nurses typifies behaviors that nurses should strive for (2), others argue that since no "shoulds" or "shalls" are used, the behaviors are written as though they are what every nurse does (29). One important function of the code is to justify differences between the nurse's personal and professional values. As citizens, we are entitled to our own opinions, which are based on our values, culture, and past experiences. But when we are acting as professional nurses, those opinions may have to be put aside and our actions must be consistent

1. The nurse provides services with respect for human dignity and the uniqueness of the client unrestricted by considerations of social or economic status, personal attributes, or the nature of health problems.
2. The nurse safeguards the client's right to privacy by judiciously protecting information of a confidential nature.
3. The nurse acts to safeguard the client and the public when health care and safety are affected by the incompetent, unethical, or illegal practice of any person.
4. The nurse assumes responsibility and accountability for individual nursing judgments and actions.
5. The nurse maintains competence in nursing.
6. The nurse exercises informed judgment and uses individual competence and qualifications as criteria in seeking consultation, accepting responsibilities and delegating nursing activities to others.
7. The nurse participates in activities that contribute to the ongoing development of the profession's body of knowledge.
8. The nurse participates in the profession's efforts to implement and improve standards of nursing.
9. The nurse participates in the profession's efforts to establish and maintain conditions of employment conducive to high-quality nursing care.
10. The nurse participates in the profession's effort to protect the public from misinformation and misrepresentation and to maintain the integrity of nursing.
11. The nurse collaborates with members of the health professions and other citizens in promoting community and national efforts to meet the health needs of the public.

Figure 6.1. Code for Nurses

Source: Code for Nurses with Interpretive Statements. American Nurses' Association, 2420 Pershing Rd., Kansas City, Mo. 64108, 1976.

with the code. For example, as individuals we do not condone murder, but if we are working with prisoners, we must put aside our repulsion for their actions and focus on their health care needs. The code is not a theoretical document, but a working framework that gives answers about ethical dilemmas. Some nurses, fearful for their personal safety when the contagion of AIDS was in question, refused to care for people with that disease. That behavior was inconsistent with the first principle of the code, which prohibits discrimination based on a person's health problem.

There are some interesting differences between the medical code for ethics and the nursing profession's statements about ethical beliefs. One difference concerns who should receive services. Independent nurse practitioners, more than nurses working in hospitals, have influence over whom they give care to. The ethical advice given by the physician's code is that the physician, except in emergencies, shall be free to choose whom to serve; the nursing code is silent on the issue. Nurses in private practice may want to consider this ethical issue of how to render their services and to whom. As employees, nurses have little freedom to choose their clients, but as more nurses are self-employed, the issue may assume greater importance.

The last statement of the code specifically speaks to the responsibility of the professional nurse to promote the health needs of the public. This advice tends to reaffirm the dilemma that community health nurses may face when they act according to the individualistic ethic by focusing on the needs of each specific client, while at the same time having an ethical responsibility to the total community. The community health nurse clearly sees the need to view the total picture, not just one client. But the code gives direction when it specifies that the nurse should attempt to meet the public's health needs by collaborating with other health professionals and citizens. This advice recognizes that there is a shared responsibility and interconnectedness.

Agency Policy

The work environment may have an impact on ethical decision making. Research thus far has been unable to support that statement, which feels intuitively correct. Murphy (20) looked at moral reasoning of nurses working in hospitals in contrast to nurses working in public health settings and found no difference. Nokes (21) studied the impact of the work environment on the ethical behavior of staff nurses working in an acute care facility, and also no significant statistical data were found. Nokes did, however, find that at least one factor, supervisor support, significantly affected nurses' ethical behavior. The problem with conducting research in this area is that both work environment and ethical decision making, and subsequently ethical behaviors, are complex and difficult to assess.

People are influenced by others in authority. The cognitive dissonance theory implies that power can be exerted to force a change in behavior (29). If the authority in the employing agency supports ethical decision making, nurses would be more likely to act ethically. On the other hand, if the focus is on rules and regulations, paperwork, and productivity, nurses may get the message that outcome is more important than process.

In contrast to nurses in the hospital setting, most community health nurses work independently. When they leave the office in the morning, they are presumed to be visiting clients, but there is no way to account for each minute of their time. Nurses know that they have the responsibility to give comprehensive nursing care to every client, but they can manage their time as they see fit. For some nurses, this freedom may prompt less than ethical behaviors, in that they may rush through the visits in order to leave the clinical area early. The agency may try to control this behavior by making all nurses account for their time. This agency response often results in resentment from those nurses who were using their time ethically.

Documentation can also result in many ethical dilemmas. Because there is no other person to validate what nurses document, they may be tempted to fabricate some items. If the agency demands certain things, nurses will be prone toward charting what the agency expects and omitting the more controversial issues when inclusion of those items may result in their having to defend their position. For example, if the home health aide reports to the community health nurse that the client, who is mentally retarded, threatens her with a knife, the nurse may face a dilemma on how to report this. On the one hand, the community health nurse has an ethical responsibility to the home health aide to take her claim seriously and intervene with the client and to discuss sedation or institutional care with the physician. On the other hand, the agency might be concerned that outside auditors might perceive continuation of the client on the program as unwise.

Another common illustration concerns medications. Every community health nurse knows that there is often a difference between the medication orders and the medications that the client is actually taking. Although this is reality, it does not look good on the chart. The home care coordinator wants to know answers, not "Well, the physician ordered Minipres b.i.d., but the patient is taking it q.d." The problem with this situation is that the doctor must be notified, and when the doctor persists in ordering the drug b.i.d., the ethical nurse has no other option but to document that the client is noncompliant. Somehow it seems simpler, although unethical, to chart that the client is taking the drug as prescribed.

Many ethical dilemmas can result when agency policies are restrictive and require doctor orders for areas that some might perceive as nursing interventions. The nurse who suspects that a client with diabetes has an unusually high blood sugar may do a finger stick to assess blood sugar. When the result is 240 mg, the nurse can intervene immediately with the client by reviewing dietary intake and determine whether the client has been watching her intake of carbohydrate foods. But if agency policy requires a doctor's order to do a finger stick, the nurse is faced with an ethical dilemma. Does the nurse not document the action? But doesn't that negate the nurse's contribution to the client's well-being? If the nurse documents the results, the nurse will be censored by the agency and perhaps be asked to rewrite the note. In deciding whether to rewrite, the nurse also faces an ethical dilemma.

One could argue that the nurse should have called the doctor for input before taking any action, but that presumes the doctor is available—a presumption that is often false. One could also accept the premise that nurses have no ability to make judgments and gather data. The nurse, working for a restrictive agency, has some options: to document only what is consistent with agency policy while giving holistic care; to give care only within the rules of the agency; to leave the agency; to try to work within the agency to change the policies. The ethical nurse will probably choose each one of these options, and others, depending on the specific circumstances.

Impact of Third-Party Payers on Ethical Decision Making

Rules and regulations, like law, are not necessarily ethical. Some believe that when a person's life-style has led to the development of a disease, such as lung cancer in the presence of a chronic smoker, insurance companies should not have to pay, or should pay less. In terms of home care, some think that the burden of providing services should be borne by a person's family rather than by the government (7). The forms created by the Health Care Financing Administration "have turned the concept of a visit into a doctored house call with a chart of procedures" (14). The focus is on skilled interventions, basically doing procedures, and caring is not valued. It is not valued because Medicare will not pay for any visit unless it is thoroughly documented that the nurse has "done something." One experienced author states: "Your staff may provide excellent skilled care but when it is not adequately documented, you will not be reimbursed" (16). She warns that every note must establish that the client is homebound if Medicare is to pay for the services.

Documenting homebound status can create ethical dilemmas for the thinking nurse. Instructing the home health aide to walk with the client outdoors to increase exercise tolerance and for a change of scenery can be well within the nursing care plan. But if this intervention is documented, the visit and perhaps all of the services will be disallowed. The nurse is again forced to chart what people want to see rather than the holistic, client-centered interventions. Many nurses in community health complain about the amount of paperwork, but one wonders if the complaint isn't the amount, but the elaborate cover-up that rules and regulations require. The nurse knows that the client requires services, and it is usually this consideration that prompts the nurse to chart consistent with the rules so that the client can stay on the program.

The purpose of the following case studies is to identify the implicit ethical dilemmas commonly faced by primary care practitioners. As has been previously stated, there is no necessarily right or wrong answer; the individual situation greatly influences the outcome.

CASE STUDY 1

Susan Farrow, 82, lives with her 64-year-old daughter, Lillian. Mrs. Farrow has diabetes and congestive heart failure. Her medical plan includes many medications and a special diet. Mrs. Farrow was recently discharged from the hospital, and the VNS is making an initial assessment. Her medical diagnosis was malnutrition and dehydration. Lillian is present during the visit, and the relationship between mother and daughter is characterized by bickering. Mrs. Farrow cannot manage her medications independently, so Lillian is in charge.

1. Why did Mrs. Farrow's fluid and nutritional input fall to the extent that she required hospitalization?
2. Is Lillian neglecting her mother's care?
3. Are there other signs of potential neglect or abuse?
4. Can Mrs. Farrow safely stay at home?
5. Is Lillian competent to manage her mother's medications?
6. Is Mrs. Farrow competent to decide where she wants to live?
7. Must Lillian care for her mother?
8. How much of a change in life-style will Mrs. Farrow and Lillian permit?

CASE STUDY 2

John Andrews, 24, is a gay man with AIDS who was recently discharged after being treated for Kaposi's sarcoma. He lives with his lover of three years, and their relationship is stable. John visits an oncology clinic for chemotherapy, and he is returning to work as a computer analyst.

1. Should John tell the occupational health nurse about his medical diagnosis?
2. Does the OHN have an obligation to tell John's coworkers about his medical diagnosis?
3. Should John abstain from sexual relations with his lover?
4. Should his lover abstain from sexual relations with others?
5. What should the OHN tell other employees when they ask about John's marks from Kaposi's sarcoma?
6. Isn't John at higher risk for work-related injuries while receiving chemotherapy and therefore a greater insurance risk?

CASE STUDY 3

Mary O'Brien is in jail for 4 years after being convicted of assault and battery. She gave birth to a daughter one month ago.

1. What right does Mary have to nurture her daughter?
2. What is in the best interests of the infant?
3. Should Mary be confined with the other prisoners?
4. Should the prison routine be adjusted to allow Mary time with her daughter?
5. Should Mary be released from prison early?
6. Should Mary be encouraged to give her daughter up for adoption?

REFERENCES

1. Allen, D., and M. Fowler, "Cognitive Moral Development Theory and Moral Decisions in Health Care." *Law, Medicine, and Health Care* 10 (1): 19, 1982.
2. American Nurses' Association. *Guidelines for Implementing the Code for Nurses.* Kansas City, Mo.: American Nurses' Association, 1980.
3. Aroskar, M. "Anatomy of an Ethical Dilemma: The Theory, the Practice." *American Journal of Nursing* 80 (4): 658, 1980.
4. Aroskar, M. "Are Nurses' Mind Sets Compatible with Ethical Practice?" *Topics in Clinical Nursing,* 4:22, 1982.
5. Aroskar, M. "Access to Hospice: Ethical Dimensions." *Nursing Clinics of North America* 20 (2):299, 1982.
6. Aroskar, M. "A Nursing Perspective on the Right of the Patient to Reject Treatment." In *Ethical Problems in the*

Nurse-Patient Relationship, ed. C. Murphy and H. Hunter. Boston: Allyn & Bacon, 1983, 138–48.

7. Bayer, R. "Ethical Challenges of the Movement for Home Care." *Caring* 3 (10):57, 1984.

8. Bayer, R. "Ethics in Home Care and Quality Assurance." *Caring* 5 (1):50, 1986.

9. Connaway, N. "My Patient Won't Follow the Medical Plan of Treatment. What Should I Do to Protect Myself—Legally?" *Home Healthcare Nursing* 3 (4):6, 1985.

10. Fromer, M. J. "Solving Ethical Dilemmas in Nursing Practice." *Topics in Clinical Nursing* 4:15, 1982.

11. Fry, S. T. "Dilemma in Community Health Ethics." *Nursing Outlook* 31 (3): 176, 1983.

12. Fry, S. T. "Ethics in Community Health Practice." In *Community Health Nursing Process and Practice for Promoting Health,* ed. M. Stanhope and J. Lancaster. St. Louis: C. V. Mosby, 1984, 77–96.

13. Gilligan, C. *In a Different Voice.* Cambridge, Mass.: Harvard University Press, 1982.

14. Hall, H. D. "Home Care and the Values of Public Health." *Caring* 4 (12):38, 1985.

15. Holleran, C. "Ethics in Prison Health Care." *International Nursing Review* 30 (5):138, 1983.

16. Holloway, V. "Documentation: One of the Ultimate Challenges in Home Health Care." *Home Healthcare Nursing* 2 (1):19, 1984.

17. Kane, F. "Keeping Elizabeth Bouvia Alive for the Public Good." *Hastings Center Report* 15 (6):5, 1985.

18. Karhausen, K. "Medical Ethics and Moral Philosophy." In *Ethical Issues in Preventive Medicine,* ed. S. Doxiadis. Boston: Martinus Nijhoff Medical Publishers, 1985.

19. Kohlberg, L. "Moral Stages and Moralization: The Cognitive Developmental Approach." In *Moral Development and Behavior, Theory, Research, and Social Issues,* ed. T. Lickona. New York: Holt, Rinehart, & Winston, 1976, 31–53.

20. Murphy, C. "The Changing Role of Nurses Making Ethical Decisions." *Law, Medicine and Health Care* 12 (4):173, 1984.

21. Nokes, K. "The Relationship Between Moral Reasoning, the Relationship Dimension of the Social Climate of the Work Environment, and Perception of Realistic Moral Behavior Among Registered Professional Nurses." Ph.D. diss., New York University, 1984.

22. Northrop, C. "Government and Legal Influences on the Practice of Community Health Nurses." In *Community Health Nursing Process and Practice for Promoting Health,* ed. M. Stanhope and J. Lancaster. St. Louis: C. V. Mosby, 1984, 97–119.

23. O'Malley, T. "Identifying and Preventing Family-Mediated Abuse and Neglect." *Caring* 5 (1):28, 1986.

24. Rest, J. R. "Longitudinal Study of the DIT: A Strategy for Analyzing Developmental Change." *Developmental Psychology* 11:738, 1975.

25. Rogers, M. E. *An Introduction to the Theoretical Basis of Nursing.* Philadelphia: F. A. Davis, 1970.

26. Smith, J. P. "The Relationship Between Rights and Responsibilities in Health Care: A Dilemma for Nurses." *Journal of Advanced Nursing* 8 (5):437, 1983.

27. Smith, S., and A. Davis. "Ethical Dilemmas: Conflicts Among Rights, Duties, and Obligations." *American Journal of Nursing* 80:1463, 1980.

28. Wagner, D., and D. Cosgrove. "Quality Assurance: A Professional Responsibility." *Caring* 5 (1):46, 1986.

29. Yeaworth, R. "The ANA Code: A Comparative Perspective." *Image* 17 (3):94, 1983.

CHAPTER 7

Research and Nursing Practice

JEAN C. KIJEK

■

OBJECTIVES

After completing this chapter, the reader will be able to:

□ Value the need for the use of research in nursing.
□ Identify the functional role of each nurse according to educational level.
□ Identify sources of nursing research.
□ Identify the way to access the literature for nursing research.
□ Identify the stages of the research process.
□ Critically analyze a nursing problem.
□ Identify strategies for facilitating the use of research in practice.

For nursing to be a credible profession and scientific discipline, its practices must be based on findings from research, questioned, critically evaluated, and verified by valid and reliable scientific methods, and its practitioners must know how to use such findings. With the increasing complexity of human systems and health care systems, the primary nurse needs to be able to use the best information and data available for practice. This information and data comes from nursing research.

In order for research to be incorporated and used in nursing practice, nurses must believe that nursing is a scientific discipline whose practice is scientific. Nurses must value existing knowledge and the development of *new* knowledge for nursing practice. In order to accomplish this task, nurses need to know how to find research, how to use research, and how to participate in the research process. In addition, nurses must constantly evaluate their practice and vigorously question it. With the increasingly limited amount of resources and the increasing competition in the health care arena, nursing will need to be able to demonstrate that its practice is both effective and efficient in terms of health care costs and health care needs. This is best done through nursing research.

Educational Level of the Nurse and the Nurse's Role in Research

At all levels of preparation, nurses have a role in nursing research. In 1981 the American Nurses' Association Commission on Nursing Research published its *Guidelines for the Investigative Functions of Nurses* (3). This document clearly outlines the responsibilities for each level of nurse from the nurse with an associate degree in nursing to the nurse with a doctorate in nursing (see Table 7.1). Although primary nurses are ideally prepared at the baccalaureate degree level or higher, understanding the potential contributions of all levels of nurses to research can enhance research.

The associate degree nurse should demonstrate an awareness of the value of research in nursing, assist in

Table 7.1
Level of Education and Nurse's Role in Research

Level of Education	Role of Nurse
Associate degree	Participant Problem identifier Data collector
Baccalaureate degree	Critiquer Utilizer
Master's degree	Practice evaluator Clinical investigator
Doctoral degree	Nurse researcher Theory developer Knowledge generator

identifying problem areas that need study, and assist in data collection. The baccalaureate degree nurse should identify research problems for scientific study, critique research, apply nursing research to practice, and share these findings with nurse colleagues. The master's degree nurse should be thoroughly familiar with the research process and facilitate the investigation of clinical problems, in addition to applying findings to practice. This nurse should conduct investigations for the purpose of monitoring the quality of nursing practice, assisted by baccalaureate degree and associate degree nurses. The nurse with a doctoral degree in nursing should be engaged in developing theoretical explanations about nursing practice and nursing phenomena, as well as in developing methods to modify or extend existing knowledge for nursing (3). He or she should serve as a consultant to all nurses. Although in reality it is not common for primary nurses to have access to a group of nurse researchers, it is important to appreciate how nurses at each level of education may be involved in their distinct investigative functions, collectively and individually, to promote the conduct of research and research utilization that will directly enhance professional practice and the care delivered to its clients.

Value of Research in Nursing Practice

Nursing research is a subject avoided by many nurses and nursing students. They fail to perceive the relationship between research and their goal of providing the highest standards of nursing care by learning all they possibly can about nursing practice and health care systems. Nursing educators attempt to stimulate interest in the research process, but they will continue to have a difficult time convincing generic students of the need for research in practice until professional practitioners embody research throughout practice. Students will fail to see the relationship between research and practice when it is clearly evident to them that nurses who are practicing daily do not use research in their work, nor is it expected of them. In fact, many nurses in practice fail to even critically question their practices or to seek new information from current journals and conferences to use in their daily practice. Fortunately many states have laws for mandatory continuing education, so more nurses are being exposed to new ideas or reviewing current practices.

Commitment of Primary Nurses to the Research Process

Because primary nurses are the basic link to the successful implementation of research in their practice, it is important for them to be committed to the use of available research findings in their practice and to the support of research in areas that need investigation. Their efforts to improve practice through research will be strengthened if they use each other to develop their ideas and if they work with nurses of all levels outside of primary nursing to develop research proposals and conduct investigations. In addition, they can make a contribution to nursing as a whole by supporting research on a larger scale. The recent development of the Center for Nursing Research at the National Institutes of Health clearly provides evidence that research in nursing is a national priority. This center was made possible by the collective efforts of many nurses and supporters of nursing.

Support of Nursing Research by Nurse Administrators and Institutions

Although a hierarchical structure is antithetical to the concept of primary nursing, as discussed in chapter 1,

in reality many nurses still practice primary nursing in institutions and nursing services that are hierarchical. Even when practiced in the community, primary nursing may still be part of a bureaucracy that has an impact on many areas, including nursing research.

Nursing research is more apt to be applied and conducted in institutions and nursing services that value it than in those that do not. The climate for research in institutional nursing is influenced significantly by the chief nursing executive. His or her beliefs about the importance of research to practice and about nursing as a scientific discipline that requires the same rigorous questioning of its principles, theories, and practices as any other practice discipline will be reflected in the philosophy of nursing at that institution as well as in the actions of the nurses.

The nurse executive can foster nursing research by using the power associated with the position to create a climate conducive to research. Some of the basic steps include setting specific goals for nursing research, providing the structure and mechanisms that facilitate research, helping to secure resources, rewarding those who do research, and supporting the use of research findings in practice (8). The value of nursing research in cost containment and quality assurance can be a strong motivator for institutional support of nursing research.

The Standards for Nursing Services published by the American Nurses' Association (ANA) (2) include two standards which strengthen the position of research in nursing:

Standard XI: A nursing service supports research in the health care field.
Standard XII: A nursing service evaluates its clinical and administrative practices.

In summary, one responsibility of the chief nursing executive is to support nursing research. Such support can be given through such means as stating a philosophy of nursing that includes research, creating a climate and structure conducive to research (which includes the writing of position descriptions for professional nurses that include some aspect of research consistent with the ANA guidelines), assisting those interested in doing research to secure the necessary resources, and rewarding those who do research.

Finding Nursing Research

In order to use research in practice and implement its findings or results, one needs to be able to obtain re-

Table 7.2
Nursing Research Journals

Advances in Nursing Science
American Journal of Nursing
Computers in Nursing
Heart and Lung: The Journal of Critical Care
Image: The Journal of Nursing Scholarship
Issues in Comprehensive Pediatric Nursing
Journal of Gerontological Nursing
Journal of Neurosurgical Nursing
Journal of Nursing Administration
Journal of Professional Nursing
Maternal Child Nursing
Nursing Research
Pediatric Nursing
Public Health Nursing
Research in Nursing and Health
Western Journal of Nursing Research

search reports and to have access to research and re-searchers. Good nursing libraries have nursing research resources such as the current journals that report research (Table 7.2), as well as copies of texts about the research process and statistical methods for health care disciplines. The library should also have access to abstracts of current research and to computerized bibliographic data bases, such as *NurseSearch* and *Medline*.

Until recently most research was conducted by academic nurse researchers and communicated to other nurses. Reported research did not necessarily address nursing practice or how to use the findings in practice. Currently there are several sources of nursing research, including conferences, universities, nursing research organizations, and research departments. Nurses need to be resourceful and seek out research. Baccalaureate graduates will have had exposure to nursing research in their basic nursing programs. In order to continue to develop their research interests and abilities, they will need to seek out other nurses who share their interest in nursing research and have a commitment to high standards of nursing practice. They will also have to identify research resources when they are employed, including like-minded colleagues to enhance their use of and access to research.

Locating Nursing Research

The first step in locating nursing research is to look at one's practice and client outcome. The primary nurse looks at his or her practice and questions it. Why is this happening? Why did this work? Will it work again? Under what kinds of conditions will it work? Will it work with different kinds of clients? Will it work for clients with different diagnoses, ages, ethnic backgrounds, beliefs, body images? For example, a nurse who is working with a family that has decided to provide home care for a client who has right-side paralysis resulting from a severe cerebrovascular accident may question how positioning affects the development of contracture deformities. He or she may ask, How long should a position be maintained, and how does it affect the range of motion of the joint? The nurse recalls that literature discusses positioning with reference to the development of pressure sores and length of time in a position but cannot recall any data about length of time and contracture formation. The nurse may think of the following questions: Does the position of the body (supine, prone, or sidelying) and the way the affected limb is positioned (flexed or extended, pronated or supinated) when sitting and lying make a difference in the range of motion of the affected joints? Does the length of time a position is maintained make a difference? Does the way one touches the limb make a difference? These kinds of questions provide the practitioner with a way to critically analyze the practice of positioning and client outcome. The critical analysis of any problem helps the inquiring nurse to generate questions and break the problem into parts, to yield some different ways of viewing it. Ultimately, critical analysis may help the nurse to guide the family in providing the best care for the client.

Another source of client care research problems is quality assurance studies. When client care process or outcome inconsistencies are identified, questions such as the ones previously stated can be used to identify some of the possible parameters of the problem or inconsistencies that need to be investigated. Then a search of the literature helps the primary nurse to determine if others have studied the problem or similar problems. The nurse may discover that there is research reported in the literature that either provides answers to the problem or assists in studying it.

Once a question or a problem is identified, a search of appropriate sources is conducted. An important aspect of this process is the critical analysis of the problem or question, to break it down into its parts so that it can be studied. In the example cited, the primary nurse might break the clinical problem into the following parts: positioning, posture, postural reflexes, range of motion, contracture formation, and prevention of contracture development. The next step is to access the printed literature on the subject. The common ways of accessing the literature are through the library's card catalogue and the major indexes, such as the *Cumulative Index to Nursing and Allied Health Literature, International Nursing Index,* and *Index Medicus.* The computerized bibliographic data bases will be useful, once the nurse has clarified and delineated the problem. In conducting a computerized search of the literature, the nurse works closely with the librarian to select the best descriptors related to the problem so that relevant bibliographic citations can be located. Otherwise, the search may yield references that are too limited or too broad.

Other valuable resources for the primary nurse are peer groups and other professional colleagues, such as clinical specialists, educators, and researchers. Faculty at local universities often have access to the most recent data on current clinical problems or know of resources for the practicing nurse. Most university faculty members will be interested in working with practicing nurses in the evaluation and conduct of research so that their research is applicable to clinical nursing in a variety of settings and can be tested in the clinical area by appropriate clinical practitioners. Often faculty members collaborate closely with clinical experts, who may be primary nurses, in defining research problems and developing clinical protocols. After reviewing the literature and consulting with colleagues, nurse faculty, and members of other disciplines and determining that no answer or valid information is available, the primary nurse and the clinical investigator or nurse researcher (if available) may develop a proposal to study the problem, either jointly or independently (see Table 7.3).

Conducting Research in Practice

A common interest as well as a fear of many practicing nurses is the whole area of nursing research, including the research process (see Table 7.4). Some of them are aware that conducting research requires a great deal of knowledge about research methods such as the design of studies, data collection (including tools and instruments), sampling, and statistical analysis, as well as substantial knowledge about the problem area being studied. Some nurses have a realistic perception of their abilities and deficits; others do not. Some are overconfident, while others do not appreciate their abilities enough. An overview of the process of conducting clini-

Table 7.3
Steps in Locating Research

Step 1	Identify the problem (contracture development in patients with cerebrovascular accidents).
Step 2	Critically analyze the problem (what is going on here?).
Step 3	Review the literature (library search, review of indexes with abstracts, computer search).
Step 4	Consult with nurse colleagues and members of other disciplines.
Step 5	If no answer or solution to problem, consult with a master's-prepared nurse (clinical specialist or educator) or a nurse researcher (university faculty).
Step 6	Assist nurse researcher or clinical specialist with proposal development.

Table 7.4
Elements of the Research Process

Problem identification
Review of literature
    Conceptual framework
    Identification of variables
    Hypotheses development
Method
    Design
    Instruments
    Sample
    Procedure
    Data analysis
Results
    Report of findings
    Discussion of findings
    Implications for practice and further research

cal nursing research may be helpful to all of these nurses.

The conceptual framework consists of the ideas upon which a clinical nursing study is based and which provide part of the context for interpreting the findings. A good place to begin selecting a conceptual framework is to turn to theorists from either nursing or related fields. Once a conceptual framework has been selected, the investigator reviews relevant literature to refine perceptions of the problem and perhaps select a way of studying it. This phase of the research process ends with the statement of the problem and hypotheses.

Once the problem (or problems) and hypotheses have been stated, the researcher designs the study in such a way that the research problem can be answered. This process involves knowing how to locate and evaluate available research instruments and tools or, if none are available, to develop them, knowing how to collect data and knowing enough about statistics to select those instruments or tools that are appropriate to the hypotheses and the type of data collected. Research design also involves sampling, being able to select enough subjects from the desired population in as unbiased a way as possible to yield statistically significant results.

After the research design has been completed and the data collected, the researcher analyzes and interprets the data and synthesizes the findings of the study in the context of the conceptual framework, previous studies, and applicability to nursing practice. This last phase is particularly important, especially for the primary nurse whose main interest is improving his or her own nursing practice.

Not all primary nurses will have the ability, interest, or time to conduct clinical nursing research. Nevertheless, they can keep abreast of what others are doing and, when feasible, participate in research according to their ability.

Critiquing Research

In order to use research in practice, one needs to be able to judge the scientific merit of the study and the generalizability of the findings. Are the findings of the study applicable beyond the sample studied? Has the study been replicated sufficiently to establish its reliability and validity? In order to be certain of the quality of the research product, one must be an astute consumer of the products of research. Duffy (5) advised that nurses must learn to sort through what is weak and what is strong. She stated that nurses must focus both on the research process itself and on the product of the endeavor. She developed the Research Appraisal Checklist (RAC), which appears in the December 1985 issue of *Nursing and Health Care* (5), to assist nurses with critiquing research and research methods. She developed the RAC from the findings of a survey designed to identify the key elements of critique criteria. The survey was conducted using selected nurse researchers who were members of the ANA Council of Nurse Researchers. The criteria are grouped into eight major research categories: (a) title; (b) abstract; (c) problem; (d) literature review;

(e) methodology, which is subdivided into subjects, instruments, and design; (f) data analysis; (g) discussion; and (h) form and style. Each statement has a rating scale from one to six, to rate each item and then arrive at a total score. The RAC presumes a knowledge of the research process.

Nurses who use research need a working knowledge of the research process, so that they can critique the process as well as the results of the study. Many texts are currently available to assist the professional nurse in reviewing the research process and critiquing research for use in practice (7, 9, 10).

Strategies for Facilitating the Use of Research in Practice

Strategies that have been described in the literature for facilitating research in nursing practice range from having nurses attend research conferences and participate in journal clubs, to appointing resident nurse researchers and forming research departments. The feasibility of these last two strategies for primary nursing, especially in small communities, remains problematic. Many nurses and certainly many small nursing services do not have the resources available to develop and support a department of nursing research. However, one must be aware of the need for nursing research and its application in practice. The primary nurse who does not have direct access to nurse researchers or clinical investigators should not be daunted. He or she can use the literature wisely and thoroughly read monthly nursing journals that contain research reports. A nurse could establish a journal club with other primary nurses to review and discuss articles and research reports that have some relevancy to their day-to-day practice and concerns. The journal club could meet weekly, with a professional nurse selecting an article about a current client care concern. One nurse would present a review of the article, critique it, and discuss its applicability to clinical practice with the others. Ideally the journal club would meet for at least an hour each week. If this is not possible, then the primary nurses could meet during one lunch hour as feasible and discuss the article over lunch. The concept of a journal club could also be a regular feature of the local district nurses' association.

One popular way for many agencies to have access to research and researchers is to develop a close association with a university nursing program. Faculty need to conduct research and need to have access to relevant populations for research. Faculty often welcome the assistance of nursing staff with various parts of the research project, including data collection. In addition, master's degree and doctoral students need to have settings in which to conduct their research, as well as access to subjects. Baccalaureate degree students need opportunities to discover problems for research and to critique research for creative application to nursing practice. A primary nurse's practice may meet these needs.

Some universities and hospitals have developed joint committees to facilitate research activities. The committees provide ways to disseminate research findings, evaluate the need for research, provide seminars on research to staff, and serve as review boards for the protection of human subjects for proposed nursing research. In addition, some worthwhile joint research projects using the clinical expertise of agency staff and the research expertise of university faculty have been developed (1, 4).

DISCUSSION QUESTIONS

1. What is the value of nursing research?
2. What is the role of the associate degree nurse, the baccalaureate degree nurse, the master's degree nurse, and the doctoral degree nurse in nursing research?
3. Discuss how you would solve a clinical problem.

4. Describe ways to facilitate the use of research in practice.

REFERENCES

1. Alley, L., P. Gray, K. Parker, and J. Beeks. "Attuning Staff Nurses to Clinical Research. *Nursing and Health Care* 8:77, 1987.
2. American Nurses' Association. *Standards for Nursing Services.* Kansas City, Mo.: American Nurses' Association, 1973.
3. American Nurses' Association. *Guidelines for the Investigative Functions of Nurses.* Kansas City, Mo.: American Nurses' Association, 1981.
4. Batra, C. "Developing a Nursing Research Program." *Nursing and Health Care* 4:18, 1983.
5. Duffy, M. E. "Evaluating Research." *Nursing and Health Care* 6:538, 1985.
6. Fawcett, J. "Utilization of Nursing Research Findings." *Image* 14:57, 1982.
7. LoBiondo–Wood, G., and J. Haber. *Nursing Research: A Critical Appraisal.* St. Louis: C. V. Mosby, 1986.
8. McClure, M. L. "Promoting Practice Based Research: A Critical Need." *Journal of Nursing Administration* 11:66, 1986.
9. Phillips, L.R.F. *A Clinician's Guide to the Critique and Utilization of Nursing Research.* E. Norwalk, Conn.: Appleton-Century-Crofts, 1986.
10. Wilson, H. S. *Research in Nursing.* Menlo Park, Calif.: Addison-Wesley, 1985.

CHAPTER 8

Negotiating the System

BARBARA J. STEVENS BARNUM

■

OBJECTIVES

After completing this chapter, the reader will be able to:

- Identify typical organized delivery systems for nursing care.
- Discuss reasons for organized nursing delivery systems.
- Identify the educational trends that have obstructed nursing's understanding of organizational settings.
- Define the terms system, subsystem, and suprasystem.
- Identify the basic components of a system.
- Identify the institutional subsystems impacting on the nursing care delivery system.
- Discuss how the institutional subsystems impact on the nursing care delivery system.
- Define the term negotiation.
- Identify the reasons for using negotiation as a tactic to achieve nursing care delivery goals.
- Identify the skills required for successful negotiation.
- Differentiate between negotiation and control efforts.
- Identify the impediments to successful negotiation by the new nurse graduate.
- Identify and discuss the negotiation needs of the primary nurse.

This chapter considers several elements that are important to the practicing primary nurse in the organizational structure. First, the organization is considered from a systems perspective, analyzing how that system may be used effectively and manipulated to produce good nursing care. Second, the tactics required by the nurse for manipulating the system are examined. Negotiating skills are stressed. Finally, special problems of the new nurse graduate are reviewed. Problems that are unique to primary nursing care are elaborated in this section of the chapter.

Negotiating

In today's health care institution there are many individuals and groups with control and authority over some component or subsystem. These parties have their own personal and organizational goals. And these goals may or may not be congruent with the goals of the primary nurse. If the nurse is to be effective in achieving goals, frequently he or she must negotiate with others. Negotiation is only one way of interacting. Other modes of interaction include submission, appeasement, collaboration, challenge, and coercion. In negotiation, one desires to reach a consensus among two or more parties on how a certain action, tactic, procedure, or principle is to be enacted, interpreted, or approached. One enters into a negotiation with the idea that the final product (the action, tactic, procedure, or principle) will arise out of agreements made by and among the negotiating parties.

Negotiation is not a proper method of interaction when

- everyone is already in agreement on how to handle the issue;
- one holds an all-or-nothing position and is unwilling to compromise on the decision; or
- organizationally, one has the power and authority to decide the issue—and intends to do so regardless of the positions held by others in relation to the issue.

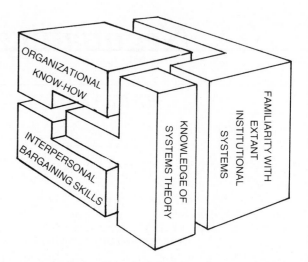

Figure 8.1. Components of Successful System Negotiation

Negotiation, then, is an alternative to total cooperation or to absolute competition in a win-lose situation. Negotiation may take place in a cooperative or competitive framework, but the end product is determined in light of the interchange that takes place during the negotiation process.

Negotiated Order Model

Negotiating in the health care organization calls for many skills and much knowledge on the part of the nurse. Chief among them are interpersonal bargaining skills, organizational know-how, familiarity with the extant institutional systems, and knowledge of systems theory (see Figure 8.1). The negotiator usually tries to get the other involved parties to agree on a product that is close to (or identical with) the one the negotiator originally desired. This chapter focuses on this sort of situation, with the nurse as negotiator of his or her own agreements, having a vested interest in the outcomes of the negotiations in light of nursing goals.

In some special instances a negotiator may be a disinterested party, not caring about the final product per se, but interested in moving parties that are far from consensus toward agreement. What the agreement *is,* is secondary to this negotiator. In formal organizational negotiations such a person is called a *mediator.* In informal relations there are also people who excel in the interpersonal influence of mediation. Sometimes nurses will find themselves mediating between others informally. Mediation between other parties is not addressed specifically in this chapter.

Negotiation Versus Control

There was a time when negotiation skills were not as essential for the nurse as they are now. The head nurse role of the recent past illustrates this point. In past decades the head nurse controlled all or most ward activities. She had strong powers: she directed all ancillary personnel as well as nursing personnel; she even had considerable authority over physician behavior on her unit. She could, for example, bar a physician from admitting clients to "her" floor if she failed to conform with her procedures. Similarly, she could fire a janitor for failing to maintain a satisfactory standard of cleanliness. Nor did the head nurse have to rely on personal charisma; she had to be obeyed and respected but not necessarily liked. She did not have to negotiate to effect her decisions; she simply exercised the power inherent in her role. She did not have to be adroit with interpersonal relations; nor did she have to support her decisions by means of extensive evaluative documentation. She simply had to act.

Whether it was good or bad, the era of absolute head nurse control is past in most institutions. In many cases authority was given away by nurses seeking to decrease their nonnursing tasks. One may argue that nurses gave away too much. Loss of control over nursing supplies, for example, may impair delivery of nursing care if supplies are hard to acquire through the regulatory systems created and managed by others. In giving away control of the support environment, nursing guaranteed that it would have to negotiate for care delivery essentials in the future. Control of the care support environment could have been retained while truly nonnursing functions were shed, but this seldom happened. No one, for example, would want to go back to the days when nursing supervisors ran to the pharmacies in the middle of the night for drugs. One might, however, differentiate indiscriminate fetch-and-carry activities from environmental support activities. Such activities as supply of equipment, client transport, clerical services, or even unit sanitation could be judged to be environmental support activities. Activities such as these could be carried out by nonnurse employees reporting to the nursing line managers, rather than by employees reporting to a non-nursing, collateral management line. Be this as it may, in most institutional settings nursing gave up control of its own environment at the same time it ceased doing irrelevant tasks. Today's head nurses, therefore, find themselves needing to negotiate for many essentials of and for care.

Like the head nurse, the primary nurses find themselves relying on interpersonal communications rather than on delegated powers in achieving many goals for the client. The complexity of this negotiating order model is revealed by contrasting the physician's mode of interaction with that of the primary nurse. The physician simply writes an "order" for the client and fully expects that others will see that the order is carried out. The primary nurse, on the other hand, may have to negotiate with several people in several subsystems in order to effect the nursing prescriptions. Suppose, for example, that the nurse wants to modify the patient's diet because of an unusual cultural pattern. The nurse may have to explore the whole operation of the dietary department in order to see how such a deviation from the norm can be effected. When the nurse finds a solution, she or he may have to negotiate with others from this subsystem in order to win support for the plan.

Suggestions for Effective Negotiating

What makes an effective negotiator? Several factors enter in. One of the most important is the negotiator's personal reputation in the organization. The nurse who has built positive and extensive communications networks in the past is in a better position to negotiate when an issue arises than one who has not done so. If the nurse knows the involved parties, and they already have a sense of his or her credibility, values, faithfulness in carrying out past agreements, the nurse is in a better negotiating position. All that a nurse does as a professional and as a person contributes to how willing or unwilling others will be to negotiate.

In addition, the effective negotiator will be one who is able to see the issue from the "sides" of the other parties to the negotiation. The nurse recognizes that their roles influence their interpretations of the issue, their degree of interest in it, and what they can and cannot do without "losing face." The nurse recognizes that these role biases are natural, and therefore uses them to advantage when possible. For example, a nurse knows that the chief dietitian is interested in seeing that clients receive food while it is still hot and appetizing, and may be able to use this shared goal (value) to negotiate a procedure of tray delivery that makes more work for the dietary department. If the nurse fails to make evident these shared goals, however, he or she may fail to get cooperation.

Similarly, a nurse must recognize that the institution's purchasing agent has little interest in client satisfaction. The agent's main interest is in showing the cost-effectiveness of a purchase. The nurse recognizes this pattern of motivation and does not stress differences in client satisfaction to get the product of choice. Instead, the nurse will find a way to argue that Product A (despite its higher initial cost) may actually be less costly in the long run than Products B and C. The effective negotiator builds arguments that take into consideration the goals and values of the other parties to the negotiation.

Negotiation is not always as simple as getting someone else to do what one wants. Often negotiation ends with a solution different from that initially imagined by either party. A successful negotiator does not become overcommitted to the initial proposal; nor does she or he forget the situation that the proposal was designed to alleviate. It may well be that a proposal other than one's own may achieve the same purpose with equal facility. Ideally, one hopes that a proposal can be found that simultaneously achieves the goals of all parties to the negotiation. The effective negotiator is flexible concerning alternative solutions, without forgetting the problem to be solved. The effective negotiator really listens to the proposals and problems of others; he or she suspends judgment and analyzes suggestions dispassionately.

The successful negotiator also gets all the facts before negotiating. After learning all the facts from his or her own perspective, the negotiator learns the "facts" from the sides of the other parties to the negotiation. If, for example, the negotiator wants to propose a change in tray-serving procedures, the nurse learns the present system and how it interfaces with other responsibilities of dietary department personnel. In learning the facts of a case the nurse also is careful to differentiate between facts and interpretations of facts. Both may be important, but confusion of facts and interpretations may lead to the wrong decision.

Many times the "facts" involve the operations of the institution. Knowledge of organizational subsystems is critical if appropriate decisions are to be made. The new graduate must acquire familiarity with ongoing practices, policies, and procedures before suggesting change.

The inexperienced nurse tends to assume that a new procedure will necessarily be better than an old one. Nursing education often has stressed change and change processes as being good. From this emphasis the inexperienced nurse may develop an unwarranted assumption that much of the status quo needs to be changed. A systems perspective helps the nurse put such notions of change in proper perspective. A systems analysis reveals the benefits of both change and continuity; it reveals effective modes of organizing as well as instances where change is needed.

Although it is quite possible that a policy, accepted practice, or procedure may become malfunctional as circumstances change, most regulations originally were devised to solve some problem or to otherwise simplify organizational life. The nurse who is sensitive to how systems work will find out what purpose was served by the old regulation before proposing an alternative. A nurse who is aware of the problem that was solved by the old regulation may make suggestions for change that achieve the present goals without reinstituting an old problem.

The effective negotiator understands trade-offs. A trade-off is achieved when one person supports another on one issue in exchange for the other party's support on an issue of interest to the first person. This may be a formalized agreement, with specific stances on issues. Trade-offs also may occur on an informal basis. In that case one relies on a sense of reciprocity and future "repayment." The nurse who has cooperated on policies and practice important to others (even if inconsequential to his or her own operations) is likely to find those people obliging when the nurse calls for their support on an issue of importance.

The effective negotiator strives to set an atmosphere of mutual problem solving. The nurse avoids placing blame for past failures in solving the issue at hand. The negotiator is future-oriented, rather than worried about who erred originally, and constructs a situation in which parties can negotiate from positions of self-respect, without recrimination or guilt. The effective negotiator knows that if a party to the negotiation feels guilty about past practices, that party may feel a paradoxical need to stand by those practices to "prove" that they were right.

Knowledge of when to negotiate and when not to is as important as the development of skill in the negotiation process. For example, the nurse who is assuming responsibility for managing other staff should not negotiate with a nurse's aide over how many patients are to be in the aide's assignment. This is a managerial decision not open to negotiation. One cannot and should not negotiate away one's own job responsibilities. This is not to say that the nurse may not consult the nurse's aide if he or she elects to do so. Asking the nurse's aide, for example, about past assignment loads might or might not be of value in making a decision concerning the assignment. Often in situations such as this nurses are forced into a negotiation because they have not learned to give clear, concise directives to subordinates. When an inexperienced nurse vacillates concerning authority, it is not surprising that subordinates challenge that authority. New graduates, therefore, must be aware that sometimes others may try to usurp their authority. Often the usurpation takes the form of negotiating (or trying to do so) over items that should not be negotiated. This example, incidentally, shows the interplay between negotiation and systems analysis. If the nurse had a better understanding of the system (in this case, the typical work-load of nurse's aides), he or she would be less vulnerable to challenges to authority.

Another danger for new graduates is the opposite extreme: refusing to negotiate when negotiation is the best tactic in a given situation. Some new graduates have been overcoached in superficial concepts of "assertiveness" and have come to think that listening to another's position on an issue is a sign of weakness. Assertiveness often is interpreted as aggressiveness. Nurses must learn to differentiate between situations that call for political management through compromise, negotiation, or trade-offs and those that require an "all or nothing" stand.

Negotiation, then, requires several abilities: (a) recognizing when negotiation is an appropriate mode of interaction, (b) analyzing the problem situation from the perspectives of all involved persons and subsystems, and (c) using effective interpersonal techniques in the negotiating process.

The System

Most nursing care is delivered in an organizational setting rather than in an entrepreneurial relationship between one nurse and one client. Hospitals, nursing homes, and home health care agencies are typical organized delivery systems for nursing. In such organizations nursing care is shared among numerous nurses so that it may be delivered on different shifts and different days. In addition to coordinating its own work, the nursing staff coordinates with other health care professionals so as to build a comprehensive health care plan for each client. In the acute care facility, for example, care must be coordinated among nurses because clients need care around the clock. Because one nurse cannot be available twenty-four hours a day, there is no choice but to coordinate, and that is an important characteristic of nursing. Even primary nursing calls for coordination between the primary nurse planner and those who will give care in his or her absence. Moreover, the primary nurse delivers care within an organization and uses the resources and practices of that organization in care planning and delivery.

Nursing, therefore, takes place in a system, an organization that is designed to achieve various goals, including those of nursing. It is natural that nursing is practiced this way, that nursing goals are achieved through organizational cooperation. It is critical, therefore, to consider the particular system in planning for and delivering nursing care. To ignore the system that constitutes the environment of nursing care is to discount a factor that has major impact on the effectiveness of care delivery. By carefully analyzing the organization from a systems perspective, nurses can enhance their ability to deliver good nursing care in that organization.

A Systems Approach

It is useful to analyze the nursing organization through a systems model. In this approach any process or phenomenon is viewed as a set of interrelated and interdependent parts designed to achieve a goal or set of goals. The nursing department of a hospital, for example, could be seen as consisting of various interdependent parts (nursing units) serving the goals of patient care delivery. That one system (nursing) can be viewed as a subsystem of a larger system (the total hospital). Similarly, a nursing unit could be viewed as a subsystem of the nursing system. A systems approach allows for systems within systems, smaller systems inside larger systems. For simplicity, the main focus of inquiry is usually called "the system." In this chapter, applying the rule, the nursing organization is hereafter referred to as the system, the total health care institution is referred to as the suprasystem, and components of a nursing organization are referred to as subsystems.

System Components

The basic components of a system are environment, input, throughput, output, goals, and feedback loops.

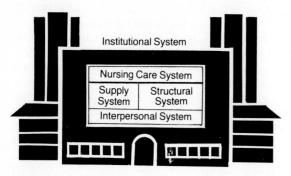

Figure 8.2. The Health Care System

Each of these elements will be discussed in relation to the nursing organization system. For convenience, a nursing organization within a hospital will be used in all of the following illustrations. Before proceeding to the illustrations, it is important to note that the components of a single system may vary, depending on the purpose of the analysis. For example, in one illustration I may perceive the subsystem components of the nursing department to be client care units. For another purpose I might conceptualize the department as consisting of various functions: care delivery, staff education, nursing administration. In yet another context I might consider the subsystems to be classes of workers: professionals, clericals, housekeeping personnel. The advantage of a systems perspective is that it is flexible in interpretation. One can look at the same organization from many perspectives. A systems view will enable one to view the inner workings and relationships of the organization in each of those perspectives. As shown in Figure 8.2, the nursing system exists within the suprasystem of the total health care institution. In turn, the nursing care system is made up of several subsystems: the logistics supply system, the organizational structural system, and the interpersonal system.

Environment.   The environment consists of those phenomena that are outside of the system itself but are vital to the system in either its functioning or its description. For example, one might describe the environment of the nursing department as the non-patient care departments of the hospital. Purchasing, admitting, laundry, dietary, and transportation departments would be part of the environment. In this example these departments interface with the nursing department but can be differentiated from it for the purpose of description. In contrast to this illustration, if one were describing the nursing

department in terms of its workers, then one might view the personnel policies, conditions of work, assignment systems, and other elements of this sort as constituting environment. Again, these elements impact on the "system," the workers, but may be differentiated from them.

Input.   In a systems model, input comprises elements that move from the environment into the system. In a nursing department focused on care delivery the most obvious input might be that of clients entering the nursing system from the community (environment). In contrast, if the nursing department were viewed from the perspective of its policies and procedures, then input might consist in recommendations from nursing committees as to which policies and procedures should be implemented.

Throughput.   Throughput (or central processing) consists of those actions that are done to or with the input. If the client were considered as input, the throughput would be those nursing acts done to or with him or her. If one were to consider the nursing department from the perspective of its workers, then the throughput might consist of those policies and practices that regulate workers, as well as the education and management that is provided for them. Throughput has the effect of converting input to output.

Output.   Output is the product of the system. In the case of the care delivery system, the most obvious product would be clients who were improved, comforted, sustained by nursing acts (throughput). Output is typically given back to the environment, as would be the case with the discharged client. In other cases the input may add to the system itself. Suppose, for example, new recruits for nurse's aide positions are viewed as input from the environment. The output of the educational process (throughput) would be fully trained aides. These outputs would be retained within the system rather than returned to the community.

Goals.   System goals represent those things one hopes to achieve through the throughput processes. In the previous example the goals would be the educational objectives identified for the aide training program. When clients are conceived as input, the goals would be drawn from various standards of care: from quality control goals, unit objectives, and other sources describing what is to be achieved for and with clients.

Feedback Loop. The feedback loop (or cybernetic component of the system) compares output and goals. If a program has identified the knowledge an obstetric client should have concerning child care before her discharge, then the feedback loop provides for testing whether or not that level of knowledge was achieved. A performance appraisal is the feedback loop that compares an employee's performance with the standards expected of one in her or his particular job category. A complete feedback loop not only compares output to goals, but also determines whether or not any deviance is within acceptable limits. If, for example, I set a goal of no client falls, a well-designed feedback loop would enable me to judge whether or not the occurrence of two falls per month was close enough to goal achievement. A feedback loop, finally, designs alterations in the system when they are required. For example, if two falls per month were determined to be excessive, then the feedback loop would determine how to change the nursing acts (throughput) to decrease the number of falls. An alternate way to bring the system into balance might be to recognize that the goal was unrealistic, and the nurse could then change the goal. The aim of the feedback mechanism is to achieve conformance between goal and system output. A complete feedback loop has three components: measurement, judgment, and alteration, if required.

Institutional Subsystems That Affect Nursing

There are several subsystems that have major impact on the ability of the nurse to deliver care. Three are discussed here: the logistics of resource supply, the structural system of organizational routines, and the interpersonal climate and interactions. These subsystems may be looked at on two levels: the institutional level and the nursing department level.

Resource Supply. The logistics of resource supply refers to the policies and practices that regulate movement of people, supplies, and equipment through the institution. When the logistics are working well, the nurse may not even notice them. However, when the nurse is unable to obtain a piece of equipment needed for client care, then the logistics come to his or her attention. Logistics may be viewed on the institutional level, for example, the movement of equipment from the materials management department to the nursing unit. Or logistics may be viewed on the nursing unit level, for example, the movement of staff from over-supplied units to those that are experiencing a personnel shortage.

In viewing the logistics subsystem as a system in itself, one might apply the following interpretation: *Goals* mediating the supply system would include (a) getting supplies (or personnel) where they are needed when they are needed, (b) accounting for use of supplies (and personnel) economically and efficiently, (c) charging for use of supplies as appropriate, and (d) returning supplies expediently to the appropriate refurbishing service. *Input* to the system would be (a) physical supplies, (b) personnel to be distributed in the system, and (c) transport equipment and space allocation. *Throughput* would consist in (a) the policies that decide how to distribute supplies, (b) cleaning/sterilizing and other preparation activities, (c) physical distribution of supplies, and (d) the monitoring systems for supplies and charges. *Feedback* would include formalized systems for reviewing supply distribution and informal systems, such as complaints of deficiencies by nurses.

Clearly nurses must know how to access the physical equipment and supplies of care. Interruption in accessibility, owing to poor supply systems or limited physical resources, impedes delivery of care. If such deficits occur, however, nurses will be in a better position to effect positive change if they understand the whole system rather than just their own perspectives. Suppose, for example, breakfast trays are invariably cold on 7 West. Rather than merely complain, the nurse may have to track the system from tray preparation to tray delivery in the client's room. Where are the breakdowns? Why do they occur? What other parties are involved? What are the constraints within which they work? The nurse takes a systems approach and gets the whole picture. He or she also learns who else must be involved in order to effect a solution. Focusing on systems change rather than on blame placing enables productive change when problems arise.

Structural-Organizational Routines. Another major subsystem is dealing with organizational routines. On an institutional level such routines might include how a client moves from admitting offices to a nursing unit, visitor policies and regulations, and purchasing procedures. Each organizational entity will have its own organizing routines: laboratory practices, housekeeping practices, pharmacy drug control practices. Some of the major organizational routines of the nursing department include client hygiene procedures, quality control systems for care, staff communication patterns, staffing and scheduling practices, client acuity systems, and nursing assignment systems.

Again, a systems view of a deficient routine goes far

in defining problems and solutions. A systems view allows for creativity in problem solving because there may be more than one way (throughput) to achieve the same goal. Indeed, different throughput may be required if differences occur in input. Take, for example, the nursing assignment system. Here we may suppose the goal to be the best possible client care. With this goal in mind it might be appropriate for an evening shift to deviate from primary nursing models to functional nursing if the input were radically reduced. Assume that three of seven nurses on a unit called in sick at the same time and that no relief staff was available. Because of the personnel shortage, it might make sense to alter throughput. In this example a judgment was made that although primary nursing was the most effective in reaching client care goals in the presence of normal resources, it was not the most efficient in a resource-deficient environment.

Interpersonal Climate.   The interpersonal climate constitutes yet another important subsystem that affects nursing. This subsystem can be viewed from the organizational perspective—how nurses interact with physicians, administrators, workers from other departments—or it may be viewed from within the nursing department itself—interactions of nursing staff on a unit, nursing staff from different units but working together on a committee, nursing staff with nursing managers. Sometimes formal policies and practices affect the interpersonal climate. Is there a joint practice committee to settle disputes between medicine and nursing? Is there a system by which a nurse may report suspected physician negligence without becoming the target of abuse for "whistle-blowing?" Labor relations, such as grievance procedures and contract negotiations, are other illustrations of formal arrangements that impact on interpersonal climate. Good structures promote good interpersonal relations; poor structures inhibit such relations.

Interpersonal climate also is formed in one-on-one and informal work group interactions. Often these relationships can best be analyzed through exploring individual roles, values accepted by practitioners of those roles, and goals accepted by these diverse parties. The use of a system model enables one to analyze problems logically, removed from the excessive emotive elements that may enter when a personal perspective is taken. To illustrate, I recently observed a situation in which the nurse's aides had developed excessive absence patterns, taking long "breaks" off the floor. The registered nurses became quite angry but responded by giving dictates

rather than by analyzing the problem. When cooler heads looked at the whole system of staff breaktime, an explanation was found. The aides felt that they were only taking "their share" of breaktime, "since the nurses did that in the back office." The solution rested in allowing the aides to know what the nurses did in the back office and demonstrating that work done there was not breaktime.

Obstructions or unresolved problems in any of these subsystems—the logistic organization, the institutional and nursing routines (structure), and the interpersonal climate—can impair delivery of nursing care. Nurses who are prepared to recognize and deal with problems in these systems are prepared to improve care delivery.

Nursing care occurs in several subsystems simultaneously. Obstructions in any of these subsystems, the supply system, the structural system, or the interpersonal environment impairs the delivery of client services (see Figure 8.3).

A systems approach is not the only way to negotiate care delivery problems, but often it does prove to be effective. It is compatible with an organizational perspective, since an organization itself is a system of interacting and interdependent parts.

The new nurse may have difficulty understanding why all good things are not immediately effected in the organizational setting. A systems perspective allows the nurse to see the problems that underlie organizational change. Such a perspective should not contribute to an attitude that change is hopeless or not appreciated. Instead, a systems model will allow the nurse to plan for effective change, considering all who need to be involved and all systems that may be affected by a change—even a subtle one—in another interfacing system.

Negotiating from the Primary Nursing Role

This section examines the negotiation needs of the primary nurse in the acute care facility. Certain similarities are evident for primary roles in other settings; in other aspects differences may be envisioned. The acute care setting is exemplified, since it represents one of the most complex settings for the primary care nursing role.

The primary nurse negotiates with at least three major groups: physicians, nursing staff, and clients. More often than not, the negotiations take place one on one rather than one on group.

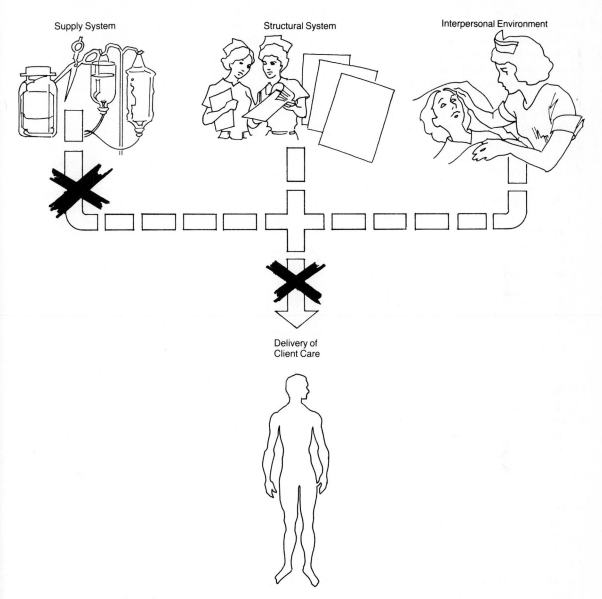

Figure 8.3. Nursing Care Subsystems

The nurse is assisted in care delivery by other nursing personnel of off-shifts and on days off. In cases where the nurse has a heavy case load, he or she may be assisted when on duty in direct care delivery. Primary nursing brings a new set of challenges to relations among nursing staff members. The professional nurse who is not the primary nurse, but who is assigned to a client's care delivery, may resent "following the orders" of a peer. This nurse may feel that subordination to the orders of another nurse demeans his or her own professional status. These feelings may be traced to the previous "team" emphasis in nursing delivery. Most nurses are able to get over such feelings when they grasp the concept of nursing accountability for practice (see chapter 4).

The registered nurse who is not a primary nurse can exemplify her or his professionalism in following the primary nurse's orders and judging when changed client status requires an adjustment in those orders. It is important to negotiate a system in which people other than the primary nurse may have input into care decisions. Usually this consists in devising input systems to the primary nurse. Further, there must be a system for changing the primary nurse's orders in case she or he cannot be reached in the event of an unanticipated change in client status. It is best that these negotiations be formalized in carefully thought out procedures.

Nursing orders (through well-developed nursing care plans) will greatly assist lower-level nursing personnel, guaranteeing a specificity of directives that often was missing when professional nurses relied heavily on word of mouth. In this sense the system of primary nursing cuts down on unnecessary negotiations by clarifying what is to be done for each client. Primary nursing also enhances care when a change is needed (or suggested). The system indicates with whom one will negotiate: the primary nurse.

In the primary nursing care model the primary nurse is the agent for negotiating directly with the physician concerning the client's needs. Because the primary nurse knows most about the client and his or her needs, this one-on-one relationship is logical. It also eliminates the danger of messages being misinterpreted when they pass through intermediaries. The one-on-one relationship also offers the best possible means for developing true colleague relations between nurse and physician. The physician comes to recognize and respect the abilities of the nurse in relation to the specific plans for his or her clients and their needs.

Often the most difficult negotiation between the primary nurse and the physician occurs when there is some disagreement about what is best for the client. Suppose, for example, the physician wants to respect a family's request that a dying client not be informed concerning his state. The nurse, on the other hand, may recognize that the client feels that "something is being kept" from him, and that this situation is creating more anxiety than an informed state would. In such cases the nurse must conduct all communications and negotiations with the physician as an equal. The nurse does not pretend to be an equal in the practice of medicine, but the nurse must clearly negotiate from the position that the nurse, not the physician, is the expert in nursing. In a case such as that given in this example, the nurse has every right to negotiate from a position of strength. Indeed, the nurse often is cast in the role of client advocate in relations with the physician. When the focus is on the needs of a shared client, interprofessional rivalries and conflicts can be subordinated to the common goal: the client's needs.

Not all nursing relationships with the client fall into the advocacy role. Sometimes the nurse also needs to negotiate with the client. Nursing has a long history of giving lip service to planning *with* rather than *for* the client; the nurse needs to assure that this commitment is real, not merely semantic. Planning with the client means that care truly is negotiated between nurse and client. The client has primacy in knowledge of his body, his life-style, and his values. The nurse has primacy in knowledge of the client's nursing and medical therapy. In negotiating with a client concerning a care plan, the nurse supplies the client with relevant information and advice for intelligent decision making on his part. The nurse ultimately respects the right of the client to make final decisions concerning his own life and health care.

C A S E   S T U D Y   1

Ms. Gamble, a new graduate, is serving as a primary nurse on 5 West, a medical-surgical unit of Memorial General. According to the system described in the nursing policy book, physicians are supposed to coordinate with the primary nurse for discussion of care for each of their patients. Ms. Gamble has had little success in implementing this system. Several of the physicians who have the greatest case loads on 5 West state that they prefer to coordinate with the head nurse rather than with the primary nurse. They say: "If we have to find the primary nurse for each patient, we waste a lot of time just finding out who that is and locating her in each case. We just don't have that much time to waste on nonproductive organizational trivia. We have a simpler method—just find the head nurse and make rounds with her. She knows what is going on with all patients anyway. She can relay any messages to the so-called primary nurse if that is required."

Ms. Gamble has discussed the problem with Ms. Levitt, the head nurse. Ms. Levitt has expressed sympathy but has yielded to the physicians' request that she make rounds with them. "What can I do when they come and take me by the hand? If I refuse, I'll have bad relations between nursing and medicine on this floor, and that will defeat the whole purpose of good patient care.

Based on this situation, do the following:

1. Identify the specific problem, or subproblems, faced by Ms. Gamble.
2. Assess the systems (logistics, organizational, personal) that are involved.
3. Suggest strategies and tactics for problem resolution.

Ms. Wright has been trying all week to teach Mr. Werth about his diabetes. (Mr. Werth is a newly diagnosed diabetic who lives alone. His level of intelligence is low, but Ms. Wright judges that he can learn to manage his disease adequately with enough careful teaching.) In order to have time to educate Mr. Werth, Ms. Wright has rushed through her other client care assignments three times this week. In all three instances the head nurse, on finding out that Ms. Wright had "finished with her baths," has sent her to another floor that is currently short-staffed. The head nurse has always empathized with Ms. Wright's intention to use the time for teaching, but she has said that "first things must come first" in a crisis staffing situation.

When Ms. Wright expressed her concern that Mr. Werth would go home in two days with little or no understanding of his disease, the head nurse responded, "Well, I know that you already spent three hours with him last week on this. We just have so much time to invest in a single patient, you know."

Ms. Wright is also concerned that this pattern of thinking about client teaching being superfluous is dominant on her unit. She has had other experiences like this one. Her inability to follow through on that important component of nursing is causing Ms. Wright to have serious doubts about her profession—or at least about its practice in this hospital.

Based on the above situation, do the following:

1. Identify the specific problem, or subproblems, faced by Ms. Wright.
2. Assess the systems (logistic, organizational, personal) that are involved.
3. Suggest strategies and tactics for problem resolution.

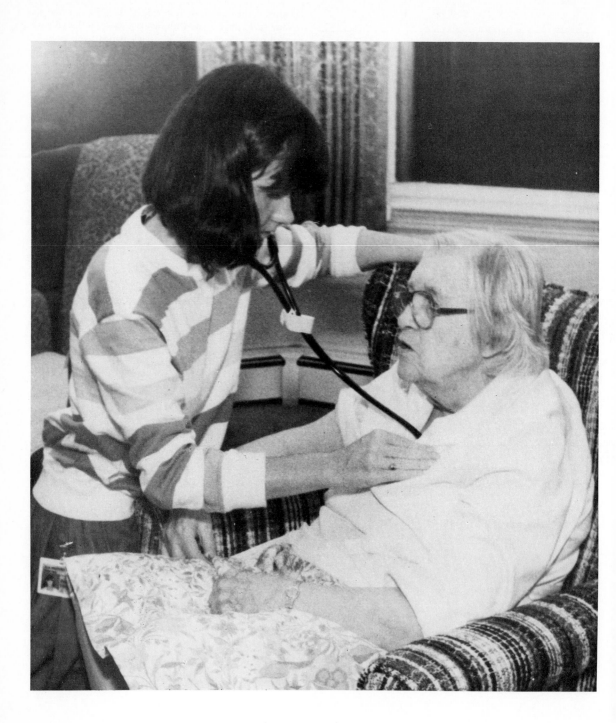

UNIT TWO

Supporting Wellness in Communities

∎

Unit two focuses on wellness in communities. It begins with assessment of a community in chapter 9 and continues in chapter 10 by placing health beliefs in a sociocultural perspective that extends beyond the familiar North American culture of the present day. Examples from diverse cultures help to illustrate how healing is largely composed of beliefs and expectations that are culturally learned and influenced by history.

In chapter 11 the need for food is developed in detail as it relates to self-care and the role of the nurse as part of a multidisciplinary health team in promoting optimum nutrition throughout the life cycle.

Chapters 12 and 13 develop the concept of wellness in specific types of communities—the school and the workplace. Unit two concludes with a discussion of home care, one of the fastest growing segments of the health care industry. Chapter 14 acknowledges and addresses the fact that home care is changing in terms of levels of care given to clients and the complexity of the system in which nurses function.

C H A P T E R 9

Nursing Assessment of a Community

S Y L V I A G E N E M E N E S H I A N

·

OBJECTIVES

After completing this chapter, the reader will be able to:

- Describe high-level wellness and its many ramifications.
- Incorporate the phases of the nursing process in an assessment of the community.
- Differentiate among the many and varied definitions of community.
- Apply the general system theory framework in studying the community.
- Identify five areas of functioning necessary in the daily life of people in the community.
- Apply the epidemiological approach, studying the incidence and distribution of morbidity/mortality in the community.
- Apply the concept of wholeness in the assessment.
- Organize the assessment according to the purpose within the defined area of study.
- Collect relevant data as a base of information pertinent to the assessment.
- Identify several sources in the assimilation of data.
- Determine the presence or lack of relevant resources in the community.

- Analyze data base information relating to the life cycle stages.
- Process and analyze data base information relating to Maslow's hierarchy of needs.
- Determine the factors that indicate the need for more data in making an adequate assessment, a systematic and continuous process.
- Identify factors related to health maintenance, prevention of disease, and promotion of health in the community assessment.
- Assess and interpret nursing needs in relation to broader community health needs.
- Correlate the identified needs/problems with nursing diagnosis.
- Comprehend the influence of value systems as a variable in the planning and implementing phases.
- Involve the community in the decision-making process of the intervention, thereby encouraging their utilization of the strategy.
- Perceive the nursing role as facilitator, coordinator, change agent, and leader in community nursing strategies.

High-level wellness for the total community is the ultimate goal in a community assessment. This is reflected in the belief that the human field and the environmental field are open systems, each influenced by the other; that they are inseparable; that they are dynamic and ever changing; and that within their relationship are determinants of wellness and illness.

In describing high-level wellness Dunn states:

> Harmony will result when the fact is faced that man is a physical, mental, and spiritual unity—a unity which is constantly undergoing a process of growth and adjustment within a continually changing physical, biological, social, and cultural environment. . . . High-level wellness can never be achieved in fragments, ignoring the unity of the whole. (2)

High-level wellness, health promotion, and health preservation of the community as a whole are within the realm of the responsibilities of the nurse, and they direct the focus of the assessment. Assessment, the initial step in the nursing process, is as relevant with a community assessment as with a client assessment. The community is perceived as the client. The assessment provides a comprehensive view of the community, an identification of its health status, plus an understanding of its uniqueness.

Applying the Nursing Process in a Community Assessment

Using the nursing process is essential in providing optimal nursing services to help achieve the goal of high-level wellness in the community. A review of the nursing process consists of the following components:

- Defining the area of study—determining the purpose of the task
- Establishing the data base—data collection
- Analyzing the data base
- Identifying the needs or problems
- Relating the needs to nursing diagnoses
- Establishing goals or objectives: short-term and long-term

- Establishing needs priorities
- Planning the nursing action or provision of services to achieve the goals
- Implementing the action or service
- Evaluating the outcomes or effectiveness of the plan or action
- Revising the plan of action based on continuous data collection, continuous evaluation, and reordering of priorities

The nursing assessment of a community is done for the purpose of determining the need for nursing action, and it involves both the collection of data pertinent to that community with an identification of its health needs, its assets and liabilities, and the resultant nursing diagnoses elicited from that data base. Analyzing the data in relation to the identified needs or problems is necessary, as they are the foundation on which goals and objectives are based and the appropriate nursing action, or provision of services, is implemented to achieve the desired outcomes, that is, to promote healthy growth or a positive change in the community. There is continuous evaluation to determine if the objectives were met, if the outcomes were successful or effective, and if revisions of the plan of action are needed. The nursing process as a systematic approach for nursing practice is used in the assessment of a community. The movement within this stratagem is constantly evolving and dynamic.

The Definition of Community

The definition of community elicits various explanations, depending on the frame of reference and within the context of the one characterizing it. Several approaches may be used; a general description of each is necessary.

Systems Approach. Defining a community using this approach entails an examination of all the parts of a system, their relationships and the purpose, content, and process of their interactions. It is analyzing the subsystem man in relation to his interactions with various subsystems of his environment. Subsystems are identified by their purpose for being, for example, educational systems, health care systems, communication systems, political systems (4, p. 436).

Functional Approach. Functional communities are defined as nongeographical groupings of people with a shared identification and a sense of belonging, for example, occupational, educational, religious communities, or groups based on common interests, resources, or needs, such as the artist community, the nursing community, and the homosexual community (1, p. 60).

Warren defines a community as related to its geographically accessible functioning components: (a) production-distribution-consumption (government, industry, religion, business), (b) socialization (schools), (c) social control (government, police, courts), (d) social participation (religious groups, voluntary groups), (e) mutual support (health departments, hospitals, social agencies) (10, pp. 9–11).

Structural Approach. In this approach, geographical or political boundaries usually organize groupings to form a community; examples include an apartment complex, a hospital, a neighborhood, a town, a state (1, p. 60).

"Community of Solution" Approach. The boundary within which to explore and resolve health problems and issues was defined by the National Committee on Community Health Services as a "community of solution." This term was created to transcend political and geographical boundaries; an example is a group of people with the same diagnosis or health-related problem (1, p. 59; 8, p. 52).

Epidemiological Approach. In this approach a community is defined in terms of the incidence and distribution of morbidity and mortality, and including the study of the determinants of disease within a human population. This involves the study of the variables: time (in terms of season or evolution), place (geographical area or setting), size (number of people), and personal characteristics (biopsychological and sociocultural attributes, which include the demographic data: birth, death, marriage, divorce rates, income levels, housing conditions, ethnic composition, educational levels, employment rates, and the occurrence of illness, diseases, and health-related problems) (7).

Wholeness Concept. Man as a unified whole interacts continuously and simultaneously with the whole of the environment; both are open and dynamic energy fields that are constantly evolving (6, pp. 92–93). This conceptual framework encompasses all of the characteristics of the preceding approaches. It implies that man may live, work, and socialize within a variety of communities, depending on his habitat and his range of interests. It extends the defining of a community to unlimited possibilities.

Determining the Purpose of the Assessment—Defining the Area of Study

The initial phase of a community assessment combines defining the area of the community to be studied and determining the purpose for the analysis; these both give direction to the investigative process and to the data collection. By providing guidelines and a focus, consideration of the preceding definitions of community assist in the decision-making process regarding the identification of the area to be studied, and the support of the specified purpose.

For the purpose of this text, an assessment of a general geographical locale is the focal setting to be studied; identifying the health status and nursing needs of that community is the purpose of the assessment. Within this proposed framework a comprehensive collection of relevant data is the next step in the process.

Establishing the Data Base

In an assessment of a community the systematic procedures in recording the collection of data are accomplished by dividing the information according to subjective and objective criteria. Subjective data consist of biased information of questionable validity and reliability that is grounded in personal sensorial observation. Objective data consist of information obtained in an organized manner; it is factual, valid, and reliable and may be used in comparative studies (1, pp. 67–73).

The objective data are further divided into two components: those of a general nature and those specifically identified as human resources or health-related services. This separation of objective data will assist the nurse in determining a community's health needs.

The assimilation of data is a continuous process, with the complexity of the collection determined by the nurse's involvement and needs.

The organization of these three categories is delineated in Tables 9.1, 9.2, and 9.3. Table 9.4 outlines the sources of information for the data base (5, pp. 94–97).

Table 9.1	Table 9.2
Subjective Data: Sensorial Observation	**Objective Data: General Variables**

Visual	Geographical area	Spatial	Geographical boundaries
	Location—urban, suburban, rural		Nonvisible—based on political structures:
	Topography		census tracts, city, county
	Visible boundaries—rivers, mountains,	Demographic	Statistical data
	highways		Age, sex, race distributions
	Functional components—location and type of		Cultural and ethnic composition and
	functional systems		distribution
	Businesses		Religious composition
	Industries		Educational achievement and literacy rate
	Municipal services—police, fire, government		levels
	offices		Per capita and family income levels
	Health care facilities—hospital, clinics,		Labor force participation—occupations
	medical doctors' offices		and rate of unemployment
	Schools		Population shifts, migration patterns
	Transportation channels and facilities		Mobility—length of residence, percentage
	Religious institutions		of "homeless"
	Parks and recreational areas		Morbidity/mortality:
	Housing—habitation, type of neighborhood		Incidence of chronic diseases
	Single dwelling, multi-dwelling		Age-specific death rate and causes
	Condition—state of repair, deterioration		Life-style patterns
	Spacing of residences: areas of density—		Family structure patterns—marital status
	clustering, areas of sparsity		Recreational and vocational interests
	People—age distribution: playing or walking on	Political	Government
	the street, talking on street corners		Legislative process and channels, relation
	Presence of animals or bird life		of federal and state to local
Sound	Noise levels		Funding mechanisms
	Type and patterns of traffic		Power of influence: business, monied
	Types of industry		interests
Taste	Food preferences—groceries, restaurants		Tax money allocations
	Water—municipal or well water	Protective	Public health laws
Smell	Noxious odors or none	Services	Environmental protection
	Types of industry		Housing—building codes, zoning codes
	Presence of gardens or flowers		Sanitation codes:
Tactile	Climate—temperature, humidity, seasonal		Solid waste collection and disposal
	patterns, altitude		Sewage disposal
	Feeling of warmth or hostility		Water purification, fluoridation
	Personality of neighborhood	Commercial	Industries of area: facilities, mobility
		Transportation	Systems available: routes and cost
		Communications	Formal
			Postal system: accessibility
			Mass media—printed material, radio,
			television—availability
			Informal
			Opinion leaders—key people, groups
			Language interpreters—availability
			Newsletters, bulletin boards

Source: The components as herein listed were developed from Carrie Jo Braden and Nancy L. Herban, *Community Health: A Systems Approach.* New York: Appleton-Century-Crofts, 1976, pp. 67–69.

Source: The components as herein listed were developed from Carrie Jo Braden and Nancy L. Herban. *Community Health: A Systems Approach.* New York: Appleton-Century-Crofts, 1976, pp. 70–73.

Table 9.3
Objective Data: Human Resources or Health-Related Services

Variables to Assess in an Agency or Service
Type of service, purpose of service, accessibility, eligibility requirements, availability, utilization, kind and number of personnel, facility adequacy, utilization of personnel, money or funding source: official—public/nonofficial—private or voluntary

Health Care Services

Curative	Preventive
Hospitals	Health department services
Outpatient departments	Occupational health
Clinics	programs
Treatment centers	Public education programs
Extended care facilities	School education programs
Home care programs	Wellness programs
Nursing homes	Maternal/child programs
Home nursing services	Parenting programs
Psychiatric facilities	Mental health care facilities
Dental services	Health maintenance
	organizations

(some facilities may provide both types of service)

Safety and Protective Services
Emergency ambulance service
Emergency medical treatment program
Respirator services
Poison control unit
Emergency disaster program
Child protective services
Adult protective services
Shelter for homeless
Social services—public assistance department
Law enforcement agency—police
Fire department
Civil defense unit
Educational programs
WIC service (Woman-infant-child nutritional program)

Social Service Agencies
Meals-on-Wheels program
Senior citizen facilities
Child day-care facilities
Family counseling services
Homemaker services
Youth group facilities

Self-help Groups
Recreational Facilities
Concerned Citizen Groups
Commercial Health Aid Programs
Weight-reduction programs
Stop-smoking programs
Childbirth education programs

Source: The components as herein listed were developed from Carrie Jo Braden and Nancy L. Herban. *Community Health: A Systems Approach.* New York: Appleton-Century-Crofts, 1976, pp. 67–87.

Table 9.4
Sources of Information for Data Collection

Subjective Observation
Tour by walk or by car
Visits to community facilities, health-related agencies
Participation on committees as nurses, as consumers
Home visits

Objective Reference materials
Maps of area
Telephone book—yellow pages directory
Directories of:
Health-related services
Self-help groups
Community resources
Voluntary organizations
Library, historical societies
Local newspaper office
Resources
Health and human resource agencies: annual reports, studies, surveys
Hospital association: annual report
Government offices:
Municipal: statistics, reports
Office of Vital Statistics: statistics
Bureau of the Census: statistics
Local and state health departments: public health laws, annual reports, sanitation codes, communicable division, public health service publications
Chamber of Commerce
County extension office, conservation office
Schools: statistics, reports
Courts: statistics
Community development or planning agencies: annual reports
Voluntary groups: reports
Professional organizations (example: American Medical Society): reports
Service groups (example: League of Women Voters): reports
Bus, train, rapid transit offices: routes and cost

Source: The components as herein listed were developed from Carrie Jo Braden and Nancy L. Herban. *Community Health: A Systems Approach.* New York: Appleton-Century-Crofts, 1976, pp. 67–87; Kathleen M. Leahy, M. Marguerite Cobb, and Mary C. Jones. *Community Health Nursing.* New York: McGraw-Hill, 1977, pp. 94–97.

Analysis of the Data Base— Data Processing

An analysis of the range of parameters in the data base reveals a community profile in which the identification of the health status and the needs of the community may be determined. It is supplementing the subjective data with the more factual and measurable objective data. The analysis is accomplished by transferring the information collected onto maps, tables, graphs, and other visual aids, thereby depicting correlations, patterns, and influencing factors.

Comparisons of the data disclose relationships and indicators of wellness or illness. With the application of the wholeness concept, an encompassing analysis provides more possibilities for identifying needs. Study of the availability of, or lack of, resources and of the patterns of utilization and coordination of services, of the application of new knowledge, of the integration of nursing services will elicit factors that influence the implementation of new strategies.

In the summarization of the data analysis, a comparison of the current health status of a community versus the desired health status reveals the existence of a health problem or a health need. The resolution of a health problem may or may not require nursing intervention— a nursing problem is identified on this basis (9, p. 230).

A nursing diagnosis defines the problem in relation to the health status. If the data analysis indicates the assumption of beneficial growth in a community as a result of a supportive nursing action, a nursing diagnosis is determined. Nursing diagnoses embracing both potential and actual health needs are dynamic and ever changing as the health status fluctuates.

Prioritizing the identified needs is the next phase in the analysis process. This ordering of needs implies focusing first on the most urgent.

Analyzing the health needs of a community in terms of age distribution and relating problems specific to life cycle stages (examples: infant, adolescent, older adult) provides a basis for prioritizing needs. Consideration of the predominant issues in the relevant age-groups correlated with the percentages of the population in that age-group determines the placing of those needs on a priority scale.

Another method, Maslow's hierarchical classification of human needs, assists the nurse in organizing health needs into priorities. Maslow conceptualized human needs in the following order of priority, beginning with the most basic need:

1. Physiologic or biologic: those necessary for life, life-sustaining: air, water, food, clothing, shelter
2. Safety, protection, or security: freedom from fear, socioeconomic needs
3. Social or affiliation: the need to be loved, to belong
4. Esteem needs: recognition and respect
5. Self-actualization: to fully realize one's potential, high-level wellness of body, mind, spirit

The most basic need must first be satisfied before advancement to the next level is possible. This arrangement of needs is not absolute: a person may be at one level with regard to one aspect of his or her life and on another level in a different aspect; also, the levels may overlap when establishing priorities (4, pp. 56–60).

Using Maslow's hierarchical framework in prioritizing a community's health needs provides a useful base and a helpful direction. As an example, Table 9.5 shows the relationship between a community's possible health needs and Maslow's hierarchy of needs.

Members in a community will vary in their ability and desire to advance in the progression of the hierarchy. (Example: A member's nutritional needs must be met before participation in a recreational program can be considered.)

If, in its totality, the community is assessed as the client, unmet needs of one member of the system affect all the other parts of the system. Therefore, to achieve the goal of high-level wellness for a community, the needs of each member of that community must be satisfied.

The meaning of high-level wellness differs for each member and for each community. The issue of values is a variable that influences the prioritizing of needs: what one member identifies as a need another may not; high-level wellness to one may not be the same to another. The impact and importance of value judgments are significant considerations in the planning and implementing phases.

After delineating health needs as they are conceived within Maslow's framework, possible ways to meet those needs are evaluated. If the resolution of a problem requires nursing intervention, a nursing need is identified. If it is perceived that a nursing strategy would promote growth or a positive change in the health status, a relevant nursing diagnosis is determined. Prioritizing the nursing diagnosis as related to this conceptual hierarchy provides direction in the next phase of the nursing process.

Table 9.5
Possible Health Needs of a Community*

Maslow's Hierarchy	
Physiologic	Adequate emergency services
	Acute medical care facilities
	Air pollution controls
	Water pollution controls
	Adequate food supplies and nutrition: WIC program, Meals-on-Wheels, soup kitchens
	Adequate housing, shelter for homeless
	Elimination of poverty, public assistance program
	Adequate sanitary and waste disposal
	Communicable disease infection controls, sexually transmitted disease program
	Insect and rodent eradication program
Safety	Child protective services
	Adult protective services
	Adequate health services: routine, preventive, specialized
	Adequate funding of health services
	Adequate access to health care: transportation
	Adequate immunization levels
	Day-care facilities
	Home nursing services
	Restorative care facilities: rehabilitation centers, nursing homes
	Long-term health care services, homemaker services
	Maternal-child programs, parenting programs
	Health education programs, wellness programs
	Mental health facilities and supportive programs
	Preventive health guidance home visits
Social	Adequate recreational facilities
	Support groups, self-help groups
	Senior citizen groups, youth group facilities
	Consumer involvement on health committees
Self-esteem	Citizen and service groups, volunteer programs
	More consumer involvement in health programs
	Adequate consumer recognition
Self-actualization	More consumer leadership in health programs

*This list of needs is not all-inclusive. One need may overlap

After Assessment

For the purpose of this text, the assessment process is completed with the discussion of the preceding elements. The data analysis provides the foundation for the planning and implementation of nursing action directed toward the achievement of the goals. Assessment furnishes the focus for completion of the nursing process.

Inherent in the planning phase is the prioritizing of the nursing diagnosis, the setting of long-term and short-term goals, and the determining of objectives. It also includes the exploration of alternative appropriate nursing actions or strategies with the resultant decision regarding the most effective and beneficial provision of service.

The implementation phase is the development and execution of the chosen intervention, followed by the evaluation of the outcomes of the action and the continuous revision of the nursing plan as indicated by ongoing data collection, evaluation, and reordering of priorities.

A community is people—they are the reason for the existence of health care. They are the ones who are most affected by the data analysis and the resulting solutions. As citizens, as consumers, their involvement and support in the planning and implementation process are essential. "Decisions made for people rather than with them have little influence or longevity" (3, p. 102). The consumer, including individual members, groups, and the community as a whole, is the determining factor in the outcome of the intervention; it is his or her response that is the key to its success or failure. Therefore, the plan of action must be congruent with his or her desires or wants and reflect his or her value system.

Integration of consumers in the nursing process enhances health planning and implementation for many reasons: the consumer can best interpret the values, preferences, and needs of the members of the community; he or she is the liaison and communicator with other citizens; he or she can inform the community regarding progress of the health action; and he or she can assist in its planning, implementation, evaluation, and revision.

into two levels. Within each level the needs are not listed in order of importance.

Source: The components as herein listed were developed from Elaine LaMonica. *The Nursing Process: A Humanistic Approach.* Menlo Park, Calif.: Addison-Wesley, 1979, pp. 56–70.

Achieving High-Level Wellness in the Community

The community is in the process of change. The health care delivery system is in the process of change. And nursing is evolving as well. The community is the new arena for nursing action. Establishing innovative health programs, both preventive and restorative, to encourage positive growth and to improve the health status of the community is accomplished most effectively in this setting. The identification of its health needs and the implementation of nursing strategies for health promotion, disease prevention, and resolution of health problems exist and come to reality in the community.

The essence of nursing originates in the health needs of the client, the "client" being a person or a community. Rather than limiting nursing care to a few, providing care to a community's needs enhances the role and responsibilities of nursing. Role implications include the demand for leadership ability with skills as a coordinator of services, a facilitator, a consumer advocate, a change agent, and a health teacher. The achievement of high-level wellness in a community provides the challenge and the opportunity for nursing to demonstrate its relevancy in today's world.

REFERENCES

1. Braden, Carrie Jo, and Nancy L. Herban. *Community Health: A Systems Approach.* New York: Appleton-Century-Crofts, 1976.
2. Dunn, Halbert L. "High-Level Wellness for Man and Society." *American Journal of Public Health* 49:789, 1959.
3. Jarvis, Linda L. *Community Health Nursing: Keeping the Public Healthy.* Philadelphia: F. A. Davis, 1981.
4. LaMonica, Elaine. *The Nursing Process: A Humanistic Approach.* Menlo Park, Calif.: Addison-Wesley, 1979.
5. Leahy, Kathleen M., M. Marguerite Cobb, and Mary C. Jones. *Community Health Nursing.* New York: McGraw-Hill, 1977.
6. Rogers, Martha E. *An Introduction to the Theoretical Basis of Nursing.* Philadelphia: F. A. Davis, 1970.
7. Ruybal, Sally E. "Community Health Planning." In *Elements of Family and Community Health. Family and Community Health, The Journal of Health Promotion and Maintenance* 1:11, April 1978.
8. Ruybal, Sally E., Eleanor Bauwens, and Mari-Jose Fasla. "Community Assessment: An Epidemiological Approach." In *Nursing in Community Health,* comp. Andrea B. O'Connor. New York: American Journal of Nursing Company, 1978.
9. Tinkham, Catherine W., and Eleanor F. Voorhies. *Community Health Nursing: Evolution and Process.* New York: Appleton-Century-Crofts, 1977.
10. Warren, Roland L. *The Community in America.* Chicago: Rand McNally, 1972.

CHAPTER 10

Health Beliefs
in Sociocultural Perspective

JUDITH M. TREISTMAN

■

OBJECTIVES

After completing this chapter, the reader will be able to:

□ Trace the development of selected health belief systems.

□ Identify differences between determinants of health in the past and present.

□ State how beliefs about conception and motherhood are determined by historical and sociocultural contexts.

□ State how concepts of illness and illness behavior are socially, culturally, and historically determined.

□ State how a layperson's and a physician's concepts of illness may differ.

□ Explain the idea that health is coping with the environment.

□ Explain the meaning of the idea that healing is a social relationship.

□ Explain the meaning of the idea that illness and illness behavior are culturally learned.

Beliefs about health and illness are shaped by a network of historical, social, and cultural factors. The illnesses that we get are not random events. How we behave when we are sick is not an idiosyncratic accident. We do not randomly choose the person who diagnoses or treats our illnesses, or the therapy we receive. The ways in which people recognize and respond to illness are determined by who they are, where and when they live, and what the neighbors think. So, too, the definition of health shifts and changes throughout history and from culture to culture. Understanding the sociocultural underpinning of beliefs about health and illness is essential for the nurse who wants to provide optimal care to clients in different settings.

We face a problem, however, in our attempt to gain this understanding. Just as it is impossible to "step into" another person's mind, to see the world as he or she sees it, it is also foolish to think that we can get inside a culture that is not our own without a lifetime of experiences. The solution to the dilemma comes not in trying to memorize a mass of unrelated details about different cultures, what the anthropologist calls a "trait list," but in learning how cultures work. This means learning how belief systems evolve and how they function.

This chapter examines some belief systems by tracing their development through history or by comparing different cultures with one another. Whenever possible we will return to the contemporary world, so that the reader has a point of reference. We can begin to meet the goal of understanding cultural diversity by questioning our own actions, observing the ways in which we do things, and by exploring the beliefs and values that support our everyday behavior. Only after we recognize the importance of our own belief system can we begin to respect the background and experiences of others.

Three little word pictures will set the discussion in perspective.

The first story is about events that took place thousands of years ago in Iraq. Archeologists working in the caves of Shanidar discovered a grave in which a middle-aged man had been buried. On examining the skeleton the scientists saw that the man had a congenitally deformed right arm. They also discovered grains of pollen, the remains of spring flowers that mourners had scattered over the burial more than forty-five thousand years ago.

The second story concerns the choices made by a forty-four-year-old woman living in Europe in 1770. The woman had tuberculosis and was pregnant. Although this was her fourth pregnancy, she had only one living child, and he was blind. One of her infants had been stillborn and the third pregnancy had miscarried. The woman's husband had syphilis. We can imagine the advice that a thoughtful counselor might give such a client today. Fortunately for us, Mrs. Beethoven lived before the science of genetics had matured.

The third image comes from the journal entries of explorers who were encountering native Americans for the first time. The Indians are described as glowing with health and being splendid of stature and bearing, graceful and fleet of movement. The irony, as we shall see, is that the very "discovery" of the aboriginal populations was to lead to their annihilation.

What can be learned from these vignettes? From the burial at Shanidar we take the lesson of caring. Human beings live in social groups that constitute units of caring. The man of Shanidar, disabled from birth, would not have survived as a solitary creature. He was able to live to a reasonably old age only with the nurturing support of others. From the little story about Beethoven we learn that quality of life is a concept that changes with historical time and cultural place, that the concept of wellness is really a set of socially situated beliefs and practices, and that a person's freedom of choice is limited by the available technology.

The explorers' journals make more sense to us when we remember that during the sixteenth century, sailors were recruited from the city slums of Portugal and Spain, where disease, squalor, and malnutrition were rampant. Thus we are reminded that each person filters his or her perception of the world through a mesh of personal experience.

How caring takes place, *who* will be cared for, whether the defective child will be exposed or cherished, *who* will be the care giver, whether a full-time specialist, an avocational healer, or a member of the family: these questions bring into play commonly held ideas and values about health and illness, about life and death.

The values and behaviors that each person learns as he or she grows up are specific to time and place. We can try to understand how these values and behaviors have come about by looking at other cultures and other historical times.

The first step is to acknowledge that the diseases of today are not the diseases of the past. For those who are uncomfortable with the notion that disease is a relative concept, this statement merely underscores the historical and cultural framework within which pathogens evolve, flourish, and disappear. The idea of relativity also helps us to recognize that in addition to the industrialized nations of the world, there are also underdeveloped and developing countries and regions.

We live among disease-experienced populations that have high levels of immunity to familiar infections, and this leads us to believe that diseases are static rather than dynamic (16). Because we assume that the diseases of the present behave much as they did in the past, we view outbreaks of specific diseases as inexplicable disasters and interruptions of normalcy. Epidemics of influenza and the epidemiclike acquired immunodeficiency syndrome are good examples of this reluctance to search out sociocultural and historical explanation.

The diseases we are familiar with are the diseases of civilization, the person-to-person diseases that are transmitted through direct contact. But for much of the human past, and certainly among the nonhuman primates, the most significant determinant of health and disease was parasitism.

Parasites are tiny organisms—viruses, bacteria, or multicellular—that find a source of nourishment in human tissues. Some parasites provoke acute disease within the host; some provoke immune reactions that kill off the parasite; and some achieve stable relations with the host. Others simply reside in the host, and the host becomes a carrier, not sick himself, but capable of infecting others. Some of these diseases of parasitism, especially malaria and schistosomiasis, will be discussed.

Man and Environment: The Disease Ecology of Agriculture

Early man—that is, hominids who preexisted Homo sapiens—evolved from primates living in the subtropical and savannah environments of Africa. Although primates are largely herbivorous, early man was probably omnivorous. When the diet began to include meat, an avenue opened for the transfer of a multitude of new parasites, including worms. The subtropics and savannahs have a particularly rich fauna of worms and protozoa. This fauna evolved along with humanity itself, and tended to intensify as human numbers intensified (16). An example of this new parasitism is sleeping sickness, a disease that has had an enormous impact on the ecology of Africa. The trypanosome, a parasite of the antelope, is transferred from host to host by the tsetse fly. Neither the host nor the fly is affected, but when transferred to humans the trypanosome causes the extreme disabilities of sleeping sickness.

In populations that are overwhelmingly infested with parasites there is almost universal anemia, lassitude, and chronic aches and pains, all of which impede food-getting activities and childbearing success. Eventually the population decreases to the point at which the "epidemic" of infection can no longer be supported. This probably happened in man's early history.

About fifty thousand years ago, when human populations expanded northward to the temperate zones of Asia and Europe, they escaped from the parasites of subtropical Africa. A new "ecology" of disease was created during the next twenty thousand years as the forests were cleared, encouraging weeds (and weed-dwelling animals like weevils, mice, and rats) to grow. The effect was to shorten the food chain, creating dense concentrations of food for select parasites (16). Animals were domesticated along with plants. People lived with or in proximity to swine, cattle, dogs, and poultry. As populations became sedentary and adopted the agricultural way of life, they also had continuous contact with human and animal wastes. Innovations, especially the introduction of irrigation technology, revolutionized simple farming villages. Larger and larger concentrations of people were supported by agricultural surpluses. Irrigation technology re-created the moist conditions of the tropics. After periods of the land being flooded with a shallow blanket of water, followed by seasons of warm, dry conditions, human populations were once again host to multitudes of parasites.

The proliferation of parasitic disease did not overtake the dramatic population increases that occurred with the development of irrigation agriculture, but it certainly did shape the concepts that people held regarding health and illness.

Schistosomiasis

Today roughly 200 million persons are host to *Schistosoma*, blood flukes transmitted by the land snail to humans, especially children. Schistosomiasis, the resulting disease, is characterized by chronic disability, endlessly recurring bouts of diarrhea, cystitis, hematomas, painful enlargement of liver and spleen, intestinal inflammation, and lifelong anemia. Health, when viewed from a world in which schistosomiasis is part of everyday life, takes on a meaning that is very different from ours.

Another revolution in health and illness came with irrigation agriculture. As populations increased in number and density, they were able to sustain bacterial and viral infections without an intermediate nonhuman host. Proximity to domesticated animals had exposed humans to a new set of pathogens; under the new ecological conditions of cities and towns, these pathogens took new forms. There is a close association between canine distemper and measles and between influenza and swine virus, and cattle harbor bacteria that give rise to smallpox and tuberculosis in humans. These disorders became the "civilized" diseases, transmitted by person-to-person contact, usually through droplets of body fluid. It has been estimated, based on contemporary experience with the measles virus, that a population of about five hundred thousand is required to sustain a viral disease through this mode of transmission.

Between 3000 and 500 B.C., the era of urbanization, incipient cities could not maintain themselves in the face of infectious disease. The only way to replace the continuous loss of population was to systematically encourage or enforce a constant flow of migrants from the countryside.

City and countryside existed in a macroparasitic relationship. Rural fertility rates soared as the maw of the city absorbed young migrants and wasted their children (16).

Malaria

Another disease of agricultural progress, malaria, currently affects 2 billion persons. In Africa 1 million children die of malaria each year; worldwide, 150 million persons contract the disease every year. This figure is probably much too low; because malaria is so common, it is grossly underreported. Adults who survive the disease are incapacitated for at least two months every year.

In 1937 the U.S. surgeon general noted that "malaria has the disastrous effect of permitting human existence while precluding the possibility of human health or happiness." That is no less true today.

Malaria is caused by a protozoa, *Plasmodium*, of which four species infest humans. The female *Anopheles* mosquito harbors the parasite. She requires a blood meal for egg production. Before withdrawing blood from the human host, the mosquito injects ripened *Plasmodia* sporozoites from her salivary glands into the victim's bloodstream. Each injection contains between one and ten thousand sporozoites. The sporozoites travel through the circulatory system, and within sixty minutes they embed themselves in the liver or bone marrow of the host. They multiply, enter the red blood corpuscles, and multiply again. Soon the red blood cell explodes and disgorges its contents into the bloodstream. By this time there are approximately one hundred thousand parasites per cubic milliliter of whole blood. Red blood cell destruction swells the spleen and causes chemical imbalances and profound anemia. Each new injection by a mosquito infects the victim again. There is no true immunity. Neonates, therefore, are susceptible shortly after birth. In regions where malaria is endemic, one-third to one-half of all infants die of the disease. Who, then, survives? Only those with genetically determined abnormalities of the red blood cell. These abnormalities, which are expressed phenotypically as sickle cell anemia, thalassemia, and probably glucose-6-phosphate dehydrogenase, confer immunity to malaria when they exist in the heterozygous state.

Eat and Be Well

Another aspect of the impact of agriculture on health and illness is nutrition. Good nutrition does not guarantee good health; poor nutrition inevitably results in poor health. In the sweeping changes from the hunting and gathering way of life to irrigation agriculture and to the present, it is possible to distinguish three major food revolutions. The first revolution involved the domestication of wheat, barley, and animals in the Near East and then Europe; rice and millet in Asia; maize, squash, and beans in the New World. At this time humans "exchanged many components of good health for opportunities to increase cultural complexity" (25, p. 150) by substituting quantity and specialization of foodstuffs for diversity. The second revolution began with the worldwide circulation of cultigens. Domesticated animals were brought to the New World, and maize, potatoes, and manioc diffused from the New World to Eurasia and the Pacific.

The third food revolution came about with innovations in food-processing technology and the centralization and commercial sale of food products. Monocropping and the industrialization of farming have created a global agricultural economy in which much of the world exports low-cost, nutritionally rich protein foods and imports expensive substitutes that are low in nutritional quality. There are many examples of this, such as the shift to mechanized reindeer herding by the Lapps (Skolts) and the one-crop economies of sugar-, coffee-, and rubber-producing countries (20).

These large-scale revolutions in food and diet have been associated with important changes in health and illness. It has been suggested that some contemporary diseases may result from disjunctions between the physiological adaptations that evolved in our hunting-gathering past and the food patterns now found in much of the world. This hypothesis states that our biology is out of step with contemporary eating patterns, despite our enormous flexibility and capacity to adapt (20). Two of the more significant effects of evolutionary disjunctions may be obesity and diabetes. The sedentary nature of contemporary life requires less energy, but this has not been matched by a decrease in caloric intake. In fact, people who live in industrialized nations consume more fat and refined carbohydrates and less fiber and complex carbohydrates than more active farmers or hunters. One example of this phenomenon may be the increasing incidence of diabetes mellitus. Although morbidity rates of the disease are stable in Europe and North America, they seem to be rising dramatically among populations undergoing acculturation. In South Africa there are forty times as many cases of diabetes among the Bantu who live in cities as there are among Bantu who live in rural areas. It has been suggested that the high rate of insulin production that served well for the hunter who required rapid metabolism and utilization of blood glucose is constantly stimulated by our high carbohydrate intake and stress levels. Thus a genetic advantage in the past may have become a precursor to disease in the present (20).

A frequently cited example of the effect of sociocultural change on nutrition and health is the increase of hypertension and cardiovascular disease among migrants from rural areas to urban centers. The evidence that dietary changes are responsible for the increased incidence of hypertension is not clear-cut, since the interplay of occupation, stress, and genetic predisposition is difficult to untangle.

Deficiency Diseases

Many of the social and economic consequences of modernization, such as migration to cities, the entrance of

women into the industrial work force, and the enforced shift from polygamy to monogamy (with the consequent rise in fertility), have decreased the length of lactation. Earlier weaning has meant that nutritional resources for infants are reduced.

Marasmus and *kwashiorkor* are examples of nutritional deficiency diseases that are manifest in childhood. Marasmus, the "wasting away" disease, involves the loss of subcutaneous fat and muscle, chronic diarrhea, anemia, and jaundice. If there is no intervention, the disease progresses to stupor and death, usually as a result of electrolyte imbalances. Infants can be salvaged, but they grow up with permanent disabilities. Because the most rapid growth of the brain occurs in the first four years of life, these children will have reduced learning capacity as well as stunted body growth.

The incidence of marasmus increases when normal social patterns are disrupted. Kwashiorkor is actually a Ghanaian word for "second-child sickness." It is found especially among just-weaned infants who are shifted to a diet that has sufficient calories to satisfy hunger but little or no protein to sustain growth (25). Kwashiorkor is the all-too-familiar face of hunger, children with water-swollen bellies and legs and matchstick arms suffering chronic anemia and mental and emotional retardation. Millions of children are afflicted with marasmus and kwashiorkor.

Hunger

Throughout human history there has been the paradox of hunger existing in a world of abundance. And yet hunger, whether it is found in pockets of poverty in the rich countries of the industrialized world or in the great famines of Africa, is a cultural artifact. We are familiar with the overgrazing of the grasslands in western America that laid the foundation for the great dust bowl of the 1930s. Similarly, deforestation of large land masses in Asia and Africa underlies much of the devastation wrought by floods. The rapid desertification that is taking place globally, the acid rain that is causing the death of Europe's forests and North America's lakes will probably bring about climatic changes that will influence food production in generations to come. The subsequent uprooting and relocation of whole populations and the disruption of exquisitely adjusted ecological adaptations that took centuries to evolve will continue to cause famine in Africa.

The Cultural Meanings of Food

In 1945 the National Research Council stated that edible food materials could be classified in several ways:

"inedible, edible by animals, edible by human beings, but not my kind of human being, edible by human beings such as self, and finally, edible by self" (quoted in 25, p. 58). There are many examples of this phenomenon, from Americans, who won't eat horsemeat, to the Bushmen of the Kalahari desert, who will eat only twenty-three of the eighty-five edible plant species available to them. *Who* eats *what* and *with whom* is determined by society and culture. Although limited by biology and environment—one cannot find grapes growing in the Arctic, nor can human digestion extract minerals from stone—the choices we make are essentially made on the basis of learned values and behavior. Again, there are many examples of this. We are familiar with the rejection of unpolished rice by most Asians, the rejection of maize by starving Europeans after World War I, and the unsuccessful introduction of fish flour into Africa.

We are undergoing enormous changes in our eating habits, in the times we eat, where we eat, and with whom we eat. It is hard to associate a chicken nugget with Old MacDonald's barnyard, or Lean Cuisine with anything. "Grazing," the world of mini-TV meals, food stalls, and the Mimosa Brunch, is one indication of the changes taking place. But we cling to food aversions that are centuries old. There are no universal proscriptions and there are no universal explanations, although many taboos seem to be associated with beliefs about death and sex roles. Others are connected to social stigmata, for example, not eating foods that are favorites of the poor (pig's ears) or signs of pollution (scavenger animals).

Food in China

Another way of looking at how food choices and nutrition are influenced by culture is to examine the network of beliefs that give symbolic meaning to food. There is no better example of this than the centuries-old tradition of Chinese cuisine. The first "cookbooks" were dietary guides to better health. They were written to instruct the elite on the correct preparation of properly balanced foods that would not disturb the body's equilibrium. Such a balance was intended to improve the internal "climate" of the body and promote longevity (4). Almost every recipe is a recommendation to physicians, ranging from tonics like venison with ginger and vinegar to ground walnuts for baldness. There was a saying in the eleventh century that "old people are generally averse to taking medicine but are fond of food." It is therefore far better to treat their complaint with proper food than with drugs (19).

Chia Ming wrote the *Essential Knowledge of Eating and Drinking* in 1368. It should be noted that Chia Ming lived to the age of 106 and died, not of ill health, but in response to an auspicious dream. There are eight chapters in the book, devoted to the fifty kinds of grains, the eighty-seven kinds of vegetables, the sixty-eight kinds of fish, the thirty-four kinds of fowl, and so on. Each food is related to the five flavors (sweet, pungent, sour, bitter, salty), the five elements (fire, water, earth, wood, metal), the five viscera (heart, lungs, stomach, liver, kidneys), the seasons, and the directions. Each food is then placed on the yin (cold) and yang (hot) continuum, and thus orchestrated to promote bodily harmony. Food, in this conception, is not seen as a system of *cures*, but as preventive medicine.

The important point to remember is that food is given meaning in all cultures, and that meaning is most often associated with beliefs about health and illness.

The First Americans

Finally, let us look at the interplay of disease, culture, and society in one of history's most horrifying and dramatic episodes, the annihilation of native Americans.

At the time of contact with European explorers, American aboriginal populations were "immunologically virginal." There were two reasons for this. Over thousands of years, warmth-loving pathogens were screened out as aboriginal populations passed from Asia across the Bering land bridge and down the western corridor of North America. Second, most aboriginal populations were too small to maintain transmission of any diseases they may have brought with them during these migrations. Smallpox, measles, and influenza had no opportunity to evolve a "working relationship" with the human populations that sustain them (25).

The best estimates suggest that there were between 100 million and 150 million inhabitants of the New World just before the Spanish conquest. The largest concentrations of people were in Mexico (25 million), Peru (10 million), and California (300,000). We know little about the health of the people in preconquest times. Physical anthropologists have analyzed the skeletal remains of forty-four persons who lived in California's Sonoma Valley some time between 600 and 300 B.C. They concluded that 40 percent of this population died before reaching the age of twenty. The oldest person was between forty-five and fifty. There was no evidence of gross pathology or malnutrition; most had died as the result of trauma or infectious processes. One-third to one-half of the adults had severe bone disease, especially arthritis of the spine (11). At another archeological site, Mesa Verde in Colorado, all but one of the people who had lived past the age of thirty-five were crippled with arthritis. At this and other North American sites, trauma, especially to the head, and pathology in the form of abscesses and periodontal disease were common. Much of the head pathology probably involved neurological impairment, such as loss of speech, paralysis, and seizures. This makes the recovery rate remarkable! Thus, for North America, the idealized descriptions of the first European explorers do not ring entirely true, but the overall picture was one of populations relatively free of disease, and of intact societies supportive of disabled people.

A somewhat different picture is beginning to emerge from analysis of the skeletal and archeological records of the Mayan civilization just before the time of the Spanish conquest. In parts of Mexico and Guatemala, evidence of increasing physical debilitation has been found. Once again, intensive irrigation agriculture encouraged the proliferation of parasites. Analysis of fragments of human cranial bones shows a loss of protein and mineral components, especially in children over the age of weaning. More than one-half of these children suffered severe iron deficiency anemia, probably caused by undernutrition and a large burden of parasites (25). Thus the Maya may have been even less prepared than other aboriginal peoples for the events of the next fifty years.

Smallpox

The first waves of smallpox (*Variola major*) washed across the Caribbean when slaves from Africa were brought to work in the mines of Cuba, Hispaniola, and Puerto Rico. Smallpox appears to have spread from ancient Egypt throughout northeast Africa, down the Nile, and along the east African coast, where it flourished in the Arab merchant settlements. Traders carried the disease to Portugal and Europe and trans-Saharan caravans brought it to west Africa. Smallpox reached Brazil on slave ships in 1560 (10).

Smallpox had killed more than one-half of the population in Puerto Rico by 1519. An African slave traveling with an expedition that rivaled that of Cortez probably introduced smallpox into Mexico. A Spanish friar wrote in 1541:

They died in heaps, like bedbugs. Many . . . died of starvation, because, as they were all taken sick at once, they could not care for each other, nor was there anyone to give them bread. . . . In many places it happened that everyone in a house died and, as it was impossible to bury the great number of dead, they pulled down the house over them in order to check the stench that rose from the dead bodies. (Quoted in 10, p. 206)

Columbus had reported from Santo Domingo that there were about one million persons on the island. By 1548 a Spanish census numbered only five hundred inhabitants. The census of 1548 for Peru listed 8,285,000 persons; in 1791 there were only 1,076,000 (10, p. 192).

Almost one-half of the population of Mexico died within six months of the introduction of smallpox. In Peru, smallpox moved by land and by sea from Central America, traveling along the thousands of miles of highways leading to Cuzco. When Pizarro arrived in Peru in 1532, the epidemic was already over, only to break out again in a few years (10, p. 211).

In North America, between 1617 and 1619, smallpox killed nine-tenths of the aboriginal population of Massachusetts and then moved along the Connecticut valley to the St. Lawrence and Great Lakes regions. In 1650 one explorer wrote: "The Hurons, as a tribe, have ceased to exist" (10, p. 235).

It is possible that the compassionate Jesuit fathers became primary carriers of the disease as they rushed from camp to camp in a vain attempt to baptize the dying. Less compassionate stories tell of the deliberate spread of smallpox by European settlers who sent "gifts" of contaminated blankets and clothing to Indian villages.

The devastation wreaked by smallpox was compounded when, in 1529, epidemics of measles swept through the Caribbean islands and Central and South America and then into North America, quickly followed by influenza. Two-thirds of the aboriginal population that survived smallpox succumbed to measles (25).

Why was there such a horror, such a holocaust by disease? The primary cause was immunological defenselessness. The foundation weakened by social disruption, the breakup of centuries-old relationships between people and environment, and the destruction of systems of values and beliefs crumbled under the attack of disease. There is little doubt that immunological depression was triggered by the stresses of rapid and overwhelming change, or that the rending apart of social systems meant that the people could not care for each other.

Being Born

With only a few disputable exceptions, all human societies connect the event of heterosexual intercourse with conception and pregnancy. In many cultures it is seen as a cumulative process in which semen and blood mix over a period of time, rather than as the result of a single act. The ancient Hebrew tradition of the Talmud says that the father contributes the white substance, sperm, and the mother contributes the red, menstrual blood. The white will constitute the bones, teeth, nails, tendons, and brain and the red will make the skin, flesh, blood, and hair of the child. In this rendering of conception, it is God who gives the shine of the face, the sight of the eyes, the hearing of the ears, the speech of the mouth, the lifting of the hands, the going of the feet, and the understanding and insight (25).

Motherhood in Sociocultural Context

Maternity is a fact of life. But maternity is also a fact of history and of culture. It shares the history of the family and of women, shifting and changing in its meanings as the family itself responds to economic and demographic changes and opportunities. The story of childbirth is the story of the transformation of a natural, biological event into an event that is culturally and socially shaped. This is a dynamic process. Because human beings can choose when to have children, or to have no children, culturally meaningful ideas about sexuality, abortion, and contraception influence reproductive behavior. The events of natality respond to historical forces and are shaped by culture. One might look to the several utopian communities of our own recent past. In the Shaker colonies of the northeastern United States, the decision was made to replace the population, not through biological reproduction, but by attracting converts. In the Oneida community of New York, reproduction was strictly controlled and permitted only in eugenically assured unions. In our own day, ultrafeminist writers have Orwellian visions not only of in vitro fertilization, but also of fetal growth and development outside the womb.

Is the urge toward motherhood something that all women, in all cultures, experience? Is the concept of motherhood a universal idealization? Do all cultures have a version of "motherhood and apple pie"? Considering the fact that childbirth is painful and dangerous, that the threat of death is always present, that, globally, 50 percent of all infants born will not survive to the age of reproduction, why do women continue to have ba-

bies? The answers to these questions are as varied as the life histories of women everywhere. Rather than trivialize the events of childbirth with stereotypic generalizations, we will just remind ourselves of the complexity of all human decision making.

All cultures have some system of explaining human physiological processes and functions. All have a gynecology and obstetrics. "Each of these arts and sciences is predicated upon the statuses and roles of mother, father, child" (13). This is another way of saying that the experience of childbirth is, in any society, dependent on the relative social status and power of women. Simone de Beauvoir, writing in 1949, made this clear:

> For it is not in giving life but in risking *Life* that man is raised above the animal: that is why superiority has been accorded in humanity not to the sex that brings forth life but to that which kills. [Women] . . . are biologically destined for the repetition of *Life*. Men transcend life by creating meaning and value. . . . It is male activity that in creating values has made of existence itself a value; this activity has prevailed over the forces of life; it has subdued Nature and Women. (1)

In addition to physiological "closeness" to nature, woman's social role consequent to childbirth identifies her with infants (who are not really human, i.e., culturally adept) and confines her to the domestic context while keeping her from realizing full participation in the public arena. A lactating mother simply doesn't run for vice-president.

The Imagery of Childbirth in Western Cultures

During the eighteenth century, women in literature simply "dropped their burdens" or were "brought to bed," but by the nineteenth century the physical act disappeared and babies just "happened": "What a miracle it was to hear its first cry!" (21). The image of passivity, however, was soon adumbrated by two metaphors that remain with us today—the images of horticulture and of the sea.

In 1895 we might have read: "She had produced the boy in the world's early manner, lightly, without any of the tragic hovering over death to give life." Birth is then compared to the "flush of the vernal orchard after a day's drink of sunlight." Nineteenth-century images are horticultural—"the delicate plant had been too deeply bruised and in the struggle to put forth a blossom it died"(6)—and nautical—"The sea moaned, more than moaned among the boulders, and below the ruins; a throe of its tide timed to regular intervals. The sounds were accompanied by an equally periodic moan from the interior of the cottage chamber; so that the articulate heave of the water and the articulate heave of life seemed but differing utterances of the troubled terrestrial Being—which in one sense they were" (9). Dickens gives us another example of the passive approach and provides a nautical image at the same time: "Do you remember, John, on the day we married, Pa's speaking of the ships that might be sailing towards us from unknown seas?" "Perfectly, my darling." "I think . . . among them . . . there is a ship upon the ocean bringing to you and me . . . a little baby, John"(5).

In the eighteenth century, childbirth had been active and physical, but by the nineteenth century it had become passive and separated from the act itself. Babies just appeared; they weren't really born: "What a miracle it was to hear its first cry" is a very different thought than "she dropped her burden."

When we consider the role of fathers in childbirth, the separation is complete. In 1913 D. H. Lawrence wrote about this. Morel, a miner coming home from the coal pit, is greeted by his neighbor. "Well," she said, "she's about as bad as she can be. It's a boy child." The miner grunted, put up his empty snap bag and his tin bottle on the dresser, went back to the scullery and hung up his coat, and then came back and dropped into his chair. "Han yer got a drink?" he asked (14).

How different from the rollicking birthing parties described by the author Henry Fielding in 1740 (7). In those days fathers-to-be gathered male friends and relatives and made merry, shielded from the actual scene of childbirth by the women who came to support the laboring woman. The men prepared mulled wine and strong ale for the mother, but they remained outside until the birth had occurred. Father entered only after the room had been tidied and mother had been washed and dressed in fresh linen. In the nineteenth century the physical aspects of the birth scene shift: Father is alone in the parlor listening to the screams and cries from above. He complains of the expense of confinement and the expenses that the new child will bring. He expresses a major psychological theme of the Victorian era, the theme of guilt. The association of childbirth suffering with sex was tied into a knotted bundle that increasingly weighed on men and women. Along with the guilt came the dissociation, separation, and, eventually, redundancy that men feel during childbirth even today.

Taboos and Restrictions

Prescribed and proscribed behaviors surround pregnancy everywhere in the world. In each culture the con-

tent of these restrictions is always in accordance with generally accepted values and ideas about health and illness. Often the pregnant woman is seen as being particularly vulnerable, especially to the actions of disgruntled kin, living or dead. It may be that the anxieties attending childbirth, inexpressible except in dreams, are given a vocabulary in terms that are recognized: the family relationships that are actualized with the birth of a "new" person. Frequently these restrictions place a woman—and the pregnant father as well—in greater dependency on the extended family. The pregnant woman who cannot lift anything above her head, who may not be permitted to work in the garden, and the expectant father who may not injure an animal or use a spear, these parents-to-be become subject to the caring attentions of the extended family. In turn the extended family becomes more and more involved with the unborn child, prefiguring the responsibilities that will be theirs after birth.

It is more difficult to interpret the myriad of food taboos that seem to be applied to pregnant women everywhere. Many of the taboos are trivial, or actually unavoidable, whereas others deny to mother and fetus the most important elements of good nutrition. It has been suggested that the dietary deficiencies are so severe in many cultures that the practice of geophagy, eating dirt, may result. It is also clear that these restrictions are frequently a planned attempt to keep the fetus small, and thus ensure an easy and safe delivery.

Certainly restrictions and taboos on activity and food weigh heavily on the already anxious and burdened woman, but in addition, when the pregnancy does terminate unproductively, the unfortunate woman must endure not only the sorrow of her loss, and considerable physical pain, but also guilt for having violated one or more of her society's rules. More often than not her culture imposes an additional sentence of gossip, scorn, and castigation. This is especially true when the imputed infringement has been social, as, for example, adultery or offense to an ancestor.

Another question should be asked: Do the restrictions and taboos reinforce sociocultural expectations of gender role? In other words, are the restrictions a reflection and perhaps an immediate symptom of women's place in society? This brings us back full circle to de Beauvoir. It is the consideration of pain, and especially pain in childbirth, that clearly demonstrates the sociocultural relationships of childbirth.

Women in traditional societies do not experience childbirth without pain or without fear. Most cultures view the "labor" of childbirth as labor in the true sense of work. However, this work is not for the pregnant woman alone. Childbirth is a community affair almost everywhere in the world. Participation may be magical, as among the Yukaghir of Siberia, who go about untying knots, opening boxes, and unbuttoning buttons to make the birth easier, or actual, when relatives, friends, and specialists participate in the birth itself.

There is a commonly held belief that labor is a voluntary act on the part of the child who now wants to emerge and join his or her kin. Often children are included in the birthing, encouraged by their elders to play noisily, enticing the baby to come out. Music, noise, and chants are also used.

Goodale (8) describes childbirth among the Tiwi of Australia. The laboring woman kneels with her legs folded under her. One woman attendant sits behind the mother with her legs supporting the mother's back, while two women flank her and the midwife squats in front. A total of twelve women and children are around the campfire during the event. The children play noisily, several women massage the mother between contractions, others support her from behind, while still others heat special leaves to be applied to the abdomen. Each person feels significant in the production of the new community member.

Pain is an expected part of labor and delivery. The Maya say that the "child is born in the center of the pain" (quoted in 25, p. 147). Pain is not seen as either a good or an evil; it is the manner in which the laboring woman deals with pain that is culturally important. In some cultures fortitude is valued, and the pains will be borne with dignity and in quiet. A blanket will be used to muffle any escaping cries, or the attendants will drown out the cries with noisemakers. Elsewhere, the louder the mother cries, the more satisfied the listeners, appreciating the hard work in which the woman is engaged and the suffering she undergoes as she gives birth to a new member of the family and community.

A word should be said about birth positions. In no culture other than our own is childbirth accomplished while the woman is supine. In fact, the Nama Hottentots believe that the child would die if the mother were to lie on her back during labor. Most common is the kneeling or squatting position. In many parts of the world the laboring woman will hold on to a rope that is suspended from above, aiding her in bearing-down efforts. In other situations she sits or kneels while supported by attendants from behind. In Europe and colonial America the most common position was to sit on a birthing stool.

Health Beliefs in Sociocultural Context

Let us pause a moment and summarize. We have said that the health concerns with which we are most familiar are relatively recent in history, and that they largely result from human manipulation of the environment. We have traced disease and dietary changes from the beginning of human evolution, through the development and spread of agriculture, and into the era of urbanization and industrialization. We have seen that concepts, expectations, and the actualities of health and disease are embedded within cultures. We have also seen that the human response to disease takes place in a social context, within families and communities. The next step will be to examine these ideas more closely, with particular reference to Western medicine.

Disease and Illness

Is illness the same thing as disease? Each of us has had the experience of leaving the doctor's office after the disease has been cured only to find that we are still symptomatic. The concept of "disease" is a concept of Western science and medicine. Scientific medicine attempts to define categories of disease in terms of evidence that will be observable to everyone. Biological criteria are used to describe these categories in order to make them universally applicable. By defining disease exclusively in terms of these criteria, an observer can decide objectively whether or not a disease is present.

However, this does not help us to understand how people behave in illness. People perceive the world selectively, according to their past experience and their social, cultural, and historical situation. Therefore, the reality of illness experienced by the sufferer is not the same thing as the disease described by the medical practitioner. How did this noncongruence come about? The foundation of much of Western science, including the model of medicine with which we are most familiar, is a system of taxonomy called Linnaean taxonomy. Taxonomy is the study of relationships. In this system the classification of diseases is correlated with the classification of pathogens, such as viruses and bacteria. Clinically observed clusters of symptoms are compared with descriptions of diseases that appear in textbooks, and diagnoses are then made. This is similar to what a butterfly collector does when he captures a specimen, notes its color, size, markings, and so on, and then leafs through the standard entomological literature until he finds a description of characteristics that are identical to those of the specimen. The collector is then able to identify, or "diagnose," the butterfly. As knowledge of anatomy and physiology proliferated in Western medicine, physicians specialized, becoming otolaryngologists, orthopedists, urologists, and so forth. Medicine began to view people as bundles of characteristics, or symptoms. Within this model, physicians were able to objectify their observations, to measure and quantify deviations from biological norms. As specialists, they had exclusive access to information and eventually came to have the exclusive function of deciding what constitutes a disease and how to treat it.

A simple example of this occurs in childbirth. Professionals involved in labor and delivery refer to the "labor curve," the stages of labor a woman goes through in delivering her child. Each stage is characterized by certain measurable quantities. The interval, duration, and strength of contractions and the dilatation of the cervix of the uterus are plotted against the axis of time. Hundreds of labors were measured for these characteristics, norms were established, and any unfortunate woman who deviated from these norms was labeled as having "complications" of labor. In the obstetric textbooks each complication is given its appropriate treatment.

A similar example is related by an anthropologist who showed films of a "normal" childbirth to a group of Mexican midwives (12). After the baby had been delivered in the filmed episode, the anthropologist stopped the action in order to conduct a discussion about birth techniques. As time passed she noticed that the audience was becoming increasingly restless. Finally, one of the midwives stood up and expressed what was worrying everyone. They were all waiting for the placenta to be expelled, a signal that the delivery was truly over. Counting the minutes of time frozen on the screen as real time, they realized that a most dangerous situation was occurring; for them, the childbirth event had very different boundaries.

We must become aware of the different models of meaning that are inherent in a culture's expression of illness. The medical texts contain little of relevance to this question. Tuberculosis presents a classic example of the disjunction. We know the pathogen, the specific bacillus, that "causes" the disease, and we know how to treat it with medicines. But what about the patterns of incidence and its effect on communities? It might be just as relevant to classify illnesses according to the social attributes of the people affected, for example, age, wealth, education, occupation, and access to health care, or even by the social effects of the illness, such as inadequate job performance or disruption in the home.

These features might tell us more about the illness than a list of characteristic symptoms.

Social Illness

There is another important effect of defining illness as disease. We overlook the illnesses that are social in nature and cause. The major killers of the young people of our society are not to be found under microscopes; nor can they be treated with pills. The leading causes of death are homicides, suicides, motor vehicle accidents, and alcohol abuse.

Noncompliance. People do not perceive illness in the same way as does the doctor who has spent years learning which features he must look for in order to diagnose and treat. The term *disease* indicates the biological dimension of nonhealth, which is the focus of modern medicine. Disease is an "objective" phenomenon that can be measured by laboratory tests, direct observation, and diagnostic methods. It is physiological deviation from normal. This contrasts with *illness,* which refers to the more subjective or psychological indications that are of concern to the people experiencing them. People don't usually come to the health professional with a disease; they come with symptoms (i.e., illness). The professional in Western medicine converts the illness to disease (15).

This means that symptoms may not have the same associations for a layperson and a doctor; they may use the same term but give it different significance. People have tummyaches, strokes, heart attacks, lumbago. This is a lay classification of illness that differs from specialist classification. To make this construction of illness more complex, not all cultures give similar meaning to symptomology. The problem that lies within the noncongruence of meaning is the failure of the practitioner's actions and behaviors to meet the client's expectations. The nurse risks losing the client's confidence and diminishes her or his ability to heal. Another effect of the noncongruence of understanding is to reinforce the dependency nature of the client-nurse relationship by introducing the concept of noncompliance. If there is no agreement on the "illness," then there is not much reason for the client to comply with a therapeutic regimen that appears to be irrelevant.

The following is a good example of lack of agreement. In a study of the meaning of the diagnosis of hypertension, respondents were asked to enumerate the causes of this illness. They redefined hypertension to mean "hyper-tension," and they listed acute stress, external and internal, as the major causative factor. The subjects, all of whom were being treated in a hypertension clinic, described these stressors as stress on the job, unemployment, the worries of everyday life, and intrafamilial conflict. If this is the model of illness that people hold, it is no wonder that the rate of noncompliance with a regimen of diuretic medications is high (3)!

The Social Context of Health Beliefs

According to Rene Dubos, health is a condition that permits an organism to adapt to its environmental situation with relatively minimal pain and discomfort, to achieve at least some physical and psychic gratifications, and to possess a reasonable probability of survival. Disease is a condition that obtrudes against these adaptive requirements and causes partial or complete disablement and physical or behavioral dysfunction (13).

Cultures represent strategies, devices, and organizational arrangements for coping with the environment by eradicating or containing disease and achieving health. As we have seen, the practices, beliefs, and technology that are designed to improve the quality of life may become the cause of disease and death.

We have discussed the impact on health of industrialization, urbanization, and occupational and geographical mobility. Changes in diet and life-style and exposure to a toxic or hazardous physical environment is an obvious pathway to illness. Less direct but equally important are the changes in social systems that automated modernization. In particular, changes in social networks (i.e., in marital status, composition of household, frequency of contact with relatives and friends, church membership, and other less formal group associations) have direct effect on health status. For example, married people have lower mortality rates than those who are single, widowed, or divorced, and widows report more morbidity than do married women of the same age cohort (2). The impact of social networks on health is striking. In a study of mortality rates among 4,486 widowers aged fifty-five or older, 213 died during the first six months after bereavement. This represents a 40 percent increase over the expected death rate of married men of the same age (2). Other studies have shown that utilization of health care practitioners and facilities dramatically increases when there is stress within a family (17).

At this point in our discussion it might be entertaining to take a figurative "trip around the world" to look at exotic therapies and healing rituals in different cultures. Although such a trip would be interesting, little would be learned. A belief system—in this case behaviors and ideas concerned with health—cannot be taken out of its unique sociocultural context. I could specify the 1,288 medicinal plants used by the North Americans, or recount a harrowing Eskimo healing technique in which the practitioner, a *shaman*, goes on a journey to the netherworld, where he physically wrestles with malevolent spirits until they divulge the cause of illness and the appropriate treatment. We might note with approval the empirical tradition behind the Navaho herbalist who gathers thirty botanical medicines, among which many are recognized by Western scientists to contain effective pharmaceutical agents. But what would we say when the decoction made from these herbs was *washed* over the client's body—and then over a half dozen friends and relatives who are participating in the ritual?

No one can deny the efficacy of indigenous (i.e., non-Western) pharmacopoeia or healing techniques, but everyone concerned would acknowledge, along with Oliver Wendell Holmes, that 90 percent of ill people would recover sooner or later, "provided nothing were done to interfere seriously with the efforts of nature" (24).

The Placebo Response

Between 70 percent and 90 percent of all health care takes place in the home, and this care is largely successful. Undoubtedly the theophylline in tea and the L-tryptophan in a glass of warm milk and honey effect many cures, but is there a dimension to healing that is outside of medicine itself?

Such a dimension is seen when the client responds to inert medical treatment. The "placebo response," as it is called, is variously credited with between 35 percent and 60 percent of the effectiveness of modern therapy. In the placebo response the client has a biological response to the form, not the content, of the treatment; in other words, the client responds physiologically to a symbolic stimulus. Two of the best documented examples of the use of placebos are in the treatment of peptic ulcers and in coronary bypass surgery for the pain of angina pectoris.

In the classic study of the placebo response, antacid therapy (Tagamet) was tested against placebo therapy for peptic ulcers. All the clients were examined endoscopically before and after four weeks of treatment. The endoscopic examination showed that 78 percent of those treated with the antacid had significant healing, whereas those to whom the placebo was administered had only 45 percent healing. But there was no difference in the success rate of each regimen: symptoms were reduced by 80 percent in both groups. In fact, the rate of symptom recurrence was lower in the placebo-treated group than in the group treated with the drug (18).

What accounts for the significant improvement measured by reported symptoms? One of three competing explanations may be offered whenever a client gets better after therapy. They are as follows:

1. The client improved because of some intrinsic property of the treatment.
2. The client improved because of the natural history of the disease (i.e., the client would have gotten better with or without intervention).
3. The client recovered because of the placebo response (i.e., the symbolic dimension of the treatment).

Probably all three factors operate at once. The health beliefs and expectations that a person brings with him or her to the practitioner largely shape the response to treatment. Beliefs and expectations can hurt and they can kill. We are, for example, aware of the vast range of pain tolerance among people. But culturally learned beliefs and expectations can also heal. They can be as effective as pills and potions. The placebo is the treatment: the beliefs and expectations that we symbolize as "hope" can stimulate a physiological response.

Two points have been made: All healing takes place in a social context and at a particular moment in history. Healing is essentially a social relationship. Satisfaction of needs, specifically the health needs of individuals, families, and communities, means meeting expectations shaped by cultural beliefs. Healing is largely composed of beliefs and expectations that are culturally learned and influenced by history.

The model derived from the cultural assessment of health needs is one that respects and utilizes what people bring to their own health care. Nursing bridges the beliefs, practices, habits, likes and dislikes, rituals and values that people assimilate as they grow up in a particular culture and society, and the beliefs, practices, rituals, and values that the nurse learns as a professional health care provider. But the essential material out of which this bridge is constructed comes from within the nurse. The nurse uses life experience and cultural "knowledge" to ask the appropriate questions and collect the information that will facilitate understanding of the client's model of health and illness. Only in this way will there be congruence between diagnosis, treatment, and outcome, and only in this way will the client be guided toward realization of the goal of self-care.

Recognition that definitions of illness and illness behavior are culturally learned, and understanding that these factors govern both compliance with plans of treatment and the ultimate response to treatment, will truly make healing a collaborative effort of nurse and client.

REFERENCES

1. Beauvoir, S. de *The Second Sex.* New York: Vintage Books, 1974, 64–65.
2. Berkman, L. "Physical Health and the Social Environment." In *The Relevance of Social Science for Medicine,* ed. L. Eisenberg and A. Kleinman. Holland: D. Reidel, 1981, 51–75.
3. Blumhagen, D. "The Meaning of Hypertension." In *Clinically Applied Anthropology,* ed. N. J. Chrisman, J. Noel, and T. W. Maretzki. Holland: D. Reidel, 1982, 297–323.
4. Chang, K. C. *Food in China.* New Haven, Conn.: Yale University Press, 1977, 87.
5. Dickens, C. *Our Mutual Friend.* London: J. M. Dent & Sons, 1908.
6. Elliot, G. *Scenes from a Clerical Life.* London: Oxford University Press, 1909.
7. Fielding, H. *The History of Tom Jones.* London: Blackwell, 1926.
8. Goodale, J. C. *Tiwi Wives: A Study of the Women of Melville Island, Northern Australia.* Seattle: University of Washington Press, 1971.
9. Hardy, T. *The Well Beloved.* London: Osgood & McIvaine, 1897.
10. Hopkins, D. R. *Princes and Peasants: Smallpox in History.* Chicago: University of Chicago Press, 1983, 171.
11. Jarcho, S. *Human Paleopathology.* New Haven, Conn.: Yale University Press, 1966, 115.
12. Jordan, B. "Studying Childbirth: The Experience and Methods of a Woman Anthropologist." In *Childbirth Alternatives to Medical Control,* ed. S. Romalis. Austin: University of Texas Press, 1981.
13. Landy, D. *Culture, Disease and Healing: Studies in Medical Anthropology.* New York: Macmillan, 1977, 287.
14. Lawrence, D. H. *Sons and Lovers.* 1913.
15. Lewis, G. "Cultural Influences on Illness Behavior: A Medical Anthropological Approach." In *The Relevance of Social Science for Medicine,* ed. L. Eisenberg and A. Kleinman. Holland: D. Reidel, 1981, 151–62.
16. McNeil, W. H. *Plagues and Peoples.* New York: Doubleday, 1976, 3–69.
17. Mechanic, D. "Effects of Psychological Distress on Perceptions of Physical Health and Use of Medical and Psychiatric Facilities." *Journal of Human Stress* 4:26, 1978.

18. Moerman, D. E. "Physiology and Symbols: The Anthropological Implications of the Placebo Effect." In *The Anthropology of Medicine: From Culture to Method,* ed. L. Romanucci–Ross et al. South Hadley, Mass.: Bergin & Garvey, 1983.

19. Mote, F. W., Yuan and Ming. In K. C. Chang, *Food in China.* New Haven, Conn.: Yale University Press, 1977, 228.

20. Pelto, P. J., and G. Pelto. "Culture, Nutrition and Health." In *The Anthropology of Medicine: From Culture to Method,* ed. L. Romanucci–Ross et al. South Hadley, Mass.: Bergin & Garvey, 1983, 177.

21. Riley, M. *Brought to Bed.* London: J. M. Dent & Sons, 1968, 1–6.

22. Schwabe, C. W. *Unmentionable Cuisine.* Charlottesville, Va.: The University Press of Virginia, 1979.

23. Tripp–Reimer, T., P. J. Brink, and J. M. Saunders. "Cultural Assessment: Content and Process." *Nursing Outlook* 3:78, 1984.

24. Weil, A. *Health and Healing.* Boston: Houghton Mifflin, 1983, 128.

25. Wood, C. S. *Human Sickness and Health: A Sociocultural View.* Palo Alto, Calif.: Mayfield, 1979, 150.

CHAPTER 11

Nutrition and Self-Care

JOSEPHINE DISPARTI

■

OBJECTIVES

After completing this chapter, the reader will be able to:

- Describe the place of nutritional care within the overall nursing care of clients.
- List specific ways in which nurses provide nutrition services.
- Identify the multiple factors that determine a person's eating behavior and the comprehensive approach necessary for nutrition intervention.
- Describe the current importance of nutrition in disease prevention, health promotion, and illness management.
- Identify and discuss the four major components of nutritional assessment.
- Describe the role of the multidisciplinary health team in providing nutrition services.
- Describe nutritional needs according to three categories suggested by Dorothea Orem—universal, developmental, and therapeutic
- Identify four important periods within the life cycle that are crucial nutritional periods, and list pertinent physical, social, psychological, and economic considerations for each period.

Nutrition is a major determinant of health, essential in disease prevention and health promotion, and mandatory in illness or condition amelioration. Therefore, those professions who focus on nutrition are making a major contribution for health. (7)

Nurses operate on the knowledge that nutrition is a decisive factor in maintaining and restoring health. Nutrition courses have long been an established part of nursing education, and nutrition-related responsibilities have traditionally been built into nursing job descriptions. There are countless examples in all settings of efforts to (a) promote health and prevent disease through the fostering of good nutritional practice and (b) ensure adequate nutrition for people who are ill or under specific medical treatments.

More than ever before, nutrition is recognized by other health care providers as being a most pertinent and promising area of emphasis. There are challenges and opportunities in using nutritional approaches in both health promotion and therapeutic intervention. The relevance of nutrition, for example, in the etiology and management of the major chronic diseases is unmistakable.

Consumers are also showing an increased interest in nutrition. For many reasons (the consumer and ecological movements, public education, changing concepts of wellness, prohibitive cost of sickness, disenchantment with medical care) people are increasingly recognizing the value of good nutrition. The opportunity exists, therefore, for nurses, and others, to be active proponents of wellness, that is, to make people aware of the relationships between their actions and life-style, and their health; to become knowledgeable about risk factors; and to assist people to make beneficial changes.

Along with these opportunities comes the pressure to keep up with the rapid developments in the field of nutrition and apply our knowledge and technology wisely. Some examples of advances in clinical care and the increasing information being made available are as follows: (a) mineral requirements are being revised; (b) interactions between diet and disease are better understood; (c) research on the relationship of food and brain chemistry is progressing; (d) sophisticated procedures, such as total parenteral nutrition, are being used that permit people to live longer; (e) technological achievements (computers, automated equipment) make it easier to obtain and analyze nutritional information; (f) research in the behavioral therapies is suggesting new treatment approaches.

This chapter underscores the importance of nutritional care in health promotion and disease prevention and treatment. It deals in general terms with what nutritional care involves, who it is important for, and how the nurse fits in.

Determining Nutritional Status

Assessment of a person's nutritional needs involves a thorough physical examination, a dietary history, laboratory tests, anthropometric measurements, and an investigation of pertinent psychosocial, economic, and cultural factors (see Figure 11.1).

The information derived in each of these areas is analyzed to determine the condition of the person's health as influenced by his or her diet and the utilization of nutrients provided by that diet. Any significant or abnormal finding indicates the need for further assessment and, possibly, nutritional intervention.

Nutrition History and Interview

The purposes of the dietary history and interview are as follows:

- To obtain accurate and complete information about a person's food intake and eating patterns
- To ascertain the variables (psychological, sociocultural, economic, environmental) that determine eating behavior
- To discover specific factors that affect the adequacy of a person's nutrient intake and utilization
- To assess nutrition needs related to presence of certain disease or illness states

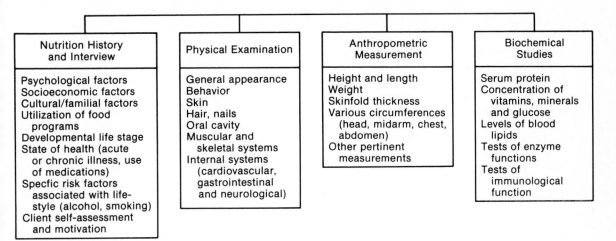

Nutrition History and Interview	Physical Examination	Anthropometric Measurement	Biochemical Studies
Psychological factors Socioeconomic factors Cultural/familial factors Utilization of food programs Developmental life stage State of health (acute or chronic illness, use of medications) Specfic risk factors associated with life-style (alcohol, smoking) Client self-assessment and motivation	General appearance Behavior Skin Hair, nails Oral cavity Muscular and skeletal systems Internal systems (cardiovascular, gastrointestinal and neurological)	Height and length Weight Skinfold thickness Various circumferences (head, midarm, chest, abdomen) Other pertinent measurements	Serum protein Concentration of vitamins, minerals and glucose Levels of blood lipids Tests of enzyme functions Tests of immunological function

Figure 11.1. Components of Nutrition Assessment

A variety of formats are used to determine actual food intake and specific food habits. Widely recommended methods are the twenty-four-hour recall, food frequency list, typical day history, and food diary. In the *diet recall* the client is asked to recall food intake for the preceding twenty-four hours—the type, quantity, method of preparation, and time eaten. The twenty-four-hour recall is useful as a screening tool for determining broad habits. Other methods need to be used to supply more complete, specific information.

Food frequencies determine how often in a certain period of time (day, week, month) specific foods are eaten. A variety of foods are included, depending on the information to be obtained, for example, adequacy of the diet and frequency of a specific category of food "intake," such as iron-containing foods.

The *food diary* is used when a careful analysis of calories and nutrient intake is needed, or when the interviewer wants to analyze the patterns of behavior and feelings associated with eating. Clients are asked to record (usually for three to seven days) the specific types and exact amounts of food eaten as soon as possible after eating, along with their feelings, behaviors, and particular habits related to the food consumption.

Each type of dietary study has advantages and disadvantages. The choice of method will depend on the purpose for which it is intended and certain characteristics of the client, such as degree of motivation and discipline, life-style, and age. The findings of the diet history are then correlated with other clinical and biochemical findings, and these become the basis for individualized

dietary counseling. (The most successful diet intervention plan will be based on modifications of the client's usual diet and current behavior patterns.)

Calculation of Nutrient Intake

The diet histories are analyzed for areas that are suggestive of deficiencies (or excesses). The two most useful tools are the basic food groups and the recommended dietary allowances. Using exchange lists of the basic food groups, the data are converted into nutritive values for carbohydrates, protein, fat, and calories and are compared with the recommended dietary allowances for the person's age and sex category.

For vitamin and mineral intake, the twenty-four-hour diet is compared with good sources of the essential nutrients (vitamins A, D, and C, thiamine, riboflavin, niacin, vitamin B_{12}, calcium, iron) to determine if they were adequately provided.

Adjustments to the diet are then recommended, for example, reducing the percentage of total calories obtained from fat or increasing foods that will provide adequate amounts of a deficient vitamin or mineral.

Diet calculations are usually the responsibility of the nutritionist or dietitian. Computers are currently being used to rapidly determine nutrient content of food intake and compare it with appropriate standards.

Interview

To complete the nutritional history, an interviewer elicits information in other areas significant to eating behavior.

Cultural Factors. Ethnic and cultural influences result in eating behaviors some of which are beneficial and others of which are harmful in promoting health. It is important, therefore, to know a person's ethnicity and degree of adherence to traditional cultural eating behaviors. This is especially true in cases where food habits of the cultural group conflict with specific therapeutic diet modifications.

Food beliefs, attitudes, health definitions, and values are all culturally defined and therefore deeply ingrained. The client may not be willing to make a recommended change when that recommendation conflicts with a strong health belief, for example, overweight as a sign of health.

Religious beliefs and practices regarding food are also important to know in assessing and counseling on diet—such things as dietary laws, prohibited foods, fasting practices, celebrations, and use of food.

Socioeconomic Factors. A person's socioeconomic situation is extremely relevant to nutrition. The amount, source, and dependability of one's income is related to the quality and amount of food that is available.

The degree of relationship with other people—friends, family members—will affect one's eating pattern. (A person living alone may have a depressed appetite and eat only quickly prepared, processed foods.) Also, the amount of physical activity is likely to be affected by interpersonal contacts.

Psychological Factors. Some important facts to get in this area are the effects of mood on eating (what purpose food serves for the person) and what food represents to the person (security, gratification, love).

General factors such as degree of self-esteem, overall emotional state, and ability to handle stress (and how much stress is present in the environment) are basic to know.

Health History

The following specific information regarding the person's state of health is needed:

- Present state of health, present illnesses (especially those relating to nutrition)
- Any handicaps relating to feeding
- Weight history
- Digestive and endocrine system health status
- Medications currently being taken

- Special (life-style) risk factors: alcohol use, smoking, drug use
- Use of any special diets or nutrient supplements

Utilization of Food and Nutrition Programs. It is determined whether the person participates in any food assistance programs (food stamps, mother and infant program, senior center lunch program) or is eligible to do so.

Food Selection, Shopping, Preparation, and Storage. Who performs these tasks? Determine the availability of food and to what degree convenience "fast" foods are used.

Client Perception and Motivation

It is crucial to understand what clients believe about their state of nutrition, what, if anything, they want to change about the way they eat, and what they have tried before.

In order to be effective, the health professional needs to know how best to help—by providing needed information? offering moral support and encouragement? The degree and reason for motivation will be important information in later planning. A care plan will clearly be different for the person who is not motivated, who is trying to please someone else (spouse, doctor), or who is intensely and personally motivated but cannot do it by him- or herself.

Clinical Examination

Certain body areas are examined for signs associated with vitamin, mineral, protein, and caloric deficiencies. Clinical findings that suggest the possibility of nutritional deficiencies are (a) deviations in growth pattern (undersize, failure to grow, appearance of obesity); (b) general appearance and behavior; (c) abnormalities of skin, hair, eyes, mouth, teeth, and muscles and skeletal deformities; and (d) signs associated with internal (cardiovascular, gastrointestinal, neurological) system problems (1).

Anthropometric Measurements

Body weight is considered one of the most useful and convenient indicators of nutritional status. Weight and height are determined and plotted on a reference graph. This is done routinely with children and with hospitalized adults at nutritional risk, to document the changes that occur during hospitalization. In children, the measurements indicate physical growth percentile; in adults, they identify overweight (over 20 percent standard) and underweight (below 20 percent standard).

Skin fold thickness measurements are helpful in assessing adipose tissue storage. The triceps area is the most accessible for measurement and believed to be representative of the body's subcutaneous fat stores (8, pp. 395–96). The skin fold thickness measurement is taken with calipers and then compared with standard measurements.

Biochemical Studies

Biochemical determinations are useful in detecting nutritional deficiencies or excesses before clinical manifestations occur, as well as in making diagnoses (i.e., confirming clinical and dietary data). Studies are done on blood, urine, feces, and, occasionally, hair, liver, and bone. Analysis of the various materials are made for: (a) nutrient levels of glucose, lipids, amino acids, vitamins, and minerals and (b) concentrations of metabolic products, such as serum proteins, hemoglobin, and enzymes, and (c) excretory substances, such as urea, creatinine, ketones, vitamins, and intermediary metabolites (8, p. 399). The significance of the abnormal laboratory findings is interpreted by the physician. The findings may be due to inappropriate nutrient intake, faulty absorption, alterations in intermediary metabolism, destruction of specific components, defective waste elimination, or nutrient drug interaction.

Planning and Intervention

After a nutrition problem is identified and understood, an intervention plan is developed by the health care providers, including, when indicated, the nutrition consultant. The purpose of the plan is to determine how the client can improve his or her nutritional state. The nutrition plan should be feasible and have measurable and achievable objectives, for example, weight loss of ten pounds in two months. Designations should be made regarding who is responsible for each aspect of the plan. The client must be willing and able to work toward the stated goal.

The plan should take into consideration the complexity and interactive nature of all the variables operating (biological, cultural, psychological, social, economic, and so on). It should represent a total, individualized approach to the nutritional problem. Ideally the health team explores with the client the nature of the problem and the resources for solving the problem, the advisability of the proposed dietary changes, and any environmental influences or conflicts.

Any theories, knowledge, skills, programs, and techniques that seem to fit the clinical situation should be used to implement the nutrition plan. There are many possible approaches: dietary measures and educational, behaviorist, psychoanalytic, self-help, drug, and surgical methods. Specific interventions include direct nutrition support services, formal or informal instruction, counseling, social and psychological support groups, individual psychotherapy, behavior modification, family therapy, therapeutic diets (restricted, supplemental), specific advocacy and referral services, and medical or surgical therapies.

The resources available in the community should be adequately understood, evaluated, and fully utilized. Some communities will have nutrition education resources, counseling services, client self-help groups, and therapeutic programs based in hospitals, health centers, departments of health, universities, and schools. When these services are not available in key health care agencies, nurses can be supportive by advocating the employment of nutrition personnel.

The activities indicated by the nutritional care plan are carried out and continually evaluated.

Evaluation

Periodically it is determined whether the client is making the expected progress toward the stated objective. If the client is not experiencing the beneficial results or is unsuccessful with the plan, the reason for the failure needs to be determined. The person's condition may have changed; there may have been, for example, insufficient motivation, incomplete knowledge of what to do, lack of support from family, or an inappropriate referral. If necessary, the plan is revised, new objectives are stated, and other activities are pursued.

Nutrition Health Team

The evaluation of a person's nutritional status, and the subsequent intervention, is best done by a team of health professionals. The basic nutrition support team comprises the nurse, physician, and nutritionist, with other disciplines included as indicated (social worker, pharmacist, physical and occupational therapist). This basic team represents the professional fields that have the knowledge and skills necessary to successfully integrate the science of nutrition into effective clinical practice. Through a collaborative process in assessing and planning intervention, two things occur: (1) the resultant assessment and care plans are more complete, since they represent the best efforts of a diverse group of health professionals, and (2) the role of each health professional is strengthened and supported.

Although each team member (nurse, nutritionist, physician) has the ability to perform the general functions required in nutrition assessment and intervention, there are distinct areas of strength, knowledge, and usual roles that are followed by each discipline.

Physician's Role. The physician is responsible for making pathophysiological correlations. He or she diagnoses medical or surgical problems, considers how nutritional status and diet are related to disease and treatment, and initiates nutritional aspects of illness management (prescribing diets, medications). Physicians also assist in motivating and educating clients by emphasizing the importance of nutrition to the curative plan of care, that is, to make explicit that the medical "prescription" is, in part, a nutritional one.

Nutritionist's Role. The nutritionist generally takes the nutrition history and makes the necessary calculations to determine the adequacy of nutrient intake. Sometimes this results in the nutritionist's writing diet orders. At other times, based on a medical order, the nutritionist develops an individualized nutrition plan reflecting the client's cultural eating pattern. He or she may work directly with clients in diet counseling or in teaching group nutrition classes.

As the specialist in the field, the nutritionist serves as a resource person to the other team members. He or she is the person who is most familiar with the latest literature in the field, the most up-to-date research, information, service programs, and health education materials.

Nurse's Role in Nutrition Intervention

The nurse applies nutrition knowledge in various ways, depending on the setting, the needs of the individual client, personal preparation and job description, and the roles of other health team members. Sometimes the nurse works independently with clients; at other times she or he works as part of a health care team, supporting or coordinating her or his efforts with other health professionals. In the role of coordinator the nurse promotes communication between health team members and facilitates a consistency of approach and coopera-

tion. Sometimes the nurse's function is to provide a specific nutrition service—for example, to perform a feeding procedure—or to consult on nutrition management problems as part of a nutrition support team, or to teach nutrition classes in a school or other community setting. The nurse integrates nutrition care into the overall nursing care of clients. Because of her broad education, her mastery of needed skills, and her continuous contact with clients, the nurse is the health professional most often able to see clients through whatever processes of change, coping, or adaptation are required. Also, because the nurse sees clients for many other reasons besides nutrition intervention, she is in a position to identify nutritional needs, provide acceptable, relevant help, and coordinate all aspects of care.

Whatever the role of nurses within the field of nutrition (specialized, technical or expanded, primary), and however these roles are being adapted to accommodate the newer needs of clients and new developments in the field, the usual functions of nursing remain: direct care giving, teaching, counseling, advocacy efforts, psychological-social support giving, and management of care.

Direct Care

Nurses continue to be directly responsible for the feeding and nourishing of clients. Assuring that clients receive adequate nourishment may involve a number of activities: recommending a diet prescription change in the hospital, administering a nasogastric tube feeding, caring for the catheter site in total parenteral nutrition, arranging for meal delivery to the homebound elderly, showing a physically handicapped person how to use a special eating utensil, directing people to supplemental food programs, and so on.

Nurses are involved with diet therapy and therapeutic nutrition for clients in all stages of illness and in all health care settings—acute care, ambulatory care, and, increasingly, in the home. The demand for specialized nutritional support services—infusion therapy and parenteral and enteral nutrition—for chronically and terminally ill patients in the home is rapidly growing.

Nutrition Counseling

The nurse is frequently confronted with a situation that calls for the initiation of nutrition counseling. Clients who have difficulty understanding and adhering to therapeutic diets present a challenge to the nurse. At the same time, other health team members and professionals look to the nurse to monitor and promote compliance with a nutrition or diet plan, often a diet restriction. The nurse directs her efforts toward helping the client change a well-established eating behavior, and ensuring the success of a therapeutic plan of care.

The preferable counseling approach is a nonauthoritarian one intended to encourage clients to assume more responsibility for their own health and increase their ability to care for themselves. The first step, then, is to find out in what area the client is having difficulty. The nurse helps the client to identify problems, explore solutions, consider the consequences of different alternatives, choose a solution, and then incorporate that solution into his or her daily living. Sometimes the nurse can suggest ways to get around the difficulties; sometimes he stresses the health benefits that are possible with the desired changes compared with the risks involved; at other times he assists clients in ways that increase their ability to practice the desired behavior. These other ways may involve advocacy activities or attempts to manipulate influential environmental factors.

Although changing a behavior, especially one having to do with food, is extremely difficult, most people will achieve some degree of success if they are helped to understand the rationale for the change and are given some guidance about making the change.

Teaching

The nurse may initiate nutrition education with individuals, families, or community groups. She may conduct formal classes or provide informal instruction in whatever situation she finds the opportunity and the need.

Often, nurses integrate nutrition instruction into structured classes for patients with a particular condition, for example, cardiac problems, diabetes, newborn care.

Individual instruction may be done on referral of a client from another health professional who has determined the need for nutrition instruction, or it may be given to clients who themselves seek nutrition information as a way to improve their health and prevent illness.

Whomever the learner(s) and whatever the content, the teaching should address the three areas in which learning occurs: cognitive, affective, and psychomotor. The goal in nutrition education is to convey information, promote positive attitudes and motivations, and assist clients to gain needed abilities or skills. Just what knowledge, skill, or attitude change is needed and how to accomplish the change depends on the individual situation. Sometimes an explanation of the need for a particular nutrient or dietary restriction is all that is neces-

sary; at other times significant interpersonal support and tangible services are required along with instruction. In many cases the six essential steps in teaching are as follows:

1. Identify the areas of information needed by the client (food sources of a particular nutrient, special diets, food groups, food exchange lists, side effects of medication, psychomotor skills, such as are needed to give insulin).
2. Determine the client's current level of understanding of the nutrition (health) problem and how to care for himself or herself (knowledge of diagnosis and care plan, food beliefs, level of knowledge, possession of needed skills).
3. Assess the client's readiness and capacity to learn (self-care readiness, acceptance of diagnosis or condition, self-care capacity, attitudes, level of education, intelligence).
4. Prepare the content in an organized, appropriate manner (have visual materials, appropriate patient education materials, and handout pamphlets and recommend reference material).
5. Communicate the appropriate information to the individual or group (consider the learning style of the person and the level of material; allow for feedback and reinforcement of content; involve significant people—family members, teachers).
6. Evaluate the client's understanding of his or her nutritional problem and mastery of the knowledge and skills needed for nutritional self-care.

Much has been written about the limits of education in directly influencing behavior. Certainly all health professionals have experienced the failure on the part of some of their clients to follow through with recommendations.

In a sense, education can do little more than create cognitive and affective conditions within individuals that are favorable to the adoption and maintenance of desirable nutritional habits and hope that these will assert themselves behaviorally against present and future counter-influences. (2)

Nurses, in addition to hoping that clients can withstand negative environmental influences, frequently try to reduce the counterinfluences through advocacy measures.

Advocacy

Nurses often engage in activities that advocate the client's and the community's needs relative to nutrition. Advocacy involves the aspects of promoting what is best for the client, ensuring that the client gets what he or she needs, and protecting the client's rights. Effective advocacy strategies operate through many channels, including the clients themselves. In fact, it is preferable to have clients act on their own behalf to actively seek what they need or want for themselves and to oppose what is harmful to their welfare or what conflicts with their rights. Nurses should therefore encourage clients to address the issues that affect them and provide assistance as appropriate.

There are many societal influences that negatively affect the nutritional state of Americans. These include powerful advertising and marketing practices that promote nonnutritious foods (often exploitive of children—sugar cereals, soft drinks, fast-food hamburgers); political lobbies of food manufacturers that fight against food regulations and public education that would negatively affect their profits; and the easy availability of harmful substances such as alcohol and cigarettes. The nurse may encourage affiliation with consumer protection, public interest, and advocacy groups that work for improved national policies, combat harmful food practices, and promote nutrition programs. (Lappa, in her book *Diet for a Small Planet,* gives a complete list of advocacy groups and organizations that work to improve nutrition in America and the world [4].) Another important strategy is to help people find an alternative to expensive, overrefined processed foods, using, for instance, food co-ops, urban gardens, and green markets.

Improved meals for schoolchildren and the initiation of nutrition programs as needed in the community are other possible goals for community action. Referral to other agencies is a major advocacy practice. Nurses need a broad understanding of the social programs and financial entitlements that provide nutrition services and supports for clients. They need to know how to negotiate these programs and entitlements for and with their clients.

Federal Nutrition Programs. Nutrition programs for the elderly are under Title III of the Older Americans Act. The purpose of such programs is to congregate meals (often in churches, schools, or community buildings), deliver meals to the homes of those who are ill and disabled (Meals on Wheels), and provide nutrition education.

National School Lunch and Breakfast programs are administered by the U.S. Department of Agriculture. Such programs grant cash and food subsidies to school programs and offer free and reduced-cost meals for children from low-income families.

The Supplemental Food Program for Women, Infants, and Children (WIC) aims to improve the nutrient intake of women prenatally and postnatally, lactating mothers, infants, and young children who are at high nutritional risk. The WIC program, designed as a preventive health care program for low-income families, provides vouchers that can be exchanged in participating stores for certain foods—for example, infant formula, milk, eggs, cheese, juice, legumes.

Under the Food Stamp Program (established by the Food Stamp Act of 1977) low-income households are eligible to receive food stamps (coupons), which can be used like money to purchase food. This program recognizes that some families do not have sufficient income to guarantee good nutrition.

The Cooperative Extension Service of the U.S. Department of Agriculture administers the Expanded Food and Nutrition Education Program. Under this program home economists and nutritionists give intensive training to nutrition aides who are selected from a given community who give practical assistance on nutrition related to families.

Although these programs do raise the level of nutrition in the people they serve, there are serious problems connected with their implementation. There are waiting lists of people who need and are eligible for the services but who don't receive them because of inadequate funding levels. Many families are never reached by existing programs. Also, during economic recession—when people need nutrition programs the most—there may be decreasing federal support and even cutbacks (freezes) in funding.

Nurses, especially primary nurses in the community, need to have a working knowledge of these programs and know how to contact the advocate agencies and the hunger task forces. People who suddenly find themselves without money for food (usually because welfare or social security checks have not been received, or have been stolen, or because benefits have been canceled) need referral to food and hunger emergency programs in a community.

One last indication for nutrition advocacy is to direct people away from fads and fraudulent programs that promise the impossible. Given the prevalence of crash diet books on the market, the controversies in the field of nutrition, and the increase in nutrition (usually weight control) programs, sometimes run by those who are not qualified, it is important for nurses to help people find sources of scientifically sound information and reliable guidance.

Nutritional Needs of Clients

When are nutrition care services indicated? Who should be assessed for possible or actual nutrition problems? Obviously, it is those people for whom nutrition is most crucial, who are at greatest risk, and who are most likely to benefit from nutrition assessment and care.

People may be at risk for nutritional problems because of the effects of certain disease states, because of the medical care they are receiving (iatrogenic malnutrition), or because of their stage of human development, physical environment, economic status, or particular habits and life-style.

A useful way to discuss the nutritional needs of clients is to consider them in the framework suggested by Dorothea Orem's categories of self-care requirements (6, p. 41). They become then (a) universal nutritional needs, (b) developmental-nutritional needs, and (c) health deviation and therapeutic nutritional needs.

Universal Nutritional Needs

Although nutrient and energy needs vary greatly from person to person, certain nutrients are required by everyone. The essential nutrients that must be supplied to the body in suitable amounts are water, proteins and the amino acids of which they are composed, fats and fatty acids, carbohydrates, minerals, and vitamins (see Table 11.1). Inadequate intake of the proper nutrients or impaired ability to digest, absorb, or utilize foods leads to nutritional deficiencies. Without an adequate diet the body is unable to maintain tissue structures, perform necessary functions, combat infection, and prevent or overcome illness.

There is general agreement that the nutritional status of Americans, although good, warrants some concern. The classic deficiency diseases have dramatically decreased in the United States because of improved nutritional knowledge, the standard of living, and the availability of enriched foods, but they have given way to "modern epidemic" diseases that are diet-related. Diet is considered a developmental fact in six of the ten leading causes of death—heart disease, cancer, stroke, diabetes, liver disease and cirrhosis, and arteriosclerosis. The

problem for many Americans is excess nutrition. The American diet is one of an imbalance of nutrients, of excessive fat, excessive calories, excessive cholesterol, excessive sodium, and insufficient complex carbohydrates.

At the same time there are still groups of people in the United States whose basic nutrition needs are not being met. The exact extent of hunger in America is unknown, but studies show that undernourishment and deficiency diseases exist among migrant farm workers, American Indians on reservations, the urban and rural poor, the elderly poor, pregnant women, and children aged six months to five years (3, 9).

Another group of people with primary nutrient deficiencies are those whose life-style or personal choices make them vulnerable (for example, fad dieters and alcohol abusers).

Overall, it appears that the food consumption habits and the life-styles of Americans may be placing many at risk for nutrition problems. In recognition of this fact the surgeon general's office has made the following recommendations for dietary changes (11):

- *Maintain or achieve ideal weight* by increasing caloric expenditure (i.e., increasing physical activity) and decreasing caloric intake.
- *Increase consumption of complex carbohydrates and decrease consumption of refined carbohydrates* by increasing intake of whole grain breads and cereals, fruits, vegetables, and legumes; substituting starches for fats and sugars; and reducing intake of soda and fruit drinks and sugar-containing foods.
- *Reduce fat, saturated fat, and cholesterol intake* by selecting low-fat protein sources, including vegetable sources; moderating use of eggs; limiting use of fats (e.g., butter, cream, hydrogenated margarine, coconut oil); and being aware of the fat content of processed foods.
- *Reduce salt intake* by limiting salt use; limiting intake of salty foods, such as potato chips, pretzels, condiments, cured meats; and determining the sodium content of processed foods.
- *If you drink alcohol, do so in moderation.* Limit consumption especially during pregnancy.

Two other concerns that involve the overall nutritional status of the U.S. population are (1) the increasing exposure to toxic metals, industrial contaminants, and food additives, and (2) the high degree of stress as-

Table 11.1
Food and Nutrition Board, National Academy of Sciences–National Research Council
Recommended Daily Dietary Allowances,* Revised 1980
Designed for the Maintenance of Good Nutrition of Practically All Healthy People in the United States

							Fat-Soluble Vitamins		
	Age (years)	Weight (kg)	Weight (lbs)	Height (cm)	Height (in)	Protein (g)	Vitamin A (µg RE)†	Vitamin D (µg)‡	Vitamin E (mg α TE) §
Infants	0.0–0.5	6	13	60	24	kg × 2.2	420	10	3
	0.5–1.0	9	20	71	28	kg × 2.0	400	10	4
Children	1–3	13	29	90	35	23	400	10	5
	4–6	20	44	112	44	30	500	10	6
	7–10	28	62	132	52	34	700	10	7
Males	11–14	45	99	157	62	45	1000	10	8
	15–18	66	145	176	69	56	1000	10	10
	19–22	70	154	177	70	56	1000	7.5	10
	23–50	70	154	178	70	56	1000	5	10
	51+	70	154	178	70	56	1000	5	10
Females	11–14	46	101	157	62	46	800	10	8
	15–18	55	120	163	64	46	800	10	8
	19–22	55	120	163	64	44	800	7.5	8
	23–50	55	120	163	64	44	800	5	8
	51+	55	120	163	64	44	800	5	8
Pregnant						+30	+200	+5	+2
Lactating						+20	+400	+5	+3

*The allowances are intended to provide for individual variations among most normal persons as they live in the United States under usual environmental stresses. Diets should be based on a variety of common foods in order to provide other nutrients for which human requirements have been less well defined.

†Retinol equivalents. 1 retinol equivalent = 1 µg retinol or 6 µg β-carotene.

‡As cholecalciferol, 10 µg cholecalciferol = 400 I.U. vitamin D.

§α tocopherol equivalents. 1 mg d-α-tocopherol = 1 α TE.

sociated with contemporary life, and its direct or indirect effects on nutrition.

Developmental-Nutritional Needs (Nutrition and the Life Cycle)

The importance of nutrition at every stage of human development is well accepted. However, there are certain periods when adequate nutrition is especially critical. The most important periods are during pregnancy, infancy, adolescence, and old age. During these critical life periods the need for specific nutrients and calories

shifts somewhat. Each stage has different physical and psychosocial factors that influence nutritional status (see Figure 11.2), and each stage has different needs in those same areas. The following discussion of each of the four life stages considers only some of the significant factors.

Taking a life cycle perspective is also useful when we consider that a person's nutritional state depends on the health status at previous states, so that a healthy adulthood (or old age) begins early in life. Furthermore, different approaches are needed for assisting people to meet their particular nutrient needs at each stage of the life cycle. This requires knowledge of the influence of

Table 11.1 (continued)

| Water-Soluble Vitamins | | | | | | | Minerals | | | | | |
Vita-min C (mg)	Thia-mine (mg)	Ribo-flavin (mg)	Niacin (mg NE)**	Vitamin B6 (mg)	Folacin†† (µg)	Vitamin B12 (µg)	Calcium (mg)	Phospho-rus (mg)	Magne-sium (mg)	Iron (mg)	Zinc (mg)	Iodine (µg)
35	0.3	0.4	6	0.3	30	0.5‡‡	360	240	50	10	3	40
35	0.5	0.6	8	0.6	45	1.5	540	360	70	15	5	50
45	0.7	0.8	9	0.9	100	2.0	800	800	150	15	10	70
45	0.9	1.0	11	1.3	200	2.5	800	800	200	10	10	90
45	1.2	1.4	16	1.6	300	3.0	800	800	250	10	10	120
50	1.4	1.6	18	1.8	400	3.0	1200	1200	350	18	15	150
60	1.4	1.7	18	2.0	400	3.0	1200	1200	400	18	15	150
60	1.5	1.7	19	2.2	400	3.0	800	800	350	10	15	150
60	1.4	1.6	18	2.2	400	3.0	800	800	350	10	15	150
60	1.2	1.4	16	2.2	400	3.0	800	800	350	10	15	150
50	1.1	1.3	15	1.8	400	3.0	1200	1200	300	18	15	150
60	1.1	1.3	14	2.0	400	3.0	1200	1200	300	18	15	150
60	1.1	1.3	14	2.0	400	3.0	800	800	300	18	15	150
60	1.0	1.2	13	2.0	400	3.0	800	800	300	18	15	150
60	1.0	1.2	13	2.0	400	3.0	800	800	300	10	15	150
+20	+0.4	+0.3	+2	+0.6	+400	+1.0	+400	+400	+150	§§	+5	+25
+40	+0.5	+0.5	+5	+0.5	+100	+1.0	+400	+400	+150	§§	+10	+50

**1 NE (niacin equivalent) is equal to 1 mg of niacin or 60 mg of dietary tryptophan.

††The folacin allowances refer to dietary sources as determined by *Lactobacillus casei* assay after treatment with enzymes ("conjugases") to make polyglutamyl forms of the vitamin available to the test organism.

‡‡The RDA for vitamin B-12 in infants is based on average concentration of the vitamin in human milk. The allowances after weaning are based on energy intake (as recommended by the American Academy of Pediatrics) and consideration of other factors such as intestinal absorption.

§§The increased requirement during pregnancy cannot be met by the iron content of habitual American diets nor by the existing iron stores of many women; therefore the use of 30–60 mg of supplemental iron is recommended. Iron needs during lactation are not substantially different from those of nonpregnant women, but continued supplementation of the mother for 2–3 months after parturition is advisable in order to replenish stores depleted by pregnancy.

Source: Food and Nutrition Board, Recommended Dietary Allowances, 9th ed. Washington, D.C.: National Research Council, National Academy of Science, 1980.

various developmental stages on nutrient needs, as well as of methods that will be effective.

Pregnancy. Nutritional practices are a major influence on the outcome of pregnancy. Mothers who are well nourished before and during pregnancy are more likely to have uncomplicated pregnancies and deliver healthy infants. Normal fetal development depends on adequate transfer from the mother of nutrients necessary for cell growth, differentiation, and maintenance. Undernour-ishment of the pregnant woman causes maladaptation of pregnancy and malnourishment (impaired development and reduced weight) of the fetus.

Low-birth-weight infants statistically have higher mortality and morbidity rates than do normal-weight infants. Inadequate nutrition has also been linked to mental retardation and birth defects. The demand for nutrients to support tissue development is great, as is the vulnerability of developing tissue to environmental stressors.

NUTRITIONAL LIFE CYCLE
Important Considerations for Critical Periods

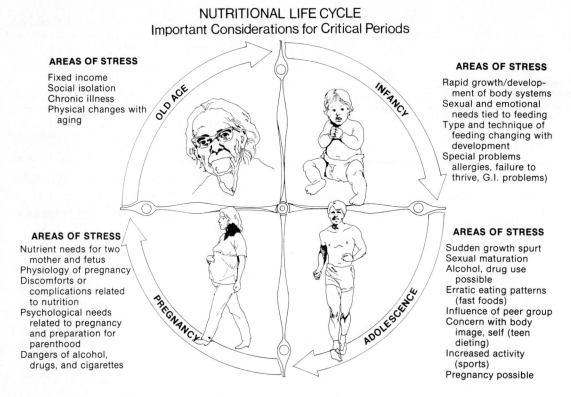

AREAS OF STRESS

Fixed income
Social isolation
Chronic illness
Physical changes with
    aging

OLD AGE

INFANCY

AREAS OF STRESS

Rapid growth/develop-
    ment of body systems
Sexual and emotional
    needs tied to feeding
Type and technique of
    feeding changing with
    development
Special problems
    allergies, failure to
    thrive, G.I. problems)

AREAS OF STRESS

Nutrient needs for two
    mother and fetus
Physiology of pregnancy
Discomforts or
    complications related
    to nutrition
Psychological needs
    related to pregnancy
    and preparation for
    parenthood
Dangers of alcohol,
    drugs, and cigarettes

PREGNANCY

ADOLESCENCE

AREAS OF STRESS

Sudden growth spurt
Sexual maturation
Alcohol, drug use
    possible
Erratic eating patterns
    (fast foods)
Influence of peer group
Concern with body
    image, self (teen
    dieting)
Increased activity
    (sports)
Pregnancy possible

Figure 11.2. Important Periods in Nutritional Life Cycle

Physical Needs. During pregnancy the placenta develops in the uterus to nourish and sustain the fetus. The hormones estrogen and progesterone that are produced affect the entire body system, not just the reproductive process. Poor maternal nutrition results in a small and ineffective placenta, and thus inadequate transfer of nutrients. Because maternal weight gain is a major determinant of fetal birth weight, a sufficient amount of calories must be consumed to ensure adequate weight gain during pregnancy. The pattern rate of weight gain is important, with the greatest weight gain occurring late in the pregnancy.

The effect of nutrients or drugs on the fetus depends on the period of fetal development. Each organ has a critical period of development, and specific nutrients are especially important at selected periods.

Other factors that contribute to low infant birth weight are alcohol consumption and cigarette smoking.

Table 11.1 shows the increased amounts of nutrients recommended during pregnancy. Pregnant women have an extra need for iron, protein, calcium, and calories.

Nutrient requirements generally are highest during the third trimester, when fetal growth is the greatest. Energy needs, therefore, are highest in the third trimester, but in general the recommended increase in calories per day is 300.

An increase of 30 g of protein per day over the nonpregnant amount is recommended. Maintaining an adequate level of essential amino acids is crucial.

Most vitamin requirements are met by modest increases in dietary intake. Folic acid (needed for rapid cell division) may be an exception (folate deficiency anemia is seen in some pregnant women).

The use of iron supplements is recommended, since the increased iron requirements cannot be met by the iron content of the usual diet or by iron stores of most women (supplementation with 30 to 60 mg per day is usually recommended).

An increase of 400 mg per day of calcium is recommended during pregnancy. Dietary intake of calcium should be adequate to prevent depletion of maternal stores and to meet fetal needs.

The requirements of the nursing mother for protein, minerals, vitamins, and energy are greater than they are in the nonpregnant state (see Table 11.1).

Support and counseling by the nurse may be needed. Alcohol, tobacco, and drugs (street, over-the-counter, or prescribed) are transferred to the infant through the milk and may produce adverse effects (see chapter 22).

Psychosocial Factors. Pregnancy may be a stressful emotional period for a woman. There may be ambivalent feelings about the pregnancy (fear of taking on new responsibilities, economic worries, uncertainty about how a baby will change marital relationships). In the case of very young women there may be a social rejection and conflict among family members. There may be emotional stress associated with hormonal changes or physical fatigue. In general, the pregnant woman needs encouragement and support to maintain her appetite and nutritional intake, despite any problems she might be coping with.

Often during pregnancy there is a feeling of well-being and the desire to learn about nutrition. The nurse can capitalize on the woman's (or couple's) interest in how the baby is developing to tie in information about nutrients and their relationship to fetal health.

Referrals may be indicated to assist or support a couple (person) through pregnancy. There may be indications to suggest prenatal classes, parenting groups, or supplemental food programs.

The following nutrition teaching points should be emphasized:

- Eat a balanced diet, allowing for the extra nutrient needs during pregnancy. Use a food guide for pregnancy that gives nutrition requirements.
- Take nutrient supplements recommended by health practitioners, usually ferrous sulfate (30–60 mg per day).
- A weight gain of 1.5 to 3 lbs is recommended for the first trimester and approximately 1 lb per week during the second and third trimesters. (If there are unusual circumstances [that is, an at-risk pregnancy], emphasize that the health practitioner's counseling and advice should be followed.)
- Do not try to reduce weight during pregnancy; do not restrict sodium intake. Discuss any diet addition or change with health practitioner.
- Do not smoke, drink, take drugs that are not prescribed (even then be informed and make sure that the drug is necessary).

- Adjust food habits as necessary to minimize gastrointestinal discomfort, but make sure adequate levels of nutrients and caloric intake are maintained.
- Consider the benefits of breastfeeding for the infant and mother.

Infancy. Infancy is a period of remarkable and rapid growth. (Most full-term infants double their birth weight by four months and triple it by one year). The demand for nutrients to support tissue development is correspondingly great. There must be adequate amounts of nutrients and energy for a sufficient number of cells to be formed and maintained.

From birth to one year of age nutrient needs change as the growth rate changes and physical development progresses within the infant. The method of feeding, as well as the amount and type of food, will change as the infant matures physiologically and developmentally. Food behavior and feeding follow the degree of development of certain skills (sitting, hand-to-mouth coordination), and the infant is able to hold a bottle, drink from a cup, or manage finger foods.

Physiological factors primarily determine the type of food and the number and volume of feedings. Because body organs are incompletely developed in the infant, there is a limited capacity to handle certain types and amounts of food. The food generally considered best for infants, breast (human) milk, has the following advantages over bottle feeding: higher digestibility, increased resistance to infection, improved maternal-infant bonding, lower cost, greater convenience, absence of preparation errors, and control of amount of feeding by the infant.

The best indicator of adequate infant nutrition is the rate of growth, that is, by appropriate gains in weight for length as documented in official city, state, or national growth parameters. (For recommended feeding schedules and infant foods, see chapter 22.)

Specific Nutrient Needs. Because infants grow rapidly, their nutrient and energy needs are great. Infants who feed well at breast or on commercial formulas, or on both, will generally take in sufficient nutrients and calories. However, the levels of certain nutrients may be low, and these should be determined.

During periods of rapid growth, the blood volume is expanding at a great rate and more iron is required to synthesize new hemoglobin. Iron status is measured by hemoglobin and hematocrit concentrations to determine the need for supplementation.

Psychosocial Factors. Because feeding is such an important part of an infant's life, it is imperative that the experience be positive. Desirable feeding practices and a pleasant emotional climate during feeding are necessary to promote a sense of security, well-being, and trust in the infant. Social contact is crucial for normal growth and development. This involves stimulating the infant by holding him or her during feeding and by cuddling, stroking, smiling, and otherwise providing a climate of warmth, security, and affection.

The associations that the infant makes with food will be carried over into adult life. Attitudes, tastes, and eating behaviors are formed in infancy. Sound feeding habits have implications for normal growth and development of the infant and lifetime psychological and emotional well-being in adulthood.

Teaching/Counseling Areas

- Encourage breast-feeding of infants. (See chapter 22.)
- Teach proper feeding of infants, whether breast- or bottle-fed (when and how to feed, formula preparation, introduction of solid new foods, promoting self-feeding, etc.). Help with feeding problems—regurgitation, vomiting, diarrhea, irritability, gulping down formula, etc. Give supplements as recommended. Assist in special needs such as determining soy-bases formulas for all ages.
- Promote a natural, pleasant environment during feeding. Facilitate positive association with food.
- Help parents to relate feeding to the changing needs and skills of the developing infant. Stress the importance of tactile and social stimulation for young infants and encouraging older infants to self-feed.
- Caution parents to avoid overfeeding in order to prevent overweight, which may carry over into adulthood.
- Consider cultural beliefs related to infant feeding. Give recommendations with these in mind. Involve all significant family members in teaching.

Adolescence. Adolescence is a nutritionally important period because a dramatic increase in physical growth and development occurs (and therefore increased nutrient and caloric requirements) at the same time that other conditions potentially interface with adequate nutrient intake. Failure to consume an adequate diet during adolescence can retard growth, delay sexual maturity, and increase vulnerability to nutrition disorders. Some ado-

lescent nutrition-related problems of current concern are obesity; cardiovascular disease (hypertension); cigarette, alcohol, and drug use; iron deficiency anemia; teen pregnancy; and anorexia nervosa and bulimia.

Physical Changes and Needs. During adolescence, there is considerable variation in chronological timing of changes in height, weight, body composition, and secondary sexual development. These changes vary from person to person, and the patterns of growth are markedly different between the sexes. The growth spurt occurs earlier in girls (ages ten to twelve) and precedes the actual entry into puberty. In boys the growth spurt begins about twelve years of age, when genitalia are well developed, and, overall, is more intense and rapid than in girls. Changes in body composition occur during this rapid growth period: in boys there are increases in lean body tissue and skeletal mass, whereas in girls there is proportionately more adipose tissue, along with an increase in muscle tissue.

Little is known about the specialized nutritional requirements of adolescents. The available information is not based on studies of adolescents. In general, however, it is agreed that the nutrient requirements are high during this period because of rapid growth and sexual maturation.

Caloric requirements for all adolescents are high but depend on the person's physiological (not chronological) age, sex, and degree of sexual maturation. Food intake needs to (a) be increased when the growth spurt is greatest (earlier for girls) and (b) allow for body size and composition. Also, in adolescence there may be increased energy need because of increased activity level (especially in sports participation and pregnancy).

Protein intake must be adequate (in amount and quality) to enable tissue synthesis and an adequate growth rate. Both males and females need additional iron to cover the expanded blood volume associated with increase in body size and expansion of muscle mass (especially in males) and to allow for blood losses of menstruation in females. Calcium is essential for skeletal growth, and requirements are high.

The nutrients most likely to be low in adolescent diets are iron, calcium, vitamin A, and ascorbic acid (10).

Psychosocial Needs. The psychosocial development of adolescents is a major influence on nutrition. As the young person strives to become more independent, he or she tends to reject parental authority (and other people who offer good nutritional advice), to experiment with life (including diets and harmful substances), to consider different beliefs and philosophies, to want time away from home and adult supervision.

The adolescent's concerns have to do with self-identity, body image, peer acceptance, intellectual achievement, physical ability, sex relationships, being normal, and fitting into society. As the adolescent struggles with these concerns, the behaviors (impulsiveness, experimenting with drugs, crash diets, excitement seeking) often put him or her at nutritional risk.

Diet Teaching/Counseling Areas

- Encourage the adolescent to eat regular well-balanced meals, stressing the need for some food in the morning, nutritious snacks. Make specific recommendations about high-energy foods that are rich in the most critical nutrients: iron, calcium, and so forth. Watch for signs of iron deficiencies.
- Present sound nutrition information; encourage the adolescent to make his or her own informed decisions and recognize personal food beliefs and values. Reinforce his or her selection of nutritious foods. Give proper advice without trying to radically change the diet pattern. Suggest foods geared to peer group acceptance. Gain the teen's participation in any formal teaching and involve friends.
- Stress the immediate tangible benefits of good nutrition—appearance, vitality, health, athletic performance, weight control, and ability to have healthy children.
- Counsel significant others (parents, teachers) regarding the need for patience with the behavior, avoiding conflict situations, making nutritious food available, and inviting friends to share meals with the family.
- Reassure the adolescent about physical and developmental changes and relate them to nutritional needs.
- Show an interest in the adolescent's personal goals or special needs. Give assistance as is needed and acceptable. Make referrals for special help that might be indicated—drug programs, clinics, counseling services, recreational or employment programs.

Old Age. As a person grows older the consequences of lifetime dietary habits become evident. Proper nutrition may help the person remain active and productive and may minimize the degenerative changes associated with aging. On the other hand poor nutrition may contribute to debilitating illness and depletion of nutrient stores. Some conditions caused by nutritional deficiencies that

may be delayed (or avoided) are osteoporosis, some forms of senility, chronic constipation, and the development of such diseases as diabetes, hypertension, heart disease, cancer, and stroke.

The results of a number of surveys conducted with older Americans show that their dietary intake of calories and certain nutrients (most often protein, iron, calcium, and vitamins A and C) is often inadequate to meet recommended allowances (5). There are multiple explanations for existing nutritional deficiencies in older people. The major problems are physical changes and social isolation.

Physiology. In aging, normal degenerative changes occur that affect numerous body tissues and physiological processes. These changes may subsequently be associated with chronic diseases. The physiological changes most relevant to nutrition are those of the gastrointestinal, renal, neuromusculoskeletal, and sensory systems.

Gastrointestinal function deteriorates with age, resulting in impairment of certain digestive and absorptive functions. There is reduced secretion by the digestive glands and of hydrochloric acid, along with decreased motility of the stomach and intestines. These changes may result in decreased appetite and inefficient bowel function (constipation).

Diminished renal function results in decreased ability to handle renal solute loads. Chronic renal insufficiency commonly causes anorexia.

With age, motor function and physical strength decrease. There is a reduction in the number and bulk of muscle fibers and a decline in the strength of the contractile process, resulting in diminished muscle strength, endurance, and agility.

Bones become less dense with age. This is related to estrogen deficiency after menopause; insufficient intake of calcium, protein, and amino acids; and generally altered bone metabolism. The effect is reduced bone formation and increased bone destruction.

The decline in motor function is especially significant because it affects the degree of activity (exercise and appetite) and the performance of self-care.

Sensory functions are affected. Partly because of the central nervous system and partly from organ changes, aging is accompanied by reduced visual and auditory acuity and changes in the ability to taste and smell. Such sensory losses result in reduced enjoyment of food, lack of appetite, impaired ability to obtain and prepare meals, and less sociability.

Nutrient Needs. Guidelines for the nutritional needs of the older population are provided by the recommended daily allowances (Table 11.1). Myron Winick summarizes the nutrient needs of older people as follows:

> There is much we still must learn about nutrition and aging but there are certain practical things we can do immediately to improve nutrition of the elderly. These include providing a balanced diet slightly reduced in calories, relatively low in fats, high in fiber, and particularly rich in iron, vitamin B_{12}, and calcium. (13, p. 33)

The caloric requirements of the elderly are lower than those of younger adults because of decreased basal metabolism and the tendency to become less active.

The nutrient requirements are not believed to differ from those of younger adults, but since fewer calories are needed, the diet must be of higher nutrient density, that is, more vital nutrients packed into fewer calories. However, these allowances need to be considered on an individual basis, allowing for such factors as interference with digestion or absorption, deficiencies in cardiovascular and renal functions, infections, and use of medications.

Protein needs are still high. Although less new tissue is being produced, the ability to absorb and digest protein is decreased. There is no general need to use multivitamin or mineral supplements.

Adequate intake of fiber is important to improve bowel function and to lessen the need for frequent use of laxatives, which prevent the body from absorbing fat-soluble vitamins A, D, and E.

Socioeconomic Factors.   An increasing number of elderly people have incomes below the poverty level. Many live on reduced, low, and fixed incomes, which directly affects the amount and quality of food purchased. The tendency to purchase high-carbohydrate, easily consumable, and generally cheaper food results in reduced intake of protein, vitamins, and calcium. Older people often refuse needed financial assistance because they associate it with charity and dependency.

An elderly person may be socially isolated because of the death of friends and family members, the difficulty in getting around to visit, the moving away of younger relatives, and the loss of social contacts at work. In general, social stimulation is decreased, which may result in lethargy and apathy toward food, overeating, or erratic food habits.

Psychological and Mental Factors.   Some older people experience periods of depression and even despair. They may have suffered multiple losses or may have serious illnesses that they are coping with, perhaps alone, without family, friends, or the necessary resources. The advantages of proper nutrition at this stage of their lives may not seem significant to them.

Organic brain changes may cause confusion and limit a person's ability to provide for nutritional needs.

Specific Nursing Intervention.   Diet counseling may include the following recommendations:

- Eat small, frequent, nutritious meals that include vegetables, sources of iron, calcium, vitamin B_{12}, and fiber.
- Use fish and poultry as low-fat sources of protein.
- Increase fluid intake to provide for adequate elimination of body wastes and to maintain kidney function.
- Try new food seasonings; decrease sodium intake and avoid canned foods.
- Eat with others, such as relatives, or peers at church or senior centers, if possible.
- Use community resources for food delivery if needed.

Counsel clients regarding specific therapeutic diet, and teach regarding food-drug interactions, right consistency of foods, and nutrition supplements.

Advise the elderly person to keep physically active. Regular activity will improve appetite, relieve depression, help maintain body weight, and benefit pulmonary and cardiac function.

Inform the elderly person of the psychosocial supports that are available. Encourage him or her to have regular social interaction with friends and family. If this is not possible, suggest that the person get involved with volunteer work or join a senior center, social club, interest group, or discussion group.

Help the client obtain specific therapies (occupational, recreational, speech), dentures, or hearing aid. Use reality orientation techniques and family counseling.

It may be necessary to refer the elderly person to various agencies so that he or she can receive special senior services, such as Meals on Wheels, transportation and shopping assistance, home visiting, nursing care, and personal health services.

Health Deviation and Therapeutic Nutritional Needs

Additional nutrition needs are related to the presence of certain disease or illness states. Pathological states (health deviations) may result from genetic or constitutional defects, acquired disease states that affect normal physiology, life-style practices, or accidental trauma.

Illness states affect a person's nutritional state in several ways—by reducing the body's ability to metabolize nutrients and by making it difficult, or impossible, for the person to eat, perhaps as a direct consequence of the pathological process itself, as in cancer. Inadequate intake of the proper nutrients or impaired ability to digest, absorb, or metabolize foods leads to nutritional deficiencies.

Nutrition plays a large role in the management of certain conditions. Sometimes, as in diabetes mellitus, diet is the principal therapeutic agent. Nutritional management is used to treat or control the disease process, to minimize the risk factors associated with the condition, or to maintain the body during acute or terminal periods of illness. Often modified diets, involving restrictions and altered amounts of specific nutrients, are indicated.

The most common restrictions probably are those of *calories, sodium* (cardiovascular diseases like hypertension, congestive heart failure; renal insufficiency), and *fat* (gallbladder disease, obesity, hyperlipemia). The amount of a given nutrient, for example, protein, is adjusted according to the condition (increased for the burn patient, decreased in renal insufficiency).

The nurse helps clients to understand the changes in nutrient needs brought on by a given health problem and helps them to make the necessary dietary adaptations. She therefore needs to be familiar with (a) the pathology of the diet-related diseases, (b) what constitutes the therapeutic diets for the specific diagnostic categories, and (c) food sources of the various nutrients.

Clients for whom nutritional intervention is most pertinent are those with hepatic disease, gastrointestinal disease, cancer, trauma, burns, renal disease, diabetes, obesity, cardiovascular disease, hyperlipemia, and allergies.

The nurse uses nutritional resources as needed for personal reference or client referrals. The specifics of a given special diet often require consultation with a nutritionist, who is best able to plan the diet.

Because of their health problems, clients will have needs and responsibilities related to diet, medication, and activity. The nurse will teach the client or family about the diet and any specialized procedures that are required, such as insulin injection, tube feeding, or colostomy care. Written guides to self-care on the particular problem—are frequently helpful to clients.

Another important aspect of diet teaching is the monitoring of food and drug interactions. Prescribed drugs may have unexpected or undesirable effects on nutritional status. Nurses counsel clients on how to take drugs properly and what side effects to watch for.

It is somewhat ironic that one group of clients who are at high risk for nutritional problems are clients of the health care system—those who are under medical treatment—especially surgery, and drug and radiation therapy. Much of the iatrogenic, or hospital-induced, malnutrition is a necessary consequence of the effort to cure disease. Some writers point out, however, a certain neglect of fundamental nutritional principles in our present-day health care:

> To a considerable extent, physician-induced malnutrition is caused by emphasis on some complex modern treatment program while fundamental principles of nutrition remain in the background. Too often physicians lose sight of the fact that antibiotics cannot replace host defenses; that sterile gauzes and sutures cannot heal wounds; or that the most advanced, sophisticated life-support system cannot revitalize the malnourished patient. (12, pp. 6–7)

The implications for nurses are twofold:

1. Nurses must continue to evaluate their part in providing nutrition support services and, when necessary, speak up for simpler, more natural, effective, and balanced means of ensuring adequate nutrition to clients.
2. Nurses need to be sure that clients and family members understand the nutritional consequences as well as potential benefits of treatments so that they can make informed choices about their care.

REFERENCES

1. Christakis, G. "Nutritional Assessment in Health Programs." *American Journal of Public Health* 63, pt. 2, suppl., 1973.
2. Hochbaum, G. M. "Strategies and Their Rationale for Changing People's Eating Habits." *Journal of Nutrition Education* 13, suppl.: 59–65, 1981.
3. Kotz, N. *Hunger in America: The Federal Response.* New York: The Field Foundation, 1975.
4. Lappa, F. M. *Diet for a Small Planet.* New York: Ballantine Books, 1972.
5. O'Hanlon, P. O., and M. B. Kohrs. "Dietary Studies of Older Americans." *American Journal of Clinical Nutrition* 31: 1257, 1978.
6. Orem, D. *Nursing: Concepts of Practice.* 2nd ed. New York: McGraw-Hill, 1981.
7. Residency Program in Social Medicine. Attitude Objectives, Nutrition Education Program. Montefiore Hospital,

Residency Program in Social Medicine, Bronx, New York, 1980.

8. Robinson, C. H., and M. R. Lawler. *Normal and Therapeutic Nutrition.* 16th ed. New York: Macmillan, 1982.

9. Schwartz-Nobel, L. *Starving in the Shadow of Plenty.* New York: G. P. Putnam's Sons, 1981.

10. Ten-State Nutrition Survey, 1968–1970. Washington, D.C.: Department of Health, Education, and Welfare, publication no. 72-8130-34, 1972.

11. U.S. Departments of Agriculture and Health, Education, and Welfare. *Nutrition and Your Health: Dietary Guidelines for Americans.* Washington, D.C.: Government Printing Office, 1980.

12. Weinsier, R. L., and C. E. Butterworth, Jr. *Handbook of Clinical Nutrition.* St. Louis: C. V. Mosby, 1981.

13. Winick, M. *Nutrition in Health and Disease.* New York: John Wiley & Sons, 1980.

CHAPTER 12

School Health

JOSEPHINE DISPARTI

■

OBJECTIVES

After completing this chapter, the reader will be able to:

- Identify the three basic components of school health programs.
- Discuss the role of the school nurse in each major component of school health programs.
- Describe the major factors that determine the nature and quality of school health programs.
- Describe how the role of the school nurse has changed over time.
- Identify several controversial issues in the delivery of school health programs and in the role of the school nurse.
- Discuss the health needs of school-age children.
- Identify four areas for research within the field of school nursing.

Defining School Health

School health is "an interdisciplinary entity encompassing personnel in health services, health education, health counseling and community health" (11).

A *school health program* encompasses all the activities that are planned, organized, and conducted by the school to maintain and improve the health of the school population.

School nursing is professional nursing directed to a special population—school-age children. "School nursing practice is characterized by nurses who assume teaching, counseling, advocacy, coordinating, consulting and care giving roles" (39).

Basic Components of School Health Programs

The basic services usually found in school health programs fall into three interrelated categories: (a) provision of health services, (b) maintenance of a healthy, safe environment, and (c) health education.

There is tremendous diversity nationwide in the types and quality of school health programs in operation. Some programs are well planned and creative, offer comprehensive health, educational, environmental, and community services, and are specifically designed for and with the participation of a particular community.

Other programs are determined by complicated mandates; that is, they consist exclusively of activities initiated to comply with multiple laws and regulatory bodies on federal, state, and local levels. One writer gives this vivid description of the state of some school health programs: "In many places the programs have become administrative nightmares and ramshackle contraptions that defy description or evaluation" (15, p. 64).

Factors That Affect School Health Concerns

The three major factors that determine the extent and quality of school health programs are:

1. the type of legal or regulatory authority for the school program;
2. federal, state, and local laws that mandate specific school program activities and school nurse qualifications; and
3. individual, local characteristics of the community and school.

It is useful to examine each of these factors separately and to consider their implications for school nursing.

School Health Organization and Administration

The legal responsibility for the organization and administration of school health services is granted to the states under the U.S. Constitution. Each state sets minimal standards and delegates the authority to administer elementary and secondary schools to localities.

There are four possible types of administration at the local level:

1. by local boards of education as a specialized program with specifically hired school health personnel;
2. by local health departments as part of a generalized health program with regular health department personnel;
3. by a combination of resources from the local boards of education and health; or
4. by a private or voluntary agent in a contractual agreement with the school district (24, p. 489).

Results of a survey published in 1979 show that the primary responsibility for conducting school health programs on the local level is placed with local boards of education in forty-five states (30). The importance of this administrative distribution is that since most school nurses are employed by school systems, rather than by health departments, they are isolated from the supports and supervision of both their profession and the field of health. School nurses are, instead, accountable to school principals or some other discipline in the educational hierarchy, who determine what the nurse's activities will be as well as the extent of the school health program.

A basic problem with most of the organizational designs is that, because school health is not the primary purpose of either the health department or the board of education, school health programs are often inadequately supported and, in the event of fiscal difficulty, are the first to suffer cutbacks.

Igoe suggests that the organizational designation may shift away from educational to health departments or school health corporations in the future if the trend continues to increase school-based health services (24, p. 489).

Federal, State, and Local Laws

Some school services are required by state, federal, or local laws, some are recommended, and others are optional, so that in the fifty states there is a wide range of resulting programs. The health services that are most often mandated by states are immunizations (forty-seven states), vision and hearing screening (twenty-seven states), physical examinations (sixteen states), and dental examinations (ten states) (12). Even when these services are required, however, there is great variation in the quality and degree of implementation. For example, the specific grades to be screened are often left to the judgment of school health personnel, and the regulations, although mandated, may not be evenly enforced.

Regarding standards in the area of safe environment, such standards exist in thirty-two states and are usually enforced by public health departments (12, p. 5). There is, again, a wide range within the standards, from minimal requirements for toilet facilities to specific standards for the entire school environment.

In the area of health education, some states legislate and develop entire "comprehensive" health education programs—master plans—that local districts further detail and implement. Of the various specific subject areas addressed, instruction on drugs, tobacco, and alcohol is most frequently required by state legislation (12, p. 4). Other commonly required subjects are safety education, mental health, venereal disease education, family/sex education, nutrition, dental care, and exercise.

An important *federal* law that is having an impact on school health programs is the Education for All Handicapped Children Act of 1975 (Public Law 94-142). This act states that handicapped children should be educated in environments that resemble, as closely as possible, those in which the handicapped child can adequately function. The requirement to place the child in the "least restrictive environment" is referred to as "mainstreaming." The law authorized funds for provision of special health services that might be needed within the school to successfully integrate the child into the regular classroom.

School Nurse Certification. Many state boards of education have mandatory certification requirements for nurses employed by school boards. These requirements are in addition to professional licensure and are different from professional (American Nurses' Association) certification. State certification is an additional legal procedure, intended to protect the public, that authorizes a person who has completed specific requirements to perform certain services in schools.

Individual Characteristics, Needs, and Desires of the Community and Local School

Ideally, school health programs are based on an epidemiological study of the needs of school-age children in a given community, and the resources, desires, and capabilities of that community. The school program should be developed with participation from the community, that is, from parents, health and other professionals, and relevant agencies (health department, mental health center, youth organizations, family service agencies, etc.). A study of the health status of the children and the services available in the community will ensure the development of a program that is data-based and consistent with the needs of the community.

Many individual factors, in addition to the health needs of the children, will influence the nature, extent, and pattern of delivery of the school health program, for example, the type of school (private, public, vocational, elementary, high school, special education), the type of community (urban/rural, wealthy/poor, large/small), the ideology and values of the residents (conservative, liberal, degree of support for education, health beliefs), the educational philosophy and objectives of the school board and educators, and the availability and acceptance of particular types of school health professionals.

Role of the School in Providing Primary Health Care Services

Just how much the schools should or can be involved in directly providing health care to children is currently a seriously considered and actively debated issue (11, 13, 37). Those in favor of the provision of primary health care in the schools stress the need, the advantages, and the opportunities of this use of schools. *Objections* have to do with economic, philosophical, ethical, and administrative concerns. School-based services are seen as further fragmenting health care, not being the proper business of educational institutions, and not being financially or administratively feasible in the current climate of cutbacks to education. There does, however, seem to be growing support for, or at least recognition of, the need to increase the school's role in providing health services for children. This support has come about for several reasons.

Children in the United States, despite many recent gains, still have many serious and unmet health needs. This suggests the need to do more than what we have traditionally done in the area of child health. It is believed that school-based health services would provide adequate health care, including preventive care, to children who otherwise would not receive such care.

George Silver, in an article urging a national comprehensive child health program, points out the low priority and protection afforded to children in the United States. "School children seem to be caught in a crossfire of professional, traditional, and political struggles—innocent victims of social attitudes and values which offer children no priority in concern or resources" (49). He adds that the child's needs take on a tertiary priority, after the protection of the family role and the preservation of the entrepreneurial nature of medical practice.

Another reason for turning to the schools to provide health services is the increasing appreciation that health and education are inextricably intertwined. A physician with the U.S. Department of Health and Human Services makes this point in the following statement:

A student who is not healthy, who suffers from an undetected vision or hearing deficit, or who is hungry, or who is impaired by drugs or alcohol, is not a student who will profit optimally from the educational process. Likewise, an individual who has not been provided assistance in the shaping of healthy attitudes, beliefs and habits early in life,

will be more likely to suffer the consequences of reduced productivity in later years. (34, p. 13)

A congressional report, entitled "Better Health for Our Children: A National Strategy," strongly recommended that efforts to improve health behavior include policies aimed at schools. Mullen, referring to the findings of that report, states:

Schools are the most important and far-reaching of our social institutions, and yet we do not make adequate use of their potential to promote health. School health curriculum, health and nutrition services, physical education, environmental health and overall climate of discipline and support are all of interest to the panel. (36, p. 20)

Another explanation for the trend toward increased provision of primary care services in the schools is the interest generated by recent demonstration projects. One such project is the National School Health Project, undertaken in 1978 by the Robert Wood Johnson Foundation. The five-year project funded a network of school health programs in four states (New York, North Dakota, Utah, and Colorado), which experimented with health care delivery systems in the schools, using school nurse practitioners. The nurses in these demonstration school clinics provided primary health services, using innovative measures such as twenty-four-hour telephone coverage, coaching children in relaxation techniques, and promoting self-care (44, 45). The findings of these programs are useful in the planning of future programs.

The Role of the School Nurse

Historical Perspective

Since the origin of school nursing in the early 1900s, many developments have shaped school health and subsequently influenced the role of school nurses. School health programs historically have reflected the changing health needs of children, the social ideology of the period, economic and political factors, and developments in the fields of public health, nursing, medicine, and education (24, p. 486; 43; 52, p. 141).

School nursing originated in 1902 within the field of community health nursing when Lillian Wald and Lina Rogers, of the Henry Street Settlement House in New York City, demonstrated that nursing services could reduce school absenteeism. The early emphasis of school nursing was on physical care and the control of contagious disease, the then principle cause of child illnesses. Control was accomplished by teaching in the areas of nutrition and hygiene and by the direct provision of health services to children in their homes and in school. The families of school-age children were helped to understand how to maintain their health, given necessary treatment, and taught how to use community resources. At the same time, the nurses attempted to improve housing and sanitary conditions in the community.

For a period of time, between 1930 and 1960, the emphasis shifted from direct health services to health education and activities such as early case-finding. This was partly due to an increasing public health orientation, but there were other factors. School systems had gained control over school health services, states increasingly mandated the specifics of school health programs, and organized medicine exerted pressure to limit the delivery of health services in the schools except for emergency care. In practice, however, the priority of tasks continued to be defined by school principals, who wanted nurses to remain available to provide first aid, to admit and exclude children from school, and to ensure compliance with mandated health regulations.

The literature contains many references to the restraints on school nursing projects. There were other problems in addition to the restrictions placed by state and local laws, local school boards, local medical societies, and the administrative directives. These include assignment of one nurse to several schools or too high a nurse-pupil ratio; lack of support services to do clerical, first aid, or subprofessional work; large number and variety of tasks required; and lack of power and acceptance (legitimacy) within the educational institution. Descriptions of the nurses in tortuous positions conjure up images of the school nurse with her "hands tied," a "millstone around her neck," "drowning in paperwork," "being pulled between the interests of the school and the needs of children," and, more recently, being "squeezed in fiscal crunches."

The picture changes again in the 1960s, during a period of social reform and activism in the United States. Increased concern on the part of the public and government for the delivery of basic health care to the underprivileged and handicapped resulted in passage of important federal legislation (Title I of the Elementary and Secondary Education Act, Social Security Act Amendments, PL 94-142—the Education of all Handicapped Children Act), which stimulated the growth of health programs and mandated funds for health services,

sometimes specifically for school health programs. Significant developments within nursing included the establishment of nurse practitioner programs, the emphasis on increased professional education, and the establishment of standards for practice for school nurses (4).

A current trend in school nursing is a return to providing primary care services in schools, using school nurse practitioners to provide that care in a cost-effective way. Some writers have noted the irony of our needing to return to our original emphasis in school nursing (40).

Florence Downs expresses her difficulty in understanding "how we nurses have strayed so far that we need to be born again under the rubric of school nurse practitioner." Downs reminds us that nursing intervention that includes treatment, self-care, and parent education, that is, a clinical, comprehensive approach, was the original essence of school nursing (15).

School Nursing Now—
Status, Image, Controversy

It is by now apparent to the reader that school nursing is not a well-understood field of practice. Even people within the health professions, including nurses, have varying degrees of understanding, confidence, and respect for school nursing as a professional position and career line (see Figure 12.1).

George Silver offers the following observation:

School nursing—despite statements and announcements in professional journals, despite outlines of proposed areas of concern and action, despite the requirement for qualification in the field, despite the training programs and degrees offered— is not yet a uniform professional calling. Retired hospital nurses, local nurses without specialized experience or orientation whose hours are congruent with their children's schooling are hired for the job. (49, p. 159)

This quote is cited not to encourage discrimination in hiring against retired nurses or nurses with school-age children, but because it addresses some important issues in school nursing. These are issues that the nursing profession as a whole is experiencing: entry-level preparation, focus (essence) of nursing service, and standardizing of practice.

Entry-Level Preparation. Nurses come to employment as school nurses from many educational routes; they may be graduates of diploma schools or community col-

Some nurse leaders argue that preparation at the master's level is necessary for school nurses because the master's degree offers a greater range of professional knowledge, enhances career mobility, and provides the nurse with an equivalent educational background to other personnel in the school system (53).

Focus of Service. The determination of the future emphasis of school nursing is a crucial, controversial matter. Leaders in the field point out that school nursing is developing in seemingly divergent directions (26). Although there is support for the delivery of primary health care services within the school, there is, at the same time, an increasing emphasis on preventive services and the recognition of the need for a comprehensive approach that combines treatment and education services.

School nurses currently practice in both generalized and specialized roles, depending on their preparation, previous experience, what their school district and community want (require), and their own priorities. (Descriptions of the role and educational programs for school nurse practitioners can be found in references 29, 45, 50.) Some nurses want to be direct providers of care; to do comprehensive in-depth assessments of physical, social, developmental psychoeducational, behavioral, and learning problems; to diagnose and manage children's problems; to provide well child care. Some school nurses do not think that the primary care school nursing role will benefit school nursing. These nurses want to move away from a medical provider model to a model that stresses health education, counseling, and consultation. Some who oppose primary care services at this time believe that the focus should be on the positive concept of wellness.

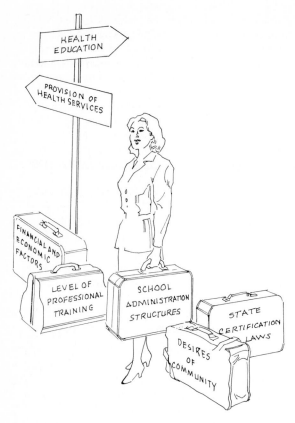

Figure 12.1. School Nursing—Which Way?

Both approaches, health guidance and health services, are essential and compatible. Both could be combined within one role—a generalized practice emphasis that would conceivably be carried out by all school nurses according to their ability and determined by the individual situation—or both approaches could be practiced by a team of nurses working together in an integrated, complementary manner. In fact, many regular school nurses have expanded skills and can provide primary care services, and many school nurse practitioners are prepared and eager to do health teaching and consultation.

Health professionals have learned that primary care is care that integrates prevention and treatment, and therefore school nurses should resist pressures to choose between the two.

leges, have baccalaureate or master's degrees, be pediatric or school nurse practitioners. Some have graduate degrees in fields other than nursing or public health, such as health education or guidance. Their experience may have been in hospitals, pediatric clinics, or public health agencies. There is, therefore, not a consensus among nurses on the proper educational requirement of a school nurse.

In 1978 more than 33,000 registered nurses were employed in school health, including 915 in nurse practitioner positions (3, p. 10). A survey in 1973 showed that more than half of the fifty states require a baccalaureate for regular or permanent certification. (19).

Some nurses believe that no specific requirement should be made, taking the position that nurses will get the education and skills they need for their particular population by attending continuing education courses and workshops to expand their knowledge and skill base.

Role Standardization.   Igoe points out that school nursing is in an extremely vulnerable position because it is so poorly understood by school boards and policy decision makers. Igoe believes that, although there is more than a single role for school nursing, "there must be greater specificity with respect to the definitions of the tasks and duties assigned to each role" (27, p. 308). Clarifying and standardizing the roles within school nursing would increase the visibility of school nursing, enable evaluation and documentation of cost benefit of services, and allow for direct reimbursement of services.

Standardization of roles on a national basis could come about in one of three ways: (a) certification by the ANA, (b) school nursing guidelines jointly developed by national nursing and school health organizations, and (c) conformity of requirements for state certification.

Health Needs of School-Age Children

Before considering the specific functions of the nurse in each area of the school health program, it is important to have an appreciation of the health needs of her clients, school-age children. What are the significant health problems and health promotion needs of school-age children? Which ones does the school nurse need to be most concerned with? Which ones are most realistic to address?

As noted earlier, there is still reason to be concerned about the health status of school-age children in the United States. Mullen points out that although the health status of children has improved, the progress has not been equal for all groups. "Sharp disparities persist in both health status and the use of health services according to family income, ethnic background, parental education, and geographic location" (36, p. 17).

Many children die needlessly and many preventable diseases disable or cause premature death and needless suffering to children in later years. Here are some frightening statistics:

- Accidents account for 45 percent of total childhood mortality.
- Black American children have a 30 percent higher mortality rate than white American children.
- Forty percent of young people between ages eleven and fourteen are estimated to have one or more of the risk factors associated with heart disease: overweight, high blood pressure, high blood cholesterol, cigarette smoking, lack of exercise, or diabetes).
- It is estimated that there are about four million cases of child abuse a year.

- By age eleven, the average American child has three permanent teeth damaged by decay.
- Americans aged fifteen to twenty-four have a higher death rate now than they did twenty years ago.
- Accidents, homicides, and suicides account for three-fourths of all deaths that occur between fifteen and twenty-four years of age.
- Homicide is the leading cause of death for a black male between the ages of fifteen and twenty-four.
- Suicide is the third leading cause of death among teenagers and young adults.
- One million adolescents under the age of nineteen become pregnant every year, which represents an annual rate of 10 percent of all teenage girls. (Birthrates for teenagers under sixteen are increasing.) (56)

Other Statistics.   Many children, as many as one-third of the 45 million school-age children, go nowhere for health care except in dire emergencies (24, p. 487). A large proportion of children live in families whose income is below the poverty level—between 16 and 25 percent for all children and approximately 40 percent for black children. Table 12.1 lists the leading causes of death of children and young adults. It is difficult to comprehend the reality of so many deaths occurring to children because of accidents, suicide, and homicide—all preventable causes.

Given the state of health of school-age children reflected in these statistics, what should be the corresponding action on the part of school nurses?

The range of the problems and needs over a large age span and the degree of seriousness are overwhelming; it is everything from cavities to cancer in younger children and from acne to drug overdose in adolescents. What can the school nurse do about poverty, discrimination, and the fact that children under fourteen kill themselves, or are killed by others? What is her responsibility? What is within her ability, power, role to change? Where does she begin? Where does she draw the line?

Some of the school nurses' possible routes of responses are suggested in the next section, where we look at the specific ways the school nurse functions to promote health and provide nursing services in each part of the school health program.

The Nurse's Role in Each Component of the School Health Program

So many factors determine the school nurse's role that it is difficult to even summarize her functions within the

Table 12.1
Leading Causes of Death of Children and Young Adults

	Children (Ages 1–14)		Adults/Young Adults (Ages 15–24)	
	Rank	Rate*	Rank	Rate*
Trauma				
Accidents				
Motor vehicles	2	9.0	1	44.1
All other accidents	1	10.8	2	18.4
Suicide	10	.4	3	13.6
Homicide	5	1.6	4	12.7
Congenital birth defects	4	3.6	7	1.6
Chronic disease				
Heart disease	7	1.1	6	2.5
Stroke	8	.6	9	1.2
Cancer	3	4.9	5	6.5
Diabetes mellitus			10	.4
Infectious disease				
Influenza and pneumonia	6	1.5	8	1.3
Meningitis	8	.6		

*Rate per 100,000 population in specified group.

Source: Data from National Center for Health Statistics, Division of Vital Statistics, 1977. Adapted from table "Causes of Death by Life Stage, 1977" in U.S. Department of Health, Education, and Welfare, *Healthy People: The Surgeon General's Report on Health Promotion and Disease Prevention* (Washington, D.C.: Government Printing Office, 1979).

areas of health services, health education, and safe environment without constant qualifications. One factor that has not been mentioned is the nurse in relation to other health professionals in the school health program. It is obvious that the school nurse's role will be different in a situation where he or she is the only health professional and one in which there are health educators, psychologists, social workers, health aides, audiometrists, school physicians, speech therapists, and so on. The

ability to be flexible, creative, skilled, and accommodative in multiple roles is a particular characteristic of this field of nursing practice. The most the author can do within the scope of this chapter is to discuss some selected functions of school nurses—in some cases summarizing, in other cases merely giving examples of the whole. Table 12.2 lists some specific functions of school nurses in the three components of the school health program.

Some themes underlie the discussion. One theme is the combining of the individual case clinical approach with a group or epidemiological approach. Another is the importance of using every activity to involve the relevant people (child, parent, teacher) in the health activity.

Health Services

In this area the nurse is involved in health appraisals, emergency care, counseling, care giving in the area of primary health care, and special services.

Health Appraisal. The purpose of health appraisal is to pick up problems when they can be easily treated and when more serious damage can be prevented.

The school nurse can use a variety of methods to identify health problems in children. Review of health records, observation of children in classrooms, playgrounds, cafeterias, working with teachers, reaching out to parents and children—all are good ways. (One author describes an organized method of observing children in the classroom [59].)

Contacts with teachers should be frequent, informal (lunches, volunteering to help with school activities), and formal (in-service programs, conferences) so that there is open communication and cooperation between teachers and nurse. Many of the health problems of children are recognizable to the classroom teacher if he or she knows what to look for. Nurses use their professional knowledge to determine priorities for screening, counseling, or educating.

One suggestion of epidemiologists is to follow-up on children who have frequent absences from school (6, 55). The absences are likely to be related to a health condition of the child (or family member) and may indicate the need for some counseling or service. In the same way, the nurse might pay special attention to the hearing ability of children with a history of frequent ear infections, or to the needs of children with asthma.

Health History. Review of health histories, although time-consuming, identify children with special needs. Often, however, histories contain limited or in-

Table 12.2
School Nursing Role Within the School Health Program

Health Services	Healthy/Safe Environment	Health Education
1. Health appraisal a. history and physical exam b. screening tests, referral, and follow-up c. review of immunizations	1. Surveillance related to a. communicable disease b. healthy environment c. safe procedures, equipment, physical facility	1. Planning a. curriculum development b. educational resources c. approaches
2. Emergency care a. trauma b. illness	2. Promotion of a healthy, enhancing environment and beneficial programs	2. Health instruction a. with individuals b. informal group discussions c. formal classroom teaching
3. Provision of primary health care a. well child care b. management of acute and chronic illness		3. Liaison with family and community
4. Counseling, health guidance		
5. Other services designed for specific health needs of children		

complete information. They are often hurriedly prepared by private physicians' office secretaries or are limited to questionnaires filled out by parents. Sometimes parents purposely withhold information out of fear that a child will be stigmatized.

A good history is extremely valuable. It would include all the basic areas (past medical history, basic review of body systems, and so on) plus a special focus on the child's immunization status, nutrition and exercise patterns, school adjustment and school academic progress, speech and language ability, health-related health practices such as drug use and smoking, special health needs (chronic illnesses) or restrictions, and the parents' or child's health concerns and goals.

With the advent of computerized record systems, the school health record is extremely important. Information regarding immunizations, screening results, follow-up, need for services, health conditions, services provided will be readily available at any time. Complete data would be available for each child as well as for program planning (28).

Physical Examination. At one time the school nurse organized mass physical examinations, prepared students for the school physician who performed the examinations, and did follow-up on the physician's findings. Now it is generally agreed that routine school physical

examinations are not justified because they are an ineffective means of case finding. However, because periodic physical examinations are frequently mandated by law (or school policy), they are still done.

When the specifics are not designated by law, recommended guidelines are available. The American Academy of Pediatrics (2) recommends periodic examinations be done for:

- children identified as having problems—high-risk children owing to socioeconomic status, poor school performance, existing handicaps, frequent absences;
- children entering school;
- children who are mid-school (grades six and seven);
- children leaving school; and
- children participating in competitive athletic programs.

When the physical examination and history are done in the school, they should be used to give information to children (or parents) about their health status and physical condition.

When the physical examination is done for children who are going to participate in rigorous sports, there should be a special assessment of particular parts of the body that may be vulnerable or stressed, depending on the sport. One school nurse, Thorne, describes how the findings from a screening examination program fit into an overall sports inquiry prevention program (54). It was found that 51 percent of the football team candidates had the potential for some type of injury. Thorne adds that many of the problems identified in that program could be corrected by exercising, stretching, and strengthening the specific body area involved.

Planned Screening Programs. Such programs have traditionally been conducted to systematically assess childrens' health status. School nurses participate in the planning, implementation, and follow-up of screening programs, but they do not necessarily conduct the screening themselves. Technicians, school aides, teachers, volunteer parents may actually do the testing after being adequately trained in the technique and use of equipment (2; 5; 17; 18; 31; 38; 60, ch. 13).

Three types of screening tests will be discussed briefly here. They were chosen because (a) they are frequently required by law (or recommended), (b) they require early detection for adequate treatment and prevention of complications, and (c) they are significant problems that affect the education and development of children.

Other screening programs that have recently been proposed and implemented in some places are cardiac screening, hypertension, streptococcal throat infection screening, communicable disease (tuberculosis), asymptomatic urinary tract infections, anemia, psychosocial difficulties, learning disabilities, and plumbism.

Screening programs may be selected when there is a need and if they are acceptable to the parents and school system. Some involve intrusive procedures (like taking blood samples) and may not be well accepted.

Vision screening detects the most common vision problems, refractive errors. These include hyperopia (farsightedness), myopia (nearsightedness), and astigmatism. Refractive errors vary in prevalence from 6 percent to 7 percent among six-year-olds, to 15 percent among fifteen-year-olds (60, p. 300). Other problems are amblyopia, strabismus, and defects in color vision.

The Snellen test (either E chart or mixed-letter chart) is the most frequently used test for visual acuity. It can be done by teachers and volunteers who are trained and supervised by the school nurse. Children in the first three grades (kindergarten through third) should be able to read the 20/40 line or better with each eye; after third grade they should be able to read the 20/30 line. Another criterion for referral is a two-line acuity difference between the right and left eyes.

Additional tests that may be used are the cover test or

Maddox rod test for muscle balance, the "plus" lens test for hyperopia, and the Ishihara test for color vision. Sometimes combination tests are used (2, pp. 93, 193–94); several have been developed using binocular viewing machines.

All children entering school should be screened if they have not had a recommended preschool eye examination. Children should also be screened if they rub their eyes occasionally, hold books too close or too far away, hold their heads tilted forward, squint or frown when trying to see, cross their eyes, have red eyes (evidence of eye irritations), have frequent headaches, or complain of blurred or double vision.

Screening for visual acuity is usually done annually. Children who wear glasses are tested while wearing their glasses, to determine if acuity is normal using the glasses. If acuity is abnormal, then investigate the last examination to determine if this is the best possible vision.

Hearing testing is one of the most significant types of screening to be offered. Hearing ability is crucial for a child's learning, speech, and personality development. Approximately 5 percent of schoolchildren fail the hearing screening test (60, p. 301).

The most common hearing losses are conductive hearing losses (caused by impacted ear wax, scarred eardrums, foreign objects, otitis media, or congenital abnormalities). Medical or surgical treatment may be indicated. Sensorineural hearing losses may be the result of inner ear defects, auditory nerve damage, or brain damage. Treatment for this type of hearing loss includes use of hearing aids, education in lip reading, and speech therapy.

The hearing test used is (individual) pure tone audiometry. The audiometer is designed to test hearing from low to high pitches in varying ranges of intensity. Generally a "sweep check" test is done to establish which frequencies can be heard when the volume remains fixed. Criteria for referral and which frequencies should be tested are determined by the professionals responsible for the program (2, p. 94).

The recommended age for the first hearing test is before age four, or whenever an indication of a hearing problem appears (ear disease, language and speech problems, inattentiveness, turning one ear to the speaker, academic difficulty despite ability).

Annual hearing testing for children in kindergarten through grade three is recommended, with follow-up tests every two to three years, including once during junior high and senior high school (2, p. 195).

Frequently hearing testing is done by specially trained

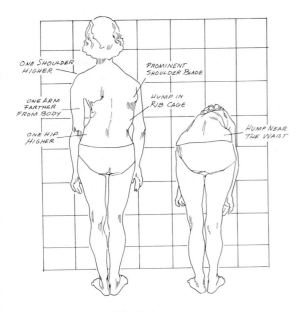

ONE SHOULDER HIGHER

ONE ARM FARTHER FROM BODY

ONE HIP HIGHER

PROMINENT SHOULDER BLADE

HUMP IN RIB CAGE

HUMP NEAR THE WAIST

Figure 12.2. Signs of Scoliosis

technicians. Some states require audiometric certification by whoever does the testing.

Scoliosis screening is an example of screening for an important orthopedic problem. Early detection of scoliosis is important, to prevent deformity and avoid major, hazardous surgery. The prevalence of scoliosis is estimated at 4.5 to 5 percent of children, with girls affected in most cases (80 percent to 90 percent) (2, p. 94).

Lateral spinal curves may develop during adolescence and progress rapidly during the adolescent growth spurt. In functional scoliosis, where there is no pathology of the spine, medical treatment may not be necessary. However, in "structural idiopathic scoliosis" there are vertebral changes that require treatment with a back brace and exercise.

Briefly stated, the screening consists of observation of the child in two positions—the Adam forward-bending position to detect any prominence of the rib cage, "rib hump," or lateral curvature, and the erect standing position, when the back is examined for any asymmetry, such as difference in shoulder and hip heights, an observable spinal curve, prominence of either scapula or hip, and any difference in size of the spaces between the arms and body and neck (Figure 12.2) (48).

Screening is recommended (annually or semiannually) in grades five, six, seven, and eight and for younger siblings of students known to have scoliosis (23). Screening can be done rapidly by the school nurse or physical education teacher.

Because it is so important to correct problems detected in these screening programs, there needs to be effective, adequate provision for follow-up. Careful tracking of the referral needs to be done and considerable effort expended to ensure that the child receives the further assessment, obtains the care or aid prescribed (glasses, hearing aid, brace), knows how to use the aid, and accepts its use; that parents can obtain the care (or equipment); and that the aids are replaced when lost or outgrown.

Children and parents may need instruction, emotional support, or financial assistance in order to follow through with the care needed. Parents and children who understand the condition, treatment, and consequences of the condition will be better able to accept and deal with the problem.

Emergency Care. It is the nurse's responsibility to help develop and implement emergency procedures. In the event of sudden illness or trauma there needs to be a clear-cut, well-known policy of what to do, including the lines of responsibility, source of the emergency care, arrangements for transportation, notification of parents, and records to be completed.

The nurse may provide the first aid care and manage the emergency, but she or he need not be the only one in the school system prepared or designated to do so. Selected personnel should have first aid certification and cardiopulmonary resuscitation training. Well-equipped first aid kits should be strategically located in such places as the school office, gymnasium, home economics class, industrial arts shops, and chemistry laboratories. Teachers should be permitted to take care of minor injuries without routinely involving the school nurse (a practice that has earned school nurses the name of "Band-Aid Betsy"). Instead of always being available to perform first aid procedures, school nurses could put their skills and time to better use by working with teachers and others to prepare them to deal with the common, generally minor problems, and by alerting appropriate school personnel to children who are at higher risk for health emergencies and informing them about the specifically indicated emergency procedures. Examples of children who may have emergencies are those with diabetes, severe asthma, convulsive disorders, emotional problems, and handicapping conditions. Adults who supervise children in the playground, at street crossings, and in other areas where accidents may occur should especially be knowledgeable in first aid procedures.

Provision of Primary Health Care. An increasing number of school programs now include the provision of well child health care and the treatment of acute and chronic illness by school nurses. It is generally school nurse practitioners who function in this role because they are recognized as having the necessary skills and their services are more likely to generate income. The school nurse identifies and manages many common, minor conditions. The most frequent conditions are respiratory, gastrointestinal, and dermatological disorders, and minor injuries (cuts, sprains). There may be nutritional problems as well as mental and emotional problems, such as hyperactivity, mental retardation, inappropriate behavior, school phobias, ulcers, and bedwetting. Complete examinations are conducted using instruments and including some diagnostic laboratory tests—throat culture, urinalysis, hematocrit, stool specimen analysis, pregnancy tests, sickle cell anemia screening. The nurse gives medication that may be indicated according to treatment protocols developed with medical consultation.

Any problem identified that requires evaluation and treatment beyond the ability of the nurse is referred.

Counseling. The school nurse is in an excellent position to both recognize the need for counseling services and provide that service for children, parents, and teachers. She represents a nonthreatening, caring, trusted adult and health professional who is an available, knowledgeable source of help. Frequently children come to the school nurse with vague physical symptoms, or to escape a stressful situation in the classroom. Many children have special problems in their home situations that are reflected in psychosomatic conditions and academic failure. They may need help, for example, to cope with the stress of living with alcoholic parents or to withstand family violence and disruption.

Other young people have concerns about normal physical development or their personal health problems. They need someone to help them understand their feelings, separate the facts from the fears, figure out their personal situation, and explore the outcomes (consequences) of alternative options. The school nurse attempts, through counseling, to help children make constructive health choices and to foster self-responsibility.

A few examples of the need for counseling are the young person who is pregnant or who wants to give up drug use or who is severely depressed because of a chronic illness or handicapping condition. Parents of the children with those problems may themselves desperately need counseling in order to help their children. Parents often react on an emotional level, feeling guilt, despair, and hopelessness. A major purpose of counseling is to inform and refer young people and their parents to professional health services in the community for the specifically identified problem.

Special Services. Some schools may have programs or provisions to meet specific needs of the school population. For example, the school nurse may have significant involvement in the delivery of health services and the education of handicapped children in the school (16). Children with such "handicapping" conditions as mental retardation, hearing and vision impairment, serious emotional disturbance, speech handicap, orthopedic impairment, and learning disability are likely to need special procedures related to their physical care, medical treatment, and special therapies. Children may need help with maintaining adequate nutrition; provisions may be needed for modified school lunches, special utensils, or even tube feedings. They may have special toileting needs that require help with bladder and bowel training or catheterizations. Special chairs, mats, and tiltboards may be needed to ensure change of position and good posture.

Services other than physical care are also important. Advocacy efforts are often necessary to see that, for example, modified physical education programs are devised or that other students understand the special needs of and offer assistance to the handicapped students. Social and emotional adjustment needs of children with handicaps are major considerations. Therapeutic and supportive services need to be available so that handicapped children can successfully adapt to life and school, and deal with their feelings. Depression is now recognized as a significant problem for chronically ill or handicapped children. Several sources discuss the importance of counseling the child and family (including the siblings) of handicapped children (10, 46, 47). Such counseling is geared toward helping people to accept the limitations, mourn the loss of normalcy, cope with negative peer group and societal reactions, and handle crisis situations positively.

Safe and Healthy Environment

The school nurse has a special appreciation of the need for accident prevention and health promotion because she has learned, through her professional training and experience, the terrible consequences that may result from carelessness or inadequate preventive action. A large part of the school nurse's role is to encourage such awareness and vigilance in others. The school nurse needs to be enthusiastic, aggressive, and persistent in her efforts with other school personnel to provide a safe and healthy school environment. She might, for example, need to insist on the removal of hazards in the playground, or that money be found for essential equipment.

A certain percentage of the accident statistics represents accidental deaths and injuries connected with school life. Two especially important areas are fire prevention measures, including rapid, safe exit from school buildings, and bus safety.

Some schools have safety committees with representation of parents, teachers, administration, school nurse, and others. The participation of teachers and students is crucial to ensure adequate awareness and cooperation. McKenzie and Williams developed a self-awareness checklist for teachers to use in assessing their classrooms as safe learning environments (35, p. 284). The authors point out that teachers have many responsibilities, and safety may not be "foremost in mind." Included in the checklist are questions that encourage the teacher to have the students help develop and discuss the classroom policies for safety and emergencies.

Schools are routinely inspected by representatives of the health department. The specific standards vary according to the local and state building, safety, and sanitation codes, but generally they deal with such areas as adequate architectural design (including adequacy for developmental characteristics of children), heating, lighting, ventilation, sanitation, food service, drinking fountains, fire exits. The school nurse should review the regulations for a safe school environment so she can be aware of violations. Because she is present in the school, she is in a good position to discover hazards or unsanitary conditions in the school environment. When there is an unusual occurrence of accidents or illness, she can investigate further to determine the cause and, in the case of communicable disease, the source of transmission.

One example of this epidemiological approach to correcting a problem is provided by the school nurse who observed that several children had an unusual eye infection. When the nurse pursued the coincidence she discovered that the common factor for all the affected children was that they were on a swimming team that practiced in the late afternoon, when the chlorine level of the pool was too low. The problem was solved when chlorine was added to the pool at midday as well as in the early morning.

The nurse needs to consider if the school environment is safe for physically handicapped children. Architectural barriers may need to be added, modified, or removed to accommodate children with mobility problems. Such modifications would include installation of ramps and elevators, widening of doors, mounting handrailings in hallways, and revamping toilet facilities to accommodate wheelchairs. Additional medical, life-sustaining equipment, such as oxygen, may be required.

Another consideration is the need to be prepared for natural disasters, such as hurricanes, floods, and earthquakes, that might occur. The specific effects of the disaster need to be understood and methods of dealing with the emergency determined beforehand.

The school nurse wants to encourage an environment that promotes health. She is interested, then, in seeing to it that the school has a nutritious lunch program, that it promotes physical fitness, and that recreation programs give all children an opportunity to participate. (Handicapped students require adaptive physical education services.) Drawing the line on where the environment ends may be difficult for the school nurse—the social environment is as important as the physical environment, and clearly the neighborhood, street, and family environment directly affect the health of children.

Health Education

The school nurse functions in various roles in the planning, promoting, and implementing of health education programs. She may act as a consultant or resource person for curriculum planning, may be counted on to coordinate instruction programs with the school, parents, and community, or may actually teach specific topics ("units") in the classroom. Again, there is no single, definite health education role for the school nurse; instead, the role varies and continues to evolve along with efforts to develop and evaluate health education programs. It is, however, a crucial area in which the school nurse can promote health.

There is much criticism in the health education literature regarding the effectiveness of health education methods and approaches now being used. Current health statistics show that problems exist, and may even be increasing, in the very areas where health teaching in schools is mandated—areas such as alcohol and drug use, nutrition, smoking, and sexually transmitted disease. Although it is unrealistic to expect schools alone to have a major impact on health statistics in those areas, there is still dissatisfaction with current methods and approaches in health education. The traditional classroom teaching model is recognized as being too limited, not always relevant to the student's experience, not tied into programs of prevention and service, and does not allow for the potent influence of the environment. Teaching of the facts alone is furthermore acknowledged as an insufficient goal for health education; instead, students are now seen as needing help to acquire the ability and motivation, as well as the knowledge, to maintain their health.

The following discussion points out some newer emphases in health education—a focus on self-care education, comprehensive approaches to health education, and the importance of a normative approach.

Several writers consider what specific concepts, skills, and attitudes children need in order to develop sound health practices. Igoe stresses the importance of self-care education and the health consumer role (25, 26). A major focus of health education, according to Igoe (and others), is to increase students' responsibility and independence for their own health care. Using this approach, nurses and teachers would need to facilitate a process of learning and decision making in children within which they can develop the awareness, commitment, and experience necessary to practice self-care.

One program, Project Health PACT, was developed at the University of Colorado specifically to orient students to a new role as participatory health consumers (42). Children at all grade levels are taught how to solve health problems and how to get the best care available—the participatory behavior and cognitive learning are progressive from kindergarten to high school (32).

Allanson states:

If we want children to rely on internal strengths to make intelligent health-related decisions and maintain healthy lifestyles, curriculum emphasis should be on building strengths which help students:
1. Recognize, cope with and reduce harmful stress
2. Develop self-discipline
3. Cope with undesired peer pressures
4. Build positive self-concepts and self-esteem
5. Understand human rights and develop self-responsibility
6. Think critically and develop decision-making skills
7. Clarify personal ethics

8. Develop both short-term and long-range life goals
9. Use school and community resources more effectively. (1, p. 559)

This quote suggests several possible approaches and topics for health education curriculum. Whatever specific health topics are selected in the health education curriculum, they should be tied into the reality of the students' life experience. The instruction will be more effective if the environment supports the instructional message, if it is relevant to the students' needs, and if the student participates in the learning experience. Allanson addresses this question of "how to" in pointing out that health topics need to be "taught in conjunction with efforts to address pressing social needs and with an effort that is complemented by strategic environmental changes, appropriate economic incentives, effective use of mass media, improved access to the health service system, appropriate changes in health laws" (1, p. 559). The same understanding of the need to approach health goals from multiple routes is seen in the report *Primary Health/Preventing Disease: Objectives for the Nation,* published by the U.S. Department of Health and Human Services (57). Objectives are established for fifteen priority areas of preventable threats to health, several pertinent to children's health. For example, the prevention and promotion measures for accident prevention are considered in the following categories: education and information, technological measures, legislative and regulatory measures, and economic measures.

Each problem affecting the current or future health of children could be looked at in the classroom in this total way, and responsibilities of the individual student, parent, school, community, and government identified. Complete analysis of a specific subject would be more interesting, more meaningful, more suggestive of actions for the future and would more likely give direction and motivation to students. It should increase the student's ability to make independent, informed decisions despite negative pressures from individuals or the environment. This is a very different approach to health education from one that is limited to didactic instruction about what to do and what not to do.

Another important area is the influence of peer pressure in school-age children. Children, especially adolescents, are vulnerable to the reactions and behavior of their age-group. Children need approval from their peer group to practice healthful behaviors and reject harmful ones. The implications of this fact have led, in some places, to a peer approach in health education programs where older students are paired with younger ones to teach in some area (smoking, drugs, pregnancy) in an attempt to reduce negative peer pressure and present positive role models (7). Blain also attempts to work with young people in groups rather than individually. This would allow the questioning of norms for the group and lend support for constructive health choices.

Other determinants of children's health behavior are obviously the home and community environment. The school nurse is instrumental in getting the participation of significant people (parents, community leaders) in health education programs. This involvement would assist in the community's learning about the existing health problems and the need to assume greater responsibility for health care maintenance of children.

The preceding has dealt with the health educational process and approaches rather than specific subjects to be included in the curriculum. Sources are available in the health education literature for curriculum topics (22, 51). Again, no ideal standard curriculum can be recommended. The specific topics are determined by law, local characteristics, needs of the school population, and the values and philosophy of the school district and community.

Free or inexpensive health education materials are available from governmental agencies, private (voluntary) organizations, professional associations, and commercial groups. It is important to use creative teaching methods and up-to-date materials that may have been developed by others. Educational packages and campaigns against specific problems (smoking, cancer, sexually transmitted diseases), along with information about health education funding and consultation sources are available from the U.S. Department of Education.

Special consideration should be given to health education for the handicapped child. Learning activities need to be planned that are consistent with the needs and possible limitations of specific children. Curricular modifications may be needed, including the instructional approach used, the content, and instructional goals.

Research Issues in School Nursing

The advancement of school nursing will depend, in large part, on a clear conceptualization of what constitutes school nursing practice and a better understanding of the needs of students and school systems.

School nurses are now engaged in research that will give them empirical knowledge in several pertinent areas. Studies are being conducted that help to clarify the activities and areas of practice within school nursing (9, 20, 21, 33, 58). Other investigators are demonstrating the value and effectiveness of school nursing efforts in various aspects of the school program (8, 14, 41). In keeping with the current emphasis on cost-effectiveness in all health services, the costs of school nursing services to children are being compared with costs of providing similar services in the community.

Other studies are undertaken to identify specific health needs of children, to better understand particular clinical conditions, and to determine the knowledge and motivation of students.

REFERENCES

1. Allanson, J. "Comprehensive School Health Education: Maltese Chicken or Phoenix." *Journal of School Health,* October 1981, 556–59.
2. American Academy of Pediatrics. *School Health: A Guide for Health Professionals.* Evanston, Ill.: American Academy of Pediatrics, 1977.
3. American Nurses' Association. *Facts About Nursing, 1980–81.* New York: American Nurses' Association, 1981.
4. American Nurses' Association. *Standards for School Nursing Practice.* Kansas City, Mo.: American Nurses' Association, 1983.
5. Anderson, C. L., and W. H. Creswell. *School Health Practice.* St. Louis: C. V. Mosby, 1980.
6. Basco, et al. "Epidemiological Analysis of School Population as a Basis for Change in School Nursing Practice." *Journal of School Health,* April 1972, 491.
7. Blain, G., and M. Brusko. "Starting a Peer Counseling Program in the High School." *Journal of School Health,* March 1985, 116–19.
8. Blazek, B., and M. S. McClelland. "The Effects of Self-Care Instruction on Locus of Control in Children." *Journal of School Health,* September 1985, 554–56.
9. Brink, S. G., S. Dale, M. C. Williamson, and P. R. Nader. "Nurses and Nurse Practitioners in Schools." *Journal of School Health,* January 1981, 7–10.
10. Buscaglia, L. *The Disabled and Their Parents: A Counseling Challenge.* Thorofare, N.J.: Charles B. Slack, 1975.
11. Buser, B. N. "The Evolution of School Health Services: New York and Nationwide." *Journal of School Health,* October 1980.
12. Castle, A. S., and S. J. Jerrick. "School Health in America: A Survey of State School Programs." Kent, Ohio: American School Health Association, 1976.
13. Cook, D. E. "The Role of Primary Health Care in the Schools." *Journal of School Health,* March 1979, 183–84.

14. De Angelis, C., B. Beeman, D. Oda, and R. Meeker. "The Comparative Values of School Physical Examinations and Mass Screening Tests." *Journal of Pediatrics* 102 (1983): 477–81.

15. Downs, F. S. "Schools: A Setting for Nursing Practice." Chapter in *Health Policy and Nursing Practice,* ed. Linda Aiken. New York: McGraw-Hill, 1981, 64–70.

16. Dunn, J. D. "A Nursing Care Plan for the Handicapped Student." *Journal of School Health,* September 1984, 302–05.

17. Eisner, V., and A. Oglesby. "Health Assessment of School Children II: Screening Tests." *Journal of School Health* 41 (7): 344–46.

18. Frankenburg, W. K. "Selection of Diseases and Tests in Pediatric Screening." *Pediatrics* 54 (1974): 608–11.

19. Frels, L. "National Survey—School Nurse Certification." *Journal of School Health,* June 1974, 340.

20. Goodwin, L. D. "The Effectiveness of School Nurse Practitioners: A Review of the Literature." *Journal of School Health* 51 (1981): 623–24.

21. Goodwin, L. D., J. B. Igoe, and A. N. Smith. "An Evaluation of the School Nurse Achievement Program: A Follow-up Survey of School Nurses." *Journal of School Health,* December 1984, 335–38.

22. Hardt, D. V. "Health Curriculum: 370 Topics." *Journal of School Health* 48 (1978): 656–60.

23. Hill, P. M., and L. S. Romm. "Screening for Scoliosis in Adolescents." *Maternal Child Nursing* 2 (3): 156–59.

24. Igoe, J. B. "Changing Patterns in School Health and School Nursing." *Nursing Outlook* 28 (1980): 486–91.

25. Igoe, J. B. "The School Nurse Practitioner." *Nursing Outlook,* June 1975.

26. Igoe, J. B. "School-Based Health Services." *Journal of School Health,* May 1979, 291–92.

27. Igoe, J. B. "What Is School Nursing? A Plea for Nurse Standardized Roles." *Maternal Child Nursing,* September 1980, 307–11.

28. Johansen, S., and J. Orthoefer. "Development of a School Health Information System." *American Journal of Public Health* 65:1203.

29. Joint Statement of the American Nurses' Association and the American School Health Association. "Recommendations of the Educational Preparation and Definitions of the Expanded Role and Functions of the School Nurse Practitioner." *Journal of School Health,* November 1973.

30. Kohn, M. A., et al. "School Health Services and Nurse Practitioners: A Survey of State Laws." Washington, D.C.: Center for Law and Policy Studies, 1979.

31. Lessler, K. "Screening, Screening Programs and the Pediatrician." *Pediatrics* 54 (1974): 512–16.

32. Lewis, M. A. "Child-Initiated Care." *American Journal of Nursing,* April 1974, 652–55.

33. McAtee, P. A. "Nurse Practitioners in Our Public Schools? An Assessment of Their Expanded Role as Compared with School Nurses." *Clinical Pediatrics* 13 (1974): 360–62.

34. McGinnis, J. M. "Health Problems of Children and Youth: A Challenge for Schools." *Health Education Quarterly* 8, no. 1 (Spring 1981).

35. McKenzie, J. F., and I. C. Williams. "Are Your Students Learning in a Safe Environment?" *Journal of School Health,* May 1982, 284–85.

36. Mullen, P. D. "Children as a National Priority: Closing the Gap Between Knowledge and Policy." *Health Education Quarterly* 8, no. 1 (Spring 1981).

37. Newton, J. "Primary Health Care in a School Setting." *Journal of School Health,* January 1979, 54.

38. North, A. F. "Screening in Child Health Care: Where Are We Now and Where Are We Going?" *Pediatrics for the Clinician* 54 (1974): 631–39.

39. Oda, D. S. "A Viewpoint on School Nursing." *American Journal of Nursing,* September 1981, 1677–78.

40. Oda, D. S. "School Health Services: Growth Potential for Nursing." Chapter in *Nursing in the 1980's: Crisis, Opportunities, Challenges,* ed. Linda Aiken. Philadelphia: J. B. Lippincott, 1982.

41. Perkin, J. "Evaluating a Nutrition Education Program for Pregnant Teen-Agers: Cognitive vs. Behavioral Outcomes." *Journal of School Health,* July 1983, 420–22.

42. *Project Health P.A.C.T.* Denver: University of Colorado School Nurse Practitioner Program, Health Sciences Center, 1980.

43. Regen, P. "A Historical Study of the School Nurse Role." *Journal of School Health* 46 (1976): 518.

44. Robert Wood Johnson Foundation. *School Health Services,* Special Report No. 1. Princeton, N.J.: Robert Wood Johnson Foundation, 1979.

45. Robinson, T. "School Nurse Practitioners on the Job." *American Journal of Nursing,* September 1981, 1674–76.

46. Rodgers, B. M., et al. "Depression in the Chronically Ill or Handicapped School-Aged Child." *Maternal Child Nursing,* July–August 1981, 266–73.

47. Safford, P. L. "Mental Health Counseling Dimensions of Special Education Programs." *Journal of School Health* 48 (1978): 541–47.

48. Sells, C. J., and E. A. May. "Scoliosis Screening in Public Schools." *American Journal of Nursing* 74, no. 1 (1974): 60–62.

49. Silver, G. A. "Redefining School Health Services: Comprehensive Child Health Care as the Framework." *Journal of School Health,* November 1981, 159.

50. Silver, H. K., J. B. Igoe, and P. R. McAtee. "School Nurse Practitioners: A Concise Description of Their Functions and Activities." *Journal of School Health,* December 1977.

51. Sinacore, J. S. "Priorities in Health Education." *Journal of School Health* 48, no. 4 (1978): 213–17.

52. Stember, M. L. "Nursing Role in School Health." Chapter in *Community Health Nursing: Keeping the Public Healthy,* ed. L. L. Jarvis, F. A. Davis, and P. Condon. Philadelphia: Davis, 1981, 141–71.

53. Stobo, E. C. "Trends in the Preparation and Qualifica-

tions of the School Nurse." *American Journal of Public Health* 50 (1969): 669.

54. Thorne, B. P. "A Nurse Helps Prevent Sports Injuries." *Maternal Child Nursing,* July–August 1982, 236.

55. Tuthill et al. "Evaluating a School Health Program Focused on High Absence Pupils: A Research Design." *American Journal of Public Health* 62 (1972): 40.

56. U.S. Department of Health, Education, and Welfare. *Healthy People: The Surgeon General's Report on Health Promotion and Disease Prevention.* Washington, D.C.: Government Printing Office, No. 79–55071, 1979.

57. U.S. Department of Health and Human Services. *Promoting Health/Preventing Disease: Objectives for the Nation.* Washington, D.C.: Government Printing Office, Fall 1980.

58. White, D. H. "A Study of Current School Nurse Practice Activities." *Journal of School Health,* February 1985, 52–56.

59. Withrow, C. "The School Nurse Takes a Look at Her Charges." *Nursing 79,* January 1979, 48–51.

60. Wold, S. J. *School Nursing: A Framework for Practice.* St. Louis: C. V. Mosby, 1981.

C H A P T E R 1 3

Occupational Health

PATRICIA MOCCIA

•

OBJECTIVES

After completing this chapter, the reader will be able to:

- Discuss the health needs of an extended labor force.
- Discuss appropriate services offered by the professional nurse in an occupational environment.
- Discuss various roles for professional nursing practice within occupational environments.
- Discuss the incidence and prevalence of occupationally related illnesses and injuries.
- List a chronology of legislation significant to occupational health and safety.
- Discuss the impact of the Occupational Safety and Health Act of 1970.
- Analyze the effects of governmental policy on the health of an extended labor force.

- Identify the different services offered by industrial hygienists, occupational physicians, toxicologists, and safety professionals.
- Analyze the interrelationships on the interdisciplinary occupational health and safety team.
- Discuss occupational health nursing as a coordinating point of the interdisciplinary health team.
- Identify common social forces that influence occupational health nursing.
- Identify common legal-political forces that influence occupational health nursing.
- Locate literature appropriate as resource material for the occupational health nurse.

Occupational health nursing is community health nursing when the community is the workplace and the client population is the labor force. Professional nurses work with men and women in varied occupational settings, ranging from coal mines to the National Aeronautics and Space Administration's space centers. Between these two extremes, people work in forests and fisheries, and in mining and construction, manufacturing, transportation, communications, public utilities, wholesale and retail trades, finance, insurance and real estate, and the government (2). In addition, this labor force can be "extended" to include such non-wage earners as homemakers, who physically and emotionally care for and socialize the nation's workers, and the unemployed, whose existence and numbers influence the expectations and behavior of the employed.

The American Association of Occupational Health Nurses defines occupational health nursing as "the application of nursing principles in conserving the health of workers in all occupations. It involves prevention, recognition and treatment of illness and injury and requires special skills and knowledge in the field of health education and counselling, environmental health, rehabilitation, and human relations" (12, p. 3). Occupational health nurses, relying heavily on epidemiology, fulfill their responsibilities by (a) direct care to the extended labor force and (b) health planning for the working population as a whole.

Professional nurses practicing within occupational settings deliver services similar to those delivered by nurses in other settings. They act as consumer advocates by educating workers about their health and the most appropriate and effective ways of promoting and protecting it; they plan for and administer health services and represent workers on interdisciplinary management teams. Occupational health nurses research general nursing concerns and take part in multidiscipline research specific to occupational health and safety, for example, the interactions between carcinogenic environmental factors and the health potentials of workers, or the influence of such inherent job characteristics as stress on the overall health status of workers and their families, or the health needs of the families of injured

or deceased workers, or the health needs of the larger community facing plant layoffs or closings.

Need for Nursing Services

The physical environment of the workplace is potentially more hostile than other communities. In 1982, 11,100 workers were killed on the job and 19 million suffered disabling injuries (18, No. 732, p. 442). There can be only the roughest of estimates as to the millions of workers who will suffer the long-term adverse effects of having been exposed to toxic substances in the course of their work (17, pp. 3–11).

Perhaps more than any other setting, the workplace, with its emphasis on performance and productivity and its predominantly healthy adult population, seems ideal for nursing self-care models and an emphasis on higher-order needs of self-actualization, self-responsibility, and affiliation. However, in addition to the concrete environmental hazards, workers are susceptible to the stress and increasing alienation that is correlated with the fragmented labor process that characterizes the contemporary workplace (8). The health risks of stress and alienation, especially to the cardiovascular system, have been well documented (17, p. 79).

Few would deny that workers have health needs specific to their place and type of employment, or that workers have health needs similar to those of the general population. But whether or not the "extended labor force" has access to the nursing expertise it needs is not as indisputable. Questions of workers' access, the nature and quality of health services, and the responsibilities for safe and healthy workplaces are part of the basic challenge for occupational health nurses.

Business Versus Health: A Basic Conflict

Resolving a basic, perhaps inherent conflict between the health of the extended labor force and the health of business is the challenge to occupational health nurses that provides the productive tension for their practice. The basic differences between business and health care will be problematic unless they are acknowledged, respected, and addressed at each step of the nursing process. Once addressed, however, the differences have at least a potential as a resource in health planning.

Extremely simplified and condensed—the purpose of business is to produce goods or services, and management, by definition, is responsible for using available resources efficiently and effectively toward that end. Workers are but one of these resources to be used, channeled, and managed in the process of production. As means to an end, workers are valued to the extent that they contribute to the process. Any management concern for workers beyond their immediate productivity is a function of (a) whether or not management recognizes workers as an essential, and not merely a necessary, resource; (b) whether or not a relationship between workers' health and productivity has been demonstrated to management's satisfaction; (c) whether or not management espouses a moral philosophy of some collective good or social responsibility; or (d) philanthropy.

In contrast, health care professionals are in the business of health, wherein workers—and their health—are not the means, but are themselves an end. Energies that would be dissipated in a confusion over means and ends, or in a debate on different value systems are directed into more productive activities by occupational health nurses, who reframe their concerns for workers' health into quantitative measures that reflect management's interests. So, for example, the occupational health nurse might identify the potential benefits of health promotion programs in terms of an increased productivity resulting from (a) a reduction in absenteeism that increases the total output, or (b) a conservation of operating costs through increasing the productivity for the amount of resources (human) used, or (c) improved morale, or (d) an overall improvement in the quality of the staff or their performance abilities (13, pp. 11–12).

Occupational Health Nursing: Theory and Practice

As with other professional challenges, those met by occupational health nurses are best approached from a scientifically based practice. In developing the knowledge base for their practice, occupational health nurses can comfortably use the four common elements from the conceptual systems that currently frame the theories underlying all professional practice: person, health, environment, and nursing (25, pp. 17–25). The first step is to identify, within each component, the similarities and differences between the general population and the specific community of workers.

Occupational health nurses must be knowledgeable about the health needs of adults, families, and communities, the meaning and value of work, the social dynamics of the working situation, and the epidemiology of occupationally related illnesses and injuries. They also need to know the constituent elements of specific occupational environments, the expected interactions of those elements and the workers, what interactions maximize health and reduce disease. In addition, they need specific knowledge and certain skills as they face the conflicts between business and health (see Table 13.1).

Person

Workers are, first of all, people and are, therefore, in continuous interaction with their environment, growing and developing as holistic beings, manifesting a complex of biological, psychological, social, and spiritual needs. This is a common statement, generally accepted by nurses in the more usual health care settings. Yet even there, where the medical model predominates, it often places nurses in the minority. There are, however, other nurses in health care settings to offer some degree of consensual validation.

But occupational health nurses, more often than not, find themselves alone, working with other professionals, managements, unions, and workers themselves, who usually have a more focused, less comprehensive understanding of people. In the context of the workplace, a person is either a human resource to be allocated and managed or a source of labor power to be used in the production of goods or services. The pervasiveness of the dehumanizing effects of such a value system makes a reaffirmation and articulation of people's holistic nature necessary for occupational health nurses.

Demographics

The Nation's Labor Force.   In the United States in 1984, 113.5 million persons, 64.4 percent of the population of 238.8 million, were workers (18, No. 624, p. 375). That year 50.8 percent of all workers were between ages twenty-five and forty-four and of these 49.5 percent were women. There were more than 12 million

Table 13.1
Comparison of Nursing Knowledge and Skills

Common to All Professional Nursing	Unique to Occupational Health Nursing
1. Nursing models	1. Epidemiology
2. Nursing research findings	2. Industrial sociology
3. Nursing philosophies	3. Organizational behavior
a. Caring	4. Management theories
b. Self-care	5. Business administration
4. Human behavior	6. Management-labor relations
a. Growth and development	7. History of occupational safety and health
b. Hierarchy of needs	8. Legislation
c. Motivation	9. Philosophy of occupational health nursing
d. Group dynamics	10. Occupationally related diseases and injuries
e. Change	11. Principles of industrial hygiene
5. Health	12. Safety principles
a. Community health	13. Principles of ergonomics
b. Primary care	14. Principles of toxicology
c. Rehabilitation	15. Skills
6. Health education	a. Policy development
a. Principles of teaching-learning	b. Collaboration
b. Teaching methods	c. Conflict resolution
7. Skills	d. Budget preparation
a. Communication	e. Consultation
b. Data collection	
c. Assessment	
d. Program planning	
e. Program evaluation	
f. Counseling	
g. Crisis intervention	
1. First aid	
2. Psychiatric emergencies	
3. Acute intoxication	
4. Disaster control	

combination of both; young adults will be choosing support networks or reference groups, deciding whether or not to form new family units and how such units will be organized. Workers in middle adulthood will be working through issues related to their own generativity, parenting, aging parents, the death of parents, the loss of youth, either career successes, failures, or plateaus. Half of these workers will be carrying the stress of societal expectations that as women, they will simultaneously maintain homes and families. Workers approaching late adulthood must integrate the realities of retirement, what being "old" in America means, the nearness of mortality (6, pp. 46–55).

Employee Profile. An employee profile is a systematic collection of specific information about the labor force in a particular occupational setting, including data about the significant external relationships of the workers. It is more focused, with a greater degree of specificity than general demographics, and identifies the unique aspects of the particular community of workers. It establishes the baseline for any nursing assessment.

At a minimum, an employee profile includes the following information:

- Number and distribution of employees by age, sex, race, and religion
- Educational levels and their distribution
- Number of employees with sole and shared parental responsibilities
- Type of domestic arrangements for child care created by employees, and their distribution according to sex
- Number of employees on full- and part-time status
- Number and distribution of employees working in areas statistically identified as high risk
- Supply and demand of similarly skilled workers within physical distances that can be traveled on a daily basis
- Supply and demand of employees in similar industries on a regional and national basis

The last two items are included as objective indicators of the value of the work to the employees and the value of the employee to the employer.

Health

From a Nursing Model. Whichever of its various definitions nurses use, health is considered a multidimensional process of community and individual activities directed toward fulfilling biological, psychological, social,

black workers, and close to 10 million Hispanic workers (18, pp. 5, 392, 396).

In general, the infamous baby boom will continue to strongly influence the policies and treatment priorities in occupational health, as will the diverse cultural norms and educational levels. Occupational health nurses can expect to work with people facing a range of developmental tasks who are likely to need education and support as they make their choices. Workers who are in late adolescence will be planning careers and deciding between work and school, or opting for some and cultural needs. The health status of the worker community and individual workers is determined by occupational health nurses making comparisons, based on both their general and specialized nursing knowledge, of presenting data with expected norms.

Necessary information includes mortality and morbidity rates, the leading causes of each, the degree of limited activity, and the age, race, and sex distribution of each (see Tables 13.2 and 13.3). Although these rates would be most helpful if they were collected for each occupation, such information is generally unavailable from government sources. For this data the occupational health nurse will have to look to other groups. Often the unions that represent specific crafts or industries will have collected it, or citizen activist groups, such as Committees for Occupational Safety and Health, the Black Lung Associations, and White Lung Associations.

Despite these limits, nurses have a considerable base from which to draw. If, for example, most of the workers in a business are between forty and sixty years old, the occupational health nurse would expect the business to be extremely concerned with its employees' productivity as workers, citizens, and social beings, and whether their "work ethic" varies, depending on whether they are blue collar or white collar (6, p. 47). Within this age-group, chronic illnesses are more common as certain biological systems become inefficient; there are musculoskeletal changes and alterations in biological rhythms, corollary changes in life-styles and activities of daily living, and a range of developmental tasks to be completed (6, p. 48).

Such a comprehensive view of health, however, puts nurses in conflict with medicine, which, despite its limited focus on the absence of illness and disease, is supposedly also concerned with health. There is also a potential conflict with employers, who, given their obvious legitimate concerns, define healthy as "being able to work." These conflicts of definitions and expectations must be resolved by occupational health nurses at both the policy level and the program level if they are to promote the overall health of workers.

From a Medical Model. The general differences between nursing and medicine as to how health is defined and what, therefore, constitutes health care are specifically demonstrated in occupational settings. Here, medicine's domination has been, until recently, reinforced by management policies that value workers in proportion to their abilities to produce goods or services. The collaboration between medicine and management developed naturally as occupational physicians who concentrated their practices on, and in some cases limited them to, the control of occupationally related illnesses or injuries thereby established the absence of either condition as evidence that a worker was "healthy," and therefore able to work.

The Physical Examination. Under the misleading name of health programs or health assessments, physicians do prescreening physicals to determine whether or not people are able to work, placement physicals to determine where they might work most efficiently, periodic assessments, monitoring and reevaluations on the worker's return from illness or accident in order to determine the ongoing compatibility between worker and job (10, pp. 23–27). Their findings are, in fact, categorized into classes 1 through 5, depending on how physically fit "for work" the employee is (7, p. 82). The clinical tests and measurements that are part of such assessments include audiometric and vision testing,

Table 13.2
Civilian Labor Force Distribution, 1984

Sex	Age (%)						
	16–19	20–24	25–34	35–44	45–54	55–64	65+
Total	7.0	14.1	28.8	22.0	15.0	10.5	2.6
Men	6.5	13.5	29.0	22.0	15.3	11.0	2.7
Women	7.7	15.0	28.6	21.9	14.5	9.9	2.4

Source: U.S. Bureau of the Census, *Statistical Abstract of the United States: 1986.* 106th ed. Washington, D.C., 1985, p. 392.

Table 13.3
Activity Limitation by Chronic Conditions, 1982

Condition	Persons Affected (%)
Heart disease	16.8
Arthritis and rheumatism	18.9
Hypertension	12.1
Impairment of back and spine	9.6
Impairment of lower extremities	8.8
Total: 32.4 million persons	
14.3%—some activity limitations	
9.9%—limitations in major activity	

Source: U.S. Bureau of the Census, *Statistical Abstracts of the United States: 1986.* 106th ed. Washington, D.C., 1985, p. 117.

specimen collection for biological monitoring, x-rays, and pulmonary and liver function studies (10, p. 27).

Within this medical model, nurses are too often distracted from health issues by expectations that they will assist the physicians in their work. In such cases the responsibilities of occupational health nurses include and may be limited to scheduling the doctors' appointments, keeping medical records, assisting in the physical examinations, performing some of the clinical tests, and planning referrals (10, p. 26).

Occupational Illness and Injury. The National Institute of Occupational Safety and Health (NIOSH) estimates that as many as 100,000 persons a year die of occupation-caused diseases (14, p. 111). According to the 1972 President's Report on Occupational Safety and Health, at least 390,000 new cases of occupational diseases are diagnosed each year (14, p. 128), and results of another federal study indicate that between 20 percent and 40 percent of cancer deaths are caused by on-the-job exposure (24).

Furthermore, it is generally agreed that any of these and other statistics for occupationally related diseases are greatly underestimated because of several factors (17, pp. 5–7). The primary reason lies in the nature of the environmental hazards and the nature of the illnesses; because most toxic exposure is of low levels and the onset of symptoms is slow and insidious, the relationship between an occupational history (see Figure 13.1) and any presenting problem is often unnoticed or unacknowledged. In addition, too few health professionals are educated to recognize and treat the relation-

ships between health and work, despite the fact that the relationships had been identified as early as the 1700s in the work of the Italian physician Bernardino Ramazzini (15). But in the early 1970s there were, at most, 20,000 occupational health nurses and only an estimated 8,000 occupational physicians for more than 112 million workers (4, p. 439).

Because acute injuries are obvious events, there is little dispute about their incidence. The most common injuries suffered by workers are burns, trauma, chemical intoxication, electrical shock, cuts, bruises, sprains, broken bones, and traumatic loss of limbs, eyesight, and hearing (10, p. 20). Nonetheless there is debate about (a) where the responsibilities for injuries lie—with unsafe practices and mistakes by the injured worker or with unsafe working conditions as maintained by the employer—and (b) who is the final authority on determining the extent and duration of the resultant disabilities—the occupational physician or the worker.

From a Worker Model. Despite the disagreements among professionals, the workers themselves are remarkably clear on the ill effects of their work. Coal miners, for example, have long recognized that "miner's asthma" or "black lung" is part of their jobs. The families of firefighters can tell whether or not that day's fires were bad ones from the amount of coughing and spitting afterward, the visible eye irritation, the impaired hearing, or the color of the sputum on handkerchiefs. (Once gray or sooty, the sputum of firefighters now displays a rainbowed reflection of the innumerable chemicals and plastic materials, known and unknown, that burn in any modern fire.) And the debilitating and harmful effects of the stress of most jobs has always been acknowledged by family members who exhort one another "not to bother Daddy (or Mommy). He (or she) has had a rough day at the office (or in the hospital, in the store, at the plant, etc.)."

This particular conflict is over who has the right to define health and illness. In the case of a respiratory disease like pneumoconiosis, for example, will the decision as to who is sick and who is well be made by a physician or the afflicted worker? When both agree, the question is moot, but a disagreement illustrates issues of power, legitimacy, and responsibility. Concerned with making a correct clinical diagnosis, medical doctors look to the germ theory and Koch's postulates, x-rays, and a series of clinical trials, including pulmonary function tests. Regardless of whether or not the physician diagnoses pneumoconiosis, the worker, without benefit of science, can tell how difficult breathing has a negative effect on

PATIENT ENVIRONMENTAL/OCCUPATIONAL HISTORY FORM

Date Taken: _____ **Patient Name:** _____

1. WORKPLACE

Current Work (i.e. carpenter, housewife, police officer, etc.)

_____

Name and address of company or employer (if any) _____

_____

How long at this job? _____

General description of work _____

_____

Any contact with dusts, fumes, vapors, gases, chemicals, radiation, pressure, excessive noise, vibration, temperature extremes?

_____

Any adverse effects noted? (Describe) _____

_____

Previous Work	Years	Description of Work	Exposures
First regular job			
Next regular job			
Next regular job			
Next regular job			
Next regular job			
Vacation jobs			
"Second" jobs			
Temporary work			
Work in military services			

2. HOME AND COMMUNITY

Are there any conditions in your home which you think may affect your health (use of aerosol sprays, chemicals or cleaning agents, recent reconstruction, etc.?

_____

_____

Does anyone in family work in a trade where hazardous materials could have been brought home (i.e., asbestos, lead, beryllium, vinyl chloride, etc.)?

_____

_____

Did you ever live near a plant, shipyard, mine, chemical (petroleum) factory, dumpsite?

_____

Did you ever live near a busy highway, street or gas station? _____

Hobbies involving adverse exposures: (furniture refinishing, arts and crafts, etc.):

_____

_____

3. CIGARETTES:

Ever smoke? _____. If yes, age started _____. On average, number/day _____.

Current smoking, number/day _____. If stopped, how long _____.

Cigars/pipe:

Ever smoke? _____. Current smoking, amount _____. If stopped, how long? _____.

4. COMMENTS:

_____

_____

Figure 13.1. Occupational History Form

Source: Adapted from the form used at Mount Sinai Hospital, New York City.

work, family life, sexual relations, involvement with communities, and activities of daily living.

In such a disagreement, or in any variation of it, the position of the occupational health nurse is clear. First, avoid being drawn into the debate or attempting to resolve it; it is a direct issue between the physician and the worker. Second, the worker's experience of the situation is the only legitimate starting point for the nurse. Third, resolving the disagreement or reducing its impact should be considered as one of several other tasks facing the worker and as such a means to health.

Environment

In understanding workers and their health and in planning and developing appropriate nursing services in the occupational setting, the nurse must be knowledgeable about certain characteristics of the environment, including (a) the physical environment, (b) the organizational relationships between management and labor, (c) legal and political factors, (d) community resources, and (e) the social and cultural norms of work, its values and ethics.

Physical Environment. Our nation's workplaces have changed dramatically since the first occupational health nurses cared for ailing Pennsylvanian coal miners and their families and the employees of Vermont marble companies in the late 1800s (1, p. 1). The early predominance of heavy industry has been gradually eroded over the past century until white-collar occupations and service industries are now characteristic. The growth has been among professional, managerial, and clerical workers, with a corresponding decrease in the blue-collar sector. Workers' health needs have undergone parallel changes from emergency first aid to protection from stress, chemical and radiation exposure, and substance abuse.

Health Hazards. Despite the medical arguments regarding the existence, nature, and extent of occupationally related diseases, there is a general consensus in the health community on the existence of certain elements in the occupational environment that are potentially harmful to workers, their families, and their communities. Health hazards are generally classified into four categories: physical, chemical, biological, and stress. Physical hazards commonly include noise, heat, vibrations, and radiation. Common chemical hazards include dust, poisonous gases and fumes, toxic metals, and carcinogens. Biological hazards include bacteria, fungi, and insects. And the hazards of stress include certain

physical chemical, ergonomic, and psychological characteristics of the environment (4, p. 73).

Interdisciplinary Collaboration. Occupational environments are most appropriately evaluated and monitored by the industrial hygienists and safety engineers with whom occupational health nurses collaborate in order to provide workers with a safe and healthy workplace. Nurses bring their unique and critically important understanding of people and their health needs to the interdisciplinary health team, where the hygienists and engineers share their specific expertise on the work environment. The difference is one of focus. Whereas nurses are expert in human behavior, the industrial hygienist and the safety engineer are expert in the environment.

Industrial hygienists (a) identify, through "walk-arounds," "walk throughs," and other survey methods, those environmental factors that threaten workers' health; (b) assess, through sampling and other means, the extent and degree of these factors; (c) either change the environment through substituting a less toxic substance, isolating the hazard with engineering controls, installing a different ventilation system, or, as a last resort, change the interaction between the environment and the worker by instituting the use of personal protective equipment (7, pp. 33–40). Safety professionals are concerned with designing a work environment that will keep accidents and loss-producing conditions to a minimum (3). Together with occupational physicians and toxicologists, the industrial hygienists and the safety personnel join occupational health nurses in collaboration that promotes a safe and healthy physical environment.

Organizational Relationship Between Management and Labor. In an economic system such as ours, management's goals are logically to maximize profits while minimizing costs. Workers are just as logically interested in maximizing wages and benefits. Because a gain for either management or labor must come from a loss of the other, the relationship is inherently adversarial. New ways of balancing both agendas and keeping both sides comparatively satisfied are always being sought.

One alternative chosen by many workers has been to form or join labor unions for the purpose of collective bargaining. Today more than 20 million American workers are unionized, although the proportion of the labor force that belongs to any labor organization is declining (see Table 13.4). Despite the decline, the potential strength of organized workers continues, as evidenced by the considerable amount of time and money spent by companies to hire "union-busting" consultants

Table 13.4
Labor Union Membership, 1950–1980

	1950	1955	1960	1965	1970	1974	1978
Number of unions	209	199	184	191	185	175	174
Total membership (× 1,000)	15,000	17,749	18,117	18,519	20,752	21,643	21,784
Percentage of total labor force	22.0	24.4	23.6	22.4	22.6	21.7	19.7

Source: U.S. Bureau of the Census, *Statistical Abstracts of the United States: 1982–83.* 103rd ed. Washington, D.C., 1982, p. 408.

in order to keep themselves union-free. (See popular handbooks and strategy manuals such as G. E. Jackson, *When Labor Trouble Strikes: An Action Handbook* [Englewood Cliffs, N.J., Prentice-Hall, 1981].)

Both management and labor are investigating newer models for humanizing the workplace and increasing productivity. American industry is drawing on international experiences and adapting Japanese labor-management theories (11), codetermination models from western Europe, and a wide range of work reform programs based on models of "participative management" (9, pp. 164–324). Theoretically, both unions and these models allow workers opportunities for becoming healthier. Each is a means for meeting affiliation needs and assuming more responsibility for one's interactions with the environment, in this case the working environment. As such, they merit the attention of occupational health nurses.

Legal and Political Factors. The occupational health nurse advocating for workers' health has strong support from the Occupational Safety and Health Act of 1970 (OSHAct), whose passage is commonly attributed to the political influence of organized labor and the citizen movements of the 1960s (4, p. 4). The OSHAct was passed by a bipartisan Congress "to assure so far as possible every working man and woman in the Nation safe and healthful working conditions and to preserve our human resources" (21). Under the OSHAct, employers "must furnish . . . a place of employment which is free from recognized hazards that cause or are likely to cause death or serious physical harm to employees." The

OSHAct established the Occupational Safety and Health Administration (OSHA) within the Department of Labor for the purpose of developing, implementing, and enforcing health and safety standards. In situations where no specific standard has been set, employers are still legally responsible for the intent of the act.

In addition, the OSHAct created NIOSH as a separate federal agency within the Department of Health and Human Services. NIOSH's responsibilities include both field and laboratory research in all aspects of job safety and health and making recommendations on standards to OSHA. NIOSH is also responsible for the Educational Resource Centers, which are regionally based, multidisciplinary educational programs that prepare specialist personnel, including occupational physicians, occupational health nurses, industrial hygienists, and safety professionals.

While the OSHAct was the first comprehensive governmental effort to protect the health rights of workers, it was preceded by a long list of equally significant legislation. Act by act the relationship between employer and employees has been defined according to (a) the general rights and responsibilities of each and (b) those specific to occupational safety and health (see Table 13.5). Together, this legislation provides a supportive context for the practice of occupational health nurses.

Deregulation and Voluntary Compliance. Some of the early promise of the OSHAct and the enthusiasm of occupational safety and health specialists have been checked by the severe budget cuts and the deregulation philosophy of the Reagan administration (1980–84). Under Assistant Secretary of Labor for Occupational

Table 13.5
Chronology of Legislation Relevant to Employer-Employee Relationship

Year	Legislation	Year	Legislation
1911	First *State Workman's Compensation Act* (New Jersey); allowed compensation for certain job-related injuries.	1947	*Taft-Hartley Act;* protected rights and detailed responsibilities of both employers and employees by defining "unfair labor practices."
1912	*Lloyd-LaFollette Act;* allowed federal employees the right to organize and lobby on their own behalf.	1959	*Landum-Griffins Act;* established rights and responsibilities of union leaders and union members.
1916	*Federal Employees Compensation Act;* compensated federal employees who were injured on the job.	1963	*Equal Pay Act;*
		1964	*Civil Rights Act;*
1920	*Immigration Acts;* controlled the supply and composition of the available labor force.	1972	*Equal Employment Opportunity Act;* together prohibited discrimination because of race, color, religion, sex, or national origin; in any term, condition, or privilege of employment.
1932	*Norris-LaGuardia Act;* restricted use of the strike injunction and prohibited "yellow dog" contracts.	1965	*McNamara-O'Hara Public Service Contract Act;* extended Walsh-Healey to cover suppliers of government services.
1935	*National Labor Relations Act (Wagner Act);* gave employees the right to organize and join unions for the purpose of collective bargaining. Established the National Labor Relations Board.	1969	*Federal Coal Mine Health and Safety Act;* established standards and provided for Black Lung Benefits Program.
1935	*Social Security Act;* ensured certain benefits, including (since 1965) health benefits, for population over sixty-five years old.	1970	*Occupational Safety and Health Act;* established the Occupational Safety and Health Administration within the Department of Labor and the National Institute of Occupational Safety and Health within the Department of Health, Education, and Welfare.
1936	*Walsh-Healey Public Contracts Act;* established safety and health standards for employers receiving government contracts over $10,000.		
1938	*Fair Labor Standards Act (Wage and Hour Act);* established minimum wage and abolished child labor.	1976	*Toxic Substance Control Act;* required testing and restrictions of certain chemical substances.

Safety and Health Thorne G. Auchter, a Reagan appointee with no history in occupational safety and health, OSHA redirected its attention—against the advice of most specialists—from inspection and enforcement to a systematic approach to "voluntary compliance" (22). The effects of this dramatic turnaround in policy on workers' health have yet to fully surface and, given the long-term effects of occupational exposures, the repercussions will be part of workers' lives and occupational health nursing for many years to come.

Community Resources. Another of the differences between health and medical models is the emphasis by health models on strengths and assets rather than on weaknesses and deficits. The health of workers is a function of many things, including the strengths, assets, and health of the general community.

Health Agencies. These include local health departments, community visiting nurses' associations, emergency medical services, trauma and burn units, preventive services and social medicine programs, voluntary health organizations (for example, the American Lung Association and American Red Cross).

Community and Public Interest Groups. In addition to religious and social organizations, the following special interest groups have strong consumer leadership and participation.

- Committee for Occupational Safety and Health (COSH): independent local organizations composed of trade unionists, workers, health and legal professionals, and educators working to provide technical support, educational programs, and preventive training

- Black Lung Association, White Lung Association, Brown Lung Association: workers and their families and friends organized to educate the general public; provide co-workers support, technical support, and legal assistance; and lobby, usually around specific occupations and diseases.
- Health PAC: an independent, not-for-profit public interest center concerned with monitoring and interpreting the health system. Health PAC (17 Murray Street, New York, N.Y. 10007) publishes reports and bulletins on occupational and environmental health issues.

Professional Groups

- American Association of Occupational Health Nurses: specialty organization with state and local chapters
- Nurses Environmental Health Watch: national organization with chapters in New York City and Austin, Texas; publishes the quarterly newsletter *Health Watch* for nurses and other health workers. The activities of the local chapters are focused on educational programs that "support, promote and conduct research in the areas of environmental concerns." (NEHW, 655 Avenue of the Americas, New York, N.Y. 10010)
- Women's Occupational Health Resource Center: works with women, trade unions, management, professionals, and government agencies on occupational safety and health issues specific to women. WOHRC, at the Columbia University School of Public Health, provides a research library and information center, technical assistance in setting up programs, and films, workshops, and courses. It also serves as a formal and informal clearinghouse for people and groups working in the field.
- Trade unions: many unions have a health and safety department that provides written materials, technical assistance, and educational programs.

Government Agencies. Both OSHA and NIOSH have regional offices that provide free assistance and information on occupational and environmental issues.

Social and Cultural Factors. Every business and industry exists within particular social environments that impact on the experiences of workers. Whether or not the industry is the "only job in town," for example, will influence workers' expectations, tolerance levels for unsatisfactory working conditions, and performance. In addition, all work in this country takes place, or does not take place, within a national social consciousness of innumerable issues. Some of the most pressing and potentially most significant issues for transforming the nation's work force include unemployment rates, an increasing poverty level and the collapse of the middle class, comparable worth, and the heightened consciousness and expectations of workers and the general citizenry.

Unemployment Rates. High unemployment rates continue to increase the value, for employed workers, of any job. In February 1984, 9.2 percent of white, 15.7 percent of Hispanic, and 20.7 percent of black workers were unemployed (20, pp. 149–56). With so many people out of work and looking for a job, those who are employed are constantly under the threat that they can easily be replaced. This factor alone intensifies the stress of any work and alters a worker's perception of his or her value and self-worth. In addition to these immediate effects, such high unemployment rates, especially among first-time and beginning workers and within black communities (see Table 13.6) will influence the future health status of workers and their communities.

Increased Poverty Levels. There are more poor people today, and they are poorer than before (37). The negative effects of poverty on individual and community health have been well documented. And few, if any, in the health community would not agree that any illness,

Table 13.6
Unemployment Rates by Race, Sex, and Age,
February 1984 (in percentages)

	White	Black	Hispanic
All workers	9.2	20.7	15.7
Men	9.6	22.0	ND
Women	8.8	19.3	ND
16–19 years old	21.1	51.4	ND
Men	22.6	53.7	ND
Women	19.7	52.2	ND
20 +	8.3	18.7	ND
Men	8.8	20.0	ND
Women	7.9	17.4	ND

ND = Not determined

Source: U.S. Department of Labor, Bureau of Labor Statistics. *Employment and Earnings,* February 1984, 149–56.

chronic condition, or injury is aggravated when one is poor.

Comparable Worth. This has been called the "issue of the '80s." If women are to be paid for their labor in wages comparable to what men are paid for similar and, in some cases, identical work, and if the grievances of the past are to be redressed, our economy will obviously have to be revolutionized. Were that to happen, changes in social relations and workers' experiences would follow.

Heightened Consciousness and Expectations. Workers have come to expect certain wages, benefits, and protection of their rights to safe and healthy working conditions. In addition, the social protests of the 1960s and 1970s and the grass-root citizen movements of the 1970s and 1980s have demonstrated a collective power to change unacceptable situations. Owing to these trends, the recent corporate attempts to have labor absorb the company's financial difficulties through "concessions" and "give-backs" of wages and benefits—including occupational health and safety programs—face a growing resistance. More and more workers are reacting in ways articulated by Machinists Union President William Winpisinger: "We in the trade union today do not have the right to give away gains and rights won yesterday. They are not ours to give away. They belong to our heritage and our progeny" (23).

Nursing

Nursing in occupational settings is similar to primary nursing practiced anywhere: it is a process, a commitment to action, and an interpersonal relationship (see chapter 1). Nursing's goals in occupational settings are derived from the profession's universal purposes—to promote health, encourage self-care, teach attitudes, and attend to human health needs—including the higher-order needs of self-actualization, self-responsibility, and affiliation. Occupational health nurses use the nursing process to identify (a) potential or actual changes in the health status of an extended work force and individual workers, (b) human and environmental factors that contribute to those changes, (c) internal and external resources for either reinforcing those factors that promote health or controlling, if not eliminating, those factors that threaten it. Their practice includes (a) working to establish conjoint relationships with workers through which both can advocate for and effect the necessary changes; (b) sharing the information and skills necessary for developing human health potentials with

worker communities; (c) coordinating services and assuring a continuity of care.

Informal and Formal Authority. Even more than usual, nursing in occupational settings is characterized by the possibilities for a fully autonomous, independent practice in which the nurse's authority and accountability are clear. But the realities of the nurse's role differ with each of the varied occupational health programs. Within a medically modeled program, nurses are likely to face the same conflicts of expectations and responsibilities that they encounter in the hospital as they work in one-nurse or multiple-nurse medical units.

Here nurses are expected—in order even to have access to workers—to assume such nonnursing tasks as medical screening and surveillance, environmental monitoring and control, record keeping, and periodic reporting to regulatory agencies. As in the hospital, professional nurses in such programs often "nurse" by "sneaking" such nursing practices as counseling and health teaching into other activities. In a NIOSH publication that discusses nursing responsibilities in a physical examination, for instance, one of the thirteen tasks listed is "use(s) every opportunity to teach good health practices" (10, p. 26). To the degree that they are successful in nursing in spite of the system, occupational health nurses are recognized by the workers as a resource and as an *informal* authority on health.

Occupational health nurses act as worker advocates when they use such authority to validate an individual worker's experience of diseases or to provide a group of workers with a consensual validation for their working experiences. By identifying recurring patterns of health and illness, nurses lend the weight of their professional opinions to workers' concerns. In the process, workers' complaints or problems become legitimate issues for management to address. In addition, advocacy activities can increase workers' self-care abilities if, in the planning and implementation of change, nurses help workers use their own skills in presenting health and safety concerns to management.

When management joins workers in acknowledging nurses' expertise in health and decides that workers' health should be incorporated into the company's goals and objectives, professional nurses are more likely to find themselves with *formal* authority. Whether functioning within a corporate structure, as a consultant, an administrator, or a manager of in-house health departments or health units, professional nurses assume responsibility for promoting the health of workers and that of their families and communities with health and wellness programs that incorporate the specific concerns of occupational health and safety.

Accountability and the Question of Confidentiality.   If the occupational health nurse learns something from the worker that concerns management, or something from management that concerns workers, where is allegiance due? As always, the nurse's direct accountability is to the consumer of services, whether the information is from management or workers. Tragic examples of misplaced accountability are found in the past policies of asbestos companies, where company managements, including, in some cases, medical and research staff, "fraudulently concealed" their information on the severe effects of asbestos exposure from the thousands of workers exposed (5). And although courts and state legislatures have since established that workers have a "right to know" about factors in their working conditions that have the potential to impact on their health (19), difficulties continue to present themselves to the nurse, since the rulings are neither universal nor uncontested.

On the other hand, when nurses identify more closely with workers, other ethical and practical decisions present themselves. For example, the nurse who is counseling a worker who has confided some problem *seemingly* unrelated to working conditions, although potentially affecting work performance, for instance, chemotherapy, must resolve several questions. Does management have a "right to know" about the health status of its employees? Can any interaction with a worker be therapeutic if a trust is betrayed? Should specific programs that count on confidentiality for their success, such as employee assistance programs, be undertaken unless it can be completely assured?

Because these professionally conflicting situations will recur, nurses can protect themselves from repeated individual dilemmas if they approach the issue on a policy level. Occupational health nurses must seek ways to shape or influence company policies so that they account for professional standards and a code of ethics. For while management might pay the nurse's salary, as does a hospital administration, both are brokering agents between the nurse and the client. Neither can assume nor interrupt the nurse's direct accountability to the client.

Collaboration and Coordination.   A change in company focus from occupational safety and health to health and wellness allows professional nurses the full range of an autonomous practice as they plan programs appropriate to workers' health needs and company and community resources (see Table 13.7). Depending on the particular health needs, the particular work environment, and the particular intervention plan, the occupational health nurse might initiate a collaborative effort that includes the usual members of an occupational safety and health team. Or if the needs are broader, the nurse might call in, for example, a health educator for smoking cessation programs, a nutritionist for weight control programs, a psychologist for alcohol or substance abuse, a nurse for stress reduction or blood pressure control, all of these, or any of many other specialists.

The professional nurse is the health care provider in occupational settings who, conceptually and practically,

Table 13.7
Common Occupational Health Programs

Wellness Oriented	Prevention Oriented
1. Stress reduction—both organizational and personal	1. Substance dependency—food, tobacco, alcohol, drug
2. Nutritional	2. Reproductive hazards—both men and women
3. Fitness	3. Vision conservation
4. Family health	4. Hearing conservation
5. Community health	5. Respiratory disease surveillance
6. Environmental health	6. Dermatitis control
7. Social affiliations	7. Immunizations
8. Political participation	8. Hypertension control
9. Retirement planning	
10. Cultural history	
11. Creative expressions	

is the logical coordinator of interdisciplinary activities. Conceptually, occupational health nurses have the necessary information on the *whole* picture; they know about the *person* who is experiencing, who is threatened by, or who is being protected from occupational disease or injury. Practically, the nurse is the provider who directly interacts with other disciplines and so provides a natural continuity for processing information. In addition, reality too often finds the nurse as the only professional available on a regular or full-time basis.

Future Directions

The history of occupational health nursing, once known as industrial nursing, found nurses in every conceivable workplace, responding to the pressing needs of workers for safe and healthy working conditions by developing a patchwork of skills through on-the-job training or education in other disciplines. Similar to hospital nurses' assuming responsibility for whatever needed to be done that no one else would do, the occupational health nurse became increasingly distracted from a primary responsibility—workers and their health needs. So, for a very common example, a nurse might return to the only occupational safety and health program available and accessible to nurses and become a safety specialist, rather than a nurse specialist. Or a nurse at a plant that was showing an abnormally high incidence of upper respiratory tract ailments among its workers would become an expert, through apprenticeship and self-instruction, at conducting "walk-throughs" and other surveys of the occupational environment.

This situation has dramatically changed for two major reasons. First, after a long struggle, nursing has secured its position as a distinct science and an autonomous profession. (Legislation in the form of nurse practice acts might still lag behind the reality, but that's more usual than not.) Nursing's full attention is turning more and more from arguing its legitimacy toward demonstrating it by testing, validating, and refining the theories underlying practice. As the knowledge base grows and practice expands, delivery of both nursing services and other professional and technical services becomes more difficult. With the real health needs of workers/clients becoming more complex and nursing practice, more comprehensive, there is simply not enough time to be "the nurse" and "the safety person" and "the person who does the surveys" and a physician's assistant and on and on.

Second, the nursing faculties in community health nursing programs and at NIOSH's Educational Resource Centers (ERCs) have made major contributions toward shaping new and future roles for the occupational health nurse. Working primarily with graduate students, nurse educators at ERCs, for example, at the University of Cincinnati, at the University of Minnesota, and at the University of North Carolina, have advanced the profession and the specialty by addressing occupational health and safety issues from nursing's conceptual systems. Along with other colleagues, they have responded to the challenges that all professional nurses face—how to develop a theoretically based nursing practice that is responsive and accountable to society's needs.

Building on the work of such pioneers as Mary Louise Brown, Jane Lee, and Edna May Klutas, and the expertise of occupational health nurses currently engaged in clinical practice, contemporary specialists are researching the relationships between people, their health, and the variable aspects of their working environments. From this combination of educators, researchers, and clinicians, occupational health nursing continues to grow and develop, anticipating and striving to meet the emerging health needs of our nation's workers.

REFERENCES

1. American Association of Industrial Nurses. *The Nurse in Industry. A History of the American Association of Nurses.* New York, 1976.
2. American Public Health Association. *Health and Workers in America: A Chartbook.* Washington, D.C.: American Public Health Association, 1975.
3. American Society of Safety Engineers. *Scope and Function of the Professional Safety Position.* Des Plaines, Illinois, 1972.
4. Ashford, N. A. *Crisis in the Workplace. Occupational Disease and Injury.* A Report to the Ford Foundation. Cambridge, Mass.: MIT Press, 1976.
5. Bale, T. "Breath of Death. The Asbestos Disaster Comes Home to Roost." *Health PAC Bulletin* 14 (3):7–21, 1983.
6. Billings, D. M., and L. G. Stokes. *Medical-Surgical Nursing. Common Health Problems of Adults and Children Across the Life Span.* St. Louis: C. V. Mosby, 1982.
7. Brown, M. L. *Occupational Health Nursing Principles and Practices.* New York: Springer, 1981.
8. Edwards, R. *Contested Terrain: The Transformation of the Workplace in the Twentieth Century.* New York: Basic Books, 1979.

9. Hunnuis, G., G. D. Garson, and J. Case, eds. *Workers' Control. A Reader on Labor and Social Change.* New York, Vintage Books, 1973.

10. Lee, J. A. *The New Nurse in Industry. A Guide for the Newly Employed Occupational Health Nurse.* Cincinnati: DHEW (NIOSH) Publication No. 78–143, 1978.

11. Main, J. "Westinghouse's Cultural Revolution." *Fortune,* June 15, 1981, 74–93.

12. National Institute of Occupational Safety and Health. *Occupational Health Nursing: Basic Theory and Update.* Cincinnati, 1980.

13. O'Donnell, M. P., and T. Ainsworth. *Health Promotion in the Workplace.* New York: John Wiley & Sons, 1984.

14. President's Report on Occupational Safety and Health. Document No. 2915-0011. Washington, D.C.: Government Printing Office, May 1972.

15. Ramazzini, B. *Diseases of Workers.* 1713. Reprint. New York: The New York Academy of Medicine, 1964.

16. "Slimmer Middle, Bigger Bottom. Reagan Rearranges Income Distribution." *Dollars and Sense,* April 1984, 1–5.

17. Stellman, J. M., and S. M. Daum. *Work Is Hazardous to Your Health.* New York: Random House, 1973.

18. U.S. Bureau of the Census. *Statistical Abstracts of the United States, 1986.* 106th ed. Washington, D.C.: U.S. Department of Commerce, 1985.

19. U.S. Department of Health, Education, and Welfare, Public Health Service. *Criteria for a Recommended Standard of Occupational Exposure.* Washington, D.C., 1972–present.

20. U.S. Department of Labor, Bureau of Labor Statistics. *Employment and Earnings,* February 1984.

21. U.S. Department of Labor, Occupational Safety and Health Administration. *All About OSHA.* Washington, D.C., 1981 (revised).

22. "Voluntary Programs to Supplement Enforcement and to Provide Safe and Healthful Working Conditions: Request for Comments and Information." *Federal Register* 47 (12):2796–801, 1982.

23. Winpisinger, M. W. "Foreword." In J. Slaughter, ed., *Concessions—and How to Beat Them.* Detroit, Labor Education and Research Project, 1983.

24. *Work in America.* Report of a Special Task Force to the Secretary of Health, Education, and Welfare. Cambridge, Mass.: MIT Press, 1973.

25. Yura, H., and G. Torres. *Today's Conceptual Framework Within Baccalaureate Nursing Programs.* NLN Publication No. 15-1558. New York: National League of Nursing, 1975.

CHAPTER 14

Home Care

MARILYN D. HARRIS

■

OBJECTIVES

After completing this chapter, the reader will be able to:

- □ List the components of a comprehensive home care program.
- □ Identify internal and external factors that affect the delivery of home health care services.
- □ Describe the levels of care that home care clients require.
- □ Describe the role of the nurse in home health care.

This chapter is an overview of home care. It is not all inclusive, nor does it deal with any one specific topic in detail.

The material in this chapter introduces the concept of home care; what it is, who provides it, what effect it has on the client and family, how it is documented and evaluated. The material also identifies some potential challenges that may be encountered in reaching established goals and examines the role of the primary nurse in arranging for and providing home care.

Home Care—Past and Present

They were dressed in identical dark blue uniforms with matching hats on their heads. In one hand each clutched a small black bag filled with first-aid equipment such as thermometers, sterile bandages, antiseptic, alcohol, ointments. They threaded their way in and out of pushcarts, through the noise and bustle until they came to Hester Street. There on the dirtiest and most crowded thoroughfare of the East Side, they caught sight of a young boy playing in the litter, who had an eye infection they considered so serious that it could result in blindness. They found out his address and set out to locate his flat knocking at every door in a building tenement at 7 Hester Street. As each door opened, they were assailed by the sour odors of rubbish-strewn rooms. They entered each home, gave an impromptu lecture on sanitation, and handed out advice. Where they found infants sick with diarrhea, a fatal malady in the hot summer months, they advised parents to buy uncontaminated milk and demonstrated the rudiments of receiving care. In one flat, they arranged for a child with measles to be admitted to a hospital. (34, p. 99)

Formal home care programs began in the United States in the late 1800s. The opening paragraph describes the activities of Lillian Wald, founder of the Henry Street Settlement House, and Mary Brewster, one of her nurses in 1893. These two nurses, along with other nurses who worked with them, established the basic principles of a Visiting Nurses Service (VNS) in New York City.

About this same time visiting nurse services were founded in other cities: Visiting Nurse Service of Philadelphia in 1886; the Instructive District Nursing Association of Boston in 1886; Chicago Visiting Nurse Association in 1889 (5, pp. 10–11; 10).

By the early 1900s an increasing number of communities had identified a need for in-home community nursing service. The minutes of the meetings of the board of directors and letters of one such association in the early 1920s show the extent of involvement in a myriad of health concerns: "sick visits, hospital and clinic visits; visits to homes of school children, social services visits, visits to schools" (44).

During the early 1900s most home care services were offered by voluntary community agencies. In 1908 Lillian Wald convinced the Metropolitan Life Insurance Company to set up a nursing program for industrial policyholders, using her Henry Street nurses to provide the service. The program was successful and led to an expansion of this type of nursing service.

A major change that affected home care services was the establishment of Medicare in 1965. This federal program made home health services available for people over age sixty-five and for those who are disabled. Since that time an increasing number of regulations have been issued that have impacted on the home health aspect of the Medicare benefit. At the same time that Medicare benefits for home care service were becoming more stringent, several changes were affecting the acute care setting, which in turn affected home care services.

The Tax Equity and Fiscal Responsibility Act of 1981 and the introduction of the diagnostic-related groups (DRGs) prospective payment system in the social security amendments of 1983 impacted on the length of stay and cost limits of acute care. As a result, some clients are discharged from the hospital at an earlier stage in the recovery period and may require a more intensive level of home care.

Table 14.1
Certified Home Health Agencies, August 1985

Type of Agency	Number
Voluntary nonprofit	525
Combination	56
Official	1,224
Rehabilitation facility-based	24
Hospital-based	1,116
Skilled nursing facility-based	139
Proprietary	1,811
Private nonprofit	795
Unclassified	8
	5,698

Source: National Association for Home Care, "Number and Type of Certified Home Health Agencies as of August 7, 1985," Report 135, August 19, 1985.

The number of outpatient surgical procedures being performed is on the rise. Some facilities that offer outpatient surgery arrange to have a home care nurse visit the client on the evening of surgery and the next morning. This nursing visit reassures the client and family and provides professional observations for the physician.

The Health Care Financing Administration (HCFA) reports that the number of Medicare beneficiaries receiving home health benefits has increased from 890,000 in 1980 to an estimated 1.3 million in 1984.

The National Association for Home Care (NAHC) data show that the number of Medicare-certified home health agencies increased from 2,864 in 1980 to an estimated 5,151 in 1984. The most dramatic increases have been in hospital-based and proprietary agencies (24). NAHC's "Report" (24) stated that, according to HCFA, there were 5,698 Medicare-certified home health agencies as of August 1985 (see Table 14.1).

As of September 1985, the following are some changes that are proposed for home care by the federal government: (a) freeze home health cost; (b) remove the Medicare waiver of liability presumption; (c) tighten eligibility; (d) change from aggregate to per discipline cost limits. "Industry and Consumer groups say the cumulative effect of the Administration's efforts will be disastrous for both providers and beneficiaries" (12).

Home health care has experienced many changes during the past 100 years. The financing of services, criteria for eligibility, levels of care required, and consumer involvement will affect the future of home care.

Home Care—What It Is

Home care—the providing of health care service to families at their place of residence—is a welcome option to institutional care for the young, the old, and everyone in between. Coordinated comprehensive and high-quality skilled and support services make it possible for young parents to bring home a newborn who needs a cardiac monitor, for a forty-year-old to receive care related to physical impairments resulting from multiple sclerosis or cancer, or for an eighty-five-year-old who has had a fractured hip to complete recovery at home.

People of all ages usually prefer to recuperate in familiar surroundings. The ability to enjoy family, friends, pets, favorite foods, familiar objects on a continuous basis, even though one is ill, is a valuable aspect of home care.

Components of a Comprehensive Home Care Program

Comprehensive home care includes a wide array of services. A brief description of each service follows.

Skilled nursing includes observation and evaluation, teaching and training clients and family members, supervision and direct care.

Physical therapy is initiated to help a client regain use of impaired muscles, increase joint motion, control pain, or regain the ability to perform activities of daily living.

Occupational therapy is appropriate when a client may have to relearn physical and general awareness skills. With instruction, and possibly an adaptive device, a person can become more independent.

Speech pathology helps the client regain the ability to communicate after an accident or illness or because of a learning disability.

Medical social service is indicated when clients find it difficult to cope with the emotional and social stresses of illness or an accident. Social workers may address housing, financial relief, family relationships, or environmental problems.

Home health aides assist clients to follow regimens prescribed by physicians, help with personal care, such as bathing, and perform light housekeeping tasks and errands.

Hospice involves a carefully developed program designed to relieve the physical, emotional, and spiritual pain of dying clients and their families. The hospice team includes nurses, physicians, clergy, volunteers, and social workers.

Nutritional support services include parenteral and enteral fluids and needed supplies.

Durable medical equipment, such as wheelchairs, hospital beds, and walkers, may be medically necessary and reasonable items for the treatment of illness or injury.

Laboratory studies, x-rays, and portable electrocardiograms are services that can be done in the home setting.

Supplies are essential to carry out the care the physician ordered. Examples are catheters, dressings, and intravenous solutions.

Transportation, either by family, automobile, or ambulance, is sometimes necessary to move a homebound client to a hospital or a physician's office for a specific reason.

Homemaker/attendant care services enable people to remain in their homes even though they need help on a short- or long-term basis. An attendant may visit for a half-hour to help a client get in or out of bed, or may stay for an extended period to help with household chores.

Volunteers may serve as friendly visitors or as members of the hospice team.

Chore services may include fixing a stair rail, installing an elevated toilet seat, or replacing a broken window.

Meals-on-Wheels organizations deliver meals (usually one hot and one cold) to homebound clients. Such organizations may be funded by community or government dollars.

Telephone reassurance services include a daily call at a predetermined time. If the person does not respond, a call is made to an emergency number to verify the client's status.

Additional services such as dental and eye care, pastoral counseling, or emergency alert systems may be available through home care agencies.

In home care it is important to know whether or not the client's physician will make home visits when office or clinic visits are no longer possible.

Pediatric home care is receiving increased attention (15, 22). Care can be provided for postpartum supervision, children in early intervention programs who need supplemental services, failure to thrive, delayed growth and development, high-risk infants (aborted sudden infant death syndrome), hospice care, hydrocephalus, burns, cardiomyopathy, and fractures.

The goal of pediatric home care is to help the child

and parents achieve an optimal level of health. Care includes monitoring the parents' level of comprehension and compliance with the prescribed regimens.

Levels of Care

The quality of a home care program and services depends on a qualified staff. Home care clients require different levels and types of care. Qualified personnel must provide various levels of care in accordance with the prescribed plan of treatments and the individual client's needs.

The *intensive level* of care requires active treatment or rehabilitation of unstable disease or injury. Without the availability and use of intensive home care service, the client would require inpatient care. Examples of clients who require this level of care are those who are ventilator-dependent and those with Hickman catheters.

The *intermediate level* of care is appropriate for clients who require treatment or rehabilitation of a relatively controlled disease or injury, for example, clients with fractures and those with cardiac monitors. Such clients do not require inpatient care.

The *maintenance level* of care is appropriate for persons who are relatively stable medically or have reached a plateau in their rehabilitation. They require assistance with activities of daily living or supportive personal care services. Examples of this level of care are clients who need a Foley (indwelling) catheter change on a monthly basis, or those who need a monthly injection of vitamin B_{12} for pernicious anemia.

Standards of Home Care

There are numerous standards that are applicable for home care agencies and personnel.

Agency Standards

Accreditation. The National League for Nursing (NLN) defines a standard as a specific level of achievement a provider must abide by in order to become accredited (27, 28). A criterion describes the value to be measured.

The NLN states that there are three major purposes of the criteria and standards of the accreditation program: (a) to assist a provider to develop, interpret, improve, and evaluate all aspects of its operation; (b) to provide the basis for accreditation decisions; (c) to assure consumers that the provider has met predetermined standards relative to quality control.

This accreditation process is voluntary for home health agencies. The accreditation decision is based on data contained in the provider's self-study report (twenty-four criteria), the report of a site visit, and supplemental information submitted to the board of review.

The self-study process is completed on a five-year basis with an interim report to the review board.

The Deficit Reduction Act of 1984 authorized the secretary of health and human services to recognize national accrediting bodies, thereby affirming the decisions of those bodies in determining whether a provider meets requirements for Medicare participation. NLN's application for deemed status has been satisfactorily reviewed by the staff of the Health Standards and Quality Bureau and the Bureau of Eligibility, Reimbursement and Coverage of the HCFA.

The Joint Commission on the Accreditation of Healthcare Organizations (JCAHO) reviews hospital-based home health agencies as part of the hospital survey process. JCAHO accreditation includes a site visit every year.

Certification.   In order to qualify for Medicare and Medicaid funding an agency must be certified by the U.S. Department of Health and Human Services. The survey process is delegated to the individual state health departments. This process includes a site visit to determine if federal, state, and agency policies are being followed.

The certification requirements are stated in the Home Health Agency Survey Report (40) and include the following: (a) compliance with federal, state, and local laws; (b) organization, services, and administration (governing body and qualified administrator, personnel policies); (c) a professional advisory committee; (d) policies related to acceptance of clients, plan of treatment, medical supervision; (e) skilled nursing service; (f) therapy service; (g) medical social service; (h) home health aide service; (i) clinical records; (j) evaluation of agency and records.

Licensure.   Individual states may have a licensure law for home care agencies. The regulations delineate specific conditions that must be met on a periodic basis in order to be licensed as a service provider. The state department of health usually has responsibility for determining that providers meet the licensure requirement.

Additional standards are imposed by various funding sources that cover home care services. Two examples

of such sources are United Way and other third-party payers, such as the area agency on aging.

The American Nurses' Association (ANA) has published Standards for Nursing Service (2), Standards of Community Health Nursing Practice (3), and a position statement in support of an increased emphasis on health care at home and the integration of home care into the health care delivery system.

Individual Standards

Certification.   Individual practitioners can be certified by state, professional, or specialty organizations. For example, in Pennsylvania a nurse practitioner can become certified by submitting required documentation to the appropriate department of state.

National certification is offered by the ANA for community health nurses. Other specialty groups also offer certification in certain areas of nursing. This national certification process usually includes a written examination and proof of completing requirements for recertification on a stated basis (9).

Licensure.   Individual states license the individual professional provider of health care services on a periodic basis. Some states also require evidence of specified hours of continuing education at the time of relicensure.

Selecting a Home Care Agency

On most occasions the client delegates the selection of a home care agency to a physician or hospital. Many times the hospital or physician makes a referral to a specific home care agency, based on past experience or contractual arrangements. Other clients in need of service may be referred by word of mouth or other social service agencies.

Printed material, such as consumer guides, can be used by clients as an aid in the selection of a home health agency (see Figure 14.1) (1, 6, 23, 26, 29).

External Changes That Affect Home Care

Home care services place a great emphasis and responsibility on the client and the family. Many of the services, such as antibiotic therapy or care of the ventilator-dependent client, are self-care programs. Clients and their families are taught how to do procedures, monitor equipment, and handle emergencies. The members of the home care team visit on a scheduled basis to provide the professional services such as changing an infuser or

The following checklist of questions should help a potential user of home health services to evaluate agency programs.

Standards

1. Is the agency licensed by the state? Have any complaints against the agency been filed with the state regulating agency (generally the state health department)?
2. Is the agency accredited by one of the following:
   a) National League for Nursing/American Public Health Association
   b) National HomeCaring Council
   c) Joint Commission on Accreditation of Hospitals
3. Is the agency bonded? Does the agency bond its employees or do the employees carry bonding for themselves?
4. Is the agency Medicare/Medicaid-certified?
5. How long has the agency been operating in the community? Can the agency provide you with references from hospital personnel or community social workers who have used or recommended the agency?

Services

1. Does the agency provide a complete written list of its services?
2. Does the agency confer with your doctor before providing services? If your doctor prepares a plan of care for you, how does the agency coordinate with the doctor on that plan and monitor its staff to see that the plan is being followed?
3. Is care available on the weekends or after regular hours?
4. What procedures does the agency use in an emergency? Are the agency personnel trained to handle emergencies?

Costs

1. Does the agency provide a written list of services and the cost for each service? Does it explain which services are covered by your private insurance, Medicare, Medicaid or other sources of financial assistance and which services you will be responsible for paying?
2. Do you sign a service agreement or a contract allowing the agency to bill your insurance company or Medicare or agreeing to cover the costs yourself? What if you are dissatisfied with the service?
3. How are the costs billed—per visit, per hour or on some other basis? Are there minimum hours or days

per week required? Do you sign a time sheet for each employee? Are you billed each week for the services you received that week?

4. If fees are on the basis of hourly or per visit charges, do those charges cover all services? Are there separate charges for an evaluation visit or employee social security or travel?
5. If you are covered by private or government insurance, will the agency handle the billing to them? If you have to pay for some or all the services, what arrangements can you make for payment?

Agency Personnel

1. Do the people whom the agency refers to you work for the agency or do you become their employer?
2. Could you be liable for an injury or accident to an agency employee in your home?
3. What kind of education, training and experience do the agency personnel have? Have they met state licensing requirements for their profession and are they certified by their professional organizations?
4. Are references required of the agency personnel before they are hired and have their references been checked? Can you see their references?
5. Will you be assigned the same person for the length of time you need care? Does the agency check with you to see if the people assigned to you are satisfactory? What happens if you complain about a person assigned from the agency? Will you get a replacement and if so, how quickly?
6. Does the agency have a full range of health service personnel on staff or does it sub-contract for any services or specialties? If it does sub-contract, how does it ensure the reliability and competence of these personnel?
7. What kind of supervision does the agency provide for the people it sends into your home? Does a supervisor come out to your home to observe the employee, to check on how he or she is carrying out your plan of care and to find out if you are satisfied with your care?
8. Does the agency provide registered nurses, licensed nurses, or both? How much education, training and experience are they required to have? Does the agency have its own testing system for its staff and requirements for in-service training?
9. Does the agency require home health aides to be licensed or certified? How much training and/or experience are they required to have?

Figure 14.1.   Checklist for Consumers

Source: National Consumer League, 600 Maryland Avenue, S.W., Suite 202 West, Washington, D.C. 20024.

administering specific medications. Support services such as a home health aide may be available for several hours several days a week. But the client or family members are expected to manage the majority of the care on a twenty-four-hour-a-day basis (19).

Why then, in view of the increased responsibility placed on client and family, is so much attention being paid to home care?

Many external changes are taking place today that influence home care, directly or indirectly, and make this an option for clients.

Reimbursement. There is an increased emphasis on home care as an alternative method of providing needed health-related services at a reduced cost. As the home care business expands and changes and reimbursement for acute care decreases, there is increased interest in home care. Hospitals, nursing homes, insurance and equipment companies, and entrepreneurs, as well as established agencies with a long history of providing in-home services, are now in the home care business.

Demographics. A majority of home care services are used by the over-sixty-five age-group. The 1980 U.S. Census Data indicate that this is a fast-growing segment of the population. Eleven percent of the population was over sixty-five in 1985. This number will increase to 20 percent by 2040. The fastest-growing segment of people is the eighty-five-years-and-over group (1.5 percent of the population in 1985, projected to 1.6 percent in 1995). Those in the over-sixty-five age-group use a major portion of the home care service.

Changes in the nuclear family, such as single parents and both mother and father employed in full- or part-time jobs, increase the need for outside help in the home. The demand for companions, homemakers, and other support services increases when someone in the family becomes ill and needs help while family members are away from the home.

Technologies. Treatments once confined to the acute care setting are now offered in the home. The table of contents from one agency's *Special Nursing Procedures and Policies Manual* included the following: (a) Care of the ventilator-dependent patient; (b) Administration of intravenous solutions; (c) Intravenous administration of chemotherapeutic agents; (d) Intravenous administration of narcotics; (e) Total parenteral nutrition; (f) Chemotherapy extravasation policy; (g) Procedure for drawing blood through Hickman or Broviac catheter; (h) Care of patients on continuous ambulatory perito-

neal dialysis; (i) Administering medications via Port-a-Cath System (45).

Performing these procedures requires a staff of professional nurses with sophisticated skills, and individual nurses as well as the administrative staff must be committed to providing skilled services on a twenty-four-hour-a-day basis in the home setting. Other necessary ingredients include in-service education and training programs, good working relationships with medical supply companies that are able to deliver ordered solutions and medications on short notice, and client/family education programs. In some instances families are "certified" to perform a procedure while the client is still in the hospital.

The availability of these technologies makes it necessary for the home care team to be alert to the environmental conditions of home care patients. Such questions as, Does the house have the required electric and water installation to accommodate some of the procedures required? or, Is the house structurally safe? are as important as being assured that the client and family can carry out the procedure safely.

These changes in procedures make it advantageous to use adult and pediatric nurse practitioners and clinical specialists to provide direct care as well as to serve as consultants to the professional staff.

Educated Consumers. An increasing number of clients who require health care services are asking necessary questions: What alternative do I have? What about a second opinion? Can I use a generic product? This increased consumer awareness and response are appropriate, since consumers are being asked to pay a larger portion of their health care costs through increased deductibles, co-insurances, or full payment for noncovered services.

Competition among health care providers and a change in marketing efforts make it imperative that consumers become familiar with the various types of agencies and services so that they can make informed decisions.

Internal Factors That Affect Home Care

There are numerous internal factors that influence home care. Several factors must be evaluated before a client is accepted on a home care program.

All home care agencies should have written policies and procedures. There should be a written policy for each service provided. The policies should address the services that will and will not be provided and who will provide them under what conditions.

Acceptance Policy.   A home health agency should have a written policy to establish criteria for assessment and planning of in-home services. The policy should list specific requirements for acceptance, such as client's residence located within a specific geographical area, if applicable; plan of treatment and follow-up are in accordance with the agency's policies; agency can provide requested service; acceptance of agency's service policies and proposed plan of care by the client and family; ability and willingness of client/family to participate in client's interim care between agency's service visits; adequate cooperative efforts by client/family to establish safety measures and a plan for medical emergencies; adequate physical facilities.

Given that a client is accepted for home care, there are additional factors that influence the ultimate outcome.

Referral Information.   The referral for home care is an important starting point. Complete and correct medical, social, environmental, and financial information is basic.

A good working relationship with hospital discharge planners or the use of liaison nurses to facilitate the smooth transfer of clients from hospital to home care is essential.

It is also important to foster a trust relationship among professionals in hospitals and home care agencies. A referral for home care provides for continuity of care. A client may have been taught and demonstrated a specific procedure in the hospital. But the conditions are different in the home. For example, a hook may replace an intravenous pole to hang irrigating solution, or an injection technique may need reinforcement "one more time" in the home setting. The presence of the nurse to observe and supervise a specific procedure for the first time in the home is beneficial for the client and family.

Ambulatory Status.   The client's ambulatory status both before and after the current illness will influence his or her outcome status. The rehabilitative process may be delayed if the primary diagnosis is a fractured hip, but the client's medical history includes a previous cerebrovascular accident that affected the same side as the newly fractured hip.

Mental Status.   It is important to determine the client's mental status before the onset of the current illness. Will this status influence the method in which care is deliv-

ered? For example, a forty-five-year-old client with newly diagnosed diabetes mellitus needs to be taught how to administer insulin. The care plan will differ, depending on whether the client has no other presenting diagnosis, as compared with the care plan when the client is mentally retarded and living in a community living arrangement.

Medical Diagnoses.   The client's admission to a home care program is probably for the primary diagnosis that is the immediate presenting problem. It is important to obtain secondary diagnoses, since these could impact on the client's ultimate outcome.

Nursing Diagnoses.   The nursing diagnoses, such as knowledge or self-care deficits, will affect the client's care requirements.

Home Environment.   It is important to evaluate the home environment from a physical and family viewpoint. Who is the care giver? Is it the spouse, who is as old as the client and who is also experiencing a physical problem? Is it a family member who works full time? Does the client live on the first or second floor? Where are the bathroom and kitchen located? Is the client shuttled from one relative to another? How does this impact on the quality of care delivered and the client's emotional status?

Client/Family Acceptance or Rejection of Illness.   The client's and family's acceptance or rejection of the client's illness will influence the care plan and the outcome. Questions to be considered are, How will or can the family contribute to the client's recovery? Will the family be willing to do interim dressing changes, turn the client frequently, do tube feedings?

As mentioned earlier, home care is many times a self-care program. The professional nurse may spend one hour with the client on an intermittent basis, perhaps twice or three times a week. During the remaining time the client or family members are expected to carry out the plan of care. Their ability or failure to carry out this responsibility will impact on the client's progress.

Coordination of Service.   The nurse is the coordinator of care. It is the nurse's responsibility to know what services have been ordered for a client and to monitor progress toward an established realistic goal.

Discharge planning begins on admission to home care services. Interdisciplinary conferences are necessary to evaluate and reevaluate the plan of treatment and to bring changes in the client's status or progress reports to the physician's attention.

The plan of care, projected time frames for attaining established goals, and plans for discharge should be discussed with the client or family from the onset of care.

Documentation of Services

"If you didn't document it, you didn't do it!" These words speak to the importance of documentation for home care services. Documentation is required to record what has been done for the client, to communicate client changes among professionals, to record telephone calls for coordination of care, and for legal and reimbursement purposes.

Clinical Record

The Medicare conditions of participation (8, 38) state that a clinical record must be maintained for every client who receives home health services. The record must contain appropriate identifying information: name of physician; drug regimen; dietary, treatment, and activity orders; signed and dated clinical and progress notes (clinical notes are written the day that service is rendered and are incorporated into the record no less often than weekly); copies of summary reports sent to the physician and a discharge summary.

An organized, legible clinical record is essential for home care services. Within an agency there should be a standardized procedure for filing of documents within the clinical record.

A clinical note must be written for each service provided. Notes are also recorded for telephone calls and conferences. These notes may be handwritten, or recorded and transcribed (18, 32, 43), depending on the agency's policy.

Plan of Treatment

On September 1, 1985, new standardized home health data element forms were initiated by the Medicare program to promote more consistent application of coverage guidelines (42). These forms are (a) HCFA 485, Home Health Certification and Plan of Treatment Data Elements; (b) HCFA 486, Medical Update and Patient Information; (c) HCFA 487, Addendum to the Plan of Treatment/Medical Update and Patient Information

Form; (d) HCFA 488, Intermediary Medical Information Request Form.

These new forms are specific and will be used by all home care agencies for clients on the Medicare program. Nurses and other disciplines must indicate the total number of visits made during a sixty-day period. The frequency of visits and a timetable for attainment of expected outcome must be included on each certification.

Client Classification System

Another important aspect of documentation is the use of a classification system to identify client outcomes. Such a system is important not only from an overall evaluation standpoint—What happened to the client? Why did it happen? How much did it cost?—but also from an efficiency standpoint. A classification system with appropriate and concise tools makes it possible for staff to collect all pertinent information. This is also valuable from a productivity viewpoint. Needed documentation can be completed and more time can be made available for client care.

Giovannetti (11) describes a client classification system as "the grouping of patients according to some observable or inferred properties or characteristics" and "quantification of these categories or measures of the nursing effort."

Several classification systems in home care have been described in the literature (4, 7, 14, 17, 35, 43, 46). One such system, the Rehabilitative Potential Patient Classification System (RPPCS) (46), will be used to illustrate how one system can be used to identify client outcome goals, to document nursing care, to evaluate the quality of care provided through periodic record review, as well as to collect statistical and financial data associated with these goals.

Daubert (7) described and implemented the RPPCS in a community health agency at the Visiting Nurse Association of New Haven. This method is copyrighted and was developed as one component of a quality assurance program to evaluate client outcomes.

In this system all clients are classified on admission into one of five groups. The classification is done regardless of the number of diagnoses per client or the mix of agency services required.

The five groups are (a) clients who will return to pre-illness level of function; (b) clients who are experiencing an acute episode of illness but have the potential for returning to pre-episode levels of functioning; (c) clients who will eventually function without agency service; (d) clients who will remain at home as long as possible with ongoing agency services; (e) clients who will be maintained at home during the end stage of illness for as long as possible with services.

Staff nurses in one agency (45) use the RPPCS to complete documentation of care. Standardized flow sheets have been developed that correspond with each of the five client classification categories. The primary nurse selects the appropriate category when the client is admitted to service. The general assessment sheet for each category of client includes those parameters that must be documented.

Standardized flow sheets also have been prepared for selected nursing diagnoses. One or more of these flow sheets are incorporated into the client's clinical record with the general assessment sheet.

Flow sheets are supplemented with narrative notes on a weekly or more frequent basis.

The client outcomes are tabulated statistically and financially by the computer. The outcomes are also evaluated by peer review of a random selection of clients' charts, both open and closed to service and through the Quarterly Record Review process that is part of the quality assurance program.

The use of a classification system to identify client outcome goals and to document and evaluate care is important for client care. The financial and statistical data generated by such a system are also used as management tools by nursing service administrators. They can be used to predict staffing needs, in-service programs, and changes in types of care required by clients.

Nursing Diagnoses

Nursing diagnoses (13, 20, 21, 32) are important components of home care nursing service. Two clients of the same age may have the same medical diagnosis, but it is the nursing diagnoses that influence the level and amount of care needed to attain the established goal.

For example, two clients, Mr. A. and Mr. B., both aged seventy, are approved for home care after surgery for a fractured hip. Mr. A. lives with his son's family in a one-story home. He has no secondary diagnosis and is able to ambulate with a walker. Nursing diagnoses for Mr. A. include impaired physical mobility and potential for injury.

Mr. B. lives in a two-story home with his sixty-eight-year-old wife, who has a history of cardiac disease. Mr. B. had a cerebrovascular accident three years ago and had not regained full use of his right arm and leg before his recent fall. Nursing diagnoses for Mr. B. include impaired physical mobility, potential for injury, self-care

deficit, sensory-perceptional alterations, impaired home maintenance management, and ineffectual family coping.

Reimbursement Issues

Home health care is a business. Even nonprofit agencies that have a history of providing care to clients, regardless of ability to pay for service, must be able to maintain a balanced budget to remain financially solvent.

In home care the primary nurse is an important part of the reimbursement picture. Home care reimbursement is unique. The source of payment for service may vary from day to day or from discipline to discipline. For example, Mrs. S.'s physician has ordered vitamin B_{12} injections weekly for Mrs. S., to treat her pernicious anemia. It is the nurse's responsibility to know the federal regulations as they apply to this medication. Usually only one injection per month can be billed to the Medicare program (39). The other three visits per month that Mrs. S. receives must be billed to another source, such as the client.

The nurse must know the regulations and must enter the correct code on the daily log sheet or other reporting format used by the home care agency for the specific data, so that the billing is correct at the end of the month.

At other times one discipline, such as therapy, may be reimbursed under the Medicare program, but another discipline may not be covered.

As of 1985 home health agencies are reimbursed on a cost-per-visit basis.

It is most important that the primary nurse be aware of the most common reimbursement sources for home care services.

Medicare

Medicare legislation was signed into law by President Lyndon Johnson in 1965. It provides for home health services for people who are over sixty-five years of age or who are disabled.

The three principles of Medicare coverage are (a) the client must be homebound, (b) there must be a plan of treatment signed by a physician, and (c) there must be certification that the client is homebound and in need of skilled intermittent services.

Primary services include nursing, physical therapy,

and speech pathology. These services can be offered on a stand-alone basis.

Ancillary services include occupational therapy, medical social service, home health aides, and supplies or durable medical equipment. These services must be offered in cooperation with one of the primary services, with one exception: occupational therapy may be continued on an individual basis but may not be the only service offered at the start of care.

Even though a client has a Medicare card, this does not guarantee automatic payment for home health care. The three stated principles must be met.

When the services rendered to a client do not qualify for Medicare coverage, the client must be notified in writing by the provider, either at the start of care or when specific services no longer qualify as covered under Medicare. Written notice must be provided by the nurse or other professional care giver. The client or a person acting on behalf of the beneficiary signs the notice. The client, physician, and agency each receive a copy of the signed notification of noncoverage of service.

If this written notice is not provided, and the agency personnel know the service provided is not covered under the Medicare program, the agency, not the beneficiary, is responsible for the cost of providing services.

Given that Medicare coverage is available, the physician must certify (sign) the client's plan of treatment every sixty days.

Medicaid

Medicaid funds come from the federal and state governments. These funds provide coverage for those clients whose income falls under a certain level, or for those who are blind or disabled. Clients must apply for this coverage.

Reimbursement for home care services varies from state to state; some are cost based, and others are an established flat fee for service. Specific services such as medical social service or supplies may be excluded from coverage. Prior approval may be required for equipment or selected supplies.

Private Insurance

The Pennsylvania Association of Home Health Agencies (30) conducted a membership survey in 1985 to determine the extent to which home health care insurance coverage is currently available. Respondents said that they had experience with approximately forty insurance companies.

The following observations could be made about current home health care coverage by private third-party payers from this survey.

- Home health care is covered by many insurers.
- Services covered are primarily skilled services, including registered nurses and physical, occupational, and speech therapists. Medical social worker, home health aides, and homemaker services generally are not covered. Some policies include coverage for equipment and supplies.
- Many policies limit coverage to a posthospital stay, to a specific number of visits per calendar year, to a specific number of hours, or to a certain amount of dollars per day.
- There is an average deductible of $100 to $200 and an average co-insurance of 20 percent for the beneficiary.
- All services must be medically necessary. Some companies require prior approval, doctor's orders, a plan of treatment, or documentation of visits.
- Although there are commonalities in coverage between and within companies, coverage varies with each contract.

Clients may not be aware that their health insurance policy includes home care benefits until this option is discussed by the nurse or agency representative (31).

Self-Pay

Many agencies offer home care services on a self-pay basis. Individuals or families are able to make arrangements for necessary or wanted services and agree to pay for them.

Some agencies, depending on their auspice or corporate structure, may offer necessary services on an adjusted fee or sliding scale basis. One example of such an agency is a voluntary, nonprofit visiting nurse association.

Additional funding may be available for home care through the local area agency on aging, office of children and youth, county and municipal governments, United Way, and grants.

The method of handling the reimbursement aspect of home care may differ from agency to agency. In one agency all identifying information may be obtained and verified before a professional visit. In other agencies the nurse may collect the needed information as part of the first nursing assessment visit.

Agencies should have a policy relevant to billing and collection of fees for services. The nurse should become acquainted with this policy as part of the orientation to the agency.

Quality Assurance in Home Care

What is quality care? How is it evaluated? Sometimes quality may be intangible, but in home care, documentation is a major component of the quality assurance process, since care is evaluated through clinical record review (16).

An agency's quality assurance program should include a myriad of tools to evaluate the quality of care provided. The following are examples of such tools.

The conditions of participation for the Medicare program require home health agencies to do two types of clinical record review: (a) At least quarterly, appropriate health professionals, representing at least the scope of the program, review a sample of both active and closed clinical records to assure that established policies are followed in providing service. (b) There is a continuous review of clinical records for each sixty-day period that a client receives home health services, to determine adequacy of the plan of treatment and appropriateness of continuation of care.

Additional evaluation tools include client questionnaires, physician questionnaires, client outcome criteria, unsolicited testimonials, periodic review of policies and procedure, evaluation of staff performances and staffing positions.

All Medicare-certified agencies are required to complete an overall evaluation of the agency's total programs once a year. All aspects of the quality assurance program are incorporated into the annual process.

The Future of Home Care

As of 1985 home health care is reimbursed on a cost-per-visit basis. The cost of providing a specific discipline (nursing, therapy) is determined in the same manner by all certified home health agencies. This uniform method of cost finding (39) applies to both community- and hospital-based agencies.

As of July 1985 the HCFA published a final notice that limits home health costs and revises the current methodology for determining those limits. This action by HCFA also establishes a single schedule of limits for hospital-based and freestanding agencies but retains an add-on adjustment to the hospital-based agencies for higher administrative and general costs owing to Medicare cost allocations.

Implications of DRG System

At least three aspects of the DRG (diagnostic-related group) system have implications for home care.

Acuity Level of Clients. Clients who are referred for home care are being discharged from the hospital sooner and require more skilled service in length of time and intensity. Home care is reimbursed on a cost-per-visit basis. The same dollar amount is paid for a visit regardless of the length of time spent with a client. The result is that the daily productivity of a nurse may decrease as the level of client care increases. This could have a negative impact on agency reimbursement (i.e., fewer visits result in fewer dollars under the current reimbursement system).

Prospective Payment for Home Care. Some type of alternate payment system will become effective in the future for home care. Several alternate methods of reimbursement are being proposed. The National Home Health Agency Prospective Payment Demonstration (47) is to be conducted under the sponsorship of the HCFA, to test alternate methods for paying for services provided by Medicare-certified home health agencies.

Three methods of prospective payments are to be tested: (a) rate per visit by discipline; (b) comprehensive monthly rate paid for each month in which clients are under the care of the provider; (c) comprehensive rate per episode of treatment. As of late 1985, the project was on hold.

Volume of Services. One study conducted by the National Association of Area Agencies on Aging in Washington, D.C., and the Southeast Long-Term Care Gerontology Center at the University of Texas found that in-home skilled nursing increased 196 percent, housekeeping services increased 69 percent, and personal care services went up 63 percent since the DRG system was implemented.

A second study was conducted by the Eastern Washington Area Agency on Aging in Spokane, Washington. The results of this study showed that the DRG system had a significant effect on the extent and range of services being provided by home care agencies.

A variety of other actions are taking place in home care. In New York State, as of August 1985, Governor

Mario C. Cuomo signed into law the following legislation: (a) a per capita state aid bill for home care; (b) a bill to conduct a home care voucher demonstration program for physically disabled self-directed persons; (c) a bill authorizing the New York State Office for the Aging to establish programs for informal care-giving training (25).

The House Energy and Commerce Committee requested the Office of Technology Assessment to undertake a study of home health care for chronically ill children as of August 1985. Several areas of focus are to estimate the number of children with chronic life-threatening illness, to assess current insurance coverage, and to assess the net costs for home-delivered services.

The American Association of Retired Persons and Prudential Insurance Company designed a long-term care/home health insurance package that began test marketing in October 1985.

Staff nurses, as well as nurse administrators, must be aware of the impact that a change in reimbursement policy will have on home care. Given a specific dollar limit, what services can be provided, in what number, and in what mix of disciplines?

In the future, dollars available, not need, may determine the level of care provided. Tonges (36) states: "In a cost-containment atmosphere, providers now must either lower their standards or find ways to provide quality care more economically." The challenge is to provide high-quality care despite dollar limitations. Creative strategies by individual nurses and home care administrators will be needed to meet the goal of quality health care in the home.

Role of the Nurse

Initial Contact

The first contact with the home care client and the family is most important. This is when the client is introduced to the service of the agency. An explanation should be given of the services ordered and how they will be delivered. Both client and provider expectation should be outlined. Clients should receive an approved printed copy of "Patient Rights and Responsibilities" (see Figure 14.2 for sample). The function of each discipline that provides service should be described. Limitations should be set. Required documents should be explained to the client and the appropriate signatures obtained.

The National Association for Home Care states the rights of the home care recipient and his family as follows:

1. The patient is to be fully informed of all his rights and responsibilities by the home care agency.
2. The patient has the right to appropriate and professional care relating to physician orders.
3. The patient has the right of choice of care providers.
4. The patient has the right to receive information necessary to give informed consent prior to the start of any procedure or treatment.
5. The patient has the right to refuse treatment within the confines of the law and to be informed of the consequences of his action.
6. The patient has the right to privacy.
7. The patient has the right to receive a timely response from the agency to his request for service.
8. A patient will be admitted for service only if the agency has the ability to provide safe professional care at the level of intensity needed. The patient has the right to reasonable continuity of care.
9. The patient has the right to be informed within reasonable time of anticipated termination of service or plans for transfer to another agency.
10. The patient has the right to voice grievances and suggest changes in service or staff without fear of restraint or discrimination.
    A fair hearing shall be available to any individual to whom service has been denied, reduced or terminated or who is otherwise aggrieved by agency action. The fair hearing procedure shall be set forth by each agency as appropriate to the unique patient situation (e.g., funding source, level of care, diagnosis).
11. The patient has the right to be fully informed of agency policies and charges for services, including eligibility for third party reimbursements.
12. A patient denied service solely on his inability to pay shall have the right to be referred elsewhere.
13. The patient (and the public) has the right to honest, accurate forthright information regarding the home care industry in general and his chosen agency in particular.

Getting proper home care for yourself or someone you love should be as important to the agency you choose as it is to you.

Figure 14.2. Patient Rights and Responsibilities
Source: National Association for Home Care, 519 C Street, N.E., Stanton Park, Washington, D.C. 20002.

A nursing assessment is completed and documented, and a nursing plan of care established, using the home care agency's established format.

Discharge planning begins on this first visit. Goals are established; an estimation of how long service will be provided is made and communicated to the client and family.

Depending on the agency's internal procedure, this could also be the time that payment for service is discussed. Who will pay? For how long? What happens then? Are services continued? Are alternate funding sources available?

The first contact with the client and family establishes the framework for home care services.

Responsibility for Health Maintenance and Therapy for Illness

Coordinator of Care. Using the Medicare standards, the nurse is the coordinator of care. The nurse coordinates nursing care as well as other disciplines that provide services to a client.

When the reimbursement system changes, it will be more important than ever, from a financial and quality of care standard, for the nurse to be aware of the cost of each service and to dertemine how the client will benefit the most from the various services that are needed. This coordinated role will be foremost as the nurse assumes the responsibility for both health maintenance and therapy for illness.

Direct Care Giver. This role includes carrying out medical and nursing procedures and administering and monitoring oral and parenteral medications.

Educator/Observer. The nurse has the responsibility to use and develop educational tools to help clients attain their mutually agreed on goals.

The nurse must be alert for environmental changes, such as loss of a spouse, pet, or appliance (hearing aid, dentures); frequent moves from one relative to another; a change in income status that could affect their progress.

Teacher. The nurse has to assess the learner and the support systems (availability, willingness, and capabilities). The nurse has to teach new information as well as correct misinformation.

Guidance Counselor. The guidance and counseling role should address current and future issues. What type of planning has been done? What should be done? What can be done?

To address current issues, the questions might be, Can the client return home to a safe environment? Can the client live alone? Questions related to future issues might be, What will happen to the client if the care giver dies? Can the family manage to care for a terminally ill client who wants to return home? What type of support systems are available? What additional services will be needed for the client to reach this goal?

Referral to Other Providers and Community Services

The following is a partial listing of organizations or materials that can be beneficial to clients and families.

- Vial of Life Program (if available in community). The patient's emergency information and medical history are recorded on a medical information form, and the form is placed in a plastic vial. The vial is secured to the right side of the refrigerator's top shelf with a rubber band. A decal is attached to the outside of the refrigerator door. This alerts the ambulance crew that a Vial of Life is inside. If such a program is not available in your community, the nurse could initiate this program. Vials could be made available through pharmaceutical companies, pharmacies, or local service clubs.
- Emergency electronic alert system. The client either wears the device or has it installed in the home. The alert system can be activated in an emergency. The operator can give rescue workers pertinent information and also notify designated persons, such as the family or a physician.
- Notification of local police and fire departments that the client is homebound and will require help in an emergency situation. Some departments may provide identification stickers for the client's window; others may provide daily telephone reassurance calls.
- Meals on wheels
- Financial referrals for health- and social-related reasons: insurance coverage, need for medication, unpaid bills
- Seek outlet for talents, such as elder craftsperson. Some people may have ability to make hand-

crafted items and there may be an appropriate outlet for such items.
- Awareness of religious interest
- Publications to be used to supplement teaching as well as to provide needed information on current illness; support groups for the future

Concerns for Physical, Social, Emotional, and Economic Status of Client and Family

Physical. The nurse provides needed services as well as arranges for additional services both through the agency and by referral. The nurse determines whether the client is complying with the regimen. If noncompliance is evident, the nurse seeks to identify the reasons why: Does the client feel better without the treatment? Is the client experiencing side effects of a medication? If so, have they been reported to the physician, and have changes been made in the regimen? Are care givers following through with interim care, administering medications, changing dressings? If not, why not?

Social. The following questions will help to elicit the social impact of the client's illness. How has this illness affected the client's and family's life-style? How have friends reacted? Why isn't the client eating meals with the family? Possibly the reason is the client's dentures are ill-fitting and he or she is unable to eat without embarrassment. (This could also influence a physical condition. Ill-fitting dentures can cause a person to avoid eating the proper foods necessary for bowel elimination. This could result in a fecal impaction.) Why is the client avoiding family gatherings? Could the reason be incontinence?

The nurse has knowledge of multiple resources that could improve the client's social interaction within the home.

Referrals to support groups may be beneficial for family members to help them cope with the social aspect of the client's illness.

Emotional. The emotional status of the client and family can be determined by asking the following questions: How does the client feel about this illness? Is there loss of self-esteem and identity? Is there an attitude of indifference on the part of the spouse, children? Are there feelings of helplessness or depression? Is there a threat to one's physical welfare because of the emotional status? Is there fear of pending hospitalization or placement? Is there need for increased independence? How

can this be accomplished? Is there need for physical contact? What are the client's strengths and weaknesses?

The nurse can assess the emotional status of the client and family, consult with the physician, and make referrals to appropriate professionals. The nurse can recognize and communicate any changes to other professionals involved with the client's case.

Economic. Illness brings with it additional bills. Many times clients and families have questions about health care costs in general. These questions can be directed to other health professionals if the nurse is unable to answer them. The nurse should be alert to economic conditions as they relate to a client's compliance or noncompliance with medical and nursing regimens.

Promotion of Continued Interaction Between Client and Care Provider

Continued interaction among clients, care givers, and professionals is essential for clients to attain their established realistic outcome goals. When the first three nursing roles (initial contact, responsibility for health maintenance and illness, and concerns for the physical, social, emotional, and economic status of the client and family) are accomplished, the client and family will be comfortable with and willing to contact the nurse and the home care agency for future services when the need arises.

DISCUSSION QUESTIONS

1. All clients are not candidates for home care services. List three factors that would preclude home care and explain why.
2. Home care is funded through various sources. List four funding sources. Describe criteria for coverage.
3. Medicare is one source of funding for home care services. List three principles of coverage under this program.
4. The nurse is the coordinator of home care services for the client. List three distinct nursing activities that could be included in home care.
5. The nurse as coordinator of care has the responsibility to know what services have been ordered by the physician and initiated for the client. List at least six services that a client may require as part of a home care program.

6. List four ways that the quality of care can be evaluated as part of a quality assurance program in home care.
7. List at least six roles that are important in home care.
8. Describe three external changes that influence home care services.
9. List three internal factors that influence home care services.
10. List and describe two types of standards for both agencies and individuals who provide home care services.

REFERENCES

1. American Association of Retired Persons. *A Handbook About Care in the Home.* Washington, D.C.: AARP, 1982.
2. American Nurses' Association. *Standards for Nursing Service.* Kansas City: American Nurses' Association, 1973.
3. American Nurses' Association. *Standards of Community Health Nursing Practice.* Kansas City: American Nurses' Association, 1973.
4. Ballard, S., and R. McNamara. "Quantifying Nursing Needs in Home Health Care." *Nursing Research* 32:236–41, 1983.
5. Benson, E. H., and J. Q. McDevitt. *Community Health and Nursing Practice.* 2nd ed. Englewood Cliffs, N.J.: Prentice-Hall, 1980.
6. Coleman, B. *A Consumers Guide to Home Health Care.* Washington, D.C.: National Consumer League, 1985.
7. Daubert, E. "Patient Classification Systems and Outcome Criteria." *Nursing Outlook* 27:450–54, 1979.
8. Federal Register. *Conditions of Participation for Home Health Agencies.* Department of Health and Welfare. July 16, 1973, 38:135.
9. Fickeissen, J. L. "Getting Certified." *American Journal of Nursing* 85 (3):265–69, 1985.
10. Freeman, R. B., and J. Heinrich. *Community Health Nursing Practice.* 2nd ed. Philadelphia: W. B. Saunders Co., 1981.
11. Giovannetti, P. "Understanding Patient Classification Systems." *JONA* 9:4, 1979.
12. Glenn, K., ed. *Washington Report on Medicine and Health Perspectives.* St. Louis: McGraw-Hill, August 5, 1985.
13. Gordon, M. *Nursing Diagnosis—Process and Application.* New York: McGraw-Hill, 1982.
14. Hardy, J. A. "A Patient Classification System for Home Health Patients." *Caring* 3:26–27, 1984.
15. Harmer, L., M. Harris, and M. Nyman. "Agency Profile: Development of a Pediatric Home Care Program." *Caring* 4:82–83, 1985.
16. Harris, M. "Evaluating Home Care? Compare Viewpoints." *Nursing and Health Care* 2 (4):207–13, 1981.
17. Harris, M., C. Santoferraro, and S. Silva. "A Patient Classification System in Home Care." *Nursing Economics* 3:276–82, 1985.
18. Harris, M. "A Tape Recording and Transcribing System to Maintain Patient's Clinical Records." *Nursing and Health Care* 5 (9):503–7, 1984.
19. Intermed Communications. Nursing Photobook. *Helping Geriatric Patients.* Springhouse, Pa.: Intermed Communications, 1982.
20. Kim, M. J., and D. A. Moritz, eds. *Classification of Nursing Diagnosis.* Proceedings of the Third and Fourth National Conferences. New York: McGraw-Hill, 1982.
21. Kritek, P. "Nursing Diagnosis in Perspective: Response to a Critique." *Image* 17:3–8, 1985.
22. National Association for Home Care. *Caring.* Pediatric Home Issue, 4 (5), 1985.
23. National Association for Home Care. *Home Care.* 1984.
24. National Association for Home Care. *Report.* Washington, D.C., #135, August 19, 1985.
25. National Association for Home Care. *Report.* Washington, D.C., #136, August 30, 1985, 5–6.
26. National Home Caring Council and the Better Business Bureau of Metropolitan New York. *All About Home Care: A Consumer's Guide.* 1982.
27. National League for Nursing. *Accreditation Program for Home Care and Community Health—1985 Revisions—Criteria, Standards and Substantiating Evidence.* New York: NLN, 1985.
28. National League for Nursing. *Policies and Procedures for NLN/APHA Accreditation of Home Health Agencies and Community Nursing Services.* New York: NLN, 1980.
29. Noese, A. E. *A Guide to Home Health Care.* Kalamazoo, Mich.: Upjohn Health Care Services, 1982.
30. Pennsylvania Association of Home Health Agencies (PAHHA). *PAHHA Insurance Survey Report.* Harrisburg, 1985.
31. Rak, K. *Home Health Line* 10:234, 1985.
32. Shamansky, S., and C. Yanni. "In Opposition to Nursing Diagnosis: A Majority Opinion." *Image* 15:47–50, 1983.
33. Sherman, S. *Community Health Nursing Care Plans: A Guide for Home Health Care Professionals.* New York: John Wiley & Sons, 1985.
34. Siegel, B. *Lillian Wald of Henry Street.* New York: Macmillan, 1983.
35. Sienkiewiez, J. "Patient Classification in Community Health Nursing." *Nursing Outlook* 32:319–321, 1984.
36. Tonges, M. "Quality with Economy: Doing the Right Thing for Less." *Nursing Economics* 3:205–11, 1985.
37. U.S. Department of HEW. *Conditions of Participation.* Federal Register, 38 (135). Section 405, 1228. Clinical Records, 18981.
38. U.S. Department of HEW—SSA. *Conditions of Participation for Home Health Agencies.* Federal Register, July 16, 1973, 38 (135), Part III.

39. U.S. Department of HEW—SSA. *Medicare Home Health Agency Manual.* HM, 11-6-66, 5/71. Section 204.4 (H) (I) (A).
40. U.S. Department of HHS. *Home Health Agency Survey Report.* OMB No: 72-R0735 SSA Form 1572, 10–73.
41. U.S. Department of HHS—HCFA. *Medicare Home Health Agency Manual.* Pub. 11. Transmitted 173, July 1985.
42. U.S. Department of HHS—HCFA. *Provider Reimbursement Manual.* Transmitted #15, May 1982. Part II. Provider Cost Reporting Forms and Instructions, ch. 3: Form HCFA 2552.
43. U.S. Department of HHS—Public Health Service—Health Resources Administration Bureau of Health Professionals, Division of Nursing. *A Classification Scheme for Client Problems in Community Health Nursing.* Hyattsville, Md. DHHS Pub. # HRA-80-16.
44. VNA of Eastern Montgomery County. Board Minutes, 1919, Abington, Pa.
45. VNA of Eastern Montgomery County. *Policies and Procedures Manual.* Abington, Pa., 1985.
46. VNA of New Haven. *Patient Classification/Objectives System Methodology Manual.* New Haven, Conn., 1980.
47. Williams, J., G. Gaumer, and R. Schmitz. *National Home Health Agency Prospective Payment Demonstration.* Cambridge, Mass.: Abt Associates, 1985.

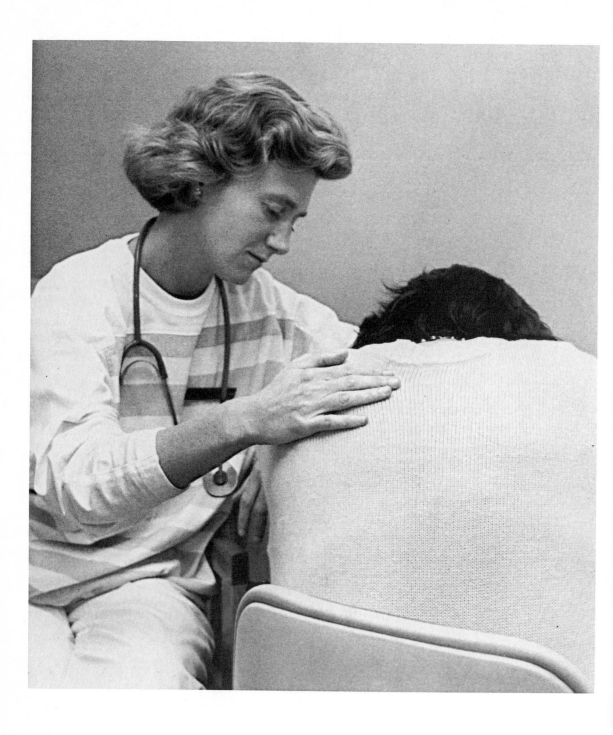

Primary Practice in Stress and Crisis

■

The content development in Unit Three recognizes the fact that an important aspect of primary nursing care is being able to deal effectively with clients and their families during stress and crisis. As the unit begins with chapter 15, the reader is introduced to concepts of stress and crisis and to nursing intervention appropriate for managing them. The author includes a discussion of one way in which nurses handle stress—burnout—and offers suggestions for preventing it. The author of chapter 16 continues with a presentation of concepts of crisis and methods of crisis intervention and an examination of suicide.

As discussed in chapter 17, a common response to stress and crisis is grief. How the nurse in primary nursing practice can assist the grieving client is presented from a cultural perspective.

The unit concludes with three problems that are characterized by stress, crisis, and grief—substance abuse, abuse in families, and cancer. Authors demonstrate how the concepts of primary nursing care can be used to move clients toward higher levels of self-care and wellness. The concluding unit chapter, entitled "Overcoming Barriers to Primary Cancer

Nursing Care," is unique. Its authors recognize that caring for cancer clients causes discomfort in nurses, resulting in personal and professional barriers that may impair the nurse's ability to function in expected roles. How to deal with these barriers is examined.

CHAPTER 15

Stress and Stress Management

ALENE HARRISON

■

OBJECTIVES

After completing this chapter, the reader will be able to:

- Define stress.
- Differentiate between stress, distress, and eustress.
- Define the term stressor.
- Identify the seven essential attachments, according to Hansell.
- Discuss possible stressors related to each of the seven essential attachments.
- Discuss the general purpose of stress responses.
- Identify the three basic results of prolonged stress.
- Identify subjective, behavioral, cognitive, physiological, health, and organizational responses to stressors.
- Identify six determinants of response to stressors.

- Discuss the role of therapeutic communications in assisting a client with a stress management program.
- Discuss factors indicative of need to refer a client for psychological counseling.
- Explain seven techniques used in stress management programs.
- Define burnout.
- Discuss factors that contribute to development of burnout in nurses and nursing students.
- Identify symptoms of burnout.
- Devise a program of prevention for burnout.
- Apply the nursing process to clients who are experiencing stress.

Stress . . . an everyday event in the lives of all in our rapid-moving, complex society. Nurses, in their roles of caring for and promoting self-care on the part of clients, have significant opportunities to assist clients to recognize and manage everyday stresses and thereby minimize stress-related health problems. Nurses in every care setting should recognize the stressors that their clients experience and help clients to develop preventive stress management behaviors.

This chapter focuses on the information necessary to identify sources and signs and symptoms of stress and to apply basic techniques of stress management in the provision of care to clients. The role of stress in the professional life of the nurse will be explored, as will techniques for the prevention of burnout.

Theoretical Definitions of Stress

The term *stress* has been used to identify a wide variety of life experiences, particularly those that are unpleasant, inconvenient, or undesired. The term has become such a common part of our vocabulary that its scientific meaning appears to have been forgotten. It is important, however, that nurses be aware of the more complete, scientific meaning of stress in order to fulfill their role in assisting clients with stress management.

According to Sorenson and Luckmann (16), in the seventeenth century the term *stress* meant "hardship, straits, adversity or affliction." By the nineteenth century it was used to mean "force, pressure, strain, or strong effort that acts upon a person or an object."

Hans Selye, a noted twentieth-century authority on physiological stress, defined *stress* as "the nonspecific response of the body to any demand made upon it. For general orientation, it suffices to keep in mind that by stress, the physician means the common results of exposure to any stimulus. For example, the bodily changes produced whether a person is exposed to nervous tension, physical injury, infection, cold, heat, x-rays or anything else are what we call stress" (14).

Although Selye originally focused on physiological re-

sponses to stress, he considered both physiological and psychological causes of stress. His phrase "or anything else" can be broadly interpreted to include psychological, environmental, or sociological sources of stress.

Engel broadened the definition of stress to specifically account for the psychological component. He stated: "Psychological stress refers to all processes, whether originating in the external environment or within the person, which impose a demand or requirement upon the organism, the resolution or handling of which requires work or activity of the mental apparatus before any other system is involved or activated."

Wolff (18) also explored psychological stress and added the consideration of social problems. He focused on the person's past experiences and nervous system as mediating factors. In his definition, stress is viewed as "the internal or resisting force brought into action in part by external forces or loads."

Hinkle (9) points to the social aspect of stress when he states that "at the present time the 'stress' exploration is no longer necessary. It is evident that any disease process, and in fact any process within the living process, might be influenced by the reaction of the individual to his social environment or to other people."

Whether a particular definition of stress focuses on the physiological, psychological, or sociological component, all researchers on stress point out that stress is a natural occurrence of living. Hoff (10), who defines stress as "tension, strain, or pressure," states that "stress is a common denominator as we move from infancy through childhood to adolescence, adulthood, and old age. Throughout life individuals are called upon to respond to stress."

Some researchers and authors differentiate between stress, eustress, and distress. Flynn (5) expands on Selye's definitions of stress: "Stress is the nonspecific response of the body to any demand, whether it is caused by or results in pleasant or unpleasant conditions. Responses to harmful demands should be called distress, while those resulting from, or in, pleasure are eustress" (p. 95). Flynn further points out that eustress can cause damage to the body, just as stress and distress do, but to a lesser degree.

Stressors of Everyday Life

The term *stressor* indicates any activity that results in a person experiencing stress. Stimuli, or sources of stress, have been identified by numerous researchers.

Dixon (3) felt that every activity a person undertakes produces some stress. He discussed physical, psychological, socioeconomic, environmental, and cultural sources of stress. Physiological sources of stress are numerous and vary from normal growth and developmental changes, normal patterns of nutrition and oxygenation, to illnesses and injuries. Psychological sources of stress include any activity that calls forth an emotional response and vary from pleasurable, enjoyable, desired experiences to experiences of grief, loss, or unhappiness. Psychological stressors also include maturational changes in roles. Socioeconomic sources of stress could be upward or downward changes in financial or social functioning or status. Environmental stressors include such things as noise, air pollution, temperature, humidity, or geographical and physical surroundings. Cultural stressors refer to the demands any culture places on people through behavioral expectations.

Sorenson and Luckmann (16) identify the following four basic sources of stress:

1. Stress arising from difficult, threatening, or rapidly changing situations
2. Stress arising from normal living activities
3. Stress resulting from planned activities and therapies, or curative stress
4. Stress from anticipation of activities or events, or anticipatory stress

In order to accurately assess the stressors a client may be experiencing, the nurse should have a framework for evaluating the person's current experiences and activities as stressors. Norris Hansell (8) developed a list of "seven essential attachments," which include the major behaviors and situations that people must have in their living environments and that can provide a framework for the nurse to assess experiences as sources of stress. According to Hansell, each of the seven attachments is necessary for a person to survive. Each category is interdependent; if any one attachment is severed, other attachments also experience damage. That is, stress in any one category can lead to stress in any other category. Together, all seven attachments include all behaviors needed to maintain a person. The seven attachments are as follows:

1. *Supports necessary to existence.* These include food, oxygen, and information provided by sensory input necessary to maintain physical and psychological functioning.
2. *The notion of identity.* This attachment refers to the person's having a clear self-identity, a valid self-picture to guide actions and behaviors.
3. *Connection with other people.* This attachment relates to the need for intimacy. Hansell says that "an individual requires a persisting attachment to at least one individual."
4. *Connection with groups.* "All persons require at least one group attachment which can assist in ongoing tasks like provision of food, shelter and recreation and which can also assist in managing episodes of unusual challenge."
5. *Connection to a social role.* People must perform at least one persisting role. Hansell elaborates on this, stating that people need to have skills, show they can accomplish tasks, interest others in helping them, and demonstrate that they can be useful to others in order to regard themselves with esteem and dignity.
6. *Money and purchasing power.* It is necessary to have a supply of money or purchasing power as a person or as a member of a family in order to obtain services and goods needed to maintain or increase security.
7. *A system of meaning.* To survive, it is necessary for a person to have a meaningful, satisfying set of beliefs that guide decisions and give meaning to experiences.

Any experience or event that influences the functioning of any of these attachments should be considered a source of stress, or a stressor. It can be seen that the stressors are many and will vary from person to person. Some examples of stressors that are related to the seven attachments are as follows:

- Acute or chronic physical conditions or environmental situations that interfere with nutritional or oxygenation status (for example, diabetes, colitis, pneumonia, emphysema, air pollution)
- The disease process itself, which may be a result of stress. It must also be recognized that the disease is a source of stress when it interferes with ability to maintain many of the essential attachments. Conditions that interfere with sensory input are, for example, excessive noise, blindness, loss of hearing, institutionalization, confinement to bed.

Table 15.1
Relationship of Stressors to Attachments

Attachment	Possible Stressor
Supports necessary for existence: food, water, oxygen, information	Change in eating patterns; difficulty in breathing; air pollution; change in activities, events, or ability to participate in social activities; increase or decrease in sensory input; excessive noise; isolation; confinement to bed; institutionalization; change in ability to receive or respond to sensory input
Notion of identity	Change to new developmental stage; change in body image resulting from growth, aging, illness, accident, surgical interventions, or emotional changes; change in professional or occupational activities or recognition; move to a new area; change in marital status
Connection with other people	Change in social, professional, or family contacts; change in marital status; parenthood; change in people living in household; death of significant other; move to a new area
Connection with groups	Change in work, religious, social, or political groups, activity, or status
Connection to a social role	Restriction of social or physical action owing to age, illness, or institutionalization; change in financial status; migration; social upheaval; personal injury; situation in which promotion or achievement is not possible; recent promotion or achievement; unemployment; retirement
Money and purchasing power	Change in financial status; unemployment; retirement; chronic poverty; change in purchasing ability; change in credit standing; loss of family unit by moving, divorce, or death
System of meaning	Inability to participate in usual rituals owing to physical, emotional, geographical, or cultural restraints

- Changes in developmental status (for example, entry into adolescence or old age, parenthood)
- Changes in family, work, or social role: geographical relocations, lack of privacy, poor housing, marriage, divorce, change of job, retirement, promotion, unemployment
- Change of church or other social affiliations

Although this list is not all-inclusive, it gives the practitioner an idea of the number of events that must be monitored as stressors. The nurse who is concerned with providing holistic care must be alert to any change in a person's ability to maintain the essential attachments and indications of stressors affecting any attachment. It should be noted that illness may be considered a stressor or a stress response.

Table 15.1 summarizes stressors related to specific attachments.

Response to Stressors

Selye's work on stress resulted in identification of a three-stage syndrome of response to stress, the general adaptation syndrome. The syndrome focuses on the body's physiological response to stress in which hormonal responses allow the body to defend tissues. Numerous and complex biological, biochemical mechanisms that either create a state of tolerance to the stressors or destroy the agents creating the stress are involved in the syndromes. Selye recognized the relationship between bodily and mental reactions and the fact that both physical and emotional stimuli serve as stressors and elicit the general adaptation syndrome. The reader is referred to a basic medical-surgical nursing textbook for a review of the specific responses in the general adaptation syndrome.

All of the responses to stress are designed to restore the person to the usual state of functioning, or to maintain homeostasis. Dixon (3) states that a person accomplishes this return to homeostasis through use of "habitual patterns of adaptation to restore, then sets about resolving the next conflict or meeting the next need. Each person learns techniques to cope with that allow him or her to carry out daily responsibilities while attempting to maintain internal consistency."

These techniques of coping may be psychological, cognitive, behavioral, or physiological strategies. If the techniques normally used are not effective, stress is pro-

Table 15.2
Possible Responses to Stress

Response	Characteristic Effects
Subjective	Anxiety, aggression, apathy, boredom, depression, fatigue, frustration, guilt and shame, irritability, bad temper, moodiness, low self-esteem, threat and tension, nervousness, loneliness
Behavioral	Accident proneness, drug use, emotional outbursts, excessive eating or loss of appetite, excessive drinking and smoking, excitability, impulsive behavior, impaired speech, nervous laughter, restlessness and trembling, insomnia, excessive sleeping, loss of sphincter control
Cognitive	Inability to make decisions and concentrate, frequent forgetfulness, decreased attention span, hypersensitivity to criticism, mental blocks
Physiological	Increased blood and urine catecholamine and corticosteroid levels, increased blood glucose levels, increased heart and respiratory rates, increased blood pressure, dryness of mouth, sweating, dilation of pupils, difficulty in breathing, hot and cold spells, a "lump in the throat," numbness and tingling in extremities, difficulty swallowing, diarrhea
Health	Asthma, amenorrhea, chest and back pains, coronary heart disease, diarrhea, faintness and dizziness, dyspepsia, frequent urination, headache and migraine, neuroses, nightmares, insomnia, psychoses, psychosomatic disorder, diabetes mellitus, skin rash, ulcers, loss of sexual interest, and weakness
Organizational	Absenteeism, poor industrial relations and poor productivity, high accident and labor turnover rates, poor organizational climate, antagonism at work and job dissatisfaction, ineffectiveness of work routine

Source: Adapted from T. Cox, Stress. Baltimore: University Park Press, 1978.

longed. Failure to discharge the physiological responses to stress has a cumulative effect on the body that leads to a chronic state of stress.

Persistent, prolonged stress has been found by researchers (2, 14, 15, 17) to lead to functional and structural damage, to lower body resistance, and to predispose the person to illness. Selye (15) cites experiments of the Swiss army that "prove that relatively brief stints of stress, below the intensity that most people ordinarily experience at some time in their lives, can provoke pathologic changes in our body. If they are repeated often or are allowed to persist for long periods, they might cause disease."

Table 15.2 summarizes possible responses to stress.

Determinants of Stress Responses

As can be seen from Table 15.2, the possible responses to a stressor are many. Not everyone responds to a par-

ticular stressor in a similar way. People respond to stressors with different behaviors and with varying degrees of response. Factors that influence individual responses to any stressor include the person's personality, coping style (previously used responses), perception of the stressor and surrounding situations, previous experience with similar situations, psychological and cognitive abilities and needs, and available supports (people and physical resources). The nurse who identifies a potential stressor in a client's life situation must make a complete assessment of these factors in order to determine the risk involved to the client and to develop an appropriate plan of action to minimize the stress to the client.

The Primary Nurse's Role in Assessment of Stress

The first step in the nursing process, assessment, is also the first step in assisting clients with stress management.

The nurse should assess the client's functioning in each of the areas identified in Table 15.2 to identify signs of a stress response. In addition to observation skills, it is important for the nurse to use therapeutic communication skills to assist the client in exploring and identifying feelings, thoughts, and areas of life functioning that might be sources of stress. The nurse must be able to use the communication process in such a way that the nurse-client relationship becomes one of therapeutic intimacy, that is, a relationship in which the client and nurse are mutually accepting and work to support the client's problem-solving process. The reader is referred to the many available texts on therapeutic communications for a review of the techniques used to develop this relationship (see chapter 3).

The nurse must be acutely aware of behaviors that indicate a need for professional psychological counseling. Extremes of behavior that make it impossible for a person to maintain personality integrity, communications with others, or self-care functions should alert the nurse to the possibility that the client is in need of psychological counseling.

Hoff (10) suggests a two-level assessment that would be helpful in determining if the client should be referred for psychological counseling. On the first level the nurse should determine risks for suicide or homicide. This assessment should consider previous history of suicidal or homicidal actions or threats, current threats and plans, lethality of plans, availability of suicide/homicide weapons included in plan, current use of drugs, including alcohol, and intactness of relationships with significant others. This assessment is critical in determining what services must be mobilized to assist the client. If there is any indication of suicidal or homicidal potential, emergency services must be used and may include the police as well as professional counselors if the threat is imminent. The nurse should be aware of her or his legal responsibility to mobilize health care professionals in response to the threat of suicidal or homicidal tendencies of the client. Failure to do so can lead to liability for negligence.

On the second level the client's ability to function in usual life roles and remain part of the usual social setting is assessed. This involves assessing personal and social characteristics that are included in a psychosocial assessment. If the person is unable to maintain role functions or is in danger of being excluded from usual social interactions, referral should be made for professional counseling.

The Role of the Primary Nurse in Intervening in Stress

Once an assessment of stress response has been made, there are a number of interventions the nurse should consider. The importance of self-care strategies in the management of everyday stress must be recognized. Relaxation techniques and meditation are tools that clients can apply themselves in adjusting to stressful environments and situations (6). The nurse can be instrumental in assisting clients to use stress management techniques.

Help Clients Identify Stress

A significant aspect of stress management is client education. Clients should learn to recognize early signs of stress or distress in order to engage in a preventive stress management program and avoid developing chronic stress and stress-related disorders. The nurse should assist clients to become more aware of signals that their bodies give when they experience stressors in the physical, emotional, spiritual, or social aspects of living. Some early stress responses include muscle tension, backaches, headache, irritability, and restlessness.

Help Clients Identify Acceptable Stress Levels

Each person must learn the level of stress at which he or she functions best. Flynn (5) points out that it is both impossible and undesirable to avoid all stress; a certain degree of stress is necessary to maintain homeostatic function and mobilize individual resources.

Clients should be aware that they can regulate the circumstances to which they must adapt at any one time. A client who is experiencing a period of stress should be assisted to examine the activities and decisions in the current life situation and determine what needs immediate attention and what can be delayed. Hansell (8) states that it is important to help the client find a comfortable pace at which to move through a stressful situation. He emphasizes that a problem-solving situation will extend over a period of time, not just one day. Many decisions require time for thought and should not be made in haste. Nor should they necessarily be made when the client's perception is narrowed because of a stressor.

Selye's (15) first guideline for minimizing distress, "find your own natural predilections and stress level," discusses the importance for every person to do a thoughtful self-analysis of desires, the amount and kind of work that is important for the person to engage in daily, and the kinds of experiences that provide meaningful release of energy. In this way the person will be aware of those activities that are likely to evoke a stress response and can determine if that level of stress is important enough to be considered desirable. Keeping a journal of activities and feelings can be a means for clients to increase their awareness of their own stress levels and of early signs that the desirable level of stress is being exceeded. In addition to noting stress levels, journal entries can be used to identify coping mechanisms that were effective and those that were ineffective in managing stress situations.

Help Clients Maintain Relationships

It is important to help the client maintain relationships with significant others. During a stress situation social supports are necessary to help the client maintain a realistic perception of the stressful event and of self and to explore alternative behaviors and actions. Selye's second and third guidelines for a code of behavior based on classification of the nonspecific adaptation mechanism provide some direction for such activities in a stress management program. These guidelines are "Learn altruistic egoism" and "Earn your neighbor's love." Altruistic egoism, giving to others while building self, assists in building self-esteem necessary to maintain a healthy self-concept. A healthy self-esteem and self-identity will allow the person to maintain internal supports necessary to prevent the progression of a stress state to a crisis state. Activities that earn the respect, support, and esteem of others, that is, that "earn your neighbor's love," are a person's most efficient way of discharging energy and building up the support groups and connections with other people, groups, and social roles necessary for survival. The nurse should assist the client in "conscious stock-taking," reviewing past achievements, successes, and coping mechanisms to help the client maintain a realistic perception of behavior, actions, and situations. This review can be done either verbally or as part of the journal used in the stress management program. The primary nurse should help the client plan ways to keep contacts open and to have regular communication and contact with significant others.

Help Clients Maintain Health Practices

The client should be helped to maintain adequate nutrition, rest, relaxation, and activity during stress situations and to recognize that these activities are necessary for successful resolution of the stress situation.

Diet and exercise aid in the management of stress in that they help the client to maintain a high level of physical health, which increases the person's ability to handle stress appropriately and avoid becoming involved in a chronic stress pattern. Diet is important in providing energy resources necessary to meet daily physiological and psychological activity requirements and to prevent stress from overnutrition or undernutrition. Nurses have many opportunities to evaluate the client's dietary patterns and to provide health teaching to assist the client to achieve adequate nutrition.

The role of exercise in management of stress is well recognized. Exercise, as a preventive measure, maintains optimum physical status. As a method of stress management, exercise provides a means of responding that alters negative stress responses. Clients may use exercise in place of negative, stress-continuing responses. Glasser (7) discusses exercise, running in particular, as a positive addiction that can strengthen the person and make his or her life more satisfactory. Nurses may review exercise and activity patterns with clients. Health teaching can be important in helping clients recognize the role of exercise in stress management.

Teach Clients Relaxation as Stress Management

A number of relaxation techniques can be taught to clients for use as part of a daily program of stress management. Numerous studies have shown that relaxation techniques successfully reduce anxiety and the perception of pain and discomfort.

The primary purpose of relaxation techniques is simply to relax the body. The simplest technique is controlled breathing. Clients can be taught to breathe rhythmically and more slowly than usual in an anxiety-provoking stress situation. This technique helps to restore a sense of control in the situation. Clients will initially need the guidance of the nurse as they learn breath control. As they gain experience with the relaxation method, they will be able to use it to intervene in stressful situations on their own. Nurses can help clients identify situations in which controlled breathing may help reduce stress. Students can be taught to use controlled breathing when they become anxious during exams or presentations. Mothers may find the exercise helpful in reducing everyday stress. Professional people may be taught to use the exercise during stressful meetings or discussions. All clients may find the technique helpful during physical examinations or treatment procedures that are discomforting.

Flynn (5) details a brief relaxation exercise for use in preventive stress management.

Breathe in a deep, centering breath.
Let it center and ground you.
Then let it blow out all the tension and anxiety in your mind-body.
Take another breath centering yourself with peaceful energy.
Blow and let go of all negative thoughts, feelings and worry.
Breathe in calm energy,
Relaxed and energetic
Calmly active
Actively calm. (5, p. 16)

She also gives directions for a progressive relaxation exercise based on Edmund Jacobsen's technique. The exercise, which is written for right-handed people, should begin with the dominant hand.

Sit or lie in a comfortable position and let your eyes close.
I take a moment to be here (allow time).
I focus my attention on my right hand and I make a fist.
Slowly and steadily I clench my fist and study the tension.
Now I let go and feel the difference.
I repeat that.
I clench my fist, tightly, feeling the tension.
I let go and enjoy the contrast in my feelings.
Now I tense my right forearm.
Studying the tension.
And let go and notice the difference.
Now I tense my bicep—tighten.
And let go.
I stretch my arm straight out and feel the tension in my arm and shoulder.
I let go and appreciate the difference.
Now I focus my attention on my left hand and I make a fist.
Slowly and steadily I clench my fist and study the tension.
Now I let go and feel the difference.
I do that again.
Clenching my fist, tightly, feeling the tension.
And I let go and enjoy the contrast in my feelings.
Now I tense my left forearm.
Studying the tension.
And let go and notice the difference.

Now I tense my bicep—tighten.
And let go.
I stretch my arm straight out and feel the tension in my arm and shoulder.
I let go and appreciate the difference.
I focus my attention on my scalp.
I tighten it.
And now I smooth it out.
I pay attention to the muscles of my forehead—I frown.
And study the tension as I frown.
I let go and notice the difference.
I raise my eyebrows and hold them for a few seconds.
And let go.
Now the muscles around my eyes—I tense them and tighten them.
And let go.
The muscles of my cheeks, I tighten them.
And release, acknowledging the difference.
Now I tighten my jaw muscles, tighter.
And let go.
I let it relax.
And now the muscles in the back of my neck—I tighten those.
I feel the tension and now I let it go.
I pull my shoulders back and up and tighten the muscles between my shoulders.
Tighten and notice the tension.
And let go.
Now I tighten the muscles of my upper back.
Tighten—and let go.
I focus my attention now on the muscles of my lower back.
I tighten them and notice the tension.
And let go.
Now the muscles of my buttocks.
Tighten—feel the tension.
And let go.
Breathing easily and calmly, deeply and efficiently.
I bring my attention to the muscles of the front of my neck.
I tighten them, bringing my chin up.
And let go.
Now I tighten my chest muscles—tighten.
And let go.
I let myself take in a good deep breath and hold it, feeling all my muscles expand.
And now I let go—letting all the breath out.
I repeat this and notice my feelings.
I tense the muscles of my abdomen.
I tighten them and notice the tension.

And let go and appreciate the relaxation.
And my pelvic muscles—I tighten them—tight.
And let go.
My thighs—I tighten those muscles.
And let go, noticing the difference.
Now the muscles of my calves and lower legs.
I tense them tighter and note the tension.
And let go.
And the muscles of my feet—tighten them.
And let go and appreciate the difference.
And now I take a moment to scan my body—
   noticing any part of my body that still needs
   relaxation.
And I tense that part and let go.
Any other muscles—I take a moment to tense them.
And let go.
And now, feeling the pleasure of this relaxation, I
   take a few moments to bring my attention back
   to this time and this place, and filled with energy
   and peace, I open my eyes, stretch, and get up (5).

Primary care nurses can teach clients to use progressive relaxation techniques. Such techniques are particularly helpful for people who experience chronic fatigue, insomnia, hypertension, and chronic pain.

Help Clients Use Meditation

Meditation may also be used as part of stress management programs. The form of activity used for periods of meditation can vary from listening to quiet music, running, walking, praying, to the more structured forms of meditations such as transcendental meditation. Whatever form it takes, everyone needs a daily period of quiet thought and reflection to balance the day's activities.

Anticipatory Guidance

Anticipatory guidance is an important principle of stress management. There are predictable life events that can prove stressful. The nurse who has a good understanding of growth and development as well as an appreciation of the client's life situation will be able to help the client plan approaches to potentially stressful events before their occurrence, thus minimizing the stress experiences.

Working with Professional Stress

Continued stress experienced by professionals can lead to a syndrome referred to as burnout. People in any profession can experience this syndrome. People in the helping professions are a high-risk group for professional stress. The emotional stress of caring for clients can be great. Decisions must be made quickly and often without complete background information. Peers and other health professionals may not be in complete agreement with decisions and plans. Clients frequently complain about care. Expectations for performance are high. Physical and psychological demands placed on the nurse as a professional person are high. Nursing students are also exposed to many stressors that can lead to professional stress syndrome. High expectations for performance in classroom and clinical settings, the demands for responsibility for other people, emotional responses to new levels of responsibility, intimate contact with clients both physically and emotionally, time pressures for classroom and clinical work, and unfamiliar environments, roles, cues, and expectations can all contribute to a high stress level.

Burnout, or professional stress, is manifested by "physical and emotional exhaustion, involving the development of negative self-concept, negative job attitudes, and a loss of concern for feeling for clients" (12). Maslach (13) further describes the symptoms as loss of "positive feelings, sympathy or respect for patients or clients." Initial symptoms may be vague and may include tiredness, emotional exhaustion, headache, gastrointestinal distress, aches and pains, increased susceptibility to illness, insomnia, and increased absenteeism (11).

In later stages of burnout the professional labels clients in derogatory ways and treats clients with little concern or care as a cynical dehumanized perception of clients develops. At this point the person may change jobs, move into administrative work, or leave the profession in an attempt to cope with the chronic stress state. Maslach further states that use and abuse of drugs and alcohol may now increase to reduce tension. The person may either stay away from work or spend increased time at work without completing the necessary tasks. It is not uncommon for professionals in a high level of chronic stress to develop feelings of personal failure in the profession and perceive themselves as incompetent practitioners.

The effects of professional stress may also be seen in family and social life as increased irritability spills over into these areas of functioning. The person may experience a greater need for solitary time and privacy in order to cope with the stress. This may be interpreted as rejection by family and friends who do not understand the professional stressors. Disruptions in relationships may follow.

Coping with Professional Stress

The principles of stress management detailed in preceding sections of this chapter are applicable to the professionals in preventing and managing burnout. Self-analysis, diet, exercise, relaxation, meditation, use of support groups, and manipulation of the number of stressful activities encountered should be part of the professional person's daily program of stress management.

Specific measures for use in stress management related to professional activities include the following.

Join a peer support group. Development of a professional support group that meets regularly on both a formal and an informal basis is a crucial component of management of professional stress. The group can be used to report successes, discuss problem situations, and share experiences, emotions, and frustrations. The peer support group can provide opportunities for exploration of expectations of self and others and possible responses to stressful professional situations. Each member of the support group can also receive feedback that is helpful in maintaining realistic self and professional perceptions. In addition, group settings allow for the use of humor, which is an important means of reducing tension and anxiety.

Alternate activities during the work day. Plan routines so that high-stress activities are followed by less emotionally and physically demanding activities. Take regular breaks. Have lunch with friends, not necessarily with co-workers. Take breaks and lunch periods away from the work area. Maintain an area in the workplace that is always available for staff to use for breaks. Avoid shoptalk during breaks and lunch periods.

Maintain professional interest, skills, and involvements. Attend in-service programs. Become involved in interesting projects and activities in the work setting or in professional organizations.

Develop interests outside professional activities. These interests can be shared with family and friends other than professional colleagues.

Set realistic expectations for your own and colleagues' actions. It is important to recognize verbally, intellectually, and emotionally that it is not possible to save or cure every client, to win every case, or to be the best in your field. It may be sufficient in some situations to help

the client to be as comfortable as possible or to live as full a life as possible within the client's limitations.

Learn to accept your own feelings. Burger (1), in discussing the effect of emotions on helping professionals, states that "emotions are the by-products of healthy, caring involvement. Once caregivers can accept the fact that they have feelings, they can begin the process of sharing them with others."

Recognize the positives. Burger suggests that focusing on satisfactions of the job and assets of clients helps prevent becoming overwhelmed with feelings of helplessness, which contribute to stress and burnout.

Educate yourself and others about the possibility of burnout, signs and symptoms of burnout, and preventive measures. Be aware of signs of burnout in yourself and colleagues. Be available as part of a support system for your colleagues. Use your colleagues as part of your support system. Let them know when you need their support.

Work with administrators in the work setting to maintain adequate staffing, flexibility in scheduling, private areas for breaks, and rewards and recognition for performance. Take an active role in the workplace to provide mechanisms for reducing stress and preventing burnout.

The following case studies are presented to help you apply your knowledge about stress and stress management techniques.

CASE STUDY 1

Paul Grey, age thirty-five, an accountant in a large urban accounting firm, is to have his blood pressure monitored weekly by the company nurse. During his regular physical examination last week his blood pressure was 168/92. As the nurse talks with Paul she learns that he and his wife have two children, Paula, age three, and Brian, age eleven months. Brian is moderately retarded and has had numerous illnesses since birth. Nine months ago Paul was given a large account to handle and as a result of his work received a promotion and a $5,000 yearly salary increase. A junior vice-president position will be open in six months and Paul hopes to receive the appointment. Consequently he has been devoting more time to work projects and has increased his social activities with colleagues who can be helpful in this quest. This has meant less time for activities with his family and church group. Paul had planned to use his hobby of furniture refinishing to help furnish the suburban home he and his wife purchased six months ago, since the furniture from their four-room apartment in the city is not sufficient. However, he finds that he is too tired when he is home to enjoy his hobby. He no longer stops at the health club to work out, as commuting takes too much of his time and he likes to be able to provide some help for his wife with Brian.

1. Identify stressors Paul has experienced.
2. Categorize the sources of stress Paul has experienced.
3. Identify and categorize Paul's symptoms of stress.
4. Propose a stress management program for Paul.

CASE STUDY 2

Mrs. Grady, a public health nurse, is reading the referral form before her first visit to Joan Prince. Mrs. Prince, age thirty-seven, gave birth to her first child, Angela, three days ago. Mr. and Mrs. Prince have been married for ten years but chose to delay having children in order for Mrs. Prince to become established in her career as an interior designer. Last year Mrs. Prince decided to become pregnant and to work on an independent, part-time basis once the child was born. She and her husband have rearranged their suburban home so that she has an office in the home. She does not plan to take any clients until Angela is three months old. Both Mr. and Mrs. Prince are delighted with their daughter and look forward to having the nurse visit their home to help them give Angela the best possible care.

1. What potential stressors can the nurse identify before her visit with Mrs. Prince?
2. Identify behavioral indications of stress that the nurse should be alert for as she does her initial assessment.
3. Discuss the role of anticipatory guidance in a stress management program for Mrs. Prince.
4. Devise a preventive stress management program for Mrs. Prince.

CASE STUDY 3

Janet Martin, R.N., has worked on the cardiac intensive care unit for six years. She transferred there after working on a general medical unit for a year. She enjoyed the challenge of working with cardiac clients, had attended workshops and in-service programs whenever possible to keep abreast of innovations in the field, gave excellent client care, and was respected by the nurses and physicians with whom she worked. She prided herself on her accumulation of unused sick time.

Six months ago she began to feel tired and headachy and to have severe back pain and frequent insomnia. Every few weeks she would have to take several days sick leave. She became very critical of the way other staff members performed and would often stay after the end of the shift to "finish up a few details." During break and over lunch she would talk with colleagues

about how unappreciative clients, physicians, and administrators were and would complain about how demanding and uncooperative her clients were, referring to them by room numbers rather than by names. Friends said that she seemed listless, apathetic, and disinterested in any social activities. Gradually they had stopped calling her, as she never had enough energy to join them. Two weeks ago she applied for a supervisory position, stating that she'd had enough of direct client care.

1. Identify symptoms of burnout displayed by Ms. Martin.
2. Discuss factors that would contribute to Ms. Martin's developing burnout.
3. Discuss the role of a support group in prevention of burnout.
4. Develop a plan for Janet to use in managing stress in her professional role.
5. Develop a plan for nurses on the cardiac intensive care unit.

REFERENCES

1. Burger, L. A. "Emotions: Their Presence and Impact Upon the Helping Role." In *Stress and Survival*, ed. C. A. Garfield. St. Louis: C. V. Mosby Co., 1979.
2. Cox, T. *Stress.* Baltimore, Md.: University Park Press, 1978.
3. Dixon, S. L. *Working People in Crisis: Theory and Practice.* St. Louis: C. V. Mosby Co., 1979.
4. Engel, G. S. *Psychological Development in Health and Disease.* Philadelphia: W. B. Saunders Co., 1962, 264.
5. Flynn, P. A. R. *Holistic Health: The Art and Science of Care.* Bowie, Md.: Robert J. Brady Co., 1980.
6. Garfield, C. A., ed. *Stress and Survival: The Emotional Realities of Life Threatening Illness.* St. Louis: C. V. Mosby Co., 1979.
7. Glasser, W. *Positive Addictions.* New York: Harper and Row, 1976.
8. Hansell, N. *The Person in Distress.* New York: Human Sciences Press, 1976.
9. Hinkle, L. E. "The Concept of 'Stress' in the Biological and Social Sciences." *Science, Medicine and Man* 1:43 (1973).
10. Hoff, Lee Ann. *People in Crisis: Understanding and Helping.* Menlo Park, Calif.: Addison-Wesley Pub. Co., 1978.
11. Maslach, G. "Burn-Out." *Human Behavior* 5, no. 9 (1976), 16–22.
12. Maslach, G. "Job Burnout: How People Cope." *Public Welfare* 36, no. 2 (1978), 56–58.
13. Maslach, G. "The Burnout Syndrome and Patient Care." In *Stress and Survival,* ed. C. A. Garfield. St. Louis: C. V. Mosby Co., 1979.
14. Selye, Hans. *The Stress of Life.* New York: McGraw-Hill, 1956.

15. Selye, Hans. "Stress Without Distress." In *Stress and Survival,* ed. C. A. Garfield. St. Louis: C. V. Mosby Co., 1979, 14.
16. Sorenson, K. G., and J. Luckmann. *Basic Nursing.* Philadelphia: W. B. Saunders Co., 1979.
17. Williams, C. E., and T. H. Holmes. "Life, Change, Human Adaptation, and Onset of Illness." In *Clinical Practice in Psychological Nursing: Assessment and Intervention.* New York: Appleton-Century-Crofts, 1978.
18. Wolff, H. G. *Stress and Disease.* 2nd ed. Springfield, Ill.: Charles C. Thomas, Publisher, 1968.

Crisis Theory and Intervention for the Nurse in General Practice

LYNN MILLER-SEIDMAN

■

OBJECTIVES

After completing this chapter, the reader will be able to:

- Define crisis.
- Describe the relationship of stress to crisis.
- Classify crisis, using Aguilera and Messick's categories for crisis classification.
- Classify crisis, using Baldwin's categories for crisis classification.
- Identify the elements of assessment of a client in crisis.
- Use Aguilera and Messick's paradigm in assessing a client for reaction to a stressful event and possible crisis state.

- Define crisis intervention.
- Identify principles of crisis intervention.
- Apply principles of crisis intervention.
- Identify high-risk candidates for suicide.
- Identify element in the assessment of a client for suicidal intent
- Apply suicide assessment principles.
- Describe the primary crisis role as "therapist" in working with a client in crisis.

This chapter is concerned with the definition of crisis, the assessment of a client in crisis, and crisis intervention theory. Crisis theory is relevant to the primary nurse because as a health care provider, the nurse is often called upon to assess a client for crisis states and, subsequently, plan, implement, and evaluate interventions aimed at restoring the client to optimal functioning. In this chapter the reader is presented with information and tools to provide care to a client in crisis. Crisis is defined and its relationship to stress is discussed. The principles of crisis are presented as they need to be used by the professional nurse. Assessment of a client for suicidal intent is described. Self-care theory is presented as it relates to crisis intervention. Finally, the role of the primary nurse as crisis intervention therapist/counselor is addressed.

The Relationship of Stress to Crisis

Gerald Caplan defines a crisis state as a "state of disequilibrium and disorganization during which one's normal coping mechanisms do not function" (3). Whenever a person enters a new situation, makes a significant life change, or takes on a new role, new demands are made on him or her. These demands create stress. The greater the number and strength of new situations and life changes occurring in a given period of time for a person, the greater the amount of stress on that person and, subsequently, the greater the likelihood that current available coping mechanisms will not operate sufficiently to maintain a state of equilibrium. When those coping mechanisms are inadequate, the likelihood of the person going into a state of disequilibrium or crisis greatly increases (4, 7). (For a complete description of stress and stressors, review chapter 15.)

Thus severity of stress in any person's life is influential in the development of illnesses for that person. Many of these illnesses are considered crises.

Information about stressors in a person's life is currently listed in the *Diagnostic and Statistical Manual III* (1980) as one of the criteria that must be used by psychi-

atric health care professionals for determining psychiatric diagnoses for clients, many of which are considered crisis states.

Each person is armed at any given time with a varying number and sophistication of coping mechanisms. Whether a person enters into a crisis state depends on the level and degree of stress that his or her coping mechanism can adequately handle without a period of disorganization.

Classification of Crisis

Aguilera and Messick (1, p. 73) have classified crises into two categories: situational and maturational. Situational crises are those that are precipitated by stressful events occurring in the course of one's life. Examples are crisis states after a disaster, the death of a loved one, marital separation or divorce, or acute severe illness.

Aguilera and Messick (1, p. 132) view maturational crises as those precipitated by the tasks and issues one must deal with in the normal growth and development process. Examples are crisis states precipitated by the trust versus mistrust task of infancy, independence/dependence issues during adolescence, or intimacy issues during young adulthood.

Baldwin (2, p. 539) classifies crises into six categories: dispositional crises, crises of anticipated life transitions, crises resulting from traumatic stress, maturational/developmental crises, crises reflecting psychopathology, and psychiatric emergencies. The rationale for developing this classification of crises, according to Baldwin, is based on some tenets of assessment in crisis intervention.

Assessment in crisis intervention is directed to the characteristics of the situation that produced the crisis (the precipitating event), the style and mode of response to that event, and the precipitant that defines the dynamic implications of the individual's inability to cope. Because of these emphases, traditional assessment techniques and psychiatric diagnosis do not "fit" the "crises model." (2)

Baldwin's classification is an attempt to develop a definitive paradigm that could be used in crisis intervention. For purposes of this chapter, Baldwin's six categories of crisis are briefly described below.

1. *Dispositional Crises*. These are periods of disequilibrium resulting from an upsetting situation for the client that leads the therapist to simply provide information to the client or family or to refer the client or family to a specific resource for information. In this situation the therapist operates at a cognitive general level rather than at a therapeutic emotional level. An example of this category of crisis is a period of disorganization that ensues after a person learns of the serious illness of a loved one. Intervention would include providing information to the person about the alternatives for treatment of the loved one.

2. *Crises of Anticipated Life Transitions*. These are periods of disequilibrium resulting from anticipated, usually normal changes that occur in the course of one's existence. One may or may not have control over these changes. An example of this kind of crisis is the client being separated or getting divorced. During these crises the therapist moves the client toward an understanding of the current and upcoming changes and the psychological implications of these transitions. Therapist and client then work on developing new coping mechanisms and using existing ones in a healthy manner.

3. *Crises Resulting from Traumatic Stress*. These are periods of disequilibrium occurring as a result of unexpected and uncontrolled stressful situations. A classic example of a client in this type of crisis is the rape victim. A client in this category of crises is often emotionally overwhelmed, leaving herself vulnerable to developing unhealthy coping mechanisms. In this situation the therapist supports the client in the use of effective coping mechanisms while helping her to understand the impact of the traumatic stress.

4. *Maturational/Developmental Crises*. These are periods of emotional disequilibrium resulting from unsatisfactory attempts on the client's part in the successful completion of those interpersonal developmental tasks essential to the attainment of emotional maturity. Examples are crises resulting from unfinished work on such developmental tasks as dependence versus independence, identity or role confusion, or intimacy versus isolation. Interventions on the part of the therapist in developmental crises are aimed at clarifying and working through the underlying developmental issue involved in precipitating the problem situation and, at the same time, helping a client to develop more adaptive interpersonal responses. This category of developmental/maturational crises, more than any of the other categories of crisis, offers the opportunity to assist a client in a successful growth experience.

5. *Crises Reflecting Psychopathology*. These are periods of emotional disequilibrium in which preexisting psychopathology significantly hinders or complicates successful resolution. Examples include people who are in periods of disequilibrium who *concurrently* suffer from severe neuroses or schizophrenia. The therapeutic aim in this category of crises is to reduce the stress on the client as soon as possible in order to prevent total decompensation. If the client is not already in long-term psychotherapy, he or she must be prepared and immediately referred for that treatment approach.

6. *Psychiatric Emergencies*. These are periods of disequilibrium in which the client's functioning is severely altered so that he or she cannot assume personal responsibility. Examples of people in such crises are clients who are acutely suicidal or in an acute psychosis. In this situation the client is clearly a danger either to himself or herself or to others. The nurse in such crises must assess the client's medical and psychiatric status and obtain necessary emergency treatment. The crisis worker then often coordinates various health care services for the client.

Regardless of how one classifies crises, the precipitation of a crisis state is very individual; that is, events or issues that might lead to a crisis state in one person do not necessarily precipitate a crisis state in another person. This is because people have varied coping mechanisms that operate with different degrees of success and sophistication. When those individual coping skills are no longer successful, a crisis state ensues.

Crisis Intervention and the Suicidal Client

Whenever one discusses crisis and crisis intervention, it is most important to address assessment of the client who is or has recently been suicidal. The client who is actively suicidal is considered to be in a crisis state and, using Baldwin's categories of classification, in a psychiatric emergency warranting hospitalization. Knowledge of these assessment skills is especially important for the primary nurse, as she is often the first caring health professional with whom the client comes in contact. This holds true especially in such nursing roles as community health nurse and school nurse. In these instances the professional nurse is responsible for assessing the suicide potential and degree of risk for the client and, subsequently, for initiating action that will maintain the client in a safe position. The determination of whether or not the client requires hospitalization is of prime importance to the client's safety.

Populations at Risk for Suicide

Certain populations are at high risk for suicide. A client who fits in one or more of these groups increases his or her potential for suicide. Groups at high risk for suicide include men, single people, people living in industrial societies, people who have experienced recent losses, the elderly, adolescents, people in nurturing professions, depressed people, people with psychoses, drug and alcohol abusers, and people with a history of suicide attempts.

When the primary nurse comes in contact with a client who may be actively suicidal, he or she needs to assess that person for suicidal intent. The following questions must be answered:

1. If the client makes contact with the nurse shortly after a suicide attempt
   a. How lethal was the attempt?
   b. Was the attempt at a time and circumstance when help was quickly and easily available?
   c. Did the client try to prevent intervention?
   d. Did the client seek assistance immediately after the attempt? Before the attempt?
   e. How much planning went into the attempt? Did the client leave a note?
   f. What was the client hoping to accomplish with the attempt? Did he or she want to kill himself or herself? Did he or she want to make others aware of his or her distress?
   g. How does the client feel about the attempt? Does he or she regret it? Would he or she do it again? How does the client intend to handle future problems?
   h. Have there been previous attempts? If so, how many?
   i. Is the client in any of the high-risk groups described earlier?
2. If the client shares with the nurses that he or she is considering an attempt but has not yet actually made an attempt
   a. Does the client have a plan? If so, what is the plan and how lethal does it appear to be?
   b. Have there been previous attempts?
   c. How strong is the client's support system? Who does he or she feel close to? On whom can he or she depend?
   d. Is the client in any of the high-risk groups mentioned earlier?
   e. What does the client hope to accomplish? Does he or she want to kill himself or herself?
   f. What is or has been going on in the client's life that has led him or her to consider suicide as a major alternative?

Based on the client's responses to these questions, the primary nurse will assess whether or not the client requires hospitalization. It is important to remember that any person who either has just made a suicide attempt or is considering taking such action, *must be referred to a professional with expertise in mental health* for further evaluation and treatment. It is essential that each nursing professional know her or his limitations and refer clients to the appropriate channels for adequate, safe, and quality health care.

CASE STUDY*

Maria, a sixteen-year-old Hispanic girl, was referred to the mental health clinic for an emergency intake by the school nurse, to whom the girl had expressed suicidal intention. Because the school nurse did not feel qualified to assess whether or not the child needed hospitalization, she referred the girl to the center and had her directly brought to the center by her mother. Maria was seen by a mental health nurse for assessment. On being questioned as to her reason for coming to the center, Maria states that her mother brought her when she learned from the school nurse that Maria had stated she had plans for killing herself. Maria then describes to the mental health nurse a rather complicated home situation: Maria's father has recently remarried a twenty-one-year-old woman, and Maria learned of this about one week before being seen at the clinic. The father has been living in Puerto Rico for the past five years, after Maria's parents had divorced. Maria is living with her mother and two younger brothers. She describes her most recent home situation (past few months) as "strangers living in the same house." Maria describes herself and her mother as "usually being close," until six months ago. Maria tells the therapist that her mother had a child approximately two years before the interview that her mother had told her was her father's child. Six months before the intake, the family had gone to Puerto Rico, and Maria had learned that this youngest child was not her father's. Maria says that her learning of this upset her mother very much, and her mother has subsequently been depressed and withdrawn. In addition, Ma-

*The author wishes to acknowledge the senior students at Lehman College who worked with clients from whom the case studies in this chapter are derived.

ria states that four months before the interview, her mother had returned to school full time, resulting in a major increase in Maria's household and baby-sitting responsibilities. Her mother has also been less available to Maria.

Concerning prior suicidal attempts and intention, Maria describes two prior suicide attempts in the family. One attempt was made by her mother approximately four years ago, and one attempt was made by Maria herself three and one half years ago. In both instances a small number of nonlethal pills were taken at such a time and circumstance that help was available and quickly sought.

At this point in the interview the nurse redirects Maria back to what seems to be the precipitating event, the news of her father's remarriage. Maria states that when she learned of the remarriage, she didn't want to love anyone. She goes on to say, however, that she also felt like killing herself about one week before that news because she "felt overwhelmed and didn't believe anyone cared about me or wanted me around." When asked about a plan and what she does when she feels this way, Maria states that she thought about taking "some pills" but then went to talk about it with her boy friend, who convinced her not to do it. She then says that she really wanted to get some attention and response from people. Maria states that she no longer wants to kill herself; she just wants to "make things better at home and doesn't know any other way to let them know." When asked what she will do the next time she feels this way, Maria states that she will talk to her mother and boy friend about it.

After the interview with Maria the nurse speaks briefly with the mother and establishes that there are grandparents nearby who are viewed as supportive and are available to help the family. Maria's mother also indicates that she will relieve Maria of some household responsibilities.

Intake assessment and recommendations are as follows: sixteen-year-old articulate female who has experienced a number of life stressor changes and transitions—divorce, recent remarriage of father to a young woman, two changes in residence, a sibling addition, and an increase in household responsibilities. Based on the interview, her recent suicidal ideation and current suicidal intent are not strong in degree, and she has some support system available to her; hospitalization is not recommended. Initially, however, four private sessions for Maria, followed by family counseling, are recommended to work on reducing current stressors, learning more effective coping mechanisms in dealing with uncomfortable situations, assisting both mother and daughter in accepting the loss of the father, and increasing both mother's and daughter's self-esteem. A contract is made with the client and family to return for counseling and with Maria to seek immediate assistance if thoughts of suicide return, without taking any self-destructive action.

Assessment in Crisis

Aguilera and Messick have developed a paradigm that shows the human organism's possible reaction to a

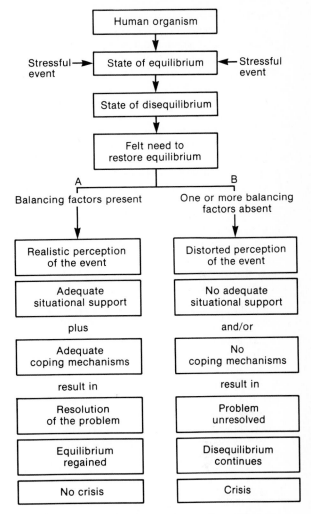

Figure 16.1. Aguilera and Messick's Paradigm: Effect of Balancing Factors in a Stressful Event

Source: Donna C. Aguilera and Janice M. Messick. *Crisis Intervention: Theory and Methodology.* St. Louis: C. V. Mosby Co., 1978.

stressful event and indicates whether or not the client will end up in a crisis state (Figure 16.1). The development of a crisis state, they suggest, depends on the balancing factors in any person's life that can influence a return to equilibrium. These balancing factors are perception of the event, available situational supports, and coping mechanisms.

Using this paradigm for crises, the more balancing factors absent in any person's life during a stressful event, the greater the likelihood that a crisis state will result. Aguilera and Messick use the paradigm in their test for the presentation of case studies on crisis. It is a helpful method of visualizing the development of a crisis in any individual case. Later in this chapter the use of this paradigm is illustrated in the presentation of a specific crisis case study. In the initial interview, then, in crisis assessment, in addition to the usual history and assessment that the primary nurse would do on any client with a problem, the crisis intervention worker needs to assess the client specifically to determine if he or she is indeed in a crisis state. The nurse needs to see if the client's usual coping mechanisms are failing and if the client is experiencing a period of disorganization. The "problem" needs to be identified; that is, what the client views as the problem that made him or her seek assistance needs to be determined. A mental status examination should be performed.

In assessing a client in crisis the nurse collects data about the characteristics of the situation that has precipitated the crisis, the response to that situation, and the degree of the client's current coping abilities. The following questions can help get at this information:

- Exactly what is the problem?
- How much has it disrupted the client's normal life-style?
- To what degree is the client able to accomplish his or her usual activities of daily living?
- What has the client discovered that makes the situation better or worse?
- What is the client's support system like?
- Is the client in touch with reality?
- Is the client suicidal or homicidal?

On the basis of the answers to the questions and issues addressed above, the nurse needs to determine the degree of emergency that exists and some initial plans for the client. The immediate determination to be made is whether or not the client requires hospitalization. Once this initial decision is made, the nurse and client are able to proceed through the crisis intervention process. If it is determined that hospitalization is not necessary, but the client is indeed in crisis, plans need to be initiated for outpatient treatment.

Crisis Intervention: Definition and Principles

Crisis intervention refers to a specific approach used in helping clients during the period of disequilibrium and disorganization termed the crisis state. It is a therapeutic approach used over a short period—usually not more than six weeks. The focus of crisis intervention is resolu-

tion of the defined problem in a healthy manner. The entire intervention process usually requires not more than ten hours of the nurse's time, including phone contacts and sessions.

A number of principles of crisis intervention are essential for the nurse to use in order to assist the client or family in successfully resolving a crisis state. These are immediate actions, establishing rapport/trust, identification and assessment of the problem, limited goal, support, problem solving, self-image, self-reliance, and closure (5).

Immediate Action. As noted earlier, clients/families in crisis are in a period of disorganization, which often means that they are in distress and, at times, in danger. Because this is such a vulnerable period in a person's life, it can result in either regression or growth on the part of the client, depending on how the crisis is handled. This necessitates immediate intervention on the part of the health professional. Generally, then, once the client has contacted the health professional he or she should be seen in less than twenty-four hours for an initial in-depth assessment of the situation.

Establishing Rapport/Trust. Because crisis intervention is a short-term process, it is of prime importance that the nurse establish rapport and a trusting relationship with the client in the shortest possible time period. *Every* contact with the client, in person or otherwise, needs to be used to demonstrate honesty, consistency, concern, and competence.

Because the client is in great distress, he or she is often more open to trusting the health professional. In addition, the distress of the client often makes him or her increasingly accessible to trying new forms of behavior or changes in coping skills. This vulnerability makes crisis a period out of which personal growth can occur. The Chinese symbol for crisis indicates both danger and opportunity (see Figure 16.2).

Limited Goal. In doing crisis intervention it is important to keep in perspective the fact that the goal in this type of therapy is, at the minimum, to restore the client to his or her precrisis level of functioning and, optimally, to enhance some personal growth. The goal needs to be kept limited so that it can be accomplishable within the limited time frame. When the client appears in a crisis state, he or she will be having enough difficulty handling limited goals without the increased complexity of handling multiple complex goals.

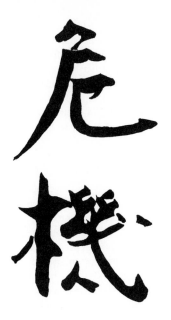

Figure 16.2.   Crisis Symbol

Support.   Most often by the time the client in crisis seeks assistance at a crisis or health center, he or she is feeling quite hopeless and helpless and totally alone. One of the initial actions of the crisis therapist is to instill hope and provide support for the client. The primary nurse communicates hope by demonstrating an attitude of caring and of confidence that, with the use of the problem-solving process, there will be a resolution to the problem the client presents. Support is initially provided by the nurse, by being available in person or by phone, or by having someone else available if the therapist is not. Frequently just the knowledge that the primary nurse is available to the client is enough to mobilize the client to begin to work on the problem himself or herself.

In addition, the primary nurse needs to investigate and use the current support system of the client and try to enlarge it. The nurse needs to find out what family, friends, neighbors, or clergy exist who might be helpful to the client during this period. Ideally, besides helping with the resolution of the crisis, new useful relationships may be established for the future.

Although it is important to provide as much support as is necessary during a crisis period, it is equally important *not* to provide more support than is necessary. Too much support fosters dependence on the primary nurse and others for that which the client can do for himself

or herself. The client should be encouraged to be as self-caring as the situation allows.

Problem Solving.   Resolving the underlying problem that precipitated the crisis is the focus of crisis intervention. The primary nurse doing crisis intervention is viewed as an expert in the process of problem solving who will assist the client through the process in order to restore equilibrium. In the initial sessions the nurse and client determine what the problem is and how to go about resolving it. Focusing on the problem helps to organize the client and helps him or her to concentrate on a concrete, workable issue, the "problem." This approach helps the client to mobilize his or her energies in a specific direction.

It is important to keep the client focused on defining and solving the problem. Feelings, however, need to be acknowledged and handled. For example, if the client has come to the primary nurse in crisis resulting from a loss, that is, a death or divorce, assisting the client in expressing his or her feelings is part of the intervention. At the same time, the nurse must help the client face the reality of the situation. In the case of the death of a loved one, the problem might be described by client and nurse as "the need to help the client through the grieving process." The reality that the loved one is gone must be faced in a factual manner, gradually and in small "doses." The expression of the client's feelings needs to be encouraged and accepted by the nurse. The client's feeling of upset must be acknowledged and accepted by the nurse. It is almost standard that the client is going to be upset in a crisis, and the cutting off of the expression of those feelings is not helpful to the client and will result in the internalization of such feelings. The internalization of these feelings usually becomes manifested in the form of lowered self-esteem. Once the client's feelings about the situation are expressed, the primary nurse needs to help the client look at the connection between these feelings and the identified problem, always with the aim of working at resolving the problem.

Self-Image.   When a client seeks professional help in a crisis state, self-esteem is lowered. The major contribution to this lowered self-esteem is the client's inability to resolve the problem without assistance. What self-esteem the client does have, then, must be protected and supported by the nurse. As the primary nurse doing crisis intervention, it is important to remain cognizant of the fact that this intervention process is brief and that shortly, in most instances, the client will again be functioning without assistance. For this reason positive self-esteem must be reinforced and enhanced. This is accomplished by the nurse in a number of ways. Tasks should be assigned to the client that are realistic and *can* be accomplished. At all times the client must be treated with respect and as a valuable human being. Positive aspects of the client's functioning need to be verbally acknowledged. The nurse's attitude must convey that the client is capable of resolving the "problem" with some assistance.

Self-Reliance. Related to maintaining self-esteem in crisis intervention is fostering self-reliance. The client needs to be encouraged to be as self-caring as possible.

Expectations for self-reliance and self-caring can be increased as the client's abilities increase. Thus, whenever possible, independence is encouraged. Again, tasks given to the client must be realistic and accomplishable. Assessing the problem, planning intervention, and implementing plans are done *with* the client, not *for* him or her, unless the client can do no part of each of these for himself or herself. The rationale for these expectations is independence. Independence must be fostered, since soon the client will again be responsible for his or her own decision making and problem solving.

Closure. At intervals, and certainly toward the end of the crisis intervention period, the client and primary nurse need to review where the client has been and what he or she has accomplished toward the resolution of the problem. This puts closure on the intervention and increases the client's self-esteem and self-reliance. In addition, it reinforces the intervention experience as a healthy, successful one that can be used in the future. The client has then gained the ability to use problem solving as a coping mechanism.

Stages of Crisis Intervention

The crisis intervention process usually proceeds through a series of steps or phases similar to those of the problem-solving process. The problem-solving process is the same process that primary nurses use in assisting clients with other health care problems.

In each of these phases the principles of crisis intervention are used. This series of steps is as follows:

- Identify the problem. Establish rapport with the client and collect data related to the problem.
- Formulate a therapeutic plan. Assess the client's strength, weaknesses, and capabilities.

- Implement the plan. Mobilize the client for some self-caring action, assist her or him to understand the problem and her or his feelings about the problem, and assist her or him in the development of effective coping mechanisms.
- Evaluate. The client and primary nurse examine what has changed and been accomplished and provide for some follow-up (1, 5).

Physical Illness/Surgery and Crisis Intervention

Because this text generally will be concerned with clients suffering primarily from a physical problem, it is important to specifically address serious physical illness/surgery from a crisis intervention perspective. Serious physical illness or injury represents a potent stressful event for the client and often provokes a crisis state. Golan suggests that all people who suffer from serious physical illness deal with stresses in three major areas: pain and loss of functional ability resulting from the disease itself, dependency and passivity with resulting regression, and separation and aloneness. She describes an overall process through which the sick person passes:

> The *onset phase,* when the illness is developing and being diagnosed; the *acute phase* of treatment including hospitalization and surgical procedures; the *recuperation phase,* which encompasses the gradual recovery of normal functions; and the posthospital *restoration phase,* including adjustment to new limitations and disabilities and re-establishment of systems, relationships. (6, p. 190)

The primary nurse's role as a crisis intervention worker with the physically ill person, at the time of diagnosis, focuses on clarifying the meaning of the diagnosis and encouraging the expression of feelings of fear and loss. The client is assisted in facing and accepting the situation and setting up realistic goals for improvement and functioning.

CASE STUDY

Ms. Morgan, a forty-year-old black widow, was referred to the mental health center by the local hospital emergency room staff. She had been the victim of an assault and robbery, during which she had sustained three fractured vertebrae. This injury had left her physically dependent on a full back brace and walker. Before the assault Ms. Morgan had been functioning well in the community, maintaining her own apartment and full-time employment. With this injury Ms. Morgan was unable to work. In addition, she needed assistance in performing the activities of daily living. Soon after the assault, Ms. Morgan began having auditory hallucinations and panic attacks.

Using Baldwin's classification of crisis, Ms. Morgan would be considered both a classification 3—crisis resulting from traumatic stress—and a classification 6—psychiatric emergency crisis. The crisis health care worker, in caring for this client, would be using both theory about management of the client in a psychiatric emergency and management of the client who is suffering from physical illness/injury that resulted in a crisis. The tasks of the primary nurse should include offering support while helping Ms. Morgan to understand the impact of the situation on her normal life-style, helping her accept the current situation, and helping her to restore and learn new effective coping mechanisms. In addition, the nurse would be involved in helping the client obtain concrete services when necessary, such as homemaking services. The nurse would assist Ms. Morgan in the understanding and acceptance of the loss of any functional ability. Feelings of separation and aloneness would need to be expressed and understood. Ms. Morgan would also need to be helped to express and accept the dependency resulting from the injury.

Specifically, in Ms. Morgan's case, she had lost her independence, at least for a period of time. She was now unable to work and needed assistance at home. In addition, Ms. Morgan expressed feelings about the loss of her femininity as a result of the use of the back brace. She was also encouraged to discuss her feelings of loss concerning not being able to independently seek out her friends and family. All of the above feelings resulted in a loss of self-esteem.

Ms. Morgan was supported and encouraged to accept her current situation while she received assistance at home from a nurse and later underwent surgery as an inpatient to correct her injuries. Eventually Ms. Morgan was placed on antipsychotic medication to alleviate her hallucinations and decrease her anxiety. She became accessible to therapeutic intervention. These interventions aimed at assisting Ms. Morgan to accept the reality of her situation, including new limitations, increase her independent functioning when possible, improving her support system and increasing her self-esteem. Shortly, as a result of therapeutic interventions and improvement in physical condition, the medication was discontinued without the recurrence of symptoms. The "problem" of how to deal with Ms. Morgan's physical injury and the resulting changes in her life-style was dealt with throughout the crisis period. Ms. Morgan was assigned tasks that were accomplishable by her, thereby increasing her self-esteem and allowing for as independent a stance as possible in her current situation. She was encouraged to contact friends and family by phone and elicit their support. Gradually Ms. Morgan accepted her current situation and began to make use of her immediate support systems. With surgery and hospitalization, Ms. Morgan's physical condition improved and she was able to function with increasing independence. Figure 16.3 is a diagram of this case study using Aguilera and Messick's paradigm for crisis.

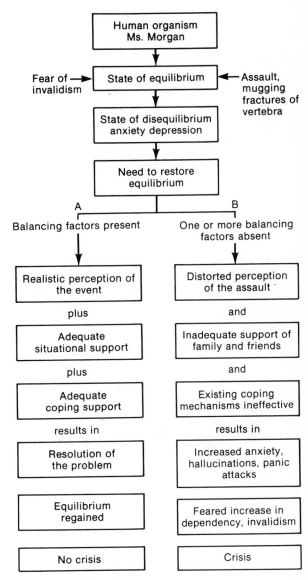

Figure 16.3. Case Study: Ms. Morgan

Self-Care and Crisis Intervention

For purposes of this chapter, Dorothea Orem's conceptual model of self-care is used in giving care to patients with a variety of problems, many of whom may be viewed as being in a crisis state (8). A brief description of Orem's model is thus presented and then applied to the client in crisis.

According to Orem, the term self-care refers to tasks accomplished toward promoting and maintaining the well-being of the person "for oneself and given by oneself" (8, p. 35). Depending on the current capabilities of the client at any given time, he or she can provide, totally or partially, his or her own self-care.

In doing crisis intervention how much self-care the client is capable of depends very much on both the class of crisis in which the professional is intervening and the degree of disorganization suffered by the client. In crisis situations that meet the criteria for Baldwin's class 6 crisis—psychiatric emergencies—generally the client is capable of almost *no* self-care. In contrast, in working with a client in a class 1—dispositional—crisis, the client may be capable of much of her or his own self-care needs. The client's current self-care abilities need to be assessed when doing crisis intervention. An in-depth examination of the self-care theory is provided in chapter 2.

The Primary Nurse in Crisis Intervention

Nursing as a profession has more and more been entering the realm of providing primary care in many wellness and illness settings. In primary nursing practice the nurse functions as both the main care planner/coordinator and care giver. This role has increasingly been used by nursing in specific crisis intervention settings, as well as in other health-illness settings, such as in mental health settings, prisons, schools, and industry, all of which are settings in which it is likely that the professional nurse would be assessing a client for a crisis state.

In each of these settings the primary nurse will often be one of the professionals responsible for implementing and following through with crisis intervention for the client or family, or both. Within this role the nurse is viewed *not* as someone who will solve another person's problem, but as an expert in problem solving and as a professional who will help the client in crisis through the problem-solving process.

When the primary nurse is operating in the capacity of principal health care provider, he or she must always be cognizant of his or her own abilities and at what point the client in crisis needs to be referred to another health professional with specialist expertise in any given area. For example, the nurse generalist who is a primary care giver should be able to assess a client for a crisis state that would be considered a psychiatric emergency, but she would probably not have the skills necessary to take that client through the crisis intervention process. The nurse would then refer this client to a specialist in the area of mental health. In contrast, the nurse generalist health care provider should be prepared to assess clients for crisis *and* do crisis intervention with those clients who are in dispositional or anticipated life transition crises.

REFERENCES

1. Aguilera, D., and J. Messick. *Crisis Intervention: Theory and Methodology.* 4th ed. St. Louis: C. V. Mosby Co., 1982.
2. Baldwin, B. "A Paradigm for the Classification of Emotional Crisis." *American Journal of Orthopsychiatry* 48:539, July 1978.
3. Caplan, G. *Support Systems and Community Mental Health Lectures on Concept Development.* New York: Behavioral Publications, 1974.
4. Dohrenwend, B. P., ed. *Stressful Life Events: Their Natural Effects.* New York: John Wiley & Sons, 1974.
5. Douglas, A. *Helping People in Crisis.* San Francisco: Jossey-Bass, 1979, 21–57.
6. Golan, N. *Treatment in Crisis Situations.* New York: Free Press/Macmillan, 1978.
7. Miller, T. W. "Life Events Scaling: Clinical Methodological Issues." *Nursing Research* 30: 316–20, 1981.
8. Orem, D. *Nursing: Concepts of Practice.* 2nd ed. New York: McGraw-Hill, 1980.

CHAPTER 17

Grief and Grieving

PAMELLA HAY HOSANG

■

OBJECTIVES

After completing this chapter, the reader will be able to:

- Discuss the essential elements of loss, grief, mourning, and bereavement.
- Define loss, grief, grieving, mourning, and bereavement.
- Describe four types of loss that can lead to grieving.
- Identify and describe the phases of grief.
- Identify manifestations of grief.
- Differentiate between normal and abnormal grief.
- Recognize manifestations of grief at different stages in the life span.
- Identify the impact of loss and grieving on children.
- Identify the impact of loss and grieving on adolescents.
- Identify the impact of loss and grieving on young adults.
- Identify the response of individuals and families to divorce.
- Identify the grief response to loss of a body part.
- Assess grieving individuals and families.
- Plan appropriate grief intervention for individuals and families.
- Discuss the importance of understanding one's own response to loss and grief.

Grief is a response to loss that occurs many times during a person's life. It encompasses much more than loss of a loved one. The response may be caused by a change in one's life-style, such as a job relocation, divorce, injury or surgery, or a child's entry into nursery school, or by the ultimate loss through death of a spouse, parent, or loved one. The depth of feeling associated with loss is directly related to the significance of the lost object to the one who loses. As we consider the number of losses each person experiences in a lifetime and the resulting trauma, we can appreciate the necessity of understanding and intervening appropriately in the grief process.

Nurses and physicians, more than any other group of workers, encounter a variety of losses in their professional practice. Because of this, it is essential for them to understand the nature of loss and the diversity of its manifestations. People seldom, if ever, seek professional help with grieving. When they do present themselves for help, it is usually for some related somatic or emotional disorder that they identify as the primary problem. Health professionals, when responding, are often required to deal not only with the grieving person, but also with the reactions of families, co-workers, and themselves.

Implications of Loss

Loss and Change

Loss implies change, and it is the disruption of familiar patterns of behavior that threatens the "reality system" and evokes a variety of emotions in people who experience loss. The reality system, according to Cheikin (2), comprises our physical reality, social reality, and personal reality of oneself and one's nature. These realities constitute our belief systems that are based on the physical world, our conception of ourselves, and the reality of our relationships with other persons, ideals, concepts, and such. When the personal reality is shaken by

the loss of a significant other, our lives must, of necessity, change.

The range of emotional responses that may occur as a result of the trauma of loss runs the gamut of human capabilities. During the initial phase, numbness, disbelief, and denial of reality are frequently experienced. These may be replaced by anger, hopelessness, a sense of abandonment, and lack of control. Later fear of future loneliness, resentment, resistance to changes in life-style, and self-perception may replace or expand some earlier manifestations. These are a few examples of a vast array of reactions and responses.

Loss and Attachment

Loss implies that a sense of attachment existed between the bereaved and the lost object. Because the potential for loss is always imminent, one might question why humans form attachments. Attachments begin from the moment of birth with maternal-infant bonding, which, according to recent postulations, has survival value for the species. When an infant is separated from its mother, to whom an attachment has developed, its cries of protest, its reaching, following, and attempts to regain her indicate its distress. If the mother does not return, the child appears to give up, although he continues to look with expectancy, until he finally accepts the loss with detachment (22). As the child grows older he learns to accept separations, but the need for love, friendship, trust, warmth, intimacy, and commitment persists. Gradually the threat of the pain of loss, separation, abandonment, fear, and loneliness diminishes. It appears also that our narcissistic belief in our own immortality creates the illusion of being in control of life's bitter experiences. When, in fact, we encounter severe loss, the realization of our own vulnerability is shattering and numbing to our sensibilities.

Loss and Pain

Loss implies pain. Losing someone or something that one has formed an attachment to is both frightening and disappointing. It shakes the foundation of one's sense of security and erodes the self-esteem. Loss disrupts one's identity in terms of one's relationship with the person or object lost. The pain is unavoidable because it is the price of commitment to that which was lost. Fear of what will be experienced in the ensuing months is reflected in the stages of grief that accompany loss. According to Davenport (5), it is our unwillingness to accept the pain of loss that sets the stage for grieving. Also, narcissistic concerns may cause the grieving person to search for failings in himself or herself that may have contributed to the loss. Finding none often leads to anger at the deceased. Occasionally the anger may be projected onto the physician, nurse, or family member.

Types of Loss

Developmental Loss

In more recent years attention has focused on developmental loss, which occurs with normal growth and development. Such losses are seen as aids to maturation. They begin during infancy and continue throughout one's lifetime. For instance, a child loses the breast or bottle when weaned, or his favored position as an only child when a sibling is born. Peretz (22), in discussing how loss can aid maturation, noted that physical, psychological, and emotional capacities are nurtured by the gratifications that infants derive from others in the environment. As infants increase their capacity for mastery, significant people expect more of them, and they must renounce certain pleasures before alternatives are well established. Although newly acquired emotional and cognitive capacities aid in withstanding frustration and integrating the experience of loss, the quality and quantity of the loss, as well as its meaning at the time, may create a negative and lasting impression on the developing personality of the child.

Adequate nurturance is essential during periods of developmental vulnerability for people to grow. Infancy and childhood are two important periods of vulnerability. Another period of increased vulnerability is old age, when defensive and adaptive skills may be diminished and loss can disrupt both emotional and physical balance.

Loss of a Valued Person

Loss may be gradual or sudden, anticipated or unanticipated. Although gradual, anticipated loss permits time for anticipatory grieving and may cause less trauma, the grief felt by the bereaved may be just as intense as when loss is sudden and unanticipated. Temporary loss, such as that experienced by a relocated adult or a hospitalized infant and its parents, can cause grieving with all its symptoms. Likewise, a fancied loss can create as much havoc as a real one (25).

Loss of Some Aspect of Self

Loss of some aspect of the self refers to changes in one's self-image perceived as a loss. Loss of positive self-attitudes regarding attractiveness, lovability, self-esteem, independence, and control, as well as loss of self-definitions such as social roles related to occupation, family position, and the status attached to these, can have marked psychological and physiological consequences on a person's life. Disfiguring surgery or trauma and debilitating illness can have equal or greater impact.

The feeling of loss is apparent in many people as they age. Loss of motor function and decreased sensory acuity usually are accompanied by increasing dependence on others. Social attitudes toward work and identity can likewise engender feelings of loss among the elderly as they approach retirement.

Loss of External Objects

Loss is experienced when one is deprived of valued external objects through theft, disaster, migration, or ruin. Loss of possessions, such as home and family treasures, as a result of some disaster, such as a flood, earthquake, or fire, leave victims with a sense of deep loss, which can lead to anxiety, depression, and difficulty remembering (4). Relocation or migration, whether planned or forced, causes significant disruption in familiar lifestyles. Uprooting from family, friends, neighborhood, or homeland requires adaptation to many unanticipated circumstances that are stressful for those involved.

Grief and Loss

Any significant loss leads to a grief response. Similarly a significant loss also leads to inherent change, and we are normally ambivalent about change. Grief reactions vary among people, depending on the amount of emotional disruption incurred by the loss. It is important to bear in mind that growth occurs with resolution.

The grief phenomenon involves resolving one's fear

for the lost object. Resolution of fear is at the heart of the grief process, according to Heikkinen (13). This fear threatens self-esteem, leading to various manifestations of grief. Thus the grieving process is meant to enhance fear resolution so that the bereaved might move away from the sense of loss toward restitution and reintegration.

During the process of grieving the bereaved may experience extreme fear, including fear of insanity. It is important to understand grief feelings that extend from the initial shock through acute distress to reintegration and that must be worked through by the grieving person. If the grieving person cannot work through these feelings, lasting emotional damage may occur.

The Ripple Effect

Evidence implies that a ripple effect is inherent in loss because each loss carries with it the threat of additional loss. For example, loss of health may lead to loss of skills, leading in turn to loss of job, loss of role as breadwinner, and real or imagined loss of respect from others. Loss of a spouse or parent may lead to loss of financial security, emotional support, and prized dreams, such as going to college. With each loss individuals and families are required to make a number of changes. Some theorists believe that our ability to adapt to losses enhances our ability to grow; thus fear of future loss is minimized by each experience with loss in normal life changes.

Because loss is a universal experience, Peretz (22) contends that it may be overlooked as a cause of disease and dysfunction. Interestingly enough, poets and writers from times past recognized the connection between loss and grief and illness and death. The expression "died of a broken heart" is familiar to us, as are the themes of withdrawal, melancholia, the jilted maiden, and death.

Phases of Normal Grief

Marris (18) and Corrazini (3) identified three phases in the grief process. The first phase is an awareness of conflict resulting from loss, which must be worked out in order to restore a vital sense of continuity to experience. The second phase involves conflict resolution, which becomes meaningful only through ambivalent exploration. The third phase is reintegration, in which the person attempts to engage with the future while resolving ambivalence between past and future.

During the first phase of grief the person responds to loss with shock, disbelief, and denial. There may be attempts to dismiss the event as a hoax or a bad dream. Restlessness may alternate with immobility as realization sinks in and grief behaviors take hold.

During the second phase there is consolidation, as awareness of the loss is conceptualized and the bereaved realizes that the loss is not a dream and there will be no reprieve.

Physiological changes affecting some or all of the body systems may occur during the first two phases as the person grapples with shock and change, and mourns for the loss of self. Changes that may occur include the following:

- Gastrointestinal disturbances, such as loss of appetite and feelings of hollowness in the abdomen
- Cardiovascular reactions, such as changes in heart rate, tightening of the chest, and shortness of breath
- Genitourinary changes, such as frequency of urination
- Respiratory responses, such as sighing, choking, and shortness of breath
- Musculoskeletal weakness with generalized exhaustion and tightening in the throat
- Neurological symptoms, including headaches (18)

Concurrently, emotional changes, such as immobility, lack of zest, apathy, restlessness with aimless movements, depression, and feelings of increased emotional distance from other people, may occur. Intense preoccupation with images of the deceased may lead to auditory and visual hallucinations. Neglect of self, obsessions with guilt, irritability, anxiety, and anger are other manifestations. The bereaved may demonstrate a disconcerting lack of warmth toward others, decreased social interactions, and, ultimately, withdrawal. The mood is usually egocentric, sometimes accusatory as the person withdraws into a cocoon of grief. The isolation that the bereaved imposes while living on memories, dreams, or illusions may make life seem futile, leading to thoughts of suicide.

Extreme conflict pervades this period and must be worked through toward grief resolution. Freud recognized the difficulty of this when he wrote:

The testing of reality, having shown that the love object no longer exists, requires that all the libido should forthwith withdraw from its attachment to this object. Against this a struggle of course arises. It has been universally observed, that a man never willingly abandons a libido position, not even when a substitute is already beckoning to him. (18)

Thus, as the bereaved strives toward resolution of conflict and grief, he vacillates through many moods through a process of reformulation.

There are no clear lines of demarcation between the three phases of grief identified by Corrazini and Marris; however, a keen observer will look for signs of readiness or transition to the third phase, reintegration. Reintegration commences at the onset of disengagement from the deceased. Some authors refer to this as leave taking. The fact of death is accepted and the bereaved is ready for adjustments or the taking up once more of purposeful relationships. Heikkinen (13) contends that resolution of fear is the core of grief work; thus once fear is overcome the bereaved is ready to accept changes.

During reintegration the bereft self moves away from emotional catharsis and anticathexis toward resolution of ambivalence between respect for the past and demands of the future. As it recovers its emotional investment, the self is imbued with new energy, each attempt being more successful than the preceding one. The bereaved is now able to establish a new relationship with the deceased whereby the person has been somehow spiritualized and incorporated within the being of the mourner. At this point thoughts of the deceased become memories that can be recalled at will. The final resolution is said to occur as the person resumes life tasks by taking new creative demands on himself or herself and others. As the bereaved moves through these phases of mourning, somatic symptoms tend to linger or disappear, depending on how grief work is managed. In Table 17.1, the phases of grief described by Marris and Corrazini, as well as those identified by other theorists, are shown.

Abnormal Grief

Most scholars who have studied grief agree that there are conventional and socially determined periods of mourning after loss that facilitate healthy or normal resolution. Yet not everyone who suffers loss shares this experience. The literature refers to aberrations as abortive or morbid grief, in which distortions of normal grief are evident (15, 18). Some of the reasons given for the occurrence are lack of support systems in society, con-

ventions of society that stipulate acceptable and unacceptable overt expressions, duration, and mourning customs, as well as preexisting personality characteristics of the bereaved. Three patterns of abnormal grief identified by Marris and others are delayed, inhibited, and chronic bereavement states.

Delayed Grief

Delayed grief is characterized by a shallow grief response—business as usual—and rapid reorganization of life activities. There is little expression of sorrow and the loss is accepted calmly. The busy activity, according to Marris, betrays itself by haste and poor judgment, or is even perversely self-destructive. It may be weeks, months, or even years before any indication of grieving is expressed. In the meantime the bereaved will concern herself or himself with a great deal of trivia in order to suppress true feelings. When subsequently a less significant loss occurs, such as the loss of a pet, it is followed by severe and seemingly unusual grief reactions. Lindemann (15) contends that the precipitating factor for delayed reaction may be a deliberate recall of circumstances surrounding the death, or it could be a spontaneous occurrence in the person's life.

Peretz (22) reminds us, however, that absence of grief immediately after loss need not be considered abnormal, as it may represent temporary shock, numbness, or denial. In fact, some people try to postpone grief temporarily, particularly if they must attend to funeral and burial arrangements. Oftentimes their emotions erupt overwhelmingly at or after the funeral.

Inhibited Grief

Some people, especially men and public figures, do not permit themselves any public expression of grief, although they grieve secretly in the privacy of home or bedroom. Others are afraid to show deep feelings of loss toward the deceased, or have a need to deny the reality of the loss. They may attempt to minimize their loss with rationalizations, such as, "She was relieved from her suffering." But those who delay or postpone grief are most vulnerable to developing physical conditions that require medical intervention, or they may develop anniversary reactions, that is, experience again the loss on an important date associated with the deceased.

In extreme instances grief is permanently inhibited and never finds expression. Subsequent to the loss, the person develops neurotic symptoms or physical disorders that are seldom recognized as displaced grief. Re-

Table 17.1
Phases of Grief and Mourning

Engel	Kubler-Ross	Marris and Corrazini	Ramsay and Happee	Degner	Kadushin	McConville
1. Shock and disbelief 2. Developing awareness of the loss 3. Restitution and recovery	1. Denial and isolation 2. Anger 3. Bargaining 4. Depression	1. Conflict 2. Resolution of conflict 3. Reintegration	1. Shock 2. Denial 3. Depression 4. Guilt 5. Anxiety 6. Aggression 7. Reintegration	1. Shock 2. Disbelief and incredulity 3. Anger 4. Weeping, sadness, helplessness or hopelessness 5. Guilt and shame 6. Disorganization of behavior (restlessness, tension, irritability) 7. A sense of continued presence of the deceased 8. Somatic manifestations 9. Reorganization	1. Anger 2. Anxiety 3. Guilt 4. Despair	1. Egocentricity 2. Aggression 3. Denial 4. Preoccupation with the dead 5. Restrictive dreams

cent investigations imply that repressed grief can lead to the occurrence of neoplasms or other disorders associated with the body's immune system. Such claims, although seemingly premature to be definitive at this time, ought to be borne in mind when a client's history is taken.

Chronic Grief

By contrast, chronic grief seems to be the antithesis of inhibited grief. Here the bereaved mourns endlessly. Yearning and despair at the loss are prolonged, and six months to a year after the loss there seems to be no respite. The bereaved settles into a lasting depression—anxious, irritable, apathetic, and obsessed by memories. The deceased is enshrined or memorialized unrealistically and life is designed to go on as usual as if the loved one were still alive. Miss Faversham, the jilted bride who sat forever at the bridal table awaiting the appearance of the groom in Charles Dickens's *Great Expectations,* is a classic example of chronic grief.

Children and Loss

Since the 1950s interest and research focusing on the meaning of death to children, their reactions to loss, and

what constitutes grief reactions at different ages have broadened. Yet this progress has yielded little toward easing the controversy in Western societies as to how to help children deal with irreversible loss, such as death of a loved one. The tendency is to deny children opportunities for learning about loss, particularly death. Parents rationalize that by avoiding discussions of the loss, they spare the feelings of the child. Such attitudes only increase the child's confusion and further hinder resolution.

Theorists have identified some of the problems that children have with loss. These include (a) incorrect assumptions about what actually happened, particularly among children under ten years of age, because their cognitive abilities are incompletely developed; (b) anxiety and apathy after the loss of a parent if practical needs normally fulfilled by the lost parent are unfulfilled (this is more evident in young children); and (c) increasing frustration and feelings of hopelessness (9).

Incorrect assumptions about what actually caused parental separation, divorce, or death in a family foster guilt and anxiety in many children. This can be disturbing for a young child who perceives himself or herself as responsible for the loss. Likewise, unrealistic explanations about death, such as "Grandma has gone away (or gone to sleep)" or "God took your brother away during the night," can not only destroy religious concepts but also create undue anxiety, nightmares, or fear of the dark. Parents and nurses are reminded that a child's level of cognition, his fantasy world, and his ability—or inability—to master abstract thinking at certain ages should be kept in mind when introducing complex concepts.

Fear of not having needs fulfilled can be very real for a child who has lost a parent. We are reminded that the person who fulfills the needs of a young child is of secondary importance to the fulfilled need, which, to the child, is crucial. Substituting a consistent surrogate parent is of primary importance in enabling a normal recovery from grief.

Basic bodily needs, such as bathing, feeding, dressing, and protection, assume primary significance to a preschool child. Furman recommends the following four important tasks to assist the child.

1. Consistency in the person or persons fulfilling the vacant role
2. Constancy of environment
3. Simple repeated explanations of what happened
4. Arrangement of the transition by the dying parent, if possible (11)

Furman also feels that helping the child to remember the lost parent with pictures and providing a substitute of the same sex as the lost parent to whom the child can respond with day-to-day problems are important and should not be neglected.

Emotional responses of children to the loss of a parent are quite similar to those of adults, but frustration and feelings of helplessness may be marked. The way in which the child is told about the loss affects the response. If the child is told about the loss with feeling, the child will respond with feeling. Some children, when told, may return to their play as if nothing happened. This does not mean that the child does not care. An apparent indifference during the first few days or weeks should be considered adaptive and should be distinguished from the child's pretense that the loss has not occurred.

Denial may be manifested in a variety of ways, such as avoiding activities previously shared with the lost parent, ignoring the fact of death or separation, avoiding any discussion of the parent, aggression, and withdrawal. Occasionally denial is accompanied by anger and guilt. Anger stems from feelings of abandonment by the parent as well as from conflicts between the magical and real world toward the parent. Intense feelings of anger may engender guilt.

It is often difficult to recognize a child's grief because external behaviors may not correspond to inner responses, and the child's lack of overt responses may lead others to presume that the child is unaffected. Sustained grief might be too much for the child's ego to bear. Professional help may be needed to help the child to cope with grief, anger, and guilt. If the child has a good relationship with the remaining parent, the difficulties may be handled within the family. When behavior problems exist, professional help is strongly recommended.

Much can be done to prevent negative reactions in children to death of a loved one. Communication between parents and children is extremely important. Honesty and appropriateness in imparting information about the illness can clarify confusing and complex information. Including children in family discussions about a crisis can also help them in adapting to the crisis as well as assure their place in the family unit. Parents should be frank with older children who are able to comprehend the meaning of terminal illness or death, and answer questions truthfully. Deception, however well meaning, is ultimately self-defeating, regardless of the intent, and should be avoided.

When the crisis centers on an ill child, parents will need guidance in coping with sibling rivalry, particularly during periods of remission, when the child appears well. It will be difficult for other children in the family to tolerate the special attention and dispensations regarding rules and limits waived for the child, and parents should be aware of this. Perceptions of favoritism will create more resentment among children if they do not understand, and even when they do understand, there may be guilt. Guilt is sometimes expressed in depression, nightmares, and reactive-aggressive behaviors that erode parents' endurance. These conflicting emotions will be extremely difficult for children and parents to manage. Preventive professional support can be most beneficial, as it increases awareness of crises the family may encounter later and provides appropriate coping mechanisms.

Grief and Adolescence

Opportunities for grieving are relatively high among adolescents when compared with other age-groups. Some potential sources of loss are associated with puberty. Adolescents experience loss of childhood as they face the complexities of the adult world. Normal physiological and emotional changes are themselves problematic. Environmental changes, such as entering high school or college, unanticipated parental relocation, and sociological changes associated with relocations, such as forming new friendships, selecting careers, choosing partners, and becoming socially and economically independent are some life events that are likely to evoke ambivalence and feelings of loss. Adolescents, being more mobile than young children, are at risk for accidental death. Automobile accidents are the leading cause of death for adolescents and young adult males, but an increasing number of adolescents die each year because of suicide or substance abuse. Adolescent pregnancy is another crisis faced by many.

Terminal illness accounts for a small percentage of deaths among teenagers, but its effect can be profound. Imminent death of an adolescent child is particularly stressful for parents, eroding their coping abilities. The problem is exacerbated by conflictive relationships between parents and adolescents.

Frequently parents of terminally ill adolescents request that the diagnosis be withheld from the child because of their own difficulties in coping. A conspiracy of silence ensues, and valuable time for intimacy and reparations is sacrificed. Adolescents may ultimately avoid discussing their own prognoses so as not to cause more hurt for their parents. If the pretense continues, adolescents may opt to face death alone. Their aloneness can be further compounded by care givers who identify with them and whose heightened death anxiety prevents therapeutic communication and support.

As time passes during a terminal illness, adolescents' networks tend to shrink. They may choose to distance themselves from family and friends. In some instances friends may choose to avoid the dying adolescent in order to cope with their own fear and discomfort. Grieving becomes difficult for all, particularly those facing death, for they grieve not only their own death, but also the loss of family and friends who are unable to say good-bye and share their sorrow, guilt, frustration, and anger.

Grieving peers of dying adolescents are particularly vulnerable and in need of support. Meyers and Pitt (19) propose a consultative approach to help school personnel cope with losses and bereavement. They believe that teachers should become more involved in helping by encouraging open discussions among students and sharing their own feelings as well. Such open dialogue is intended to enhance understanding of loss, emotional responses, and coping behaviors. Ongoing preventive counseling can be incorporated into health education curricula with the collaboration of guidance counselors, school nurses, and teachers in high schools and colleges.

Loss of Body Image

Loss of a body part or function can generate as much grief as the death of a loved one. Because loss is determined by the meaning the bereaved attaches to the loved object, loss of an external body part, such as an arm, eye, or breast, loss of skin owing to massive burns, or loss of one's hair owing to chemotherapy can erode the victim's ego, causing severe grief. Similarly surgery such as colostomy, cystectomy, and hysterectomy that results in loss of an internal organ and function causes grief, although the loss in such instances usually represents a choice between survival and death.

Awareness of one's self begins during infancy through external tactile, kinesthetic, and internal sensations. Later we develop a conceptual and perceptual self-image that results from the image of our body formed in our minds. Intactness of the body image is essential to ego integrity. When the body image is suddenly altered by accident or radical surgery, the person is vulnerable to psychotic or delusional behavior. A prime example of this is the phantom limb syndrome experienced by persons after amputation.

In any society disfigurement connotes being different. In our society, where much emphasis is placed on beauty, physical differences and possible rejection can evoke much anxiety, depression, low self-esteem, denial, anger, withdrawal, depersonalization, or thoughts of suicide. Frequently perceptions of the altered selves are distorted. Emotional reparation depends on the person's ability to come to terms with reality. This involves realistic acceptance of the new body image and adapting to it. Adaptation may take months.

Grieving Divorce

Since 1962 the divorce rate in the United States has more than doubled. Approximately one divorce occurs for every two marriages (8). Not only are couples traumatized by the experience, but children are often left emotionally bruised by parental conflict and separation. They feel hurt, confused, embarrassed, and angry. Often they feel guilty and responsible for the separation.

It is difficult for many children to adjust to the loss of

family structure and vital relationships. Emotional problems, learning difficulties, and increased delinquency are manifestations of faulty coping mechanisms.

Grief Assessment

The first step in treating grief is to assess the grief state and process. It is essential to establish a comprehensive data base by taking a physical, psychological, and social history. The following points should be considered:

- Obtain an objective description of the loss.
- Elicit the person's and family's perception of the loss and how they are responding.
- Assess the developmental and maturity levels of the person and family.
- Identify the family's personal resources—financial, educational, health, and psychological.
- Identify the family's internal resources—integration and adaptability.
- Determine what social support systems are available, type and adequacy of support systems, such as family members, friends, and community agencies, and assess the person's and family's willingness to use them.
- Identify coping techniques or mechanisms available and operational—past experiences as well as current measures.

It is often difficult to assess grief soon after the loss has occurred because the grieving person uses a variety of mental mechanisms to ease pain during the acute phase of grief. Mechanisms used depend on the person's personality, age, level of maturity, culture, and perception of society's demands. Denial, suppression, repression, substitution, and regression are some of the mental mechanisms that can make assessment difficult.

Intervention

Because many people seek professional help for physical and emotional problems that they do not associate with grief, the first step in intervention is to determine whether or not the person is grieving. Treatment can then be initiated and referrals made as necessary. Physiological disorders may require medical intervention and counseling. Emotional disorders, depending on their severity, may be treated by a primary nurse

with expertise in bereavement counseling, a clergyman, a counselor, a psychologist, or a psychiatrist. The primary aim of grief intervention is to help the person and family work toward final resolution and maximum recovery.

Frequently all that is necessary is an opportunity for the person or family to verbalize feelings and receive validation that their responses to grief are normal. Grieving persons often feel a loss of control and may have illusions of seeing or hearing the dead person or perceiving a body part if the loss relates to trauma or surgery. These responses could lead to anxiety and fear of mental illness. Helping clients to understand that these are common, transient, normal responses relieves their anxiety and restores confidence in their ability to cope effectively.

When loss of a body part due to surgery is anticipated, preoperative preparation of the client and family begins as soon as they are aware of the diagnosis and surgery. They are encouraged to verbalize their feelings, ask questions, and express doubts. Establishing a warm, supportive relationship with the client and family facilitates openness. It is best to adopt the role of listener and facilitator at these discussions so that the client and family can begin to mobilize their own coping mechanisms. Clues to the client's and family's ability to adapt are their willingness to express their feelings regarding the loss and change and to participate in rehabilitation.

After surgery, a rehabilitation plan that includes the family as well as the client is implemented. Counseling continues until an optimal level of coping with the loss and change is achieved. Major disruptions of body image may require intensive psychotherapy as well as occupational, vocational, and physical therapy. The client's acceptance of the new body image and the attitudes of professional staff, family, and friends are most important. The course of recovery may be erratic, but with adequate support systems clients can overcome their loss.

An understanding and supportive attitude toward the client and family can enable them to deal effectively with conflicting feelings. Clients are encouraged to express negative feelings, such as ambivalence, guilt, anger, and hostility, even if these evoke anxiety, embarrassment, and pain because repressing them denies the significance of the loss. Explanations of the feelings are given to increase understanding of normal grief reactions.

In Table 17.2, Corrazini provides some useful guidelines for counselors working with grieving persons.

Openness in communicating with the bereaved per-

Table 17.2
Tasks for Counselor and Bereaved
for Effective Grief Therapy

Counselor	Bereaved
Remain open to the loss	Perceive the openness
Be empathic	Express feelings
Encourage reminiscing	Reminisce
Insist on the loss	Acknowledge the loss

Source: J. G. Corrazini, "The Theory and Practice of Loss Therapy," in *Bereavement Counseling,* ed. B. Schoenberg et al. Westport, Conn.: Greenwood Press, 1980, 75.

haps will be most difficult to achieve because of personal difficulties in dealing with grief and cultural mores that shape personalities of care givers. Western cultures do not permit inordinate grieving. Shortly after the loss, partial or full recovery is expected. If this does not occur, associates tolerate the grieving persons for a short period of time before avoiding them completely. Yet a grieving person is unable to put away grief and must mourn the loss until resolution occurs. Family, friends, and nurses must allow the grieving person to acknowledge loss rather than suppress it.

Besides family and friends, support services are available in most communities. Clinics, churches, counseling centers, mental health centers, crisis centers, and special interest groups such as Parents Without Partners are some examples. Clergymen traditionally have provided counseling for grieving individuals and families within their parishes. In addition, a number of informal community groups exist. A serious drawback to many voluntary agencies is their lack of permanent or qualified staff. Committed people with experience and expertise in human relationships and professionals from the helping professions often contribute a great deal to such organizations, but limitations are still evident.

Self-Understanding and Grief

It is essential for nurses, counselors, and others who work with grieving persons to be in touch with their own feelings about loss. Fears regarding change, and reluctance to resolve previous losses of their own are two indications that a professional may not be ready to assist

someone else in dealing with loss. Heikkinen identified the following indicators that professionals have failed to overcome their fear of loss:

- Failing to work on their own personal growth
- Shying away from loss issues faced by clients
- Prolonging the number of counseling sessions with clients far beyond the number required for client change
- Using one counseling approach for all clients
- Ending the counseling contact without a proper termination ceremony (13)

One response to unresolved personal difficulties in dealing with loss observed among nurses and physicians is avoidance. The situation is more difficult when persons who are dying are not informed about impending death. The provision of direct care to such persons produces tension and awkwardness because the constraints imposed by not revealing information create an unrealistic milieu. In an effort to cope, nurses distance themselves from dying persons, resulting in apparent depersonalization. Such behaviors compound the social isolation of dying and limit the opportunities the dying person has to achieve closure through interacting with significant others (1).

A paradox that nurses and physicians share is being part of a culture that avoids or denies death, yet expects them to respond to the needs of the dying and their grieving families with sensitivity, understanding, and a lack of anxiety. Significant attempts to assist professionals to deal with their own fears of loss and death are relatively recent. The importance of preparing for this cannot be minimized, for as Peretz expressed so succinctly, "Patients need help in dying just as they often do in living" (22).

DISCUSSION QUESTIONS

1. Identify some behaviors that would lead you to suspect that a client is experiencing unresolved grief; classify the major physiological and psychological manifestations. Develop a questionnaire that would assist you in your assessment.
2. Many somatic disorders have their origins in unresolved grief. What actions could you take as a primary nurse in dealing with such clients?
3. Consider yourself in this situation: A recent suicide of an adolescent not only has left a void among staff and clients on your unit but has also left you feeling depressed. You have also observed a number of be-

havior changes among clients and staff members. Yet everyone has avoided discussing the effect of the suicide on them. You decide to initiate a grief workshop.

    a. Describe observed behaviors that would lead you to conclude that your action is necessary.

    b. Analyze your reactions to the death and give some possible reasons for your feelings.

    c. Describe the participants you plan to include in the workshop and your rationale for including them.

    d. Identify your goals and strategies for implementation.

4. Parents of terminally ill children often experience great difficulty in sharing their grief with their children or in discussing the child's imminent death. Describe a plan that could assist parents who are experiencing this problem. Identify your own difficulties if faced with this task and analyze the problems.

REFERENCES

1. Benoliel, J. Q. "Nurses and the Human Experience of Dying." In *New Meanings of Death,* ed. H. Feifel. New York: McGraw-Hill, 1977.
2. Cheikin, M. "Loss and Reality." *Personnel and Guidance Journal* 59:355, 1981.
3. Corrazini, J. G. "The Theory and Practice of Loss Therapy." In *Bereavement Counseling,* ed. B. Schoenberg et al. Westport, Conn.: Greenwood Press, 1980.
4. Crabbs, M. A., and E. Heffron. "Associated with Natural Disaster." *Personnel and Guidance Journal* 59:379, 1981.
5. Davenport, D. "A Closer Look at the 'Healthy' Grieving Process." *Personnel and Guidance Journal* 59:332, 1981.
6. Degner, L. "Death in Disaster: Implications for Bereavement." *Essence* 1:69, 1976.
7. Engel, G. "Is Grief a Disease?" *Psychosomatic Medicine* 23:18, 1961.
8. Fetsch, R. J., and J. Surdam. "New Beginnings: Group Techniques for Coping with Losses Due to Divorce." *Personnel and Guidance Journal* 59:395, 1981.
9. Frears, L. H., and J. Schneider. "Exploring Loss and Grief Within a Wholistic Framework." *Personnel and Guidance Journal* 59:341, 1981.
10. Freihofer, P., and G. Felton. "Nursing Behaviors in Bereavement." *Nursing Research* 25 (5):332, 1976.
11. Furman, R. "A Child's Reaction to Death in the Family." In *Loss and Grief,* ed. B. Schoenberg et al. New York: Columbia University Press, 1970.
12. Headington, B. J. "Understanding the Core Experience: Loss." *Personnel and Guidance Journal* 59:338, 1981.
13. Heikkinen, C. A. "Loss Resolution for Growth." *Personnel and Guidance Journal* 59:327, 1981.
14. Kubler-Ross, E. *Death: The Final Stage of Growth.* Englewood Cliffs, N.J.: Prentice-Hall, 1975.
15. Lindemann, E. "Symptomatology and Management of Acute Grief." *American Journal of Psychiatry* 101:141, 1944.
16. McCain, C. "How to Work More Comfortably with Grief: Your Own and Your Patients'." *Nursing Life* 1:52, 1981.
17. McCubbin, H. I., et al. "Family Stress and Coping: A Decade Review." *Journal of Marriage and Family.* 42:861, 1980.
18. Marris, P. *Loss and Change.* Garden City, N.Y.: Doubleday, 1975.
19. Meyers, J., and N. W. Pitt. "A Consultative Approach to Help a School Cope with the Bereavement Process." *Professional Psychology* 7:559–64.
20. Nagy, M. "The Child's View of Death." In *The Meaning of Death,* ed. H. Feifel. New York: McGraw-Hill, 1959.
21. Parkes, C. M. *Bereavement: Studies of Grief in Adult Life.* New York: International University Press, 1973.
22. Peretz, D. "Development, Object-Relationships, and Loss and Reaction to Loss." In *Loss and Grief: Psychological Management in Medical Practice,* ed. B. Schoenberg et al. New York: Columbia University Press, 1970.
23. Ramsay, R. W., and J. A. Happee. "The Stress of Bereavement: Components and Treatment." In *Stress and Anxiety,* ed. C. P. Spielberger and J. G. Sarson, vol. 4. London: John Wiley and Sons, 1977.
24. Raphael, B. "Mourning and the Prevention of Melancholia." *British Journal of Medical Psychology.* 51:303, 1978.
25. Rochlin, G. *Griefs and Discontents: The Forces of Change.* Boston: Little, Brown, 1965.
26. *Webster's Third International Dictionary,* ed. P. Babcock. Springfield, Mass.: G & C Merriam Co., 1967.

CHAPTER 18

Substance Abuse

ALICIA GEORGES

■

OBJECTIVES

After completing this chapter, the reader will be able to:

- Define substance abuse, tolerance, physiological dependence, alcoholism, alcohol abuse, withdrawal, delerium tremors, intoxication, psychological dependence, and addiction.
- List commonly abused substances as defined in this chapter.
- List various sources of data used for the epidemiological estimate of the problem of substance abuse.
- Describe the physiological and psychological manifestations of alcohol, opiate, barbiturate, marihuana, cocaine, and hallucinogen abuse.
- Identify the economic impact of substance use and abuse.
- Describe the consequences of substance

abuse in terms of morbidity, life expectancy, and quality of life.
- Describe various patterns of substance abuse and their social consequences.
- Identify the psychological and physiological needs of the substance abuser.
- Describe acute and habilitative care required for the substance abuser.
- Identify modalities for rehabilitation of the substance abuser.
- Identify the self-care responsibilities of the individual, family, and community in relation to substance abuse.
- Delineate ethical and legal responsibilities of the nurse as primary care coordinator for the client, the family, and the community.

The abuse of various chemical substances has become commonplace in American society. The substances abused include such things as tobacco, over-the-counter drugs, prescription drugs, and the illegal psychoactive drugs. This chapter focuses on some stimulants and depressants, such as cocaine, marihuana, alcohol, barbiturate sedatives, and tranquilizers. It also addresses concerns and issues that have evolved because of the use and abuse of these substances in communities across America. The role of the professional nurse is defined as it relates to the care of clients, families, and communities affected by the outcomes of substance abuse in their environment.

It is estimated that there are 10 million alcoholics, 18 million persons who have used cocaine, and 50 million persons who have smoked marihuana, and the numbers continue to increase. Men and women of all ethnic and socioeconomic groups are represented (14, 15, 17). The number of women who are substance abusers has increased since the 1970s. Some researchers attribute this increase to the infusion of more women into the work force and the changing definitions of femininity. Conflicts in sex roles and participation in multiple roles also are contributing factors to the increase of women substance abusers (4).

According to Research Triangle Institute, alcohol abuse cost the nation $116.7 billion in 1983. The Institute also reported that diminished work productivity resulting from alcohol abuse accounted for $65.5 billion of the cost in 1983 (5). The National Institute on Drug Abuse reported in 1984 that the economic cost of alcohol and drug abuse was more than four times greater than that of cardiovascular diseases. Data from the Eunice Kennedy Shriver Center highlighted the significance of fetal alcohol syndrome, the third most common cause of mental retardation. Each year, between 3,700 and 7,400 U.S. babies are born with fetal alcohol syndrome (18).

Although alcohol abuse cost the nation $89.5 billion in 1980, only $1.3 billion from all public, private, and third-party sources was spent to combat the problem—a sixty-nine to one ratio. Forty-five percent, or $585 million, of that amount was from federal sources (18).

The National Association of State Alcohol and Drug Abuse Directors, Inc. has estimated that, in 1984, states spent 11.5 percent of total available public and private funds on efforts to prevent alcohol and drug abuse, while, in contrast, spending 80 percent on treatment programs (18).

The attraction of accruing large sums of money in a relatively short period of time by the sale of such illegal substances can lead to competition and associated violence. Another area of consideration is the loss of tax dollars from the nontaxable income generated from the sale of illegal substances.

Alcohol, however, is taxed heavily and is a good revenue producer for most states. The use of alcohol has had a tremendous impact on the national economy. State legislatures have always used taxes on alcoholic beverages to generate income for state budgets. This measure is indicative of the degree to which the sale of alcohol has been inextricably intertwined with our socioeconomic superstructure.

The cost to the community in terms of caring for those who have physiological and psychological problems directly related to the abuse of substances can be measured by hospital days, morbidity and mortality rates, and the incidence of criminal activity. Studies have revealed (1) that drugs, particularly alcohol, influence criminal behavior. The dual role of rehabilitation for the criminal offender who is also a substance abuser is extremely costly to society. The average annual per capita cost of incarceration is $30,000 for an offender without a substance abuse problem. The cost of incarceration coupled with the attempt to rehabilitate the substance abuser is generally prohibitive, and thus the rehabilitative aspect is usually neglected or eliminated. Major corporations have had to bear the cost of lost work time resulting from the inability of the substance abuser to function appropriately. Some corporations, in an attempt to salvage the working substance abuser, have had to institute costly programs.

Nature of the Problem

Etiology

Substance abuse relates to many factors, each equally important in its effect on the individual. There is usually more than one causative factor. We are a drug-using society. We are all encouraged by the media and peer pressure to solve problems through the use of drugs. Problems such as boredom, isolation, social alienation, and discrimination, not to mention physiological problems of pain and malaise, are all prime candidates for "solution" through the use of drugs.

Physiology and Chemical Reaction of Ethanol

Alcohol is absorbed from the gastrointestinal tract into the bloodstream. The amount and kind of alcoholic beverage ingested may influence how rapidly the alcohol is absorbed. The use of carbonated beverages or additives retards absorption.

The metabolism of alcohol begins in the liver. Alcohol dehydrogenase oxidizes the alcohol to acetaldehyde. The acetaldehyde is further metabolized in the liver or carried to the tissues, where it is converted to acetyl-coenzyme A, of which the acetate portion can be oxidized to carbon dioxide and water. The key in the metabolism of the alcohol is the activity of the alcohol dehydrogenase. The energy produced during the metabolism of alcohol is not stored, and therefore must be used immediately (16).

The kind and amount of alcohol ingested and the time span in which it was ingested determines the blood alcohol concentration and the effects on the nervous system, as well as subsequent signs and symptoms throughout the body. Four to five ounces of whiskey drunk by an average person who weighs about 150 pounds in a period of one hour would give a blood alcohol concentration (BAC) of about 0.10 in two hours (12).

Using the above estimate as a guideline, we can begin to project some possible changes within the system. At blood concentration levels of 0.02 to 0.03 the person does not display any signs of impairment. At 0.05 to 0.06 the person is again, not intoxicated, but some changes in fine motor skills occur. At 0.08 to 0.09 some impairment of gross motor coordination skills occurs, and at 0.11 to 0.12 definite impairment exists. Legal intoxication states occur at 0.15 BAC because of definite impairment of physical and mental control. Higher concentrations cause additional problems, with 0.60 causing death (12).

The primary action of alcohol (ethanol) is that of a central nervous system depressant. Alcohol causes immediate changes in brain function and directly affects the thalamus; the medulla; the frontal, parietal, and occipital lobes; and the cerebellum. Changes in equilibrium, coordination, sensation, fine motor skills, body temperature, and speech patterns can be predicted to some degree with the consumption of alcohol. Continued and persistent use of large quantities of alcohol affects all the body systems and organs. Chronic drinking of alcohol for more than ten days may cause an improper protein synthesis, which will lead to impaired metabolism in the neurons, with subsequent damage to the brain cells, and the person has evidence of loss of or poor memory and a decreased learning capacity. Nutritional deficiencies, primarily folate, may lead to niacin deficiencies, which cause dermatitis, gastrointestinal problems, and severe intellectual impairment. The nutritional deficiency also contributes to the impaired production of the enzymes needed for myelination, which causes the formation of lesions in distal peripheral nerves, leading to peripheral neuropathies (8). Severe vomiting, which may occur with excessive use of alcohol or a decrease in vitamin B_1 intake, may result in thiamine deficiency, which then interferes with the Krebs-Henseleit cycle. Impairment of this cycle may lead to damage of brain cells, since the waste product of protein deamination, ammonia, cannot be properly converted to urea. Thiamine deficiency may also impair the mechanism that produces the fatty acids needed to synthesize and maintain cerebral myelin. This in turn will probably cause petechial lesions and hemorrhages to develop in the brain. The alcohol abuser may develop Wernicke's or Korsakoff's syndrome. The signs and symptoms manifested in these syndromes include diplopia from palsy of the third or fourth cranial nerve, hyperactivity, delirium from stimulation of cortical and thalamic lesions, severe recent memory deficit, possible deficit in insight and judgment, and confabulation to cover for the memory deficit. Another pathophysiological manifestation in the neurological system is demyelination of the optic nerve. The client may have painless blurred vision, decreased visual acuity, and scotomas. The metabolism of ethanol produces high levels of acetaldehyde, which remains in the cerebellum. This concentration of the acetaldehyde in the cerebellum may lead to corticocerebellar lesions and degeneration, progressing to cerebral atrophy, which results in broad-based and unsteady gait, impaired coordination, and fine tremors. Interference with biochemical substances, particularly destruction of serotoninergic neurons, decreases ion serotonin, which in turn produces long periods of wakefulness and aberrations in rapid-eye-movement sleep. The sleep disorders that occur may also lead to periods of depression (8). Toxic effects of alcohol (0.20 BAC) produce changes in myocardial cells. There is a leakage of cardiac electrolytes, such as potassium and phosphate, and cardiac enzymes, and a decrease in fatty acid uptake with an increase in the extraction and accumulation of triglycerides. The resulting signs and symptoms are a decrease in the rate of contractions and decreased left ventricular pressure, which reduces cardiac output. Cardiomyopathy occurs, which increases the likelihood of the alcohol abuser's developing congestive heart failure and cardiomegaly. The use of large amounts of alcohol may produce some other cardiac signs and symptoms. The effects produced are indirectly attributed to the action of the ethanol within the system. Some of the effects are altered fluid balance, hypokalemia, hypomagnesemia, alcohol withdrawal reactions, hyperlipemia, and pericardial effusion and congestive heart failure seen with persons who drink large amounts of beer. Electrocardiographic changes are noted: low, wide, inverted T waves, depressed ST segments, and prolonged QT interval related to the hypokalemia and hyperlipemia. The hypomagnesemia, which evolved from increased excretion of magnesium in the urine, may eventually lead to myocardial necrosis. The necrosis occurs because of impaired oxidation. The decrease in magnesium may also increase central nervous system irritability, which in turn may increase cardiac stress. Hyperlipemia, an increase in blood lipids, results in atherosclerotic changes. A rebounding phenomenon occurs when there is an increase of alcohol in the bloodstream. First, there is a decrease in antidiuretic hormone levels; as the level of alcohol in the blood decreases, the pituitary secretes a large amount of antidiuretic hormone, which causes fluid retention and possibly congestive heart failure (8).

Folate deficiency occurs with the chronic use of alcohol and results in interference of amino acid and DNA production, which in turn causes disorders in cell division. Because of the ineffective cell production, immature red blood cells may be produced, leading to anemia, thrombocytopenia, leukopenia, and megaloblastic hematopoiesis. The leukopenia increases the alcohol abuser's susceptibility to infection and he or she is more likely to contract tuberculosis and have frequent bouts of upper respiratory tract infections and pneumonia (8).

The liver is the primary site for metabolism of alcohol. The conversion of ethanol to acetaldehyde occurs by way of oxidation in the alcohol dehydrogenase enzyme system. The process produces hydrogen-bound nicotinamide-adenine dinucleotide, which eventually interferes with the production and synthesis of lipids and glycogen formation. Hepatic fat becomes easily evident in the alcohol abuser. Some structural changes may also occur in the liver that interfere with the normal oxidation of fatty acids, eventually leading to ketogenesis and ketoacidosis. The same structural damage also increases the metabolism of drugs and alcohol, which results in an increased tolerance for some of the commonly abused substances, (alcohol, sedatives). Along with the fatty liver, inflammation may occur. This is frequently described as alcoholic hepatitis. The fatty liver, coupled with the inflammation of the liver, over time may produce necrosis of the hepatic cells, leading to scarring and, eventually, fibrosis of the liver. This phenomenon is called cirrhosis. The cirrhotic process, with obliteration of the hepatic central veins, causes a collection of hepatic lymph in the peritoneal cavity, leading to portal hypertension and ascites. The sustained use of alcohol may produce an increase in gastric acid secretion and frequent vomiting. This causes the development of esophagitis. This disorder may escalate into other problems. One is Mallory–Weiss syndrome, which is a mucosal laceration at the gastroesophageal junction (8). Painless hemoptysis may occur with this. The chronic use of alcohol, combined with heavy smoking, increases the risk of developing cancer of the mouth, pharynx, and esophagus. Those particularly at risk for cancer of the esophagus are nonwhite males (3). An impaired mucosal cell barrier may result in back digestion of gastric acid with erosive gastritis, and, eventually, gastric ulcers. The folate deficiency noted earlier disrupts small intestine function and causes malabsorption of nutrients. The increased secretion of gastric acid and secretin with the chronic use of alcohol stimulates pancreatic secretions. This causes upper abdominal pain, nausea, vomiting, and ileus, and is usually diagnosed as acute pancreatitis. Chronic pancreatitis is caused by duodenal spasm and spasm of the sphincter of Oddi, which increases biliary and pancreatic intraductal pressure. This produces chronic pain and results in an exocrine deficiency. This deficiency is manifested by fat malabsorption with resultant weight loss, steatorrhea, malabsorption of vitamin B_{12}, and glucose intolerance (diabetes mellitus) (7).

Specific data are now available that documents the detrimental effects of alcohol on a fetus. Because there is no safe level of alcohol consumption during pregnancy, pregnant women are advised to refrain from consuming alcohol. The following are some specific effects on fetal development that have been identified (9, 10):

- Central nervous system deficiencies—mild to moderate mental retardation, microcephaly, irritability in infancy
- Growth deficiencies—prenatal retarded intrauterine growth, postnatal failure to thrive
- Abnormal facial characteristics—short palpebral fissures, flat or absent groove above upper lip, thinned upper lip, receding jaw in infancy
- Abnormalities in other systems—heart abnormalities, joint defects, abnormalities of the external genitalia, kidney defects, birth marks

Specific Effects of Drugs

Cocaine.   This substance has gained notoriety in the United States because of its cost and the frequency of use by many Americans. Street names for cocaine include "snow, snort, coke." Cocaine has a direct effect on the mucous membranes and is absorbed and distributed throughout the body. It is a powerful central nervous system stimulant. The duration of action is short-lived, usually twenty to forty minutes. The user of cocaine may experience exhilaration, euphoria, well-being, confidence, increased energy, suppression of fatigue, increased ability to continue physical and mental activities. Some users indicate that in small doses, it acts as an aphrodisiac. Some signs and symptoms of abuse are excitability, anxiety, talkativeness, increased pulse rate and blood pressure, and dilated pupils. Long-term use may cause tissue necrosis leading to perforation of the nasal septum, lingering depression, disturbances in sleep patterns, inability to concentrate, and increasing nervousness when the immediate effects have subsided. Whether cocaine is addictive is debatable. Some professionals do not believe it is because it does not result in withdrawal crises, such as delerium tremens seen in alcoholics (11, 13). The psychological consequences of use and abuse are great.

Heroin ("H, horse").   This opiate has major effects on the central nervous system and the gastrointestinal tract. Heroin, like all narcotics, reduces pain and may cause drowsiness. One of the dangerous effects of heroin is its depressive action on the respiratory center in the brain. The depression of the respiratory center can result in the abuser having shallow respirations and apnea and becoming at risk for respiratory arrest. When a large dose of heroin is injected, nausea and vomiting can oc-

cur as side effects of the drug. Nausea and vomiting, coupled with the slowed respiration, predisposes a user to aspiration of the vomitus. This may occur because of the user's diminished ability to stay awake and breathe effectively. The decreased respiration or cessation of respiration is indicative of overdose. Another area of the brain adversely affected by heroin is the hypothalamus. The resultant effect is a fluctuation in body temperature and fluid retention (12).

Normal functions of the gastrointestinal tract are decreased when heroin is present in the body. Normal peristalsis is less frequent. Ingested food moves more slowly through the gastrointestinal tract. Because food moves more slowly in the gastrointestinal tract, water is reabsorbed in larger-than-normal amounts. The result of this action is constipation.

Heroin users report experiencing euphoria when they inject the substance into their bloodstreams. However, data from various sources have documented that many heroin users have not injected a large enough amount of the drug to induce the effect they perceive. Effects of the drug are directly related to dosage. The potency of the drug is not usually ascertained by the user. Additives are widely used in the preparation of heroin for sale. Injection of the drug is always potentially dangerous, and the additives themselves may be harmful.

Heroin withdrawal produces specific signs and symptoms. Some develop within four hours after discontinuation of the drug; others occur up to thirty-six hours later. The user experiences a craving for the drug, yawning, diaphoresis, rhinitis, teary eyes, dilation of the pupils, goose bumps, tremors, hot and cold flashes, pain in the bones and muscles, increased blood pressure, increased temperature, increased pulse and respiratory rate, and weight loss. The intensity of the withdrawal symptoms varies with the individual user and the amount and strength of the heroin used.

Barbiturates.   Barbiturates depress the central nervous system and produce effects that range from mild sedation to coma. The most frequently abused barbiturates are those that are short acting, such as secobarbital and pentobarbital. The effect of barbiturates is similar to that of alcohol. Barbiturates are absorbed from the stomach. If used with alcohol, they are absorbed more rapidly. The liver cannot metabolize barbiturates, and therefore they are found unchanged in the urine of the user (19). Depending on the dose, barbiturates may produce a calm, relaxed state, impaired judgment, decreased alertness and reaction, or coma. Unlike some other substances, the lethal dose of barbiturates is the same for abusers and nonabusers alike. The side effects of barbiturates are slowed reactions, lethargy, and respiratory depression. Mortality usually results from severe respiratory depression or aspiration of vomitus.

Hallucinogens.   Hallucinogens are stimulants that affect the autonomic nervous system. Detoxification occurs in the liver. Somatic symptoms occur a few minutes after use, beginning with vertigo, nausea, some weakness, drowsiness, concurrent desire to laugh and cry, progressing to perceptual changes, such as distortion of visual and auditory stimuli. The effects may clear after twelve hours (11).

Marihuana (cannabis sativa).   Also known by the street names "pot, ganja, grass," marihuana is the most often used and abused of any illegal psychoactive drug. Unlike alcohol and some other abused substances, it is not eliminated rapidly from the body. The active component in marihuana is tetrahydrocannabinol (THC). Because of its high solubility in fat and low solubility in water, THC is not completely metabolized. The THC along with other residues are tightly bound to the fat and are slowly excreted by the bile (15). The transport, digestion, and excretion of fat-soluble substances are undertaken by the biliary system. Therefore, elimination of THC occurs slowly through the kidneys, intestines, and feces. It can be detected in the urine up to one week after use, even if the person smoked only one cigarette (15). Although there are no conclusive data regarding long-term use of marihuana and its effects, definitive information is available about some effects. The Institute of Medicine of the National Academy of Science, in its 1982 report on marihuana and health, indicated the following: an increase in heart rate, changes in the respiratory tract, impairment of psychomotor performance; some persons were noted to have difficulty with short-term memory and might experience anxiety and panic reactions; some male users were found to have a decrease in the number and motility of sperm; some females had cessation of menstruation; specific information about long-term effects on fertility is not yet known (15).

Risk Factors

Who is at risk for substance abuse? Can we identify some specific qualities that would alert us to potential substance abusers? Valliant, in his study of alcohol-ism, found that ethnicity and having an alcoholic parent were strong predictors of subsequent alcohol use (20). Some common variables found in abusers of various substances are low self-esteem, inability to cope with life stressors, being easily influenced by peers, availability of the substances, and lack of positive role models in the environment. Users of one substance are at risk for the use of others. Using alcohol to enhance barbiturates, or using alcohol to potentiate the effects of methadone, is not uncommon.

Prevention and Screening for Early Intervention

The potential substance abuser can be identified by using the data available about those people who are at risk for the problem. Counseling of children of parents who are substance abusers, particularly alcohol abusers, should be done as soon as the problem of abuse is identified by the health professional. Discussion with children in primary grades regarding the effects of chemical substances is not a revolutionary idea. This may deter them from trying the substance. The decision regarding trying a substance later in life may be partly based on the information they receive at that time. Peer group sessions that advocate the problem-solving approach to aid in the development of healthy coping mechanisms can be used. The professional nurse can be a catalyst in a group session in the primary grades by encouraging group participants to identify how they can best handle their problems of coping with daily life stressors. The nurse can stimulate the group to develop new or more effective coping mechanisms. Getting youngsters to express and deal with feelings is important, since suppression of feelings may be a basis for seeking the use of a chemical substance later on in their lives. Some people use chemical substances in an attempt to decrease anxiety. The professional nurse can aid a client in the identification of those factors in one's environment that cause the buildup of anxiety. The client can be encouraged and aided in the development of self-esteem and health coping mechanisms. Again, this can be done through group sessions with people who have healthy coping mechanisms and are positive role models for the client.

Involvement in the political and legislative processes is an important role for the professional nurse to undertake. It is a professional responsibility to identify those legislative measures that are counterproductive and encourage or support the use and abuse of chemical substances. Developing school and community programs that help youngsters, teenagers, and adults develop healthy coping skills is another pursuit. Such programs might include "rap sessions," recreational programs, or special interest groups to decrease social isolation and idle time. Locating funding for the creation and maintenance of such programs is a professional responsibility.

The nurse must always be vigilant and focus on identification and case finding. Early detection and intervention for the youngster who may have started to drink beer with his classmates in the eighth grade, or tried a few marihuana cigarettes, are extremely crucial. The primary responsibility of the professional nurse at this stage is to prevent complications of the problem and establish a sound treatment plan. Assessment of the factors that precipitated the use of the substance must be undertaken. Selection of an individualized treatment plan that will minimize the physiological and psychological consequences will require patience on the part of the professional and commitment to change behavior from the client. Inclusion of the family or significant others is paramount at this time. The physiological effects of the substance abused should not be minimized. Treatment should be well coordinated by the professional nurse. Prevention of complications is the goal of intervention at this stage of early intervention.

Nursing Intervention in Acute and Chronic Phases

Assessment

Health History.   The nurse, as the primary provider of care to potential substance abusers, substance abusers, and their families and significant others, must use her skills in interviewing. It is extremely important that the health history for these clients be complete. The nurse must create an environment to facilitate openness. To do this, the interview and the gathering of data must be done in a nonjudgmental manner.

Client Profile.   The initial step in the health history should be the client profile. These data include the client's name, address, date of birth, sex, and race. The educational background, religious affiliation, ethnic group that client and family prefer to be identified with, and socioeconomic status are also included. Particular attention should be given to eliciting information about habits such as smoking, nail biting, use of caffeine. The nurse then needs to address in detail use of chemical

substances: the kind used, frequency of use, when started, amount used, under what circumstances substances are used, reactions to use, reactions to nonuse. Family members or significant others could be used as validators regarding this information.

Family History.   This is an important facet of the health history. Information given and that not known or shared by the client are of equal importance. The family constellation, role of parents and grandparents, siblings, and other relatives, should be determined. Family illnesses, particularly problems with substance use and abuse, should be ascertained. Other significant information regarding specific disease entities, particularly those that may have a familial or genetic tendency, should be addressed. Of particular importance are those diseases or problems that may have been sequelae of an abuse problem but not so identified by family members. The relationship of the client with other family members and interactions between and among family members should be noted.

Past Medical History.   This is another area of the health history that is important for the primary nurse to obtain. All hospitalizations, reasons for the hospitalizations, specific diagnosis, or at least problems that the client presented with at the time of the hospitalization are significant. Many times clients may not be aware of the complete diagnosis but are aware of the reasons for their hospitalization. Names of hospitals and health providers are also necessary data. Past treatment regimens and the client's response to the treatment should be noted. This might also be an opportunity to identify the role of family members during the treatment or hospitalization. What specific follow-up or posthospitalization plan was carried out by the client? What role, if any, did the family assume in this period? Specific medication dosage and frequency and how the client responded to same and used the medications are valuable information that the nurse will need. What other medications has the client used, both over-the-counter and prescribed? Has the client misused or abused any of these medications?

History of the Present Problem.   This part of the history taking attempts to identify the chief complaint, or the reason the client is now seeking care from the health care provider. The reason the client is seeking assistance should be restated. Is he currently using any chemical substance? If so, how much and what kind of chemical? Does he believe that the substance use is causing him a problem at this time? How does he describe his problem? Specific symptoms should be described by the client. The symptom should be analyzed by the primary nurse. What is it? When did it start (onset)? What has been the course since onset? What precipitated the symptom? What has aggravated the symptom? What has relieved the symptom? Have any other symptoms surfaced since the initial onset? The nurse should then review all body systems, with emphasis on those that are directly affected by the use of the substance, such as the neurological and gastrointestinal systems.

The Mental Status Assessment. This assessment should be done at this junction, before starting the physical examination. Placement at this point is important because it allows the nurse to look over some of the information elicited in the client profile that needs further expansion. It also gives the nurse an opportunity to arrange the data in an organized format, since the mental status assessment includes both subjective and objective data. The seven areas that need to be assessed are (a) level of awareness; (b) appearance and behavior; (c) speech and communication; (d) mood or affect; (e) disturbances in thinking process, disorganization of thought process, disturbance in content of thought, problems with memory; (f) problems with perception, (g) abstract thinking and judgment (2). The nurse may have obtained some of this information during the earlier part of the interview. The problem identification will be done at a later time.

Physical Assessment.   The next step in the assessment of the problems of the substance abuser is the physical assessment. A cephalopedal examination is necessary for the client with a substance abuse problem, in the attempt to identify problems that the client may have reported during the history and to focus on those systems that are particularly susceptible to the substance abused. The following systems require particular attention.

Integumentary.   This system should be checked for the presence of vascularity, dryness, moisture, signs of recent trauma, presence of edema, cyanosis, changes in hair distribution, changes in nailbeds, areas of inflammation and infection, scarring, recent or old track marks. These areas are assessed because of pathophysiological changes that may occur. Hematologic abnormalities may occur with substance abuse and the changes may be evidenced in the skin. Substance abusers may have frequent accidents. Some substance abusers may have cardiovascular changes that may be evidenced in hair distribution and nail changes also.

Musculoskeletal.   This system should be assessed for range of motion of joints, muscle for tone, and gait. Because substance abusers may experience frequent falls

or accidents, a restriction may be present because of the trauma. Gait and muscle tone may be affected because of changes or a deficit in the neurological system.

Respiratory.   The thorax should be auscultated for the presence of normal breath sounds or adventitious sounds. Because of poor nutrition or aspiration of materials when under the influence of the drug, pneumonia may develop. Also, in many substance abusers, particularly intravenous drug abusers (IVDA), there may be a lowered immune response (see chapter 34).

Cardiovascular.   Auscultation of anterior thorax to identify normal heart sounds and extra heart sounds is also warranted. The substance abuser is at risk for the development of cardiovascular disease. Cardiomyopathy or subacute bacterial endocarditis may cause changes in heart sounds and other perfusion problems, such as changes in the skin and nailbeds noted earlier.

Abdominal.   This system is examined to identify bowel sounds, distension, presence of fluid or gas, pain or tenderness (only light palpation may be possible in the presence of liver tenderness). Substance abusers may encounter problems with elimination, diarrhea, or constipation.

Genitourinary.   The substance abuser may experience oliguria, polyuria, frequency, dysuria, hematuria. The costovertebral angle should be tested for tenderness.

Gynecological.   A vaginal examination should be performed to identify the presence of any infections, since the substance abuser, particularly the IVDA, may be more susceptible to infections because of a lowered immune response.

Neurological.   All cranial nerves, reflexes, and cerebrum and cerebellar functioning should be examined. Chemical substances abused are central nervous system depressants and cause specific changes within the system.

Diagnostic Tests

The diagnostic tests performed regarding substance abuse are usually done to identify the effects that the substance may have had within the system. Alcohol (ethanol) presence in the blood can be determined by testing. Seldom is such testing used to diagnose alcoholism. Its major usage has been for law enforcement purposes to determine intoxication levels, particularly if persons operated motor vehicles while impaired by alcohol. Liver function tests to determine fat metabolism, protein metabolism, bilirubin metabolism, serum enzymes, and excretory function are done if liver damage is suspected. Careful examination of the nares may be undertaken to determine the degree of destruction of mucous membranes in the person who inhales cocaine. Again, this is done if and when the client presents with a problem in this area. Urine is examined for the presence of THC. All this indicates is use of marihuana sometime before the test was done. Barbiturate levels in the bloodstream can also be ascertained.

When there is liver damage in the substance abuser, fat metabolism may be decreased, protein metabolism (i.e., total serum protein) may be normal, but albumin may be decreased. Blood urea nitrogen may vary and serum prothrombin time and blood ammonia may be increased. Bilirubin metabolism, serum enzymes, and liver excretory function are invariably increased (6). It is the responsibility of the primary nurse, along with the staff physician to determine the necessity for these tests. This determination is made on the basis of the findings of the health history and physical examination. The primary nurse must explain the purpose of the tests to the client or family members. In some settings it might be the responsibility of the nurse to do the venipuncture or obtain the urine specimen. The nurse also needs to explain the specific procedure to the client. The findings of the diagnostic tests should be clearly explained to the client and the family members, with the specific reasons for the change in the normal findings.

Nursing Diagnoses

The nursing diagnoses are determined after the information gathered during the history and physical examination is sorted and grouped. The nursing diagnosis takes into account not only the problems identified in the physical examination, but also potential problems that might be related to developmental or situational aspects in the client's life. Nursing diagnoses related to substance abuse include the following:

Alteration in bowel elimination: Constipation or diarrhea
Potential for infection
Impairment of skin integrity: actual or potential
Disturbance in sleep pattern
Potential for injury: trauma or drug overdosage
Alteration in patterns of urinary elimination

Ineffective individual coping
Ineffective family coping: compromised
Disturbance in self-concept: self-esteem, role performance, or personal identity
Impaired social interaction

Alterations in thought processes
Sensory-perceptual alterations
Social isolation
Powerlessness

Spiritual distress

The primary nurse must decide which of these diagnoses take priority. The decision must be based on those that might lead to life-threatening situations, the meeting of basic needs, and the desire of the client or family or significant others.

Planning and Implementation

The professional nurse who provides care for substance abusers and their families or significant others must be concerned with the multiple factors that are present with drug use. Substance abusers may not be willing to share information with the professional nurse regarding their abuse of a substance. Some kinds of substance abuse may be viewed by society as socially deviant behavior, and therefore carry with them negative connotations. Another factor is that many of the chemical substances abused must be obtained through illegal channels. This might force the user and abuser of the substance to interact with a "criminal element in our society." Health professionals, in most instances, are viewed by the substance abuser as belonging to that section of society that would neither condone nor engage in the abuse of chemical substances or deviant behavior. Because of the tendency of the substance abuser to be evasive, and because of the pervasive abuse of substances across all socioeconomic levels, the professional nurse faces a challenge in obtaining a valid profile of the substance abuser in many situations. Another area that must be taken into account is the denial on the part of the abuser and family members or significant others that the person is having a serious problem. Helping the substance abuser and family members to become self-caring requires an innovative but caring approach by the professional nurse. Such an approach requires knowledge of the various substances, their effects and consequences, the pattern of use, and the alterations in behavior that evolve when the drug is used. Assessment of the individual and family includes the person's and family's readiness for self-care and their capabilities.

The nurse, client, and family must determine what specific behaviors are necessary to resolve the problems identified, or the nursing diagnoses. Short- and long-term goals must be established before any actions are undertaken. Alteration in nutrition, resulting in a debilitated state, would have abstinence from the drug as a long-term goal. The short-term goal may be to decrease the use of the drug and improve nutritional intake in the next thirty days. This would be necessary for those who abuse amphetamines and opiates, since amphetamines decrease appetite and opiates interfere with digestion. The alcoholic would also have to resort to abstinence in order to improve his or her nutritional state.

Alterations in bowel elimination—constipation or diarrhea—or alterations in patterns of urinary elimination are caused by fluid imbalance related to abuse of chemical substances. Opiates can cause fluid retention. The use of cocaine or hallucinogens increases cardiovascular activity, which might cause diaphoresis. Acute or chronic pancreatitis in the alcoholic may cause vomiting. Urinary infections may occur. Abstaining from using the drug must be both a long-term goal and a short-term goal, with the client paying particular attention to the proper intake of fluids during the next thirty days.

Disturbances in sleep patterns may result from the abuse of a chemical substance. The long-term goal of abstinence itself, however, might cause a disruption in the sleep pattern. Persistent drinking may lead to periods when the alcoholic may be unable to account for his time. He may be asleep for long periods or be constantly awake. During withdrawal, or detoxification, the substance abuser may experience insomnia. Recognizing this as a symptom that will eventually subside and not requesting medication constantly for this problem are steps in becoming self-caring.

Periods of physical activities appropriate to age and general state of health must be properly spaced. The family's role is that of support and encouragement in the development of realistic activities that might involve the client.

Social isolation, disturbances in self-concept, impaired social interaction, powerlessness, and alteration in thought processes all must have abstinence as a long-term goal. The short-term goal must also include abstinence and involvement in a treatment modality. The substances abused all affect the central nervous system. Most cause some alteration in perception. Some, such as the hallucinogens, might cause a person to be more talkative or to laugh inappropriately. The inability to communicate appropriately with others is a common corollary of substance abuse. Participation in a treatment program in which the abuser will begin to identify along with others when and why he uses and abuses a particular chemical substance is of utmost importance. The role of the family is to continue to support abstinence and to attempt to establish clearer communication with the client. This might necessitate the involvement of family members in a treatment process if they wish to have the family remain intact.

Potential for injury would involve abstinence in most cases, or not becoming involved in activities that would put the person or others at risk, for example, operating a motor vehicle after drinking in excess or using other chemical substances that alter behavior and motor activity. The abuse of the substance itself poses a danger to the life and well-being of the abuser because of the deleterious effects on the body systems. It also affects the well-being of significant others with whom the abuser interacts. Withdrawal from such substances must be done under controlled conditions for the most part. Avoidance of any of the commonly abused substances during pregnancy is imperative. The frequent infections, possible cardiovascular complications, and the criminal or violent activity that might be associated with obtaining illegal substances are all hazards to the abuser.

Two of the primary tools that the professional will use during the time that care is being provided to a client and the family are teaching and counseling. The primary nurse will be responsible for teaching the client and the family about a nutritionally balanced diet and about the signs and symptoms that might occur because of withdrawal from any of these drugs, allowing the client and family members to discuss their feelings regarding the use and abuse of the chemical substances and the effects they have had on the family dynamics. The primary nurse must be cognizant of the available community resources, not only for the treatment of the client, but also for family members. The primary nurse must be cognizant of the relapse rate of substance abusers, particularly alcoholics, so that support can be provided to the client and family during that period of time.

Of utmost importance is the primary nurse's being in contact with feelings that she might have regarding drug use. Trust in the care giver must be developed early in the interventive process. The substance abuser will quickly lose confidence and trust in the primary care giver if she herself is involved in using the substances the client is abusing while caring for him.

Evaluation

In the care of the client and family experiencing a substance abuse problem, the long-term goal is abstinence. The primary nurse, after providing care for the client and establishing realistic goals, must determine if the actions being taken are workable. The specific nursing diagnoses must be reviewed. The goals and actions must be analyzed. Is the client free from drugs? If so, how long has he remained drug free? Were there any complications noted during the period of contact with the primary care provider? Did the client continue in the treatment modality recommended? Did the family participate in the treatment? Have any of the potential problems identified earlier surfaced? Is the client able to express the factors that precipitate his or her abuse of substances? Working with a substance abuse client in the hopes of attaining abstinence is a slow and arduous process. The primary nurse must evaluate the goal of abstinence and self-care activities at thirty- to sixty-day intervals. For instance, has the client improved her nutritional status, has she gained weight? What is the condition of her skin? Has she had any accidents related to possible neurological problems?

Complications

Because most of the chemical substances abused are central nervous system depressants and stimulants, the health care provider must be prepared to deliver acute emergency care. The common effect of overdose of most chemical substances is respiratory arrest. The priority in treatment of a person in respiratory arrest is to establish an airway, establish breathing, and maintain circulation. The treatment after this initial intervention depends on the substance that has been used.

If it has been established that the person has overdosed by using an opiate—which might be difficult to ascertain unless someone is available to give an adequate history—a narcotic antagonist, usually naloxone, 0.4 mg to 0.8 mg, is administered intravenously by the physician. The neck vein is usually used, since it may be the most accessible. An increased level of consciousness with pupil dilation should be immediate if the overdose was due to an opiate. If the client responds by waking up and moving or kicking his or her extremities, a continuous infusion of dextrose 5% in water is begun. Chronic opiate abusers will respond to naloxone with signs and symptoms of withdrawal (21). Withdrawal from opiates in and of itself is not life-threatening. Most care givers treat this complication symptomatically. The signs and symptoms produced are directly related to the specific action that the opiate has on the central nervous system and the gastrointestinal tract. Therefore, such

signs as diarrhea, nausea, hot and cold flashes, muscle twitching, bone aches, and insomnia are present because the centers that control these phenomena are no longer depressed.

The role of the professional nurse, in many situations, is supportive. She or he will have to decide if the signs and symptoms are such that use of a prescribed medication is indicated for relief. The professional nurse has to be cautious about not substituting another "drug" on which the client will become psychologically or physiologically dependent.

Barbiturate overdose poses a different kind of problem for the health care provider. After the client's airway, breathing, and circulation are stabilized, the stomach contents are removed by means of a large-lumen gastric tube. Measurement of arterial blood gases and pH and analysis of blood barbiturate levels are carried out simultaneously. Gastric lavage is performed after an endotracheal tube has been inserted. It is generally accepted that some kind of saline solution is used for lavage. This is followed by the instillation of activated charcoal (21).

Withdrawal from the substances abused must be carefully monitored by the health care provider. For the barbiturate abuser, withdrawal is a medical emergency. Sudden cessation of the use of these drugs will result in a series of reactions, convulsions being the most prominent (21). Therefore, withdrawal must be done gradually and slowly, under medical supervision.

One of the complications of IVDA is acquired immunodeficiency syndrome (AIDS), a disease that has mystified epidemiologists. It is known, however, that IVDAs are at risk. The use of contaminated needles among IVDAs has fostered the transmission of the disease. Anyone presenting with infections of unknown cause who uses intravenous drugs will more than likely be worked up to rule out AIDS. Another disease entity that is often seen in the abuse of intravenous drugs is hepatitis B, which, for many IVDAs, is a chronic state of illness. Hepatitis B surface antigen is usually positive for this group of clients and some institutions follow strict precautions when caring for them. The focus, however, is to prevent transmission via blood and other body fluids. Therefore, special attention must be given to the screening of the IVDA when he or she presents for any type of examination that would entail withdrawing blood for laboratory testing. Needles or other equipment used for an invasive procedure must be disposed of under strict conditions. In some states these materials are incinerated. Maintenance of proper asepsis is a mandate for the professional nurse and all others caring for the client.

Withdrawal from alcohol may escalate into a medical emergency if an adequate assessment of the abuse of this substance is not done by the professional nurse and others providing care. The withdrawal syndrome may begin with mild tremors of the hands, progressing to the extremities and trunk within a few hours after the last drink and up to two days later. The tremors may be controlled with chlordiazepoxide (Librium) (21). Seizures may occur during this period. The seizures may be managed symptomatically, but the client's safety must be assured. The professional nurse must exercise good judgment to assure that the client is protected. Delirium tremens poses an additional problem. This is a medical emergency, although some of the symptoms may be classified as psychosis. The client may have visual and auditory hallucinations and exhibit overall shaking of the body, extreme restlessness, and agitation. Immediate treatment should include a combination of tranquilizers and sedatives. The client must be closely observed to prevent injuries to himself and to ensure that the desired effect of the medication is occurring.

The most serious complication is the polyabuse of chemical substances. Damman and Ousley noted polyabuse among women, and although no typical polyabuser was identified, they did note that the polyabusers they studied lacked the educational and occupational background usually associated with the middle class (5). It is not uncommon to encounter an abuser of alcohol who also abuses barbiturates, or an abuser of heroin who is also using cocaine, tranquilizers, and other sedatives. This leads to problems in management for the health provider, if there is an overdose of any of these substances. Deciding which antagonist to use becomes a more difficult task.

Ethical and Legal Issues Related to the Problem

There are some questions and concerns that must be voiced about some of the chemical substances that are abused. The first is alcohol (ethanol). What is the responsibility of society and government regarding the legal use of a drug, knowing the detrimental effects that it has on those who abuse it? What is the responsibility of the manufacturer to the public who uses the product? Does anyone have the right to tell another what he or she could or should consume? What is the responsibility

of society to those persons who are at risk, who knowingly use a product that will inevitably cause problems that society will have to pay for? Because some of the chemical substances abused are illegal, other issues may arise for the professional nurse. Is the health professional responsible for reporting a client's source of drugs if this is revealed during an interview? If the health professional uses a drug such as marihuana and enjoys the euphoria or altered perceptions that result, can he or she objectively discuss with the client the possible adverse effects of a substance that is being abused? The issues raised with these questions have been debated and will continue to be debated in our society.

CASE STUDY

Thomas Brown is a forty-two-year-old married account executive and father of two sons, ages sixteen and fourteen. Mr. Brown graduated from a college with a bachelor's degree in business administration. He started to drink when he was thirteen years old.

At age eighteen, when he went away to the state university, his drinking continued, particularly on weekends, at sporting events and after exam times. Being the one to drink the most beer at college parties was not unusual for Mr. Brown. His friends usually told him of his funny antics, since he passed out so many times and could not remember the events that had occurred. He had a few car accidents on his way back to the dorm, but never anything that involved law enforcement officers.

After college, Mr. Brown joined a rapidly growing company where he was required to meet clients frequently for lunch or dinner. Although he was able to remain sober during these business contacts, the bartender occasionally had to help him to a cab afterwards.

Mr. Brown married his childhood sweetheart when he was twenty-four. For a while he managed to control his drinking, but after the birth of their first child, it began to escalate, and his relationship with his wife deteriorated. Drinking now began to interfere with his business. Finally, after a second child was born, his wife left him.

Now alone, Mr. Brown continued to drink, and after a few months of an erratic work record, he was confronted by his employer because of the ever-present odor of alcohol on his breath. He was told to resolve his problem or he would be fired. Mr. Brown became despondent over the possible loss of his job; he left his office that evening and went to the bar near the office before taking the train back to his community. After getting home, he found that his alcohol supply was low and took his car out of the garage to drive to the liquor store. Because he had been drinking for a few hours prior to coming home, his coordination and reaction times were impaired. He did not notice a stop sign and kept driving through the intersection, crashing into a tractor-trailer truck that had the right of way. Mr. Brown sustained a blow to his head resulting in a four-inch laceration above the right eye as well as other injuries. He was brought into the emergency room by ambulance, and the ambulance attendant reported that the odor of alcohol was very strong when the patient was removed from his car. The physician sutured the laceration on his head and took x-rays.

Mr. Brown is being admitted to the medical unit for observation. When you see him, it is four hours after he was first brought into the hospital. He appears frightened and slightly nervous.

1. What is the initial observation that must be made by the nurse who will be caring for this patient?
2. Should the fact that he was drinking when the accident occurred be mentioned by the nurse? What specific questions should be asked by the nurse?
3. What specific areas should be examined on the nurse's initial physical exam of the patient?
4. What specific precautions should be taken with the patient?
5. What intervention could a primary nurse have initiated early in the course of this family's problems to help prevent family dysfunction and deterioration?

REFERENCES

1. Ball, J., et al. "The Impact of Heroin Addiction upon Criminality." In *Problems of Drug Dependence*. Rockville, Md.: National Institute of Drug Abuse, 1979, 163–79.
2. Barry, P. *Psychosocial Nursing Assessment and Intervention*. Philadelphia: J. B. Lippincott, 1984, 110.
3. Blume, S. "Epidemiology and Characteristics of Drug and Alcohol Use." In *Research Developments in Drug and Alcohol Use,* ed. R. Milman. New York: New York Academy of Science, 1981, 4–15.
4. Cahill, M., and B. Volica. "Male and Female Differences in Severity of Problems with Alcohol at the Workplace." *Drug and Alcohol Dependence* 8:143, 1981.
5. Damman, G., and N. Ousley. "Female Polydrug Abusers." In *Poly Drug Abuse: The Results of a National Collabora-*

tive Study, ed. R. R. Wesson et al. New York: Academic Press, 1978, 59–95.
6. *Diagnostics,* Nurse's Reference Library. Springhouse, Pa.: Intermed Communications, 1983, 110–19, 452–54.
7. Einstein, S. *Drugs in Relation to the Drug User.* New York: Pergamon Press, 1980, 192–243.
8. Estes, N. J., and M. E. Heinemann. *Alcoholism: Development, Consequences and Intervention.* St. Louis: C. V. Mosby, 1982, 136–84.
9. *Fetal Alcohol Syndrome: Task Force Report to the Governor.* New York State Division of Alcoholism and Alcohol Abuse, November 1979.
10. Finnegan, L. "Effects of Narcotics and Alcohol on Pregnancy and the Newborn." In *Research Developments in Drug and Alcohol Use,* ed. R. Milman et al. New York: New York Academy of Science, 1981, 362.
11. Gay, G. "Psychedelics and Cocaine." In *Drugs in Relation to the Drug User,* ed. S. Einstein. New York: Pergamon Press, 1980, 244–73.
12. Girdano, D., and D. Dusek. *Drugs: A Factual Account.* Redwood City, Calif.: Addison-Wesley, 1980.
13. Goode, E. *Drugs in American Society.* New York: Alfred A. Knopf, 1984, 189–90.
14. Lieber, C. "Alcoholism Medical Complications." In *Research Developments in Drug and Alcohol Use,* R. Milman et al. New York: New York Academy of Science, 1981, 132.
15. *Marijuana and Health: Report of a Study by a Committee of the Institute of Medicine.* Washington, D.C.: National Academy Press, 1982.
16. Metzler, D. E. *Biochemistry: The Chemical Reactions of Living Cells.* New York: Academic Press, 1977.
17. *National Institute on Drug Abuse Report,* 1982.
18. *Prevention of Alcohol Abuse in American Families: Fact Sheet.* U.S. House of Representatives Select Committee on Children, Youth and Families. May 1985, 1.
19. Smith, D., et al. "Clinical Approaches to Acute and Chronic Intervention in the Sedative Hypnotic Abuser." In *Drugs in Relation to the Drug User,* ed. S. Einstein. New York: Pergamon Press, 1980, 192–243.
20. Valliant, G. F. *The Natural History of Alcoholism: Causes, Patterns and Paths to Recovery.* Cambridge, Mass.: Harvard University Press, 1983.
21. Warner, C. *Emergency Care Assessment and Intervention.* St. Louis: C. V. Mosby, 1978, 173–204.

CHAPTER 19

Abuse in Families

MARJORY J. MARTIN

.

OBJECTIVES

After completing this chapter, the reader will be able to:

□ Describe the characteristics of abusive families.

□ Identify early signs of abusive behaviors.

□ Apply the nursing process in working with victims of abuse.

□ Use assessment guides in the health appraisal of victims of abuse at various age levels.

□ Formulate nursing care plans based on the nursing assessment.

□ Design nursing interventions at three levels of care.

□ Identify evaluation measures in working with abusive families.

□ Perceive the need for multidisciplinary cooperation.

□ Compare the legal and ethical dilemmas faced by the primary care nurse in working with families where abuse is suspected and where it is identified.

□ Recognize societal forces that contribute to the problems of abusive families.

This chapter focuses on patterns of abuse within the family, to help the primary nurse identify the early indicators of abusive behaviors through health appraisal and apply the nursing process at the primary, secondary, and tertiary levels of prevention.

The Problem

The primary care provider encounters incidents of abusive behaviors among family members in a variety of situations in institutions and community settings. Assaultive and abusive behaviors are known at all age levels and in all social and economic strata. Child abuse, battering of spouses, and maltreatment of the elderly are common occurrences. Only a small percentage of the incidents of abuse are called to the attention of health care providers, social welfare agencies, or law enforcement agencies. Fontana describes maltreatment of children as the "world's most desperate problem" (5). Physical, emotional, and medical neglect as well as outright inflicted abuse initiate a cycle of dangerous crippling of individuals and families that is passed from generation to generation.

The battered child syndrome, first identified by Kempe (17) in the early 1960s, is one of the leading causes of death and disability in the pediatric age group. National recognition of the prevalence of the problem as a well-identified aggregate of symptoms led to the passage in 1967 of laws relating to child abuse in all states of the union. Recognition of the magnitude of the problem led to the creation of the National Center on Child Abuse and Neglect through the Child Abuse and Treatment Act of 1974 (PL93-247). The activities of that agency have focused on the development of policies and programs for the prevention, identification, and treatment of child abuse and neglect. Since that time research efforts have been directed toward the understanding and treatment of this complex health problem. Since the identification of the battered child syndrome, attention has been focused on other types of abuse in families, such as the battered spouse, sexual abuse between family members, and maltreatment of the elderly.

The problem of abuse within families is complex and involves individual characteristics of family members, family structure and dynamics, and sociocultural factors. Individual family members, both abused and abuser, may have personality characteristics that make them prone to aggressive behavior. Intrapsychic conflicts, hostility, displacement of anger, tendencies toward sadism, and frank psychosis are examples of psychological variables that may lead to abusive behavior.

The family is a basic unit of society and as such functions to nurture and support its members. Sadly, the abuse of children, spouses, and the elderly occurs most often within the intimate confines of the family unit. The intense emotional links between family members as well as their proximity are seen as factors that evoke hostility (11). The intense relationships of nuclear family members, as well as the rapid changes in family structure from the extended family to single parenthood and dual-career families, contribute to difficulty in providing adequate support to members and to disharmony in family life.

Societal characteristics such as large-scale unemployment, poverty, racism, and culturally sanctioned use of physical punishment in the home and institutional settings must be considered as significant in the perpetuation of abusive behavior in the family. Failure on the part of the government to provide adequate financial and social support to childbearing families contributes to declining family strength and cohesiveness.

In this chapter, abuse within the family is viewed within the framework of human growth and development. The application of the nursing process in life stages of family development is seen as appropriate for the diagnosis and treatment of actual and potential problems of abusive behavior.

The primary care nurse, in providing assistance to families through episodes of maturational and situational crisis, can reduce and prevent the occurrence and recurrence of abusive behavior. At the same time the primary care nurse needs to recognize the existence of psychological and social pathology that requires a restructuring of individual family values and the initiation of social programs in the larger society. The primary nurse, acting as an independent practitioner or in conjunction with other members of the health care team, has a significant contribution to make in the identification and control of the difficult and pervasive problem of family abuse.

Characteristics of Abuse-Prone Families

Behaviors related to neglect, maltreatment, and abuse are known to exist in families at all social and economic levels. No specific cultural or ethnic group has been identified as having a propensity for abusive behaviors. Life circumstances, however, make some families more vulnerable than others, depending on their position in relation to the dominant social group, their stage of development in the life cycle, and the nature of natural and community support systems. The primary care provider can be alert to actual and potential problems of abuse in the following family situations:

- Families in which parent spouses or caretakers were themselves abused, neglected, or maltreated
- Families in which there is marital strife with frequent separations and reconciliations
- Families in the childbearing stage of the family life cycle with the birth of siblings less than a year apart or with multiple births
- Families who are isolated with few natural support systems (family and friends) and who are alienated from community support systems
- Families inclined to religiosity and moralizing
- Families with low educational levels and few financial resources
- Families with a history of alcohol or other drug abuse

History of Abuse.   Studies of abusive behaviors in families have consistently demonstrated the perpetuation of aggression from generation to generation (16). Abusing parents have been subjected to abuse and neglect in their own childhood. The absence of effective role modeling plays an important part in domestic violence. In spouse abuse where the woman is the victim, the history shows that the perpetrator had a father who was abusive and the wife had a mother who was abused (26). In a study cited by Finlay, 54 percent of the men and 37 percent of the women who engaged in domestic aggression also abused their children. Of 150 women victims of abuse,

45 percent reported that at least one child in the home was also a victim of the man's assault (4).

Marital Strife.   Marital stress, frequent separations, accidents, and change of residence are characteristic of abusive families. Dell Martin points out that fear dominates the lives of abused women (20). There is a fear of staying in a dangerous environment and fear of leaving because of threats of retaliation. Remorse on the part of the perpetrator and the victim's loneliness or lack of resources lead to a pattern of separation and reconciliation. The fear of isolation and abandonment and not being able to make it on one's own creates a dilemma for the abused wife. Where there is marital discord, children may be used as scapegoats.

Childbearing.   It is well established that childbirth constitutes a natural developmental crisis in the life of a family. Closely spaced children without adequate support systems can be a stressor that leads to child abuse. One study indicates that families with twins experienced a significantly higher incidence of child abuse and neglect than did those with single births (28). The study also reveals that mothers felt that health professionals did not provide adequate education or support after the birth of their infants.

Support Systems.   Single parents and young parents with no family nearby are more prone toward abusive behaviors. Abusive families have been noted to be isolated nonjoiners with few natural or organizational sources of support. It is imperative, therefore, that the primary care provider inquire about the availability of families and friends during the prenatal and postpartum periods.

Religiosity and Moralizing.   Families who are obsessively religious may adhere to the "spare the rod and spoil the child" ethic and rely mainly on corporal punishment as a mode of discipline. The cultural scripting of patriarchy and male dominance have also been cited as perpetuating aggressive modes of interpersonal relationships in family life (9). Parents who have a poor understanding of normal behavior at stages of child growth and development or who are inclined toward moralism may use physical punishment inappropriately. A parent may strike a small child for behavior that may reflect a normal exploratory phase, and healthy assertiveness may be misinterpreted as aggression or disobedience requiring control with a belt, paddle, or hairbrush.

Low Educational Levels. Families with members who have low educational levels are more susceptible to economic changes that lead to unemployment. Lack of education and vocational training leaves people poorly prepared to compete in a tight job market, and subsequently they are subjects for potential abuse. A lack of education may be the cause of a poorly developed self-concept, leaving the family provider with a low level of tolerance for frustration and a high level of defensiveness. The inability to provide for the family and the difficulties in applying for public assistance may trigger abusive behavior.

Substance Abuse. Families who use drugs and alcohol are apt to be irritated by the demands of children and other dependent family members. Under the influence of an addictive substance, a family member may lose control and resort to impulsive, assaultive behavior. In the case of spouse abuse, it has been proposed that alcohol intoxication is not the cause of battering, but an excuse to release what is otherwise unacceptable behavior (22). The expenditure of funds to support an addictive habit rather than to provide for needs of family members can be a form of abuse.

The task of assessing the characteristics of individual family members, their habits and ways of relating to one another is not always easy. The primary care nurse, in the home and in the hospital setting, is in an excellent position to observe family interactions. Too often opportunities for diagnostic observations are missed because of preoccupation with an assigned task. Closer attention to family dynamics and interrelations may provide important clues to the potential onset of abusive actions.

Women's Movement. Shainess contends that as a result of the women's movement, women have become more assertive. This healthy assertiveness may elicit assaultive behavior on the part of the husband. She cites the case of a professional woman who, in addition to her professional responsibilities, was expected to, and did, assume full responsibility for household management and childrearing. She was also expected to be sexually available at the spouse's will. During the course of therapy she became more assertive and requested assistance from the spouse. This triggered an inordinate amount of rage and assault. The ultimate resolution was a dissolution of the marriage (31).

The women's movement, with women entering the work force in larger numbers and entering predominantly male occupations, also triggers incidents of as-

sault. Not infrequently the woman's decision to return to school for professional training creates conflicts that lead to aggressive behavior and ultimate severing of relationships.

Symonds discusses the traditional attitudes toward women victims of violence and the psychological patterns that operate in people who experience violent acts. She explodes the myth of female masochism and denounces Freud's theory of unconscious wishes to be punished. Symonds proposes a new model of women victims with the psychology of catastrophic events and victimology as the new paradigm for studying battered and abused women (32).

Sexual Abuse of Children. Sexual abuse of preschool and school-age children is being reported with more frequency than in the past. There has been an increased awareness on the part of health care professionals and school personnel regarding the incidence of sexual abuse of children. Child victims of sexual abuse are usually known by or related to the abuser. Studies reveal characteristic patterns of family dynamics in child abuse (24, 25).

Nakashima and Zakus (25) describe two types of families that are incest prone, classic and multiproblem. In the classic typology the family presents a picture of stability and domestic tranquillity, and is characterized by early marriage of long duration, absence of extramarital affairs, patterns of rigid control by the father, and limited family contact with the outside world.

In the multiproblem family the characteristics are parental inadequacies manifested in child abuse and neglect, acting out behaviors, truancy, aggression, assault, and murder; drug dependency and alcoholism; sexual promiscuity and pregnancies outside of marriage. In multiproblem families the incest is a "minor theme in the pathological chaos of the multi-problem family" (25).

Mrazek and Kempe (24) further describe characteristics of family relationships in which incest occurs. In father-daughter incest the oldest daughter is the most vulnerable. The mother is passive, dependent, sexually cold, and avoidant of sexual relationships. The mother unconsciously condones the relationship through denial and through abdication of the maternal role to her daughter. In mother-son incest the mother has unstable relationships with men, there are frequent separations, and multiple marriages and divorces. The mother uses the son for sexual gratification in the absence of a lover.

In brother-sister incest the youngest sister with several older brothers is "at risk." There is little or no documentation of mother-daughter, sister-sister, or brother-brother incest. Father-son incest may occur if there is sexual estrangement in the marriage or if the father has unrevealed or unrecognized homosexual tendencies. Incidents of multiple family sexual relationships occur more frequently in multiproblem families (24).

Herman and Hirschman studied forty women who had incestuous relationships with their fathers during childhood. They were compared with twenty women who had close relationships with their fathers but the relationships were seductive rather than incestuous. Of those who experienced overt incest, there was a higher incidence of runaway, suicide attempt, and pregnancy during adolescence. In many of these families the mother was disabled, chronically ill, or battered. There was a high frequency of violence in the fathers (12).

The results of this small sample would indicate that the damaging effects of interfamilial sexual activity may be related to other factors in family life as well as to the incestuous act itself. There are cross-cultural variations in what is considered to be incest, and anthropologists have indicated that all societies have some form of incest taboo. Another question to be considered is the degree of eroticism that is tolerated within the family unit and the point at which sexual activity within the family is identified as sexual abuse or incest.

The Nursing Process Applied to Abusive Families

The major steps in the nursing process have applications in work with abusive families in both the hospital and community settings. Goals that are established are realized through problem-solving, educative, and crisis intervention approaches. The seven steps in the nursing process are as follows:

1. Establish a meaningful, working relationship.
2. Assess the health status of the family and individual members.
3. Formulate a nursing diagnosis.
4. Establish goals for health and for nursing care.
5. Select and implement nursing interventions.
6. Evaluate the outcomes of nursing actions.
7. Reestablish new goals.

Establishing a Relationship

The problems of abusive families are often multiple and complex. In addition to the propensity to resolve con-

flicts through physical, verbal, and emotional attack, families may have additional problems in communication, characterized by distancing. The resolution of interfamily conflicts often depends on the willingness of family members to communicate with and establish a working relationship with health care providers. The course of action may be long and difficult and may involve changing very basic patterns of behavior and altering lifelong, ingrained habits. In many cases abusive persons have been so isolated that they have not been able to place their trust in anyone. The primary care provider, therefore, must draw on interpersonal, therapeutic, and communication skills to establish a working relationship with family members. Freeman describes a working relationship as one that "is consistent with the demands of a particular situation and that creates a climate which fosters the required action, whether the action is to help the family or to protect the community" (6). Freeman characterizes a working relationship as one that contains the essential elements of trust, empathy, and outreach.

In abusive families the members must *trust* that the health care worker is acting in the best interest of the family. This may be difficult in working with those who have been damaged by their own life experiences. Nevertheless every effort must be made to convince parents and caretakers that the professional is genuinely concerned about the family's well-being as well as the well-being of the victim, and that the ultimate purpose in offering help is to keep the family together and improve family functioning.

Empathy may be established by indicating to the family that the health care provider is able to see the problem from the family's point of view. The problems of handling a difficult infant, stresses related to overcrowding, financial problems, and the burden of caring for dependent members must be recognized. Empathy may be expressed both verbally and nonverbally. Verbal expressions of empathy reflect the feelings that aroused the abusive actions. "The baby's crying must be very upsetting to you." Or, "Caring for your mother must be very tiring after working all day." Nonverbal empathy may be expressed by attitude, facial expression, and an emotional identification with the feelings that are being disclosed.

In *outreach* the health provider takes the initiative in raising issues with the family rather than waiting for the topic to arise. The worker structures the interview in such a way that the need for assistance becomes apparent and the offer of help is extended. For example, if the close spacing of births is a contributing factor in the abusive situation, the worker may raise the issue of contraception and arrange for an educative intervention.

A *working relationship* implies educative and problem-solving approaches without resorting to coercive methods. When situations occur (as is the case of abusive behaviors) in which the use of authority is necessary, whenever possible the health care worker will minimize the legal process in the total health care plan.

Assessing Family Members

The assessment phase of the nursing process defines the nature of the health problem and determines the possible effect of nursing interventions in alleviating the problem. With abusive or potentially abusive families, the assessment focuses on the health appraisal of both the abused and the abusive members, and the evaluation of family dynamics. See Table 19.1 for guidelines for nursing assessment.

Development Assessment. Formal developmental testing is essential to the total health appraisal of the infant or child when abuse is suspected. Formal testing provides an opportunity to identify specific areas of delay in development, to observe the child's behavior, and to observe interactions with the evaluator. The primary care provider may administer a developmental scale, such as the Denver Developmental Screening Test, the Bayley Scales of Infant Development, or the Yale Modified Gesell Test. Although the administration of developmental scales does not require formal training in psychometrics, the evaluator needs skill and precision in the administration and interpretation of the tests.

Rodehoffer (29) reports the following characteristic behaviors of abused children during the testing procedure:

- Hypervigilance—a state of constant readiness for unexpected events
- Fear of failure—extreme anxiety when faced with a difficult task
- Difficulty in attending to instructions—highly distractable and unable to focus attention
- Verbal inhibition—difficulty with word finding and organization of thoughts
- Passive-aggressiveness and resistance—superficial cooperation with underlying obstructive maneuvers

The following specific areas of development should be considered:

- Nutrition—history of poor feeding patterns, forced feeding by parent, anorexia, failure to thrive, poor weight gain

- Sleep disturbance—frequent periods of waking; may begin at about age two with the onset of dreams; punished for waking parents; night terrors
- Enuresis—bed-wetting and daytime accidents well beyond expected age for control
- Bowel control—failure to gain control at expected age
- Thumb-sucking—prolonged and excessive thumb-sucking or other oral patterns
- Temper tantrums—frequent periods of rage, throwing self on floor, kicking, biting
- Other—excessive masturbation, stuttering that may have invoked punishment, aggressive behavior toward other children, hitting, throwing objects

A study of infants aged twelve to twenty-six months referred because of documented abuse found low scores on the Bayley Scales, lack of sustained attention, and reaction of anger, frustration, and withdrawal (7). Abused children show uneven performance; that is, they may perform up to their age level in psychomotor tasks but show delay in language development. Careful interpretation of test results is important in avoiding premature conclusions about retarded development. Rodehoffer indicates that it is misleading merely to add up scores and determine a developmental quotient (29).

The results of the developmental evaluation may be used as a guide in the treatment plan. The form used for the Denver Developmental Screening Test is especially useful in parental guidance. The form indicates expected behaviors at various age ranges. It helps the parent or caretaker to understand age-appropriate behavior. McKittrick points out that a child may be punished for behavior that is appropriate to the child's developmental stage but that is not seen as appropriate by the caretaker (19). A review of the developmental schedules with the responsible adult can aid in understanding expected behavior in language, adaptive, motor, and self-help activities. Parents can learn that difficult periods of development are transitional, and they can better tolerate the "terrible twos" if the end is in sight.

Nursing Assessment—School Age Child and Adolescent

History. The abused child or adolescent may have a long history of maltreatment, or the abuse may be related to a developmental stage of teenage rebellion. The younger child, if abuse has occurred during the pre-

Table 19.1
Nursing Assessment—Infant and Preschool Child

General History	Information taken from parent, caretaker, or health records
Obstetric	Unplanned or unwanted pregnancy, complications of pregnancy, prolonged and difficult labor, cesarean section, precipitous delivery, prematurity, multiple birth
Neonatal	Low Apgar score, separation from mother because of prematurity, congenital anomalies, or other complications
Postnatal	Failure to thrive, poor weight gain, difficulties in feeding and sucking, colic, excessive crying, frequent upper respiratory tract infections
General Appraisal	
Weight	Below the third percentile
Temperature	Subnormal owing to lack of body fat; heat loss owing to exposure or immaturity
Head	Lacerations, abrasions, subdural hematoma; bald spot or flattened head owing to static positioning; skull fracture
Nose	Bruises or fractures; nasal discharge or congestion
Face	Facial expression indicates distress; lack of expression owing to passive withdrawal; forlorn expression. (Lack of social smile at six weeks may indicate early neglect or failure of bonding.)
Cry	Excessive crying; high-pitched, shrill cry may indicate central nervous system damage or drug addiction (withdrawal). Weak, whimpering cry may indicate lack of nourishment or distress.
Skin	Multiple bruises, lacerations, or burns at varying stages of healing. Type of burn may indicate the form of abuse, e.g., doughnut burns on palms or soles from cigarette, glove burns on hands and feet from immersion in boiling water; erythematous areas around buttocks may be an immersion burn or ammonia burn from unchanged diaper. Cyanosis may be present owing to injury to larynx or thorax. Teeth marks may be from animal or human bites.
Extremities	Limitation of range of motion owing to dislocation or fracture. Fracture of the long bone occurs when the infant is picked up by the limb and flung. Spiral fractures may result from twisting an extremity.
Thorax	Fractured ribs; funnel or pigeon breast owing to malnutrition or disease
Respiration	Shallow, irregular retractions, periods of apnea, labored breathing owing to injury or choking
Abdomen	Pain on percussion, distended abdomen owing to malnutrition or injury; ruptured spleen
Genitalia	Bruised, swollen, lacerations owing to sexual abuse; vaginal discharge, ruptured hymen
Neurological	Sustained moro reflex, hyperactive reflexes
Immunization	Incomplete or total lack of immunization

school period, may enter school as a handicapped child with brain damage or mental retardation. The older child may have a history of school failure, delinquency, or merely a failure to make friends or form close associations. Rebellious behavior may be manifested as defiance of family rules, sexual exploration, substance abuse, or truancy. The teenager may have a history of attempted suicide. A study by Teicher and Jacobs revealed that a suicidal teenager had a characteristic biography that included broken homes, rejection by parents, family fights, and isolation from any meaningful relationships. The isolation and lack of family communication is evidenced by the fact that most teenage suicides occur at home with parents in the house (33).

The medical history of the abused adolescent may reveal frequent hospital admissions or emergency room treatment. There may be a history of congenital anomalies, chronic illness, or repeated accidents. The account of an accidental injury may not fit in with the type of injury sustained.

Health Appraisal. Physical examination may reveal evidence of physical abuse, such as lacerations and bruises at varying stages of healing. X-ray may reveal new fractures or old, healed fractures. The health appraisal may also reveal significant findings on mental status assessment. Obsession with appearance, anorexia nervosa, and obesity may be related to interfamilial conflicts. The presence of sexually transmitted disease or teenage pregnancy may not only cause anxiety and depression in the adolescent, but also incite the wrath of and instigate physical abuse by parents or caretakers. The health provider who suspects abuse or sees evidence of abuse in the history or on health appraisal will do well to look into the family dynamics and interfamilial conflicts that are adversely effecting the health status of the adolescent.

Nursing Assessment—Adult Family Member (Abused Spouse)

History.   Abused women are frequent users of emergency services, psychiatric services, and gynecological services (14).

The primary care provider working in these services should be especially alert to actual and potential incidents of nonaccidental injury, sexual abuse, and mental abuse arising from interfamilial conflicts. As in child and adolescent history taking, the adult member may give information about the source of injury that is discrepant. In the case of a battered spouse there is a repetition of similar injuries (15). Healed injuries may indicate a delay in seeking medical assistance because of fear of retaliation. The health history may reveal frequent episodes of depression or a history of alcoholism or other substance abuse. There may be an account of frequent separations and reconciliations.

Health Appraisal.   Physical examination may reveal a variety of presenting symptoms indicative of assault. The battered woman may complain of frequent headaches, chest pain, lower abdominal pain, breast pain, nervousness, or choking sensations. Evidence of assault may be manifested in multiple bruises at varying stages of healing, broken jaw, skull fracture, broken arms and legs. There may be burns from cigarettes or from scalding liquid and lacerations from knives, razors, or other sharp objects. Bald spots may be due to pulling out of hair during altercation. In the physical examination special attention should be paid to the pregnant woman who has bruises around the breast and abdomen.

In performing the health appraisal the primary nurse must avoid expressions that reflect shock, even though the battering may be severe. It is essential to express concern and to pose questions in a nonjudgmental way. Houghton suggests "desensitizing" the language used in history taking and restoring a sense of dignity to the injured person (14).

Nursing Assessment—Elderly Family Member

History.   Elderly abused family members may present a history of frequent emergency room visits or hospitalizations. There may be a long history of dependence on their children because of illness or financial need. The elderly abused person may have been an abusing parent. Observations of family interaction during history taking may give clues to actual or potential abuse.

Health Appraisal.   The physical examination may reveal unexplained bruises, lacerations, and fractures. There may be an emaciated appearance, dehydration, and pressure sores. Soiled clothing, unwashed hair, and unwashed body may be evidence that the elderly person is left alone, is isolated, or is ignored by family members. Abuse may also be manifested in the withholding of food and medication, points that require attention in the total appraisal. Other forms of abuse that have an adverse effect on the mental status as well as physical well-being are physical restraint, deprivation of autonomy, exclusion from family functions, and financial exploitation.

The problem of abuse of the elderly is of no small dimension. Hickey and Douglass found that 60 percent of health care practitioners interviewed had discovered incidents of neglect and abuse (13). Vigilance on the part of the primary nurse in the home and hospital may prove the incidence to be higher.

Formulating a Nursing Diagnosis

In formulating the nursing care plan, family and multidisciplinary involvement should be considered. In formulating the care plan, family participation and validation are necessary for goal attainment. Family strengths are identified and used before nursing or other professional activities are delineated. Self-care concepts and self-determination should keynote the care plan. All family resources should be analyzed before authoritative actions are taken.

The primary care provider who encounters incidence of actual or potential abuse will, of necessity, work with members of other disciplines such as social workers, physicians, and law enforcement representatives. Although the differentiation of roles lies in the expertise required in a given situation, all disciplines should work together toward a common end. The goals and objectives established through the care plan should be common to all disciplines. There may, however, be interdisciplinary conflicts regarding the best course of action. These conflicts should be resolved in interdisciplinary conference before actions are taken. Unresolved conflicts of professional health workers may be detrimental to the family and to the outcome of the care plan. In the instance of child abuse, for example, the common goal is to safeguard the victim, to promote healing, and to prevent further abuse. The action taken to achieve these goals may not be totally agreed on. There may be disagreement relating to the family treatment plan—family therapy, home visits, or foster care placement. It is important that the best interests of the parent and child are not sacrificed to the vested interests of a particular discipline.

The developmental framework of families provides effective guidelines for formulating nursing diagnoses and structuring nursing care plans. Duvall describes developmental tasks that arise at various stages in the life of the family (1). Failure to accomplish developmental tasks leads to discontent and disruptions in family life, often taking the form of abusive and violent behaviors. Deviations from developmental tasks provide guidelines for interventions at a primary and secondary level.

The developmental framework provides a basis for evaluating family dynamics and for formulating a diagnosis and care plan (see Table 19.2). It is recognized that the categories are not definitive, and that there is a great deal of overlapping in developmental phases. In some families, for example, there may be teenage children and an unexpected midlife pregnancy. This situation may contribute an additional stress point in terms of another family member. At the same time it may help the teenager in transition from a child-dependent role to potential parenthood. Age categories are not absolute. There is, for example, a recent trend toward later-year childbearing. Adjustment for family developmental stages can be made for midlife progenitors.

Selecting and Implementing Nursing Interventions

Nursing actions applied to families when there are actual or potential abusive behaviors are based on thorough and accurate assessment and well-formulated nursing care plans. The care plans are implemented at three levels of prevention: primary, secondary, and tertiary. Pringle points out the importance of primary prevention in child abuse, stating that early intervention is likely to be more effective than crisis intervention. Pringle adds that the intervention must promote the interest of the victim, and every effort should be made to prevent reinjury (27). These principles may be applied to victims of abuse at any age level, including the abused spouse and the elderly victim.

Primary Prevention. Primary prevention measures focus on the interfamilial interactions during the prepathogenic period. Primary prevention includes health promotion activities and specific protection measures that are directed toward the developmental process. Health promotion requires the analysis of agent-host-environmental interactions that promote family wellness or that leave families vulnerable to the development of pathology.

There are indications that interfamilial violence is rooted in culturally determined theories and practices of childrearing. It has been estimated that more than 90 percent of American families use physical punishment in the discipline and training of children. Harsh physical punishment, together with lack of impulse control, leads to abusive behaviors. The battered child of today becomes the battering adult of tomorrow. Interruption of an intergenerational cycle of violence is a problem of major proportions.

In addition to culturally sanctioned use of physical force as discipline, certain societal forces create another causal dimension. The prevalence of poverty among minority groups, high infant mortality and morbidity rates of nonwhite populations, poor educational systems, and other forms of discrimination point to society as well as to parents, guardians, and caretakers as perpetrators of violence (10).

The complexity of the problem should not discourage the primary nurse from initiating and participating in primary prevention measures aimed particularly at high-risk groups. Primary prevention measures may include the following:

- Initiating and conducting parenting classes and family life education in outpatient clinics, schools, churches, and community centers
- Conducting classes in child growth and development for young parents, baby-sitters, and other caretakers
- Promoting widespread dissemination of contraceptive information and encouraging availability of effective contraceptive devices
- Supporting legislation to liberalize contraception and family planning policies
- Teaching stress reduction techniques in clinics, schools, and occupational settings
- Establishing networking systems for families at various stages of development
- Initiating classes on interpersonal relations and conflict resolution

Table 19.2
Phases of Family Development—Tasks and Variance

Developmental Task	Variance
Establishment Phase	
Establish a home	Substandard housing; living with relatives; overcrowding; frequent change of residence
Manage income	Impulsive spending; unable to budget to stretch salary; inadequate income
Establish a satisfactory marriage relationship	Sexual conflicts; inconsistencies; jealousy
Maintain family relationships	Socially isolated; few friends or relatives nearby; lack of social support system
Expectant-Childbearing Phase	
Arrange for care of new members	Unprepared for infant; no materials for basic needs—feeding, clothing, sleeping
Adapt home to accommodate children	Children are an intrusion on adult spatial arrangements; emphasis on order and compulsive cleanliness
Safeguard health of mother and infant	Delays prenatal care; uses drugs and alcohol; smokes excessively
Foster growth and development of infant	Irregular feeding; poor weight gain; little developmental stimulation; uses physical punishment; fails to keep clinic appointments; erratic immunization
Relating to the community	Avoids contact with health care providers; family is isolated, "nonjoiners"
Plan and control childbearing	Lack of knowledge of or refusal to use contraception; short interpregnancy interval to detriment of mother's health; reliance on ineffectual birth control methods

The ultimate resolution of problems of family violence primarily lies in social policies and the provision of legislation to support adequate family income and promote family health and stability.

Secondary Prevention. Secondary prevention measures are aimed toward early identification of deviations from developmental tasks and of abusive behaviors, and prompt intervention at incipient stages of family conflicts.

The primary care nurse is in an excellent position to initiate secondary prevention measures through contacts with families at risk in prenatal and postpartum clinics, well-child clinics, schools, and other health care settings.

Secondary prevention measures may include the following:

- Screening in prenatal clinics for clients at risk for potential abuse, with special attention to:
  —Unplanned or unwanted pregnancies
  —Teenage pregnancies
  —Single-parent pregnancies
  —Pregnant clients without family support systems
- Screening in obstetrical units during labor and delivery and the postnatal period, with special attention to:
  —Husband and wife interactions suggesting conflict or distancing
  —Premature births, multiple births, cesarean sections
  —Separation of mother and infant because of prematurity, and other reason
  —Signs of postpartum depression
  —Parental reaction to infant's crying
  —Early signs of delayed development or failure to thrive

Table 19.2 *(continued)*

Developmental Task	Variance
Preschool—School Age Phase	
Provide facilities for growth and development	Few toys; restrictive play activities
Maintain social control	Harsh childrearing practices; use of "hairbrush" discipline
Create effective communication patterns	Conflicts over methods of discipline; unable to discuss problems without argument; reacts to differences with hostile silence or abuse
Provide sex education	Fosters myths about sexuality; punishes for sensual behavior; promotes shame and guilt over sexuality; masturbatory activity harshly punished
Maintain community affiliation	Avoids contact with school and community agencies; contacts limited to calls from authority for disciplinary actions
Teenage and Young Adult Phase	
Promote sense of responsibility	Inconsistent in demands—easy one day, bears down the next; few or no assigned responsibilities; ignorant of whereabouts at late hours
Arrange for economic independence	Allowance inadequate to meet basic needs; encourages illegal means of financial gain
Maintain social control	Uses physical punishment as discipline; at odds with authority; protects antisocial behavior
Recognize and accept growing sexuality	Alarmed at development of secondary sex characteristics; unable to control feelings of sexuality toward offspring; engages in incestuous activity
Maintain satisfying marriage relationship	Distancing, frigidity, coldness, aloofness or open conflict; unable to work out conflicts without violence
Release young adults and accept new members	Restricts social relationships; resents potential mates of offspring; promotes guilt at suggestion of leaving home
Middle Years Phase	
Reaffirm marital bonds	Conflicts intensify when children leave home; resorts to alcohol or drugs
Provide supportive assistance to aging members	Expresses hostility and resentment toward aging and dependent members; deprives of basic needs and uses physical and emotional punishment

- Screening during the preschool period with special attention to:
  - Delays in language, adaptive, or self-help behaviors
  - Interactions with other children characterized by withdrawal or aggressive behavior
  - Problems in feeding, toilet training
  - Unusual fears
- Screening during the school-age period with special attention to:
  - Absenteeism, truancy, frequent illness, and accidents
  - Frequent encounters with school authorities
  - Health-related problems, pregnancy, sexually transmitted disease
  - Changes in academic performance and personality changes
- Screening in the adult period with special attention to:
  - Repeated visits to gynecology clinics, mental health clinics, and emergency services
  - Requests for tranquilizers or sleeping pills
  - Alcohol and other substance abuse
  - Fearfulness, evasiveness, and depression
  - Homes with elderly dependent members

In addition to the screening procedures in secondary prevention, the primary care nurse initiates prompt treatment through direct intervention, multidisciplinary team effort, and referral. Secondary prevention measures are means of dealing with abusive behaviors in the early stages and are primarily supportive. Examples of supportive services are housekeepers for mothers with young children, for families with elderly dependent members, or for families with an absent parent. Head Start programs, day-care centers, foster home care, visiting nurse services, and self-help groups are but a few examples of resources that can be used to prevent the proliferation of conflicts within families.

Tertiary Prevention.   Tertiary prevention measures are implemented after the abusive behaviors have been identified. The goal in tertiary prevention is the restoration of the victim of abuse to a high level of wellness and the prevention of the recurrence of abusive behaviors in the family. The primary care nurse engages in tertiary prevention measures in the hospital, home, and community settings. Nursing interventions aimed at the client as an individual may be ineffective. In cases of abuse, family-centered nursing care is essential. Nursing interventions focus on direct care of the victim, family crisis intervention, and referral. The complexity of the problem of abuse frequently calls for a team effort, most often involving physicians, social workers, and law enforcement representatives.

Nursing Care in the Hospital Setting.   When the victim of abuse is a child, nursing care in the hospital setting will promote restoration of wellness through the following measures:

- *Direct care* of injuries and promotion of healing
- *Psychological support* through creation of a warm and consistent environment, assistance in verbalizing feelings, use of toys and drawings to express feelings
- *Observation* of family interactions to identify areas of stress
- *Encouragement* of positive family relationships; encouragement of parental participation in care
- *Communication* with family about findings of physical examination, developmental assessment, and other diagnostic examinations; informing family of child's progress, projected length of hospital stay, plans for discharge; interpreting the need for ongoing treatment
- *Strengthening* positive parent-child relationships;

encouraging parents' participation in care; giving encouragement and support; helping families to deal with their reaction to the crisis
- *Educative* influence by interpreting child's behavior and reactions, explaining level of growth and development, initiating parent-education classes; providing a role model for care
- *Referral* for assistance; encouraging parental acceptance of help from social workers and other members of the health care team; preparing the family for mandatory reporting of the incident, for referral to a protective agency, and for the possibility of court involvement; referring to self-help groups or other community groups

The primary nurse in the hospital setting is in an excellent position to initiate interventions and to plan programs to prevent further abuse. Specific intervention will vary with the age of the abused patient (whether infant, child, or adult), but the goals will be similar in protecting the abused person and restoring him or her to an optimal level of functioning. A goal of equal importance is assistance to the perpetrator of abuse, the prevention of recurrence, and the strengthening of the family unit. Conducting group discussions, initiating self-help groups, promoting educative programs are all appropriate interventions planned and carried out by the primary nurse. Such activities may be jointly planned with other disciplines as appropriate.

When caring for sexually abused children, the nurse first determines the extent of the abuse and whether or not it is part of a pattern of more extensive abuse. In families where incest is an isolated incident in an otherwise intact stable family, treatment modalities focus on addressing the family issues that foster the sexual abuse. Mrazek and Bentovin (23) indicate that the therapist must be "intrusive" and determined to participate in the family system so that it can be modified.

Treatment programs in sexual abuse are most effective when children and parents are included. Children must have an opportunity to express their feelings in a safe setting with understanding adult role models. At the same time, therapy sessions for parents focus on explorations of reasons for sexual abuse and means of preventing future abuse. Giarretto describes the Santa Clara program, which uses lay and professional support groups. The treatment plan includes individual counseling, family therapy, self-assessment, confrontation, and self-help. The self-help groups focus on self-assessment and identification, self-management, and self-determination. Members strive for the ability to control behavior and direct their lives into more meaningful activities. The program reports a high number of marriages saved, with 90 percent of the cases free of incestuous activities (8).

When the victim of abuse is an adult, the focus of care is, as with the child, on the restoration of wellness. The hospitalized battered woman, in addition to suffering from physical wounds, will experience fear, guilt, shame, and humiliation. She may be concerned for the safety of other family members as well as for her own safety. Nursing interventions include the promotion of healing of the psychological wounds as well as the physical wounds. Alleviation of feelings of shame and humiliation and the restoration of human dignity through empathetic care are essential. As the abused client recovers, an exploration of family dynamics and observation of spouse interactions will help the nurse to establish realistic goals with the client. The educative process includes explanation of the legal implications of the battering incident and information about community resources such as women's shelters and public assistance. The nurse's interventions should focus on the exploration of alternatives and the strengthening of the client's confidence in her own decision making. Whether or not to separate from the abusing spouse is a serious decision. Elbow emphasizes the importance of not urging a woman to leave home before she has the strength to take the step (2). The safety of the client, however, is the most important consideration in planning interventions.

During the acute phase of the crisis, while the victim is hospitalized, the offending spouse may feel shame and remorse. This period of vulnerability may be the appropriate time for referral for counseling, psychotherapy, or self-help groups. Communication with other members of the health care team is essential in establishing goals that are in agreement with all concerned.

Nursing Care in the Home Setting. Community health nurses and social caseworkers are the link between the hospital team and the family in the home setting. Referrals may be made to existing community agencies, or the nurse may be part of the crisis intervention team. Tertiary prevention measures are aimed at returning the victim of abuse to the home and promoting a safe environment that is conducive to the well-being of the victims at any age.

In order to be effective in working with the family, the nurse builds on a trusting relationship in preparation for further interventions. She demonstrates a helping attitude and gains understanding of family dynamics and family coping mechanisms. In addition, the nurse pro-

motes acceptance of all phases of treatment through interpretation of the goals of the treatment plan.

The family may view the community nurse as a "neutral" person who is not involved in the legal process. In order not to violate the feeling of trust, it is important that the nurse convey to the family the understanding that feelings will be communicated to other members of the health care team.

When the victim is a child, the community nurse may continue interventions initiated in the hospital setting. These interventions will focus on promoting optimal growth and development and reducing parent-child conflicts.

The community health nurse may be prepared for long-range goals and home visits over a long period of time. Visits intermittently spaced over a period of one to three years is often indicated. Unfortunately the constraints of agency policy and matters of payment may prohibit the implementation of nursing intervention that the primary nurse prescribes.

Alternative Care. If the family is not prepared for the return of the child to the home, if the home is unsuitable, or if the parents are not amenable to treatment, foster home care may be recommended. In child abuse, uncontrollable battering because of psychotic personality disorder in the family may be cited as reasons for placement. Reasons for placement are not always so obvious. Runyan (30) studied the records of the North Carolina Central Registry to determine which characteristics were influential in the decision to place the child in foster care. Referrals from law enforcement agencies were more likely to result in foster care placements and families who lived in poor or ghetto neighborhoods were more likely to have foster care of the child recommended. Primary care providers and crisis intervention teams must become aware of these tendencies toward social bias in formulating care and treatment goals. Nursing interventions in the home may include play therapy, early developmental training, health guidance, family counseling, and family therapy. It is important that all family members, especially young children, be included in the therapeutic process.

Outcomes of foster care placement have not always been favorable. Separation from parents and significant family members can be as harmful to children as return to the natural family. Fanshel (3) points out that even seriously impaired parents are important to their children, and that social agencies tend to treat abusive biological parents as society's discards once children have been placed in foster care. He indicates that in New York City, the average length of time for children in foster care placement is 4.8 years, and that 50 percent of the children receive no parental visits. He suggests that social agencies have failed in making an effort to rebuild families, and that blacks, Hispanics, and native Americans have suffered most from the failure of communities to deliver mental health and addictive services and to help families overcome deficits in income, housing, and social services.

Martin cites the case of a six-year-old girl who began being abused at age twelve months. The initial injuries were mildly handicapping, but the decision was made for placement. In a five-year period she had thirteen home changes, resulting in severe emotional disturbance (21). It is the responsibility of health care workers to choose, to the extent that it is possible, the least detrimental alternatives and to try to avoid iatrogenic abuse.

Evaluating Outcomes and Reestablishing Goals

The purpose of the evaluation phase of the nursing process is to determine whether the goals of the nursing care plan have been accomplished. In primary prevention measures, for example, the plan may include the establishment of parent-education programs in a high-risk community with a large population of young families. Evaluation of the plan will involve measurement of not only the knowledge gained by the program participants, but also the impact on the community in terms of decreased incidence of child abuse.

In secondary prevention measures the early identification of family instability may lead to a goal of strengthening family ties. The identification of closely spaced pregnancies may indicate a need for family-planning education. The measure of the effectiveness of the intervention will depend on the extent to which the family has remained together or the extent to which pregnancies have been more reasonably spaced. In both instances the ultimate measure is the prevention of abusive behaviors among family members.

In tertiary prevention interventions evaluation will depend on the type and extent of abuse and the goals that have been established. In young children, for example, maltreatment and neglect may result in mild developmental delays. Enrollment in a preschool program or early developmental training in the home may restore the child to an age-appropriate level of functioning. If the damage is more severe, full restoration may be an unrealistic goal. A more limited goal may be realized through a special program for the handicapped. The important factor is to strive for the highest level of functioning that can be achieved.

An indication of successful intervention for the abused spouse is the extent to which the abusive behavior has been discontinued or the victim is able to become self-supportive and independent of the abuser. For the abused elderly, successful outcome may be measured by the degree of freedom from abuse, the degree of autonomy gained, and the freedom to continue to utilize potential. For the incapacitated elderly, adequate family support or protective placement may be a realistic means to prevent further abuse.

The most common causes of failure to reach stated goals and objectives are (a) unrealistic goals and objectives, (b) failure to include the family in the care plan, and (c) ineffective or inappropriate interventions. When goals are not achieved, reassessment is indicated in order to establish new and more realistic goals. In the case of spouse battering, for example, if the original goal was to maintain family unity and the perpetrator did not respond to treatment, the goals would be changed to provide safe harbor for the spouse and children.

Beyond the prevention or cessation of abusive behaviors, the measure of effectiveness of interventions is the extent to which families are able to perform developmental tasks at life stages. Nursing interventions during maturational and situational crises can be useful in preventing and alleviating family conflicts. Nurses are in strategic positions to interview families during critical events such as pregnancy, parenthood, and stages of child development. Their contacts with families in hospitals, clinics, and the home can be used to strengthen family bonds during childbirth, school admission, illness, and death. Nurses have yet to realize their full potential in strengthening family life during crisis and developmental phases.

The Legal Aspects of Abuse in Families

Although it is not within the scope of this chapter to discuss the intricacies and complexities of the legal aspects of abuse in families, it is essential that the primary care provider be familiar with the laws of the community. All states have laws relating to child abuse, neglect, and domestic violence, and several have legislation covering elder abuse.

Child Abuse

The purpose of the law is to protect children and to prevent further maltreatment or abuse, not to punish parents. Inherent in the law is the concept that in most cases, the best way to help abused children is to help their families. Maltreatment and abuse are danger signs and are symptomatic that a family is in need of help. Reporting and referral are the first steps in providing help.

The law may require that certain people, in their professional capacity, report suspected abuse or maltreatment of any child under the age of eighteen. Examples of professionals who are required to report are nurses, physicians, teachers, social workers, hospital admission personnel, and law enforcement officials. A report must be made by telephone immediately, followed by a written report within forty-eight hours. Any other person may report if there is reasonable cause to believe that a child is suffering as a result of abuse or maltreatment. A person, official, or institution participating in good faith in the making of a report has immunity from civil or criminal liability.

Abuse includes sexual abuse, physical beatings, cutting, burns, or physical dependency on addictive drugs at birth.

Maltreatment includes malnutrition; lack of adequate food, clothing, shelter, medical care, or supervision; and serious emotional injury.

Educational neglect refers to children who are not attending school in accordance with compulsory educational laws. Failure of parents to ensure regular and prompt attendance, keeping children out of school for inappropriate reasons, and lack of interest in academic achievement are examples.

Supervisory neglect refers to children being left alone or with an inadequate caretaker, or being exposed to hazardous conditions. It includes allowing children to roam or to be away from home for extended periods of time without knowledge of their whereabouts.

Abandonment is desertion by a parent whose present whereabouts are unknown and who apparently has no intention of assuming parental responsibilities.

When child protective laws are invoked, the trusting relationship between the primary care nurse and the family may be impaired. The nurse must be prepared to confront the family's anger and hostility even when good intentions and offers of help are explained. Therapeutic modalities, inner strength, and self-confidence are essential in this difficult situation.

Family Violence

A victim of family violence can ask the family court for an order of protection. The order can state conditions of behavior to be followed for a specified period of time by the victim or the abuser, or both. It can require that a person stay away from the home, or give proper protection to the spouse and children. In the event of violence the offended person has a right to bring the case before the family court or the criminal court.

Difficulties in dealing with problems of family violence are illustrated in the experiences of a police officer:

As a police officer, I have experiences almost daily with battered women. The police jargon for these calls for service are 1052s. The fact that these calls are the most dangerous for us to respond to is constantly reinforced in our training sessions. All too often what starts out as an intervention in a domestic disturbance ends up with both combatants redirecting their hostilities toward us.

One can imagine the difficulty a woman has in relating the abuse she has suffered to strangers when, in most cases, she hasn't dared share with her own mother. When a woman decides to have her husband or boyfriend arrested, this does not necessarily terminate the abuse; it may exacerbate the problem. If the battering constitutes a simple assault, the only police action is to issue a summons similar to a traffic offense. This enables the offender to go back home in a short time. When the assault is more serious, the perpetrator is formally arrested and housed in a detention facility. Before the case is presented at arraignment the district attorney attempts to convince the complainant to agree to mediation. Mediation is the process where certain crimes are decriminalized to reduce the heavy case loads in the courtrooms.

If the victim agrees to mediation, the couple will go before an arbitrator, who usually makes some monetary awards for the beatings received. Most women I have talked to have never received these awards, since the husband or boyfriend has no means of financial support. If she refuses the mediation, the case will be heard by a judge, and nine times out of ten it will be transferred to family court, regardless of the couple's marital status. It seems to me that our present system of criminal justice is more concerned with reducing case loads than curtailing the large incidence of battered women. (18)

In elder abuse, legislation typically defines physical, psychological, and financial abuse as assault, neglect of care, threats, isolation, and theft of money or property.

Mandatory reporting is required in some states. Legal mandatory reporting in child abuse may lead to ineffective protective services for children and may violate the rights of parents as well, especially those who are innocent or are ignorant of childrearing methods. The ambiguity of complicated legal issues in both child and spouse abuse can be seen in the involuntary removal of children from their parents in the light of strong evidence that foster care is a poor alternative and that abuse exists in all forms of public institutions. For abused women, the alternatives of temporary shelter and prolonged poverty are equally undesirable. And statutes protecting the elderly may reinforce the perception of the older population as in need of protection. The answers lie not in the legal process but in an alteration of societal values, with adequate financial and social support for families together with educational and preventive programs.

DISCUSSION QUESTIONS

1. State three significant characteristics of abuse-prone families.
2. Identify at least four early signs of abuse in infants and preschool children; in adolescents; in the elderly.
3. Outline the deviations in family developmental tasks that may lead to abusive behavior.
4. State three important considerations in formulating the nursing care plan in actual and potential problems of abuse.
5. Compare the legal and ethical dilemmas faced by the primary care nurse in working with families where abuse is suspected and where it is identified.

REFERENCES

1. Duvall, E. *Marriage and Family Development.* 5th ed. Philadelphia: J. B. Lippincott, 1977.
2. Elbow, M. "Theoretical Considerations of Violent Marriages." *Social Casework* 58:515–26, 1977.
3. Fanshel, D. "Decision Making Under Uncertainty: Foster Care for Abused or Neglected Children." *American Journal of Public Health* 71:685–91, 1981.
4. Finlay, B. "Nursing Process with the Battered Woman." *Nurse Practitioner* 6 (4):11–13, 1981.
5. Fontana, R. *The Maltreated Child.* Springfield, Ill.: Charles C. Thomas, 1979,.6.
6. Freeman, R. *Community Health Nursing Practice.* Philadelphia: W. B. Saunders, 1970.

7. Gaensbauer, T., Mrazek, D., and Harmon, R. "Emotional Expression in Abused and Neglected Infants." In *Psychological Approaches to Child Abuse,* ed. N. Frude. Totowa, N.J.: Rowman and Littlefield, 1981, 120–35.
8. Giarretto, H. "A Comprehensive Child Sexual Abuse Treatment Program." In *Sexually Abused Children and Their Families,* ed. P. Mrazek and C. Kempe. New York: Pergamon Press, 1981.
9. G.I.D. "Unraveling Child Abuse." *American Journal of Orthopsychiatry* 45:347–55, 1975.
10. Gil, D. *Violence Against Children: Physical Child Abuse in the United States.* Cambridge, Mass.: Harvard University Press, 1970.
11. Goode, W. "Force and Violence in the Family." *Journal of Marriage and the Family* 33:624–36, 1971.
12. Herman, J., and L. Hirschman. "Families at Risk for Father-Daughter Incest." *American Journal of Psychiatry* 138:967–70, 1981.
13. Hickey, T., and R. Douglass. "Mistreatment of the Elderly in the Domestic Setting: An Exploratory Study." *American Journal of Public Health* 71:500–07, 1981.
14. Houghton, B. "Domestic Violence Training: Treatment of Adult Victims of Family Violence." *Journal of the New York State Nurses Association* 12 (4):25–31, 1981.
15. Iyer, P. "The Battered Wife." *Nursing* 10:52–55, 1980.
16. Justice, B., and R. Justice. *The Abusing Family.* New York: Human Sciences Press, 1976.
17. Kempe, C. H., et al. "The Battered Child Syndrome." *Journal of the American Medical Association* 49:105–12, 1962.
18. Lee, V. Personal communication.
19. McKittrick, C. "Child Abuse: Recognition and Reporting by Health Professionals." *Nursing Clinics of North America* 16:103–15, 1981.
20. Martin, D. *Battered Wives.* San Francisco: New *Glide,* 1976.
21. Martin, H., and C. Kempe, eds. *The Abused Child.* Cambridge, Mass.: Ballinger Publishing Co., 1976.
22. Moore, D., ed. *Battered Women.* Beverly Hills, Calif.: Sage Publications, 1979.
23. Mrazek, P., and A. Bentovin. "Incest and the Dysfunctional Family System." In *Sexually Abused Children and Their Families,* ed. P. Mrazek and C. Kempe. New York: Pergamon Press, 1981.
24. Mrazek, P., and C. Kempe, eds. *Sexually Abused Children and Their Families.* New York: Pergamon Press, 1981.
25. Nakashima, I., and G. Zakus. "Incest: Review and Clinical Experience." *Pediatrics* 60:696–701, 1977.
26. Parker, B., and D. Schumacher. "The Battered Wife Syndrome and Violence in the Nuclear Family of Origin: A Controlled Pilot Study." *American Journal of Public Health* 67:760–62, 1977.
27. Pringle, M. "Toward the Prevention of Child Abuse." In *Psychological Approaches to Child Abuse,* ed. N. Fruse. Totowa, N.J.: Rowman and Littlefield, 1981, 220–34.
28. Robarge, J., Z. Reynolds, and J. Groothius. "Increased

Child Abuse in Families with Twins." *Research in Nursing and Health* 5:199–203, 1982.

29. Rodehoffer, M., and H. Martin. "Special Problems in Developmental Assessment of Abused Children." In *The Abused Child,* ed. H. Martin and C. Kempe. Cambridge, Mass.: Ballinger Publishing Co., 1976.

30. Runyan, D., C. Gould, D. Trost, and F. Loda. "Determinants of Foster Care Placement for the Maltreated Child." *American Journal of Public Health* 71:706–10, 1981.

31. Shainess, N. "Psychological Aspects of Wife Battering." In *Battered Women,* ed. M. Roy. New York: Van Nostrand Reinhold Co., 1977, 111–19.

32. Symonds, A. "Violence Against Women: The Myth of Masochism." *American Journal of Psychotherapy* 33 (2):161–73, 1979.

33. Teicher, J. D., and J. Jacobs. "Adolescents Who Attempt Suicide." *American Journal of Psychiatry* 122:1248–57, 1966.

CHAPTER 20

Overcoming Barriers to Primary Cancer Nursing Care

CONSTANCE H. ENGELKING

and

NANCY E. STEELE

■

OBJECTIVES

After completing this chapter, the reader will be able to:

- Recognize emerging trends in cancer control and cancer care that affect nursing practice.
- Identify phenomena that distinguish the cancer experience as unique.
- List four major factors that influence or determine the needs of clients with cancer and their families.
- Describe three stages of cancer.
- Discuss how cancer client/family need may change during the course of the illness.
- Describe five functional expectations of the primary nursing role in cancer care.
- Recognize behaviors that are indicative of

discomfort in caring for clients who have cancer, and their families.

- Distinguish between attitudinal, cognitive, and interpersonal barriers to cancer nursing care.
- Identify at least two cancer care barriers within each of the three specified categories.
- List elements basic to the development of strategies to resolve the identified barriers to cancer nursing care.
- Identify at least one potential resolution strategy for each barrier that can be applied in his or her own clinical setting.

Cancer is a major health problem in the United States today. A large segment of the population is or will be afflicted with this potentially disabling and often terminal chronic illness. In 1986 cancer was expected to occur in 930,000 more Americans and to cause 472,000 deaths (55). The American Cancer Society has projected that one out of four Americans will develop the disease in their lifetime and that two out of every three families will be affected (53). Yet the outlook for cancer clients continues to improve.

Significant progress has been made toward a better understanding of the biology of cancer and its treatment. The recent discovery of oncogenes, the annual addition of new antineoplastic drugs, and the sophistication of treatment techniques such as new drug delivery systems, bone marrow transplantation, monoclonal antibody production, and biological response modifiers have all contributed to that progress. As a result, survival for the person with cancer has been prolonged. In the 1930s less than one in five cancer clients were alive five years after diagnosis. Today one in three clients treated for cancer lives for at least five years (51), and many survive more than ten (26). Overall, cancer death rates have declined since 1960, and the realization of cures in a significant number of clients with such cancers as acute lymphocytic leukemia, testicular and cervical carcinomas, and various lymphomas has given rise to an attitude of cautious optimism among cancer specialists (51).

Although successful in prolonging life and providing hope of cure, advances in cancer therapy have compounded the cancer problem by imposing an entirely new set of concerns on those afflicted and society as a whole. The client and his or her family are directly faced with the task of adapting to the disease-imposed alterations in their lives while facing the unpredictable course the illness will take. Society, in a broader sense, is faced with a growing population of uncured cancer clients for whom costly health care is necessary during extended periods of time (14). Nurses, as the primary providers of that health care, must facilitate the process of adaptation for the person with cancer and his or her family in a continuous and cost-effective manner to enhance the quality of survival. Because they move through a variety of health care settings during the course of their illness, however, the provision of continuity to clients with cancer becomes a difficult issue. Baird suggests that the only real stabilization is provided through continuity in nursing care, and that the introduction of the primary nursing concept has been a facilitator in this regard (1). Rendering primary care to those affected by cancer is often the responsibility of the professional nurse in general practice.

The purpose of this chapter is to provide information that will assist the generalist in assuming a primary role when caring for the cancer client and family unit during different stages of the disease and in various health care settings. Rather than examining the pathophysiology of cancer or the efficacy of the anticancer therapies, this chapter examines common personal and professional barriers that may impair the nurse's ability to function in this role and suggests strategies for overcoming these barriers.

Cancer Prevention and Early Detection in Primary Nursing

Cancer prevention and early detection activities are a mandated element of modern health care delivery. In a climate of cost reduction and the subsequent decline in available health care resources, disease prevention is the most cost-effective strategy for dealing with the dilemma of matching limited resources to existing health care need. Cancer prevention activities save direct, indirect, and economic costs of considerable magnitude. Further, because low tumor burden is known to be associated with disease responsiveness and curability, the best weapon against morbidity and mortality when cancer does occur is early detection (49).

Although the benefits of engaging in cancer prevention and detection activities are obvious, such wellness behaviors are not routinely practiced by the public for various reasons. It is well known, for example, that cigarette smoking is a serious health hazard that is implicated as a causative factor in the development of lung, esophagus, and head and neck cancers and is associated with the occurrence of other cancers as well. Yet one-third of the population in North America continues to smoke despite the accessibility of smoking cessation programs (31).

With regard to breast cancer, Greenwald and associates found that tumors discovered by means of purposeful breast examination were, on average, 20 percent smaller than those found accidentally, concluding that deaths owing to breast cancer could be reduced significantly by using this technique (49). Despite the convenience, low cost, and effectiveness of breast self-examination in detecting breast cancer, however, studies have shown that a limited number of women regularly perform breast self-examination (BSE). A 1979 study conducted nationally revealed that 75 percent of women reported practicing BSE once that year, with only 24 percent stating that they practiced it monthly (40). Reasons for low BSE performance rates include a lack of concern about breast cancer, a lack of knowledge, and a perceived sense of inadequacy with regard to practicing the technique correctly. Other factors include the fear of discovering cancer and the threat that diagnosis poses to one's life (29).

Increased cure rates in testicular and cervical cancers have been attributed, respectively, to testicular self-examination (TSE) and the Papanicolaou test (Pap smear), since both techniques facilitate diagnosis before the development of symptoms indicative of advanced disease (16). As in breast cancer prevention, participation in these activities is not universal. Kegeles has found that although many women are knowledgeable about and have Pap smears performed for cervical cancer, those at highest risk (nonwhite, older, less educated, low income) have the poorest screening rates. Similarly, a 1978 survey of male college students revealed that 75 percent had no knowledge of testicular cancer and none knew how to perform TSE (58).

The successful incorporation of cancer prevention and early detection behaviors into a person's established life-style patterns is a complex task, requiring a belief in personal susceptibility to serious illness and education in specific health care skills. Both the health promoting behaviors and the responsibility for following through with them must be taught (32). Several factors place the nurse in a strategic position to provide such education to the public. First, nurses are perceived by the public as being authoritative sources of medical information, as health educators and as role models (4). Because of

this public perception, nurses can be influential teachers of health-enhancing behaviors. Second, health education is inherent in the primary nursing role. Consequently, nurses are prepared educationally and expected by their employers to take on that responsibility. Finally, nurses have contact with the well family members and friends of their patients as well as their own families, neighbors, and friends, thus expanding potential case-finding and teaching opportunities. According to Valentine, because of their numbers and the hours of contact with clients, nurses have greater potential for influencing health behavior than any other health professional (58).

Although the nurse seems the ideal professional to take on primary and secondary cancer prevention activities, Glasel notes that these are not customarily incorporated into the daily clinical practice of most nurses (20). This notion is supported by the findings of Stillman's study, in which 87 of 142 women reported learning BSE technique from a physician, whereas only 4 of those women felt that they had been taught by a nurse (56). Two surveys conducted by the American Cancer Society support Glasel's observation. In one, a large public survey, only a small percentage of respondents reported that information about cancer came from a nurse. In the other, an inventory of nurse knowledge about the seven warning signals (Table 20.1), only two of eighty-one acute care nurses were able to identify all seven signals (23).

In addition, nurses themselves do not typically engage in behaviors to reduce their personal risk for cancer. Numerous examples of nurse nonparticipation in personal cancer prevention strategies and potential public impact exist in the literature. In studies examining the incidence of smoking in health professionals, for example, it has been found that nurses smoke at a rate greater than other health professionals, despite their reported awareness of smoking as a health hazard and agreement

Table 20.1
Cancer's Seven Warning Signals

Change in bowel or bladder habits
A sore that does not heal
Unusual bleeding or discharge
Thickening or lump in breast or elsewhere
Indigestion or difficulty in swallowing
Obvious change in wart or mole
Nagging cough or hoarseness

that they have a role as exemplars for the public (28). Findings in relation to BSE practices are similar. Studying the BSE practices and attitudes of ninety-three registered nurses in a community hospital setting, Cole and Gorman found that although all nurses rated BSE as important, approximately 70 percent did not practice BSE, performed the technique sporadically, or used incorrect technique (4).

Although many nurses may believe that their personal health habits are separate from job-related activities, an association between the two has been demonstrated in the area of cancer prevention. In their study of nurse counseling behaviors, Dalton and Swenson found that nurses in North Carolina who smoked were less likely to counsel clients and family members as to the ill effects of smoking (6). Another example of impact to nursing practice can be seen in Sawyer's study of eighty hospital-based nurses, which revealed a significant relationship between the nurse's personal BSE practices and her assessment of her client's performance. Almost 100 percent of nurses who examined their own breasts monthly included questions regarding BSE performance in their patient interviews, whereas this line of questioning was included in the client interviews of less than half of those nurses who were themselves noncompliant with routine BSE (49). When a nurse who does not engage in health-enhancing behaviors encourages others to change their eating habits, stop smoking, or incorporate self-screening exams into their daily routine, the stage is set for conflict, and credibility is lost (41).

Credibility, a key element for fulfillment of the educational component of the primary nursing role, is also lost when the nurse is not the initiator of health teaching for the consumer. Consequently, nurses are faced with the challenge and the responsibility of acquiring the knowledge and skills necessary to carry out the mandate defined in standard I of the Outcome Standards for Cancer Nursing Practice (see Table 20.14), to become involved in cancer prevention. The first step in this endeavor is to examine personal health practices, to identify deficits and analyze underlying attitudinal or cognitive causes for noncompliance. Once that has been accomplished, each nurse must build a prevention/detection knowledge base, using the wide range of resources that exist. Frank–Stromberg's table of common adult cancers (Table 20.2) provides an excellent summary of prevention, screening, and detection considerations for nursing practice. The American Cancer Society's early detection guidelines (Table 20.3) are an additional resource for teaching.

Dynamics of Cancer Patient Need

People who have cancer experience a wide range of physical, emotional, spiritual, socioeconomic, and environmental needs. It is the nurse who considers all these factors in developing a holistic plan of care. It is the nurse who has the longest contacts with clients and their families and who delivers intimate types of care in all settings. Consequently, it is the nurse who is in a strategic position to identify specific client/family problems, to plan and carry out interventions that will satisfy their needs. To accomplish this, the nurse must have knowledge of the cancer client's potential needs and an appreciation for how those needs may change throughout the client's illness experience.

Much of the need demonstrated by people experiencing cancer and their families is related to the dramatic alterations in life-style patterns to which they must adapt. According to Van Scoy-Mosher:

> The suffering of the cancer patient and family is associated with the terrible disruptions in individual and family life that occur: the loss of role and function, the disturbances in body image, the physical and emotional isolation, and the overwhelming sense of loss of control over one's destiny. . . . [Herein] lies the role and unique function of the . . . nurse. (50)

The described disruptions in life-style that occur as a consequence of cancer create health care needs similar to those associated with other chronic illnesses. Parsons (46) suggests, however, that cancer imposes additional needs. Describing it as a special disease that is perceived differently from other diseases with similar prognoses, she postulates that unique stresses are experienced by persons with cancer as a result of their own and others' perceptions of cancer's meaning (46).

What creates these unique stresses? Van Woerdt states that "symptoms acquire specific meaning largely within the context of the threat of death" (63). Supporting that philosophy is the observation that clients with cancer frequently interpret the temporary fatigue and weakness associated with anticancer therapy as a sign of approaching death, despite the fact that their disease may be responding to treatment. Similarly, the families of such clients may be unable to differentiate between treatment side effects and symptoms of disease progression. Because cancer is perceived in our society as an

Table 20.2
Common Adult Cancers: Prevention, Screening, and Detection

Type of Cancer	Preventive Health Practices	Screening Recommendations	Pertinent History Questions	Detection — Early Signs and Symptoms	Detection — Primary Diagnostic Techniques
Skin cancer	Avoid overexposure to sunlight. Use sunscreens and wear protective clothing.	Self-examination	Changes in moles? Unhealed sores?	Changes in moles Skin lesions Sores that will not heal	Biopsy of lesions
Lung cancer	Do *not* start smoking. Stop smoking.	None	Smoking history: Packs per day? Filtered? Style of smoking? Smokers' cough? Years smoked? (Pack years = packs per day × years smoked) Bronchitis, emphysema, asthma, or hay fever? History of pneumonia? Wheezing or coughing? Expectoration of sputum? (odor, amount, color) Shortness of breath? Last chest x-ray?	Persistent cough Hemoptysis Dyspnea Wheezing Thoracic pain Respiratory infection nonresponsive to antibiotics	Chest x-ray

Colorectal cancer	Diet: low in animal fat, high in fiber Test stool at recommended intervals. Obtain annual digital rectal exam.	Age 40 and over: Digital rectal exam every year Stool guaiac test every year after 50 Proctoscopy (after two initial negative tests one year apart) every three to five years after 50 (more frequent exams if at high risk)	Family or personal history of colorectal cancers, polyps, or colitis? Diet high in fat? Diet low in fiber?	Change in bowel habits Anemia Rectal bleeding Vague abdominal pain Rectal pain Anorexia Weight loss Decreased diameter of stools	Rectal exam Proctosigmoidoscopy Fiberoptic colonoscopy Barium enema with air contrast
Breast cancer	Practice monthly breast self-exam (BSE).	20 to 40 years: Professional exam every three years BSE every month Baseline mammogram between 35 and 40 years 40 years and older: Professional exam every year BSE every month Mammogram every one to two years (40 to 49 years) Mammogram every year after 50	Lumpy or cystic breasts? Sore breasts or swollen breasts? Breast infections? Scaly or itchy nipples? Color changes in breast? Sores or open wounds on breast? Practice BSE and how often? Last menstrual period?	Painless lump or mass in breast Dimpling Flattening of nipple Nipple discharge Abnormal breast contour Peau d'orange Erythema Ulcerations	Physical exam Mammography Biopsy

Source: M. Frank–Stromberg, "The Role of the Nurse in Cancer Detection and Screening," *Seminars in Oncology Nursing* 2(3): 193, 1986.

Table 20.3
Guidelines for the Early Detection of Cancer in People Without Symptoms

Ages 20–40	Age 40 and Over
Cancer-related checkup every three years	Cancer-related checkup every year
Breast*	Breast
Exam by doctor every three years	Exam by doctor every year
Self-exam every month	Self-exam every month
One baseline breast x-ray between ages 35 and 40*	Breast x-ray every year after 50; between ages 40 and 49, one every one or two years as recommended
Uterus	Uterus
Pelvic exam every three years	Pelvic exam every year
Cervix†	Cervix
Pap test after two initial negative tests one year apart, at least every three years‡	Pap test after two initial negative tests one year apart, at least every three years
	Endometrium§
	Endometrial tissue sample at menopause if at risk
	Colon and rectum‖
	Digital rectal exam every year
	Stool slide test every year after 50
	Proctologic exam after two initial negative tests one year apart and every three to five years after 50

Note: Cancer-related checkups should include the procedures listed above plus health counseling (such as tips on quitting smoking) and examinations for cancers of the thyroid, testes, prostate, mouth, ovaries, skin, and lymph nodes. Some people are at higher risk for certain cancers and may need to be tested more frequently.

*A higher risk of breast cancer is characterized by a personal or family history of breast cancer, never giving birth, or having the first child after age 30.

†A higher risk of cervical cancer is characterized by early age at first intercourse and multiple sex partners.

‡This includes women under age 20 if sexually active.

§A higher risk of endometrial cancer is characterized by infertility, obesity, failure of ovulation, abnormal uterine bleeding, and estrogen therapy.

‖A higher risk of colorectal cancer is characterized by personal or family history of colon or rectal cancer, polyps in the colon or rectum, or ulcerative colitis.

Source: M. Frank-Stromberg. "The Role of the Nurse in Cancer Detection and Screening." *Seminars in Oncology Nursing* 2(3): 193–94, 1986.

acute disease process leading to immediate death (45), death thoughts may pervade the illness experience for both clients and their families.

Additional phenomena that distinguish the cancer experience as unique have been identified. These include the use of multimodality therapy that may produce both acute and chronic toxicities, the frequent participation in clinical trials to test new treatment approaches, and stage-related symptom complexes that have the potential to change dramatically (61). All of these factors determine not only the needs that cancer clients and their families experience, but also the severity and duration of that need. The nurse must be cognizant of the uniqueness of the disease and must intervene to assist the client

and his family in managing the special stresses that result throughout the course of the illness.

Stages of Cancer

The complexity of client/family needs often changes dramatically as the person with cancer passes through distinct phases during the illness experience. These stages are primarily determined by the natural history of the particular cancer. Although there is a common thread of need, each stage is characterized by a different set of client/family concerns and problems to which the nurse must respond. Various stages of cancer are described in the literature (8, 46), but three emerge as primary time periods: (a) the diagnostic stage, (b) the intermediate stage, and (c) the end stage (Figure 20.1) (11).

Diagnostic Stage. This stage extends from initial awareness of symptoms through the diagnostic workup and selection of a definitive treatment plan. Procedures such as surgical biopsies, tumor marker assays, x-rays, and scans necessary to determine the existence and extent of cancer in a person constitute the workup. Some of these tests may be performed in an ambulatory care setting, whereas others require hospitalization. For example, the initial evaluation of a person with a persistent cough and progressive shortness of breath will probably take place in a doctor's office. In addition to physical examination, chest x-rays, or scans, it will probably be performed on an outpatient basis. If a lung lesion is found, the client will be admitted to the hospital for bronchoscopy, or perhaps mediastinoscopy, to make a definitive diagnosis. At this point, treatment recommendations are made and the client enters another stage of disease.

Intermediate Stage. The next period is a complex and prolonged period that may involve multimodal therapy, with potential outcomes being cure, disease control, or progression. Edstrom and Miller suggest that this may be the longest period in the cancer experience (11). Aggressive anticancer therapy designed to eradicate disease is balanced with supportive therapies such as hyperalimentation, antibiotic therapy, or administration of blood components. This phase of the cancer experience

may include periods of remission, alternating with episodes of severe illness, tumor recurrence, or metastasis to other parts of the body. Multiple hospital admissions, as well as outpatient visits, are often required, depending on the individual client's response to the prescribed treatment. A client with lymphoma, for instance, may receive much of his chemotherapy in an ambulatory care setting during the intermediate stage. If this client should develop superior vena cava syndrome secondary to disease progression, chemotherapy would be interrupted. The client would require immediate hospitalization and emergency radiation therapy. When the acute episode had passed, this client could resume outpatient treatment with a new chemotherapy regimen. If treatment is no longer successful in achieving disease control, however, the client moves on to the next and final stage of cancer.

End Stage. This stage is characterized by progressive disease leading to death. A person with advanced cancer that does not respond to treatment is considered to be terminally ill (37). This terminal phase may last for weeks or months. The goal of medical and nursing care during this stage is to continue to prevent or minimize distressing disease-induced symptomatology, using whatever means necessary (e.g., palliative radiation to relieve bone pain). Clients may be cared for at home or in a chronic care facility with periodic admissions to an acute care hospital. A client with advanced colorectal cancer, for example, may be hospitalized for treatment of dehydration, nausea, and vomiting secondary to gastrointestinal obstruction. If the obstruction cannot be relieved, the client and family may opt to continue infusional therapy as a comfort measure either at home or in a chronic care facility, depending on the resources available to them.

How does cancer client need change according to stage of disease? Using the framework described by Kim and Moritz (30) and, later, Gordon (22), it is possible to identify nursing diagnoses that describe problems common to clients as they pass through the three stages of cancer. This framework is used to illustrate the dynamic nature of client/family need because nursing diagnosis is synonymous with client/family problems and will, therefore, serve as a standard method of articulating nursing, rather than medical, need throughout. During each stage of disease, clients will encounter new problems and concerns. Some problems, however, may persist from stage to stage. Table 20.4 illustrates that primary diagnoses often remain the same throughout the illness experience but that the causes associated with

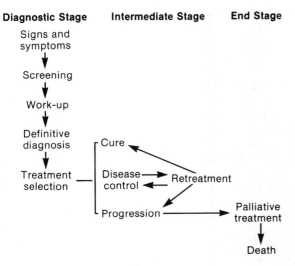

Figure 20.1. The Process of Cancer

Table 20.4
Potential Nursing Diagnoses for Cancer Stages

Diagnostic Stage	Intermediate Stage	End Stage
Knowledge deficit r/t method and/or purpose specific diagnostic tests	*Knowledge deficit* r/t selected anticancer therapy (i.e., chemotherapy or radiation therapy) and/or goal of therapy	*Knowledge deficit* r/t symptom control strategies (i.e., pain management)
Anticipatory anxiety (mild to severe) r/t the possibility of cancer diagnosis	*Anxiety (mild to severe)* r/t fear of life-threatening effects of and/or poor tumor response to anticancer therapy	*Anxiety (mild to severe)* r/t fear of abandonment by health care team
Ineffective family or individual coping r/t the situational crisis of impending cancer diagnosis	*Ineffective family/individual coping r/t the situational crisis* of financial depletion	*Ineffective family/individual coping r/t the situational crisis* of exhaustion of supportive capacity
Sleep pattern disturbance r/t personal/family stress induced by possible cancer diagnosis	*Sleep pattern disturbance* r/t personal/family stress induced by treatment-related anxiety	*Sleep pattern disturbance* r/t fear of death
Anticipatory grieving r/t expected change in life-style patterns and/or loss of personal control induced by chronic illness	*Anticipatory grieving* r/t expected increase in degree of life-style changes and/or losses	*Anticipatory grieving* r/t expected loss of life

Note: r/t = related to

those diagnoses may differ according to the particular stage of disease. The nurse must be prepared to individualize the detail of planned client care according to either specific problems or the cause of the problem, and hence the stage of disease.

Type and Extent of Cancer

Client need, however, is not solely determined by the stage of cancer. The type and extent of cancer are other important factors that influence the specific needs a client or his family members will experience. This is because it is the nature of different tumors to behave differently and respond to different anticancer therapies. Numerous nursing diagnoses related to the physical sequelae of specific tumor types and the extent of disease can be identified. Examples are listed in Table 20.5. This is not to say that knowledge of the type and extent of cancer in a person yields an automatic list of problems to be applied to every client situation. Rather, knowledge of potential problems faced by the client and his family assists the nurse in identifying functional pattern areas that need to be explored more intensively during the client/family assessment interview.

Anticancer Treatment

Another factor that acts as a determinant of client/family need is the type of anticancer therapy selected for

treatment. There are four primary methods for treating cancer: surgery, chemotherapy, radiation therapy, immunotherapy. These modalities may be applied simultaneously or sequentially to the treatment of a specific cancer. The goal of cancer treatment may be to cure or control the disease, or to alleviate distressing symptoms. The needs of the client and family that emerge during treatment periods depend not only on the specific therapy used and its related side effects but also on the client's current physical and emotional status and prior health patterns. Frequent and systematic nursing assessment is needed to identify those clients who are at risk for or who have developed treatment-induced symptomatology. Such as assessment would lead to the formulation of nursing diagnoses similar to those presented for each treatment modality in Table 20.6. When nursing diagnoses explicitly define the client's treatment-related needs as well as the cause of those needs, nursing strategies can be designed to enhance the client's physical and emotional tolerance of a recuperation from cancer therapy.

Need Perception/Coping Ability

The presence of physiological symptomatology is not a sufficient predictor of a person's needs in and of itself. The person must perceive his dysfunction or difficulty to be incapacitating in order for it to be so (64). The

Table 20.5
Potential Nursing Diagnoses for Types and Extent of Cancer

Type of Cancer	Local Disease	Metastatic Disease
Breast cancer	*Alteration in Nutrition: potential for more than body's requirements* r/t high incidence of weight gain in post-mastectomy patients receiving adjuvant chemotherapy.	*Alteration in comfort* r/t impaired skin integrity of chest wall
	Impaired mobility of arm r/t postoperative pain, axillary tissue fibrosis and fluid accumulation.	*Potential for injury* r/t weakness and bone pain.
Lung cancer	*Potential for infection* r/t ineffective airway clearance, lung mass obstruction.	*Impaired thought processes* r/t brain metastasis.
	Decreased activity tolerance r/t imbalance between oxygen supply and demand induced by lung mass.	*Ineffective breathing pattern* r/t malignant pleural effusions.
Colorectal cancer	*Decreased Activity tolerance* r/t rectal bleeding, fatigue, weight loss	*Impaired nutritional intake* r/t GI obstruction, nausea, vomiting.
	Potential alteration in bowel elimination: constipation r/t decreased activity, low fluid intake, low roughage diet postoperatively.	*Discomfort* r/t ascites.
Ovarian cancer	*Sexual dysfunction* r/t surgically induced menopause.	*Impaired urinary elimination* r/t ureteral obstruction.
		Discomfort r/t ascites.
Acute leukemia	*Potential for infection* r/t neutropenia.	*Self-care deficit* r/t decreased energy, fatigue.
	Potential for injury: bleeding r/t thrombocytopenia.	*Alteration in cardiac output* r/t hemorrhage.

Note: r/t = related to

Table 20.6
Nursing Diagnoses for Cancer Therapy Methods

Surgery	*Anticipatory grief* r/t loss of a body part or function *Potential impaired skin integrity (wound healing)* r/t anorexia, debilitation, cachexia *Disturbance in sleep pattern* *Alteration in comfort: pain* r/t anxiety, fear of outcome of surgery, fear of inability to resect tumor
Chemotherapy	*Potential for infection* r/t chemotherapy-induced neutropenia *Nutritional deficit* r/t anorexia, nausea, vomiting, taste changes *Impaired skin integrity* r/t chemotherapy-induced stomatitis *Home maintenance management deficit* r/t lack of information about side effect management
Radiation therapy	*Potential ineffective breathing pattern* r/t radiation-induced tracheal edema *Fluid volume deficit* r/t active loss of fluid in diarrhea induced by pelvic irradiation *Altered urinary elimination* r/t radiation induced cystitis *Fear* of radiation treatments r/t knowledge deficit about procedure and effects

Note: r/t = related to

premise that perception is an important factor in the determination of client need is supported by Parsons, who found the total physical needs of twenty clients with metastatic cancer to be "few and remarkably lacking in seriousness or urgency despite an obviously severe degree of illness" (46). She attributed this to the clients' perceptions of their illness, as well as to their coping abilities. Friedman identifies ten common coping strategies used by people facing cancer: (a) information gathering, (b) seeking support from others, (c) placing faith in health professionals, (d) denying/escaping, (e) engaging in tension-reducing behaviors, (f) defining the meaning of their illness and living their lives to the fullest, (g) preparing for death, (h) returning to work, (i) placing blame for the illness on something or someone, and (j) relying on past coping strategies (17).

Development of Cancer Nursing

To meet the cancer client's changing needs along the continuum of his illness, a special body of cancer nursing knowledge and related clinical skills has developed. As a result, the subspecialty of cancer nursing has emerged (24). The advent of this nursing specialty has occurred, to a large extent, according to Hubbard and Donehower, in response to the rapid growth of clinical trials and the widespread use of sophisticated methods of cancer treatment (27). The development of this field of nursing has been furthered by the conduct of clinically oriented nursing research. Through this research a knowledge base specific to cancer nursing practice has been established and is constantly growing. Problems, needs, and concerns unique to people experiencing cancer have been described. The efficacy of standard nursing interventions has been evaluated, and new nursing strategies for patient problem management identified. Thus a distinct core of cancer nursing knowledge and expertise is developing (44), which serves as a foundation for basic and advanced oncology nursing education.

Currently, educators and oncology nurse specialists who have mastered the knowledge and are proficient in cancer nursing are preparing other nurses to render comprehensive cancer care. For the most part, however, these professional nurses practice in major cancer research centers or on oncology units in community hospitals. Yet when one considers the size of the population affected by cancer and the multiple settings in which these people receive care, it is apparent that the relatively small number of nurses qualified to practice cancer nursing cannot deliver state of the art primary nursing care to all those in need.

The Generalist as Primary Nurse in Cancer Care

More than 85 percent of clients with cancer are now receiving treatment in their own communities (57). As a result, the generalist nurse in virtually every community health care setting is responsible for the care of clients with cancer at some point during their illness experience. Because cancer care is becoming increasingly complex in these settings, the nurse's role is changing. Basic nursing education does not adequately prepare nurses to either recognize or resolve the unique problems experienced by cancer clients and their families. B. Given notes that baccalaureate programs in nursing education include "theoretic and clinical content basic to general nursing practice and little specific content that meets the needs of cancer patients. . . . This preparation is a basic and general preparation and does not make nurses expert in cancer care" (19). Despite this lack of knowledge, the general practitioner in the role of primary nurse may be expected to function as deliverer of skilled care, coordinator of services and community resources, teacher, counselor, and supporter for those clients with cancer (1). Although specific nursing behaviors are associated with each of these role functions, as outlined in Table 20.7, in practice they are overlapping and complementary. To successfully implement all of these aspects of the primary nursing role, generalist nurses practicing in community settings must possess a fundamental knowledge base regarding the process of cancer, principles of cancer treatment, and common client/family responses to this illness. Positive personal attitudes toward the client with cancer and toward cancer nursing care must be developed. Generalists must become adept in the use of available clinical tools that apply the concepts of nursing process and nursing diagnoses to oncology client care. Thus equipped, professional nurses can fulfill the demands of the primary nursing role.

Barriers to Cancer Nursing Care

The first step in assuming the role of primary nurse to clients with cancer is to examine one's own perceptions and acknowledge those factors that may hamper assumption of that role. We are aware that inhibitors to nursing the cancer client exist because nurses, like other

Table 20.7
Role of the Primary Nurse in Cancer Care

Role Component	Nursing Behavior
Deliverer of skilled care	Engages in symptom management strategies
	Administers chemotherapeutic drugs
	Monitors client responses to treatments
Educator	Teaches client/family about disease, therapies, and self-care strategies
	Instructs collaborating health professionals about special procedures/approaches to client/family care
Coordinator of resources	Facilitates access to appropriate hospital/community resources (e.g., American Cancer Society)
	Acts as liaison among health team members, client, and family members
	Communicates resource information to client/family
Counselor	Actively listens to client/family concerns and perceptions of illness experience
	Assists client/family to develop realistic hopes/future goals
	Facilitates active participation by client/family in decision-making process
Supporter	Acts as advocate for client/family
	Respects client/family decisions

Source: Adapted from S. Baird. "Nursing Roles in Continuing Care: Home Care and Hospice." *Seminars in Oncology* 7(1): 28, 1980.

health professionals, frequently exhibit both verbal and nonverbal behaviors indicative of discomfort with the role. Major manifestations of that discomfort include verbal negativism and avoidance behaviors. Verbal negativism is expressed by either direct or indirect statement. Nurses may flatly acknowledge their own inadequacy or dislike for caring for clients with cancer, or they may imply these feelings in less direct ways. For instance, nurses frequently comment on their own inability to work exclusively with clients who have cancer and question the ability of those who do. Remarks such as "Isn't it depressing to work with cancer clients?" are classic. In conjunction with this, nurses may express an inordinate level of admiration for their colleagues who choose to specialize in cancer nursing, implying that they themselves are not cut out for what they perceive to be difficult and depressing work. Verbal negativism can also be extrapolated from angry discussions among nurses regarding the disparity between acuity level and staffing when there are a large number of cancer clients on a nonspecialty nursing unit. A frequent solution to this problem is to accept noncancer client admissions, regardless of acuity, in lieu of cancer clients. The rationale is that caring for clients with illnesses other than cancer is less stressful. Interestingly, it is not often that one "needs relief" from chronic cardiac clients, even

though mortality rates in the United States are higher for heart disease than for cancer (59).

Avoidance is manifest in a wide range of nonverbal behaviors. Examining the phenomenon of avoidance by nurses caring for cancer clients, Wegmann operationally defined nonverbal avoidance as the placement of a physical barrier between the nurse and the client. This may be accomplished in several ways. Assigning these clients to rooms far from the nurses' station uses distance as a physical barrier. Closing the door to their rooms or pulling the curtain around their beds screens them from the nurse's view (59). Other avoidance behaviors include those that limit the nurse's direct contact with the client or family. Delaying answering client calls, postponing or delegating major portions of care to ancillary staff members, and rigidly limiting visitors, especially when they are family members, are all examples. Glaser and Strauss labeled the phenomenon of limiting client/family contacts "expressive avoidance" (21). These verbal and nonverbal behaviors inhibit the generalist nurse's assumption of a primary nursing role when caring for clients with cancer.

What causes these behaviors? Why do they interfere with cancer nursing care? How do they inhibit assumption of the primary nursing role? We postulate that multiple overlapping barriers do exist, and we categorize them as attitudinal, interpersonal, and cognitive (Table 20.8). Analysis of these barriers may enhance awareness of their existence, and therefore stimulate the initiation of resolution strategies in the nurse. Such strategies may grow out of Donovan and Pierce's suggestion that nurses who possess knowledge about cancer and a philosophy of life compatible with cancer nursing, and who receive satisfaction and peer support, are able to render quality care to clients with cancer (62).

Attitudinal Barriers

It is well established that the attitudes we have about a particular subject or experience influence our behavioral response to it. Positive attitudes tend to produce positive behaviors and vice versa. The existence of negative attitudes and stereotypical perceptions of the cancer client on the part of nurses is equally well documented (10). A common perception held by health professionals, in general, is that a person with cancer is "terminally ill," regardless of the type and extent of disease. Similarly, nurses, despite advancements in the field of oncology, continue to identify cancer with death and are reluctant to change that negative perception. Carol Reed–Ash summarizes these attitudes:

> Many professionals feel the work of cancer nursing is too hard, requiring complex physical and psychosocial skills. They also feel it is frustrating,

unrewarding and depressing because of the patient's acuity of illness, the complexity of the treatment modality and the common perception that all cancer patients will die (47).

These perceptions and subsequent attitudes are important to this discussion because perception of a disease influences the care that is delivered to the client who has that disease. Attitudes can be either constructive or destructive, and they can have a dramatic effect on the practice of nursing, especially with regard to the nurse-client relationship (13). A pessimistic attitude about the outcome of cancer may lead to failure on the part of the nurse to take steps toward the prevention or early detection of problems that may be amenable to nursing intervention and are certainly the responsibility of the primary nurse (15).

Consider the following example: A nurse caring for a client with acute myelogenous leukemia administers mycostatin, prescribed by the physician to manage the client's oral candidiasis. She does not, however, plan or carry out a nursing regimen for oral care. Crusty debris in the client's mouth prevents the antifungal medicine from directly contacting the oral mucosa. The client's candidiasis worsens, resulting in increased oral pain, decreased oral intake, and, ultimately, systemic Candida infection. If the nurse in this clinical situation had had positive attitudes about the impact of her care on the client's well-being, she may have assigned higher prior-

Table 20.8
Inhibitors to Cancer Nursing Care

Attitudinal (Self-focused)	Interpersonal (Multifocused)	Cognitive (Client/Family-focused)
Failure to recognize/handle personal reactions to cancer Frustration Anxiety Stress Burnout Failure to define personal philosophies/goals Nursing Death and dying Cancer care	Difficulty establishing/maintaining effective communication patterns Physician Client/family Other	Difficulty making specialized assessment of cancer client needs Difficulty deriving appropriate nursing diagnoses Difficulty selecting appropriate interventions Teaching approach Resource mobilization Symptom control strategies Difficulty following through Coordinating multiple services Referral decisions Difficulty evaluating care Identifying Communicating Client/family responses to interventions

ity to the need for meticulous oral hygiene. Consequently, she may have engaged in oral care strategies that enhanced the client's comfort, increased his ability to eat and drink, and, ultimately, prevented dissemination of his candidiasis.

Two major factors that may stand in the way of developing and maintaining positive attitudes about caring for clients with cancer are listed in Table 20.8. The first is the nurse's failure to acknowledge and deal with her own reactions to cancer and her failure to render care to those who have cancer.

Many nurses have had personal experiences with cancer that may negatively affect their perceptions of this disease and its treatment, particularly if those experiences have not had positive outcomes (52). Cancer often represents overwhelming loss—loss of independence and the ability to be productive, loss of personal control, loss of self-esteem, or loss of life. Recall of painful past experiences could easily interfere with a nurse's ability to be objective if she associates her own loss experiences with those of her client. Without resolving negative feelings about her own experiences with cancer, she may be unable to render effective nursing care. Further, the nurse may have a personal belief pattern established as part of her cultural or religious background that is not compatible with aggressive and unconventional cancer treatment approaches or, conversely, with decisions to withhold treatment. Because our values guide our practice, personal recognition of one's own belief system is necessary to prevent the delivery of care that meets our own needs rather than those of our client or "succumbing under pressure to dehumanizing practices."

Finally, cancer may represent to the nurse an incurable illness with an unpredictable course that produces in clients a syndrome of unresolvable problems. This focus may subsequently result in little job satisfaction and in an array of feelings that create negative attitudes that ultimately lead to burnout. She may experience guilt at rendering treatments that produce a high incidence of morbidity for her client; or at having failed her client, who dies despite treatment; or perhaps at "abandoning" the family network, in which she participated intimately, when her client dies (42). If her goals have a cure focus, she may feel angry and frustrated if her client does not respond to treatment. Or she may feel impotent at her inability to change the outcome of her client's illness. Because it is not always possible to know what the outcome of disease and treatment will be, she may be stressed by her uncertainty as to what message to give her client and family (36). In the face of continuous ex-posure to the labile emotions and turmoil experienced by clients with cancer and their families, such feelings may be heightened in the nurse.

The other impediment to positive attitudes is the nurse's failure to define her personal philosophy, first about nursing and then about cancer care, death, and dying. Without a philosophy and goals encompassing those aspects of her work, the nurse lacks direction and a sense that her "interventions (or doing nothing) have meaning and purpose for [herself] and her clients." Moreover the ideals that comprise the nurse's philosophy will, to a large extent, determine her approach to ethical problems (18). Without a well-defined philosophy, then, the nurse's efforts to resolve ethical dilemmas, which seem endemic to cancer nursing, may be futile. This sense of futility in caring for clients with cancer and in successfully dealing with the ethical problems that arise severely hampers the development and maintenance of positive attitudes in nurses who render cancer care.

Resolving Attitudinal Barriers

Developing a philosophy compatible with cancer nursing is a necessary first step in the process of eliminating attitudinal barriers. The ability to develop one's philosophy and professional goals grows out of introspective activities that elucidate personal value-belief patterns that may be incompatible with cancer nursing. Once aware of her own beliefs in relation to cancer, the nurse must consider and resolve, in her own mind, the "cure-versus-care" dilemma described by Benoliel (2). This dilemma relates to the ultimate goals that one wishes to achieve for clients as a result of his or her nursing practice. As outlined in Table 20.9, it is characteristic of the cure goals to have a disease focus, whereas the care goals focus more on the client as a person. Both the cure goals and the care goals are fundamental and complementary in the delivery of health care. However, the emphasis in our health care delivery patterns has traditionally been placed on cure, rather than on care, by nurses as well as physicians (35). Because cancer is often a chronic illness, with an uncertain outcome, the cure goals may be unachievable and would, therefore, nurture frustration in the care giver who feels responsible for meeting those goals.

While the nurse participates in efforts to cure the client by executing the physician's prescribed medical regimen, she is directed by the state nurse practice act in some states to diagnose and treat human responses to illness rather than the illness itself. It is, therefore, in-

Table 20.9
Complementary Health Care Goals

Cure Goals	Care Goals
Concerned with diagnosis and treatment of disease process	Concerned with assessments and interventions on behalf of well-being of client
Deals with objective aspects of care	Deals with subjective meaning of disease experience and effects of treatment on the client
Relates to instrumentation and "doing to" people	Relates to respect for the needs of the client and "doing with" people
Physicians primarily responsible for implementation	Nurses primarily responsible for implementation

Source: Adapted from J. Q. Benoliel. "Overview: Care, Cure and the Challenge of Choice." In *The Nurse as Caregiver for the Terminal Patient and His Family,* ed. A. Earle et al. New York: Columbia University Press, 1976, 9–32.

consistent with the legal definition and not within the scope of nursing practice for the nurse to philosophically assume primary responsibility for curing the client. Rather, she is free to direct her energy and attention to the caring aspects of health care delivery. Such goals may be more achievable for this client population and, subsequently, more professionally satisfying for the nurse. Assisting the client to control persistent nausea and vomiting through dietary counseling or distraction

techniques, for example, is more within the scope of nursing practice than curing his gastric cancer with chemotherapy. The care goals here would certainly be more realistic and achievable than the cure goals for the nurse.

The other product of introspection on the part of the nurse is to identify negative feelings or stress-induced potential for burnout generated by her personal experiences with cancer or professional contacts with those who have cancer. Because awareness of personal manifestations of stress and burnout is consistently recommended as a first step in managing the phenomenon (43), Table 20.10, which summarizes associated assessment parameters, may serve as a simple inventory for the nurse to evaluate her own stress level on a regular basis. A more comprehensive self-inventory, as well as specific stress management strategies, appears in chapter 15.

Another valuable activity in this endeavor is to attempt to organize relevant personal feelings by putting them in writing. Keeping a daily or weekly journal of cancer care experiences and referring to it is one method of accomplishing this. Such a journal can assist the nurse to highlight positive experiences and may, at the same time, lend increased understanding to those experiences deemed negative. Selecting a mentor with background in the field of oncology is certainly not essential to the achievement of this goal, but it may be helpful in the self-assessment process. For example, joint analysis of negative experiences recorded in the journal may provide insight for the nurse as to how those situations might have been handled or viewed differently to yield

Table 20.10
Recognizing Burnout

Physical Signs	Cognitive Signs	Psychological Signs
Exhaustion/fatigue, severe lack of energy	Impaired decision-making or problem-solving ability	Negative alteration of self-image; attitudes toward co-workers
Prolonged "cold" symptoms	High-level rigidity to new programs or concepts	Depression, anger, withdrawal
Shortness of breath	Inflexibility in relation to change	Excessive levels of frustration
Weight loss or gain	Excessive complaining/fault finding	Viewing clients as "troublemakers," negative labeling of clients/families
Sleep/rest disorders		Inability to emotionally detach oneself from the job
Excessive irritability		Guilt over taking time off from work

Source: M. Ogle. "Stages of Burnout Among Oncology Nurses in the Hospital Setting." *Oncology Nursing Forum* 10(1):31–32, 1983.

more positive client outcomes or nurse perceptions. Similarly, a mentor may assist in identifying professionally satisfying experiences initially overlooked by the nurse, thus creating a source of positive feedback that otherwise would not have existed.

Selecting and participating in educational programs that emphasize the development of positive attitudes toward cancer nursing care is still another avenue to the resolution of negative feelings about cancer. The objectives of a model program designed by Craytor and colleagues to reduce nurse resistance to involvement in cancer care and to improve the nurse's perception of herself as cancer care giver appear in Table 20.11. This program is based on the principles of adult learning and is intended for those who can independently seek out and build on positive cancer care experiences. It is designed as a group learning activity; however, many of the activities outlined could easily be pursued on an individual basis. Because the need for introspection is reflected throughout the module, a mentor who is able to provide feedback at each milestone would be particularly useful here as well.

Another way to achieve and maintain positive personal attitudes toward cancer nursing is to keep abreast of current developments in cancer treatment and related nursing interventions. Progress in both areas expands the options available to cancer clients and, in doing so, provides a basis for realistic hope in the nurse as well as in clients and their family members.

Taking advantage of networking opportunities with nurses who demonstrate a high level of professional and personal satisfaction in cancer nursing is an important way of encouraging that sense in oneself. Having role models helps the person feel that she is not alone. Examples of such opportunities include involvement in local American Cancer Society unit or division activities as well as in specialty nursing organizations like the Oncology Nursing Society.

Cognitive Barriers

The cognitive barriers to cancer nursing care are related to both attitudes toward the cancer client and the level of cancer-specific knowledge the nurse possesses. These barriers have a direct impact on the care delivered to clients experiencing cancer and to their family members. Eliezer (12) suggests that a lack of knowledge about cancer and its treatment supports the perception that all cancers are hopeless and inevitably painful (12). If the generalist nurse has received limited instruction specific to oncology, she is likely to have this perception of the cancer client's clinical situation. As previously mentioned, this perception has a negative influence on the quality of nursing care delivered. Craytor (5), Dickinson (9), Morrow and associates (39), and Brown (3) have all found that rather than arising from an aversion to the client, reluctance in cancer care is probably related to the nurse's feelings of inadequacy about or frustration in caring for the client and his family. These feelings arise not only from an actual lack of knowledge and skills, but also out of the resulting fear of being unprepared to meet the challenge. This fear can prevent nurses from thoroughly assessing or treating symptoms reported by the client.

A classic example of the interrelationship between cognitive and attitudinal barriers is the nurse who is caring for the client whose pain is uncontrolled by analgesics. Without the appropriate knowledge and clinical experience, the nurse may be reluctant or unable to identify factors that influence the client's pain, and thus to prescribe nursing interventions that will increase the client's comfort. Instead, the nurse may fail to respond appropriately to a client's expressions of discomfort or may rely solely on physician-prescribed analgesics to treat the client's pain. If these analgesics are ineffective, a pattern of failure and frustration can develop in the nurse. The inability to successfully control the client's pain may lead to or reinforce negative attitudes on the part of the nurse toward caring for all clients in pain or all clients with cancer. Removing cognitive barriers in this situation by expanding the nurse's knowledge regarding pain assessment, effective manipulation of analgesic regimens, and the use of nonpharmacologic strategies could enhance the nurse's ability to effectively care for clients who are in pain. Ultimately the nurse may develop more positive attitudes toward cancer client care based on this positive experience.

Resolving Cognitive Barriers

By examining the cognitive barriers and potential resolutions within the context of the nursing process, it is possible to identify those associated with each process component, as shown in Table 20.8. Assessment, the first step of the nursing process, is essential to identify or predict client/family problems with accuracy. Because the complexity and severity of a cancer client's problems can be overwhelming to the nurse, an organized assessment approach that includes cancer-specific information is a necessity. Factors such as type and extent of cancer, the specific anticancer therapy prescribed, and both client and family perceptions of the

Table 20.11
Model Program for Resolving Attitudinal Barriers to Cancer Nursing

Objective 1

The nurse will identify at least one reason for his/her reluctance, if any, to care for cancer patients.

Objective 2

The nurse will compare and analyze his/her descriptions of a cancer patient with the responses of 100 nurses in an acute hospital. In a group discussion, the nurse will describe the meaning of cancer to him/her, including personal experiences with patients, family members, and/or friends with cancer.

Objective 3

The nurse will identify sources of personal satisfaction in working with cancer patients and their families.

Objective 4

Given a choice of responses to the question, "the most difficult problem in working with people who have cancer is . . . ," the nurse will specify some category that reflects his/her knowledgeability about the needs of cancer patients and their families.

Objective 5

The nurse will visit a Chemotherapy Clinic or a Radiation Therapy Clinic and talk briefly with a patient, another nurse, and a physician. Following the visit, the nurse will write down, evaluate, and discuss each participant's perception of the particular patient's situation.

Objective 6

The nurse will identify positive changes in his/her willingness to care for cancer patients.

Objective 7

The nurse will select at least one physical and one psychosocial care area related to giving cancer care in which he/she would like additional knowledge. The nurse will actively demonstrate an interest in these areas by taking additional learning modules or engaging in other learning experiences related to them.

Objective 8

Given a patient with cancer, the nurse will write down his/her own perceptions, perceptions of the physician, the patient's family, and the patient in regard to (a) diagnosis, (b) extent of the disease, (c) prognosis, (d) effects of treatment, (e) ability to cope, (f) changes in the family situation, and (g) special problems of the patient.

Objective 9

The nurse will find out about and report on five articles and/or television or radio programs in the popular media. He/she will discuss the effect of these on patients' attitudes, and the relevance of knowing about such material in giving cancer care.

Objective 10

Given a patient situation where teaching seems to be required, the nurse will devise a nursing plan for teaching information related to prevention, early diagnosis, and/or treatment. The plan will include (a) an assessment of the patient's learning needs, (b) a listing of pertinent learning materials, (c) sources of factual and theoretical information, and (d) a method of evaluating the intervention.

Objective 11

The nurse will discuss and explore his/her own feelings toward death and dying and compare these to feelings of other nurses.

Objective 12

The nurse will differentiate between empathy for and identification with a patient.

Objective 13

By talking to a terminally ill patient and his/her family, the nurse will identify their expressed needs and reactions to the environment. He/she will devise a nursing care plan to try to meet these needs.

Objective 14

The nurse will identify co-workers with a different role in his/her working environment and define the role. He/she will discuss ways in which these roles enhance or detract from a cooperative working relationship among the co-workers, and possibilities for constructive change.

Objective 15

The nurse will begin to expand his/her professional role by implementing exercises designed to improve the attitudes and feelings of others involved in his/her working environment. In so doing, he/she will give positive reinforcement to others.

Objective 16

The nurse will initiate and attend a supportive problem-solving weekly or biweekly group of 5–7 nurses, residents, interns, social workers, ministers, rabbis, and/or other staff to discuss and air concerns about and reactions to patients, patient problems, staff misunderstandings, and floor rules and policies. (Contact and include some skilled and trusted group leaders if possible and desired.)

Objective 17

The nurse will identify ways in which other members of the health care team can contribute to patient care problems.

Objective 18

Given a biographical case report, the nurse will assess the nursing care problems and devise an appropriate nursing care plan.

Source: J. K. Craytor. and M. L. Fass. "Changing Nurses' Perceptions of Cancer and Cancer Care." *Cancer Nursing* 5(1): 44, 1982.

meaning of cancer are an integral part of nursing assessment because they give rise to a unique set of needs within the client/family network. Because these needs are different from those seen in a general medical/surgical population, as previously discussed, they may be unfamiliar to the generalist nurse. Further, the generalist is likely to structure her assessment of the person with cancer according to standard nursing history forms, which might give a broad overview of need but do not cue her to collect data as to cancer-related symptomatology. The nurse, then, may have difficulty identifying important predictors of potential need or recognizing the significance of an actual problem. The nurse may also have difficulty organizing and translating thoughts about client need into concise and meaningful terms. The incomplete data base generated would stand in the way of deriving appropriate nursing diagnoses, and hence planning appropriate interventions.

A way to eliminate this barrier to cancer client/family needs assessment is to use clinical tools that have been designed to assist the nurse in evaluating the special needs of clients with cancer. These data collection instruments facilitate the nurse's ability to gather information most relevant to the cancer client's illness experience. One example of a specialized assessment guideline is the Cancer Nursing Assessment Tool devised by Miaskowski and Neilson and the Prechemotherapy Nursing Assessment Guidelines developed by Engelking and Steele (Appendixes 20 A and 20 B).

When the employing institution or agency has already established data collection tools, such as an admitting data base or nursing Kardex, the resolution may be to modify the existing tool(s) by integrating interview questions that highlight problems, concerns, or risk factors unique to the cancer client population. For example, when assessing a client's pattern of bowel elimination, Gordon's Functional Health Pattern Assessment Model (22) directs the nurse to collect information about the client's normal bowel pattern, the current frequency and character of his stool, and any associated discomfort. When using this model to evaluate the cancer client, the nurse must interject questions regarding cancer-specific causes, such as the presence of an abdominal mass or the use of vinca alkaloids in the client's chemotherapy regimen. The answers to these questions are necessary for the nurse to plan strategies to anticipate and prevent constipation for her client.

In addition to identifying specific problems, nursing assessment should reveal information as to the extent or severity of those problems. The use of a scale, numerical or otherwise, that identifies degrees of severity provides the nurse with a mechanism for exploring symptoms manifest by her client and standardizes the data she collects. Terms such as fair or poor do not tell us enough about the status of a client's oral mucosa to derive a diagnosis, and to subsequently plan nursing interventions that would fit the problem. If, however, the nurse has a rating scale to use as a guide, like the one found in Table 20.12, she is better equipped to describe in detail alterations in the integrity of her client's oral mucosa, and hence plan oral care strategies that have a greater chance of success in resolving the problem.

The use of cancer-specific assessment models permits the generalist nurse to assume the role of primary care giver for cancer clients and their families by directing her to collect data that reveals needs and problems unique to the cancer experience. The formulation of nursing diagnoses that reflect the client's stage of cancer, type and extent of disease, and prescribed anticancer therapy, as outlined in Tables 20.4, 20.5, and 20.6, is facilitated by her ability to conduct a focused nursing assessment. The Outcome Standards for Cancer Nursing Practice developed by the Oncology Nursing Society may be used as a framework for organizing assessment data and selecting appropriate nursing diagnoses (44).

Once actual and potential client/family problems have been diagnosed, the process of planning and delivering client care begins. A lack of knowledge and skill in the areas of symptom management, client/family education, and resource mobilization for clients with cancer is a major difficulty for the generalist nurse. Scientific and empirical information about the characteristics and nursing management of symptom complexes that occur in the context of cancer have been generated dur-

Table 20.12
Mucositis Rating Scale

0 = pink, moist, intact mucosa without pain or burning
+1 = generalized erythema ± pain or burning sensation: scalloping or ridging of tongue/buccal mucosa
+2 = isolated small ulcerations and/or white patches
+3 = confluent ulcerations with white patches >25% mucosa
+4 = homorrhagic ulcerations over >25% of mucosa

Source: Adapted from Oncology Nursing Society Clinical Practice Committee Standardized Nursing Care Plan for Stomatitis.

Cancer Nursing Assessment Tool

Name	Phone	Age
Address	Marital Status	
	Physician	

Date	Time	From ☐ Home Other
Via ☐ Ambulatory ☐ Wheelchair ☐ Stretcher		Information From:

PRESENTING PROBLEM (Quote patient's chief complaint)	
HISTORY OF PRESENT CANCER PROBLEM (Description of chronology, duration of symptoms, understanding of conditions)	
PAST AND PRESENT CANCER TREATMENT SURGERY (type, date)	None ☐
RADIATION THERAPY (Area radiated, number of courses)	None ☐
CHEMOTHERAPY (drugs, dose, routes, effects, schedule, access devices)	None ☐
OTHER THERAPIES (Immunotherapy, Hyperthermia, Imagery, Alternative therapies)	None ☐
OTHER ILLNESSES AND/OR HOSPITALIZATIONS (Date and reason)	
FAMILY HISTORY OF CANCER	
ADAPTATION TO PAST HEALTH PROBLEMS	
EXPECTATIONS AND/OR CONCERNS ABOUT ILLNESS AT PRESENT TIME	
HEALTH MAINTENANCE HABITS (Physical exam, exercise, BSE, Pap smear, Proctoscopy, Testicular exam, Mammography, X-ray, dental, Prostate exam, Hemocult)	
ALLERGIES (Food, drugs, other allergens & reactions)	
MEDICATIONS OTHER THAN CHEMOTHERAPY (Name, dosages, frequency, home remedies, over the counter preparations)	
KNOWLEDGE OF MEDICATIONS	

Source: C. Miaskowski and B. Neilson. "A Cancer Nursing Assessment Tool." *Oncology Nursing Forum* 12(6):38–41, 1985.

Appendix 20 A (continued)

VENTILATORY INTEGRITY shortness of breath, dyspnea on exertion, paroxysmal noctural dyspnea, cyanosis, cough, sputum production, fatigue, tracheostomy, aids to breathing.	Respiratory Rate;
	Smoking:
	Breath Sounds:
	Category WNL ☐

CIRCULATORY INTEGRITY rhythm, pulse deficit, chest pain, palpitations, intermittent claudication, color of extremities, edema, neck veins, varicosities.	Blood Pressure: Pulse
	Category WNL ☐

NUTRITION dysphagia, anorexia, stomatitis, nausea, vomiting, weight loss, changes in taste, food preferences, dietary patterns, nutritional supplements, feeding devices, hyperalimentation.	DIET:
	Food Preparation By:
	Food Intolerances:
	Height: Weight:
	Alcohol Intake:
	Dentures: Upper ☐ Lower ☐ Both ☐ None ☐
	Oral Exam:
	Category WNL ☐

INTESTINAL INTEGRITY pain, constipation, diarrhea, distention, tarry stools, change in bowel habits, blood per rectum, hemorrhoids, colostomy, ileostomy, appliances, liver breadth, spleenomegaly.	Normal Pattern:
	Last B.M.:
	Aids for Bowel Functioning:
	Hemocult:
	Bowel Sounds:
	Category WNL ☐

RENAL–URINARY INTEGRITY frequency, burning, color, hematuria, nocturia, retention, polyuria, incontinence, flank pain, aids to urination, dialysis, appliances, catheter.	
	Category WNL ☐

COMFORT Pain Description - location, duration, periodicity, severity, aggravating factors. Relief Measures - medication, biofeedback, meditation, TENS, visual imagery, diversional activity, music therapy.	Sleep Pattern:
	Pain Description:
	Relief Measures:
	Category WNL ☐

(continued)

Appendix 20 A (continued)

PROTECTIVE MECHANISMS Skin Integrity — change in wart or mole, color, swelling, turgor, abrasions, petechiae, scars, ulcers, photosensitivity, pruritis, desquammation, temperature, extravasation.	
	Category WNL ☐
Immune/Hematologic — chills, fever, rigors, petechiae, nosebleeds.	Temperature:
	Evidence of Bleeding:
	Evidence of Infection:
	Blood Values: Hct Hgb Platelets
	WBC
	◉
	Category WNL ☐
SENSORY - PERCEPTUAL INTEGRITY — orientation, memory loss, personality changes, syncope, vertigo, convulsions, headache, numbness, tingling, alterations in heat and cold sensation.	Level of Consciousness:
	Pupils:
	Category WNL ☐
VISION — visal disturbances, diplopia, blurring, tearing.	Eye Glasses? Yes ☐ No ☐ Contact Lenses? Yes ☐ No ☐
	Glass Eye? Yes ☐ No ☐
	Degree of Visual Acuity:
	Category WNL ☐
HEARING — tinnitus, vertigo, pain, discharge.	Hearing Aid? Yes ☐ No ☐
	Degree of Hearing Loss:
	Category WNL ☐
SPEECH — language barrier, aphasia, dysarthria.	
	Category WNL ☐
MOBILITY lethargy, gait, muscle weakness, paralysis, deformities, joint swelling, physical tolerance, muscle atrophy, tremors, range of motion, range of ambulation, fractures, set-up at home to assist mobility.	Muscle Strength: RUE LUE
	RLE LLE
	Level of Independence:
	Use of Aids: None ☐ Walker ☐ Cane ☐ Wheelchair ☐
	Other
	Category WNL ☐
SEXUAL INTEGRITY menses, contraception, pregnancies, breast changes, gynecomastia, impotency, changes in sexual activity, changes in sexual desire, changes in sexual performance.	LMP: Last Pap Smear:
	Breast Exam:
	Testicular Exam:
	Category WNL ☐

Appendix 20 A (continued)

COPING INTEGRITY anxiety, anger, depression, body image changes, affect, self-esteem, stress, role changes, communication patterns, counseling	Spirituality:
	Ethnic Background:
	Category WNL ☐
SOCIAL INTEGRITY	Occupation:
	Education:
	Family - Significant Other:
	With Whom Does Patient Live?
	Family Support Systems:
	Impact of Hospitalization on Family:
	Economic Resources:
	Previous Use of Community Agencies:
ANTICIPATED TEACHING NEEDS (Based on knowledge deficits assessed)	
	None ☐
DISCHARGE PLAN	Anticipated Discharge to:
	Possible Need for Follow-Up Care (Check all that apply): ACS ☐ Hospice ☐ Reach to Recovery ☐ Ostomy Association ☐ Laryngectomy Association ☐ Social Service ☐ Counseling ☐
	Other:
	Discharge Plan:

Additional Comments:

Signature_____R.N.

Appendix 20 B

Prechemotherapy Nursing Assessment Model: Guidelines for Nursing Assessment of the Patient Receiving Cancer Chemotherapy [a]

Part I: Physical Status

Potential Problems	Assessment Parameters/Signs and Symptoms	Drug and Dose Limiting Factors
Hematopoietic System 1. Impaired tissue perfusion related to chemotherapy-induced *anemia*	• Hgb g (norms 12–14; 14–16) Hct % (norms 32–36; 36–40) • Vital signs (↓BP ↑pulse ↑respiration) • Pale skin color (face, palms, conjunctiva) • Fatigue or weakness • Vertigo	Hgb < 8 g Hct < 20% and blood transfusions not initiated
2. Potential for *infection* related to chemotherapy-induced *leukopenia*	• W.B.C. (norm 4500–9000/mm³) • Pyrexia/rigor, erythema, swelling, pain any site • Abnormal discharges, draining wounds, skin/mm lesions • Productive cough, SOB, rectal pain, urinary frequency	W.B.C. < 3000/mm³ Fever > 101°F • Hold all myelosuppressive agents (Exceptions may include leukemia and lymphoma)
3. Potential for *bleeding* related to chemotherapy-induced *thrombocytopenia*	• Platelet count (150,000–400,000/mm³) • Spontaneous gingival bleeding or epistaxis • Presence of petechiae or easy bruisability • Hematuria, melena, hematemesis, hemoptysis • Hypermenorrhea • Signs and sx intracranial bleed (irritability, sensory loss, unequal pupils, headache, ataxia)	Platelet count ≤ 100,000/mm³ • Hold all myelosuppressive agents (Exceptions may include leukemia and lymphoma)
Integumentary System *Impairment of skin integrity* related to chemotherapy-induced *mucositis* of mouth, nasopharynx, esophagus, rectum, anus, or ostomy stoma	Mucositis Scale [b] 0 = pink, moist, intact mucosa; absence of pain or burning +1 = generalized erythema with or without pain or burning +2 = isolated small ulcerations and/or white patches +3 = confluent ulcerations with white patches on 25% mucosa +4 = hemorrhagic ulcerations	+2 mucositis • Hold antimetabolites (esp. Methotrexate, 5-FU) • Hold antitumor antibiotics (esp. Adriamycin, Dactinomycin)

Gastrointestinal System

Discomfort, nutritional deficiency and/or fluid and electrolyte disturbances related to chemotherapy-induced:

A. Anorexia
- Lab values: albumin and total protein
- Normal weight/present weight (% of body weight loss)
- Normal diet pattern/changes in diet pattern
- Presence of alterations in taste sensation
- Presence of early satiety

B. Nausea and vomiting
- Lab values: Electrolytes
- Pattern of n/v (incidence, duration, severity)
- Antiemetic plan
  - Drug(s), dosage(s), schedule, efficacy
  - Other (dietary adjustments, relaxation techniques, environmental manipulation)

- Intractable n/v × 24 hours if I.V. hydration not initiated

C. Bowel disturbances
1. diarrhea
- Normal pattern of bowel elimination
- Consistency (loose, watery/bloody stools)
- Frequency and duration (no./day and no. of days)
- Antidiarrheal drug(s), dosage(s), efficacy

- Diarrheal stools × 3/24 hours
  - Hold antimetabolites (esp. Methotrexate, 5-FU)

2. constipation
- Normal pattern of bowel elimination
- Consistency (hard, dry, small stools)
- Frequency (hours or days beyond normal pattern)
- Stool softener(s)/laxative(s), efficacy

- No. B.M. × 48 hours past normal bowel patterns
  - Hold vinca alkaloids

D. Hepatotoxicity
- Lab Values: LDH, SGOT, SGPT, Alk Phos, Bilirubin
- Pain/tenderness over liver, feeling of fullness
- Increase in nausea/vomiting or anorexia
- Changes in mental status
- Presence jaundice
- Presence high-risk factors:

Hepatic metastasis	Concurrent hepatotoxic drugs
Viral hepatitis	Graft vs. host disease
Abdominal XRT	Blood transfusions

- Evidence chemical hepatitis
  - Hold hepatotoxic agents (esp. Methotrexate, 6-MP) until differential dx established

Respiratory System

Respiratory dysfunction related to chemotherapy-induced pulmonary fibrosis

- Lab values: PFT's CXR
- Respiration (rate, rhythm, depth)
- Chest pain
- Nonproductive cough
- Progressive dyspnea
- Wheezing/stridor
- Presence high-risk factors:

Total cumulative dose of Bleomycin	Age > 60 years
Preexisting lung disease	Concomitant use of other pulmonary toxic drugs
Prior/concomitant XRT	Smoking hx

- Acute unexplained onset respiratory symptoms
  - Hold all antineoplastic agents until differential dx established

(*continued*)

Appendix 20 B (continued)

Part I: Physical Status (continued)

Potential Problems	Assessment Parameters/Signs and Symptoms	Drug and Dose Limiting Factors

Cardiovascular System
Decreased cardiac output related to chemotherapy-induced:
A. Cardiac arrhythmias
B. Congestive heart failure
	• Lab values: cardiac enzymes, lytes, ECG, ECHO, MUGA
	• Vital signs
	• Presence of arrhythmia (irregular radial/apical)
	• Signs/sx C.H.F. (dyspnea, ankle edema, nonproductive cough, rales, cyanosis)
	• Presence high-risk factors:
	  Total cumulative Prior/concurrent medias-
	  doses anthracyclines tinal XRT
	  Preexisting cardiac Bolus administration
	  disease higher drug doses
		Acute sx C.H.F. and/or cardiac arrhythmia
		• Hold all antineoplastic agents until differential dx established
		Total dose Adriamycin or Daunomycin > 550 mg/m^2
		• Hold anthracyclines

Genitourinary System
Impaired renal function related to chemotherapy-induced:
A. Hemorrhagic cystitis
B. Glomerular or renal tubule damage
C. Hyperuricemic nephropathy
	• Lab values: BUN, creatinine clearance, serum creatinine, uric acid, electrolytes, urinalysis
	• Color, odor, clarity of urine
	• 24 hour fluid intake and output (estimate/actual)
	• Presence of hematuria; proteinuria
	• Development of oliguria or anuria
	• Presence high-risk factors:
	  Preexisting renal disease
	  Concurrent treatment with nephrotoxic drugs (esp. aminoglycoside antibiotics)
		Hematuria
		• Hold cytoxan
		Serum creat > 2.0 and/or Creat clear < 70 ml/minute
		• Hold *cis*-platinum, streptozotocin
		Anuria × 24 hours
		• Hold all antineoplastic agents

Nervous System 1. *Impaired sensory/motor function* related to chemotherapy-induced: A. Peripheral neuropathy B. Cranial nerve neuropathy	Presence of: • Paresthesias (numbness, tingling in feet, fingertips) • Trigeminal nerve toxicity (severe jaw pain) • Diminished or absent deep tendon reflexes (ankle and knee jerks) • Motor weakness/slapping gait/ataxia • Visual and auditory disturbances	Presence of any neurologic signs and symptoms • Hold vinca alkaloids, *cis*-platinum, hexamethyl amine, procarbazine until differential dx established

2. *Impaired bowel and bladder elimination* related to chemotherapy-induced *autonomic nerve dysfunction*	Presence of:
	• Urinary retention
	• Constipation/abdominal cramping and distention
	• Presence of high-risk factors:
	  Changes in diet or mobility
	  Frequent use narcotic analgesics
	  Obstructive disease process
		Presence of any neurologic signs and symptoms
		• Hold vinca alkaloids until differential dx established

Part II: Performance Status
Modified Zubrod Scale

Patient Classification	Defining Characteristics
0	Normal activity; no evidence of disease
1	Disease symptoms present, but able to carry out ADL
2	OOB > 50% of time; requires occasional assistance
3	OOB < 50% of time; requires specialized care
4	Bedridden, requires complete care or assistance with all aspects of care

Part III: Psychosocial/Cognitive Functioning[c]

Potential Problems	Assessment Parameters
Anxiety related to disease and treatment	• Potential Etiology Fear of treatment procedure (i.e., pain of injection) Fear of potentially life-threatening complications; poor rx response Concern about potential/actual changes in body image (i.e., alopecia) Concern about potential/actual changes in life-style or role Communication difficulty with health care provider(s) Financial/occupational concerns • Subjective Data Verbalization of fears, concerns, feeling nervous • Objective Data Physiologic manifestations: Voice tremors/pitch changes — Diaphoresis Increased vital signs — Tremors/headaches Increased muscle tension — Anticipatory nausea/vomiting Behavioral manifestations: Fixed perceptual focus (excessive attention to rx detail) — Scattered perceptual focus (inability to concentrate) Pacing, crying, handwringing — Increased verbalization

(continued)

Appendix 20 B (continued)

Part III: Psychosocial/Cognitive Functioning (*continued*)[c]

Potential Problems	Assessment Parameters

Ineffective individual coping secondary to the need for cancer chemotherapy	• Potential Etiology
	  See identified etiologies for "Anxiety . . . " and "Knowledge Deficit . . . "
	  Hx of ineffective problem-solving abilities and/or coping behaviors
	  Lack of kinship and social support network(s)
	• Subjective Data
	  Verbalization of inability to cope with chemotherapy-related fears or side effects
	• Objective Data
	  Inability to request or accept information or assistance in coping with chemotherapy-related fears or side effects
	  Inappropriate or exaggerated behaviors (e.g., anger, hostility, agitation, apathy, dependency)
	  Deterioration of established pattern of communication with health care providers/significant others
	  Demonstrated withdrawal from social relationships and/or activities, occupational/role responsibilities

Ineffective family coping secondary to their family member's need for cancer chemotherapy	• Potential Etiology
	  See identified etiologies for "Ineffective Individual Coping . . . "
	  Preestablished pattern of family conflict
	  Impaired family communication pattern
	• Subjective Data
	  Patient expresses or confirms concern or complaint about significant other's response to patient's illness and rx
	  Significant person describes or confirms inadequate understanding or knowledge base regarding chemotherapy, which interferes with effective supportive behaviors
	• Objective Data
	  See Objective Data for "Ineffective Individual Coping . . . "
	  Exacerbation, family conflicts or tension
	  Display of disproportionate protective behavior to patient's abilities or need for autonomy

Knowledge deficit related to chemotherapy

- Potential Etiology
  Lack of exposure
  Lack of recall
  Cognitive/perceptual limitation
  Difficulty communicating with health care provider(s)
  Information misinterpretation
  Conflicting information given
  Impaired readiness for learning related to fear, anxiety, denial, disinterest
- Subjective Data
  Verbalization of lack of knowledge/understanding of chemotherapy regimen or required self-management activities
- Objective Data
  Inadequate performance self-management activities:
  Failure to recognize/report occurrence of treatment complications
  Inaccurate follow through on instruction for management of drug-induced side effects
  Failure to obtain prescribed tests/keep appointments

[a]Copyright 1982, by C. Engelking and N. Steele.
[b]Adapted from the Oncology Nursing Society Clinical Practice Committee: Guidelines for nursing care of patients with altered protective mechanisms.
[c]Adapted from Kim and Moritz: Classification of Nursing Diagnoses: Proceedings of Third and Fourth National Conferences. *Oncology Nursing Forum*, 1982, 69–73.
Note: Because this is a general guide, nor all assessment parameters will apply to every patient. Some may weigh more heavily than others depending upon the disease itself, the particular drugs and dosages, as well as individual factors. Therefore, the nurse using these guidelines to assess a patient prior to chemotherapy administration must modify her assessment to address each individual situation.
Source: C. H. Engelking and N. E. Steele. "A Model for Pretreatment Nursing Assessment of Patients Receiving Cancer Chemotherapy." *Cancer Nursing* 7 (June 1984), 205–08.

ing the past decade by cancer nursing research and careful anecdotal documentation. This information has been organized into clinically applicable models of nursing care delivery. The medical/surgical nurse can function skillfully in the role of primary nurse for clients with cancer by using available guidelines to establish an individualized plan of care for each of her clients. Yasko's Symptom Management Model (66), for instance, addresses the common areas of potential physical dysfunction that may potentially confront the client with cancer. Based on nursing process, this model clearly delineates nursing assessment, planning, and intervention for each identified dysfunctional area listed in Table 20.13.

Another valuable reference to guide the nurse in selecting appropriate interventions for the cancer client/family unit is the Oncology Nursing Society's collection of standardized nursing care plans (38). Organized according to the ten outcome standards shown in Table 20.14, the sixty-four protocols prescribe management strategies for a wide range of common disease- and treatment-induced problems that fall within the realm of nursing. Examples include nursing prescriptions for client/family knowledge deficits regarding chemotherapy, internal or external radiation therapy, impairment of skin integrity resulting from malignant skin lesions, altered nutritional status related to gastrointestinal mucositis, ineffective individual and family coping, and grieving.

Because the survival of people with chronic illnesses like cancer depends to a great extent on their ability to engage in self-care, client/family education and resource mobilization are a major focus for the nurse in her symptom management approach. The outcome standard for information requires that "the client and

family possess knowledge about the disease and therapy in order to attain self-management, participation in therapy, optimal living, and peaceful death" (45). This clearly defines the nurse's role as educator in cancer care. The generalist nurse, however, may have difficulty fulfilling this responsibility because of her own lack of knowledge about effective symptom management strategies. To reduce the impact of this cognitive barrier on her practice, the generalist can determine the required content of client/family teaching sessions by referring to prepared treatment- or symptom-specific teaching guides, or to specific client teaching points incorporated into standardized nursing care plans (38). Relying on her assessment of the individual client's learning needs and on her basic knowledge of client education principles, the nurse can use these teaching guides to establish and carry out a teaching plan designed to meet her cancer client's needs.

Resource mobilization, so essential to self-management, demands that the nurse be skillful in determining the human and material resources that exist within the client/family network. Without this determination the nurse may inaccurately assume that a client or family is able to cope alone with current and anticipated problems, or she may overutilize external support services, including her own care, unnecessarily. Answering questions as to the role of significant others surrounding the client, the assistance obtained from these people in past crises, and the strengths and limitations of this network is essential. This information allows the nurse to identify client/family resources and deficits as well as their desire and ability to actively enlist the help of others. This assessment, coupled with an awareness of the cancer care resources available in the client's community, will allow the generalist nurse to assume a primary role in helping cancer clients and their families develop, organize, or sustain their natural support systems. Client/family education and resource mobilization assist clients to participate actively in all aspects of their care. Through these interventions the primary nurse may help to relieve the sense of powerlessness and loss of control often associated with the diagnosis of cancer.

Successful follow-through of a holistic plan of care depends on the nurse's ability to make appropriate referrals to other health care providers and to coordinate the multiple services required for comprehensive care.

Two types of referral may be made by the primary nurse. In one the nurse may seek consultative advice from a colleague in nursing or from another health team member. The consultant may or may not have direct contact with the client but will suggest ways in which a

Table 20.13
Dysfunctional Areas Addressed in Yasko's Symptom Management Model

---

Bone marrow suppression
Chronic pain
Cutaneous manifestations
Gastrointestinal toxicities
Respiratory system dysfunction
Sexual/reproductive dysfunction
Urinary system dysfunction

Source: J. Yasko. *Guidelines for Cancer Care: Symptom Management.* Reston, Va.: Reston Publishing Co., 1983.

Table 20.14
Outcome Standards for Cancer Nursing Practice

Standard Number	Topic	Standard	Outcome Criteria
I	Prevention and early detection	The client and family possess adequate information about cancer prevention and detection.	The client and family— 1. recognize factors that place an individual at risk and may lead to cancer, such as use of tobacco, improper nutrition, and immunosuppressive agents. 2. state cancer's warning signs. 3. identify a plan for seeking health care assistance whenever any alteration in health status occurs. 4. describe applicable cancer self-detection measures.
II	Information	The client and family possess knowledge about the disease and therapy in order to attain self-management, participation in therapy, optimal living, and peaceful death.	The client and family— 1. describe the state of the disease and therapy at a level consistent with their intellectual and emotional states. 2. participate in the decision-making process pertaining to the plan of care and life activities. 3. identify appropriate community and personal resources that would provide information or services. 4. describe appropriate actions for highly predictable problems, oncologic emergencies, and major side effects of disease or therapy. 5. describe the schedule when ongoing therapy is predicted. 6. describe plans for integrating valued activities into daily life.
III	Coping	While living with cancer, the client and family manage stress within their individual physical, psychological, and spiritual capacities and their value systems.	Within a level consistent with physical, psychosocial, and spiritual capacities and their value system, the client and family— 1. use appropriate resources for support in coping. 2. communicate feelings about living with cancer. 3. participate in care and ongoing decision making. 4. identify alternative resources when present coping strategies do not provide support. 5. state accomplishable goals.
IV	Comfort	The client and family identify and manage factors that influence comfort.	The client and family— 1. report alterations in comfort level. 2. identify measures to modify psychosocial, environmental, and physical factors that influence comfort and enhance the continuance of valued activities and relationships. 3. state the source of pain, the treatment, and the expected outcome of the proposed intervention. 4. describe appropriate interventions for potential or predictable problems of the pain and sleep management program.

(continued)

Table 20.14 (continued)

Standard Number	Topic	Standard	Outcome Criteria
V	Nutrition	The client and family manage nutrition and hydration that facilitate optimal health and comfort in the presence of disease and treatment.	The client and family— 1. identify foods that are tolerated and those that cause discomfort or aversion. 2. state measures that enhance food intake and retention. 3. select appropriate dietary alternative to provide sufficient nutrients when usual foods are not tolerated. 4. state methods of modifying consistency, flavor, or amounts of nutrients to ensure adequate nutrient intake. 5. state dietary modifications compatible with cultural, social, ethnic practices. 6. state foods and fluids that provide optimal comfort during the terminal stage of illness.
VI	Protective mechanisms, such as immune, hematopoietic, integumentary, and sensory-motor systems	The client and family possess the knowledge to prevent or manage problems related to alterations in protective mechanisms.	The client and family— 1. list measures to prevent skin breakdown, mucosal trauma, infection, and bleeding. 2. identify signs and symptoms of infection, bleeding, or sensory-motor dysfunction. 3. contact an appropriate health team member when initial signs and symptoms of infection, bleeding, or sensory-motor dysfunction occur. 4. state measures to manage infection, bleeding, or sensory-motor dysfunction.
VII	Mobility	The client and family maintain an optimal mobility level of the client consistent with the disease and therapy.	The client and family— 1. state the cause of the immobility, the treatment, and the outcome of the treatment. 2. describe an appropriate management plan to optimally integrate the alteration in mobility into life-style. 3. describe optimal level of activities of daily living in keeping with disease state and treatment. 4. identify health services and community resources available for managing changes in mobility. 5. use measures to aid or improve mobility. 6. demonstrate measures to prevent the complications of decreased mobility.

VIII	Elimination (alterations in elimination may include fecal and urinary diversions, fistulas, diarrhea, constipation, bladder insufficiencies, incontinence, or fecal or urinary obstruction)	The client and family manage alterations in elimination to be consistent with activities of daily living.	The client and family— 1. state appropriate actions if changes in elimination patterns occur. 2. describe the relationship between adequate elimination and physiologic integrity. 3. identify and manage factors that may affect elimination, such as diet, stress, physical activity, and neurogenic conditions. 4. develop a plan for managing an altered elimination route within personal life-style.
IX	Ventilation	The client and family recognize factors that may impair ventilatory function and can intervene with measures that may enhance optimum ventilatory capacity.	The client and family— 1. state plans for daily activity that demonstrate maximum conservation of energy. 2. list measures to reduce or modify pulmonary irritants from the environment, such as smoke, dry air, powders, and aerosols. 3. describe the effect of environmental extremes on ventilatory function and oxygen utilization. 4. state effective measures to maintain a patent airway. 5. identify reasons for altered ventilation, such as decreased hemoglobin, infection, anxiety, effusion, and obstructed airway. 6. identify an appropriate plan of action should altered ventilation occur. 7. develop a plan for managing an altered airway.
X	Sexuality	The client and partner can identify aspects of sexuality that may be threatened by disease and can enumerate ways of maintaining sexual identity.	The client and partner— 1. identify potential or actual alterations in perception of sexuality or sexual function. 2. identify alternate methods of expressing sexuality.

Source: Clinical Practice Committee of Oncology Nursing Society and American Nurses' Association Division on Medical/Surgical Nursing Practice. Kansas City: American Nurses' Association, 1979.

primary nurse might resolve a specific client problem. The consultant, in this instance, does not assume the role of implementation. For example, a generalist may ask an oncology nurse to recommend standard nursing measures to supplement pharmacologic interventions designed to control cisplatin-induced nausea and vomiting. If these standard measures should not be effective, the nurse may consult an oncology clinical specialist to recommend modifications to the antiemetic plan to produce the desired effect.

In the other type of referral the nurse actually delegates a portion of her client's care to another person. She may identify a client or family need that she thinks can be better met by another member of the health team for various reasons. For instance, a primary nurse may be uncomfortable addressing the issue of sexuality with a young man diagnosed to have testicular cancer and may ask a psychiatric clinical nurse specialist to do so. Or she may refer to a dietitian to give a client information about nutritional supplements, or to a social worker to assist a family in applying for financial assistance. The nurse with a strong professional identity is able to make this type of referral without giving up her role as primary care giver. Role uncertainty on the part of the nurse may result in the inappropriate or ineffective use of other health care providers. If the nurse relinquishes to others all responsibility for dealing with various aspects of a client's care, such as emotional distress or discharge planning, she may not be viewed as primary care giver for that client. Consequently, eliciting adequate data from the client or family in order to formulate nursing diagnoses and a plan of care may be difficult for her. Or she may behave as a subordinate, not initiating and carrying out a plan, but rather following the directions of others. And finally, the client, family, and other health team members may not seek her advice or heed her recommendations for care.

Because no one person can meet all the needs of people who have cancer, professionals must rely on one another in order to deliver continuous comprehensive care. The primary nurse might prevent uncertainty about her role from interfering with her ability to collaborate with others by examining her potential role and defining realistic self-expectations in cancer care situations. Some simple but concrete measures can accomplish this.

First, the nurse must realize that she cannot and need not be the primary care giver for every client to whom she delivers care. Circumstances may dictate that other nurses or other professionals will fill that role. Ideally the nurse should match her availability and skill to client/family need when selecting primary care cases. Then she can make a conscious decision and professional commitment to assume a primary role in their care. Once she has selected her case(s), the nurse must articulate to her clients how she might help them as primary care giver. If the client is to receive chemotherapy, for instance, she might explain that she will conduct pretreatment assessments each time the client is seen in the outpatient department for therapy and will collaborate with the physician to establish a plan of care similar to the one shown in Figure 20.2. This lets the client and family know what to expect of her and allows them to decide how they can best use her knowledge and skill. When her role has been clarified, the primary nurse can make referral decisions jointly with the client and family, based on their needs and her ability to meet those needs, as well as a knowledge of the role and potential contribution of other professionals.

When these steps have been taken, the nurse quite naturally falls into the role of coordinator of care. Her close contact with the client and family and collaborative relationship with other involved professionals enables her to anticipate and avoid either a gap in care or a duplication of services. Clients with cancer often need the services of various health care providers and community agencies. The nurse can interpret the role and activities of each of these to her clients and provide guidance as to how they can obtain a specific service or get

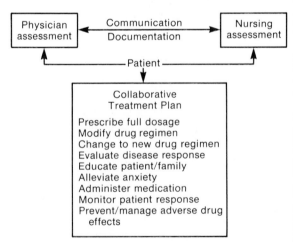

Figure 20.2. Development of Collaborative Treatment Plan

Source: C. Engelking and N. Steele. "A Model for Pretreatment Nursing Assessment of Patients Receiving Ca Chemotherapy." *Cancer Nursing* 7 (June 1984).

answers to certain questions. Through this coordination the nurse provides the client with cancer and his family with the information and support necessary for them to make appropriate use of all care givers and strengthen their sense of control over the situation.

Evaluation is the last component of the nursing process and the phase during which the nurse will formally identify whether or not the intended goals of care have been met. This determination will direct the nurse to continue, modify, or discontinue interventions previously outlined in her nursing care plan. The most important parameter for making these determinations is demonstrated client/family behaviors. Established standards of care provide a mechanism for measuring those behaviors against a desired minimum level of achievement in the client or his family members.

A valuable document available to assist the generalist nurse in evaluating the efficacy of her care to clients with cancer is the Outcome Standards for Cancer Nursing Practice. These standards were developed by the Clinical Practice Committee of the Oncology Nursing Society and endorsed by the American Nurses' Association in 1979 (45). The standards cite ten potential high-need areas for the cancer client population and identify the level of functional ability expected in clients and family as a result of nursing assessment and intervention. The outcome criteria included for each of the ten standards are written as observable behaviors in the client and family that can be used in measuring or evaluating attainment of the standard. The ten standards and their accompanying outcome criteria can be found in Table 20.14.

Using the coping standard to illustrate how these standards assist in the process of evaluation, one can see that the five concrete behaviors cited operationalize the term coping and provide a goal to work toward. Client/family failure to demonstrate those behaviors will cue the nurse to revise her plan. If a client or family member is unable to use appropriate resources for support after the nurse has given verbal information about available resources, for instances it is obvious that her plan did not work. The nurse, then, is directed to modify her intervention, perhaps by providing a written list of resources or by making agency contacts herself on behalf of her client.

Because expected or desired client/family outcomes are used to evaluate the efficacy of prescribed nursing intervention, an important consideration when establishing these outcome criteria is their feasibility—or the likelihood of achieving them through nursing care. For instance, prevention of stomatitis is not a realistic goal for a client who has received high-dose chemotherapy. However, reduction of oral discomfort and minimizing the risk of secondary infection are both desirable and achievable outcomes of nursing intervention. Finally, communicating nursing care goals and progress made toward those goals with other health professionals provides an opportunity for the generalist nurse to demonstrate her accountability as a primary care giver.

Using the resources discussed in this section to remove cognitive impediments to cancer care will expand the cancer nursing knowledge base of the general nurse practitioner and prepare her to assume a primary role in cancer patient care and a collaborative role as a member of the cancer care team.

Interpersonal Barriers

Interpersonal barriers are a common problem in the face of cancer and may be particularly inhibiting to the delivery of cancer nursing care. The emotional turmoil generated by a diagnosis of cancer can seriously hamper interpersonal relationships not only between clients and their family members, but with involved health care providers as well. This occurs largely in response to the perceived threat of suffering, loss, and death inherent in the cancer diagnosis. Untested assumptions as to one another's capacity for dealing with the diagnosis and its implications contribute to this phenomenon. Herein lies a primary role for the nurse when caring for clients facing cancer, and their families. The nurse can provide an environment in which people affected by cancer can explore their feelings. Through the process of communication she can help clients and families make informed decisions about complex problems, prepare her clients for potential consequences of cancer or cancer treatment, and collaborate with other professionals to plan the client's care (34). Carrying out these communication-dependent responsibilities requires that the nurse establish close relationships with clients and their families. Indeed, the nurse's regular presence at the client's bedside and consistent contact with family members provide her with an excellent opportunity to do so. This opportunity, however, may pose a serious threat to the nurse both personally and professionally.

Developing close relationships with people who are experiencing cancer may awaken in the nurse feelings of sadness, frustration, and fear, as well as a recognition of her own mortality. These deeply personal reactions may interfere with her ability to function therapeutically (7). In addition, her professional confidence may be shaken because of her inability to effectively assist her client in resolving psychological distress. As one nurse has stated: "I feel for most of the patients, but honestly, I haven't any idea what's best to do. If someone is depressed or is disturbed, what do you say? What can you do? You can't handle it the way you handle physical pain." (7)

Confirming this nurse's personal observation are the reports of several authors that nurses who are knowledgeable about cancer and secure in meeting the physical needs of people with cancer are, nonetheless, unsure of their interpersonal techniques and communication skills. They are uncomfortable being with clients without performing a physical task and are hesitant to form relationships with cancer clients and their families (9).

Reluctance on the part of the nurse to enter into anything more than a superficial relationship with clients and families is a major barrier to primary cancer nursing care and one component of the Nontherapeutic Interpersonal Nurse Behavior Cycle shown in Figure 20.3. Welch postulates that both external and internal factors inhibit the nurse's ability and motivation to develop therapeutic interpersonal relationships with clients and family members, as shown in Table 20.15. External factors are those imposed by the institution or agency in which the nurse practices and by her co-workers. Traditionally, little energy is devoted by hospital or nursing administrators toward creating a milieu conducive to the development of interactive skills in the nurse. Such

interventions are deemed low priority and are not rewarded, as are the more concrete nursing tasks. Role models for staff nurses to emulate are often lacking, and retrospective analysis of interpersonal encounters is not promoted. Conflict among professionals often arises when there is disagreement as to the type and amount of information shared with the client and his family, or when lines of communication have not been clearly delineated. Lack of peer support and strained interpersonal relationships among staff contribute to an already difficult situation.

Internal factors that interfere with relationship development arise in the nurse herself and are closely intertwined with attitudinal inhibitors. In addition to feelings of inadequacy in the area of communication skills, other fears are common. The fear of behaving unprofessionally or losing composure in difficult client/family interactions, for instance, often prevents the nurse from initiating dialogue with clients or family members that might reveal painful emotions. The fear of emotional attachment to clients facing cancer is a frequent result of the nurse's sense of fatalism about the outcomes of cancer. Remaining superficially involved, then, protects her from feelings of helplessness or negligence evoked by the inability to cure her client's illness. These external and internal factors combined are a powerful force in deterring nurses from building working relationships with cancer clients and their families (2, 34, 60).

An actual communication skill deficit in the nurse is another major interpersonal barrier and the second component of the behavior cycle in Figure 20.3. Although gaps in basic nursing education are partially responsible, a primary reason for the existence of this deficit is limited clinical experience. This problem is compounded when the nurse shies away from developing interpersonal relationships with cancer clients and their families for the reasons cited previously. In doing so she limits her opportunities to practice the interactive skills she may have learned in a classroom, or to apply those skills to the cancer patient population. A nurse who does not possess a repertoire of communication skills from which to draw and sophistication in the use of those skills when engaged in difficult client/family interactions is at a serious disadvantage as primary care giver. She will be unable to develop a helping approach on behalf of her client's well-being, forced, instead, to resort to nontherapeutic responses to protect herself. Rather than meeting her client's needs, then, she is caught up in meeting her own.

The nurse's inability to recognize the emergence of nontherapeutic patterns of communication in the client-

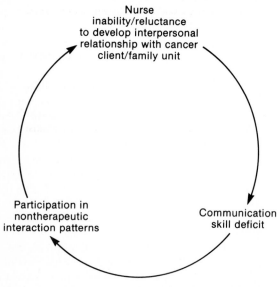

Figure 20.3. Nontherapeutic Interpersonal Nurse Behavior Cycle

Table 20.15
Inhibitors of Therapeutic Nurse/Client Interpersonal Relationships

External Factors	Internal Factors
Low priority or reward for interactive skills	Fear of behaving unprofessionally/losing composure (e.g., crying)
Lack of nursing role models in the system	
Discrepancies between nurse-client-physician lines of communication	Fatalistic attitudes about cancer outcomes
Disagreement about type or amount of information imparted to client/family members	Fear of emotional attachment to client/family
	Feelings of inadequacy in communication skills
Strained interpersonal relationships in staff	
Lack of peer support for interpersonal relationship development	

Source: Adapted from Deborah Welch. "Promoting Change in Patterns of Nurse Communication." *Nursing Administration Quarterly 5* (1981):77–81.

family-professional network poses a third major interpersonal barrier, which completes the behavior cycle. Because communication is the vehicle by which interpersonal relationships are established and maintained, relational difficulties are generally manifested as verbal and nonverbal communication problems. Nurses who are unskilled at diagnosing these problems may have difficulty effecting the role of primary care giver, and may in fact become nontherapeutic participants in these faulty interaction patterns.

Rogers and Mengel describe a series of interpersonal reactions that are symptomatic of one ineffective communication pattern that they have labeled the denial/protection syndrome (48). In this pattern the responsibility for facilitating dialogue about the illness experience is dispersed diversely, leaving no one fully accountable and providing everyone with a convenient avenue for avoiding the subject of cancer. A common indicator of this syndrome is evident when family members complain that the physician is not providing them with adequate information, while at the same time they have not arranged to be available when he makes his daily hospital rounds. Nor have they scheduled an office visit to discuss their concerns. If they have been physically present, evidence of this syndrome may be found in passive client/family behavior during their interaction with the physician. They do not seek clarification of difficult points or pursue concerns raised by the information provided. Or perhaps their anxiety has prevented them from hearing the physician's message at all.

The denial/protection syndrome may also be operative when blame for a client's depression is placed on the physician who openly shares the facts. The family, here, feels that it was insensitive on the part of the physician to divulge information about the diagnosis, prognosis, and treatment options to the client because, they believe, he or she "was not ready to hear it" or "couldn't handle it." In such situations the nurse is usually the professional selected by client or family member as the "sounding board." Often, however, she does not recognize the opportunity for her intervention. Rather, she feeds into this nontherapeutic pattern by becoming angry or disappointed with the physician before she fully evaluates the situation. This response on the part of the nurse impairs her ability to engage in productive discussion with either the physician or the client or family member and to provide guidance toward problem resolution for them.

Another ineffective interaction pattern occurs when people surrounding the client operate under the belief that "hope is the main ingredient for the patient's remaining happiness and that hope cannot coexist with the knowledge of the severity of their condition," (48) and blatantly withhold the truth from the client. Shields refers to the phenomenon of withholding information as the "conspiracy of silence," describing silence as a destructive force out of which grow distortions of reality, misunderstanding, and feelings of betrayal (52). This pattern can arise between physician and client either when the physician elects not to inform the client of his diagnosis, or, more commonly today, when the physician has told the client his diagnosis but fails to discuss the client's symptomatology within the context of cancer. It can happen between the client and his family members when the family chooses not to address the subject of cancer with the client, attributing his health problems to some other related cause. It is not uncommon for the client's physician and family to enter into collusion when the family insists that the physician withhold the diagnosis from their loved one. In this situation the physician feels free of responsibility for the deception because the family has made the decision to withhold information and because all agree that they are operating in the client's best interest.

The nurse, too, may be drawn into this system of closed communication by the traditional role perception that all discussion regarding a client's diagnosis is left to the physician. This perception prevents both nurse and client from acknowledging the reality of the situation (15) and, according to Yarling, places the nurse in "triple jeopardy" (65). As a participant, she must first behave in a way that contradicts what she believes is morally right for the client. Second, she must lie to her client to protect the physician, the institution, and, ultimately, her job security. Last, she is bound to carry through the deception day after day at the client's bedside. Under these circumstances she cannot possibly assume the role of primary care giver for this client and his family.

Henrich and Bernheim describe other patterns of closed communication, including empty reassurances, denial of feelings, superficial advice giving, and generalization (25). In all of these patterns, verbal cues from the client or family are met with responses that stifle the interaction. Empty or false reassurances, such as "Things will be better tomorrow," although well intentioned, only block in-depth exploration of client/family problems, concerns, or anxieties and communicate to them that their message is being ignored. Moral imperatives like "Don't be sad. Look at the bright side" deny the validity of the client's true feelings. This subsequently guarantees perpetuation of those undesirable feelings. Superficial advice like the frequently heard "Take one day at a time" may be unachievable for the client in the face of unresolved anxieties and would, therefore, only foster frustration in him. Finally, generalizations such as "Everyone feels afraid before they get chemotherapy" turn the focus of the interaction away from the uniqueness of an individual client's situation. When the nurse falls into these patterns, her chance to intervene as primary care giver by creating an environment in which client/family feelings can be explored and conflicts can be resolved is lost.

Interrupting the Nontherapeutic Interpersonal Nurse Behavior Cycle will enable nurses caring for cancer clients to feel clinically competent and realize a subsequent

sense of satisfaction from their interpersonal interventions with clients and their family members.

Resolving Interpersonal Barriers

An important beginning in resolving interpersonal barriers is to acknowledge feelings of discomfort generated by interactions with cancer clients or their families and then to examine why those feelings arise. Because it is often difficult for nurses to pinpoint the basis for uncomfortable feelings, the use of a structured self-inventory like the one found in Figure 20.4 could help to stimulate awareness in this area. This particular inventory identifies common anxiety-producing questions or statements posed by clients and family members who are experiencing cancer. It calls for a discomfort rating on a simple five-point Likert scale and some narrative notes describing associated fears to which identified discomfort may be attributed. After inventory completion, several considerations will make the exercise more meaningful from a problem resolution standpoint. First, for each statement or question, determining personal reasons for the assigned rating is essential. Perhaps the nurse imagines that she will induce client reactions such as hysteria or depression if she should respond to a delicate question the "wrong" way. Or maybe she fears that she will incur the physician's wrath if she unknowingly responds with contradictory information. Whatever the reason, it should be articulated verbally or in writing. Second, it is important to think out what the client's true motivation for posing the question or statement might be, and to realize that this is a personal perception that requires client/family validation in order for it to be accurate. Third, one must keep in mind that responding to every client question with "the" right answer is neither expected nor realistic. Often silent presence or simply assisting a client to better phrase his concerns is adequate to meet the need. Finally, rather than determining whether responses to client/family questions or statements are right or wrong, thinking of them in terms of being helpful or not helpful can make these nurse-client-family interactions less threatening to the nurse's sense of competence in the interpersonal aspects of her care. Table 20.16 provides a quick summary of the questions to consider when analyzing discomforting interactions. This exercise can easily be expanded to the clinical practice setting by consciously tracking the frequency of actual client/family contacts similar to those listed in the inventory, or by jotting down other encounters that created discomfort during the work day. These can be reflected on using the questions in Table 20.16

Personal Responses to Interactions with Cancer Patients and Families

Directions: 1. Read each item that might occur while you are talking to a patient or family member.
2. Estimate your discomfort level by circling a representative number on the scale.
3. Jot down your immediate reactions/concerns about what might happen in each situation.

Situation	Discomfort Level					Reactions/Concerns
	Least				Greatest	
The Adult Patient Asks:						
1. What is my diagnosis? My doctor hasn't said anything.	1	2	3	4	5	
2. My doctor said I have a tumor. Is that cancer?	1	2	3	4	5	
3. Have you known other people getting the same treatment as I am?	1	2	3	4	5	
4. Do you think I'm going to die?	1	2	3	4	5	
5. How will I look after a radical neck operation?	1	2	3	4	5	
6. Why doesn't this wound heal?	1	2	3	4	5	
7. Why do I have this terrible smell? Do you think the cancer is getting worse?	1	2	3	4	5	
8. How much pain am I going to have?	1	2	3	4	5	
9. How much longer do I have to live?	1	2	3	4	5	
10. It's not fair that I have cancer. . . . Why am I being punished?	1	2	3	4	5	
11. I don't want to see anyone. They all feel sorry for me.	1	2	3	4	5	

Figure 20.4. Self-Assessment of Interpersonal Resolution Strategy
  Source: Westchester County Medical Center, Department of Nursing, Self-inventory. Valhalla, N.Y., undated.

as a guideline for analysis at a later time. Sharing such encounters with colleagues is a potential source of growth as well. Often the mere act of recognizing the cause of uncomfortable feelings can prevent them from hindering interpersonal relationship building.

Table 20.16
Communication Discomfort Considerations

Why does this statement/question make me feel uncomfortable?
Why is my client posing this statement/question?
Is my assumption about this client's motivation a valid one?
Do I have to respond to this client's statement/question with an answer?
Would the most helpful response to my client's statement/question be verbal or nonverbal?

Once areas of discomfort have been elucidated, developing or refining a repertoire of communication skills on which to draw during cancer client/family interactions is necessary. Table 20.17 lists seven basic interactive skills that can be used in various combinations to render nurse-client-family interactions therapeutic. Like the physical skills performed by nurses, developing sound communication skills requires practice to achieve mastery. Practicing each skill individually in the clinical setting while performing a routine physical task like a bed bath or passive range-of-motion exercises is a way for the nurse to build confidence in her ability to effectively use interactive skills. A description and examples of each skill appear in Table 20.17.

Two additional strategies will help make communicating with clients facing cancer less threatening for the nurse and, at the same time, more effective in meeting the client's needs. One is to continually test assumptions

Table 20.17
Basic Therapeutic Communication Skills

Skill	Description	Example
Attending	Posture	Nurse sits close to and faces client; may use physical touch
	Eye contact	Makes eye contact when appropriate
	Accurate verbal follow-through	"I see," "um-huh"
Encouraging verbal communication	Open questions	"How do you think you might react if you find out you have cancer?"
	Minimal leads	"And then . . . "; "Can you tell me more?"
Paraphrasing	Determine and restate cognitive content	"You say your pain is caused by the cancer in your spine?"
Reflection of feeling	Identify emotional content and validate with client	"You feel angry because your treatment has been delayed, is that right?"
Summarization	Select priority concepts and tie together	"So, you've said you are confused and upset about this change in your chemotherapy treatment and you want the doctor to talk to you again when your wife is present."
Confrontation	Express observed discrepancies between client's statements and behavior	"You've often said how much you miss seeing your children when you're in the hospital, but you've asked your husband not to bring them here to visit."
Self-disclosure	Share personal reaction to client/family interaction	"It makes me feel sad to see you so upset."
	Reveal relevant personal experience and/or feeling	"I can understand what you mean. I often felt angry when my mother had cancer and needed so much of my time."

Source: Adapted from W. White et al. Hospice Education Program for Nurses, 1981.

about client responses to their illness experience and motivations for their actions or statements. Recognizing that it is natural to make assumptions about others that may not be correct and validating those perceptions with the client before acting or responding eliminate stereotypical responses and communicate concern about the client as an individual. For example, it is common to assume that a person who has just been told he or she has cancer will be upset and need comforting. If, however, this particular person prides himself or herself on the ability to face crises independently and head on, a nurse who assumes a comforting approach may not be well received by this client. In addition, the act of validation is in and of itself therapeutic because it provides the client or family member an opportunity to hear what they have said and to correct misconceptions on the part of the nurse.

The other important strategy is to establish a specific goal for each nurse-client-family interaction before entering into it. This strategy not only raises the nurse's consciousness as to the use of communication as a therapeutic tool but also gives her direction, helps to make the interaction more productive, and allows for evaluation of its effect. Eliciting information from a client as to the effectiveness of previously prescribed analgesics, for instance, is a much different goal than teaching him how to use relaxation techniques to control pain. Knowing what she wants to achieve before initiating the dialogue will enable the nurse to purposefully plan her communication strategies to produce the desired effect. In the first situation the nurse may use open questions or paraphrasing to help the client describe his pain experience; in the other she may self-disclose to introduce the concept of relaxation as a pain management technique.

The primary nurse can make a significant difference in the quality of life for people with cancer. As indicated earlier in the chapter, the first step in assuming the role of a primary nurse is to examine one's own perceptions and acknowledge those factors that may hamper fulfillment of that role. This derives from the belief that overcoming barriers to primary nursing care requires an intimate understanding of one's own attitudes, values, and philosophy of care. Knowing oneself is as important as mastery of the knowledge and skills of cancer nursing in order to meet the needs of clients and their families.

REFERENCES

1. Baird, S. "Nursing Roles in Continuing Care: Home Care and Hospice." *Seminars in Oncology Nursing* 7(1):28–29, 1980.
2. Benoliel, J. "Overview: Care, Cure and the Challenge of Choice." *The Nurse as Caregiver for the Terminal Patient and His Family,* ed. A. Earle, N. T. Argondizzo, and A. H. Kutscher. New York: Columbia University Press, 1976, 9–32.
3. Brown, J. K. "Intervention to Change Nurses' Perceptions in Cancer Nursing Care." Unpublished Master's Thesis, University of Rochester, Rochester, N.Y., 1977.
4. Cole, C., and L. Gorman. "Breast Self Examination: Practices and Attitudes of Registered Nurses." *Oncology Nursing Forum* 11:37–39, 1984.
5. Craytor, J. K., J. K. Brown, and G. R. Morrow. "Assessing Learning Needs of Nurses Who Care for Persons with Cancer." *Cancer Nursing* 1:211–20, 1978.
6. Dalton, J., and I. Swenson. "Nurses and Smoking: Role Modeling and Counseling Behaviors." *Oncology Nursing Forum* 13:45, 1986.
7. Davitz, L., and J. Davitz. "How Do Nurses Feel When Patients Suffer?" *American Journal of Nursing* 75(9): 1505–10, 1975.
8. Derdiarian, A. "Psychosocial Variables in Cancer Management: Considerations for Nursing Practice." *Concepts of Oncology Nursing,* ed. D. Vredevoe et al. Englewood Cliffs, N.J.: Prentice Hall, 1981, 39.
9. Dickinson, A. R. "Nurses' Perceptions of Their Care of Patients Dying with Cancer." Unpublished Doctoral Dissertation, Columbia University, New York, 1967.
10. Donovan, M., and S. Pierce. "The Meaning of Cancer." *Cancer Care Nursing.* New York: Appleton-Century-Crofts, 1976, 16–22.
11. Edstrom, S., and M. Miller. "Preparing the Family to Care for the Cancer Patient at Home: A Home Care Course." *Cancer Nursing* 4:49, February 1981.
12. Eliezer, N. "The Need for Support Systems for Staff on Oncology Units." *Cancer Nursing Update,* ed. R. Tiffany. London: Bailliere Tindall, 1981, 126.
13. Elkind, A. K. "Nurses' Views About Cancer." *Journal of Advanced Nursing* 7:43–50, 1982.
14. Engelking, C. "An Exploratory Study of Ten Factors Which Influence or Determine the Home Care Needs of Cancer Patients." Unpublished Master's Thesis, San Francisco State University, May 1980.
15. Fanslow, J. "Attitudes of Nurses Toward Cancer and Cancer Therapies." *Oncology Nursing Forum* 12(1):44, 1985.
16. Frank-Stromberg, M. "The Role of the Nurse in Cancer Detection and Screening." *Seminars in Oncology Nursing* 11:197–98, 1986.
17. Friedman, B. "Coping with Cancer: A Guide for Health Care Professionals." *Cancer Nursing* 3, April 1980.
18. Gadow, S. "Ethical Issues in Cancer Nursing: A Model for Ethical Decision-Making." *Oncology Nursing Forum* 7(4):44, 1980.
19. Given, B. "Education of the Oncology Nurse: The Key to Excellent Patient Care." *Seminars in Oncology Nursing* 7(1):71, 1980.
20. Glasel, M. "Cancer Prevention: The Role of the Nurse in Primary and Secondary Cancer Prevention." *Cancer Nursing* 8:5–8, 1985 (Supplement).
21. Glaser, and A. Strauss. *Awareness of Dying.* Chicago: Aldine, 1965.
22. Gordon, M. *Nursing Diagnosis Process and Application.* New York: McGraw-Hill, 1982.
23. Green, P. "The Role of the American Cancer Society in Cancer Public Education." *Seminar in Oncology Nursing* 11:206–07, 1986.
24. Henke, C. "Emerging Roles of the Nurse in Oncology." *Seminars in Oncology Nursing* 7(1):5, 1980.
25. Henrich, A., and K. Bernheim. "Responding to Patients' Concerns." *Nursing Outlook* 29:429–31, July 1981.
26. Herter, F. P. "A Surgeon Looks at Terminal Illness." *Psychosocial Aspects of Terminal Care,* ed. B. Schoenbert et al. New York: Columbia University Press, 1972.
27. Hubbard, S., and M. Donehower. "The Nurse in a Cancer Research Setting." *Seminars in Oncology Nursing* 7(1), 1980.
28. Johnson, J. *The Challenge to Action in Anti-smoking Efforts.* American Cancer Society Professional Education Publication, 1981, 4–6.
29. Kelley, P. "Self-examination for Breast Cancer: Who Does Them and Why?" *Journal of Behavior Medicine* 2:31–35, 1979.
30. Kim, M. J., and D. A. Moritz, eds. *Classification of Nursing Diagnoses: Proceedings of the Third and Fourth National Conferences on Classification of Nursing Diagnoses.* New York: McGraw-Hill, 1981.
31. Knudsen, N., S. Schulman, J. van Den Hoek, and R. Fowler. "Insights on How to Quit Smoking: A Survey of Patients with Lung Cancer." *Cancer Nursing* 8:145, 1985.
32. Love, R. R., and S. Olsen. "An Agenda for Cancer Prevention in Nursing Practice." *Cancer Nursing* 8:329, 1985.
33. Marston, M. V. "The Use of Knowledge." *Role Theory,* ed. M. Hardy and M. Conway. New York: Appleton-Century-Crofts, 1978, 215.
34. McCorkle, R. "Communication Approaches to Effective Cancer Nursing Care." *Cancer Nursing,* ed. L. B. Marino. St. Louis: C.V. Mosby, 1981.

35. McCorkle, R. "Oncology Nursing: A Challenge Not to Be Taken Lightly." *Oncology Nursing Forum* 4(4):1, 1977.

36. McElroy, A. "Burnout: A Review of the Literature with Application to Cancer Nursing." *Cancer Nursing* 5(3):211–17, 1982.

37. McGinty, C., and L. Weinstein. "Standard for Care of the Terminally Ill." *Cancer Nursing* 2:491–92, December 1979.

38. McNally, J., J. C. Stair, and E. Sommerville. *Guidelines for Cancer Nursing Practice*. New York: Grune and Stratton, 1985.

39. Morrow, G., J. Crayton, J. Brown, et al. "Nurses' Perceptions of Themselves, Cancer Nurses, Typical and Ideal, and Cancer Patients." *Percept Mot Skills* 43:1083–91, 1976.

40. National Cancer Institute. *National Survey on Breast Cancer: A Measure of Progress in Public Understanding*. Bethesda, Md.: U.S. Department of Health and Human Services, Pub. No. 81–2306, 1980.

41. Nevidjon, B. "Cancer Prevention and Early Detection: Reported Activities of Nurses." *Oncology Nursing Forum* 13(4):76, 1986.

42. Newlin, N., and D. Wellisch. "The Oncology Nurse: Life on an Emotional Roller Coaster." *Cancer Nursing* 1:448, 1978.

43. Ogle, M. "Stages of Burnout Among Oncology Nurses in the Hospital Setting." *Oncology Nursing Forum* 10(1):31–32, 1983.

44. *Outcome Standards for Cancer Nursing Education: Fundamental Level*. Oncology Nursing Society Education Committee, 1979.

45. "Outcome Standards for Cancer Nursing Practice." *Oncology Nursing Society*, July 1978.

46. Parsons, J., ed. "The Needs of the Cancer Patient." *Nursing Digest* 5(2):v, 3, 11, 1977.

47. Reed-Ash, C. "The Cancer Unit." *Cancer Nursing* 3:181, June 1980.

48. Rogers, B. J., and A. Mengel. "Communicating with Families of Terminal Cancer Patients." *Topics in Clinical Nursing* 1:55–61, 1979.

49. Sawyer, P. F. "BSE: Hospital-based Nurses Aren't Assessing Their Clients." *Oncology Nursing Forum* 13:44–48, 1986.

50. Scoy-Mosher, C. Van. "The Oncology Nurse in Independent Professional Practice." *Cancer Nursing* 1:22, February 1978.

51. See-Lasley, K., and R. J. Ignoffo, eds. *Manual of Oncology Therapeutics*. St. Louis: C.V. Mosby, 1981, 1.

52. Shields, P. "Communication: A Supportive Bridge Between Cancer Patient, Family and Health Care Staff." *Nursing Forum* 21(1), 1984.

53. Silverberg, E. *Cancer Source Book for Nurses*. New York: American Cancer Society, 1982.

54. Silverberg, E. "Cancer Statistics 1984." *CA-A Cancer Journal for Clinicians* 34(1):10–11, 1984.

55. Silverberg, E. "Cancer Statistics, 1986." *CA-A Cancer Journal for Clinicians* 34(1):9, 1986.

56. Stillman, M. J. "Women's Health Beliefs About Breast Cancer and Breast Self Examination." *Nursing Research* 26:121–25, 1977.

57. Thaney, K. "The Nurse in a Community Hospital Setting." *Seminars in Oncology Nursing* 7(1):18, 1980.

58. Valentine, A. "Behavioral Dimensions of Cancer Prevention and Detection." *Seminars in Oncology Nursing* 11:202–03, 1986.

59. Wegmann, J. "Avoidance Behaviors of Nurses as Related to Cancer Diagnosis and/or Terminality." *Oncology Nursing Forum* 4(3):8–14, 1979.

60. Welch, D. "Promoting Change in Communication." *Nursing Administration Quarterly* 5:77–81, 1981.

61. Welch, D., J. Follo, and E. Nelson. "The Development of a Specialized Nursing Assessment Tool for Cancer Patients." *Oncology Nursing Forum* 9(1):38, 1982.

62. Whelan, J. "Oncology Nurses' Attitude Toward Cancer Treatment and Survival." *Cancer Nursing* 7:376, October 1984.

63. Woerdt, A. Van. *Communication with the Fatally Ill*. Springfield, Ill.: Chas. C. Thomas, 1966, VIII.

64. Wu, R. *Behavior and Illness*. Englewood Cliffs, N.J.: Prentice Hall, 1973, 160–61.

65. Yarling, R. R. "Ethical Analysis of a Nursing Problem: The Scope of Nursing Practice in Disclosing the Truth in Terminal Patients." *Supervisor Nurse*. Reprinted in Hospice Education Program for Nurses, DHHS Pub. No. HRA, Md., 1981, 81–127.

66. Yasko, J. *Guidelines for Cancer Care: Symptoms Management*. Reston, Va.: Reston Publishing, 1983.

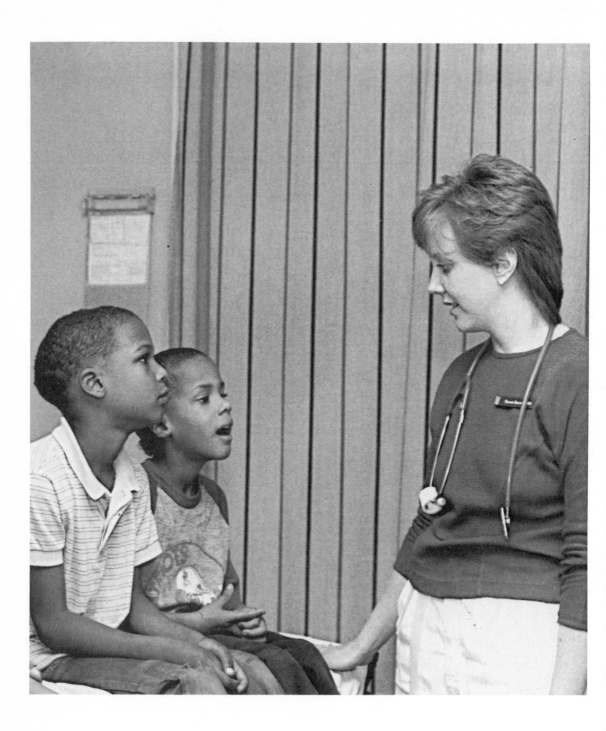

UNIT FOUR

Primary Nursing with Parents and Growing Families

■

Unit four deals with the growing family and some of the problems encountered in various situations related to child-rearing. It begins with family planning, chapter 21, and breast-feeding, chapter 22. The author of the chapters 23 through 25 addresses problems that are very much in the forefront of American attention today—working mothers, older parents, and nontraditional families. The nurse's role in applying concepts of primary nursing to these problems is amply illustrated. Chapter 26 explores the problems and challenges of caring for a family with a chronically ill child, and chapter 27 addresses sudden infant death syndrome (SIDS).

CHAPTER 21

Family Planning

LINDA K. HUXALL

■

OBJECTIVES

After completing this chapter, the reader will be able to:

- Name the most popular reversible form of contraception in the United States.
- Name the most popular type of contraception in the United States.
- Discuss the mode of action, effectiveness, and common side effects of the following: combination oral contraceptives, progestin-only oral contraceptives, intrauterine devices, condoms, spermicides, and diaphragms.
- Differentiate between the two types of oral contraceptives by composition, pill schedules, and effectiveness.
- Name the absolute contraindications for using oral contraceptives and intrauterine devices.

- Describe the five types of postcoital contraceptives and when they must be used to be effective.
- Instruct patients on the correct use of condoms and spermicides.
- Discuss two noncontraceptive benefits of condoms, spermicides, and diaphragms.
- Describe the cervical cap and three advantages and disadvantages of this contraceptive.
- Describe the vaginal contraceptive sponge.
- List four advantages and disadvantages of the natural family planning methods.

The decision to delay or limit childbearing is based on a complex interaction of socioeconomic conditions and pressures, folklore and myths, conscious and unconscious motivational factors, and emotional attitudes toward sex and childbearing. With the introduction of highly effective, inexpensive contraceptive methods, more access to birth control facilities, and an increasingly permissive society, many of the former barriers against contraception have been reduced or removed.

Nurses, more than ever before, are finding it necessary to be well informed about this subject. This is true for nurses working as primary care providers of family planning, as well as for those in hospitals and offices, and those acting as the "neighborhood consultant." Every nurse has the responsibility to increase this aspect of self-care by way of counseling and teaching.

Oral Contraceptives

Oral contraceptives (OCs) are the most effective and most popular reversible contraceptive agents available today. Eighty-five percent of reproductive-age women in the United States have few absolute contraindications to using OCs (11).

There are two basic types of OCs, combination and progestin-only, in use today. Combination pills contain both an estrogen and a progestin and are taken each day for twenty or twenty-one days, followed by no more than seven days without medication, to allow for withdrawal bleeding. Many companies have added seven placebos (or pills containing iron) of a different color to the twenty-one-pill cycle so that the woman takes a pill every day. Withdrawal bleeding occurs while the woman is taking the placebos (the newer biphasic and triphasic OCs are combination pills). The progestin-only pills contain a low dosage of progestin and are commonly known as "mini-pills." These pills are taken continuously whether or not bleeding occurs.

Table 21.1 is a list of the oral contraceptives, from the most estrogenic to the least estrogenic, that are currently available in the United States. Any such chart has

several shortcomings. First of all, different estrogens and progestins do not have the same potency per microgram or milligram of dosage. And the balance of these hormones is also important, since one compound may overshadow the other. For example, some progestins are more antiestrogenic than others (Table 21.2). Finally, any pill, once ingested, falls prey to the user's individual chemistry, including the amount of hormones produced by the adrenal glands.

Mode of Action and Effectiveness

Basically, combination OCs suppress the hypothalamic-anterior pituitary-ovarian system, thus preventing normal cyclic production of hormones. Ovulation is, therefore, suppressed in most cases. Pills containing 0.05 mg (50 μg) or less of estrogen probably suppress ovulation only 95 to 98 percent of the time. The close-to-100 percent effectiveness of the lower-dose pills is due to the strong contraceptive effects of the progestins in addition to the inhibition of ovulation (10).

The constant presence of the progestin in the combined OCs produces a cervical mucus that is thick, scanty, and hostile to sperm. It also artificially induces a mixed proliferative (estrogen)-secretory (estrogen-progestin) type of endometrium that does not easily support implantation. When taken correctly, combination OCs are almost 100 percent effective (10, 11). Oral contraceptives containing less than 0.05 mg of estrogen and lower doses of progestin are less effective than this, especially when even a single pill is missed.

Mini-pills do not always suppress ovulation because of their lack of estrogen and low dose of progestin; rather, they act to produce the secondary effects of the combination pills. In well-controlled studies in which mini-pills were taken at the same time each day, every day of the month, they were 97 percent effective (11).

In determining the effectiveness of any contraceptive, a distinction must be made between theoretical effectiveness (perfect usage without error) and actual use effectiveness (Table 21.3). Many women take their pills erratically, do not remember missing pills, or may believe that they are taking them correctly. As a result,

Table 21.1
Oral Contraceptives

Trade Name (Number of Pills)		Estrogen	Mg/Tab	Progestin	Mg/Tab
Combination Pills					
Enovid-E (20, 21)		Mestranol	0.10	Norethynodrel	2.5
Enovid 5 (20)		Mestranol	0.075	Norethynodrel	5.0
Enovid 10 (20)		Mestranol	0.06	Norethynodrel	10.0
Ovulen (21, 28)		Mestranol	0.10	Ethynodiol diacetate	1.0
Norinyl 2 (20) } Ortho-Novum 2 (20) }		Mestranol	0.10	Norethindrone	2.0
Demulen (21, 28)		Ethinyl estradiol	0.05	Ethynodiol diacetate	1.0
Norinyl 1+80 (21, 28) } Ortho-Novum 1/80 (21, 28) }		Mestranol	0.08	Norethindrone	1.0
Ovcon-50 (28)		Ethinyl estradiol	0.05	Norethindrone	1.0
Norlestrin 1 (21, 28, 28 Fe*)		Ethinyl estradiol	0.05	Norethindrone acetate	1.0
Norinyl 1+50 (21, 28) } Ortho-Novum 1/50 (21, 28) }		Mestranol	0.05	Norethindrone	1.0
Ovral (21, 28)		Ethinyl estradiol	0.05	Norgestrel	0.5
Norlestrin 2.5 (21, 28, 28 Fe*)		Ethinyl estradiol	0.05	Norethindrone acetate	2.5
Ortho-Novum 10 (20)		Mestranol	0.06	Norethindrone	10.0
Loestrin 1.5/30 (28, 28 Fe*)		Ethinyl estradiol	0.03	Norethindrone acetate	1.5
Brevicon (21, 28) } Modicon (21, 28) }		Ethinyl estradiol	0.035	Norethindrone	0.5
Ovcon-35 (28)		Ethinyl estradiol	0.035	Norethindrone	0.4
Demulen 1/35 (21, 28)		Ethinyl estradiol	0.035	Ethynodiol diacetate	1.0
Norinyl 1+35 (21, 28) } Ortho-Novum 1/35 (21, 28) }		Ethinyl estradiol	0.035	Norethindrone	1.0
Ortho-Novum 10/11 (21, 28)†		Ethinyl estradiol	0.035	Norethindrone	0.5 (1–10) 1.0 (11–21)
Lo/Ovral (21)		Ethinyl estradiol	0.03	Norgestrel	0.3
Nordette (21)		Ethinyl estradiol	0.03	Levonorgestrel	0.15
Loestrin 1/20 (28, 28 Fe*)		Ethinyl estradiol	0.02	Norethindrone acetate	1.0
Triphasic Combination Pills					
Triphasil (28)	6	Ethinyl estradiol	0.03	Levonorgestrel	0.05
Tri-Levlen (28)	5	Ethinyl estradiol	0.04	Levonorgestrel	0.075
	10	Ethinyl estradiol	0.03	Levonorgestrel	0.125
	7	Inert	—	—	—
Tri-Norinyl (21)	7	Ethinyl estradiol	0.035	Norethindrone	0.5
	9	Ethinyl estradiol	0.035	Norethindrone	1.0
	5	Ethinyl estradiol	0.035	Norethindrone	0.5
Ortho-Novum 7/7/7 (21)	7	Ethinyl estradiol	0.035	Norethindrone	0.5
	7	Ethinyl estradiol	0.035	Norethindrone	0.75
	7	Ethinyl estradiol	0.035	Norethindrone	1.0
Mini-Pills					
Nor-Q. D. (42)		None		Norethindrone	0.35
Micronor (35)		None		Norethindrone	0.35
Ovrette (28)		None		Norgestrel	0.075

*Fe—last seven pills contain iron.
†Also called biphasic.

Table 21.2
Comparison of Endocrine Properties of Progestins in Oral Contraceptives

	Estro-genic	Andro-genic	Progesta-tional
Norethynodrel (Enovid) (Enovid-E)	+ +	0	±
Norethindrone (Norinyl) (Ortho-Novum) (Ovcon)	0	+	+
Norethindrone acetate (Norlestrin)	0	+	+
Ethynodiol diacetate (Ovulen) (Demulen)	+	+	+ +
Norgestrel (Ovral)	0	+	+ + + +

0 — Inactive
± — Very weak
+
+ +
+ + +   } Active to Very Active
+ + + +

Parenthetical terms are brand names of oral contraceptives that include the hormone listed directly above.

higher failure rates may be observed in the clinical setting. Such rates may be difficult to assess, since many women are reluctant to admit having taken their pills incorrectly until they are assured that they are not pregnant. The low-dose pills (less than 0.05 mg of estrogen) have a slightly increased failure rate (24).

Side Effects

From a woman's standpoint, the side effects of OCs can be divided into symptoms that mimic pregnancy and symptoms that are related to the menstrual cycle. Some of the most common "pseudopregnancy" symptoms, which are related to the estrogen content, include nausea, vomiting, fluid retention (with cyclic weight gain), headaches, vertigo, breast enlargement and tenderness, chloasma, and nonpathogenic leukorrhea. Fatigue, depression, oily scalp and acne, and increased appetite with steady weight gain are usually related to the progestin (Table 21.4).

Most women taking OCs experience changes in their menstrual cycle. There is less menstrual blood loss, which reduces the risk of iron deficiency anemia by 50 percent (17). The menstrual cycle is often very predictable and of shortened duration. Spastic dysmenorrhea and premenstrual tension are also significantly reduced.

Other health benefits of OCs include a 50 percent reduction in the risk of endometrial cancer and significant reduction in various types of benign breast disease, and functional ovarian cysts are nearly eliminated. Endometriosis and menorrhagia are also usually relieved by combination pills. In addition, OCs appear to protect women from developing ovarian carcinoma, rheumatoid arthritis, and salpingitis (17).

Breakthrough Bleeding and Amenorrhea

Hypomenorrhea is a fairly frequent complaint among OC users. Many women want their pills changed, or they simply stop taking them, for this reason. There is a deep conviction by some that a certain amount of bleeding is necessary for good health. Moreover, if a woman is not told to expect a light flow, she often fears that she is pregnant and stops taking her pills . . . and thus becomes pregnant.

Hypomenorrhea is fairly common when OCs with potent antiestrogenic progestins such as norgestrel (Ovral) and norethindrone acetate (Norlestrin) are used. The low-dose pills, with 0.05 mg or less, also produce diminished bleeding. About 1 percent of women will have amenorrhea while taking these low-dose pills because the estrogen content is too low to support endometrial growth (24). This condition is not dangerous.

Low-dose pills produce more breakthrough bleeding than the higher-dose combination pills. Irregular bleeding usually disappears by the third cycle, as the endometrium readjusts from its thick state to the relatively thin state induced by the hormones in the OCs (24). Nonetheless, users should always be carefully questioned regarding their pill-taking schedule. The spotting may be caused by missed pills, and counseling is needed, rather than a change of pills. A second type of breakthrough bleeding can occur after many months of pill use and is caused by progestin-induced deciduation (that is, the endometrium is fragile because it is shallow).

Ortho-Novum 10/11 (see Table 21.1) is the first of the phasic OCs. Although the estrogen level remains constant at a low dose throughout the cycle, the progestin level increases. Breakthrough bleeding and spotting

Table 21.3
First-Year Failure Rates of Birth Control Methods

Method	Lowest Observed Failure Rate*	Failure Rate in Typical Users†
Tubal ligation	0.4	0.4
Vasectomy	0.4	0.4
Injectable progestin	0.25	0.25
Combined birth control pills	0.5	2
Progestin-only pill	1	2.5
IUD	1.5	5
Condom	2	10
Diaphragm (with spermicide)	2	10
Sponge (with spermicide)	9–11	10–20
Cervical cap	2	13
Foam, creams, jellies, and vaginal suppositories	3–5	18
Coitus interruptus	16	23
Fertility awareness techniques (basal body temperature, mucus method, calendar, and "rhythm")	2–20	24
Douche	—	40
Chance (no method of birth control)	90	90

*Designed to complete the sentence: "Of 100 women who start out the year using a given method, and who use it correctly and consistently, the lowest observed failure rate has been _____."

†Designed to complete the sentence: "Of 100 typical users who start out the year employing a given method, the number who will be pregnant by the end of the year will be _____."

Source: R. A. Hatcher et al. *Contraceptive Technology 1986–1987.* 13th rev. ed. New York: Irvington Publishers, 1986, 102.

is also a problem with this pill. The latest OCs, the triphasics (see Table 21.1), are also low-dose estrogen pills, with less progestin in three varying amounts. Although there are fewer metabolic effects related to the progestin in these triphasics, spotting and breakthrough bleeding are the same or even slightly increased over the popular low-dose combination OCs (10).

Doubling up on pills to correct either type of breakthrough bleeding is seldom effective and often confuses pill schedules. This is especially true for those who are on the "Sunday schedule," which is explained later in this section, or those who take the triphasic pills. If the problem of breakthrough bleeding is unacceptable, the recommended therapy is to change to a pill with more estrogen (10, 24).

Mini-pills always produce changes in the menstrual cycle. Bleeding is frequently very unpredictable. In fact, the most common reasons for discontinuing this type of pill are irregular bleeding and lack of cycle control. The mini-pill may, nevertheless, be a good choice for women who cannot take estrogen.

Contraindications

Although combined OCs are safe contraceptives for most women, they are not appropriate for every woman. Absolute contraindications for these pills include a history of thromboembolic disorder, cerebrovascular accident, or coronary artery disease; liver dysfunction, including hepatic adenoma; pill-related migraine headaches; undiagnosed breast masses; known or suspected estrogen-dependent neoplasms; known pregnancy; hypertension (diastolic 90 or above on three sep-

Table 21.4
Oral Contraceptive Side Effects: Hormone Etiology

Estrogen		Androgen	Progestin	
Excess	Deficiency	Excess	Excess	Deficiency
Nausea, vomiting	Irritability, nervousness	Increased appetite	Increased appetite	Late breakthrough
Edema, leg cramps	Hot flashes	Hirsutism	Steady weight gain	bleeding
Vertigo	Early and midcycle	Oily skin, acne, rash	Tiredness, fatigue	Heavy flow and
Fluid retention	spotting	Increased libido	Depression, change in	clots
Cyclic weight gain	Hypomenorrhea	Cholestatic jaundice	libido	Delayed onset of
Headache	Amenorrhea		Oily scalp, acne	flow
Breast tenderness,			Loss of hair	
enlargement			Decreased length of	
Chloasma			menstrual flow	
Leukorrhea			Decreased vaginal	
Increase in			secretions	
leiomyoma size			Headache	
Uterine cramps			Breast tenderness,	
Contact lenses don't			enlargement	
fit			Hypertension (?)	
Thromboembolic			Cholestatic jaundice	
disorders				
Hypertension (?)				

arate visits, or 110 or above on a single visit); and undiagnosed abnormal vaginal bleeding (10, 11, 13).

There has been much publicity in recent years regarding the relationship between OCs, smoking, and vascular disease (5, 16, 17, 21, 24). It is therefore prudent to use the lowest acceptable dose of estrogen to reduce this risk. The consensus is that women over thirty who smoke and are at risk because of hypertension, diabetes, obesity, or elevated lipids and lipoproteins, or who have a strong family history of coronary artery disease, probably should not use combination OCs. Certainly those over forty who smoke or are at risk should not do so.

It appears that the low-dose pills containing less than 0.05 mg of estrogen, or the mini-pill can be used by some diabetics with few changes in their glucose metabolism (22, 23). From a medical standpoint, however, OCs are not the contraceptive of choice for diabetics but may be used when these women cannot or will not use other contraceptives.

Women with previous histories of irregular menstrual cycles, as well as sexually inactive young teenagers, should *not* be given OCs to regulate their periods. Such women have hypothalamic-pituitary-ovarian dysfunc-

tion or, in the case of young teens, immature development of this pathway. OCs will suppress this system rather than correct any endocrine disorder.

Blood pressures should be routinely taken every six months for women taking OCs. Less than 5 percent have developed blood pressure readings above 140/90 in the large studies that have been done in the United States and England, and any increase is usually mild and reversible (11).

Other conditions, listed in Table 21.5, may be relative contraindications for using OCs. In addition, OCs should be discontinued at least four weeks before any type of surgery that will involve an increased risk of blood clotting or prolonged bed rest, because the estrogen in OCs increases the risk of blood clots.

Patient Teaching

Because there are so many OCs, each with different packaging and schedules, patient teaching is of prime importance. One should never assume that a woman will understand how to take the OCs correctly. Many women have been on several different kinds of pills and

Table 21.5
Checklist for Oral Contraceptive Users

History

Menstrual

- Last menstrual period
- Dysmenorrhea
- Hypermenorrhea
- Hypomenorrhea
- Irregularity
- Premenstrual tension

Pregnancy

- Reproductive outcome
- Infertility
- Presently nursing
- Chloasma
- Gestational diabetes
- Jaundice
- Toxemia

Overall

- Acne
- Breast cancer
- Diabetes mellitus
- Epilepsy
- Gallbladder disease
- Hyperlipemia
- Hypertension
- Liver disease
- Migraine disease
- Severe depression
- Sickle cell disease
- Thrombophlebitis
- Cervical/Uterine cancer
- Uterine myomata
- Hyperthyroidism
- Contact lenses
- Previous trouble with pills
- Recurrent yeast infections

Examination

Physical Examination

- Blood pressure
- Weight
- Thyroid palpation
- Heart, lungs auscultation
- Breast examination
- Abdominal palpation
- Pelvic examination
- Skin examination
- Peripheral vascular status

Laboratory

Most Patients

- Cervical pap smear
- Cervical gonococcal culture
- Serology
- Blood count
- Urinalysis

Some Patients

- Glucose tolerance
- Lipid profile

have used various schedules. For example, if the woman is not told that the last seven pills in a twenty-eight-day pill package are placebos, she may very well take all twenty-eight pills and then stop for seven days. The triphasic pills, which are three and four different colors, have added to patient confusion.

Because so many OCs are now designed to be started on a Sunday, I recommend teaching the "Sunday sched-ule" to all women taking twenty-one- or twenty-eight-day pills. The initial cycle of pills is started the first Sunday after menses or first trimester abortion. It is usually wise to wait until the second Sunday after delivery to begin pills for postpartum patients who are not breast-feeding, owing to their greater amount of bleeding. Not only is the Sunday schedule easy to remember, but it has an extra bonus: there is never bleeding on a weekend, when women are more apt to be active.

Abortion facilities continue to report a number of clients who have been taken off OCs to allow their bodies to "rest." Unfortunately they often believe that they cannot get pregnant easily or are offered little or no alternate contraceptive information. This situation is appalling and should not occur.

Summary

Because of their convenience and, most of all, their high degree of effectiveness, OCs will probably continue to be the most popular form of reversible contraception. With careful screening to determine women who are at risk, individualized selection of the lowest acceptable dosage for each patient, and periodic follow-up to detect problems, nurses can help ensure that OCs will be as safe as they are convenient and effective.

Hormonal Postcoital Contraceptives

There is currently no perfect "morning-after" pill—nor is there likely to ever be one. Modern technology has, however, developed several options for those women who have been exposed to one episode of unprotected intercourse during a single cycle. Hormonal postcoital contraceptives are discussed in this section, and postcoital intrauterine device (IUD) insertion is included under IUDs.

Combination Oral Contraceptives

Recent studies have shown that Ovral can be used for postcoital contraception. Two Ovral tablets are taken within seventy-two hours of intercourse and two more are taken twelve hours later. Studies have demonstrated a failure rate of less than 2 percent. There are few adverse side effects, such as nausea, and although there is no *absolute* proof of complete safety to either the woman or the offspring if she should be pregnant, thousands of women have taken comparable dosages of

Ovral in a different situation: if a woman who has been using Ovral as her regular OC misses two consecutive tablets, she doubles up and takes two tablets right away and two tablets the next day (10). So it would appear that this pill has a high degree of safety and effectiveness.

High-Dose Oral Estrogens

High doses of estrogens taken for five days have been used as postcoital contraceptives since the 1960s. Nausea is more of a problem with estrogens than with Ovral, which is taken for a shorter period of time and at a lower dose. Antiemetic drugs are frequently necessary when taking estrogens in this manner. As with Ovral, the high-dose oral estrogens must be started within seventy-two hours; they are more effective if started within twenty-four hours after intercourse (10).

High-Dose Progestins

Several progestins have been used as postcoital contraceptives in research centers. They may be available for more widespread use in the near future.

Mifepristone (RU 486)

The newest postcoital contraceptive, RU 486, is being called the "abortion pill" by the news media. It contains a steroid compound that blocks the body's use of the hormone progesterone, thus inducing the shedding of the endometrium. It is 85 percent effective if taken within ten days of a missed menses. It occasionally causes prolonged uterine bleeding that requires medical intervention. This drug is expected to be approved for general use in France and Sweden in 1987 but will probably not be released in the United States for several years.

Long-Acting Progestin Injections

The most commonly used injectable progestins being used for contraception are medroxyprogesterone acetate (Depo-Provera) and norethindrone enanthate (Noristerat). Although these medications are being used in more than eighty countries, the U.S. Food and Drug Administration (FDA) has yet to grant approval for their use as a contraceptive (10). (They are, however, approved by the FDA for treating bleeding disorders.)

Injectable progestins are highly effective in preventing pregnancy and have to be given only two or four times a year. Their chief disadvantage is that they seriously disrupt the menstrual cycle; irregular menses with amenorrhea is common. In addition, the return of fertility after discontinuation may be delayed. If these drugs are approved for contraceptive use in the United States, they will be used mostly by women in their late childbearing years who want no additional children.

Intrauterine Devices

The 1980s have seen the rapid demise of IUDs in the United States. The Dalcon Shield was removed from the market by the FDA in 1975. Schmid stopped production of its Saf-T-Coil in 1982 for economic, not medical, reasons. Lippes Loops were marketed until 1985. Then, in 1986, G. D. Searle & Co. withdrew its Tatum-T and Copper-7 (CU-7) from the market because of costs stemming from lawsuits. Litigation has made future product liability insurance virtually unobtainable.

The Progestasert-T is the only IUD currently being marketed in the United States. However, since millions of U.S. women still have the other IUDs, and since this form of contraception is more popular worldwide than even oral contraceptives, material will be presented.

Reports in the lay and medical press associating IUDs with serious morbidity and mortality have created the impression that this form of contraception should be avoided. However, the risks involved with IUDs are of a low order of magnitude, both in absolute terms and when weighed against the benefits for its users. For reversible contraception, IUDs are second only to OCs in effectiveness. IUDs have no untoward systemic effects and have the advantage of being coitus-independent. Over time IUDs are also less expensive than OCs.

The two basic categories of IUDs are nonmedicated and medicated. All are biologically active, since they create a change in the endometrium and the endometrial environment. The presence of an IUD results in endometrial infiltration by leukocytes, which produces an endometrial environment that is spermicidal and blastotoxic and inhibits implantation (12). IUDs also probably increase local production of prostaglandins, which also inhibits implantation (10).

Nonmedicated IUDs are made of a soft plastic. The two available for general use in the United States were the Lippes Loop and the Saf-T-Coil. Medicated IUDs were the Copper-7 (Gravigard) and the Copper-T

(Tatum-T). The Progestasert-T is still being marketed in the United States.

Medicated IUDs are slightly more effective than non-medicated IUDs but must be replaced at definite intervals (Table 21.6). Copper IUDs have a fine copper wire wrapped around the plastic stem, which increases the device's effectiveness. There is, however, no systemic effect. The Progestasert-T contains the natural hormone progesterone in its upright stem. The constant release of this hormone increases the effectiveness by means of a local effect on the endometrium.

Timing and Factors to Consider

The single most important factor to consider when choosing an IUD is the competence of the nurse or physician who inserts it and his or her familiarity with the IUD selected. For women who do not have a regular physician, family planning and Planned Parenthood clinics would be good choices. A careful history should be taken and an examination and appropriate laboratory tests must be done (Table 21.7) before the IUD is inserted.

Some conditions may contraindicate the use of an

Table 21.6
Comparing Intrauterine Devices

Nonmedicated	Medicated
Lippes Loop/Saf-T-Coil	*Copper-7/Copper-T*
• High effectiveness	• Higher effectiveness
• Low serious side effects	• Better acceptance among nulliparas owing to less insertion pain
• Higher degree of use	• Less cramping and blood loss
• Several sizes available	• Postcoital contraceptive
• Ease of insertion	• Replacement every 2 to 3 years
• No periodic replacement	• Higher cost
• Low cost	*Progestasert-T*
	• Higher effectiveness
	• Less menstrual loss than with Cu-7 but more spotting
	• Less dysmenorrhea
	• Replacement every year
	• Highest cost of all IUDs

Table 21.7
Checklist for Intrauterine Device Use

History	
Menstrual	*Gynecological*
• Last menstrual period	• Recurrent pelvic infection
• Dysmenorrhea, severe*	• Recent pelvic infection
• Hypermenorrhea	• Multiple sexual partners
• Polymenorrhea	• Ectopic pregnancy
• Abnormal uterine bleeding	• Valvular heart disease
	• Abnormal Pap smear
	Overall
	• Anemia
	• Allergy to copper

Examination	Laboratory
Pelvic Examination	*All Patients*
• Pregnancy	• Cervical Pap smear
• Acute cervicitis	• Cervical gonococcal culture
• Cervical stenosis	• Serology
• Very small uterus	• Hemoglobin/Hematocrit
• Bicornuate uterus	
• Endometriosis	*Some Patients*
• Endometrial polyps	• Sedimentation rate
• Uterine myomata	• Rapid pregnancy test

*May not contraindicate Progestasert-T.

IUD, while others must be treated before one is inserted. Absolute contraindications include women with recurrent or recent pelvic infection (not vaginal infection), a previous ectopic pregnancy in women wanting future pregnancy, valvular heart disease, or known or suspected pregnancy. Because of the increase in menstrual bleeding with IUDs, women with anemia, endometriosis, or endometrial myomata also should not use these devices. The cause of such problems as hypermenorrhea, polymenorrhea, other types of abnormal uterine bleeding, polyps, and abnormal Pap smears should be found and treated before IUD insertion is considered (12).

The ideal time to insert an IUD is during the menstrual period. This helps assure that the woman is not pregnant; in addition, the cervical canal is more patent at this time, which makes insertion easier.

For safety and to reduce expulsion, most IUDs should be inserted eight to twelve weeks postpartum and a full twelve weeks after a cesarean section (12). The copper IUDs can be inserted earlier (four to eight weeks postpartum) without concern for increased risk of expulsion (18). Although some clinicians insert an IUD immediately after first trimester-induced abortion, others prefer to wait two to three weeks, or until the next menstrual period. Many clinicians prefer to wait a full month after removing an IUD before inserting a second one (the concern is one of infection). They may also want to wait at least three months and have a normal sedimentation rate after any episode of proven pelvic inflammatory disease (PID) (10, 18).

Side Effects

A woman who is considering having an IUD inserted should be told of the probability of increased menstrual bleeding and intermenstrual spotting. Approximately 15 percent of women will have their IUDs removed for these reasons. Iron supplementation is probably wise for all IUD users.

Cramping and pain are fairly common side effects of IUDs, especially in nulliparous women, owing to their smaller uteri and tighter cervical openings. Insertion pain can be reduced by the use of a paracervical block. Nulliparous women report less cramping with the Copper-7, and the Progestasert-T may actually decrease cramping during the menstrual cycle.

Partial or complete expulsion of the IUD may also occur. Each user must learn how to check for the device's string and be told that if ever she cannot feel it or it suddenly feels longer, she should use another method of contraception, such as condoms and spermicides, until the IUD has been checked by a clinician. A follow-up visit after insertion should be scheduled after the next menstrual cycle, since most problems related to expulsion occur during this time.

Complications and Risks

There are three especially serious complications or potential risks associated with IUD use: uterine and cervical perforation, infection, and pregnancy (failed IUD).

Although uncommon, perforation usually occurs at the time of insertion. Perforation is generally related to the experience of the clinician, which is why it is important to have the IUD inserted by someone who is familiar with the particular device. Cervical perforation may occur as an IUD is being expelled. Fortunately the availability of ultrasound and laparoscopy has greatly aided in the management of such complications (14).

Studies have provided strong evidence that IUD users are more likely than nonusers to develop pelvic inflammatory disease (PID). PID is the most serious complication related to IUD use. Nulliparous women under the age of twenty-five who have a history of PID and those with multiple sexual partners are most likely to develop PID with or without an IUD. Therefore, women with IUDs should immediately report the following symptoms: new development of menstrual disorders, abnormal vaginal discharge, fever, chills, abdominal or pelvic pain, and dyspareunia. If PID is suspected, the IUD should be removed (14).

Although the failure rate for IUDs is low, every potential user must understand what is likely to happen if she should become pregnant with an IUD in place. The chances of a spontaneous abortion occurring with the IUD in the correct position are approximately 50 percent. If the string is visible, a nontraumatic removal of the IUD will reduce the chances to 25 to 30 percent. However, women must be told that a therapeutic abortion should be considered because of the risk of serious infection with the IUD in place and the high percentage (5 percent) of such pregnancies being ectopic. "Flu-like symptoms plus pregnancy in a woman with an IUD very likely mean sepsis. Think 'sepsis' not 'flu' when a pregnant woman with an IUD presents with fever, chills, myalgia and headaches" (10).

Patient Teaching

Because some women have a fair amount of pain or nausea immediately after IUD insertion, they should arrange to have someone take them home, rather than come to the health center alone. And if the cramping is not relieved by rest, a heating pad, or over-the-counter analgesics, they may have the IUD removed.

The woman should learn how to feel the strings that protrude two inches or so into the vagina before leaving the health center. She should be told to check for the strings frequently during the first months postinsertion and then after each period or any time she has abnormal cramping while menstruating. Menstrual pads and tampons should also be checked because expulsion is more likely to occur during menses.

It is wise to use a second method of contraception, such as condoms and spermicide, for the first few months after IUD insertion. This adds extra protection during the time when most expulsions occur. Many women will want to always add a second method of contraception to midcycle, to increase the overall effectiveness.

If a woman misses a period, or thinks she may be pregnant, she should seek medical assistance immediately.

The user should, of course, learn the IUD danger signals, described earlier.

Postcoital IUD Contraception

The Copper-T and the Copper-7 were the IUDs of choice for postcoital contraception. As with hormonal morning-after contraceptives, IUDs used in this manner were intended for those women who had one episode of unprotected intercourse during any single cycle. The copper IUD needed to be inserted within five days—preferably before then—in order to prevent implantation (10). IUDs should not be placed in women who may already be pregnant.

Postcoital IUD insertion, especially with the Copper-7, has been used extensively with rape victims. However, a word of caution is necessary. When the risk of sexually transmissible infection is high, the benefits of using an IUD instead of hormonal morning-after contraceptives must be carefully considered.

Barrier Methods and Spermicides

The Condom

The most commonly used mechanical barrier contraceptive is the condom, also called a sheath, skin, safe, prophylactic, or rubber. Condoms are made of rubber, processed collagenous tissue, or skin from the caecum of young lamb intestines. They fit over the erect penis and act as a barrier to the transmission of semen into the vagina. Rubber condoms are straight-sided or tapered, lubricated or nonlubricated (wet jellies or dry powders). Some have nipple tips (safety reservoirs) to hold the semen. Condoms are available in a variety of colors.

The condom currently represents the only reliable contraceptive, short of vasectomy, in which the male has the responsibility for prevention of pregnancy. A properly used high-quality condom can be as much as 80 to 90 percent effective. The use effectiveness rate approaches that of OCs when a vaginal spermicide is used with the condom (10).

Side Effects and Complications. A small number of men and women are allergic to rubber and should therefore use another type of condom. The major complaint of condom users is decreased sensation in the male; some men are unable to enjoy intercourse and may even be unable to maintain an erection. Condom application can be made part of the sexual foreplay. This should be stressed, since many couples feel that condoms detract from rather than enhance intercourse (13).

Noncontraceptive Benefits. Besides providing protection from pregnancy, the condom has the following benefits:

- Condoms are used in the treatment of premature ejaculation, since they reduce glans sensitivity. Further, the slight tourniquet effect helps some men to maintain an erection for a longer period of time.
- Some infertility problems are caused by antibody formation to the partner's sperm. Condoms prevent the release of sperm antigens into the vagina, which results in lowered antibody titre.
- The condom provides protection against some sexually transmitted diseases that cause infertility and may reduce the incidence of cervical cancer in some women. The use of condoms is highly recommended to help reduce the spread of acquired immunodeficiency syndrome.
- Condoms are inexpensive and easily accessible to sexually active teenagers (10).

Patient Teaching. When instructing in the use of the condom, one must caution that it should be rolled onto the erect penis *before* penile-vaginal contact. Withdrawing the penis before ejaculation and then using a condom is not only risky and unsatisfying; it also does not provide contraception, since the preejaculate fluid contains sperm. One-half inch of empty space must be left in the tip. The penis should be withdrawn soon after ejaculation to prevent semen spillage; the man should hold onto the condom during withdrawal. If the condom tears or comes off in the vagina, contraceptive spermicide should immediately be used.

Condoms will remain in good condition for about five years if they are stored in a cool, dry place. They should not be carried around in a wallet, as body heat can cause the rubber to deteriorate. Petroleum jelly (Vaseline) should *never* be used with a condom, since it will also cause the rubber to deteriorate and break. Acceptable lubricants include contraceptive spermicides, K-Y Jelly, and saliva.

Vaginal Spermicides

Spermicidal preparations are available as foams, creams, jellies, suppositories, or tablets. All consist of an inert base, which holds the spermicidal agent in the vagina, against the cervix. The chemical effect of the spermicidal agent immobilizes and kills sperm. Some spermicides are designed to be used alone, such as foam, suppositories, and tablets, whereas others are to be used with diaphragms and cervical caps.

Effectiveness rates are difficult to state because of the wide gap between average-user effectiveness and perfect-user effectiveness. Used alone, spermicides average no higher than 60 to 70 percent effective (13, 15). One should not become disinterested in this type of contraception because of its lower effectiveness rate. Spermicides are safe to use, available without a prescription, and inexpensive. Furthermore, they provide a high degree of effectiveness when used with condoms, and they are an excellent backup method for OCs and IUDs.

Side Effects and Complications.   A small percentage of men and women are allergic to this chemical method of contraception and experience burning, itching, or a rash. Couples who have oral-genital sex note that these chemicals have an unpleasant taste. Sometimes suppositories and tablets fail to melt or foam completely (10, 13).

Noncontraceptive Benefits.   Noncontraceptive benefits include the following:

- The use of chemical and barrier contraceptives is associated with a lower incidence of cervical gonorrhea. Foams have proved to be gonococcidal in in vitro studies; this may stem from their ability to lower vaginal pH (15).
- Most vaginal spermicides inhibit the growth of *Candida albicans* (yeast) and *Trichomonas vaginalis*.
- Recent research has shown that spermicides may play a major role in inhibiting the transmission of herpes virus (15).
- Spermicides provide vaginal lubrication.

Patient Teaching.   Every man and woman should be taught to use condoms and spermicides effectively, as this is the very essence of self-care. It is important to read the labels carefully when choosing a vaginal spermicide. Some are intended to be used alone, and others are intended for use with diaphragms or cervical caps. Consumers also need to be cautioned about confusing one of the feminine hygiene products or K-Y Jelly with spermicides, as they are usually stocked next to one another in pharmacies.

Following the instructions listed below will increase the effectiveness of vaginal spermicides:

- The manufacturer's instructions should be carefully read. The woman should practice using the product before she needs it.
- The correct amount of spermicide should be inserted: one full applicator of Emko (17 ml), Emko Pre-fil (10 ml), Because (17 ml), or Dalkon (17 ml), or *two* full applicators of Delfen (10 ml) or Koromex (10 ml) (10).
- Spermicides must be used before intercourse—the couple should not practice withdrawal—but should not be inserted more than twenty to thirty minutes before intercourse. They are also more effective if the woman remains in a horizontal position.
- If the couple has intercourse again, more spermicide should be inserted.
- If the woman must douche, she should not do so for at least eight hours after the last act of intercourse.

The Diaphragm

The diaphragm is a dome-shaped rubber cap surrounding a flexible metal rim. The three most commonly used diaphragms are the arching spring, the coil spring, and the flat spring. All types come in a variety of sizes. When the diaphragm is correctly placed, it rests anteriorly against the soft tissues posterior to the symphysis pubis, posteriorly within the posterior vaginal fornix, and laterally against the vaginal walls (Figure 21.1) (8).

It should be used with contraceptive jelly or cream made especially for use with diaphragms. Foams should not be used; they may damage the rubber and do not provide an adequate sealant.

The diaphragm is an excellent contraceptive method for those women who cannot or do not want to use OCs or IUDs. Although the diaphragm has recently become more popular with consumers and nurse practitioners, the medical profession in general does not promote this method (1, 7, 8). Many physicians have had little actual experience in fitting diaphragms, and even if they do have experience, they may consider the time required for proper instruction of the patient excessive and uneconomical (10).

The theoretical effectiveness rate of the diaphragm is 97 percent; the actual effectiveness rate is 83 percent. The lower actual-use effectiveness rate can be attributed

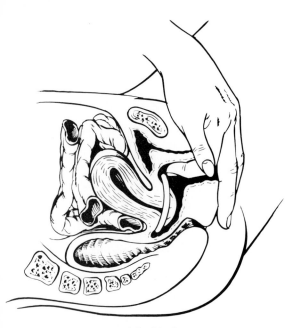

Figure 21.1. Placement of the Diaphragm

to misuse of the diaphragm because of inadequate instruction in its proper use (7).

Side Effects and Complications. Hypersensitivity to either rubber or spermicides would contraindicate the use of diaphragms. In addition, uterine prolapse, cystocele, rectocele, and other vaginal-uterine abnormalities may make diaphragm fitting difficult or impossible (8). Women who have recurrent urinary tract infections should probably not use the diaphragm, as there is some indication that diaphragm users develop cystitis and urethritis more frequently than do women who use other contraceptives (10).

Noncontraceptive Benefits. As with other barrier methods, the diaphragm used with spermicide grants some protection against sexually transmissible infections. And this method may be used during menses to provide a barrier so that blood does not escape during intercourse.

Patient Teaching. Personal experience as a nurse practitioner supports the viewpoint that proper teaching and fitting for a diaphragm requires more time than most other contraceptive methods. One should expect to spend at least an hour for the initial visit. Several follow-up visits are essential if the diaphragm is to be used effectively.

The instructions for using the diaphragm are complex and lengthy and will not be given here. Rather, the reader is referred to either of the excellent articles by Gara or Gorline (7, 8). The success of the diaphragm depends to a great extent on proper instruction.

The Cervical Cap

The cervical cap is generating interest (2, 3, 9). This "miniature diaphragm with a tall dome" (10) is a thimble-shaped cup that fits over the cervix and is held in place by suction between its rim and the surface of the cervix. Although popular in Europe, the cervical cap is currently available in the United States through a limited number of centers that are specially licensed to distribute it. (An informational packet about the cervical cap is available from the National Women's Health Network, 224 7th Street S.E., Washington, D.C. 20003, for $5.00. It includes a list of known providers.)

The advantages and disadvantages of the cervical cap are outlined in Table 21.8. With thorough client instruction, time for proper fitting, and practice with follow-up, the cervical cap is an effective method of contraception (3). It remains to be seen whether this method will gain widespread use in the United States.

Vaginal Sponge

The vaginal contraceptive sponge, is a soft, disposable polyurethane foam sponge that contains a spermicide. It can be inserted up to twenty-four hours before coitus and should be left in place for six hours after last intercourse. This type of barrier method prevents pregnancy in three ways: (a) the spermicide kills sperm; (b) the sponge blocks the cervix; and (c) the sponge traps and absorbs the sperm. Its effectiveness approaches that of the diaphragm (10). One important advantage is that it may be purchased over the counter.

Natural Family Planning Methods

Natural family planning methods (also called "fertility awareness") (10) include rhythm, the basal body temperature method, the cervical mucus method (ovulation or Billings method), and the symptothermal method. All of these methods educate people about the normal changes that occur in fertile women.

These methods help to identify a number of signals of cyclic fertility. A record of menstrual dates, basal body temperature patterns, mittelschmerz (pain at ovulation),

Table 21.8
Advantages and Disadvantages of the Cervical Cap

Advantages	Rationale
1. Does not require daily client involvement	1. Cap can be left in place up to 7 days provided it retains contraceptive cream
2. Woman learns more about her body	2. Teaching the woman requires that she identify her cervix
3. Nonhormonal and noninvasive	3. Cap is applied to the exterior of the cervix
4. Convenient for coitus and foreplay	4. Nothing is required of either the woman or her partner at this time
5. Oral sex more enjoyable than with other barrier methods	5. No spermicidal creams or jellies in the vagina

Disadvantages	Rationale
1. Not all women can be safely fitted at present	1. Depends on the angle, shape, and size of cervix
2. Not manufactured in USA	2. May not be cost effective since it is expensive to import
3. Lack of knowledgeable health care providers	3. Few are aware of the cervical cap and fewer can fit them correctly
4. Time it takes to teach this method ranges from 30–90 minutes	4. Depends on many variables: woman's comfort with her own body and sexuality, her manual dexterity, and her motivation
5. Usage depends on individual female's anatomy	5. Short fingers and long vaginas make it very difficult for some women to use the cap

Source: D. A. Canavan and C. A. Lewis. "The Cervical Cap: An Alternative Contraceptive." *JOGN Nursing* 10:271, 1981.

cervical mucus pattern and ferning, spotting, breast tenderness, and position and consistency of the cervix are signals that many women can relate to their own menstrual cycles (6, 10, 20). All of these methods are aimed at predicting the time of ovulation and the fertile days of the menstrual cycle. The advantages and disadvantages of natural family planning methods are outlined in Table 21.9.

The amount of information necessary to fully understand each of these methods is beyond the scope of this chapter. The reader is referred to the texts by Hatcher (10) and Nofziger (20) for detailed information and instruction on each of these methods.

Unreliable Methods of Contraception

Some techniques that are used to prevent conception are totally unreliable. Included among these are withdrawal (coitus interruptus), douching, various positions during intercourse, and homemade preparations.

Withdrawal fails because the preejaculate of the man contains sperm. This method is also less than satisfying to both parties involved. And although the man may intend to remove the penis before ejaculation, this is often physically and emotionally impossible.

Douching with any preparation immediately after intercourse is a losing race for the woman. Sperm will be inside the uterus before she reaches the bathroom, since sperm travel their course in about ninety seconds. The flow of the douche fluid toward the cervix may even hasten the transport of the sperm toward the uterus (13). In addition, many women do not know how to douche correctly. They do not hold the labia closed around the douche tip to allow the fluid to "unfold" the vaginal rugae. And last, products intended for douching are not necessarily spermicidal. Folk methods that involve the use of such substances as Clorox and Lysol can damage the vaginal mucosa.

Sterilization

Sterilization refers to surgery that is performed to prevent the fertilization of an ovum. Such surgery can be performed on a man or a woman and is almost always

Table 21.9
Fertility Awareness Methods

Advantages	Disadvantages
1. Safe	1. Must keep extensive records for several cycles before you can use method.
2. Free or inexpensive	2. Require substantial initial and some ongoing counseling
3. Acceptable to many religious groups that oppose other contraceptive methods	3. May restrict sexual spontaneity.
4. Extremely helpful either for planning or avoiding pregnancy	4. Some women are unable to identify clearcut cervical mucus and BBT* patterns even with diligent charting
5. Teach women (and sometimes men) about the menstrual cycle	5. Should pregnancy occur, risk is somewhat greater that an old egg will have been fertilized
6. Acceptable method of teaching teenagers about reproductive physiology in sex education programs (noncontroversial)	6. Women with irregular cycles may have difficulty with the calendar and BBT* techniques.
7. Encourage couples to communicate about family planning	

*Basal body temperature.
Source: R. A. Hatcher et al. *Contraceptive Technology 1986–1987.* 13th rev. ed. New York: Irvington Publishers, 1986, 240.

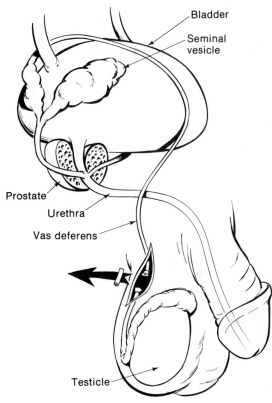

Figure 21.2. Vasectomy

irreversible. Virtually 100 percent effective, sterilization is the most commonly used method of fertility control for married couples in the United States who are over thirty years of age.

Vasectomy, the sterilization operation for men that blocks the vas deferens to prevent the passage of sperm, is a simple procedure that is often done in a physician's office under local anesthesia. Through small scrotal incisions each vas deferens is identified and ligated at two points, with transection between the points of ligature (Figure 21.2). The cut ends are usually cauterized (19).

Nearly all operations intended to sterilize women interrupt the continuity of the fallopian tubes. Tubal ligation can be accomplished by ligation with sutures, coag-

ulation, or mechanical blocking with clips, bands, or rings. These procedures can be done through the abdomen or through the vagina. If a significant pathological condition of the uterus coexists with a desire for sterilization, hysterectomy may be performed.

The permanence of these methods makes them undesirable for some people, especially those who maintain a large part of their identity through the fact that they know they are capable of reproducing.

DISCUSSION QUESTIONS

1. Consider how you would increase the self-care ability of a woman who wanted to use effective contraception. What type of questions would be appropriate to ask?

2. Mrs. Shafer is a thirty-five-year-old mother of three. She has been taking an oral contraceptive for the past five years. On her visit to the office today she asks, "I'm tired of taking these pills. I don't want

any more children. What should I do?" What choices does she have? Should she continue to take pills?

3. You find your fifteen-year-old sister crying. She tells you that she has been having intercourse with her boyfriend the past few months. She is crying because she is fearful of getting pregnant and does not know if "those rubbers are any good or not." What do you say to her? Do you think she will stop having sex?

4. Your best friend has recently broken up with her boyfriend. In an attempt to prove her desirability, she has been dating and having intercourse with several men. When you go to visit her one evening, you find her ill. She says, "Oh, I only have the flu. I am running a bit of a fever and have cramps." She has had an IUD for over a year and has had no problems with it. What do you do?

REFERENCES

1. Berlin, L. E., W. H. Dotterer, and E. S. Henriques. "Increase in Diaphragm Use in a University Population." *JOGN Nursing* 8:280, 1979.

2. Canavan, D. A., and C. A. Lewis. "The Cervical Cap: An Alternative Contraceptive." *JOGN Nursing* 10:271, 1981.

3. Cappiello, J. D., and M. Grainger–Harrison. "The Rebirth of the Cervical Cap." *Journal of Nurse-Midwifery* 26:13, 1981.

4. Cuckle, H. S., and N. J. Wald. "Evidence Against Oral Contraceptives as a Cause of Neural-Tube Defects." *Obstetrics and Gynecology* 59:547, 1982.

5. Darney, P. D. "What's New in Contraceptives?" *Contemporary Ob/Gyn.* 19:81, 1982.

6. Deibel, P. "Natural Family Planning: Different Methods." *American Journal of Maternal Child Nursing* 3:171, 1978.

7. Gara, E. "Nursing Protocol to Improve the Effectiveness of the Contraceptive Diaphragm." *American Journal of Maternal Child Nursing* 6:41, 1981.

8. Gorline, L. L. "Teaching Successful Use of the Diaphragm." *American Journal of Nursing* 79:1732, 1979.

9. Hastings-Tolsma, M. T. "The Cervical Cap: A Barrier Contraceptive." *American Journal of Maternal Child Nursing* 7:382, 1982.

10. Hatcher, R. A., et al. *Contraceptive Technology 1986–1987.* 13th rev. ed. New York: Irvington Publishers, 1986.

11. Huxall, L. K. "Today's Pill and the Individual Woman." *American Journal of Maternal Child Nursing* 2:359, 1977.

12. Huxall, L. K. "Update on IUDs." *American Journal of Maternal Child Nursing* 5:186, 1980.

13. Huxall, L. K., and S. Sawyer. "Counseling Regarding Birth Control Methods." In *Human Sexuality for Health Professionals,* ed. M. U. Barnard, B. J. Clancy, and K. E. Krantz. Philadelphia: W. B. Saunders, 1978.

14. Keith, L. G., G. S. Berger, and D. A. Edelman. "Clinician's Guide to Using IUDs Safely." *Contemporary Ob/Gyn.* 19:159, 1982.

15. Keith, L. G., G. S. Berger, and M. A. Jackson. "Perspective on Vaginal Contraception: A Method for the 1980s." *Contemporary Ob/Gyn.* 19:63, 1982.

16. Meade, T. W. "Effects of Progestogens on the Cardiovascular System." *Obstetrics and Gynecology* 59:776, 1982.

17. Mishell, D. R., Jr. "Noncontraceptive Health Benefits of Oral Steroidal Contraceptives." *Obstetrics and Gynecology* 59:809, 1982.

18. Mishell, D. R., Jr., and A. Roy. "Copper Intrauterine Contraceptive Device Event Rates Following Insertion 4 to 8 Weeks Postpartum." *American Journal of Obstetrics and Gynecology* 143:29, 1982.

19. Niswander, K. R. *Manual of Obstetrics Diagnosis and Therapy.* Boston: Little, Brown, 1980.

20. Nofziger, M. *A Cooperative Method of Natural Birth Control.* 2nd rev. ed. Summertown, Tenn.: The Book Publishing Company, 1978.

21. Porter, J. B., et al. "Oral Contraceptives and Nonfatal Vascular Disease—Recent Experience." *Obstetrics and Gynecology* 59:299, 1982.

22. Skouby, S. O., L. Molsted–Pedersen, and C. Kuhl. "Low Dosage Oral Contraception in Women with Previous Gestational Diabetes." *Obstetrics and Gynecology* 59:325, 1982.

23. Spellacy, W. N. "Carbohydrate Metabolism During Treatment with Estrogen, Progestogen, and Low-Dose Oral Contraceptives." *Obstetrics and Gynecology* 59:732, 1982.

24. Speroff, L. "A Brief for Low-Dose Pills." *Contemporary Ob/Gyn.* 17:27, 1981.

CHAPTER 22

Breast-feeding

NANCY JACKSON

■

OBJECTIVES

After completing this chapter, the reader will be able to:

- Name two professional organizations that have stated their commitment to promote breast-feeding.
- State the position of the American Academy of Pediatrics' Committee on Nutrition on milk consumption during the first year of life.
- List five advantages of breast milk over formulas for infants.
- Compare breast milk with formula in regard to protein, fat, and immunoglobulins.
- State three myths about breast-feeding.
- List two factors highly related to successful breast-feeding.
- List the three most common reasons mothers stop breast-feeding and switch to infant formula.
- Define areola, colostrom, "let-down" reflex, tail of Spense, Montgomery's glands, and engorgement.
- Explain the physiology of lactation.
- Explain how the supply-and-demand concept applies to breast-feeding.

- Counsel an antepartal client and her partner on the decision of how to feed their newborn.
- Teach a new mother how to breast-feed, demonstrating comfortable positioning, use of rooting reflex, and ways to remove the baby from the breast.
- Counsel a new mother about common areas of concern related to breast-feeding, for example, role of father, use of medication while breast-feeding, engorgement, returning to work.
- Plan nursing intervention that would promote successful breast-feeding for a new mother.
- Plan nursing strategies at the community level that would promote breast-feeding.
- Identify areas related to breast-feeding and nursing care that need further research.
- Describe how breast-feeding promotes self-care in the new mother.
- Apply concepts of crisis intervention theory to a new mother attempting to breast-feed her infant.

Breast-feeding has been chosen as a topic for this text because it highlights the many roles of the primary nurse. Planning care, teaching, advocacy, and acting as a change agent are all important in giving primary nursing care to a new breast-feeding mother.

The breast-feeding mother can easily become lost in the bureaucracy and technology of the health care system today. Specialization has led to an obstetrician or midwife, and antepartal, labor and delivery, and post-partum nurses being responsible for the mother's care, while a pediatrician and newborn nursery nurse are responsible for the baby. The obstetrical health care providers are concerned about breast-feeding only so far as the mother's comfort and well-being are concerned; the pediatric health care providers may view breast-feeding from a nutritional angle and focus only on the baby. A primary nurse would look at the "whole picture" and see how the mother's needs and the baby's needs are inseparably bound.

Primary nursing involves caring and promoting self-care for clients, as well as for their families and communities. The primary nurse of the breast-feeding mother is responsible for planning the care that each client needs. This may involve teaching, shared decision making, and referrals to other resources to aid the client. Although every situation is different, depending on the individual client, the primary nurse's role as planner and coordinator of care remains the same.

Primary nursing for the breast-feeding mother may also include working as an advocate and a change agent to facilitate her care. Hospital practices such as routine medication administered during labor and delivery, separating the mother and baby immediately after birth, fixed four-hour feeding schedules, and hospital-distributed samples of infant formula all need to be examined to determine their effect on the individual breast-feeding mother.

In working with a new breast-feeding mother, the primary nurse may find her client in crisis. The new role of mother may prove overwhelming to her. The primary nurse should assess coping skills and may need to help the mother develop new coping mechanisms to avert a crisis. The primary nurse can help the mother gain a realistic perception of her new situation, mobilize supports (partner, friends, relatives, lay groups that support breast-feeding), and regain equilibrium. Because these goals cannot all be accomplished during a brief hospitalization, referral and follow-ups are often necessary.

Teaching a new mother to breast-feed is a wonderful example of promoting self-care. For as a mother learns how her breast functions and how to nurture her child, she is also learning about herself and how to care for her own body.

Nurses meet potential nursing mothers in a variety of settings. Because women often decide in the first trimester, or even before they are pregnant, how they will feed their babies, it is never too early to bring up the subject of feeding preference.

As scientific evidence that breast milk is superior to formula accumulates, it is no longer accurate for the nurse to tell new parents that formula and breast milk are equally good for infants. The nurse who is counseling people on feeding choices must be knowledgeable about both types of feeding and be able to answer accurately questions that may arise concerning both options.

Few areas related to health are as highly personal as food and food preferences. So while nurses need to know their clients' health beliefs and practices, they also need to be aware of their own beliefs and how they can influence their nursing practice. Even though many health organizations now endorse breast-feeding, the nurse needs to take care that she does not overwhelm the client with her own preference. Feeding choice for a newborn should be an informed decision made by the parents after they have all the facts on the subject. It is the primary nurse's responsibility to know these facts and present them to the parents, who may subsequently assume responsibility for decisions concerning the health of their family.

Advantages of Breast-feeding

"Ideally, breast milk should be practically the only source of nutrients for the first four to six months for most infants" (9). This statement, which appeared in a joint publication by the Nutrition Committees of the Canadian Pediatric Society and the American Academy of Pediatrics, has important implications for nursing.

Research now shows that breast milk's unique properties make it highly favored over processed cow's milk formulas for human infants (28, 36). Based on these findings, nurses who are involved in any setting with children and families need to consider ways they can encourage breast-feeding. Goals should include the following:

- Educating clients, communities, and health care workers about the benefits of breast-feeding
- Helping couples make informed decisions about how they will feed their newborns
- Teaching new mothers how to breast-feed
- Creating a hospital environment that is supportive of breast-feeding
- Making referrals to support groups that specialize in helping breast-feeding mothers

For centuries breast-feeding constituted the only source of human infant nutrition. Only with the domestication of the cow, goat, and water buffalo, about 500 B.C., was there even an alternative (23). As technology advanced, and formulas were developed that made artificial feeding a safe alternative, bottle feeding became the "modern" way to feed infants. The technology emphasized a scientific approach, implying that a precisely calculated formula developed in a laboratory must be best for babies.

Advertising campaigns that accompanied formula development were quite successful. By 1956 only 21 percent of babies discharged from American hospitals were breast-fed, and this number decreased to 18 percent by 1966 (25, 26). There were regional differences in the prevalence of breast-feeding, but at that point most mothers who chose to breast-feed did so for financial reasons—formula costs money—so it was mothers in the lower socioeconomic group who still breast-fed their babies.

Since the 1970s there has been a resurgence of interest in breast-feeding. Nursing a baby is not a reportable event, so statistics are hard to acquire; however, according to one formula manufacturer's report in 1975, 33 percent of mothers were breast-feeding one week postpartum (30). This figure jumped to 43 percent in 1977. Some hospitals now report breast-feeding rates as high as 65 to 75 percent.

This percentage varies with the geographical region, indicating the influence of culture and socioeconomic background. It now seems that breast-feeding mothers come from better educated, upper socioeconomic groups, perhaps because they have better access to the facts about breast-feeding. The increase in breast-feeding rates in this group is also consistent with the "back to nature" health consciousness that was so prevalent in the 1970s.

Mothers from lower socioeconomic groups may qualify for social programs that supply infant formula; this may decrease the mother's incentive to even consider breast-feeding. Usually these programs include provisions for the breast-feeding mother and her extra caloric needs; however, the health care workers often overlook mentioning this option.

Another reason for the previous decrease in breast-feeding may be lack of role models. When breast-feeding was the norm there were plenty of role models who could hand down the "art" of breast-feeding through the generations. If a new mother has had no contact with breast-feeding and gets little encouragement from her family and friends, she will probably change to bottle-feeding when she encounters her first problem with breast-feeding. Neighborhood acceptance of artificial formula and manufacturers' persuasive advertising for their products may supply the support the insecure mother needs. Breast-feeding needs the same sort of vigorous advertising campaign and network of support that bottle feeding has had if it is going to continue to thrive.

Scientists and organizations that encourage breast-feeding usually cite at least five reasons breast milk is superior to processed cow's milk formula.

Nutritional and Biochemical Properties

Human breast milk and cow's milk have different compositions. Human milk is best for human babies and cow's milk is better suited to the needs of calves. Realizing this, formula manufacturers have tried to duplicate human breast milk but have not been too successful. Heat treatment, homogenization, and the addition of carbohydrates to cow's milk improved, to some extent, its usefulness and tolerance by infants, but protein and ash (mineral) levels were too high and the fat was poorly absorbed (9).

Fats from human milk are better absorbed by infants than those of cow's milk. Efforts to increase fat absorption in formulas by replacing buttermilk with vegetable oil have been successful; however, this alteration removes most of the cholesterol from the formula.

Human milk is high in cholesterol. Although adults

are warned to avoid excessive cholesterol, it may play an important role in infant nutrition. Rapid growth during infancy means membranes are being formed that have high cholesterol requirements (3). Some animal studies indicate that breast-feeding and a high intake of cholesterol as an infant may induce enzymes that subsequently metabolize cholesterol better, and thereby result in lower serum cholesterol levels later in life (9).

Cow's milk contains more than three times as much protein as human milk. This is not so surprising when one compares the rate of growth of a calf with that of a human. The calf requires a high-protein diet for quick growth that will allow early independence from its mother. A human infant grows much more slowly, not reaching full size or independence until adolescence. Thus a high-protein diet is not needed; excessive protein intake may actually stress the infant's kidneys. Whereas physical growth is slow, the brain and central nervous system are developing rapidly in infancy, so adequate nutrition at this stage is crucial.

Despite its seemingly low-protein concentration, breast milk satisfies the needs of a growing infant. The amino acid composition of human milk is particularly suited to the metabolic peculiarities of the newborn. Seventy percent of human milk protein is the easily digestible whey protein. Cow's milk protein is 80 percent casein, which is harder for human infants to digest (4). Thus, even though the formula-fed baby takes in more protein, he is unable to use it all. The breast-fed baby actually digests a larger amount of protein because it is so well suited to his body.

Breast-fed babies were once thought to need an iron supplement after the first few months of life because breast milk has a low iron content. However, more recent studies show that iron in human milk is sufficient to meet iron requirements of the exclusively breast-fed, full-term infant until he is four to six months old. The Committee on Nutrition of the Academy of Pediatrics recommends starting an iron-fortified cereal by four to six months for exclusively breast-fed babies (8).

Heat-treated formulas with iron also supply enough iron for adequate absorption. Infants fed only pasteurized cow's milk too early in life are prone to iron deficiency because that milk is a poor source of iron.

Obesity Later in Life

The relationship between infant feeding practices and obesity in adulthood is not clear. Conflicting results have been reported (11, 22, 34). Animal studies suggest that early overfeeding increases the cellularity of the adipose tissue; but there is also evidence that fat cell multiplication in humans continues throughout life (5). In either case excessive weight gain and over-feeding should be avoided throughout infancy and childhood.

Breast-feeding may aid in preventing obesity in infants and developing healthy eating habits. The breast-fed infant determines how much he drinks; when full, he stops. Studies show that milk samples from nursing mothers at the end of a feeding (sometimes called hindmilk) contain much higher levels of lipids and protein than at the beginning of the feeding; this change in composition may satiate the baby or in some way signal a cessation of feeding (18). A bottle-feeding mother may consciously or unconsciously coax her baby to finish that last ounce of formula, whether baby wants it or not.

Mothers who breast-feed also seem to introduce solid foods into the baby's diet at a later age. The addition of solids greatly increases caloric intake and nutritionally is not needed until the infant is four to six months old (9).

"A fat baby is a healthy baby" is a myth that is difficult to dispel. But if fat babies do become fat adults, with the hypertension and cardiovascular disease associated with obesity, then the need for primary prevention is evident. Breast-feeding may be a good beginning.

Antiinfective Properties

A newborn's immune system is immature, and his ability to respond effectively to infections is poor. Every infant receives passive immunity through the placenta that provides protection against some viruses, bacteria, and toxins for several weeks after delivery. But babies who are breast-fed receive colostrum, the first "milk" that is produced after delivery.

Colostrum is a yellowish, creamy fluid that is rich in host-resistance factors. It contains immunoglobulins that help the baby cope with the assault by foreign agents on his previously sterile body.

Two to five days after delivery the colostrum is replaced with true breast milk, which also contains immunoglobulins. The antibodies isolated in breast milk react against a variety of microorganisms, such as *Escherichia coli,* streptococci, staphylococci, and polio and influenza viruses. The antibodies appear to promote normal bacteria colonization and inhibit growth of certain pathogens (15).

Other immunological properties of breast milk are complex and not fully understood. Macrophages found in human breast milk appear to prevent necrotizing enterocolitis, a devastating disease found in premature low-birth-weight infants, but uncommon in breast-fed babies (2). *Lactobacillus bifidus,* a growth factor, is also present in human milk in higher amounts than in cow's milk. This factor lowers the pH of the stool in breast-fed infants and creates an acid environment that inhibits the growth of *Shigella, E. coli,* and yeast (14).

As might be expected, research on the morbidity rates of bottle-fed and breast-fed babies points to lower infection and hospitalization rates for breast-fed babies. Cunningham found that breast-feeding was associated with significantly less illness (gastrointestinal and respiratory) during the first year of life, especially if breast-feeding was continued beyond four and one-half months of age (10). Another study showed that babies who were exclusively breast-fed for the first three months had a significantly lower incidence of infections that required hospitalization (13).

These studies were done in upstate New York communities where poor sanitation and poverty are not outstanding problems. In countries or communities where sanitation is poor, education levels are low, and poverty exists, the risk of illness for infants is much higher. The proper sterilization of formula and bottles is less likely to occur and infant morbidity is high. Breast-feeding is a healthy alternative in such situations; it not only eliminates contamination of the milk source from poor sanitation but also provides immunity to prevent infection.

Antiallergic Properties

Proteins in milk from domestic animals may be allergenic for infants. Breast milk spares the infant's gastrointestinal tract from exposure to outside food antigens that may cause a local reaction.

Evidence suggests that allergies later in childhood (such as asthma and eczema) are more prevalent in bottle-fed infants than in breast-fed babies (24).

This would be particularly useful information for parents with a strong family history of allergies who are making a decision about how to feed their newborn.

Economic Factors

Breast-feeding is less expensive than bottle-feeding. Even when the extra calories and protein that a lactating woman requires are considered (about 500 calories per day over prepregnant intake), formula is still more expensive. Based on present-day prices, the additional food a nursing mother requires costs one-third to one-half the amount she would have to spend on formula (23). (This is based on the U.S. economy. The formula is even more expensive in comparison to national food sources in some other countries.) Hidden expenses with bottle-feeding include glass bottles (which break and have to be replaced), sterilizing equipment, and time required to buy the formula and prepare it.

Maternal-Infant Bonding

Early and prolonged contact between a mother and her newborn can be an important factor in mother-infant bonding and in the development of a mother's subsequent behavior to her infant (27). Breast-feeding maintains many types of contact between mother and infant—tactile, visual, and olfactory—that seem to enhance mothering behavior. Although bonding and closeness are possible with bottle feeding, breast-feeding offers an extra closeness for both mother and infant. Some mothers report an intense feeling of satisfaction and a reduction of stress when breast-feeding.

Anatomy and Physiology

A review of anatomy and physiology of the breast is necessary to understand lactation. The adult female breast consists of glandular tissue, supporting connective tissue, and protective fatty tissue (Figure 22.1). The glandular tissue is composed of fifteen to twenty-five lobes divided by connective tissue bands and arranged

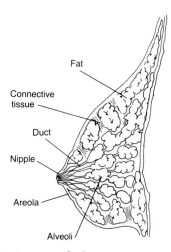

Figure 22.1. Anatomy of a Breast

radially around the centrally located nipple. Each lobe is then divided into twenty to forty lobuli, and each lobulus is subdivided into ten to one hundred alveoli. The alveoli are the secretory units of the breast (21).

There is some projection of the mammary gland tissue into the axillary region; this is known as the tail of Spence. The tissue is more noticeable during lactation (21).

The nipple is perforated by fifteen to twenty-five small openings, each an excretory duct from one of the lobes. The nipple also contains sensory nerve endings and is well supplied with sebaceous glands, but has no hair. The nipple consists of smooth muscle, which contracts on thermal, tactile, or sexual stimulation, inducing firmness and prominence (21).

A circular, pigmented area known as the areola surrounds the nipple. It ranges in color from pink in fair-skinned women to dark brown in others (21). During pregnancy the areola darkens and is enlarged. Montgomery's glands in the areola are large sebaceous glands that become enlarged during pregnancy and lactation, so that they look like small pimples. They secrete a substance that lubricates and protects the nipples during breast-feeding. After lactation these glands recede to their former size and appearance (21).

Milk Delivery

The other part of the lactation process involves delivering the milk, or getting it out of the breast. Although this seems simple, it is actually the result of a complex neurohormonal response, sometimes called the "let-down" reflex (originally a term used by dairy farmers) (Figure 22.2).

Milk is collected in the alveoli of the breasts, and the sucking of the infant on the nipple precipitates the let-down reflex, also known as the milk-ejection reflex. The sensation of sucking is transmitted to the hypothalamus, which stimulates the secretion of oxytocin by the posterior pituitary. Oxytocin is then released into the bloodstream, flows to the breasts, and causes contractile tissue that surrounds the alveoli to contract and express milk from the alveoli into the mammary ducts (16). After milk is in the ducts it is easily removed from the breasts by compression of the areola (not just the nipple). This can be accomplished by the infant's sucking, through manual expression of milk, or by a breast pump.

This complex neurohormonal response causes milk to

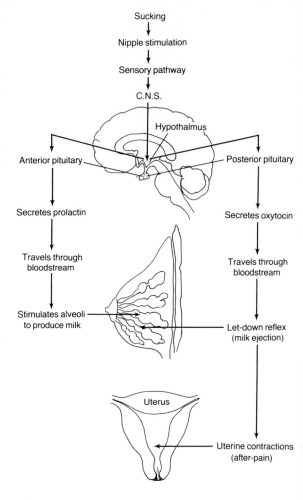

Figure 22.2. Lactation Process

flow in less than one minute after the baby begins to suck. The let-down reflex affects both breasts at once, so the breast not being sucked may drip some milk while the baby is nursing at the other breast.

Oxytocin also causes uterine contractions, known as afterpains. They are usually more pronounced in the multiparous woman. Some authorities think that putting the baby to breast on the delivery table cuts down on blood loss and decreases the chance of postpartum hemorrhage because of these oxytocin-induced contractions (19). Breast-feeding mothers also have a faster involution than bottle-feeding mothers because of the uterine contractions associated with oxytocin.

Psychological factors can influence the let-down reflex in a positive or negative way. Pain, fear, cold, fatigue, and anxiety can all inhibit the reflex, whereas hearing the baby cry or just looking at the baby can stimulate the let-down reflex. Some mothers report having the milk-ejection reflex occur when they are talking about their babies or just thinking about them. Clearly emotions play an important role in this aspect of lactation.

When distractions are inhibiting the let-down reflex, simple adjustments should be tried to make the mother more comfortable. This may mean providing more privacy, a warmer temperature, decreasing her pain or discomfort, or allaying her anxiety. If efforts fail, there is synthetic oxytocin (Sintocinon) that comes in 2-ml or 5-ml nasal spray bottles. One spray in one or both nostrils several minutes before breast-feeding is sufficient to initiate the let-down reflex.

Nursing Techniques

Contrary to common belief, breast-feeding is not totally instinctive for the new mother. It is a skill that must be learned. The beginner frequently believes that she needs several extra hands to hold the infant properly and get her breast to the baby's mouth. The nurse is usually the health worker in the best position to be of assistance.

It must be remembered that the new lactating mother is often in crisis. No matter how well prepared she was for the delivery, it was still a new, physically demanding experience. She may have received medication for pain, or may be experiencing discomfort from an episiotomy. Her anxiety or elation are also distractions that make it harder to concentrate on learning the new skill of breast-feeding. The nurse can assist her in decreasing stresses and finding coping mechanisms to resolve the crisis.

Positioning

The most basic factor to be considered in teaching the new mother to breast-feed is positioning, to enhance her and the baby's comfort. Pillows are often helpful in the beginning. The first feeding may take place on the delivery table, where a side-lying position will be used. To feed from the right breast, the mother will lie on her right side with the baby cradled in next to her with her

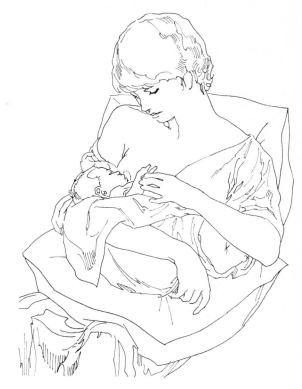

Figure 22.3. Sitting Position for Breast-feeding

right arm. The mother can use her left hand to guide her breast to the baby's mouth (Figures 22.3 and 22.4).

Sitting up in bed or in a chair is the usual position for nursing a baby. The first few days after delivery the mother may have pain from an episiotomy and may

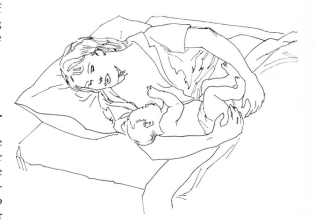

Figure 22.4. Side-lying Position for Breast-feeding

need to assume a comfortable position, and thus have the baby handed to her. A pillow on the mother's lap will bring the baby up to a comfortable level for feeding and decrease strain on the mother's back. An armchair or rocker can provide the same sort of arm support for the mother. Any physical or emotional environmental distraction may affect the mother's let-down reflex. The nurse can be instrumental in reducing the number of distractions.

Rooting Reflex

The newborn has a rooting reflex that can be used to the mother's advantage. When the cheek is stroked the baby will turn his head in that direction. When the baby is in a comfortable position for nursing, have the mother lightly touch his cheek with her nipple. The baby will automatically turn toward the nipple and grasp it in his mouth.

Sucking Position

Care must be taken to see that the baby grasps part of the areola region as well as the nipple (Figure 22.5). This is necessary for adequate milk expulsion; sucking on the nipple alone will not completely empty the breast and the infant may get frustrated and tug at the nipple. This will cause trauma to the nipples, which may already be sore.

Breaking Suction

If the baby is just hanging off the nipple and not getting an adequate flow of milk, it will be necessary to remove

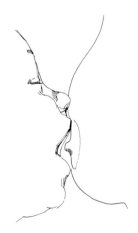

Figure 22.5. Infant at Breast

him from the breast and start again. Never pull the baby off the breast, for he will hang on and nipple tissue will be damaged. Suction must be broken before the baby is removed from the breast for any reason. This is accomplished by slipping a (clean) finger into the baby's mouth or gently squeezing the baby's cheeks together until his mouth opens.

Assuring Breathing

Care must be taken to keep the infant's nostrils free and not let them press up against the breast during feeding. This will allow him to suck continuously and not have to stop to breathe. When the mother's breast is very full, during morning feeding or when the breast is engorged, she may need to press in her breast around the baby's nose with her fingers to allow him to breathe and drink at the same time. This is not usually necessary; repositioning the infant may also solve the problem.

Frequency and Duration

How often the baby nurses the first few days and for how long vary widely. Some care givers limit the time at the breast, hoping to gradually toughen the nipples and decrease trauma to the nipple from sucking. They recommend five minutes on each breast every three to four hours. This routine frequently coincides with hospital routine when infants are kept in a central nursery and limits suckling time and the stimulation of the breast for prolactin and milk production. A vicious cycle may follow with poor let-down reflex, breast engorgement, pain, and difficult feedings, which often leads to unsuccessful lactation.

Rooming-in or a flexible hospital routine favors demand feeding with nearly unlimited infant time at the breast. This philosophy is based on the idea that mother-infant bonding is of utmost importance. The newborn may nurse as often as every two hours, providing adequate stimulation for milk production and prevention of any engorgement owing to the frequent feedings.

Nurses need to assist the new mother during the initial feedings. Not only will they be able to help in positioning and answering questions, but they can also obtain important assessment data about the mother's lactation, the mother's breast-feeding skills, and the infant's feeding habits. Because most mothers remain in the hospital for only two to four days after delivery, there is limited time to gather this information and make any needed intervention.

Common Concerns

Breast Care

Nipple preparation during pregnancy for breast-feeding, by nipple rolling, breast massage, friction with a towel, or regular airing, may be of some use. One limited study found it more effective for fair-skinned women than for women with darker pigmentation (1).

Breast care after delivery is important, whether the mother is breast-feeding or not. A good, supportive bra is needed, as breast size increases dramatically after delivery. This enlargement is due to engorgement, a swelling of the breasts that occurs three to five days after delivery, as the true milk becomes available. Swelling may extend into the axillary region, where the breast glandular tissue known as the tail of Spence is located. (Engorgement is less of a problem when newborns are fed frequently on a demand schedule.) After the initial engorgement the breasts decrease in size but remain larger than their prepregnancy size until the baby is weaned.

Clean and dry are the key words in breast care. Washing hands before and after nursing is recommended. No soap should be used on the breasts because it irritates the nipples. Plain water is adequate for cleaning the breasts.

After feedings, the nipples should be dried with a clean towel before the bra is put on again. Plastic nipple shields or plastic pads to line bra cups may keep leaking breasts from showing, but they allow moisture to collect around the nipple and invite infection.

Extreme soreness and cracking of nipples may be alleviated by heat lamp treatments for thorough drying of nipples, followed by application of pure lanolin. This type of ointment doesn't have to be washed off before the baby drinks again. Most nipple soreness lasts for only a few days.

An understanding of lactation and engorgement makes it clear that giving a supplemental bottle of water or formula to the baby when the mother's breasts are engorged and sore is the wrong approach. Unless the engorgement is relieved, by either manual expression or infant suckling, the problems will only escalate. Extreme unrelieved engorgement can lead to stasis, inadequate milk drainage, and subsequent infection.

Mastitis

Nurses and nursing mothers need to know how to differentiate between engorgement and mastitis. Engorgement is a generalized swelling of both breasts that occurs several days after delivery, when true milk production begins. It is sometimes associated with low-grade fever (21). Frequent nursing, with proper drainage of all alveoli, will decrease the engorgement.

Mastitis is an infection of the breast that produces local redness, heat and tenderness, and fever and malaise. Usually only one breast is affected. This infection is seldom seen in the hospital because it usually occurs several weeks postpartum (21).

Mastitis is treated with antibiotics and an analgesic. Ice packs or heat applied to the breast may provide some comfort. Increased fluid intake and strict bed rest are also recommended. The baby should continue to nurse, starting on the unaffected side while the affected side "lets down." It is important to completely empty the infected breast by feeding, pumping, or hand expression (21).

Diet

Lactating women require about 300 to 500 extra calories daily, depending on their nutritional status and age. Well-balanced meals with plenty of protein and dairy foods and a vitamin and mineral supplement are usually enough to support lactation.

Even if the mother is malnourished, the baby will not be nutritionally deprived. Nutritious milk will still be produced at the expense of the mother's health. Being conscientious about her diet while lactating is something the nursing mother needs to do for her own health.

Vegetarians can successfully breast-feed their babies and maintain their own health. Vegans (strict vegetarians who eat no animal products) need to take vitamin B_{12} supplements. Vitamin B_{12} is found in all animal protein but not in vegetable protein. Most pediatricians discourage vegans from breast-feeding unless they are willing to add eggs and dairy products to their diets while breast-feeding (4).

Rest

The new mother, whether she is breast-feeding or bottle-feeding, should be told well before delivery that she will experience fatigue after the birth of her baby. Many mothers are unrealistic in thinking that they will easily resume their normal activities as soon as the baby is born. The healing process, getting up for night feedings, and the stress of taking on a new role all contribute to fatigue.

If the mother is aware that fatigue may occur and plans accordingly, she may be able to prevent some of it. Accepting help from friends and relatives, cutting down on housework and on social and work-related obligations, and resting during the day are all ways to help the new mother avoid fatigue.

Effect of Breast Size

Breast size has no effect on the success of breast-feeding. Women with small breasts have the same lobule and duct system as women with large breasts; the only difference in their breasts is the amount of fatty tissue, which has no effect on milk production.

Inverted Nipples

Normal and flat nipples erect with the slightest bit of pressure. A truly inverted nipple will retract when the areola is pressed between the thumb and forefinger. Inverted nipples need not preclude breast-feeding, especially if breast preparation is begun six weeks before delivery, before any great engorgement occurs.

Treatment involves massage and stretching exercises for flat or mildly inverted nipples. Truly inverted nipples respond to nipple shields, which are intended to shield the nipple while the baby is nursing. However, they may cause more trouble than they alleviate because the baby cannot empty the breast as well and engorgement worsens. They are most effective for inverted nipples if the rubber nipple tip is removed and the base only (a plastic ring) is placed over the areola, inside the woman's bra. The pressure of the ring on the areola will cause the nipple to become erect. A regimen of nipple shield and exercise is recommended.

There are several types of nipple shields. A shield used to prevent nipple damage during engorgement may in fact increase engorgement because the baby cannot suck on the nipple too well with the shield in place and the breast is never completely emptied. Shorter, more frequent feedings are more effective in decreasing nipple soreness and engorgement than is a nipple shield. The new mother, who is just getting used to holding and feeding her baby, often feels like she needs a third arm to get everything done. Positioning a nipple shield is just one more thing for her to worry about. A nipple shield should be used as a last resort for sore nipples because most infants resist returning to the mother's nipple after

the shield has been used. All-rubber nipple shields pull on the breast and should not be used; shields with glass or plastic rings and rubber nipples are preferred.

Breast Pumps

Several types of breast pumps are available, ranging in size from small suction cup devices to elaborate electric machines that can pump both breasts simultaneously. The type used depends on the frequency and purpose of pumping. A mother who wants to store some breast milk once in a while, to be given to the baby in her absence, can probably manage with manual expression or a small suction cup style. Women with premature or ill babies, or those who have to be separated from their infants but need or want to continue breast-feedings would be candidates for a faster, more efficient method.

Supplements

A new mother who is working to establish her milk supply should probably avoid supplemental bottles until her supply is well established. This may take a few weeks. It should be remembered that the baby's frequent sucking at the breast stimulates milk production. Supplemental bottles suggested by a well-meaning doctor or relative to an anxious new mother will not only undermine her confidence, but also decrease the production of milk.

Supplemental feedings are needed when the baby and mother have to be separated for a feeding. If breast milk has been expressed and saved, it can be given in a bottle. Otherwise, an infant formula is recommended for supplemented bottles until the infant is one year old. The baby's pediatrician will recommend a formula for supplementation.

Once lactation has been established, the breast-feeding mother is not "tied" to her baby. Regular supplemental bottles of breast milk or formula can be given by the father or baby-sitter. Many mothers report that their infants will not take a bottle from them. The familiar feel of the mother and the smell of her breast milk presumably make the baby want his "usual" feeding from her.

Lawrence (21) recommends using a powder formula for supplemental bottles if breast milk is not available. Because it can be made one feeding at a time and has a long shelf life, there is little waste. The powders are made at lower temperatures than the liquid formulas, so there is no carmelizing of sugars and denaturing of proteins. The powder mixed with warm water goes quickly into solution.

Sucking Techniques in Breast-feeding and Bottle-feeding Babies

Some breast-feeding babies have difficulty even taking breast milk from a bottle. There is a logical explanation for this: the sucking mechanism is quite different for each method.

In breast-feeding, the baby draws the mother's nipple into his mouth, against the hard palate. His cheek muscles are contracted and there is much jaw motion. The tongue moves in a posterior manner and the squeezing of the breast, areola, and nipple against the hard palate is the main element of sucking.

A rubber nipple from a bottle strikes the baby's soft palate. His tongue must move forward to control the flow of formula, and cheek muscles are relaxed.

A breast-fed baby can learn to drink from a bottle too, but patience is required by the person holding the bottle. The breast-fed baby is used to having to suck vigorously to attain his milk. The different mechanism in bottle-feeding may cause him to gulp down too much milk too fast, since the milk flows so easily from the bottle. Most breast-fed babies learn to drink from bottles too. Parents will be more patient in "teaching" the breast-fed infant to drink from a bottle if they realize that it is a new technique for the baby to master.

It must also be mentioned that each baby has his own individual feeding style, whether he's being breast-fed or bottle-fed. Some babies are fast eaters and gulp down the milk, almost gagging with each swallow; others are slow and methodical. Still others fall asleep during the feeding and never seem too interested in eating. As the infant develops, the parents become intimately familiar with the baby's eating style. This is important for parents to realize. They shouldn't be surprised when a second child has a different style of eating than their first child. Once the baby's feeding style is established, a change in it may be significant. Parents should be aware of this.

Teething

Most babies get their first teeth between four and seven months of age. Around this time they may have the urge to bite the mother's nipple at the end of a feeding. A very definite response from the mother—"No," "Ouch," or "Stop"—and pulling the breast away from the baby's mouth are usually enough to make the baby stop biting for good.

It is certainly not necessary to stop breast-feeding because the baby is teething. Some babies become irritable when they are teething, and many mothers report that nursing them is one of the few things that calms them during this time.

Breast-feeding After a Cesarean Birth

Women who have had cesarean births can certainly breast-feed their babies. Breast-feeding's side effect of oxytocin release that speeds involution may even be an extra help to such women. Women who have had cesarean births may need more nursing support, for example, in positioning the baby, since they will not be mobile as soon after delivery as women who have had vaginal deliveries.

Extra care should be given to help them find a comfortable position for feeding. Initially a lying position may be necessary if a spinal anesthetic was used. They may need more help handling the baby, especially in a rooming-in situation. The type of anesthetic given during the cesarean section may initially affect the baby's sucking. These mothers may need extra encouragement and support during the first few days of nursing, until the baby's suck improves.

How to Tell Whether the Baby Is Drinking Enough

The new breast-feeding mother can get anxious about whether the baby is drinking enough milk. Frequently it is the father or another relative who poses the question. In either case, such an idea is a direct challenge to the mother's competence to provide for her newborn. She must be instructed specifically on how to tell whether her baby is getting an adequate intake, so she can relieve her own anxieties and respond to her family's concerns.

The following criteria should be used in evaluating adequate intake:

- Six or more wet diapers each day, with pale yellow urine and normal bowel movements (normal for *that* baby—this varies widely in breast-fed infants)
- Weight gain documented at periodic checkups. Daily weighings at home are not recommended, since there is too much room for variations that could increase the parents' anxiety.

• The baby's schedule—is he asleep and awake for reasonable time periods for his age? Does he nurse in a relaxed manner, or cry fitfully?

As the baby grows, his parents become familiar with his habits. But during the first few weeks it is particularly helpful for parents to have some guidelines.

Parents will be more confident if they are taught how to assess their baby and when to seek additional help from the health team.

Stools of a Breast-fed Baby

Stools of breast-fed babies are quite different from those of formula-fed babies. New mothers should be aware of this to avoid unnecessary alarm.

Dark green meconium constitutes the first stool. After that the stool is golden-yellow to greenish yellow with no unpleasant odor. The stool is usually loose; constipation is not found in breast-fed babies.

Initially the baby may have a small bowel movement with every diaper change. This is not diarrhea in a breast-fed baby. Each infant will have his own schedule for bowel movements, and it may vary from week to week with the same baby. Some breast-fed babies will go several days between bowel movements. This is not constipation, since the movement is not hard and dry. It is just that baby's unique schedule.

Breast Swelling in the Baby

The small amount of milk sometimes found in a newborn's breast is known as witch's milk. This is common in both male and female infants and results from stimulation of the infant's mammary glands by the same placental hormones that prepare the mother for lactation. After the baby's birth the hormones are no longer present until puberty, when they again stimulate mammary gland growth (21).

Nothing should be done for the swollen breasts, as the milk is gradually reabsorbed. Massage may irritate or infect the breasts.

When to Start Solid Foods

Social pressures and aggressive advertising by baby food companies are responsible for early introduction of solid foods.

Women who are successfully breast-feeding their infants are seldom in a rush to start solid foods. They seem to enjoy feeling totally responsible for their babies' nutritional well-being. But at about four to six months the normal infant begins to lose his iron stores, and iron-rich solid foods are indicated. This is the recommendation of the American Academy of Pediatrics' Committee on Nutrition (7).

Iron-fortified cereal is usually the first solid given to babies. It is recommended that new foods be introduced one at a time at weekly intervals, so that allergic reactions to new foods can be noted.

New mothers should be encouraged to read labels and know exactly what they are feeding their infants. Many commercial baby foods no longer contain added salt and sugar, and the mother should look for these types of canned foods. Babies can also be fed pureed table food from the family menu as long as any strong seasoning is added after the baby's portion is removed.

One reason sometimes given for starting solid foods early is that they help the baby sleep through the night. If this is true (it has not been determined), it may be because the solids contain more calories than milk does and are a form of overfeeding. This is not a positive habit to establish.

Leaking Breasts in Mothers

Many women complain of leaking breasts for the first few weeks after delivery. Leaking can result from engorgement or from the let-down reflex, which may be stimulated by infant sucking or a strong emotion. It affects both breasts. The breast not being sucked may begin to leak. This can usually be stopped by applying pressure to that breast while the baby nurses at the other breast. The mother needs to be reassured that leakage from engorgement will last for only a short time.

Embarrassing wet spots on blouses and dresses can be avoided by placing nursing pads or a folded handkerchief in each bra cup. Anything with a plastic lining should be avoided, as plastic traps moisture and increases the risk of infection.

Breast-feeding Adopted Children

It is possible to breast-feed an adopted child by induced lactation. This is breast-feeding without prior pregnancy. When a mother wishes to nurse her adopted child the goal is usually to achieve a mother-infant relationship that may also have some nutritional benefits. If it is made clear from the start that the baby may continue to need supplementation, and that the goal of the mother is nurturing, not nutrition alone, she will not be disappointed.

Preparation for lactation should begin several months before the infant's arrival and should consist of nipple and breast stimulation, supplemented maternal diet, and occasional use of hormones and Lact-Aid. The same technique may be used to promote relactation in a mother who didn't breast-feed or who stopped breast-feeding and wants to nurse her child again.

Lawrence devotes an entire chapter to this subject in her excellent book (21).

Breast-feeding and Contraception

Breast-feeding does delay the onset of menstruation but is not considered a reliable means of contraception. Frequent sucking suppresses ovulation; so a rigid schedule of breast-feeding with early introduction to solid foods and supplemental bottles would be less apt to delay menses. In nonindustrial societies where breast-feeding is ad lib around the clock, the return of menses may be delayed as long as twelve months.

Couples who are serious about preventing conception should be advised to seek the traditional methods of contraception and not rely on lactation as a contraceptive.

The use of birth control pills during lactation is a controversial issue. Besides the known risks of pills (thromboembolism and hypertension), their effects on milk production and content, uterine involution, and infant growth and development need to be considered. Research has shown that some birth control pills decrease milk production and alter its content, but it is too soon to tell about long-term effects of pills on infants (21). Couples are probably best advised to use another means of contraception until the infant is weaned.

Role of Father and Other Children

Some women feel guilty about wanting to breast-feed their infants because the father would be "left out." These women need to be supported, and have the benefits of breast-feeding reinforced so they can share this information with their partners. Women's bodies are designed to carry the fetus and feed the infant. If men are concerned about this, their feelings should be explored.

The father's role in breast-feeding is important. A supportive, helpful partner boosts a nursing mother's confidence. There are plenty of baby-oriented chores the father *can* participate in; he needn't feel like he gets all the drudgery and his wife gets to play with their baby. Comforting, rocking, and giving supplemental

bottles after four to six weeks are just a few ways a father can help to nurture his child.

Some fathers may openly or unconsciously reject their wives' breast-feeding because they view it as a sexual involvement between wife and baby. Such feelings need to be discussed, for breast-feeding is less likely to be successful without the constructive involvement of the father.

Mothers may feel awkward breast-feeding in front of their older children, especially if these children were not breast-fed. In general, the child will reflect the parents' view on breast-feeding. If the mother acts embarrassed and nurses the baby in private, the older children will be learning that there is something shameful about breasts and breast-feeding. An open, matter-of-fact attitude is more likely to gain acceptance by the older children. They also will be learning a cultural tradition. Young children who grow up in a community where breast-feeding is the norm will be more accepting of breast-feeding when they are parents (Figure 22.6).

Breast-feeding in Public

A well-fitting nursing bra is recommended for the breast-feeding mother. Nursing bras are designed so

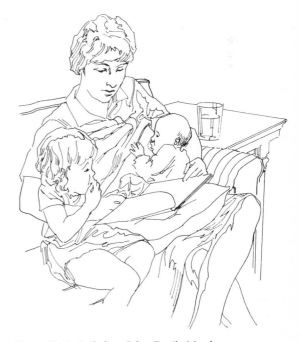

Figure 22.6. Including Other Family Members

that each cup can be unsnapped and let down, exposing the breast for nursing. Different styles and types of snap-type openings are available. Most large mail order catalogs and department stores carry nursing bras.

Two-piece outfits allow women to breast-feed more discreetly. Instead of opening the buttons on a blouse, pull the blouse up from the waist and drape a baby blanket across the baby to cover the exposed part of the mother's abdomen. As the mother gains confidence and skill in nursing and handling her newborn, it becomes easier to nurse discreetly.

Feeding Time

Some women reject the idea of breast-feeding because they think that it will take too much time. Mothers who have successfully breast-fed immediately see the flaw in this logic, for it is bottle-feeding that demands more time.

Besides shopping for bottles, nipples, bottle brushes, refill bags (for some types of bottles), and formula, the mother has to prepare and sterilize the formula and bottles. Night feedings involve a trip to the kitchen to warm up a bottle while the hungry baby screams. Traveling requires bottle bags with prepared formula packed in ice (so it won't sour) or buying the expensive bottled formula.

Day feedings, night feedings, and travel for the breast-feeding mother are much easier than for the formula-feeding mother. The milk is ready at the right temperature whenever it is needed. No special equipment is necessary.

Older children can be included in feeding times too. It needn't be just a time for mother and baby. A child over two years old can usually hold a book and turn pages so the mother can read while she feeds the baby (this is true with breast-feeding or bottle-feeding, but the breast-feeding mother is more apt to have a free hand).

Environmental and Personal Pollution

Mother's milk can carry a variety of potentially harmful pollutants to an infant. PCBs (polychlorinated biphenyls) and DDT and other pesticides are some of the environmental contaminants that can transfer from the mother's body fat to her milk. However, unless the mother is known to have had frequent exposure to these pollutants through diet (eating fish from PCB-contaminated waters) or occupation (heavy chemical fumes associated with some factories), they are not a contraindi-

cation to breast-feeding. This is the type of information that might be uncovered during the nursing health history. Women who are concerned about chemical contaminants in breast milk can contact their state health departments for information on testing breast milk.

The breast-feeding mother herself has control over some other potential contaminants of her milk. Nicotine, from smoking, is transferred to breast milk, as are alcohol, caffeine, and most prescription and over-the-counter drugs. Women who are nursing should consult their physicians before taking *any* drug. Lawrence includes a chart on the effects of specific drugs on breast milk in her book (21).

Caffeine sources include coffee, tea, chocolate, and cola drinks. Caffeine levels in the mother's blood and milk are about the same. A breast-feeding mother who consumes a lot of caffeine will be passing it on to her baby. The baby may accumulate caffeine and act jittery. It is easy to see how a destructive cycle can then begin: the mother must stay awake to comfort the jittery baby who will not sleep, so she drinks some more coffee to help her stay awake. This is once more passed on to the baby at the next feeding.

Most mothers do not have to eliminate caffeine from their diets, but it might be considered if the baby is having trouble sleeping and frequently acts irritable.

Aftereffects of Medications During Labor and Delivery

It is generally recognized that mothers and babies do best if there is minimal use of medication during labor and delivery. This is not always possible, so the effects of the medication on both mother and infant in relation to breast-feeding must be considered.

Barbiturate drugs administered to a woman during labor have been demonstrated to have an adverse effect on the baby's sucking reflexes for as long as four to five days (17). This is important information for the nurse and the mother to know. The nurse can encourage the mother to be patient if her baby isn't sucking well, and the mother won't think that she's doing something wrong if she knows that it may take the baby a little longer to begin sucking effectively.

Mothers who have had cesarean sections may have other complications that affect their well-being. This is especially true of an unplanned section, when there may have been a long and difficult labor, blood loss, infection, or toxemia. At all times medications should be short-acting so that they are quickly (within four hours) excreted by the mother (21). They should be given immediately after breast-feeding so that they reach their peak level before the next feeding is due.

Nursing mothers must be informed that many medications transfer to their milk, and that it is best to check before taking any prescription or nonprescription drug.

Adjusting to a Work/Social Schedule

Many women choose not to breast-feed because they plan to return to work within a few months after delivery, or they fear they will be too tied down and be unable to go out without the child. Having a baby does drastically alter one's life, no matter what feeding method is selected; but nursing the baby need not tie down the mother any more than bottle-feeding.

Once the new mother's milk supply is established, she can skip feedings and the baby-sitter can give the baby either formula or expressed breast milk in a bottle. If this is done occasionally on a random basis, the mother may have some mild engorgement and will probably feel more comfortable wearing some sort of absorbent, nonplastic nursing pad in her bra. But if the mother starts back to work on a regular schedule and breast-feeds morning, late afternoon, and evening only, her body will respond to the decreased sucking time and, accordingly, produce less milk.

Some mothers prefer to express milk at work at the regular feeding times, refrigerate it there, and have the baby-sitter feed the infant this milk the next day. This requires a work situation that allows enough time to express the milk (a ten-minute coffee break is adequate), access to refrigeration, a motivated mother, and a supportive work environment (29). More often the baby is switched to formula during the hours the mother works and breast-feeding continues when she is at home.

Breast-feeding is not an "all or nothing" commitment once milk production has been established. Nursing mothers need not feel tied down to their infants. This is important information for mothers to have when they are making decisions on how to feed their babies.

Babies who are breast-fed for just three to four months still gain the immunological, antiinfective, and bonding benefits of breast-feeding. The mother with a three- to six-month maternity leave needs to know this.

Weaning

Weaning is the transfer of an infant's dependence on mother's milk to dependence on another form of nourishment. Mothers vary greatly on when they want to begin this process, some after a few weeks and others when the baby is much older.

It is not necessary to totally wean the baby if the mother is returning to work or school. Partial breast-feeding, usually morning and night feedings with formula during the day, is often suited to the working mother.

Gentle, gradual replacement of one feeding at a time with solid foods or a bottle of formula is the recommended way to wean. Sudden weaning is often hard on both the mother, who may suffer engorgement, and the baby, who may be unaccustomed to drinking from a bottle.

Manual Expression and Storage of Breast Milk

There are several reasons the nursing mother may want to hand express some of her breast milk. One may be to initiate the milk flow during engorgement so the baby can grasp the nipple. If mother and child are to be separated, the mother may want to leave some breast milk in a bottle, to be fed to the baby.

The manual expression of breast milk is a skill that requires practice. Mothers need encouragement so they don't get discouraged if they are not immediately successful.

The following steps are recommended:

· Wash hands.
· With a hand cupping the breast, place the thumb above the nipple on the edge of the areola and the forefinger below the nipple on the edge of areola, and squeeze them together (Figure 22.7).
· Do not press toward the nipple.
· Bearing in mind the anatomy and physiology of the breast and its duct system, rotate the thumb and forefinger around the breast to reach all the lobuli.
· Collect the milk in a clean wide-mouth cup or glass and store it in a closed container in the refrigerator or freezer.
· Sterilization of the collecting cup is recommended if the baby is less than one month old.

Breast milk can be safely kept for twenty-four to forty-eight hours if refrigerated. A standard refrigerator freezer is adequate for storage for up to two weeks. Milk stored in a deep freezer at 0 degrees Fahrenheit can be kept for more than two years (29).

Mothers should be informed that milk freezes in layers but will readily mix when thawed. Frozen milk

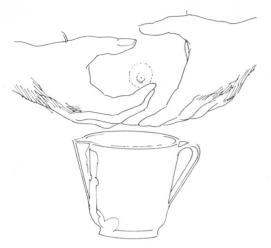

Figure 22.7.   Manual Expression of Milk

should be thawed under cold running water, as boiling water will curdle the milk.

Contraindications to Breast-feeding

Several medical conditions contraindicate breast-feeding, and breast-feeding is contraindicated for mothers who are taking certain medications. A mother with a diagnosis of breast cancer should not breast-feed her baby so that she may complete treatment immediately. Mothers with hepatitis B virus or cytomegalovirus should not breast-feed, since their infants may be at risk for these infections. β-hemolytic streptococcal disease in an infant can infect the mother's breasts and milk, causing mastitis in the mother and reinfection of the infant. Bilateral mastitis seen in such cases is a suspicious sign, and cessation of breast-feeding is recommended (21).

Because of advances in drug therapy, active tuberculosis is not necessarily a contraindication to breast-feeding any longer (21). If the mother's treatment begins in pregnancy and the infant's treatment begins at birth, no period of separation is needed. Both mother and infant need to be observed and monitored regularly for drug toxicity.

Another contraindication to breast-feeding is a personal one. Some mothers may be too anxious, embarrassed, or scared, or just "not interested" in breast-feeding. The health professional must respect these feelings. Some mothers may become more interested and change their minds when they are told the facts about breast-feeding. However, the health professional shouldn't pressure the mother into a decision she isn't comfortable with.

Breast-feeding Premature and Low-Birth-Weight Babies

Breast milk is also recommended for most premature babies. Those with extremely low birth weight may require additional nutrients, such as protein, but the colostrum and its antiinfective and antiallergic qualities are particularly important to the premature infant who is at risk for necrotizing enterocolitis. If the infant cannot suck, the colostrum can be manually expressed or pumped from the mother and given to the infant by gavage tube. For premature infants who are able to suckle, the close body contact is most welcome.

Mothers of premature or low-birth-weight infants who desire to breast-feed require extra support. Frequent feedings are usually needed, and if the infants have a poor sucking reflex, or if a pump is being used, it can be difficult for the mother to maintain a large milk volume.

Lact-Aid.   The Lact-Aid device is an effective way of nourishing the premature infant and allowing the mother to establish a milk supply. Lact-Aid was developed for mothers of adopted children, but it is also effective for the premature or sick infant who is unable to nurse regularly from the breast.

The Lact-Aid bag is filled with formula and hung around the neck of the mother (Figure 22.8). A small tube runs from the bag to the mother's nipple. As the baby sucks at the breast and stimulates milk production, he is rewarded by the supplemental formula. The amount of formula may gradually be decreased until the baby is nourished solely by the breast milk.

The formula in the bag is heated to body temperature by its position between the mother's breasts. The tubing is so narrow that it causes no discomfort to the infant's mouth or the mother's nipple. This system has been quite effective in helping mothers in special circumstances to establish a milk supply.

Multiple Births and Breast-feeding

It is possible to breast-feed twins and even triplets. Because these babies often have low birth weights, they may particularly benefit from the protective advantages of colostrum and breast milk. The breast-feeding

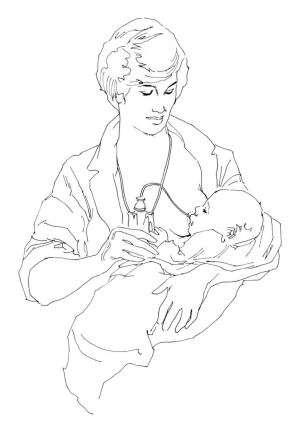

Figure 22.8. Lact-Aid Feeding

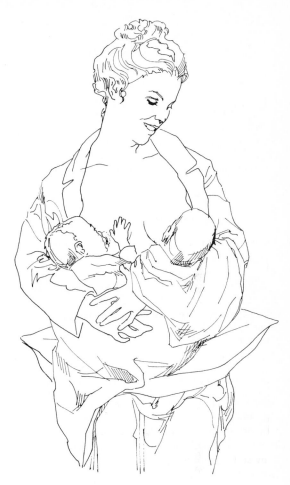

Figure 22.9. Breast-feeding in Multiple Births

mother of twins needs extra rest and calories. She will also require extra help initially in finding a comfortable position if she decides to try simultaneous feeding (Figure 22.9).

Breast-feeding twins or triplets is a time-consuming commitment, especially if the babies are fed separately. A supportive spouse and extra household help are almost necessities. Regional twin and triplet groups may also be helpful to these new parents.

Research

With the resurgence of interest in breast-feeding there has been a corollary increase in research on the subject. Of particular interest to nurses should be factors that encourage breast-feeding and reasons mothers give for

stopping breast-feeding. These can then be incorporated into nursing strategies for promoting breast-feeding.

Factors That Encourage Breast-feeding

The two most important factors in successful breast-feeding seem to be (a) emotional support from spouse, family, and anyone else involved with the mother (this would include hospital personnel) and (b) correct information about breast-feeding.

The following factors are associated with longer duration of breast-feeding:

- Rooming-in—easy access to baby and demand feeding allowing mother to build up her milk supply and gain confidence with feeding while still in the hospital

- Hospital nurses—helpful, knowledgeable nurses who can teach mothers how to breast-feed, answer their questions, and be supportive
- Time of introduction to solid foods—later introduction is associated with longer duration of breast-feeding; early introduction (before four months) decreases baby's sucking time and may decrease mother's milk supply
- Response of pediatrician—if the doctor suggests a supplemental bottle every time the mother has a question, the mother will decrease duration of nursing (6).

Reasons for Stopping Breast-feeding

The three most common reasons why mothers stop breast-feeding are (a) lack of milk (or fear of lack of milk), (b) maternal fatigue, and (c) breast or nipple complication (6). These reasons for stopping breast-feeding will be considered separately and it is shown how anticipatory guidance could prevent these problems.

Lack of Milk.   The typical new mother is discharged from the hospital three days after delivery. Her milk doesn't come in until two to five days after delivery. In the hospital she has had rich, creamy colostrum flowing from her breasts. She just gets home and it suddenly changes to a thin, almost bluish fluid (the normal consistency and appearance of breast milk). Of course she's going to think something is very wrong unless she's been told to expect this change. (This is related to correct information and knowledgeable hospital nurses—both positive factors in prolonging breast-feeding.)

Well-meaning relatives and others who are in close contact with the new mother may increase her concerns by dwelling on her inability to accurately measure the baby's intake. Unless the mother is strong enough to defend her feeding preference and knows the signs of a well-nourished newborn, she will probably give in to a supplemental bottle. A supplemental bottle decreases the baby's sucking time at the breast and therefore causes milk production to decrease. If the mother is concerned about her milk supply, she should increase her fluid intake and increase the baby's sucking time to promote milk production.

Maternal Fatigue.   Many new mothers are unprepared for the fatigue they may experience after they are discharged from the hospital. They may assume that they can easily resume work, social, and household activities without considering the healing process their bodies are undergoing. Discussing the possibility of such fatigue in advance of delivery and discharge may help the mother be more realistic in her expectations.

One suggestion might be for the mother to rest while the baby naps. If the baby doesn't nap regularly, the father or a friend could take the baby out of the home for an hour so the mother could get some undisturbed rest. This may be harder to arrange if there are other young children in the home.

When neighbors and friends offer help, advise the mother to accept it. A casserole donation or a trip to the grocery store is a small favor that a friend can perform and that can save the new mother time and energy.

Household help rather than help with the baby is usually more useful to a new mother. The first few weeks after delivery the mother needs to rest and get to know her child. All other chores should have low priority.

Breast or Nipple Complications.   Mothers should be informed that their breasts may be engorged in the days after delivery. They will feel heavy and warm owing to increased circulation, pressure from the milk, and the swelling of breast tissue. Nipples may also be sore, especially when the baby first begins to suck. This condition is normal and doesn't last for too long. Mothers who don't realize this and think that they will feel this way as long as they breast-feed will, understandably, discontinue nursing.

Inadequate milk drainage can lead to inflammation and infection, so it is important to let the baby suck despite nipple soreness. Warm towels or a warm shower may help, but the most relief will come from emptying the breast. In extreme cases engorgement is so severe that the nipple is flattened and the baby has difficulty grasping it. Manual expression of a little milk can help the baby get started.

Nipple care during engorgement is important. No soap should be used during bathing. Keep nipples clean and dry. Pure lanolin, which does not have to be removed before feedings, may be soothing.

It is easy to see how a new mother who is home alone with these problems might switch to bottle-feeding if she did not have correct information or know of a source where she could receive help. A knowledgeable, reassuring person at the other end of the telephone may be all the anxious mother needs to help her with these normal questions about breast-feeding.

Appropriate nursing intervention at several stages during pregnancy and postpartum will alleviate many potential problems when the mother goes home. Antepartal nurses, hospital delivery room, nursery, and post-partum areas, and pediatric and community health nurses all have a role in teaching and supporting the breast-feeding mother.

In order to assist the new mother who wants to breast-feed, the nurse must be knowledgeable about the subject. Results from a wide variety of recent studies show that mothers who received reliable information from health workers were more likely to initiate and continue breast-feeding (6, 35). Nurses have contact with new mothers in all stages of pregnancy and are in an ideal position to promote breast-feeding.

Another important research finding is that information and education programs aimed at hospital staff are often as effective in increasing breast-feeding rates as direct education of new parents (31–33). This outcome is understandable; when health workers are informed and supportive, their enthusiasm for breast-feeding can be contagious. When staff can easily handle questions that may arise for the breast-feeding mother and not suggest a supplemental bottle as the panacea for all problems, then the new mother will be more relaxed and confident learning this new skill.

It is interesting to note that formula manufacturers give demonstrations to hospital and clinic staff, leave samples of their products, and advertise their products. There is no formal organization or company "selling" breast-feeding, though many professional organizations now endorse the practice. So health workers must take the initiative in giving breast-feeding equal time. Attractive, well-written literature about breast-feeding in antepartal clinics and doctors' offices, and posters of infants breast-feeding are just a few ways to accomplish this. Health workers need to help advertise breast-feeding.

Nursing Intervention

Nurses have some specific responsibilities in supporting the breast-feeding mother and child. They begin in the prenatal period, when most parents make a decision on feeding preference, and end when the child is weaned.

The primary nurse in each setting—antepartal clinic or private doctor's office, labor and delivery, postpartum-nursery setting, or community—will plan with the mother the care she feels the mother needs. Other disciplines—medicine, social work, or lay support groups—may be involved in parts of the care plan, but the nurse remains the coordinator of the planning. She needs to develop some sort of follow-up in her plan, whether it

is to be done directly by her or through a home health agency or community support group.

The following list details possible nursing interventions at three levels of prevention for parents, health personnel, and the community. A different approach may be necessary for each individual client, and no *one* nurse will be complete in all of these interventions.

Intervention on the Primary Level

For the Parents

- General health maintenance
- Adequate nutrition
- Counseling on feeding choice
- Teaching—anatomy and physiology of the breast, and nipple preparation
- Family acceptance of breast-feeding, gaining support of other children in family
- Anticipatory guidance about need for rest, breast soreness, and management of breast-feeding

For the Health Worker

- Teach about breast-feeding and ways to promote it
- Help mothers prepare for drug-free deliveries

For the Community

- Provide information on breast-feeding in school health education classes
- Increase community awareness about benefits of breast-feeding through posters and articles in local newspapers

Intervention on the Secondary Level

For the Parents

- Support and teaching for the mother—positioning, how-to skills, need for rest, diet and fluids, breast care
- Encourage early feedings—in delivery room, if possible
- Promote close contact for bonding
- Group classes about breast-feeding to encourage discussion and bring up questions the mothers may have

For the Health Worker

- Recognize the effects of drugs used during delivery and plan strategies to decrease their use
- Encourage rooming-in and family-centered care using primary nursing

- Encourage immediate and continued contact between mother and child

For the Community

- Support groups—La Leche groups, nursing mothers
- Improve community facilities that are helpful to nursing mothers, e.g., stores with chairs in women's room to facilitate nursing, day-care facilities near workplaces so mothers can return to work earlier and still continue to breast-feed their babies

Intervention on the Tertiary Level

For the Parents

- Information on weaning from breast to cup or bottle

For the Health Worker

- Consult with lay support groups promoting breast-feeding

For the Community

- Groups of mothers who have successfully breast-fed their children act as educators of peers

DISCUSSION QUESTIONS

1. You are the nurse in a prenatal clinic, counseling Ms. S., a twenty-two-year-old primigravida who is sixteen weeks pregnant. When you inquire about how she plans to feed her baby, she tells you that she is undecided and asks you to explain the pros and cons of bottle- and breast-feeding. How would you respond? Consider the following points in your answer: (a) awareness of own bias toward bottle- or breast-feeding, (b) facts about each feeding method, and (c) recommendations of appropriate readings or community groups to help the woman make her decision.

2. Ms. H. has had an emergency cesarean section for fetal distress and delivered a healthy seven-and-a-half-pound daughter. She successfully breast-fed her son four years ago and was looking forward to breast-feeding again. You are the nurse with her in the recovery room and postpartum area and she voices this concern to you. "I was looking forward to breast-feeding this baby too. Now because of having a cesarean section, I guess I won't be able to."

How would you respond? Include the following points in your answer: (a) benefits of breast-feeding after a section, (b) effects of oxytocin, (c) extra help needed in positioning baby for feeding during first few days, (d) may need more help at home after discharge than with first child, and (e) baby's sucking reflex may be diminished for several days owing to maternal anesthesia during section.

3. Ms. J. is an enthusiastic new mother who is looking forward to breast-feeding her new son. Everything goes smoothly the first few days after delivery. On the morning of their discharge the baby has trouble feeding because Ms. J.'s milk has begun to come in and her breasts are engorged. You are the nurse on the unit. You arrive on the morning of discharge to find the baby crying and Ms. J. getting increasingly anxious because the baby won't suck. Nervous Mr. J. suggests a bottle of formula to get the baby quieted down and relax his wife. How would you respond? What follow-up would be appropriate? Include the following points in your answer: (a) importance of support and correct information, (b) use of supplemental bottles before milk supply is established, (c) relationship of anxiety and let-down reflex, (d) importance of informed spouse, (e) household help after discharge, and (f) support group for new mothers and breast-feeding mothers.

4. You are a public health nurse making a newborn home visit through the county health department to Ms. W., a thirty-year-old legal secretary who has been home from the hospital for ten days with her first child, a healthy six-and-a-half-pound boy. When you arrive for your 11:00 A.M. appointment you find the apartment disheveled and Ms. W. in her nightgown. When you introduce yourself and ask how things are going, she bursts into tears, saying, "I can't seem to manage. The baby is fine and nursing well, but I don't have time to do anything else. I'm usually such an organized person, but now I barely make it through the day. I've had to cancel two lunch dates and an appointment at the hairdresser's. I'm lucky if I can just get the house cleaned, keep up with laundry, and get dinner on the table by the time my husband comes home. I was looking forward to a relaxed maternity leave, but so far I haven't relaxed a bit." How would you respond? Include the following points in your answer: (a) realistic expectations of life with a newborn, (b) household help after discharge, (c) support group for new/nursing mothers, and (d) reasons women stop nursing—fatigue.

5. Ms. L. is a sixteen-year-old single woman who lives with her parents. She has recently arrived home with her healthy six-and-a-half-pound daughter, whom she is breast-feeding. You are the nurse visiting Ms. L. at home through a special program for adolescent parents. Ms. L. reports that she is afraid she is running out of milk. When you ask why, she tells you: "In the hospital my milk was so creamy and rich-looking, now it's so thin. My mother gets on the bathroom scale with the baby after every feeding and tells me the baby isn't gaining any weight. Mom says she couldn't breast-feed me because her milk dried up. She says it runs in our family. I was looking forward to breast-feeding until September, when I go back to school; of course, I'd have to stop then." How would you respond? Include the following points in your answer: (a) two parts of lactation, (b) role of anxiety in let-down reflex, (c) ways to promote milk production (diet, adequate fluids, frequent sucking by infant), (d) ways to tell if the baby is feeding adequately, (e) community support groups for nursing mothers, (f) educating the rest of the family about breast-feeding, and (g) use of supplemental bottles and breast-feeding simultaneously.

6. Ms. K. is a twenty-six-year-old woman who delivered a healthy seven-pound daughter three days ago. Her labor and delivery were slow, and she was heavily medicated during the delivery. Ms. K. is breast-feeding her baby, as she did her three-year-old son, but confides to you, her nurse, that the newborn is not drinking much. "She falls asleep at my breast, and even when she sucks, it is not too vigorous—not at all like my son was." You also note that Ms. K.'s breasts are slightly engorged. How would you respond? Include the following in your answer: (a) effects of medication during delivery on baby and sucking reflex, (b) different sucking styles of babies, and (c) ways to prevent engorgement or complications from engorgement.

REFERENCES

1. Atkinson, Leslie D. "Prenatal Nipple Conditioning for Breast-Feeding." *Nursing Research* 28 (5):267–71, 1979.
2. Beer, A. E. "Immunologic Benefits and Hazards of Milk in the Maternal-Perinatal Relationship: Natural Transplantation of Leukocytes During Sucking." *Ross Conference Pediatric Research* 68:48–53, 1975.
3. "Breast-feeding—New Evidence It's Far More Than Nutrition." *Medical World News,* February 5, 1979, 70.
4. Brody, Jane. *Jane Brody's Nutrition Book.* New York: W. W. Norton, 1981, 346.
5. Brook, C.G.D., and J. Dobbing. "Fat Cells in Childhood Obesity." *Lancet* 1:224, 1975.
6. Cole, Judith. "Breastfeeding in the Boston Suburbs in Relation to Personal-Social Factors." *Clinical Pediatrics* 16:352–56, April 1977.
7. Committee on Nutrition, American Academy of Pediatrics. "Commentary on Breast-feeding and Infant Formulas, Including Proposed Standards for Formulas." *Pediatrics* 57:278, 1976.
8. Committee on Nutrition, American Academy of Pediatrics. "Iron Supplementation for Infants." *Pediatrics* 58:765, 1976.
9. Committee on Nutrition, Canadian Paediatric Society and American Academy of Pediatrics. "Breast-feeding—A Commentary in Celebration of the International Year of the Child." *Pediatrics* 62:597, October 1978.
10. Cunningham, A. S. "Morbidity in Breast-fed and Artificially-fed Infants." *Journal of Pediatrics* 90:726, 1970.
11. Eid, E. E. "Follow-up Study of Physical Growth of Children Who Had an Excessive Weight Gain in First Six Months of Life." *British Medical Journal* 2:145, 1961.
12. Eiger, M., and S. Olds. *The Complete Book of Breastfeeding.* New York: Workman Publishing, 1972.
13. Fallot, Mary E., John L. Boyd III, and Frank Oski. "Breast-feeding Reduces the Incidence of Hospital Admissions for Infection in Infants." *Pediatrics* 65:1121–24, June 1980.
14. Goldman, A. S., and C. W. Smith. "Host Resistance Factors in Human Milk." *Journal of Pediatrics* 82:1082–90, June 1973.
15. Grams, Kathryn Effken. "Breast-feeding: A Means of Imparting Immunity?" *American Journal of Maternal Child Nursing* 3:343, November–December 1978.
16. Guyton, Arthur C. *Textbook of Medical Physiology.* Philadelphia: W. B. Saunders, 1981, 1034.
17. Haire, D. B. *The Cultural Warping of Childbirth.* Seattle: International Childbirth Education Association, 1972.
18. Hall, B. "Changing Composition of Human Milk and Early Development of an Appetite Control." *Lancet* 1:779, 1975.
19. La Leche League International, Inc. *The Womanly Art of Breastfeeding.* Franklin Park, Ill.: Interstate Publishers, 1958, 9.
20. Ladas, Alice K. "How to Help Mothers Breastfeed." *Clinical Pediatrics* 9:702–5, December 1970.
21. Lawrence, Ruth. *Breast-feeding: A Guide for the Medical Profession.* St. Louis: C. V. Mosby, 1980, 18.
22. Lloyd, J. K., O. H. Wolff, and W. S. Whelen. "Childhood Obesity: A Long-term Study of Height and Weight." *British Medical Journal* 2:145, 1961.
23. Mata, D., and Sc. Leonardo. "Breast-feeding: Main Promoter of Infant Health." *American Journal of Clinical Nutrition* 31:2058, November 1978.

24. Matthew, D. J., B. Taylor, and A. P. Norman. "Prevention of Eczema." *Lancet* 1:321, 1977.

25. Meyer, H. "Breast Feeding in the United States." *Clinical Pediatrics* 7:708–15, 1968.

26. Meyer, H. "Breast Feeding in the United States: Extent and Possible Trend." *Pediatrics* 12:116–21, 1958.

27. Newton, N. "Psychologic Differences Between Breast- and Bottle-feeding." *American Journal of Clinical Nutrition* 24:993, 1971.

28. "Recommendations for Action Programmes to Encourage Breast Feeding." *Acta Paediatrica Scandinavica* 65:275, 1976.

29. Reifsnider, E., and S. T. Myers. "Employed Mothers Can Breast-feed Too!" *American Journal of Maternal-Child Nursing* 4:256–58, July–August 1985.

30. *Ross National Mothers' Survey.* MR-77-48. Columbus, Ohio: Ross Laboratories, 1978.

31. Slopper, K. S., E. Elsden, and J. D. Baum. "Increasing Breast-feeding in a Community." *Archives of Disease in Childhood* 52:700, 1977.

32. Slopper, K. S., L. McKean, and J. D. Baum. "Factors Influencing Breastfeeding." *Archives of Disease in Childhood* 50:165, 1975.

33. Smart, J. L., and F. N. Bamford. "Breast-feeding: 'Spontaneous' Trends and Differences." *Lancet* 2:42, 1976.

34. Swict, M. de, P. Fayers, and L. Cooper. "Effect of Feeding Habit on Weight in Infancy." *Lancet* 1:892, 1977.

35. Wood, C.B.S., in discussion with S. Sojolin. "Present Trends in Breastfeeding." *Current Medical Research and Opinion* [Suppl.] 4:24, 1976.

36. World Health Organization. Twenty-seventh World Health Assembly. "Part I: Infant Nutrition and Breastfeeding." *Official Records of the World Health Organization* 217:20, 1974.

CHAPTER 23

Working Mothers

NANCY JACKSON

.

OBJECTIVES

After completing this chapter, the reader will be able to:

- State four reasons why more mothers are employed outside the home now than in the past.
- Discuss research findings on the effects of a mother's working on family life, relationship with spouse, welfare of children, and the life satisfaction of the woman.
- Explain five types of child care arrangements and the advantages and disadvantages of each type.
- List psychological and physical signs of stress exhibited by working mothers.
- Name two psychological factors that determine whether eustress or distress occurs.
- Recognize specific stresses that can affect the mother who works outside the home, the mother who works as a nurse, and the mother who works as a homemaker.
- Plan primary nursing care for a working mother, her family, and her community.
- Apply crisis intervention theory to a client who is a working mother.
- Demonstrate the use of the self-care concept in giving nursing care to a working mother.

The primary nurse should be aware of social changes that can influence the individuals, families, and communities where she works. One major change that is affecting more families every year is the increasing number of mothers working outside the home.

According to the 1980 U.S. Census Bureau report "Trends in Child Care Arrangements of Working Mothers," almost half of all women who had children under six years old were in the labor force (29). The women's movement, economic conditions, the increased divorce rate, and the trend toward smaller families have all contributed to the rise in the number of working mothers.

This chapter focuses on the special stresses and health needs of working women and their families. It looks at how the mother's working affects family life, the relationship with her spouse, the welfare of the children, and the satisfaction of the woman herself. Special attention will be given to the working mother who is a nurse, as this subject may be particularly relevant to the reader.

Although the focus of the chapter is on the mother who works outside the home, it is recognized that *all* mothers are working mothers; the unique stresses and needs of the mother who opts to remain at home with her children will also be investigated.

Nursing intervention for all of these types of working mothers is discussed, with emphasis on anticipatory guidance and self-care.

Issues in Maternal Employment

Effects on Family Life

The effects of maternal employment on family life and household management have become a major research interest. Szinovacz notes that most studies show that the wife's employment is consistently shown to increase the husband's participation in household chores and to further egalitarian roles and relationships between spouses. She believes, however, that research designs and interpretations may have been oversimplified, and that no causal link exists between female employment and the couple's division of labor (27).

Studies that differentiate between task allocation and responsibility for management consistently report that although husbands of employed women help with household chores, the responsibility for managing the household remains with the wife (2).

For the mother who returns to work soon after the birth of her first child, the changes involved may revolve mainly around child care responsibilities. Household chores are probably already divided equitably. Decisions for the working parents include what type of child care best suits their needs, who will stay with the child in the morning until the sitter arrives or who will take the baby to the sitter's, who picks the child up or arrives home to relieve the sitter, and who is responsible for child care if the sitter is ill. Added child care responsibilities may require a reallocation of other household tasks.

The woman who has been home with children for several years and decides to return to work often has a hard time delegating household chores. As a housewife she probably was totally in charge of child care, meals, cleaning, laundry, and errands. A family-based approach with cooperation from all members is really necessary for reorganizing the way the family will have to function when mother is no longer around to run the household single-handedly.

The reorganization problem frequently causes the most stress for a mother who is returning to work. She may attempt to take on a new job in addition to all of her former responsibilities. She will then have to spend a good part of her evenings and weekends finishing the housework. It is easy to begin to resent the other family members if they don't make some adjustments and help out with the family chores. Planning ahead and finding new ways for the family to function may avoid some of these stresses.

A change in the way a family functions can be a marvelous lesson for the children involved, if the change is presented positively. Even young children enjoy being treated as participating family members and will help out for the benefit of their family.

Family members may assume new roles when both parents are working; for example, if Mother has to be at work at 7:00 A.M., Father may start being responsible for the children's breakfast and getting them off to school. Children will see more role flexibility in their parents, and this may decrease their own sexual stereotyping. The children themselves may learn new skills and talents when they help out with meal preparation and household tasks. It is important for all members of the family to realize that they are going to have to help out more if they want to share in the enjoyment of having an increased family income.

A single working mother often has no one with whom she can share the responsibility of child care and household tasks. This mother may need to investigate neighborhood resources and find other mothers who can share getting children to school or doing errands. Older children of single mothers may become a great source of help.

Effects on Male-Female Relationships

There is little definitive research on the effects of maternal employment on the spousal relationship. The women's movement's support of working mothers and the economic climate have both contributed to greater acceptance of working mothers by men. It is no longer a threat to most men's egos to have a wife who works and helps in the support of the family. Many men are relieved of the burden of being the sole breadwinner. As long as a mutually agreeable arrangement for performing household tasks can be found, maternal employment is viewed positively by spouses.

An issue that is getting more attention lately is the stress that can occur in a relationship when the woman's income is higher or her job is more prestigious than that of her spouse. Although these situations are still the exception rather than the rule, they do require people to confront the stereotypic notion that men are responsible for the family income.

Effects on Welfare of Children

One area of great concern for working mothers is the effect their absence and the presence a substitute care giver will have on their children. Giants of psychiatry and psychology such as Bowlby, Erikson, and Freud, all attest to the critical role the mother plays in the psychological development of a healthy child (5, 9, 11). Yet the belief concerning the harmful effects of working mothers on preschool children is strongly based in soci-

etal and psychoanalytic tradition, neither of which has ever involved much empirical evidence.

Advocates of working mothers are now challenging these traditional beliefs and are attempting to scientifically document their findings. Hoffman (14) and Howell (15) have found no compelling empirical evidence that a mother's working per se harms her child, prevents attachment formation with her child, or that a mother has to be the principal caretaker of her child.

Several other studies done in the late 1970s documented strong attachment formation between working mothers and their children. But Yudkin and Holme (32) suggest that it may be the mother who loses out when the child is left with a substitute care giver; while the child learns to trust and relate to the substitute care giver, the mother misses out on the parent-child interaction.

Moskowitz, Schwarz, and Corsini (20) found that boys were more negatively influenced in their attachment formation by substitute care givers than were girls. Gold and Andres "found that sons of working mothers tended to have lower IQ scores than sons of mothers who remained at home" (12).

In her extensive review of the effects of maternal employment on preschool children, Smith found little to support the notion that it is quality time spent with a child that is important. Lack of a standardized definition of quality time and lack of a measurement instrument for this idea make it a difficult concept to research (26).

In their review of day-care research, Belsky and Steinberg draw several conclusions that are based on research at high-quality day-care centers. They found this form of child care had neither a salutory nor a deleterious effect on the intellectual development of the child. It did not disrupt the child's emotional bond with his mother, and it increased the degree to which the child interacts, both positively and negatively, with peers (4).

Dr. Helen Lerner, a nurse researcher, studied the cognitive skills and behavior of children using Bayler's Scales of Infant Development. She found no significant developmental difference between children of mothers who worked outside the home and children of mothers who did not (31).

The research available on the effects of maternal employment on preschool children is still limited. There are few studies on the differences between part-time and full-time maternal employment. Most research is done in university-based or specially funded programs that are generally thought to be optimal child care settings. Little is known about the effects of in-home child care, which is the most common in the United States. So for most children the effects of substitute care givers are unknown.

There is a larger body of research on the effects of maternal employment on the school-age child, but it offers few conclusive answers. According to Propper (22), a mother's working had little relationship with her children's academic or personality development, although children of working mothers had more household responsibilities. Etaugh (10) reports that maternal employment seemed to be negatively related to achievement in boys and either unrelated or positively related in girls. Daughters of working mothers tend to have less stereotypic views of roles for men and women and are more inclined to have higher career aspirations (3, 7).

Smith suggests further research in this area needs to take into consideration the early experiences of the children (at what age did their mothers begin working and was it part-time or full-time), the type of preschool educational exposure the child had, and the mother's role in the educational experience (26). Other variables to consider might be one- or two-parent homes and whether the mother is working for financial need alone or for pleasure or challenge.

Effects on the Women

It is difficult to evaluate the effects of working on the women themselves because there are so many kinds of women working in so many different jobs. Birnbaum's study showed that professional working mothers gain self-esteem and have a higher sense of competence (even in the area of child care) and fewer identity problems than women with the same background who opted for full-time mothering (14). The psychological value and challenge of work for women may be true for professional women, but the picture may be quite different for the average working woman.

Recent research on ordinary working women has not painted such a positive view of the psychological benefits of work for women. Eighty percent of all working women who are not professionals hold factory, service, or clerical positions and live a limited existence—one that is often neither challenging nor exciting. Most of these women work because of financial necessity (28).

A national survey of 150,000 women found the average worker to be a lonely person in a dead-end job, seething with frustration over her situation. Family life and children only deepened her dissatisfaction because they created more problems regarding housework and child care. About 50 percent of the respondents stated that their jobs were boring and did not use their skills, and the same number had no chance to train for better jobs. Almost 55 percent of the women reported they had no leisure time (28).

Despite these drawbacks, many women still prefer to combine motherhood and a job. In Bryant's study of 1,522 adult women in the United States, half of the women responded that the ideal life would be to remain at home when their children were young but to combine homemaking and a job after the children reached school age. Only one in ten women under thirty-five years of age wanted to be a homemaker for life (6).

A study conducted by Brown University of 3,000 students from six prestigious East Coast colleges indicates that many young women now say that they would pick family over career. About 77 percent of the women said that mothers should work not at all or only part-time until their children were five years old. Eighty-four percent of the men agreed with them. "Even some of the most career-minded women said they planned to take time off from their professions to raise children, even if it meant jeopardizing advancement" (17).

Only time will tell if these women will feel the same way when they are actually confronted with the decision of whether to interrupt a career and take at least three to five years off to start a family. The reality of losing tenure or missing out on promotions may lead them to reconsider their responses in the college survey.

One study that does have importance for both professional-managerial and clerical-technical groups was conducted on white, two-parent families. In this investigation McCroskey found that there was a positive relationship between personal life satisfaction and child care satisfaction for mothers in both occupational groups (18).

There are important implications for nursing in all of this research related to maternal employment. The primary nurse is in an ideal situation to promote self-care in the mother and, with anticipatory guidance, help her and her family adapt successfully with minimal stress.

Child Care

Because satisfaction with child care is such an important factor in most women's lives, it would be helpful for the primary nurse to be aware of the different types of care available in most communities and the benefits and drawbacks of each type. The nurse will then be better able to help the client make an educated decision on what type of child care best suits her needs.

Sharing with Spouse. This arrangement requires that parents have complementary schedules so one of them is always home to care for the child.

Advantages

- Child cared for by own parent
- Child care expenses eliminated

Disadvantage

- Parents may need to work opposite hours and thus have little time to spend with each other. This may strain their relationship.

One-to-One Care in the Home. The arrangement involves one care giver who comes in daily (or lives in) to care for the child.

Advantages

- Consistent one-to-one relationship for the child
- Convenient for the parents because care giver does the traveling
- No change in arrangement needed if child is ill
- Care giver will often have household responsibilities, such as marketing and laundry, that will assist parents

Disadvantages

- Most expensive type of care
- Back-up needed if care giver is ill
- May limit socialization as baby gets older if care giver doesn't arrange for visits with other children
- May be difficult to find a person to work the long hours sometimes needed in this arrangement
- Parents need to feel comfortable with the care giver and agree with her values and style of handling their child. This can be difficult and can change with time; for example, a care giver may be excellent at stimulating and caring for infants and toddlers but may not be good at encouraging more independent behaviors as the child grows.

One to One or More in the Sitter's Home. With this arrangement the parent takes the child each day to a baby-sitter's home. Often the baby-sitter cares for several children at the same time or has children of her own.

Advantages

- Usually less expensive than one to one at home
- Child may have more social contact than if at home with care giver

Disadvantages

- Back-up arrangement is needed if sitter or child is ill
- Parents must travel to the sitter's with the child. This can be time-consuming, especially in cold weather when boots and snowsuits are needed.
- Child may be exposed to several other children each day, increasing the risk of infections

Family Day Care. This arrangement involves taking the child to the home of a person who has been licensed to care for children in her home (this means that she and her home meet certain safety and health regulations).

Advantages

- Reassurance that care giver has been licensed by a sponsoring agency
- Same as one to one in sitter's home

Disadvantage

- Same as one to one in sitter's home

Day-Care Center. Day-care centers may be private or public and vary widely on the types of programs offered. Some businesses and hospitals are finding that providing day care at the workplace is conducive to retaining employees. Most centers, even if they are for infants, have an educational component; centers for the three-to-six-year-old group usually combine nursery school-kindergarten curriculum and child care.

Advantages

- Age-appropriate socialization and education provided for the child
- Usually administered and staffed by professionals with early childhood education backgrounds
- Often open year-round for long hours that can accommodate the parents' needs
- When teachers are ill, it is the center's responsibility to provide substitutes—the center remains open

Disadvantages

- Back-up care needed if child is ill
- May be expensive, although for the older child it includes the cost of nursery school
- May not be conveniently located

After-School Programs. These programs have grown out of the need created by more and more mothers joining the work force. They are generally located in elementary schools or community centers and run from about 3:00 P.M. to 6:00 P.M., to cover the time between dismissal from school and when parents return from work. Designed for the school-age child who is too young to safely spend these hours alone at home, these programs offer a variety of activities such as sports, arts and crafts, cooking, and dance.

Advantages

- Safe, stimulating atmosphere for school-age children of working parents
- Reduces the number of latchkey children (those who go home to an empty house after school and stay there alone until a parent arrives from work)

Disadvantages

- May be expensive
- Alternate arrangement needed if child is ill

Stress and Working Mothers

When Hans Selye described stress he called it a nonspecific response of the body to any demand (25, p. 66). He saw stress showing itself as a specific syndrome that is nonspecifically induced, and called the response the general adaptation syndrome (25).

Selye differentiated between distress, the unpleasant or harmful variety, and eustress, the pleasant, challenging type of stress. He noted that during both eustress and distress, the body undergoes virtually the same nonspecific responses to the various positive or negative stimuli acting on it. However, the fact that eustress causes much less damage than distress graphically demonstrates that it is "how you take it" that determines, ultimately, whether one can successfully adapt to change (25). (Review chapters 15 and 16.)

There is abundant and often contradictory research on the stressor effects of executive responsibilities relative to those of subordinate employees in various occupations. However, here, as in all considerations of stress manifestations, the stressor effect mainly depends on the way a person is conditioned to react to it. This explains the seemingly contradictory findings about whether it is more distressful or eustressful to be the boss or to be bossed. Some people are happier being leaders, others followers; so it is people who are channeled into the wrong leader-follower position who experience the most distress (25).

Posner and Leitner put forth a theoretical model proposing that although stress is stimulated by both pleasant and unpleasant challenges, there are two moderating psychological factors that determine whether eustress or distress occurs. The two psychological factors are the predictability and controllability of the challenging event (21).

According to this theory, events that people cannot control and cannot predict will have the greatest pathogenic stress reaction. There is less stress reaction if either control or prediction is present, and much less stress reaction if both control and prediction are present. The theory proposes that the executive who decides to stay late at the office to work up an idea that may get him a promotion has control over the decision and can predict (he is forewarned). So even though he is working extra hours the stress is a challenge and can clearly be labeled eustress. But his secretary, whom he has asked to stay late to type up his report, has no control over the situation and may or may not have been able to predict this request (staying late on occasion may have been in the job description). The secretary is more likely to experience distress.

This theory is particularly relevant to the 80 percent of women who hold factory, service, or clerical jobs. Although they may have some degree of prediction about the job, they probably have little control and are apt to experience distress.

Stress and the body's response to it have been identified as major pathogenic factors in peptic ulceration, surgical shock, hypertension, cardiovascular diseases, and many other medical problems, as well as many psychological disorders. Prevention and early treatment of stress effects clearly are important to the health of the public.

Motherhood Mandate

Much of the stress on working mothers can be traced to what Russo calls the "motherhood mandate." According to Russo, "motherhood is on a quantitatively different plane than other sex roles in our society. It is a mandate that pervades our social institutions as well as our psyches" (24). The mandate basically requires that a woman "have at least two children and raise them 'well.'" She can, however, become educated, work, and be active in public life, as long as she first fills this obligation. The kicker in this scheme is the definition of "well." A "good" mother must be physically present to fulfill her infant's every need. As the child enters school, a mother may pursue other activities, but only those permitting her to be instantly available if her child should "need" her (24).

It is easy to see how a working mother would have a hard time living up to this mandate. Most women's response to the inability to conform to this mandate is *guilt*. No matter how independent, liberated, or successful the working mother may be, on some level she seems to feel guilty about leaving her child to go to work.

Even women who are solely financially responsible for themselves and their children and truly have no choice but to work report feeling guilty about not being always available to their children. They realize that they have no alternative, but they still feel guilty. Mothers who *could* afford to remain at home with the children for the early years but who have outside interests or career aspirations and want to work feel guilty too. The motherhood mandate is most pervasive.

Role Conflict

Many working mothers are thought to suffer from role conflict—the uncertainty between whether to stay home as a homemaker or to work outside the home. But Hall thinks that working mothers are really experiencing role overload. According to Hall, the strains from work and home "have been traditionally seen as the woman's responsibility, and if she chooses to work, it was similarly seen as her responsibility to find means of coping with them" (13).

Some research confirms that working mothers experience more strain and stress than do women who remain home with their children. In her doctoral dissertation Robison defined strain as a reaction to an accumulation of role demands. She found that employed mothers, especially those with preschool children, demonstrated more strain than did housewives (23). But other studies conducted at Wellesley Center for Research on Women show that staying at home was never unstressful, and that some women experience less stress when they enter the work force. An interesting job may provide gratification and act as a buffer against the stresses at home. In one study, women reported that the mother and homemaker roles were more stressful then their workplace roles (8).

Numerous stresses may be specific to the work that the mother does. The following are some examples:

Noise: constant high noise levels for factory workers, typists, keypunch operators, laundry workers

Heat: some factory and laundry workers may work in constantly warm environments

Radiation: high levels of radiation may exist for x-ray technicians, dentists, radiologists, or nuclear power plant workers, or in some laboratories

Physical exertion: job requirements for such women as nurses, physical therapists, firewomen, or policewomen may include lifting or carrying heavy objects or people

Postural requirements: jobs that require a lot of sitting or standing can lead to back strain or poor circulation and may lead to development of varicose veins, hemorrhoids; writing and typing can lead to writer's cramp and tenosynovitis of wrists

Chemicals: workers in contact with anesthetic gases, organic solvents, and halogenated hydrocarbons, including anesthesiologists, some factory or laboratory workers, artists, photographers, beauticians

Microbial hazards: health care workers and hospital workers who care for persons with infectious diseases are at risk for contracting the diseases

Temporal stresses: any worker with strict deadlines, or workers doing slow or monotonous work; people who frequently rotate shifts

Another stress that affects the working mother is concern over her child care arrangements. Many mothers report that they worry about their children's well-being while they are separated.

Sexual harassment is said to affect up to 80 percent of working women at some point in the working career. This is another stressor that women must cope with (19).

Much concern and research about the effects of occupational stresses on working women focus on the effects of the stressors on pregnant women and the fetus. Figure 23.1 shows the potential adverse effects of job exposures on reproduction or on the ability to have healthy children. These hazards may affect either parent before conception or even after birth.

The effects of all these stresses that the working mother is experiencing may be extensive. The most frequently reported symptoms are fatigue, mild depression, frustration or anger from lack of leisure time or time for self, marital strain, and insomnia. As more women enter the work force there will be a corresponding increase in stress-related diseases among women. Health care workers should be aware of the need to pre-

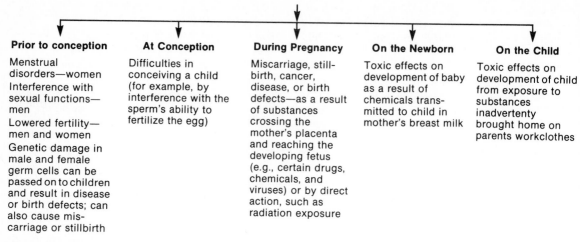

Figure 23.1. Chronology of Potential Adverse Effects of Job Exposures on Reproduction or on the Ability to Have Normal Healthy Children

Source: From A. Hricko. Working for Your Life: A Women's Guide to Job Health Hazards. Labor Occupational Health Program/Health Research Group, 1976.

vent stress-related diseases, such as hypertension, cardiovascular disease, and ulcers, in their patients who are working mothers.

Superwoman Syndrome

There is a need in many mothers, fostered by the motherhood mandate, to try to become superwoman. This syndrome involves being the best mother, wife, and worker. Some women do manage to live up to this title, at least for a while, but it is often at the expense of their own mental and physical health. These women may need help and support from health care workers in setting priorities, compromising, and promoting self-care.

Working Mothers with Unique Stresses and Needs

A few categories of working mothers have unique stresses and needs.

Single Working Mothers. Single working mothers may be totally responsible for themselves and their children. They may have the stress of a recent separation or divorce, in addition to the normal stresses of work and children. Crisis intervention is often needed to help these women mobilize their coping skills and find community resources to assist them and their children.

Another variation of the single mother is the *displaced homemaker.* This is usually an older woman whose children are grown and who is forced by divorce or the death of her spouse to enter the working world. This woman may still be in crisis, mourning the death of her spouse or her marriage, but has to find a job and learn to support herself (1). Crisis intervention is also needed for such displaced homemakers.

Homemakers. The needs of this group of working mothers are often ignored by themselves and by health care workers. Women who opt to stay at home with their children and spend their time doing household tasks are also under numerous stresses. Besides the physical exertion from housework, they are exposed to many of the same chemical and noise hazards as women in the workplace. Soaps, detergents, bleaches, polishing agents, cleaning solvents and their fumes can all have toxic effects on the homemaker who is exposed to them. Noise levels from a vacuum cleaner, dishwasher, and stove exhaust are comparable to some factory noise levels.

But the most pervasive stress associated with being a homemaker seems to be the sense of isolation and the perception of low status associated with the job. This perception is probably intensified as more mothers join the work force. Twenty years ago there was at least some social support for women who remained at home.

Ironically, the movement to support working mothers has been so successful in some ways that it has left the full-time homemaker feeling like a relic. She may be very defensive about staying home with her children, even if she intends to do this for only a few years.

One of the hardest aspects of being a homemaker is the lack of a schedule and the constant interruption that having children can involve. There is no job description and no formal training for the position, and most women set their own standards on what they expect from themselves. For some women this autonomy is an advantage of the homemaker job, but others miss the more classic rewards that are inherent in most work situations—a paycheck, evaluations, promotions, and vacations. In either case, the sense of isolation and the boredom and monotony of many of the tasks can lead to loneliness, depression, and a sense of low self-esteem.

It is a common supposition that because of all the labor-saving appliances that are now available, the homemaker of today spends fewer hours at her job than her grandmother did. Studies show that this is not true. In 1924 women spent about fifty-two hours each week doing housework and this number rose to fifty-five hours in the 1960s. Vanek's explanation for this is multifaceted. She proposes that although women now spend less time producing food and clothing, they spend the time shopping for these items; time devoted to laundry has increased despite automatic appliances and permanent press fabrics because people now have more clothes than in the past and wash them more often. The amount of time spent on child care has greatly increased, as mothers are now careful to develop their children socially and emotionally in addition to the traditional concerns of health, discipline, and cleanliness (30).

The superwoman in the working mother has a counterpart in the homemaker. She is known as Supermom and can be identified by her boundless energy for doing things for her husband and children. She, too, may ignore her own needs and eventually suffer the stressful consequences.

Nurses. Nurses are susceptible to all the usual stresses of working mothers but have some unique stresses in their profession. They may have physically demanding jobs that involve long hours with a lot of standing and lifting of patients. Emergency room nurses and those working in intensive care may also experience a fast pace. The job of a nurse is also emotionally demanding, as it frequently involves working with people in crisis, such as those experiencing death or illness in the family. The nurturing role of the nurse may be similar to her nurturing role as mother or wife at home, for example, the pediatric nurse who works with ill toddlers all day and then goes home to her own young children, or the nurse on the oncology unit whose husband is home with terminal cancer. Both of these nurses are at risk for role overload and need guidance to cope with the demands of both roles.

Nurses as a group have a lot of responsibility (the predictable factor) and little authority (the control factor), which can lead to distress. Another stress affecting nurses is the relatively low remuneration they receive in proportion to the work they perform.

The shifts and shift rotations that many nurses work are also stressful to their circadian rhythms and their personal lives. One study emphasized that peptic ulcers are particularly common among shift workers, probably because night work is especially fatiguing and conducive to mental distress. Adaptation does tend to occur after a while, especially when shift work does not provoke social problems. Rotating shift work probably produces the severest disturbances in corticoid and adrenaline production (25, p. 374).

All of these stresses can lead to a syndrome found in the caring professions known as burnout. Day-care workers, teachers, social workers, doctors, and the clergy, as well as nurses, are all susceptible to this "occupational tedium." It generally leaves its victims exhausted and physically ill. They may lose their feelings of sympathy and respect for patients and peers and try to avoid work. They may be depressed and develop a drug dependency (16).

Causes of burnout can be both personal (high expectations of self, high need for approval, unrealistic goals) and structural (too large a client load, unreasonable work schedule, lack of authority, lack of feedback on work performed). In either case, burnout is a reality for the nursing profession and is a stress that should be addressed on both a personal and an organizational level.

Planning Nursing Care for the Working Mother

The practitioner of primary nursing will come into contact with working mothers in a variety of settings (see the case studies at the end of the chapter). Frequently the working mother will not even be the primary patient with whom the nurse is working; but as a member of the family, her needs and problems cannot be overlooked.

In a crisis situation involving a working mother, the

primary nurse is equipped to help the family maximize its coping skills and regain equilibrium. But it is more likely that the primary nurse will encounter the working mother in a situation where primary prevention will be the focus. Unfortunately such opportunities are too often overlooked by health care professionals, who are accustomed to focusing on "problems" and "illness." The practitioner of primary care nursing is in an excellent position to be supportive of the working mother and assist her and her family to develop healthful self-care behaviors.

The primary nurse's many roles in relation to the working mother are outlined in Table 23.1. The role of the nurse in case finding with this group of women cannot be overlooked; indeed, part of the problem with the working mother is that she often puts her own needs last. The nurse must be an advocate for her.

One fact that cannot be overlooked when dealing with any stress-related illness, or the prevention of a stress-related illness, is the importance of exercise in the reduction of stress and the promotion of physical well-being. Morse and Furst (19) cite the following seven purposes of exercise:

1. Strengthening of muscles and tendons
2. Promotion of cardiac fitness
3. Allowance for communication and companionship (if a group activity)
4. Diversion from stress or problems
5. Provision of physical outlet for stress
6. Enhancement of relaxation
7. Prevention of disorders related to inactivity

Exercise of almost any type can be recommended as a way to reduce the stress in the working mother's life. Some types of exercise (biking, swimming, hiking, jogging) can be group activities that the whole family can participate in.

Because women who are working are, by definition, a basically "healthy" group, it may be tempting to overlook the potential stresses that occur in their lives. The primary nurse should view this "healthy" person as a challenge and help her to maintain or improve her level of health. Anticipatory guidance and promotion of self-care activities are ways the primary nurse can achieve this goal.

Caring for the working mother highlights the primary

Table 23.1
Nursing Care Plan for Working Mothers

Primary Prevention	Secondary Prevention	Tertiary Prevention
For Mother		
Anticipatory guidance on child care and changing needs of children	Early recognition of signs of too much stress—headaches, backaches, hypertension, cardiovascular changes, depression	Assist client to develop new coping skills
Health maintenance		Referrals for employment counseling
Promote self-care behaviors:	Referrals for treatment as necessary	Community resources to aid working mother, e.g., child care and after-school programs
—regular exams	Prevention of sequelae of stresses	
—schedule time for fun exercise	Crisis intervention with family	
For Family		
Education on the benefits of role flexibility within the family	Assist family members to make role changes needed to adapt to change, e.g., mother returning to work, new baby	
For Community		
Advocate increased awareness of needs for quality child care	Advocate flexible hours for jobs when it's possible—10:00–6:00 instead of 8:00–4:00 would help out mothers with school age children	
Advocate longer clinic and office hours to accommodate working mothers (early A.M., evenings, and weekends)	Advocate job sharing—where two people share the salary and benefits of one position—can work out well for part-time workers	

nurse's role in case finding and planning health care. Often the primary nurse is not directly involved with all aspects of the care given. Referrals to other health care providers or to community resources may be required to meet the working mother's needs. But the primary nurse is the coordinator of this care and is accountable for follow-up to ensure that the woman's needs are met.

CASE STUDY 1

Mrs. R., a thirty-two-year-old attorney, has a six-month-old son. You are the nurse at the gynecologist's office where she has an appointment to change her method of birth control.

You notice that Mrs. R. looks tired and ask her how her new routine of working and motherhood is going. She tells you that she enjoyed her one-month maternity leave and returned to work part-time for a few months and gradually worked back up to full-time one month ago. She hired a baby-sitter to come to her home daily to care for the infant and do light housekeeping tasks. This has worked out quite well, and she and her husband are pleased with the way the sitter handles their son.

When you ask about the change in birth control method, Mrs. R. tells you why she wants to switch from an intrauterine device to a diaphragm and then adds, "Not that it makes much difference—who has the time or energy for a sex life anymore?"

Further inquiry leads Mrs. R. to confide in you that she is exhausted when she returns from work each evening and is not always as enthusiastic about caring for her son at this time as she thinks she should be. Weekends are spent catching up on errands and shopping and there seems to be little leisure time for her and her husband, either individually or together.

Mr. R., who is also an attorney, travels a lot in connection with his job. Although he is supportive of his wife's working and does help out with household tasks and child care, he is often out of town for two or three days each week.

The past week has been particularly difficult for Mrs. R. because her husband has been away and her son has been getting up several times each night with teething problems. Mrs. R. explains to you that she's exhausted from being up with the baby during the night and then putting in a full day's work at a demanding job. She is in tears by this time and is looking to you for some help.

a. Identify some stresses in Mrs. R.'s life.
b. What nursing care can you plan for this woman and her family?

CASE STUDY 2

Mrs. L. is a forty-year-old mother of three children, ages ten, eight, and six years. Before having children Mrs. L. worked as a secretary, but she has been home full time with her children for the past ten years. You are the nurse at the HMO where she has come in for an employment physical. She tells you that she is in a training program for computer programmers.

When you inquire about her new job she informs you that she enjoys her work and everything at home has been running smoothly since she started the training program two months ago. But then she adds, "We'll see what happens when school starts and my husband starts his teaching job. He's been caring for the children all summer and it's been marvelous—of course, the house isn't as clean as it was when I was home all day, but I manage to catch up with that and the laundry on evenings and weekends. I am concerned about when school starts. My oldest child will be bringing the younger two home each afternoon and staying with them until my husband gets home at five o'clock. They'll be alone for about two hours every day. I'm not too pleased with this arrangement, but hiring a baby-sitter for those hours would just take too much of my salary."

a. What are the stresses and potential stresses in Mrs. L.'s life?
b. What would you include in planning nursing care for her and her family?

CASE STUDY 3

Ms. N. is a twenty-four-year-old single mother of two children, ages two and a half and five years old. She works as a file clerk for a municipal agency. You are the nurse at the day-care center that her children attend. Ms. N. has taken the morning off so she can be present when the two children receive their annual physical examination.

When you ask Ms. N. how she's managing with her work and the children, she replies, "Well, life will be much easier now that both children can attend the day-care center. I used to have to take them to different places each morning. By the time I got them up, dressed, fed, and dropped off, I'd feel exhausted. My biggest problem right now is that my sister, who used to live near me, is moving far away. I used to count on her to cover for me if one of my kids was sick, or something. I was hoping to start night school so I could get a better job, but now I don't think I could manage."

a. Identify the stresses in Ms. N.'s life.
b. Plan nursing care for Ms. N.

CASE STUDY 4

Mrs. B. is a twenty-eight-year-old nurse who works as a night supervisor on a busy medical-surgical unit at a large urban teaching hospital. She has worked the 11:00 P.M.-to-7:00 A.M. shift for the entire five years of her marriage. Mr. B. is an accountant who works from 9:00 A.M. to 5:00 P.M. The B.'s have found that their complementary schedules have still allowed them to spend adequate time together. They usually have breakfast together each morning as Mrs. B. is arriving home and Mr. B. is leaving for work. Mrs. B. sleeps during the day and is awake to enjoy the evening hours with her husband before she leaves for work.

Mrs. B. is five months pregnant with her first child when you meet her at the gynecologist's office where you are the nurse. When you ask about her plans to return to work, she tells you about the conflicts she is feeling—wanting to be both full-time worker and mother; how will they fit the baby into their schedules as they now stand, and what types of child care might be best suited to their needs?

a. Identify stresses in Mrs. B.'s life.
b. What would her nursing care include?

CASE STUDY 5

Mrs. A. is a thirty-five-year-old woman with two children, ages five and six years. Before becoming a mother Mrs. A. had worked for eight years as a flight attendant. After the birth of their first child she and her husband both agreed that she should quit her job and be at home full time with the children. The couple agree that they'd rather do without some luxuries that an extra income might allow to have Mrs. A. with the children.

You are the nurse at the children's school and meet Mrs. A. when she comes to pick up a neighbor's child who has become ill during school. Her facial expression and hostile voice indicate to you that Mrs. A. is angry. When you ask her about this she blurts out, "Yes, I *am* angry—not at you, or this child, or even her parent. It's just that I'm about the only full-time mother left in our neighborhood and most of the other mothers have asked if I'll cover for them in an emergency. Now how do you say no to that? But this is the third time this month I've had to pick up someone else's sick child. The last time I ended up catching whatever it was the child had, and my whole family got ill!"

Further discussion reveals that Mrs. A. is a basically happy woman who has enjoyed mothering her children. Sometimes she resents her neighbors, who she thinks take advantage of her ("You'd think I had nothing better to do than let in their repairmen and sign for their packages from United Parcel"). Mrs. A. does admit to being lonely at times, since both children are in school all day and she sometimes misses the excitement of her former work, which involved traveling and meeting so many people.

Mrs. A. also tells you of her desire to eventually begin work-

ing again when her children are several years older. But she admits to being totally at a loss for ideas for a job ("Flight attendants' hours are just too irregular and I'm really too old for that").

a. Identify the stresses in Mrs. A.'s life.
b. What nursing intervention would you plan for her?

REFERENCES

1. Bagby, Beatrice H. "Displaced Homemakers in the Midst of Crisis." *Journal of Home Economics,* Summer 1979, 24.
2. Bahr, S. J. "Effects of Power and Division of Labor in the Family." In *Working Mothers,* ed. L. W. Hoffman and F. I. Nye. San Francisco: Jossey-Bass, 1974, 167–85.
3. Baruch, G. "Maternal Influences upon College Women's Attitudes Toward Women and Work." *Developmental Psychology* 6:32–37, 1972.
4. Belsky, J., and L. D. Steinberg. "The Effects of Day Care: A Critical Review." *Child Development* 49:929, 1978.
5. Bowlby, J. A. *Attachment.* New York: Basic Books, 1969.
6. Bryant, M. "Attitudes of Adult Women." Washington, D.C.: Government Printing Office, 1977.
7. Conway, C. Y., and M. L. Niple. "The Working Patterns of Mothers and Grandmothers of Freshman at the Ohio State University, 1955 and 1965." *Journal of the National Association of Women's Deans and Counselors* 29:167, 1966.
8. Darnton, N. "Women and Stress: On the Job and at Home." *New York Times,* August 6, 1986, C1.
9. Erikson, H. E. *Childhood and Safety.* New York: W. W. Norton, 1963.
10. Etaugh, C. "Effects of Nonmaternal Care on Children: Research Evidence and Popular Views." *American Psychologist* 35:309, 1980.
11. Freud, Sigmund. *An Outline for Psychoanalysis.* New York: W. W. Norton, 1949.
12. Gold, D., and D. Andres. "Developmental Comparisons Between Adolescent Children with Employed and Unemployed Mothers." *Merrill-Palmer Quarterly* 24:243, 1978.
13. Hall, D. T. "Pressures from Work, Self and Home in the Life Stages of Married Women." *Journal of Vocational Behavior* 6:121–32, 1975.
14. Hoffman, L. W. "Maternal Employment: 1979." *American Psychologist* 34:859–65, 1979.
15. Howell, M. C. "Effects of Maternal Employment on the Child," pt. 2. *Pediatrics* 52:327–43, 1973.
16. Lavendero, Ramon. "Nursing Burnout: What Can We Learn?" *Journal of Nursing Administration* 11:17–23, November/December 1981.
17. "Many Young Women Now Say They'd Pick Family over Career." *New York Times,* December 28, 1980, 1, 24.

18. McCroskey, J. D. S. "Working Mothers and Child Care: The Context of Child Care Satisfaction for Working Mothers, with Pre-school Children." Ph.D. diss. University of California, Los Angeles. Dissertation Abstracts International, 1980, 1776-A.

19. Morse, D. R., and M. L. Furst. *Women Under Stress.* New York: Van Nostrand Reinhold Co., 1982.

20. Moskowitz, D. S., J. C. Schwarz, and D. A. Corsini. "Initiating Day Care at Three Years of Age: Effects of Attachment." *Child Development* 48:1271, 1977.

21. Posner, I., and L. A. Leitner. "Eustress vs. Distress: Determination by Predictability and Controllability of the Stressor." *Stress* 2:10, Summer 1981.

22. Propper, A. M. "The Relationship of Maternal Employment to Adolescent Roles, Activities and Parental Relationships." *Journal of Marriage and the Family* 34:417, 1972.

23. Robison, E. "Strain and Dual Role Occupation Among Women." Ph.D. diss., City University of New York, 1977. Dissertation Abstracts International, 1977, Order No. 77-28, 227.

24. Russo, N. F. "Overview: Sex Roles, Fertility and the Motherhood Mandate." *Psychology of Women Quarterly* 4:7, 1979.

25. Selye, Hans. *The Stress of Life.* Rev. ed. New York: McGraw-Hill, 1978.

26. Smith, Elsie J. "The Working Mother: A Critique of the Research." *Journal of Vocational Behavior* 19:196, 199, October 1981.

27. Szinovacz, Maximiliane. "Women Employed: Effects on Spouses' Division of Household Work." *Journal of Home Economics,* Summer 1979, 42.

28. "The Deep Discontent of the Working Women." *Business Week,* February 5, 1979, 25–29.

29. U.S. Census Bureau Report. "Trends in Child Care Arrangements of Working Mothers." 1980.

30. Vanek, Joann. "Time Spent Doing Housework." *Scientific American* 231:116–20, November 1974.

31. "What If Mother Works?" *On Campus,* October 1985, 11.

32. Yudkin, S., and A. Holme. *Working Mothers and Their Children.* London: Michael Joseph, 1963.

CHAPTER 24

Older Parents

NANCY JACKSON

∎

OBJECTIVES

After completing this chapter, the reader will be able to:

- State seven reasons why more women are having children when they are over thirty-five years old.
- State what ages are considered optimal, physically, for a woman to bear a child.
- Define maternal mortality, complication of pregnancy, obstetrical complication, prematurity, low birth weight, amniocentesis, sonography, fetoscopy, and infertility.
- Discuss maternal risks associated with advanced maternal age.
- Discuss risks to the infant associated with advanced maternal age.
- Discuss paternal age as a risk factor in pregnancy.
- Describe amniocentesis and fetoscopy and their uses.
- List ten genetic diseases and abnormalities that can be detected by amniocentesis or fetoscopy.
- State three causes of infertility in women.
- Describe three ways to treat infertility in women.
- State two causes of infertility in men.
- Describe two ways to treat infertility in men.
- Describe the role of the genetic counselor.
- Compare the role of the genetic counselor with the role of the primary nurse.
- Discuss the nurse's role in supporting the couple who is having amniocentesis.
- Plan primary nursing care for the expectant couple over thirty-five.

There has been an upward shift in the age at which women are having children. From 1979 to 1980 first-order birthrates increased 8.5 percent for women aged thirty to thirty-four and 8.3 percent for those aged thirty-five to thirty-nine, while the total birthrate increased only 3.1 percent for the same period. This is consistent with the trend in the past few years. From 1975 to 1980 the first-order birthrate advanced 60 percent for women aged thirty to thirty-four and 37 percent for those aged thirty-five to thirty-nine, whereas it rose only 22 percent for women aged twenty-two to twenty-nine (18).

Some women are opting to delay starting a family and others decide to enlarge their families at a later date. The reasons for these decisions are considered in this chapter, as well as the implications for the primary nurse. The chapter focuses on the role of the primary nurse when working with older parents.

Couples are opting for parenthood at a later age for several reasons. More young adults are spending their time going to college and establishing careers, postponing marriage and family. Men have been following this pattern for a longer time than women, but now that women are more career-minded, there is a larger group of women over age thirty-five who are bearing children. The women's movement's support of career planning for women has definitely had an impact on birth statistics.

Another influence on the age of parenting is the availability of more reliable methods of contraception, which allows couples to have more control over when they will start a family. Some people make this decision early in their relationship, but as they near the age when the decision is irrevocable, they change their minds; or couples who already have children may decide that they want one more before they are too old.

Because family size is decreasing, people seem to be thinking more about how they want their children to fit into their lives; they often opt to spend several years enjoying "adult life," getting settled in a job, and becoming financially secure before starting their small family.

The rising life expectancy for Americans makes the decision to have children at an older age less of a disadvantage now than it was several generations ago. At that time couples in their forties who gave birth to a child couldn't expect to see that child reach his or her twentieth birthday. This is not true today, when life expectancy for both men and women is over seventy years.

Another reason more women are giving birth at later ages is the high rate of divorce and remarriage. Often those who are having children later in life are starting "second families," where one or both members of the couple already have children from a previous marriage.

Infertility also plays a part in the increasing rate of childbirth in women over thirty-five. About one in five American couples are infertile (8). The American Fertility Society claims that specialists can help about 70 percent of these couples (8), but the time it takes to diagnose and treat the problem makes it more likely that these parents will be over thirty-five years old.

Another group who are having children when they are over thirty-five are single women who have decided that they may never marry and want children before their time runs out. These women usually are self-supporting and put a lot of thought into the decision to raise a child alone.

Advances in antenatal diagnosis through amniocentesis and fetoscopy have also played a role in delaying parenthood for some couples. The security they feel in being able to have the fetus checked for some of the abnormalities associated with advanced parental age has led them to put off having children until later.

How Old Is "Older"?

There is surprisingly little consensus on what age is "old" for a woman to be having a child. Conservative health professionals may label any woman over thirty-five as being at high risk for herself and the child. More liberal practitioners regard pregnancy as a normal process and don't consider such women at high risk unless there are specific reasons to suspect complications, such as chronic disease, extreme obesity, or former obstetrical-gynecological problems.

For the purpose of this chapter, a maternal age of at least thirty-five years has been selected to mean "older." This coincides with the medical standard for recommending amniocentesis, which is based on statistical evidence showing a significant rise in birth defects, mainly Down's syndrome, above maternal age thirty-five.

Not even a generation ago a woman over thirty-five having her first child was called an "elderly primigravida." But as health practitioners have seen an increase in the number of older women who have uneventful, successful pregnancies, their former cautious, often pessimistic, feelings have changed.

Many health professionals find that their older patients are well educated about their pregnancy, in good shape physically, and tremendously motivated to have a healthy pregnancy. These are, after all, often women who have consciously delayed having a child and planned their own lives first. They may have less ambivalence about parenthood than a twenty-two-year-old pregnant woman, who may be giving up or delaying career plans to have a baby.

Risks of Pregnancy for an Older Woman

Older parents and health practitioners both need to be aware of the risks of pregnancy and know which risks are increased after maternal age thirty-five. Both maternal risks and risks to the infant will be considered. It must be emphasized that at *any* age a woman's pregnancy is affected by her medical history and general health.

The two main types of maternal risk are maternal mortality and complication of pregnancy. The maternal death rate of women of all ages in the United States has dropped dramatically from 376 deaths per 100,000 live births in 1940 (16) to 12.3 per 100,000 in 1976 (15). This decline is the result of a number of factors, including better control of postpartum hemorrhage and infection, better nutrition, and increased emphasis on prenatal care.

The age breakdown for maternal mortality for 1976 shows the lowest rates in the late teens and early twenties. The rate rises steadily with age, showing the woman over forty at a much greater risk than a woman of twenty (15). There is no way of relating these statistics to primiparas and multiparas, as the National Center for Health Statistics does not classify mortality rates by parity.

Another startling finding in the maternal mortality rates is the differences in the rates by race. At any age up to forty years a nonwhite woman was twice as likely as a white woman to die in childbirth. Because the National Health Statistics are classified not by social class but only by race, researchers rely on race as the indicator of income status. This method too clearly points out the differences in pregnancy outcome of white and nonwhite mothers. One must extrapolate the combination of factors associated with low socioeconomic status that can produce such a dramatic difference in maternal mortality rates. These factors include poor nutrition, substandard housing, previously existing health problems, such as anemia, and limited access to quality health care. (These same poverty-related factors also relate to infant mortality, to be discussed subsequently.)

The other type of maternal risk, complication of pregnancy, can result from previously existing disorders or can be strictly obstetrical. Pregnancy can aggravate previously existing conditions, such as diabetes, hypertension, kidney disorders, anemia, malnutrition, obesity, thyroid disorders, and cardiovascular disorders. Changes of pregnancy, such as weight gain and increased blood volume, may worsen these chronic disorders and eventually affect the pregnancy as well.

Diabetes can be used as an example to show how a previously existing disease can affect a pregnancy and how pregnancy can affect a disease. A diabetic's risk of toxemia is three to four times greater than that of a nondiabetic woman; she is also more likely to have infections. Hydramnios (excessive amniotic fluid) occurs ten times as often in diabetic pregnancies, and major congenital anomalies (all types) are diagnosed about four times as often as in nondiabetic pregnancies. The chance of the mother's undergoing a cesarean section is also greater, since it is often planned for in the thirty-seventh to thirty-eighth week, to avoid preeclampsia or because the large babies often produced by diabetic mothers warrant a cesarean delivery (9).

The pregnancy also has an effect on the diabetes. Hyperemesis and nausea associated with the first trimester can make insulin and diet management difficult and increase the chance of acidosis. In most pregnant diabetic women there is a significant increase in insulin requirements, and both mother and newborn are apt to suffer from hypoglycemia after labor. Infections, such as pyelonephritis and vaginitis, are much more common and serious in pregnant diabetics; headache is manifested by about 10 percent of diabetic mothers, beginning in the latter half of the pregnancy (9).

Although diligent prenatal care and a closely monitored delivery and postpartum can prevent or lessen these complications, the diabetic woman should be aware of the potential problems her disease and the pregnancy pose. The diabetic woman, in particular, needs to make a well-informed choice about pregnancy, since the adverse effects of diabetes are cumulative (3).

Other complications of pregnancy are ectopic pregnancy, spontaneous abortion, hemorrhage, infection, toxemia, and prolonged labor. It is important for the health care provider and the patient to be aware of which complications are associated with advanced maternal age.

An ectopic pregnancy occurs when the fertilized egg is implanted outside the uterus, usually in the fallopian tube but occasionally in the abdomen, cervix, or ovary. There appears to be no direct relationship between maternal age and ectopic pregnancy (3).

Spontaneous abortion, commonly known as miscarriage, occurs naturally; it is not induced. Spontaneous abortion that occurs early in pregnancy usually stems from errors in fertilization or defective ova and sperm. During the first twelve weeks of pregnancy the risk of spontaneous abortion is about 3.5 times greater for women over thirty-five than for women in their twenties (17).

Toxemia, hemorrhage, and sepsis are all complications of pregnancy carried to term. The likelihood of the first two, but not the third, increases with maternal age. Because the likelihood of hypertension increases with age, an older woman who becomes pregnant runs a greater risk of developing toxemia. All hypertensive women do not develop toxemia—they are simply at greater risk. There is some evidence that older women run a greater risk of toxemia regardless of their blood pressure (3).

Hemorrhage associated with placental abnormalities is related to both maternal age and parity. Placenta previa, in which the placenta is situated low in the uterus and blocks the cervix, occurs more often in older mothers who have borne several children. Age is the more significant factor, however, since women over thirty-five are 3.5 times more likely to have placenta previa, regardless of parity. Abruptio placenta, in which a normally placed placenta becomes prematurely separated from the uterus, is associated with parity, not age. Abruptio placenta occurs three times as often among women with five or more children as among primigravidas (7).

Postpartum hemorrhage, usually caused by failure of the uterus to contract after delivery, does not appear to be related to maternal age itself, but to factors such as multiple births, prolonged labor, and many past pregnancies. Maternal age alone does not make the woman at high risk for postpartum hemorrhage (13).

Older women seem to be more prone to prolonged or dysfunctional labor. A large study in 1967 showed that women between ages twenty-five and twenty-nine had an abnormal fetal presentation 18 percent of the time; this figure rose to 31 percent for women aged forty to forty-four. But there is evidence that the *duration* of labor is not necessarily longer for older women. There is also evidence that some of the increase in dysfunctional labor and complications may be iatrogenic—caused by obstetricians who treat their older patients more conservatively, giving them heavy sedation that interferes with normal labor and proceeding with cesarean section when indications were not clear (3).

A summary of maternal risks associated with advanced maternal age indicates that nonwhite women and women with previously existing illnesses are at higher risk during pregnancy. The older pregnant woman is also at risk for spontaneous abortion, toxemia, placenta previa, and abnormal fetal presentation.

Risks to the Infant

There are three areas of medical risks for infants: infant mortality, prematurity (low birth weight), and birth defects. Of these, infant mortality and prematurity pose a more serious threat to infants of very young mothers (3). The third area, birth defects, should be of greatest concern to the older mother.

Mothers between the ages of thirty-five and thirty-nine face about the *same* risk of losing their infants once they are safely born as do mothers in their early twenties. This pattern holds true when all birth orders are combined. Older prospective first-time parents should know that when figures are disaggregated by birth order, the firstborn infants of women over thirty are somewhat more at risk than subsequent offspring (3).

The figures above refer to averages. When infant mortality rates are broken down by race, nonwhite infants have a mortality rate nearly double that of the white infant mortality rate. As with maternal mortality rates, this wide difference is thought to be caused by such factors as poverty, poor nutrition, lack of prenatal care, and environmental differences.

Premature babies, those born before 266 days of gestation, and low-birth-weight babies, those who are less than 2,500 grams at birth, are more common among very young mothers. Women between ages thirty-five and forty-four are only slightly more at risk for bearing a premature infant than women in their twenties and early thirties. But again, social and economic circumstances play a part in predicting prematurity and low birth weight, as do the mother's personal habits, such as diet, smoking, and alcohol intake.

Approximately one out of every sixteen babies is born with a birth defect (1). Comprehensive statistics on birth defects are difficult to ascertain, for much depends on what is being counted—and when. Only about half of all birth defects are detected and diagnosed at birth, and because it is not mandatory to report defects on birth certificates, most statistics are incomplete. Furthermore, many defects do not become evident until later in life. For example, deafness may not be diagnosed until age two, and minimal brain damage may go unnoticed until a six-year-old is found to have learning problems in school (3).

Although birth defects can be caused by a number of factors, such as viruses, toxic medications, environmental pollutants, or radiation, chromosomal abnormalities should be of primary concern to older parents. Most chromosomal abnormalities are incompatible with life, and the fetuses usually abort spontaneously early in the pregnancy.

The chromosomal abnormality most closely associated with advanced maternal age is Down's syndrome, or trisomy 21. It is currently estimated that incidence of Down's syndrome increases from 1 per 2,000 live births among women at age twenty, to 1 in 800 in the early thirties, to 1 in 300 in the late thirties, to 1 in 20 live births among women over forty-five (12). These dramatic age-related incidence rates for Down's syndrome show that there is a growing need for genetic counseling and prenatal diagnosis by amniocentesis.

Paternal Age

Little is known about the risks to children born of older fathers. Research relating paternal age to Down's syndrome is inconclusive and often contradictory. Other chromosomal abnormalities, known as fresh gene mutations, are associated with advanced paternal age (13, 14). Two examples of fresh gene mutations are achondroplasia, a type of dwarfism, and Marfan's syndrome, which affects vision and height and often includes cardiac anomalies.

One theory as to why older men produce more fresh gene mutations is that, whereas a woman is born with a complete supply of eggs, a man produces sperm throughout his adult life. This allows for continual chance for error, possibly caused by environmental and occupational factors, such as radiation and toxins. Jones and associates found that the probability of a man's fathering a child with a fresh gene mutation increases tenfold between ages thirty and sixty, but the absolute level of risk is still *very* small (10).

Antenatal Testing

Amniocentesis

Antenatal diagnosis of chromosomal, biochemical, and multifactorial genetic defects can now be relatively safely done through amniocentesis. This procedure is widely used and is of particular importance to older parents, since advanced maternal age is associated with a higher rate of chromosomal abnormalities.

Although amniocentesis itself is a straightforward, simple procedure, it may raise ethical and emotional questions that both health care providers and patients must address. The procedure and its impact on the individual family must be understood in order to give comprehensive nursing care.

The optimal time for amniocentesis to be done is in the fourteenth or fifteenth week of pregnancy. At this time there is a large enough volume of amniotic fluid for sampling and the tests can be completed before the twentieth week of pregnancy. Enough time still exists if the results should reveal a problem and the parents decide to abort the fetus.

Amniocentesis is usually done in conjunction with ultrasonography, which uses sound waves to produce an image of the fetus. A clear visualization of the fetal position immediately before amniocentesis helps the physician performing the procedure to select a position for aspiration that avoids the placenta and the fetal head (5).

One study of 800 women showed a statistically significant reduction in the frequency of bloody taps and an increase in the proportion of successful and informative taps when ultrasonography was used before amniocentesis. This study also found that ultrasonography itself provided useful information for helping to identify fetal abnormalities and multiple gestation and for management of the pregnancy (2). Ultrasonography also makes it possible to accurately measure fetal head size, which is well correlated with fetal age (5). This information is useful if the mother is uncertain about the date of conception and a cesarean section is planned.

Procedure. Before amniocentesis a local anesthetic, such as lidocaine (Xylocaine), is injected near the amniocentesis site, which has been determined by ultrasonography. A needle with a stylus is inserted through the abdominal wall into the amniotic sac to obtain a sample of amniotic fluid. The procedure is carried out under full aseptic technique to ensure an uncontaminated sample and prevent infection in the mother and fetus.

Composition of Amniotic Fluid. Usually about 12 to 24 ml of fluid is aspirated, about 10 to 15 percent of the 175- to 225-ml volume that is normally present at that point in the pregnancy (6). Parents may need to be reassured that the sample volume will be replaced, as amniotic fluid has several points of origin. Some fluid is secreted by the upper respiratory tract, some diffuses through the skin, some from the membranes of the amniotic sac, and the largest quantity from the urine secreted by the fetus (5).

The amniotic fluid contains living and dead fetal cells. Some have sloughed off the fetal skin, some are in the urine and the respiratory tract secretions, others are from the placenta, the umbilical cord, and the amniotic sac. In genetic content they are all fetal cells, however, since they all derive from the fertilized ovum (5). In multiple gestations each fetus may have its own amniotic sac, so it is necessary to sample fluid from each sac (5).

Testing of Sample. The amniotic fluid sample is tested for three types of disorders—chromosomal, biochemical, and multifactorial genetic defects. The vast majority of amniocenteses are performed because the fetus is at risk for a chromosomal abnormality—Down's syndrome owing to trisomy 21 in advanced maternal age or the birth of a prior child with a chromosomal abnormality (6).

One part of the amniotic fluid sample is placed in tissue culture flasks and incubated, so the living cells in the fluid multiply (5). This takes between two and four weeks. If the cells fail to grow in culture, a repeat amniocentesis is necessary to obtain a new sample. (Parents should be aware that this does happen with a small percentage of samples.)

As the living cells divide, their genetic material is condensed into chromosomes (5). The chromosomes are then stained with dyes that selectively bind to certain parts of individual chromosomes to produce characteristic patterns of banding. Close examination of the chromosomes will reveal any disorder, usually an abnormal number of chromosomes but sometimes a major structural defect in a single chromosome. The most common disorder is trisomy 21, in which each fetal cell has three, rather than the usual two, chromosomes designated number 21. Trisomy 13 also involves an extra chromosome, number 13, and almost always results in spontaneous miscarriage. If carried to term, the baby's head and brain are severely deformed and the child will probably die before age six months (5).

Another type of information that examination of the chromosomes reveals is the sex of the child. This is useful in identifying sex-linked disorders, such as hemophilia and Duchenne's muscular dystrophy. A woman with a defective X chromosome is a carrier and will pass the sex-linked defect on to half of her children. Statistically this means that half her sons will have the disease and half her daughters will be carriers. Because the disease has a 50 percent incidence for the sex at risk (the male), the indication for amniocentesis is quite strong (5).

The second test that the amniotic fluid sample undergoes is for biochemical disorders, known as inborn errors of metabolism. The inborn error is usually a deficiency of a certain enzyme. It is caused by a mistake in the gene that specifies the structure of the enzyme. Although the precise gene and its location cannot be detected, the defect is revealed by biochemical assays of the amniotic fluid or cells. The assay will show abnormal rates of enzyme activity, abnormal metabolites, or normal metabolites in abnormal concentrations (5).

Most of the inborn errors of metabolism entail severe, debilitating diseases that are currently incurable and have symptoms that cannot be alleviated. About seventy-five biochemical disorders, each of them quite rare, but collectively the source of much human suffering, can now be diagnosed by amniocentesis (5).

One example of a biochemical disorder is Tay–Sachs disease, caused by a deficiency in the enzyme hexosaminidase A. The result is a disorder that allows a fatty substance known as ganglioside to progressively accumulate in cells of the nervous system. The consequences of this abnormal accumulation include blindness, paralysis, dementia, and death before age five. Carriers of Tay–Sachs disease are uncommon in the general population, but the incidence may be as great as one person in thirty among Jews of eastern European origin. Tay–Sachs disease is one of several diseases that can be screened for carriers in the adult population. If two known carriers conceive a child, there is a one in four chance that the child will have the disease. Amniocentesis is indicated to detect the presence of the disease in the fetus (5).

The third type of test performed on an amniotic fluid sample is for multifactorial genetic defects. The incidence of certain fetal malformations is correlated with high levels of alpha-fetoprotein (AFP), both in the amniotic fluid and in the mother's blood.

The type of defect associated with an elevated AFP level usually involves the neural tube, the embryonic structure that becomes the central nervous system. Defects include anencephaly, encephalocele, and spina bifida. Occasionally these disorders can be diagnosed by ultrasonography too.

It is generally recommended that pregnant women who have previously delivered a child with a neural tube disorder, or who have family members with such a disorder, have the AFP level in their amniotic fluid measured. The fetuses of such women are known to be at greater risk for having a neural tube disorder than are those of the general population (5).

Alpha-fetoprotein maternal blood levels and amniotic fluid levels vary markedly with the age of the fetus. Accuracy of fetal age is vital in interpreting the results of AFP levels, so ultrasonography is indicated. Even so, there are false-positive results and some indication that an elevated AFP level may be associated with an anomaly other than a neural tube defect (6).

In England and the Scandinavian countries large-scale AFP screening programs for pregnant women have already been instituted. The U.S. Food and Drug Administration and the National Institutes of Health at this point have not recommended such a program and are awaiting the completion of further studies. It is the practice of many physicians and hospitals, however, to obtain an AFP level on every sample of amniotic fluid.

Fetoscopy

Fetoscopy is now being used at a few centers in the United States. It involves the use of a fiber-optic scope passed through a cannula into the anterior wall of the uterus. Originally designed to observe the fetus for defects, it is now also used for taking fetal blood samples and biopsies for diagnosis of some diseases that cannot be identified by amniocentesis. The procedure, which is done in conjunction with ultrasonography, carries a 5 percent risk of inducing abortion (6).

Amniography

Amniography involves the injection of a radiopaque dye into the amniotic sac through the amniocentesis needle.

The dye outlines the fetus and is soon swallowed by the fetus, which allows visualization of structural deformities, such as meningoceles, gastrointestinal obstructions, and diaphragmatic hernias. This procedure is becoming outmoded by noninvasive ultrasonography, which can be extremely reliable in experienced hands (6).

Risks and Concerns of Amniocentesis

Studies show that the overall risk of spontaneous abortion from amniocentesis is less than 0.5 percent. This procedure raises the natural rate of miscarriage at sixteen weeks from 3 percent to 3.5 percent. Although the risk is small, it may exceed the statistical chance of giving birth to a child with a detectable disorder (6). Parents need to consider this before deciding to have the procedure.

One of the conflicts associated with amniocentesis is that the results will put the parents in a position where they will have to decide whether or not to terminate the pregnancy. Although many parents make this decision at the same time they opt for the procedure, others are not as certain. They may just want to know in advance if they will have a child with a particular disorder. Health professionals working with families who are having antenatal diagnosis need to be aware that each family is different in its approach to the procedure and its reaction to the results. The health professional's role is to be supportive during this stressful time and allow the parents to make the decisions.

As the field of fetal therapy advances, the results of amniocentesis and fetoscopy will lead to the treatment in utero of more detectable disorders. Certain vitamin coenzymes and thyroid hormones can now be administered to the fetus that is identified by biochemical assay as needing them (6). As more treatments are developed, parents who undergo amniocentesis and fetoscopy will no longer be facing only a "terminate or don't terminate" decision; treatment will also be an option in some disorders.

Although couples may find the amniocentesis procedure itself stressful, often the implications of it are even more anxiety-provoking. Testing the fetus for possible defects places the couple in the position of candidly facing the possibility of having a less than perfect baby. Often the couple has a specific reason to fear that a disorder will be revealed, as in the case of a couple whose previous pregnancy has resulted in a child with a defect, or a couple with a strong family history of birth defects that can now be identified by amniocentesis.

The option for amniocentesis and the data it gives the parents may add more stress to the pregnancy. Couples will have to discuss with each other their feelings about how to deal with the results of the amniocentesis. What if the fetus has trisomy 21? What if it has a treatable thyroid deficiency? Should we ask to be told the sex of the child, or wait and be surprised? These are all questions that parents will ask each other, and their answers may differ. An informed, neutral health professional, such as a genetic counselor or a primary nurse, can help the couple cope with these important considerations.

Genetic Counseling

The growing field of prenatal diagnosis and treatment has led to the growth of a previously small branch of health workers who are trained in human genetics. It is their job to obtain a complete genetic and medical history from the couple, emphasizing such features as familial disease, causes of death, and frequency of spontaneous abortion and stillbirths. Blood samples are taken from the couple and, occasionally, from significant relatives. This information is entered on a chart called a pedigree.

The genetic counselor then discusses the findings with the couple, explaining any special risks they face for bearing a child with a predictable disorder. The compilation of the pedigree is ideally done before pregnancy or early in the pregnancy, thus giving the couple ample time to weigh a decision regarding amniocentesis. If the results of amniocentesis indicate that the fetus has a disorder, the counselor might again become involved in giving information about the specific defect that might assist the couple in deciding whether or not to terminate the pregnancy.

All health professionals who deal with couples undergoing genetic counseling and amniocentesis need to possess the communication skills that will enable them to discuss this highly sensitive and emotional subject. Parents who are informed that the child they are expecting is defective are often hostile, depressed, blaming, withdrawn, guilty, or angry. It is a stressful time for the marriage. A skilled genetic counselor, primary nurse, or physician needs to work with the rest of the health team to assist the parents to survive the crisis and make decisions they can live with. This becomes even more of a challenge when partners differ on what they think should be done.

Parents at risk for having a child with a disorder iden-

tifiable by amniocentesis need to know how life with such a child will differ from life with the idealized "perfect" child. A counselor can help them with this and assist them in dealing with their feelings about having an afflicted child.

The development of antenatal diagnosis has raised new ethical and medicolegal questions. Medical literature is now encouraging obstetricians to practice "defensive medicine" in order to protect themselves from malpractice suits. "Defensive medicine" involves ordering every type of test that could possibly be warranted in a situation, frankly discussing with parents the possibilities of bearing a defective child (sometimes followed up by a certified letter summarizing the discussion), and being extremely conservative in managing labor and delivery. This has resulted in a higher rate of cesarean sections. Practicing obstetrics in this manner can only have a detrimental effect on the doctor-patient relationship and certainly helps to increase health care costs. But many doctors believe that it is the only sensible way for them to practice, in light of recent court cases in which parents have won lawsuits against obstetricians after the birth of a child who suffered from a defect that could have been diagnosed by amniocentesis. Continued advances in antenatal diagnosis and treatment will probably only increase the practice of "defensive medicine."

Multiple Births

The incidence of twinning and other multiple births rises with maternal age and parity. The incidence of fraternal twins, the type that results from two eggs fertilized separately, peaks among women aged thirty-five to thirty-nine and then declines. The potential medical risks associated with multiple births include toxemia, prematurity, low birth weight, hemorrhage at delivery, and malpresentation of the fetus at birth. To the extent that the frequency of multiple births increases with maternal age, the associated risks also increase for the older mother (5).

Infertility

As noted earlier, infertility has led to an increase in the number of older parents. The time it takes to diagnose the fertility problem and treat it makes it more likely that the couple will be over thirty-five. It is important for the primary nurse to be aware of the major causes and treatments of infertility so she can understand what the couple with a history of infertility has been through in order to conceive a child.

A couple is considered infertile if they haven't conceived after one year of trying. At this time the couple is referred to a fertility specialist, usually an obstetrician, urologist, or endocrinologist. A lengthy interview that includes questions on menstrual patterns and sexual habits for both partners is then conducted. Tests are done on a sperm sample taken from the man to determine the number and quality of sperm, and the woman has a pelvic examination to check for gross abnormalities. The woman then keeps a temperature chart to determine if and when she ovulates. She may also have a postcoital cervical mucus specimen examined to see if the mucus is thin enough for the sperm to pass through it. An endometrial biopsy and hysterosalpingography may also be indicated. (In hysterosalpingography dye is injected into the uterus, fallopian tubes, and ovaries and x-rays are then taken.) These workups should lead to the discovery of the source of infertility and indicate what treatment is required.

There are several reasons for a low sperm count. Blockage of the vas deferens may result from venereal disease or vasectomy. Although the blockage resulting from vasectomy is considered permanent, in some instances it may be corrected by microsurgery, although positive results are not certain. Blockage resulting from venereal disease can also be treated with some success by microsurgery. Varicose veins in the scrotum, known as a variocele, can also be surgically repaired. The sperm itself may have low motility or an immature count or may just be low in number.

A sperm sample that has a low count but good motility can be concentrated, and the woman can be artificially inseminated with her partner's sperm. In situations where the sperm count and motility are too low for conception, artificial insemination from a donor may be the course taken. Sperm bank donors are thoroughly screened for the presence of genetic disorders. They are matched with the infertile man for such factors as physique, hair and eye color, and complexion.

Female infertility is often more complex and harder to treat. Failure to ovulate, which accounts for about 20 percent of female infertility, is usually caused by a hormonal imbalance, involving gonadotrophin-releasing hormone (GnRH) from the hypothalamus and follicle-stimulating hormone and luteinizing hormone from the pituitary gland. The fertility drug Clomid, a synthetic hormone, stimulates the release of GnRH and should start the ovulation cycle. If the problem is with the pituitary-released hormones, Pergonal is the drug of choice. Sometimes both drugs overstimulate the ovaries, causing several eggs to be released, which results in multiple births.

Blockage of the fallopian tubes can result from infections such as pelvic inflammatory disease and venereal disease, adhesions from previous surgery, endometriosis, or unknown causes. Occasionally hysterosalpingography may clear the blocked fallopian tubes when the dye is inserted. If this fails, delicate surgery must be performed to reopen the tubes.

Women with hopelessly damaged fallopian tubes may be candidates for in vitro fertilization (IVF), a procedure that has been growing in use since the first IVF baby was born in England in 1978. A woman undergoing IVF takes Pergonal after menstruation to stimulate ovulation that will yield several eggs. At the correct time in her cycle (determined by blood tests and ultrasonography) the eggs are removed with the aid of a laparoscope and placed in a Petri dish. The partner's sperm are added to the dish and the mixture is incubated for thirty-eight to forty-eight hours. After this time the fertilized eggs should have begun to divide into several cells. Fertilized eggs are selected and carefully inserted into the woman's uterus, where implantation should occur. In vitro fertilization is still being done on a limited basis, but its use is expected to increase.

Adoption

Some couples whose infertility problem cannot be successfully treated turn to adoption. Fewer healthy American babies are put up for adoption now, owing to legalized abortion and moderation of the social stigma experienced by a woman who wants to keep her out-of-wedlock baby. This shortage makes it difficult for the couple who wants to adopt. Years of applying to adoption agencies, being scrutinized by social agencies, and being on waiting lists can make the adoption process stressful.

Often parents who have surmounted infertility problems or waited through the lengthy adoption process are extremely anxious, particularly during the newborn period. Fear of losing this long-awaited child may be intense. Health professionals must remember the exceptional time and effort that these parents have expended on achieving parenthood, and treat them with understanding.

Developmental Implications for Parenting

Based on the low incidence of low-birth-weight babies and a low incidence of maternal complications, medical authorities say that the ideal time for a woman to give birth for the first time is between ages twenty-five and twenty-nine. Little is known, however, about what age is ideal for the parenting that occurs after the birth.

In a small study done on white professional couples living near a large metropolitan area, Frankel and Wise found that older mothers with established careers were generally more accepting and less conflicted in the parenting role than younger professional women (4). These mothers saw their past as enhancing their experience with their children; they believed that their greater maturity and sense of competence were definite advantages in parenting (4). The study also showed that older fathers took on a larger share of child care responsibilities and expressed enjoyment in parenting and time spent with their children (4). The financial security that the older couples enjoyed allowed them more freedom in the selection of child care and education for their children.

Disadvantages of older parenting identified by the older women were less energy and less freedom to space children. Children born to older parents have less chance of a long relationship with their grandparents. This is also cited as a disadvantage of postponing parenthood. Older mothers also tended to be more anxious about their children, especially when they were young (4). This situation is similar to that of parents who adopt or conceive after a long period of infertility; the amount of energy, time, and planning that went into producing the child makes the fear of loss all the more intense.

Young mothers in Frankel and Wise's study more often experienced isolation, restlessness, and a harder time relinquishing career and social plans. They were more apt to stress the sacrifice that motherhood entails and expressed concern about the added financial burden of having a child (4).

As more couples delay starting their families, it is likely that more research will be done on the subject. There are many variables that make it a complex issue; for example, is it the first child for *both* parents? Is it a late child born many years after originally having children? Is it a second marriage in which half-siblings are involved? Will both parents be working full time or part-time?

What *is* clear now is that more couples are postponing having children until they are in their thirties; that these parents are producing healthy children with the help of good prenatal care, antenatal diagnosis, and parent education for pregnancy and child care; and that these parents, like all parents, have special needs that can be addressed by the primary nurse.

Nursing Care

The primary nurse in almost any setting is apt to encounter an older new mother who is either pregnant or in the postpartum period. At any point where contact is made, there are specific roles for the primary nurse caring for the older parent.

Teaching

Older new parents have specific learning needs. Many are well read in the areas of pregnancy, labor, and delivery, but they still need clarification on some points and have special questions. Older mothers who have had children at an earlier age may comment on the changes in maternal care over the intervening years—more emphasis on nutrition, exercise, midwives, and birthing rooms; increased rates of cesarean sections; and participation of the father.

Older parents need to know the routine pregnancy, labor, and delivery information, as well as specifics that relate to them—amniocentesis, fetoscopy, risks to mother and fetus in older parenting, indications for a cesarean section and what to expect if one is done.

Support and Anticipatory Guidance

Older parents may need extra support during the prenatal, labor and delivery, and postpartal periods. The pregnancy may be a long-awaited event because of infertility or planned postponement. In either case they are likely to be anxious about some aspect of the pregnancy—carrying the fetus to term, adapting to having a new person in the family, rearranging their life-style to accommodate work, child, and a social life. Older parents may question their ability to learn parenting skills, and the primary nurse can be both a support and a teacher in this situation.

Sometimes the new parents are so anxious or naive that they don't consider some areas that the experienced primary nurse knows they should be concerned about.

It is the responsibility of the nurse to speak to these concerns, in a nonthreatening way, to help the parents anticipate the decisions or situations they will be encountering. Some examples of areas that parents tend to overlook that the nurse might bring up are assistance for the new postpartal mother at home, breast-feeding after a cesarean section, birth control, altered roles in the marriage, ambivalence of mother about changing work pattern, and adjustment of older sibling to newborn.

Older parents who will be undergoing amniocentesis and fetoscopy also need special support. Parents need to know exactly what the procedure entails and the risks involved. Anticipatory guidance with these tests includes explaining length of time for results (often a cause of anxiety itself), open communication between partners on their feelings about results, and whether or not to be informed of the child's sex when they are told the results of amniocentesis.

When giving emotional support to a couple who is making these decisions, the nurse should help them explore their options. The nurse in this situation needs to be aware of her own feelings about amniocentesis and abortion and must realize that everyone doesn't agree with her. An open-minded viewpoint is needed to successfully counsel and give support to such parents.

Crisis Intervention

Parenthood as a crisis state has been well documented in the professional literature (11, p. 111); however, the older couple may have developed a greater sense of maturity and have had the opportunity to develop stronger coping systems. However, although the coping mechanisms used by the older parents may have worked previously, they may not apply to this new situation. One of the feelings that older parents comment on is the loss of control over their lives that comes with the newborn. The idealized sleeping infant with adoring parents is not always the accurate picture. A baby who has colic night after night can make even the most confident, prepared parents feel frustrated, angry, and helpless.

Le Masters states that the more prepared a couple is for parenthood, the less of a crisis state it will cause (11). The primary nurse giving anticipatory guidance to new parents can help them develop coping strategies for the new conflicts, or potential conflicts, in their lives. Sometimes, as in the case of the colicky baby, just knowing that other babies and parents have gone through it and survived can help the anxious parent. Other areas that might be less apt to develop into crises if discussed beforehand are fatigue, altered roles in the marriage, child care arrangements, career changes necessitated by the child's birth, and loss of leisure time.

Advocate and Change Agent

The primary nurse working with older parents may be in the position to exercise her role as advocate and change agent. Some health workers have a prejudice toward older parents and treat them needlessly conservatively and may even allow their biases to affect the parents. Terms like "elderly primigravida" and *over*-concern about expectant mothers who are over thirty-five increase the parents' anxiety and undermine their self-confidence.

The primary nurse is in a position to make policy changes as needed and influence her co-workers to encourage support for the older parents. Nurses can be advocates in such work-related benefits as maternity leaves, flexible hours, and on-the-job day care.

Referrals

The primary nurse may need help from other health team members in planning care for the older parents. At every stage of the pregnancy and postpartum there may be necessary referrals. Early in the pregnancy a genetic counselor may be indicated for a couple undergoing amniocentesis. Childbirth separation classes, parenting classes, a Lamaze group, a visiting nurse after discharge from the hospital, a mothers' support group or community child care resource are all possible referrals for the new parents. Each of these referrals may provide a service that can supplement the care the primary nurse has planned.

Follow-up

An integral part of the delivery of primary nursing care must be follow-up on the care given. Sometimes this takes the form of evaluating the care that you, the primary nurse, have actually given, or it may involve contacting the other health workers or agencies to which the client was referred. Follow-up is the only way of ensuring that the planned comprehensive care has actually been delivered. The primary nurse is accountable for her referrals and needs to be sure that her client's needs were met by these other services.

DISCUSSION QUESTIONS

1. You are the nurse in an obstetrician's office. One of your patients is Ms. R., a thirty-five-year-old computer programmer. She and Mr. R. have been married for eight years and have purposely put off having a child so they could both finish graduate school, buy a home, and travel. Ms. R. is now fifteen weeks pregnant with their first child and is scheduled for an amniocentesis next week. Ms. R. is visibly anxious when discussing the procedure and asks you, "Why does it take so long to get the results? We didn't want to tell our parents about the pregnancy until we knew the baby was O.K." How would you respond to Ms. R.?

2. Ms. L., age thirty-five, is being seen at a neighborhood mental health clinic. She has been suffering from depression since the recent death of her newborn infant, who suffered from Down's syndrome and had severe cardiac anomalies. You are the primary nurse in the clinic and Ms. L. confides in you: "My husband and I always planned to have a family. Now we never will. My girl friends told me that all my children would probably have Down's syndrome since the first one did. Maybe we should adopt." What would you include in Ms. L.'s nursing care?

3. You are the primary nurse on a postpartum unit caring for Ms. J., a forty-two-year-old lawyer who has just delivered a healthy eight-pound baby boy, her first child. Mr. J., also a lawyer, and his fourteen-year-old daughter from a previous marriage are visiting Ms. J. Both Mr. J. and his daughter take turns holding the baby and obviously enjoy the experience. After they leave, Ms. J. comments, "They certainly seem comfortable with a newborn." You ask, "Do you feel *uncomfortable*?" Ms. J. shares with you her anxieties about caring for the child at home: "It took me five years to get pregnant. After all that time I just started focusing on the process and not the result—the baby. Now that he's finally here I feel so nervous and unsure of myself. I should be happy that John and my stepdaughter are so experienced—she's the favorite baby-sitter in our neighborhood; but instead I resent them. I've always been a capable person in my career, and now I feel at a loss about caring for a little eight-pound person." What nursing care would you plan for Ms. J.?

REFERENCES

1. Apgar, V., and J. Beck. *Is My Baby All Right? A Guide to Birth Defects.* New York: Trident Press, 1972.
2. Chandra, P., et al. "Experience with Sonography as an Adjunct to Amniocentesis for Prenatal Diagnosis of Fetal Genetic Disorders." *American Journal of Obstetrics and Gynecology* 133:519, March 1, 1979.
3. Daniels, P., and K. Weingarten. "A New Look at the Medical Risks in Late Childrearing." *Women and Health* 4:11–12, Spring 1979.
4. Frankel, S. A., and M. J. Wise. "A View of Delayed Parenting: Some Implications of a New Trend." *Psychiatry* 45:220, 1982.
5. Fuchs, F. "Genetic Amniocentesis." *Scientific American* 242:48, June 1980.
6. Golbus, M. S. "The Current Scope of Antenatal Diagnosis." *Hospital Practice,* April 1982, 181.
7. Hellman, L. M., and J. A. Pritchard. *Williams Obstetrics.* 17th ed. New York: Appleton-Century-Crofts, 1984.
8. "Infertility: New Cures, New Hope." *Newsweek,* December 6, 1982, 102.
9. Jenson, M. D., R. Benson, and I. M. Bobak. *Maternity Care—The Nurse and the Family.* St. Louis: C. V. Mosby Co., 1977, 260.
10. Jones, K. L., et al. "Older Paternal Age and Gene Mutation: Data on Additional Disorders." *Journal of Pediatrics* 86:86, 1975.
11. Le Masters, E. E. "Parenthood as Crisis." In *Crisis Intervention: Selected Readings,* ed. A. Parod. New York: Family Service Association of America, 1975.
12. Miller, W. A., and R. W. Erbe. "Prenatal Diagnosis of Genetic Disorders." *Southern Medical Journal* 71:202, 1978.
13. Murdock, J. L., B. Walker, J. G. Hall, et al. "Achondroplasia: A Genetic and Statistical Survey." *Annals of Human Genetics* 33:227, 1970.
14. Murdock, J. L., B. Walker, and V. A. McKusic. "Parental Age Effects on the Occurrence of New Mutations for the Marfan Syndrome." *Annals of Genetic Medicine* 35:331, 1972.
15. National Center for Health Statistics. "Advance Report—Final Mortality Statistics, 1976. *Monthly Vital Statistics Report,* March 30, 1978, 26 (12, Suppl. 2).
16. Nortman, D. "Parental Age as a Factor in Pregnancy Outcome and Child Development." *Reports on Population/ Family Planning* 16:1–52, 1974.
17. Shapiro, S., and M. Abramowicz. "Pregnancy Outcome Correlates Identified Through Medical Record-Based Information." *American Journal of Public Health* 59:1629, 1969.
18. U.S. Department of Health and Human Services. "Advance Report of Final Natality Statistics, 1980." *Monthly Vital Statistics Report,* November 1982, 1–4.

CHAPTER 25

Special Families

NANCY JACKSON

.

OBJECTIVES

After completing this chapter, the reader will be able to:

- Describe trends in family life in the 1980s.
- Identify five types of families that are at risk for stress.
- Apply crisis intervention to a family in stress.
- Apply self-care concepts to a family in stress.
- Plan nursing intervention for the primary nurse working with a family in stress.

This chapter explores the role of the primary nurse in caring for the nontraditional family. Families included in this discussion are those experiencing divorce, single-parenthood, remarriage, stepparenting, and adoption. Concepts related to crisis intervention, stress, and self-care are applied to these nontraditional families and implications for the primary nurse are discussed.

The types of families selected for discussion in this chapter represent the results of some social changes that have occurred during the 1970s and 1980s. These social trends include increasing rates of divorce and remarriage and increased infertility rates, leading to more adoptions. It is important to note that these nontraditional families are not necessarily susceptible to any more *long-term* stress than the so-called traditional family (Mom, Dad, and children living together). But crisis intervention and self-help measures during the transition period can assist a family in making a successful resolution of the crisis.

Although great emphasis is placed on collecting emotional and social data on clients, it is important that the primary nurse not assume a causal relationship between these data and objective findings. For example, a five-year-old girl who begins having enuresis two weeks after her father moves out may have a bladder infection, and *not* emotional problems because of the change in the family. The second-grade boy who is still not reading should be screened for learning disabilities, not assumed to be distracted by the recent remarriage of his mother and his new home situation.

Health care workers need to be aware that the stigma formerly attached to nontraditional families is rapidly decreasing as their numbers increase. In fact, there are some strengths that the nontraditional family may have that can enhance its coping ability. Health care workers must look for the strengths and work with them to assist the family, and not be guided by their own possibly negative feelings about the family's structure.

Divorce

As divorce and remarriage rates continue to climb, the American family is rapidly changing. Single parents, stepparents and stepsiblings are all becoming more common. The trends have emotional, economic, and legal implications for individuals, families, and communities.

The primary nurse should recognize divorce as a stress that can have a holistic impact on a family. Besides the physical separation of having a parent move out of the house, the family may be experiencing other changes, such as the financial burden of maintaining two residences, the mother returning to work, negotiating a visiting schedule for the absent parent, or the presence of another partner for one or both parents. As familiar patterns of family life are altered, all the members will need help in adjusting to the changes.

The impact of divorce on children is a subject of interest to researchers but one that is difficult to study, owing to the number of variables involved. The age of the children, the circumstances surrounding the divorce, the degree of contact with the noncustodial parent, and the presence or absence of stepparents are all factors that can affect children experiencing divorce.

In her article "Divorce—A Child's Perspective," Hetherington reviews research on divorce's effect on children (6). She recognizes that divorce is often a positive solution to destructive family functioning but sees both parents and children as being at high risk for emotional and physiological problems during the transition period after separation.

Other findings cited in Hetherington's work include the varying responses to divorce by children of different ages (6). Infants may be affected the least, whereas a young child is unable to accurately assess the situation and may be self-blaming, seeing himself as the cause of his parents' separation. This may be particularly true for a preschool boy in the oedipal stage of development, who may in fact have wished that his father would leave the household. The older child and adolescent have better judgment and reasoning ability and, although still feeling initial anger and hurt from the divorce, better developed coping mechanisms to handle the new situation. Children of these age-groups are also characteristically involved in more activities outside the home, which add a sense of stability to their lives during their parents' divorce.

The results of many studies indicate that male children have a greater and longer-lasting response to parental divorce than do female children (6). This has been measured in terms of developmental deviations, behavior disorders, and problems in interpersonal relationships. Interpretation of these results is difficult. It may be that boys suffer more from loss of their father (who historically has been the parent to leave the home in family separations), or it may be that boys receive less positive support and nurturance and are viewed more negatively by mothers, teachers, and peers, as Hetherington found in her 1978 study (7). This study also found divorced mothers of boys reported feeling more stress and depression than divorced mothers of girls.

The only thing that is certain about the research on divorce is that more research is needed to clearly identify the factors useful in predicting the effect of divorce on children and parents. As more fathers assume custodial care of their children after divorce, it would be most useful to compare the effects of paternal care on children, especially males, with the effects of maternal care on children.

There are several common problems associated with divorce to which families must adjust. Frequently there is a decrease in finances, as a second dwelling is needed for the parent who moves out. A decreased income may change former family patterns, such as private school, vacations, household help, or regularly dining out. These changes are more apt to be noticed by older children, who are aware of the family's life-style. An at-home mother may need to go back to work to support herself and her children, if her husband has not provided for them. The disruption in the family's routine may prove harder for children to adjust to than the actual divorce.

Open conflict between parents as they discuss future arrangements for the children may prove threatening to children. When parents have previously kept their arguing private, it may be upsetting to children to hear them overtly expressing hostility. On the other hand, some children almost need to hear their parents argue to help them accept the reality that their parents don't get along (especially if children have previously been protected from parental conflict). In either case, children may feel that they have to choose one parent to remain loyal to and, of course, find this a painful choice. This can also lead to children playing one parent against the other, a skill at which the manipulative child may excel.

As family patterns are restructured after divorce, the custodial mother may find herself relying on her children for assistance and emotional support. Older children may be pushed into a caretaker role for younger siblings and be encouraged to function more independently. Although this may be a practical solution to the mother's immediate needs, the childhood of that older child needs protection, lest the child be pushed into a role that he or she cannot or should not be expected to fill.

Nursing Interventions

When divorce is thought of as a situational crisis, it becomes clear that the primary nurse needs to assess the situation. This may involve referring the client or family to a short-term crisis intervention center, or directly handling the crisis herself.

In either case, assessment of the situation and planning therapeutic intervention are the initial steps. The client may need assistance in identifying previously used coping mechanisms, such as talking with certain friends or relatives and exercise; or the client may need guidance in finding new coping mechanisms, if previous ones are no longer feasible or adequate.

Direct, goal-oriented intervention is needed for the person or family in crisis (1). New coping behaviors and support systems that might have been overlooked in the past include neighborhood school, and church groups that could assist with child care, after-school, and social needs. Extended family as a support may be an underused resource for some people.

In the midst of crisis the divorcing parent may lose sight of the fact that eventually the most realistic, and usually the best, situation for the children is to maintain contact with both parents on a regular basis. If this can be focused on early in the divorce, it may prevent some of the game playing that parents sometimes go through in working out custody and child visitation rights.

One of the latest and most welcome additions to the area of human relations is the idea of divorce mediation. Coogler and co-workers point out that the details of divorce settlement—child custody and support, alimony, property division—can turn a couple into legal adversaries, and actively escalate anger, hostility, and distrust (3). Divorce mediation by a neutral third party provides an alternative to the adversarial model. It promotes cooperation and compromise to arrive at resolution of conflicts in a rational manner. In the process of mediation the couple also learns that this same rational approach can be used in their daily lives for more constructive resolution of differences. The divorce mediator is a resource person that might be used for the family who is undergoing separation and divorce.

Another appropriate referral for the divorced parent might be a self-help group. Most communities now have groups such as Parents Without Partners, which provide interaction with others in similar circumstances. These groups may be useful for both parents and children, who may both need peer group support.

Health care providers working with clients who are undergoing divorce would benefit from the message of Janine M. Bernard's article on "The Divorce Myth" (2). This myth is an underlying cultural belief that divorce has the inherent power to make people unhappy; the reverse is the widely held belief that marriage has the inherent power to make people happy. The fact is that many couples are better off divorcing and children are better off in single-parent families than they are in households that are filled with hostility or apathy. The optimism and hope offered by the health care worker can assist the individual or family experiencing divorce to make the transition period a constructive one and plan for the future.

Remarriage and Stepparenting

A logical outgrowth of increasing divorce rates is an increase in rates of remarriage and the formation of new family relationships. Stepparents, stepchildren, half-siblings, and stepgrandparents are all possibilities when remarriage takes place. Adjustment to remarriage seems to depend a great deal on the degree of resolution of the previous divorce. If a person has learned from the divorce, developing coping skills and more constructive ways to resolve conflicts, the remarriage is more apt to be successful.

Goetting reports that when neither spouse had a child from a previous marriage, the remarried couple resembled families of first marriage and most norms of first marriage applied (5). The addition of children from a previous marriage seems to add conflict and potential crisis in a remarriage.

Remarriage produces some problems for both the stepparent and the stepchild. While welcoming the stability of living in a two-parent family again, the stepchild may feel disloyal to the absent natural parent if he seems too enthusiastic about the remarriage. The stepparent may have many preconceived notions about how a stepparent should and shouldn't act.

Turnbull and Turnbull's "10 Commandments of Stepparenting" are as follows:

1. Provide neutral territory—a new residence, especially important if children from two marriages are being combined.
2. Don't try to fit a preconceived role—don't be phoney and saccharine sweet. Children lose respect for someone they can manipulate.
3. Set limits and enforce them—discuss discipline of children before marriage and support each other.
4. Allow an outlet for feelings by the children for the natural parent—don't make the child feel disloyal for still loving the absent natural parent.
5. Accept ambivalent feelings from stepchildren—this is natural in all human relationships.
6. Avoid mealtime misery—the time when the family is all together shouldn't be spent arguing over the menu and who cooked.
7. Don't expect instant love.
8. Don't take all the responsibility—the child has some too.
9. Be patient—there is a transition period of months or years.
10. Maintain the primacy of the marital relationship—demonstrate to children that disputes can be settled within a family. (9)

Stepparenting may become more difficult the older the child is at the time of the remarriage. Adolescents often seem to have a lot of resentment toward stepparents and have difficulties adjusting to the new management. Lutz's study on adolescent perception of stepfamilies reports that issues related to divided loyalty and discipline were perceived to be the most stressful aspects of stepfamily living (8).

Nursing Intervention

In providing nursing care to the individual or family undergoing remarriage, anticipatory guidance is indicated. Helping parents and children develop new coping skills and predicting potential sources of conflict are important goals.

The tone of cooperation and compromise set by divorce mediation is useful in conflict resolution of remarriage problems too. If the known areas of conflict are identified as loyalty to natural parents, and discipline, these are issues that should be dealt with openly and candidly even before the remarriage occurs. Acknowledging the issue and making active plans to resolve the problems should set an optimistic tone for the relationship.

If it is too late for anticipatory guidance, and the family is already in the midst of a crisis, referral to a crisis intervention center is indicated. There are also growing numbers of self-help groups for stepfamilies—for both parents and children. Sometimes talking with others going through the same conflicts can help a family discover new methods of resolving their differences.

Adoption

Although the family that adopts children may go on to become a traditional family, the transition period surrounding the adoption can cause a lot of stress and a need for crisis intervention.

It is ironic that while adoptive couples may have to wait *years* for a baby to become available, when it finally happens they may have only a few weeks or days to prepare. The nine-month gestation period that biological parents experience helps them prepare for the baby's arrival. Besides the practical details of buying equipment and clothes and preparing a room for the baby, there is a psychological preparation that is also experienced by the expectant parents. They may actively fantasize about their new role and what kind of parents they will be. Besides this, there is a social preparation—neighbors and relatives are extra attentive, and the couple may meet other expectant couples at childbirth education classes and expand their community involvement to include new friends.

Adoptive parents frequently go through the long wait alone, after they have made initial arrangements for the adoption. Some parents who adopted through agencies later stated that they were reluctant to express fears or ambivalent feelings (that are perfectly normal for new parents), lest the agency decide that they were not prepared for parenthood.

The message here for the primary nurse is that adoptive parents need encouragement and help in adapting to parenthood. The usual childbirth education—parenthood preparation classes that many parents attend—may be inappropriate for adoptive parents. They have been found to benefit from the special version of parenthood class that includes traditional infant care instruction, selection of a pediatrician, discussion of what equipment is needed, as well as concerns specific to being adoptive parents. Topics specific to adoptive parents include psychological aspects of adoption, dealing with tactless questions and comments from others, explain-

ing adoption to the child, and issues related to sealed and open adoption records (4).

Special parenthood classes for adoptive parents also serve to identify a peer group of adoptive parents. Although parents will not want to limit friendships to this group, they may find continued contact with other adoptive parents helpful. This may be particularly useful when the child is told that he is adopted and several other adopted children can be identified for him. It may be less stressful for everyone involved if there are other adoptive families who can share their experiences.

Adoption of children from other countries may present other kinds of stresses. In their article on adopting Korean babies, Coyne and Flynn point out the need for more attention to cultural differences in childrearing (4). They note that their daughters spent the first several months of their lives in Korea, where infants are strapped to their mothers' backs and are accustomed to a lot of motion. Korean babies are patted on their stomachs to soothe them and tapped on the face for a response. Korean songs are sirenlike and high pitched. This contrasts greatly with the silent, protective atmosphere that Americans try to provide for their babies. Unfortunately these women learned too late about the cultural differences in childrearing, and their daughters responded to their care with withdrawal and frequent crying.

The primary nurse is in a position to offer anticipatory guidance and crisis intervention to the couple adopting a child from another culture. She may be a resource person for the childrearing practices of different cultures. This would help ease the transition period that the adoptive family goes through.

DISCUSSION QUESTIONS

1. You are the school nurse caring for nine-year-old Tom F., who has come to your office for the third day in a row complaining of a stomachache. On the previous two days an hour of resting on the cot in your office seemed to relieve Tom's problem. A consultation with the teacher revealed no classroom problems. Mrs. F. cannot be reached at home by phone. When you ask Tom where his mother might be, he replies, "She had to go back to work since my dad moved out. She can't pick me up at three o'clock anymore and I have to go to my dumb neighbor's house after school. I hate it." What would your nursing care for Tom include?

2. You are the primary nurse at the Employee Health Service at an insurance agency. Forty-five-year-old Mr. J. comes into the office with a severe headache. His blood pressure is elevated 26 mmHg over the previous reading one year ago. An interview with Mr. J. reveals that nine months ago he married a woman with three teenaged children. After the initial "honeymoon" period of living together, the three stepchildren are now acting out in school and at home. Family tensions have increased and two of the children are talking about moving to live with their father. This upsets Mrs. J. because she doesn't think that they will receive needed supervision from him. What would you include in your nursing care for Mr. J.?

3. You are the nurse in a pediatrician's office doing an assessment on two-month-old baby boy H. Mrs. H. informs you that he was adopted directly from the hospital when he was eight days old. She reports that she and her husband are thrilled to have a child after twelve years of trying to conceive one themselves. Mrs. H. seems anxious about her son and hovers over him as you inspect the baby. All findings are normal, but you notice dirt and dried formula behind the baby's ears and retraction of his foreskin reveals some old lint from his diaper. When you ask Mrs. H. if she regularly retracts the foreskin during bathing, she looks embarrassed and tells you she really doesn't know how to bathe a baby and that she's just been giving him little sponge baths. What would your nursing care for Mrs. H. include?

REFERENCES

1. Aguilera, Donna C., and Janice M. Messick. *Crisis Intervention.* St. Louis: C. V. Mosby Co., 1974, 21.
2. Bernard, Janine M. "The Divorce Myth." *The Personnel and Guidance Journal,* October 1981, 67.
3. Coogler, O. J., Ruth E. Weber, and Patrick C. McKenny. "Divorce Mediation: A Means of Facilitating Divorce and Adjustment." *The Family Coordinator,* April 1979, 255.
4. Coyne, Ann, and Laurie Flynn. "Infant Adoption." *Children Today* 9:4, November/December 1980.
5. Goetting, Ann. "The Six Stations of Remarriage: Developmental Tasks of Remarriage After Divorce." *Family Relations* 41:213, April 1982.
6. Hetherington, E. Mavis. "Divorce—A Child's Perspective." *American Psychologist* 34:851–57, October 1979.
7. Hetherington, E. M., M. Cox, and R. Cox. "The Aftermath of Divorce." In *Mother-Child, Father-Child Relations,* ed. J. H. Stevens, Jr., and M. Matthews. Washington, D.C.: National Association for the Education of Young Children, 1978.
8. Lutz, Patricia. "The Stepfamily: An Adolescent Perspective." *Family Relations* 32:374–75, July 1983.
9. Turnbull, Sharon K., and James M. Turnbull. "To Dream the Impossible Dream: An Agenda for Discussion with Stepparents." *Family Relations* 32:228–30, April 1983.

CHAPTER 26

The Chronically Ill Child

HELEN LERNER

•

OBJECTIVES

After completing this chapter, the reader will be able to:

□ Describe the effect of chronic illness on the child and the family.

□ Discuss the principles of primary nursing management of the child with a chronic condition.

□ Identify the physical, psychosocial, and emotional needs of the chronically ill child and his family in the community and in the hospital.

□ Describe the nursing intervention in each of the above settings.

□ Discuss ways in which nursing interventions foster normal growth and development.

□ Evaluate the nursing care given to a child and family in terms of meeting the child's and family's physical, psychological, and social needs.

Primary nursing is an effective means of helping families who have children with chronic illnesses. This chapter describes the problems and challenges to the nurse in caring for families of children with chronic illness. The chronic conditions of asthma and cerebral palsy are used as examples of chronic illness.

Overview of Chronic Illness in Children

Illness of a long-term nature profoundly affects the child, family, and community. Some cultures accept tragedy without question. A birth of a child with a defect or brain damage may be seen as God's will. The parents may believe that they have been chosen especially to raise this child. In the United States we generally want to know why a particular event has occurred.

The feelings of parents who have a defective child are similar to those of parents whose infant has died. Such parents experience a loss to which they must adjust, and as long as the child lives they will have a reminder that this is not the child they dreamed of. The feelings that accompany loss of the perfect child vary in sequence and duration at each of the stages of grief. The length and depth of each stage depends on the personality structure, the previous life experiences, the extent of the baby's deformity, and the quality of the child's response to parental care. Emotional support from key people is also important in helping the parents resolve their grief (20).

The parents need time to work through their feelings. It is difficult for parents to go through the grieving process and make the adjustment to the handicapped child on their own. They need support also from professionals to develop a healthy relationship with their child. For further information on handling grief, the reader is referred to chapter 17.

The child's need for a healthful environment and a family support system that fosters growth and development and enables him to reach his maximum potential is the same as for other children. In addition, assistance is required, for the child to lessen the disabling nature of the illness, and for the family to cope with the child's additional needs. The community requires input from nurses to include the child as a valuable and functioning member.

Chronic diseases in children can take many forms (Figure 26.1). Mattson refers to chronic illness as a disorder with a protracted course that can be progressive and fatal or can be associated with a normal life span despite impaired physical or mental functioning (16). Such diseases may have periods of acute exacerbation that require medical attention. They may interfere with the child's physical and emotional growth and normal development.

Role of the Nurse

Nurses are important professionals in the care of chronically ill children. Nurses are becoming more and more involved with the primary care of families. They are taking responsibility for caring for families on a long-term basis and are in a unique position to care for families over a period of time. There are several reasons for this. First, nurses have contact with families throughout the life cycle in a variety of settings. The community health nurse sees families with newborns who have just been discharged from the hospital, as well as older children and older adults. The community health nurse is able to see these families on a long-term basis and can follow them throughout their involvement with different health care facilities. Nurses in clinics or health care centers also have the opportunity to follow families from the birth of an infant through adolescence and beyond. They have this opportunity both through their coming in for periodic assessments and care and through home visits that the nurse makes. Hospital nurses on pediatric units also have frequent contact with families who have chronically ill children. They often have deep involvement with the family and have been with them through numerous crises and are very much trusted by the families. The nurse on the pediatric unit is an important source of data for those caring for the child and family

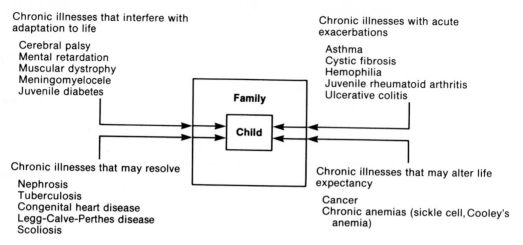

Chronic illnesses that interfere with
adaptation to life

  Cerebral palsy
  Mental retardation
  Muscular dystrophy
  Meningomyelocele
  Juvenile diabetes

Chronic illnesses with acute
exacerbations

  Asthma
  Cystic fibrosis
  Hemophilia
  Juvenile rheumatoid arthritis
  Ulcerative colitis

Family

Child

Chronic illnesses that may resolve

  Nephrosis
  Tuberculosis
  Congenital heart disease
  Legg-Calve-Perthes disease
  Scoliosis

Chronic illnesses that may alter life
expectancy

  Cancer
  Chronic anemias (sickle cell, Cooley's
    anemia)

Figure 26.1. Chronic Disease in Children

in the community, and the community nurse serves as a resource person to the pediatric nurse during periods of hospitalization.

Second, the nurse has a role in both health and illness care. The nurse is interested in both the manifestations of the disease process and in helping the child and family to cope with the disease. The nurse is also interested in other needs of the child and family, such as health maintenance and promoting family functioning in order to provide as normal an environment for the child as possible. Thus the nurse is able to focus on the child and the family and their method of coping with the disease process as it affects all aspects of their lives.

Third, nurses are able to work with many other professionals. Their education in the hospital and community has brought them in contact with physicians, social workers, teachers, physical and occupational therapists, and speech pathologists. Having experience working with other professionals has enabled the nurse to understand the contributions each can make to the child's care. Thus appropriate referrals can be made to meet many of the child's and family's needs.

Fourth, the nurse has been educated to provide counseling and teaching for families. Much of the care involved in chronic illness involves communicating with families, imparting knowledge about the disease process and health maintenance, teaching families about the kinds of care the child needs, and assisting the child and family to provide self-care and function as independently as possible.

For the above reasons the nurse is an important and

valuable caretaker for the child who has chronic disease. Many commonalities in providing nursing care for the child with chronic disease and his family are applicable no matter what the particular disease process. Nursing knowledge is especially important in three areas: the child and his or her growth and development, the family, and the community.

Growth and Development

The impact of chronic disease on a child's growth and development at an early age can be seen through behaviors of the parents and children. Infants with chronic disease are often subjected to repeated hospitalizations, resulting in separation from their parents. This disrupts the child's life at a time when he has limited powers to cope. The child undergoes many frightening procedures and experiences and has little ability to comprehend what is happening to him. Often repeated hospitalizations interfere with the attachment process. The parents have less of a chance to feel comfortable with caring for a child who may require more care than a child without a chronic condition. Repeated separations may cause the child to become even more fearful of separation from the parents.

Preschool children have little ability to understand what causes their illness. Often they interpret the illness and the pain they experience as punishment for perceived misbehavior. Preschool children also suffer from repeated separations from their families. According to

Mattson, such separations are destructive unless a strong and therapeutic alliance is forged between the parents and staff (16). The nurse's role in forging this alliance is knowing the possibility of the problem of separation and what it engenders. In the nursing process the nurse assesses plans and intervenes to prevent difficulties. Nurses must be alert to the potential traumatic effect of the separations and allow the parents ample time for visiting and opportunity to care for their child. Providing information that can be understood and preparing the child and family for procedures are essential. Nurses must also help the parents provide for the child's developmental needs both at home and in the hospital. At a time when the child is learning so many new skills and is developing rapidly, his opportunity to use these skills may be curtailed because of frequent hospitalizations and episodes of illness. If the child is not given an opportunity to practice new skills, he will regress. The child may often be angry and frustrated, since he is striving for autonomy at this age. Play can be an effective intervention, and the nurse can help the child cope with these frustrations through play. Situations can be created in which the child is allowed to practice new skills in order to maintain gains he has made in growth and development.

Older preschool children and young school-age children are just beginning to come into contact with their peer group. In a study of four- to eight-year-old children, Teplin and associates noted that by four years of age, children with handicaps were already aware, to some degree, of differences between themselves and their peers (28). The parents of handicapped children indicated that relationships with nonhandicapped children were important positive factors in their children's emerging self-concepts.

An older school-age child is better able, because of his cognitive development, to understand the cause of his illness. The major task of this age-group is developing a sense of industry that requires a degree of independence from the parents and a positive self-image. Hughes found that the consequences of illness and the causes of illness were of most concern to school-age children (10). The loneliness or the threats that were experienced as a by-product of the illness left the children with little energy to deal with other issues, such as establishing new relationships. The children had fears and fantasies that seemed to be an exaggeration of the fears and fantasies of all children. Their greatest concern was to be like others and to be accepted by others. This was often difficult because their outlets for verbal and social expression were limited, and physical expression was often restricted.

Mattson notes that by about the age of six or seven, a child can use his cognitive functions of memory and language to provide a beginning understanding of his illness (16). He begins to accept limits and responsibility for care and learns to find satisfaction in a variety of motor and intellectual activities that help him both to release and to control his emotions.

Older children are in a better position to use their cognitive abilities to comprehend their illness and its cause. They need frequent, simple, concrete explanations of what is happening with their bodies, and they need frequent validation that they understand what is happening to them.

If a child feels secure at home, he is ready to venture out into the community. This normal goal of independence for a school-age child is equally important for a child with a chronic illness.

The child normally moves outside the family to build relationships with peers. He learns new social roles and how to care for himself. These normal activities may be more difficult to accomplish for the child with a chronic illness. Often the child may be sent out of the neighborhood to a different school and is thus removed from what is familiar to him.

Even if the child remains in the neighborhood school, he is made to feel different in other ways. Because of the chronic illness the child may have more absences from school, which may interfere with his learning. Thus he may be behind his peers in schoolwork. He also may feel different because he looks different, or because he takes medicine on a regular basis, or because he needs to eat special foods. The child may also require periodic hospitalizations, which are stressful for him and his family. These hospitalizations may result in regression in the child's independent status, which he may resent. He also dislikes being away from peers, and hospitalization may increase his isolation from them. Parents may have trouble setting limits for the child during an acute episode of the illness. Nurses need to help the school-age child use each hospitalization as positively as possible and to cope with the child's behavior in ways that encourage growth and development. The nurse can do this by promoting self-care and independence in the child. The nurse can also encourage the child to keep in touch with peers and assist the parents in helping the child keep up with schoolwork. It is important to get the child to express his concerns and to listen to them.

The problems of healthy adolescents can be overwhelming for both the adolescent and the parent.

Chronic disease adds an extra stress to the situation. Jelneck describes cultural goals for adolescents as, first, the ability to accept their physical selves with all the changes going on and focus on their good points without dwelling on their imperfections; second, learning emotional control, which is the balance between childish expression and suppression of their feelings; and third, the development of social maturity, or the ability to develop good interpersonal relationships (12).

All of these cultural goals are more difficult for adolescents with chronic illness to accomplish. The ability to accept the physical self is compromised when the adolescent's physical appearance may be different from that of his peers. The adolescent may be concerned about physical problems that are in addition to the usual human imperfections.

Adolescents with chronic illness may also have more difficulty learning emotional control. They may have experienced more emotional stress because of repeated bouts of illness and, because of frequent hospitalizations, had less of an opportunity to express these emotions. Repeated hospitalizations also frequently cause regressive behaviors that do not contribute to the adolescent's learning to express his feelings in a maturer way.

The adolescent often uses defense mechanisms so that he does not have to deal with the reality of his illness. The ones most frequently seen include denial, intellectualization, regression, and projection. Denial helps the adolescent separate himself from his anxiety. The risk is in not seeking health care or complying with the therapeutic regimen. The adolescent who uses denial is also not alert to danger signs or complications of his illness.

The adolescent also often uses his intellectual functioning to deal with his concern about the disease. He may read extensively and use technical terms in speaking with health professionals. He may not ask questions and will use his intellectual knowledge to keep a distance between himself and his disease.

Regression is a common occurrence. The adolescent takes on the behavior of an earlier stage that enabled him to cope and uses it to cope with the present. However, this does not help him grow into adulthood.

The adolescent may also project the blame for his illness onto others. Both his projection and rejection result in his accepting no responsibility for his independence or self-care or for learning more about his condition.

Nursing intervention includes permitting adolescents to make some of the decisions regarding their care. For example, adolescents can make their own appointments for health care visits. At least some of the visit should

be conducted without the parent in the room. The adolescent should also be involved in setting up his own home care regimen.

Continuance of normal growth and development is especially important in adolescence. Jelneck advises against the use of TV as recreation (12). Reading or activities that involve the adolescent as more than a passive participant are recommended. In this way interests and hobbies are developed. The adolescent should be encouraged to join special interest groups and interact with teenagers who do not have disabilities. Groups of adolescents with the same disability are also helpful, but encouraging the adolescent to participate with his whole peer group is an important factor in his development. The adolescent with a chronic illness, like any other adolescent, must plan for a vocation and learn how to manage his sexuality. It may be more difficult for the family to release control when the adolescent has a chronic illness, so the nurse must give the family support and encouragement. The most important part of the care of the chronically ill adolescent is promoting his normal growth and development and his successful transition to adulthood.

Family

Some say that members of a family with a chronically ill child suffer sorrow throughout their lifetimes. Solnit and Stark note that the persistence of the effect of the living child who requires care for a long time will remind the mother of her loss and evoke guilt (24).

Olshansky used the term chronic sorrow to describe the persistent effect of the feelings of loss even though the initial period of mourning over the "dream" child passes (18). This is particularly true if the child is not expected to live or fulfill many of life's expected tasks, such as getting an education, being employed, or raising a family.

Jackson speaks of chronic sorrow as following the same stages as acute grief, except that it is prolonged. Parents are not necessarily immobilized, but can carry on their daily activities and receive satisfaction from their child. The sorrow varies in intensity and is never completely resolved as long as the child lives (11). Early identification of chronic illness and counseling of family members usually improve the care that the child receives and minimize the negative psychosocial impact that the chronic disease has on the family. The health care providers, in their initial contact, set the tone for the family's future care. The health care provider must understand that decisions made about the child and his illness are ultimately made by the family. The family reacts to the child and his illness according to its culture and beliefs. Sometimes this causes problems for health professionals who come from differing cultural backgrounds and beliefs. For example, a Haitian family had a child who was born with microcephaly. The health professionals in the hospital suggested that the family institutionalize the child. The family meanwhile had made plans to return to the rural area of Haiti that was previously their home so that the child would remain with them and grow up with the family. Doctors and nurses tried to explain to the parents the advantages of institutionalization, but the parents remained committed to their original plans. The frustrated health care professionals felt that they had not accomplished their goal. The family did not understand why they were being pressured to institutionalize their child.

All families will go through a mourning process when informed that their child has a chronic illness. The length, depth, and nature of the mourning process will depend on the parents' personality structure, the previous life experiences, and the seriousness or extent of the illness.

In order for the family to function at its best, the parents have to overcome their sorrow and feelings of guilt. Parents who can successfully adapt can encourage self-care, enforce realistic restrictions, and promote normal growth and development in their child.

Many families undergo marital stress because of the chronic illness. Parents have less opportunity to seek social outlets because of the child's constant need for care and the unavailability of reliable baby-sitters, coupled with the financial strain owing to expenses for health care. Often there is a general withdrawal from outside activity. Breslau and associates studied mothers of disabled children and compared them with a control group. It was found that the presence of a disabled child in the home had a negative effect on the mother's psychological functioning—these mothers were at risk for psychological distress. A critical factor in the distress was the impact of the condition on the child's daily functioning in terms of the care that was required from the mother. The more dependent the child, the more psychological difficulties the mother experienced (3).

Fathers have had a peripheral role in research ostensibly because they are at work and do not have the opportunity to communicate with health professionals as frequently as mothers do. Although both parents may be included in discussions in the beginning, when the crisis is over the father receives less support and information from health care providers. McKeever reports that fa-thers were deeply affected by their child's chronic illness. They felt numbness and shock when the illness was diagnosed, but they thought it was their duty to support their wives. Most also believed that they could not leave their jobs for another in a different location unless they were assured of comparable health care facilities (14).

Nine out of ten fathers said that they only went out alone with their wives once a month and reported little involvement in community activities. They reported their wives as the main source of comfort and did not use groups. They were fearful of the children's future and the children's ability to survive as independent adults.

McKeever's study points out the need for nurses to include the father in the care of the family and, if necessary, to plan for special time to give counseling and information about the disease and its manifestations so that the father is knowledgeable and can answer questions that his child may ask. The nurse also needs to help the parents plan time away from the child. Referrals to agencies that provide suitable baby-sitters or respite care are important.

The other children in the family have many needs that must be recognized. The impact of chronic illness on siblings is often overlooked unless the nurse makes certain to include it as part of her assessment. This aspect must be addressed as part of the health maintenance of the family. Times when the child is acutely ill are not appropriate times for extensive family counseling. The community health nurse has an excellent opportunity to speak with the siblings and find out their concerns. She can also include them in planning the child's home care and praise them for their assistance in coping with the family crisis. The community health nurse should also be aware of signs of maladjustment, such as frequent somatic complaints, school problems, and isolation from peers. Parents may need help in planning special time to be with their well children.

The community health nurse is in an excellent position to communicate with the school nurse and keep the school informed of the family's status so that the teachers can observe the effects on the other children in the family and assist them with coping.

Craft notes that there are often signs that another child in the family is having difficulties with adjustment. These signs include (a) somatic distress, such as constant fatigue and gastrointestinal symptoms; (b) preoccupation with the image of the sibling who is ill; (c) self-blame in search of a cause for the illness; (d) irritability, impatience, and withdrawal from social relationships; and (e) inability to maintain normal functioning (6).

The above problems can manifest themselves when a sibling is hospitalized. The nurse in the hospital should encourage frequent communication from the other children in the family. If the other children are unable to visit, letters, tapes, and phone calls are important. If a child is able to visit his sibling in the hospital, he should be prepared by his parents and the nurse for what to expect when he sees his brother or sister. Any kind of equipment or devices should be clearly explained. Other facets of the hospital environment should also be explained to the child, such as the paging system and the uniforms and outfits that various personnel wear. Children should be prepared for the sight of other children with intravenous infusions, bandages, drainage tubes, and traction.

Chronic disease is a family health problem involving all members of the family. In planning the care of the child the nurse must also make provisions for meeting the needs of the family.

Community

Nurses have several important functions in the community. They are to educate members of the community about health and illness, to encourage the community to provide services that meet the needs of all children, to alert communities to the needs of chronically ill children, and to identify resources that are particularly helpful to chronically ill children and their families.

Nurses provide information about health and illness. Members of the community should understand the causes of illness and which diseases are communicable. In this way old myths about "evil spirits" or "bad blood" causing an illness can be dispelled. Nurses should encourage all groups in the community to have contact with chronically ill children. When the children attend schools and day-care centers, nurses have a responsibility to educate the teachers and the children about why this child is "different." They can explain the child's special needs and point out ways in which many other children are themselves different.

Nurses should also make sure that the teacher feels comfortable with what must be done while the child is in class and what will happen if the child suddenly becomes ill. Nurses can point out resources in the community where the teacher can obtain additional information if there is a need.

Nurses might also speak to parents' groups about the needs of chronically ill children. They can be a resource for these groups within the community. They can be a support for the families with chronically ill children and can point out to other parents the benefits that their healthy children may get from attending school with children who are chronically ill.

Nurses should also be concerned with making sure that community facilities are accessible to all children. Federal laws concerning access for the handicapped have lead to many changes in different facilities. For example, there is now access for wheelchairs in many schools and recreation centers. Community centers should be assessed by the nurse. Is there access to activities at a local community center? Do playgrounds meet the needs of a child with a motor problem? Are the playgrounds or play areas located where there is so much pollen or pollution that they would be unsuitable for a child with asthma? Do recreation leaders understand the needs of a child with chronic illness? Will they include the child in the recreational group and feel comfortable meeting his needs? Is a child with a chronic illness encouraged to participate in whatever community activities he is able?

Nurses, both in the hospital and in the community, should be able to identify community resources that will aid the family. Many diseases have national foundations that study the particular disease entity, such as cerebral palsy, cystic fibrosis, and muscular dystrophy. These foundations provide many kinds of information and services for affected children and their families, ranging from information on where the most current research is taking place to sites where parent groups are meeting and where parents can obtain respite care.

There are other resources in the community that may be important to the family, such as social service agencies or agencies that serve handicapped people. Social service agencies may be able to provide homemaking services, help with housing or finances, and offer counseling. Agencies that serve the handicapped may prove helpful in obtaining needed equipment and acquainting the family with special services available to the community.

Nurses should alert communities to the needs of chronically ill children. They are an important minority and the community stands to lose if they are not encouraged to participate in community life. Nursery schools and day-care centers can be helped to include chronically ill children in their programs. Teachers can become acquainted with their special needs and with the fact that their greatest need is to be full participating members of the community and to grow and develop as normal children.

In planning for the future, communities that are aware of the needs of chronically ill children and their families can make policies that meet the needs of all community members and that encourage the development of all children and their families.

Asthma

To illustrate the role of the nurse in the health care of a child with a chronic condition with episodic exacerbations, asthma will be used as an example.

Overview of the Condition

Allergic conditions account for one-third of all chronic conditions in children under age seventeen. These conditions also represent one-fourth of all days lost from school owing to chronic illness. Asthma is probably the most frequent allergic manifestation that results in chronic illness. Although the pediatric death rate from asthma is low—roughly one per thousand—the morbidity remains high. Because of the high morbidity, the children's social, emotional, and intellectual growth can be disrupted. This disruption plus the financial burden can put a strain on a family (4).

Asthma stands alone among the chronic diseases with regard to its high degree of reversibility. There is excellent response to proper therapy (13).

The current consensus is that allergic disease is inheritable. If a child has two parents with allergic disease, the child has a 75 percent chance of being allergic. If one parent is allergic, the child has a 60 percent chance of becoming allergic (4). The nurses' efforts in prevention are directed at minimizing the disease in those children who are at risk.

All parents should be familiar with their own histories and with the possibility of their child developing allergic disease. This should be part of the history that a nurse takes with every pregnant woman. Parents with a history of allergic disease should be advised to breast-feed their babies. In a recent study, infants with a positive allergic history developed allergic disease equally when fed cow's milk or soy-based formula. Infants who were breast-fed developed allergic disease at a much lower rate. Breast-feeding in the first three months of life, in addition to avoiding environmental allergens, appears to play a role in preventing or minimizing the occurrence of allergic disease (9).

If the mother does not want to breast-feed, a hypoal-lergenic formula may be used. A soybean formula is not always the best substitute, since the soybean is a member of the pea family, and frequently peas are implicated in allergies.

Nursing Care of the Child with Asthma

In order for the nurse to participate in the child's treatment plan, a thorough assessment is made. The nurse bases this assessment on her own data, as well as on information that is available from other professional contacts and the family. The kind of contacts she makes depends on the child's age and developmental status. For infants and toddlers, the nurse obtains most of the data from the child's pediatrician and the parents. As the child gets to preschool and school age, the nurse can also obtain data from teachers and recreational workers who have contact with the child as well as from the child himself. Such people will be able to relate what the child's usual response to stress is, how life-style is affected by illness, and what the usual response is to medications and treatments. In addition, the nurse should get some information regarding the child's school performance and attendance. Often many children with asthma do not do well in school because of frequent absences. The child can also be affected by the medication in class. Medications can cause the child to feel drowsy or to have gastrointestinal disturbances or headaches. According to Sedlack, the nurse should obtain the usual data from a health history and a physical examination. In addition, the nurse should obtain the following information: What kind of problem is the child having with asthma? How can you tell when the child is getting sick? What physical and environmental conditions precipitate an attack? Who handles the child's care when it is an emergency? What is usual treatment for the child's acute asthmatic attack? What medication does the child take on a regular basis? (24).

It is also important to ascertain whether the parents know what allergens or other factors cause the child's asthma. The asthma may also be caused by a strong emotional component. Situational stress or poor relationships with parents or siblings may often precipitate an attack in the absence of other factors such as allergens.

What kinds of diagnostic tests have been done? Skin testing is done to aid in determining if there are hypersensitivities to certain substances that may trigger asthmatic symptoms.

The scratch test is also used. The skin is scratched with a needle and a solution containing the allergen is applied to the scratch. If the patient is hypersensitive to the allergen, a wheal will form at the spot where the solution was applied. The reaction should take place within fifteen minutes. This test will help to determine what allergens may be precipitating symptoms so that the child can try to avoid these substances. This test also gives the physician information that would influence the decision to use immunotherapy.

Nursing Intervention Related to Self-Care Responsibilities

The self-care responsibilities of the child with asthma and his or her family are numerous. The child will have asthma for his entire life, and the nurse needs to assist the family in developing ways to incorporate the necessary care into the family's life-style (19).*

The need for air is frequently the greatest concern when the child is acutely ill. It is important for the parent and child to be aware of the signs of an impending asthma attack so that they can seek treatment as soon as possible. Sometimes it is possible to avert the attack at home by removing the child from the allergen if he is beginning to show some difficulty in breathing. Medications and postural drainage are helpful. Those who care for the child should be well versed in the signs and symptoms of an asthma attack and what to do for it.

Because of frequent asthma attacks the child may have diminished breathing capacity. Often the nurse must suggest breathing exercises for the child. This can take the form of a game, such as having the child blow out a candle or having him blow a piece of paper out of someone's hand.

The need for water is also important for asthmatic children and is often closely related to the need for air. One of the effects of asthma is the production of thick tenacious secretions. The child needs to drink large amounts of fluid to loosen these secretions and facilitate coughing them up. A good amount to aim for is approximately three quarts a day (29). A child with asthma should always have an adequate fluid intake and should be encouraged to drink extra fluid at all times. Parents should inform people who care for the child, both in and out of the hospital, about the child's favorite fluids so that they can encourage fluid intake.

Food can be the focus of some of the asthmatic child's problems. Many children with asthma are allergic to certain foods. During infancy foods should be added to

*The self-care responsibilities described in this chapter are based on Dorothea Orem's work.

the diet much more slowly when there is an allergic history. Foods that are highly allergenic, such as eggs, milk, wheat, chocolate, and shellfish, should be started late or not at all. The parents should be cautioned to read the labels of all prepared foods as well, since many of them contain foods or additives that may be allergenic. A good example of this is orange juice, which is often used in the preparation of baby foods.

The child must be taught what foods he can and cannot eat. This often creates a problem for a preschool or school-age child who is anxious to eat what the other children eat. Sometimes it is possible to give the child an acceptable substitute. It is important that the child not be made to feel different from his peers.

If the child attends a school or a day-care center where meals are served as part of the program, there needs to be a notice on a bulletin board or on the refrigerator in the kitchen that states the food allergies of particular children. The nurse has an important role in making sure that the parents inform the school or day-care center of a child's food allergies, verifying that the staff understands the importance of the child's avoiding those foods.

For asthmatic children the provision of care associated with elimination is similar to that for other children. With an increased fluid intake they will probably have fewer problems with constipation, and the increased fluid intake will help to prevent urinary tract infections. Teachers may need to be reminded that because of increased fluid intake, the child may need to make more frequent trips to the bathroom.

Maintaining a balance between activity and rest is important for the child. Often if a child becomes dyspneic during a given activity, he is discouraged from attempting this activity again. The reasons for his dyspnea need to be explored so that it is possible for the child to attempt the same or a similar activity at another time. For example, medication given before the child plays might prevent episodes of dyspnea. If the child plays outside, he may be more likely to become dyspneic at certain times of the year than at others. For example a child who plays in the leaves in the fall may have an asthma attack because of the mold present. Perhaps the child could play in another area that is free of fallen leaves. Activity should be encouraged, since it is important that the child learn to cope with his environment. Children with asthma often engage in sedentary activities because they fear that more strenuous activity will bring on an asthma attack. Children need to be encouraged to participate in as many activities as they can.

Rest may often be interfered with in the child with

asthma because attacks may occur at night. The child's bedroom should be allergy-proofed, and pets and people who are smoking should not be permitted there (see Table 26.1). Toys and furniture that collect a great deal of dust or themselves have allergenic properties, such as wool or down, should be avoided in the child's room. Curtains should be replaced with window shades. If at all possible, an air filter should be used with the heating system. Because sudden changes in temperature may bring on an attack, it is helpful to have a small cotton rug or slippers by the child's bed so that when he gets up in the morning, he will not have to put his feet on the cold floor and thus precipitate an attack.

Maintaining a balance between solitude and social interaction may present a problem for an asthmatic child who, because of his illness, has frequent absences from school. The child may also be limited in where he can go because of his allergies. He may not be able to visit some friends because they have dogs or cats or items in the house that are allergenic. This often limits the opportunities for the child to be independent from the parents.

Also, the child may have frequent hospitalizations because of asthma attacks and become further isolated from his peer group. Both the nurse in the hospital and the nurse in the community can encourage contact between the child and his peers while he is in the hospital, and between the child and the school so that he can keep up with his schoolwork and not fall behind his class.

The child with asthma should be encouraged to join activities that center around personal interests and to find children with whom he can interact in activities that

Table 26.1
Allergy Proofing the Home

Areas in and Around Home	What to Avoid	What Is Needed
Child's bedroom	Stuffed chairs, wool or nylon rug, down pillows or quilts, wool covers, stuffed toys, plants, smoking, pets, old wallpaper, venetian blinds or other window coverings that collect dust	Painted wood or metal furniture, washable cotton rug (particularly by bed), cotton blankets, toys of wood or plastic that can be easily cleaned, air conditioning unit (if possible), painted walls
Playroom	Reservoirs of water, fish and turtle tanks, basement or damp areas, pets with dander, peeling plaster, smoking, fireplace, chalk and blackboard	Easily cleanable and dustable surfaces, low humidity, plastic or painted wooden toys, materials such as cotton, and synthetics (e.g., Dacron), paints, crayons
Kitchen	Poorly stored food that attracts insects or mold, poorly rinsed or damp sponges, poor storage of food that easily gets moldy (cheese, mushrooms, fruits), frying, smoking	List of foods that child is allergic to, broiling and roasting of foods, good storage arrangements for foods
Bathroom	Proximity to child's bedroom, towels or clothes that dry slowly, disinfectant with strong smell, smoking, mold on shower curtain or tile	Clean with mold-retardant cleaner, put damp articles in dryer or area where drying is quicker, keep shower area and tub free from mold
Outdoors	Plants that child is allergic to, weeds, exhaust fumes, stables, kennels	Dry area, free of animals, plastic or metal equipment

Source: Adapted from Charmaine Jennings. "Controlling the Home Environment of the Allergic Child." *American Journal of Maternal Child Nursing* 7:376–81, December 1982.

do not depend on school performance and athletic skills and who will accept him for his unique talents.

Prevention of hazards for the allergic child are the same as those for a normal child of the same age, with some additions. Environments with allergens pose a hazard for the allergic child. The nurse needs to help the family identify these hazards in places where the child will be spending significant amounts of time. The chalk dust in the classroom may cause some difficulty at school. Being in a room with wool carpeting or stuffed chairs can bring on an attack. Open windows through which pollen or pollutants can enter a room can create problems for the child. If the family is alert to these hazards, they can be prevented or at least minimized.

Perhaps one of the most difficult hazards to deal with is a beloved pet. Is is difficult for the child and the family to part with a dog or a cat, even though it may be causing the child difficulty. The nurse might suggest that the animal be kept outside if possible and that the child have minimal contact with the pet. If the allergy is mild, restricting the animal from sleeping areas and avoiding direct contact might be adequate. Frequent grooming and bathing of the animal are essential. Goldfish or turtles, which may be allergenically acceptable, are poor substitutes for something soft and furry.

Promoting maximum human functioning and development is the ultimate goal in caring for a child with a chronic illness. Infants and toddlers may be frequently hospitalized with asthma. These constant separations from family are difficult for both the parent and the child. Because of frequent illness, the child misses out on many experiences that are necessary for growth and development. The toddler may not get an opportunity to practice developmental and self-care skills, such as toilet training, without the interruption of repeated hospitalizations. The older child may have difficulties in school because of frequent absences. The child may miss out not only on academic work, but on social experiences as well. Other children, as well as teachers, may become frightened when he has an attack.

The nurse must make the family aware of the child's growth and developmental progress and praise the family for the efforts that they have made to give the child as normal an existence as possible. The nurse should tell the parents how to arrange for rooming in at the hospital and encourage them to stay with the child as much as they want and are able. The nurse should also encourage limit setting, which is a normal requirement for children of all ages, and help parents in their efforts to have the child do as much as possible for himself.

It is important for the family and the child to see the child as an essentially normal child who has asthma. The child's strengths should be emphasized, and he should be praised for the things that he does well. Efforts that the child makes to provide self-care should be especially praised.

The parents and the nurse must recognize that the prospect of an attack, which is ever present, is frightening to a child. It is well known that asthma attacks can be brought on by stress. Chronically ill children, especially adolescents, have repeated periods of stress.

Action should be taken to foster specific human development. Such action does not differ from that taken with healthy children. The nurse must remind the family to provide the child with the same stimulation and activities that other children receive.

The integrity of human structure and functioning needs to be maintained and promoted. Children with asthma need to know certain facts about their illness so they can participate in their health maintenance and promotion. They need to know the symptoms of asthma; what medications they are taking and the medications' side effects; how to prevent upper respiratory tract infections, since these will worsen the asthma; and what he is allergic to and how he can avoid these allergens. This information should be given to the child by the nurse and the family and should be frequently reinforced.

The child should be encouraged to ask questions and take an active part in all his visits to health care providers.

Attending to deviations from normal is an important part of the child's health care. In asthma the most important of these is the use of medications to prevent an attack. Asthma is much easier to control when it is treated preventively than when therapy is started after an attack.

The basic group of medications used around the clock are methylxanthines. Of these, theophylline is the most widely used. Preparations are available in several forms, such as tablets, capsules, suspensions, and elixirs. The child's age and body weight are important criteria in determining the dose. The dose should be changed as the child grows and matures, and the family should be aware of this. The child's drug regimen should be carefully monitored to avoid toxic reactions, and the child and family should know the signs and symptoms of toxic reactions: nausea, nervousness, urinary frequency, and dizziness (4).

Another drug that is frequently used in asthma therapy is cromolyn sodium. This drug's main value is prophylaxis in exercise-induced bronchospasm. It can be used before athletic events.

Prednisone is used for some children who suffer from chronic asthma. However, side effects have always been a problem with this drug. The drug can be administered in low doses in aerosol form, or it can be given on alternate days, to minimize side effects (23). Prednisone works directly on the respiratory tract and avoids adrenal suppression.

The child and his family should know the expected effects of the medication and recognize when it is not effective. When such occasions occur, they should know where to seek help. The family should know, when the child is away from home, who is responsible for giving the medication or who is supervising the child and seeing that the medication is being taken at the prescribed time and in the prescribed dose.

The child with asthma should be encouraged to lead as normal a life as possible. He should still recognize the fact that he has a chronic disease, make whatever adjustments are necessary to this condition, and continue to participate fully in life as a person of his particular age. This can be done only if both he and his family are knowledgeable and fully informed about his condition.

Cerebral Palsy

To illustrate the role of the nurse in the health care of a child with a chronic disease that requires habilitation of all aspects of a child's life and remains relatively unchanged during the child's life, cerebral palsy is used as an example.

In 1980 the prevalence of cerebral palsy in the United States was 4.6 percent in infants with birth weights under 1,500 grams. The prevalence rates for cerebral palsy in the population are sensitive to changes in the probability of survival among infants of very low birth weights. A decrease in the mortality of this group probably leads to a modest rise in neurological impairment (20).

The causes of cerebral palsy are those incidents that occur during the mother's pregnancy and during the intrapartum and neonatal periods. During the prenatal period poor nutrition, chronic disease, infections, bleeding, and the use of toxic substances, such as drugs, are contributing factors. During the intrapartum period interference with the fetal oxygen supply by maternal blood loss, drugs used during labor, tetanic uterine contractions, interference with placental blood supply, and complications of delivery may be causative factors. The most significant events contributing to cerebral palsy are prenatal infections, intrauterine toxins, and complicated perinatal asphyxia associated with low birth weight (20).

Nurse's Role in Prevention

Prevention includes nursing intervention during the prenatal, intrapartum, and neonatal periods. All expectant mothers should be advised to seek early prenatal care. The nurse can ensure that such care is delivered by providers who communicate their concern for the mother's needs as well as a caring atmosphere that will encourage the mother to keep all appointments. The nurse should also promote good nutrition; she should make sure that the mother knows what a good diet consists of and has the means to obtain it. This may require referral if additional resources are needed.

During labor and delivery the nurse must be alert to possible complications. Through supportive nursing care the need for drugs can be reduced. With frequent observations the nurse is more alert to any possible abnormalities that may occur and early intervention can be provided.

During the neonatal period close observation of the newborn is essential, particularly for low-birth-weight infants. The nurse should carefully assess the infant for abnormalities, especially if there is a history of high risk, such as a history of genetic defects, diabetes, or a previous infant born with anomaly to this mother. The infant should be observed for signs of neurological damage such as apneic spells, poor vasomotor and body temperature control, decreased or absent reflexes, seizures, poor sucking, and hypotonia (7).

Prevention in older children involves other aspects, such as the prevention of accidents and poisonings, which may lead to central nervous system damage, or infections, such as meningitis or encephalitis. The nurse must often go to the issues that are dealt with in health maintenance for young children. Immunizations are important to prevent diseases such as measles, which can lead to encephalitis. Informing parents of the importance of early recognition of the signs of illness and when to seek care can prevent the child from developing a serious illness with sequelae. Teaching a mother how to take a child's temperature and read the thermometer will help in detecting a fever early and preventing the child from suffering the effects of high fever.

Prevention of falls and motor vehicle accidents will

lessen injuries such as skull fractures, which may cause neurological damage. Safety packaging for medications and other substances aids in preventing poisoning, which may also contribute to neurological insults.

Because the child will have to cope with cerebral palsy for the rest of his life, the attitude concerning his self-sufficiency that is given to him by his parents is of the utmost importance. The nurse must assist the family in providing care and helping the child to meet his own self-care needs.

Assessment of the Child with Cerebral Palsy

In order to provide nursing care, some basic issues of assessment should be considered. The nurse should concentrate on what the child can do; therefore, she should assess the child's activity pattern related to self-care needs. What age-appropriate self-care can the child do? What is the child's pattern of the activities of daily living? A physical and developmental assessment will help to determine the areas in which the child is strong and the areas in which he needs assistance. Such an assessment also enables the nurse to determine the areas to focus on when caring for the child and family.

Nursing Care Related to the Universal Self-Care Needs

The first need is for air. Many children with cerebral palsy have frequent respiratory tract infections. Often this is due to their immobility. Because they cannot move about, secretions tend to collect and provide an excellent cultural medium for bacterial and viral growth. Parents need to help their child move more frequently or move him if he cannot move himself so that the secretions can be shifted and coughed up if possible. Children with cerebral palsy may also have weak muscles in the upper trunk, and this makes it difficult for them to cough effectively. Sometimes postural drainage done by the parents is helpful in clearing the secretions.

The second need is for water. This may be a fairly difficult need to satisfy, particularly for the young child. Many children with cerebral palsy have difficulty sucking and swallowing at birth. Many times they will have to be tube-fed. When young children are cared for at home, they might find it difficult to swallow liquids. Liquids often cause choking, and aspiration may occur. This is frightening to both parent and child, and after a bad experience the child may refuse liquids. The parent may help the child by giving liquids in very small amounts, with the use of a spoon, or giving foods that

have a high water content, such as Jello. Even with this assistance the problem may persist.

The child should be held upright during a feeding. If the child tends to choke when liquids are given from a bottle, perhaps liquids could be given from a teaspoon so that the child can have a small amount to swallow. Stroking the underside of the chin and the throat encourages swallowing. When the child is able to handle small amounts of liquid, then he can try larger amounts and drink from a cup or a bottle. Older children are encouraged to remember to drink water daily. They may forget that they are thirsty, or they may have to ask someone for water. The value of drinking water every day should be stressed.

The third self-care need, the need for food, plays an important part in every child's life. It is especially important in the early years because the feeding experience forms the basis for the early parent-child relationship. Children with cerebral palsy have varying needs for food. Those who have limited mobility need fewer calories. Overfeeding causes weight gain and thus may interfere with the little mobility that the children have. On the opposite side, children with athetosis may require more calories than normal because of involuntary movement.

Feeding the child with cerebral palsy may present several problems. Before the parent attempts feeding, the nurse should evaluate the amount of head and trunk control the child has. It is best for the child to be fed in an upright position to minimize the possibility of aspiration. Before he can sit himself, his body should be supported in the sitting position.

Tongue thrust usually persists for a longer period of time in these children. It may be necessary to hold the child's lips closed to facilitate his swallowing.

Many parents keep children with cerebral palsy on soft diets for an extended period. This discourages the children from chewing. The longer a child remains on soft baby foods, the more difficult it will be for him to make the transition to solid food. The use of peanut butter or chocolate on the lips and tongue will encourage movement of the lips and tongue, and thereby foster chewing movements. An important move toward normalcy is making the child's eating habits as much like those of other children as possible.

Self-feeding is an important goal for the child with cerebral palsy. The child must have established several skills before he is ready to attempt self-feeding. He must be able to sit by himself and grasp an object and bring it to his mouth. This stage is difficult for many families because it is extremely messy. It is also this way with a normal child, but a child with cerebral palsy may be somewhat older when he is able to begin self-feeding, and the family may find this difficult to manage. Bibs and plastic protectors are important. Plenty of soap and water and damp cloths should be available for the aftermath. As with normal children, it is often easier for the parents to continue feeding the child. The parents must be informed by the nurse of the many disconcerting aspects of the child developing the skill of self-feeding. The parents should be encouraged to verbalize their concerns. It must also be emphasized that this is an essential part of the child's normal development.

Providing care associated with elimination is directly related to satisfying the need for food and water. Many children with cerebral palsy are troubled with constipation. They do not drink enough water and may get little roughage in their diet, particularly if their diet consists of soft foods past the time that this is appropriate. In addition, many children with cerebral palsy have poor abdominal muscle tone, and thus lack the ability to use abdominal pressure to defecate. The nurse can help the parents by encouraging whatever changes in the diet are possible to include more fluids and roughage. Proper positioning of the child while he is toileting will enhance the effectiveness of the abdominal muscles. A seat with good back support at a height where a child can rest his feet on the floor is often helpful.

Many children with cerebral palsy suffer from severe diaper rash. They need their diapers changed frequently, which is often difficult to do because of the children's tendency to scissor their limbs or because of frequent involuntary movements. The use of protective ointments is helpful, as well as exposure of the diaper area to the air. Because of low fluid intake the urine is concentrated and irritating. Efforts need to be made to increase fluid intake.

Toilet training is difficult for the child with cerebral palsy. The ability to hold in or release urine and stool is related to the child's motor development. Children with cerebral palsy have delayed motor development and are usually not ready to be toilet-trained until much later than normal children. The same signs of readiness, such as being uncomfortable when wet and being able to hold urine for longer periods of time, are as important for the child with cerebral palsy as they are for normal children. Children who have cerebral palsy may take varying amounts of time to be toilet trained, as do normal children.

Maintaining a balance between activity and rest is an important consideration in the family's care of the child with cerebral palsy and in their life-style. Infants and young children with cerebral palsy cannot move around by themselves and will remain inactive and immobile unless specific efforts are made to involve them in activities and encourage action. The nurse should take a careful history of how the child spends his day. Activity must be encouraged. Once the nurse knows the pattern of the child and the family, she can offer suggestions. The child can be moved to different areas of the house to observe activities. If the child is relatively immobile, he can be placed in different positions to stimulate the use of many muscle groups. The nurse can help the parents arrange some time during the day to promote movement, perform passive range-of-motion exercises, or do exercises to strengthen certain muscle groups. Usually a child who has been active during the day will sleep better at night. The nurse should help the parents provide a bed or crib that is comfortable for the child with cerebral palsy and that provides good alignment and support for his body.

Maintaining a balance between solitude and social interaction for the child with cerebral palsy rests on many of the same principles as maintaining the balance between activity and rest. Often the child cannot seek social interactions if he is by himself in a room and is immobile. If the child is quiet and does not make many demands, this may increase his solitude. Frequently the child prefers to be with other children in the family. The nurse may encourage the parent to see that the child has the opportunity to interact with other family members. The parents may also need to establish some specific times during the day when they can focus on interaction with the child.

Setting up or maintaining interaction with the child can be difficult. Children with cerebral palsy often don't respond as well to social interaction. They may have strabismus and have difficulty maintaining eye contact. They may rear back when held, and they don't react to hugs and holding as normal children do. It becomes difficult for parents to continually attempt to interact with the child if they are rebuffed. The nurse should prepare the parents for the difficulties that they may encounter and suggest other ways, such as touching, stroking, or talking with the child, that may provide a better interaction.

The prevention of hazards to human life and human functioning is an important goal for anyone who cares for children. Those who care for children with cerebral palsy have special problems in meeting this goal. First, children with cerebral palsy, because of their delayed development, may be unable to communicate as well as other children. They may not be able to express what is happening and they may have some difficulty understanding what they are told. They may need direct supervision beyond the age that normal children need such supervision.

Developmental delay or motor problems result in their having less experience with life situations than other children the same age have. They may not be able to recognize danger when it arises. The nurse must help the parents understand the child's need for supervision in accordance with his functional level and the necessity of exposing him to as many situations as possible that are common for other children.

The nurse must also assist the parents in understanding the implications of the child's motor handicap. A child who cannot crawl or move his limbs may not be able to get away from a dangerous situation even when it is recognized.

The promotion of normalcy in accord with human potential and human limitations for a child with cerebral palsy is the overriding goal of his care. This should be frequently repeated to the parents. The child has needs first as a child of his particular age. Direct efforts may have to be made to satisfy these needs, whereas a normal child can satisfy these needs himself. The need for interaction has previously been mentioned. Initiating play may require similar efforts. Just providing toys may not be adequate. Steele points out that it is important for a child to be put in a position where he can manipulate toys. The toy cannot just be presented; it must be placed in the child's vision, rubbed against his body, and placed in his hand. Different toys should be presented to the child so he will be motivated to reach out (26).

Promoting normalcy of the child also enables him to develop a realistic self-concept, fosters development, and maintains and promotes human functioning. The child develops a realistic self-concept when he is successful in what he does and receives positive feedback from those around him. One way that the nurse is able to promote such a self-concept is to enable the child to become involved in a school or day-care program that satisfies his needs. Children with cerebral palsy need to be involved in this sort of program from a very early age. Raising a child with cerebral palsy is a difficult task and the parents need all the help they can get. In such a program a child will have access to specialists, such as occupational or physical therapists, a speech therapist, and teachers who are specially trained to work with children who have cerebral palsy. The nurse can assist the parents by helping them realize the benefits that a child will receive from such a program. She can also help them to identify the community resources that might have infor-

mation about special programs. Once the child has been accepted in a program, the community health nurse can facilitate communication between the staff of the program and the parents. In order for the child to receive the greatest benefit from the program, the parents should be involved with what the child is learning so that this can be reinforced at home. Federal law currently mandates educational programs for all children from birth.

The parents may find it difficult to give the child a realistic self-concept because they are so involved with the child's handicap that they do not recognize his strengths. They may view the child's handicap as a stigma and feel guilty that he is not "normal." The parents may need to have the child's positive characteristics pointed out to them and have developmental progress identified as he accomplishes specific tasks. Raising a handicapped child can be extremely difficult and frustrating. Parents need a great deal of positive reinforcement that they are doing a good job and that the child is doing well. They need constant support and appreciation of their efforts. The nurse must help raise their self-image so that they can support a positive self-image in the child.

Taking action to foster human development is an important process for all families with handicapped children. Specific plans can be made for the areas of development that are appropriate for the child's particular functional level. The nurse should periodically assess the child's development, using a screening test such as the Denver Developmental Screening Test. By doing this the parents can be informed about the child's level in different areas, such as gross motor, fine motor, language, and social development. It also provides an objective measure of accomplishment. The nurse can then suggest certain areas for the parents to concentrate on and advise them of ways that they can stimulate the child's development.

Through health maintenance the family takes action to maintain and promote the integrity of human structure and functioning. The child with cerebral palsy frequently has so many appointments and people involved with care and management that the routines of well-child care are forgotten. It is not unusual to see children with cerebral palsy who have been followed by numerous specialists but who have not had their immunizations. The nurse should pay attention to this aspect of health maintenance, since the nurse may be the most appropriate one to coordinate care. All children need to receive immunizations against communicable disease. Because of neurological abnormalities and seizure disorders, the child with cerebral palsy may need to receive these immunizations in divided doses. The diet should be updated as he grows and develops, and routine screening tests, such as hemoglobin and hematocrit, urinalysis, and tuberculosis screening, should be performed on a regular basis. Parents need anticipatory guidance in terms of safety that is adapted to their child with his special needs in mind. He should have periodic physical examinations that cover all the major body systems. Parents need to learn to care for minor illnesses, such as respiratory tract infections and gastrointestinal disturbances, that, with the relative immobility of a child with cerebral palsy, could become serious problems if not recognized early and treated adequately.

Attention to deviations from normal is important in the child's total care. Two deviations are of particular significance in the care of the child with cerebral palsy. Because there are many problems with the limbs, contractures and deformities are common. It is therefore important that the child be maintained in proper body alignment at all times. The nurse can help the parents achieve this by showing them proper methods of positioning and teaching them range-of-motion exercises. The parents can also be made aware of the early signs of contractures and muscle stiffness and can be taught appropriate preventive exercises. The nurse is advised to confer with the physical therapist concerning ways that muscle contractures and deformities can be prevented. The nurse can then help the parents follow through with these recommendations. The nurse can also perform periodic physical assessment to identify problems in the early stages.

Another deviation common to children with cerebral palsy is seizures. Coughlin points out that children and their parents need to know what seizures are and what action needs to be taken when they occur. They need to know how anticonvulsants work and understand that when seizures no longer occur, it does not mean that the child no longer has a need for anticonvulsants, but that the anticonvulsants are working effectively and must not be stopped. The parents and the child, if appropriate, must be aware of the side effects of the medications and the symptoms they might observe (5). The nurse should explain that periodic blood and urine tests are needed to determine if untoward side effects are occurring. The family should be informed that seizures are more likely to occur when the child is ill with fever or overtired. Teenage girls are at increased risk for having seizures during the premenstrual period. Drinking alcoholic beverages also increases the risk of seizures. Bright lights, particularly strobe lights, are likely to induce seizures; with children who are prone to seizures, even the flickering lights of television may precipitate a seizure.

Legal and Ethical Issues

Many difficult legal and ethical issues are involved in caring for very sick premature infants who will probably develop cerebral palsy. There has been a great technological revolution in the provision of neonatal care. Infants who would have had no chance of surviving years ago are now being saved. By being able to preserve life we have raised a multitude of other issues that are significant for infants, their families, health professionals, and society as a whole.

Approximately 6 percent to 10 percent of infants born each year are premature. Most of them do well; 75 percent survive and between 70 percent and 80 percent of those cared for in neonatal intensive care settings do well and have minimal, if any, sequelae. However, figures for complications rise significantly with decreasing birthweight, especially for infants who weigh less than 800 grams (5). These infants are also at greater risk for developing cerebral palsy.

Cost is a factor. In 1976 it cost an estimated $15,000 to equip one neonatal intensive care unit (NICU) bed, not including nurse and physician costs. Most infants cared for in the NICU require extended hospitalization. The allocation of money for NICU beds diverts funds from other purposes. More attention is focused on the technology available for treating prematurity than on research to find ways to prevent premature birth. Parents must deal with the high cost of neonatal intensive care as well as the disruption in their lives and the difficulty they may have being able to relate to the infant after being separated from him both by his stay in the NICU and by the tubes and devices that come between them. Parents who do not get an opportunity to bond with their infants are at a higher risk for becoming abusive parents.

The decision to treat or not to treat handicapped or very small infants causes many problems for families, nurses, and physicians in the NICU. Many complex ethical issues go into that decision, including the quality of life for the child, the economic and psychological cost of care, and the obligation to obey the law. Choosing death is viewed as an act of love by some families (27). Some parents who are aware of the prognosis may have the deep religious conviction that they should allow the child to die, but they sense staff bias and feeling and may keep their opinions to themselves (1). Health professionals are often more comfortable with aggressive treatment and seek genuine satisfaction in lowering morbidity and mortality. They may also have difficulty keeping their personal biases out of their counseling, and this may inadvertently affect parental responses. In many instances it is difficult to predict the quality of life that the child may have, and this makes the decision even more agonizing.

There is also concern that parents are receiving the information about their child's complex condition when they are greatly stressed. They may have insufficient information to know what is in the child's best interest. It is difficult for professionals to decide how much discretion to give to the parents because of this. One study reported that parents who participated in the decision to withdraw medical care from their infants did not experience more grief than those who did not participate in such a decision (8).

Under current laws it is probable that parents, physicians, and nurses who are involved in decisions to withhold treatment are at risk for civil and criminal liability (2). It is unlikely, however, that health professionals acting in good faith would be held liable for providing urgent medical care to an infant without a parent's consent (22).

Recommendations for Research

Providing care for the chronically ill child and family is an extremely demanding task for the nurse. Families need someone to coordinate the multitude of health services required and to promote and support self-care activities over time. The nurse's ultimate goals for the family are the stimulation of normal growth and development and the achievement of maximum family functioning under the stresses inherent in learning to live with a chronic disease.

Nurses need to engage in and support research efforts that will generate new knowledge related to ways of accomplishing their primary goals and contribute to a better understanding of chronic illness in children. One area that needs to be studied is the effect of a child's chronic illness on the father and other siblings in the family. This is beginning to be studied, but more knowledge is needed to help nurses work more effectively with the entire family. The effect of multiple hospitalizations on the child's growth and development is also of concern, as are ways that the nurse can intervene to lessen the stress of hospitalization for children who are repeatedly hospitalized. The effects of early intervention on

the child with cerebral palsy have been studied, but there is a need to document the specific contribution of nursing intervention.

DISCUSSION QUESTIONS

1. You are a primary nurse who has just taken responsibility for a family with a preschool child who has cerebral palsy. What potential nursing problems does the child have? What potential nursing problems does the family have? Consider your own strengths and weaknesses as a primary nurse in relating to a child with cerebral palsy and his family. What problems within yourself might require work on your part?

2. You are the primary nurse caring for a five-year-old child with moderately severe asthma. You are planning your teaching and counseling for the child and parents as they relate to the impact of asthma on the developmental needs of the child. What areas of content would you include for the child? What would you include for the parents?

3. When you are visiting the mother of a chronically ill child, the mother tells you that her eight-year-old child (the older brother of the ill child) has been acting out in school. What is an appropriate response to this bit of information? What nursing intervention might you use immediately? What nursing intervention might you plan on an ongoing basis for this family?

REFERENCES

1. "A Children's Physician: Non-treatment of Defective Newborn Babies." *Lancet* 2:1123, 1979.
2. Benfield, D. C., et al. "Grief Responses of Parents to Neonatal Death and Parent Participation in Deciding Care." *Pediatrics* 67:315–20, March 1981.
3. Breslau, N., et al. "Psychological Distress in Mothers of Disabled Children." *American Journal of Diseases of Children* 136:682–86, August 1982.
4. Buckley, R. "Advances in Asthma and Allergy." *Pediatric Nursing* 5:39–41, 1979.
5. Coughlin, M. K. "Teaching Children About Their Seizures and Medications." *American Journal of Maternal Child Nursing* 4:161–62, 1979.
6. Craft, M. J. "Help for the Family's Neglected Other Child." *American Journal of Maternal Child Nursing* 4:297–300, September–October 1979.
7. Denhoff, E. "Cerebral Palsy 1982: The State of the Art." *New York Medical Quarterly* 3:146–52, 1982.

8. Duff, F. "Counseling Families and Deciding Care of Severely Defective Children: A Way of Coping with Medical Vietnam." *Pediatrics* 67:315–20, March 1981.

9. Gruskay, F. L. "Comparison of Breast, Cow, and Soy Feedings in the Prevention of the Onset of Allergic Disease: A Fifteen-Year Prospective Study." *Clinical Pediatrics* 2:486–91, August 1982.

10. Hughes, M. "Chronically Ill Children in Groups: Recurrent Issues and Adaptations." *American Journal of Orthopsychiatry* 52:704–11, October 1982.

11. Jackson, P. L. "Chronic Grief." *American Journal of Nursing* 74:1289–90, July 1974.

12. Jelneck, L. J. "The Special Needs of the Adolescent with Chronic Illness." *American Journal of Maternal Child Nursing* 2:57–61, 1977.

13. Leffert, F. "Asthma: A Modern Perspective." *Pediatrics* 62:1061–69, December 1978.

14. McKeever, P. T. "Fathering the Chronically Ill Child." *American Journal of Maternal Child Nursing* 6:124–28, 1981.

15. Malseed, R. T. *Pharmacology: Drug Therapy and Nursing Considerations.* Philadelphia: J. B. Lippincott, 1982.

16. Mattson, A. "Long-term Physical Illness in Childhood: A Challenge to Psychosocial Adaptation." *Pediatrics* 50:801–11, November 1972.

17. Oehler, J. *Family Centered Nursing Care.* Philadelphia: J. B. Lippincott, 1981.

18. Olshansky, S. "Chronic Sorrow: A Response to Having a Mentally Defective Child." *Social Casework* 43:191–92, 1962.

19. Orem, D. *Nursing Concepts of Practice.* 3d edition. New York: McGraw-Hill, 1985.

20. Paneth, N., et al. "Cerebral Palsy and Newborn Care. III. Estimated Prevalence Rates of Cerebral Palsy Under Differing Rates of Mortality and Impairment of Low Birth Weight Infants." *Developmental Medicine and Child Neurology* 23:801–6, December 1981.

21. Pi, E. "Congenitally Handicapped Children and Their Families—Long- and Short-term Intervention." *Pediatric Basics* 31:10–14.

22. Robertson, J. A. "Passive Euthanasia of Defective Newborns: Legal Considerations." *Journal of Pediatrics* 88:883, 1976.

23. Section on Allergy and Immunology. "Management of Asthma." *Pediatrics* 68:874–79, December 1981.

24. Sedlack, K. "Helping the Asthmatic Child in School." *American Journal of Maternal Child Nursing* 3:207–10, July–August 1978.

25. Solnit, A., and M. Stark. "Mourning and the Birth of a Defective Child." *Psychoanalytic Study of the Child* 16:523–26, June 1962.

26. Steele, S. *Health Promotion of the Child with Long-Term Illness.* 3d edition. East Norwalk, Ct.: Appleton-Century-Crofts, 1983.

27. Steinfels, M. O. "New Childbirth Technology: A Clash of Values." *Hastings Center Report* 8:9–12, 1978.

28. Teplin, S. W., et al. "Self Concept of a Young Child with Cerebral Palsy." *Developmental Medicine and Child Neurology* 23:730–38, 1981.

29. Weiczorek, R. R., and B. Rossner. "The Asthmatic Child: Preventing and Controlling Attacks." *American Journal of Nursing* 79:258–62, February 1979.

Sudden Infant Death Syndrome

THERESA McCOY CLIFFORD

■

OBJECTIVES

After completing this chapter, the reader will be able to:

- Define sudden infant death syndrome.
- List the epidemiological factors of sudden infant death syndrome.
- Describe how crisis intervention theory and techniques can be applied to parents and siblings who have experienced the sudden death of their infant.
- List the self-care needs of families who have been affected by sudden infant death syndrome and identify appropriate primary nursing intervention.

Sudden infant death syndrome (SIDS) describes the sudden and unexpected death of apparently healthy babies. This diagnosis is arrived at by exclusion, meaning that no other cause of death is found during a thorough autopsy.

Etiological Theories

The exact cause of SIDS is unknown. Many theories have been proposed, but none have been substantiated. For thousands of years the death of an infant who died suddenly and unexpectedly was attributed to a mother or a wet-nurse rolling over on the infant during sleep. This was exemplified in 1 Kings 3: 19-20: "Then one night she accidentally rolled over on her baby and smothered it. She got up during the night, took my son from my side while I was asleep, and carried him to her bed; then she put the dead child in my bed" (6). Other forms of suffocation, such as that from obstruction owing to an enlarged thymus (11), from bedclothes (29), or by burying the face into the mattress, have been reported but have since been discounted.

Another theory suggests that infection may be a causative factor. Approximately 5 percent of cases of sudden infant death may be due to infant botulism (3).

Schwartz (18) proposed that an inherited prolonged Q-T interval resulted in cardiac irregularities and cardiac arrest, but this was refuted by Steinschneider (21).

Other possible explanations such as choking, child abuse, and allergy have been disproved on autopsy.

Researchers continue to pursue the cause of SIDS. To date, prolonged apneic episodes or idiopathic protracted apnea is the strongest theory in the literature. Steinschneider, in 1972, was the first person to conduct research on the apnea hypothesis (20). During his monitoring of five infants for recurrent apneic episodes, two died suddenly and without reason. All five infants experienced both brief and prolonged apneic episodes. From this he hypothesized that prolonged apnea, especially related to sleep, may be the main pathophysiological mechanism in some cases of SIDS.

Sleep Apnea

All infants have irregular breathing patterns that include short periods of apnea. Three types of sleep apnea are described by Guilleminault and co-workers (7):

1. Upper airway or obstructive apnea, in which the chest and diaphragm move but no air moves in or out of the nose. This causes greater oxygen desaturation and earlier and severer cardiac changes (e.g., bradycardia) than central or diaphragmatic apnea.
2. Central or diaphragmatic apnea, in which chest movement stops.
3. Mixed central and obstructive apnea. Bradycardia and oxygen desaturation are also associated with this type.

In the first few months of life, infants are obligate nose breathers. Therefore, if they have nasal obstruction (23) from congestion or some other cause, this could lead to respiratory distress or obstructive apnea, which produces the greatest and the most dangerous physiological changes, as noted above. Researchers are currently studying anatomical reasons for obstructive apnea, such as oropharyngeal occlusion by the tongue (19, 25), closure of the glottis owing to stimulation of the superior laryngeal nerve (22), and gastroesophageal reflux that may cause upper airway obstruction (9).

Since the cause of SIDS is unknown, it cannot be prevented. Prolonged sleep apnea is the most prominent hypothesis in the literature and continues to be investigated.

Incidence and Risk Factors

Sudden infant death syndrome is a significant health problem that warrants attention. Each year in the United States approximately 7,000 infants die of SIDS (15). The age range is between one month and one year (15), peaking between two and four months.

Epidemiological studies (26) have revealed the following data:

- Sixty percent of SIDS deaths occur in males.
- Peak incidence is between two and four months of age.
- There is no relationship with position in the family.
- Incidence is higher in multiple births; high in twins; higher in triplets.
- Incidence is high with subsequent siblings.
- Risk increases in low-birth-weight infants and premature infants.
- It occurs more often between midnight and nine o'clock in the morning than at other hours.
- It occurs more during winter months.
- It crosses all socioeconomic groups, but it is more prevalent in families with poor social conditions.
- There is no relationship to breast- versus bottle-feeding.

These epidemiological factors are associated with SIDS, but it cannot be said that all premature infants, or all twins, or all small-for-gestational-age babies will have prolonged sleep apnea and subsequently succumb to SIDS.

Nursing Care Related to SIDS

Primary nursing is based on the concept of a single nurse having total responsibility and accountability for each client. The primary nurse is responsible for assessing the client's needs; for planning, implementing, and evaluating his nursing care; and for collaborating with the other disciplines that are caring for the client. The primary nurse will not necessarily give all the care she plans for each client, but will delegate duties to other trained care givers as indicated. She is responsible for seeing that the care plan is followed by others providing the care (13). The primary nurse is accountable for her plans and actions. In the nursing care plan the primary nurse sets priorities of assessment and intervention in relation to prevention, treatment, and rehabilitation.

Primary Prevention

"Primary prevention on a community basis has the goal of reducing the incidence and prevalence of diseases in the population" (8) by helping people to maintain their health. According to Parad (16), the goal of primary

prevention is to promote an active state of positive health and to prevent problems before they develop. This can be accomplished by promoting health education, assuring adequate nutrition and housing, and so on.

In relation to primary prevention of SIDS, health education in the community is important, especially for women of childbearing age, including adolescents. The program should include the following:

- Importance of early prenatal care
- Good, adequate nutrition
- No smoking, alcohol, or drugs
- Proper personal hygiene
- Exercise
- Rest
- Early signs of complications
- Reproductive changes and signs of labor
- Childbirth education
- Care of newborn

Education to promote prenatal health is important because many victims of SIDS were premature or small for gestational age at birth. Pregnant adolescents and women with multiple births have a high rate of delivering infants with these risk factors. It is hoped that primary nurses can reduce these risk factors through education, which will lower the rate of SIDS.

Proper, uncrowded housing is another important area of primary prevention for SIDS. Victims of SIDS usually have a mild upper respiratory tract infection (4, 26), which might be prevented with adequate housing and subsequent reduction in the spread of infectious disease. Some specific housing factors that need to be addressed by the primary nurse are adequate heat and hot water, proper ventilation, number of persons per room, and presence of pests and rodents. Referrals may need to be made.

A controversial issue faced by primary nurses is whether or not to discuss SIDS in prenatal education. Some nurses believe that since it cannot be prevented, it should not be discussed unless prospective parents introduce the topic. Other nurses think that the subject should be included because parents ought to be aware of the risk factors as an incentive to comply with their own prenatal care. Previous knowledge of the disease might also reduce the immediate guilt and misinformation that is common when a SIDS death occurs. Each primary nurse must make her own decision regarding the inclusion of this topic in prenatal education based on current information and her own principles and ethics of practice.

Secondary Prevention

Secondary prevention is the early diagnosis and prompt treatment of a problem, disorder, or disease in order to reduce mortality and prevent complications. It includes individual and mass case finding, screening surveys, and selective examinations of the population at risk (8). It can also include voluntary submission to screening tests and examinations of selected primary prevention clients.

Currently, there are no reliable screening tests for identifying infants who will succumb to SIDS. Studies (12) done regarding risk factors showed a high false-positive rate (90 percent to 99.16 percent) and low sensitivity (18 percent to 50 percent). Therefore, the presence of risk factors alone cannot predict occurrence with any degree of certainty.

Although the cause of SIDS is unknown, some infants are at higher risk than others. A primary nurse must take a careful history, including prenatal, natal, and postnatal care, problems, and complications; history of apnea in the infant or siblings; identification of risk factors that may be present; and family history of SIDS.

Infants at Risk. Infants at risk include babies with infantile apnea ("near-miss" SIDS), subsequent siblings of SIDS infants, and premature infants with recurrent apnea unresponsive to theophylline therapy (17). What can be done for these infants? A complete evaluation of the infant at risk includes pneumography, which records heart rate and respiration during twelve hours of sleep; electrocardiography; electroencephalography; SMA6; and SMA12; and measurement of arterial blood gases. If there is indication of regurgitation, vomiting, choking, or difficulty breathing, a barium swallow should be performed to rule out gastroesophageal reflux (17).

Home Apnea Monitoring. Candidates for home apnea monitors include all babies with infantile apnea ("near-miss" SIDS), subsequent siblings who have an abnormal pneumogram, and premature infants with recurrent apnea unresponsive to theophylline (17).

Reisinger considers home apnea monitoring secondary prevention because it signals a prolonged apneic episode necessitating prompt intervention of mouth-to-mouth resuscitation (artificial respiration) or cardiopulmonary resuscitation, which will, it is hoped, prevent the infant's death.

Apnea monitoring at home is a controversial issue. Professionals and parents who are in favor of apnea monitoring think that now there are fewer technical problems than previously and that more devices are available. Parents may feel more relaxed having the monitor because when the alarm is activated after twenty seconds of apnea, they can immediately start mouth-to-mouth resuscitation. Apnea home monitoring cannot prevent SIDS, but it can be used in the management of infants who are at risk.

The Academy of Pediatrics does not currently endorse apnea monitoring at home. They and other professionals believe that the devices are too expensive and give off too many false alarms. Also, the alarms may not be heard over ordinary household noises, monitoring may increase the parents' anxiety level, parents must organize their lives around the monitoring, and parents may not be able to successfully resuscitate their infant.

Because each infant and family unit is different, apnea monitoring management should be considered on an individual basis.

Grieving Families. Early identification of a grieving family in the emergency room is another form of secondary prevention in SIDS. Immediate, brief, preventive intervention is vital for the mental health of a family who experiences such a sudden loss. The primary nurse can serve as the communicator between the infant and the family. Some parents prefer to stay in the waiting room while the emergency room staff tries to revive the infant. The primary nurse, in this situation, would communicate all that was being done for the infant. Some parents want to see what is being done for their infant. In this situation the primary care nurse should be assertive in meeting the parents' needs and allowing them to be present in the examination room. This calls for collaboration with the other health professionals involved in the case. The parents need someone who is assertive and authoritative, acts as their advocate, and communicates with them. These are important characteristics in the primary care nurse.

The parents need direct and simple communication. For example, "Is there someone I can call for you?" They need the primary care nurse, a familiar person, to be there when the physician gives the announcement of death. Because the primary care nurse has been providing continuity of care to this family, she should ask the family members if they would like to say good-bye and hold their infant. She should allow the family to cry, scream, express their feelings.

The infant had been part of that family for a short time, but it had been an integral part. Each parent and each sibling had a unique relationship with the infant. Because the family is a continuously interacting system, each relationship, mother-father, mother-infant, father-infant, sibling-infant, mother-sibling, father-sibling, influences the family as a whole. The entire family will need help to separate from the infant and face the reality that he or she is not going home.

Because the primary care nurse usually establishes a relationship with the family, it is important for her to be present if explanation about an autopsy is given. Autopsies, when done, are under the jurisdiction of the medical examiner. (In New York City, autopsies are performed on all cases of SIDS.) If an autopsy is required, identification of the infant's body must be made by a parent or someone who knows the infant. It is important to explain to the parents that the body is not mutilated. An autopsy is a respectful, surgical procedure to determine the cause of death.

Tertiary Prevention

In tertiary prevention the goal is to reduce the number of disabilities in the population at risk (8). With SIDS this can be done through adequate crisis intervention of the grieving family and the identification of the need for intensive individual or family therapy. It is of vital importance that the primary care nurse know her own limitations with crisis intervention and when to make a proper referral to a more experienced health professional. For further information about grief and crisis intervention, refer to chapter 17 and chapter 16.

Table 27.1 summarizes SIDS and the three levels of prevention.

Nursing Care Related to Treatment and SIDS

The following is a typical scenario of the discovery of a victim of SIDS.

A three-month-old infant is taken to the pediatrician for a well-child visit. The infant appears healthy except for a slight cold. The doctor prescribes normal saline nose drops four times a day as needed. The baby does fine the rest of the day. At 11:00 P.M. he is breast-fed, burped well, held by his father, and placed in his bassinet on his stomach with his head turned toward the right side. At 6:00 A.M. his parents wake up. The infant slept through his 4:00 A.M. feeding without making a sound. The infant is discovered with his face turned toward the left side; he is not breathing and he feels

Table 27.1
Prevention of Sudden Infant Death Syndrome

Level of Prevention	Assessment	Intervention
Primary	Identify community need for education—prepregnancy and prenatal	Educational program in schools, hospitals, and clinics; short segments on television and radio
Secondary	Need for reliable screening tests; early identification of infants at risk through history and evaluation; early identification of grieving family in emergency room	More research on SIDS; diagnostic studies (pneumogram, EKG, EEG, electrolytes, blood gases); home apnea monitoring; immediate crisis intervention; home visits; counseling; work with siblings
Tertiary	Identify need for further rehabilitation in the population at risk	Long-term individual or family therapy in ambulatory setting or in hospital

cool. The mother grabs the infant and tries mouth-to-mouth resuscitation; the father calls for an ambulance.

How would you, as primary care nurse, deal with this situation when the family arrives at the emergency room?

To deal with this family effectively, the primary care nurse must organize her thinking and set priorities.

I. Initial Assessment
   A. Triaged as a priority case needing life-support intervention until death is determined.
   B. Subjective data obtained through a thorough history
      1. What happened? Who found the infant? What did he or she do? Time of discovery? Where was the baby found? In what position was he found? Who last saw the infant alive? What time?
      2. Description of the events preceding the discovery of the infant. Anything unusual that day? Illness? Any medication given? Was in-

fant well and healthy when put to bed?
When did the baby eat last? What did he
eat?

   3. Who is providing the information? Does the
story seem consistent with what you observe?

C. After the initial shock of the infant's death,
gather more pertinent history.
   1. History of apnea
   2. History of past illnesses, hospitalizations,
allergies, immunizations
   3. History of upper respiratory tract infection
   4. History of SIDS in family
   5. Prenatal, natal, postnatal history
   6. Feeding, sleep, developmental history

D. History should be obtained in a nonjudgmental
manner.

II. Physical Assessment

A. The examiner needs to differentiate between
SIDS and child abuse or neglect.

B. Objective data obtained through inspection,
auscultation, palpation, and percussion of the
infant
   1. Inspection
     a. Does the infant appear to be well devel-
oped?
     b. Is the child small for age?
     c. Does the child appear malnourished?
     d. Are there visible signs of injury, e.g.,
burns, lacerations, scars, head trauma,
swelling, bruises, fractures?
     e. What is the infant's overall appearance?
If infant is found face down, there may
be pallor from the pressure. Some areas
of body may appear bruised from the
pooling of blood. Is the infant cool to
touch? Is there any drainage from nose
or mouth?
   2. Auscultation
     a. Is there a heartbeat?
     b. Are there respirations?
   3. Palpation may be difficult if rigor mortis has
set in (approximately three hours after
death).
     a. Are there any masses? Organomegaly?
Fractures? Lesions?
   4. Percussion may also be difficult.

C. The examiner must remain objective at all
times. There should be no blaming of parents.
They should be given every benefit of the doubt
until all facts are in, including autopsy results.

III. Impression of Given Scenario Is SIDS

IV. Plan

A. Immediate crisis intervention in emergency
room
   1. This is vital in working with the family. At
this time the family is in great emotional turmoil after losing their infant. They are unable to problem solve as they did before the
crisis.
   2. The ultimate goal of this immediate crisis
intervention is to provide a climate with
open channels of communication so that the
family can use its own resources and reach
out to support systems in the community.
This will enable them to start to deal with
their own grief and the grief of their other
children for the deceased infant.

B. Steps in crisis intervention (1)
   1. Assessment
     a. Elicit how family coped in the past with
death. Who can help with the other children? Who can you call for them? Who
can they talk to—one another, members
of the clergy, someone else?
   2. Plan intervention
     a. Parents are usually in shock, and may
use denial and disbelief to cope with their
loss. They may not hear a word anyone
says to them. By being present with them
and assisting with communication between the family and the other professionals the primary care nurse can communicate to the family that she is
someone who cares; caring is the essence
of nursing.
     b. Allowing them to cry, scream, with-
draw—however they express their feelings—is important. This means that you
accept them as they are. This requires
open communication. The primary care
nurse may not express her feelings in the
same manner as the family, but there is
acceptance that each person is different.
This is the beginning of trust in the relationship.
     c. Be direct, realistic, and goal-oriented,
and assist them in immediate problem
solving. They may need help in understanding why an autopsy must be performed, in order for them to sign the

consent. The rights of the parents and the deceased infant should be protected by the primary care nurse at all times.

3. Intervention
   a. Implement the plans above.
   b. A grieving family may need to be told, "It is O.K. to cry and express how you feel."
4. Evaluation and anticipatory planning
   a. Continued crisis intervention for four to six weeks
   b. Home visits by the primary care nurse or the public health nurse (referral)
      1) Assess how family members are resolving their grief and their knowledge of the entire event.
      2) Reexplanations may be needed; they may start to hear you now.
      3) You may have to deal with anger and hostility toward health providers. "The pediatrician said he was fine. He let him die. You doctors and nurses don't know anything," etc.
      4) Be a good listener. Listen for guilt and self-blame.
      5) The first home visit should be soon after the infant's death. The next day is best. If this is not possible, a visit should be made within one to two weeks.
      6) Cliches like "things will be fine," "soon you'll be back to normal," "you'll get over it" should be avoided. The pain of the loss will always be present; it is hoped that it will be less intense for each member of the family as they work out their grief. Grief work is a gradual process. The family has accomplished a great deal when they can talk about their memories and about the baby's death.
   c. Importance of sibling counseling
      1) If the parents want to protect their children from the pain and are unable to discuss the infant's death with their children, then the primary care nurse must do the counseling or make a proper referral.
      2) How the child views death depends on his developmental stage.
         a) Infancy and early preschool to age

three—most children are unable to comprehend death. The child is present-oriented. Parents need to give love and attention at this age.
         b) Preschool, between ages three and five—death is temporary, reversible; it happens on television but it will never happen to them or anyone they know.
         c) Latency, between ages five and nine—death is final; all living things will die except for themselves. As with their superheroes, they will also escape death. They may have nightmares.
         d) Preadolescence and older, from approximately age ten and on—death is final, irreversible; all living things will die, including themselves (28).
      3) How to tell a child about death depends on the child's developmental level.
         a) Infancy to early preschool to age three—he will not understand any explanation of death. Give reassurance, love, attention. Do familiar things with him.
         b) Preschool, between ages three and five—he needs attention and interest in him. He knows something is wrong, but he is still egocentric.
         c) Early latency, between ages five and seven—he may be able to understand the idea of death but may think that his sibling will return.
            CHILD: Is brother still in the hospital?
            NURSE OR PARENT: No, brother died.
            CHILD: Why did he die?
            NURSE OR PARENT: We don't know why he died. (*To allay guilt feelings*) You didn't do anything to make brother die. Mommy didn't do anything to make brother die. Daddy didn't do anything to make brother die. Sometimes people die and we

just don't know why. We are very sad that brother died. We will miss him very much.

d) Preadolescence, ages eight to twelve—answer the child's questions honestly and directly. He will understand that his sibling is not coming back.

e) Adolescence, age thirteen to adulthood—the adolescent may ask some peculiar questions about death because he is working through many conflicts within himself. He is in search of self and of life (10).

4) Give honest, simple answers at all developmental levels. The description above is a guideline of children's understanding of death. Some children comprehend at an earlier age and some at a later age.

5) Avoid answers like "Brother died in his sleep." The sibling may think, "If I go to sleep, I, too, will die" (30). If no one talks to the child, he will fantasize that it was something he did, said, or thought that caused his brother's death. He will be burdened with a great deal of guilt.

6) As children understand death, it will help to include them in the funeral process for working out their grief. If a child does not want to participate, do *not* force him; he needs more time to mourn.

7) Sometimes children will act out, break toys of the dead infant, or hoard all his toys and not let anyone touch them. The younger sibling is keeping them until his brother returns to play with them. Some children hold onto the toys because they don't want to let go of their sibling's memory.

8) When the child can talk about things that the infant did, e.g., when he laughed and talked to him, when he cried all night long, and can look at pictures of the infant, then he is working through his grief of the loss of his brother or sister.

9) In helping children to understand and cope with death, remember four key concepts: (a) be loving, (b) be accepting, (c) be truthful, and (d) be consistent (30).

d. Marital counseling is necessary.

1) There is a breakdown in communication between the parents.

2) Talking about the death is too upsetting; therefore, there is no discussion.

3) Father remains stoic and hard to the death; he feels the pain but does not show it; he goes away from the home, increases his work load or other activities.

4) Mother cries often, feels empty inside, talks frequently about the baby, sometimes as if the infant were alive.

5) Both parents need to be involved in the local SIDS chapter.

6) Father needs to be involved in the grieving process.

7) Subsequent children (24)

a) Parents face the question "Should we have another child?"

b) A subsequent child will not be able to replace the infant that died. Each child is unique and his own person (5).

c) Parents need to accept the loss of their infant; having another infant immediately will not speed up the mourning process.

d) Review two important facts:
i. SIDS cannot be predicted or prevented.
ii. SIDS is not hereditary (24).

e) Some couples have difficulty with sexual activity; counseling about this is important.

f) Some women have spontaneous abortions with the next pregnancy; they now have to grieve the loss of an unborn child. The primary nurse needs to make appropriate referral if abnormal grief and depression occur.

g) Some couples want another child but do not want to take the chance of a recurrence of SIDS.

They may choose foster care or adoption as an alternative. Remember, there is no guarantee that these children will not succumb to SIDS.

h) When a mother becomes pregnant, she must keep open communication with the primary care nurse and the obstetrician regarding *all* her questions and fears.

i) When the baby arrives home, the mother must keep open communication with the primary nurse and the pediatrician regarding questions and concerns.

j) Parents need to be reminded that infancy is an important time for them and the infant. They need to enjoy observing their child's growth and development.

k) Parents need to have their self-confidence built up in order to avoid overprotection of all their children.

l) The issue of apnea monitoring must be discussed, pros and cons presented, and a decision made for its use with their subsequent child.

e. Prompt and proper referral can mean the difference between mental health and mental illness for some parents (27).

When dealing with a family experiencing SIDS, other nursing concepts for intervention must not be overlooked, for example, locus of control, which deals with how a person interprets the cause and effect of behavioral outcomes or reinforcements. A person who believes that what happens to him is primarily due to his own actions is said to have an internal locus of control. A person who believes that what happens to him is primarily due to outside forces, luck, chance, or powerful others, or is unpredictable because of the complexity of the situation, is said to have an external locus of control (2).

With the intervention of a family experiencing SIDS, it is important to identify the locus of control because it will direct the nature of the nursing intervention.

Orem (14) states that "self-care is the practice of activities that individuals personally initiate and perform on their own behalf in maintaining life, health, and

Table 27.2
Orem's Three Basic Nursing Systems Applied to SIDS Families

1. Wholly compensatory nursing system	Family is devastated by the loss of the infant; cannot make any decisions on their own.
2. Partly compensatory nursing system	As the family members move along with crisis intervention, they have less need for the nurse. They are able to make some decisions on their own. They are learning ways to cope with their loss, since they have had no experience with the death of an infant.
3. Supportive-educative nursing system	a. Support given through home visits b. Guidance in assisting parents in telling children of the death of their sibling c. Opportunities provided for all family members to interact and discuss the loss of their infant, sibling. d. Teaching done when necessary after assessing the family's need and past experiences. These four items assisted the family to regain their effectiveness as self-care agents. The nurse became a consultant. The family became self-sufficient.

well-being." Self-care is a requirement of every person, including children. If self-care is not maintained, illness, disease, or death may result.

People who are in need of nursing are those with deficiencies in their current or projected capability for providing self-care or dependent care in relation to the qualitative and quantitative demand for care (14). Families experiencing SIDS may be in need of nursing because they have deficit relationships between the projected ability to perform daily activities on their own behalf and their demand for care because of immobilization after the sudden death of their infant.

Orem (14) describes three basic nursing systems (Table 27.2):

1. In the wholly compensatory nursing system the nurse compensates for a client's total inability to perform self-care.
2. In the partly compensatory nursing system the nurse compensates for some of the client's self-care, since the client can perform some self-care actions.
3. In the supportive-educative nursing system the nurse ultimately acts as a consultant, since the client is self-sufficient.

Nursing Care Related to Rehabilitation

The main focus of the primary care nurse as far as rehabilitation of families experiencing SIDS is to promote individual functioning at the same or a higher level as before the death.

As far as social welfare is concerned, the primary nurse must assess the family's basic needs. If the family is not worrying about food, clothing, and shelter, then they can work on the task at hand—the successful completion of the mourning process.

Knowledge of community resources with regard to SIDS is vital for these families (see Table 27.3). This helps with their reaching out to the community for additional support systems.

Table 27.3
Community Resources for Sudden Infant Death Syndrome

Resource	Purpose
National Sudden Infant Death Syndrome Foundation 2 Metro Plaza, Suite 205 82 Professional Place Landover, MD 20785 (Check telephone directory for local chapters.)	Helps parents and other family members cope with the loss of an infant to SIDS through counseling, parent support groups, home visits, education; provides education and literature to the community; promotes research in SIDS
Council of Guilds for Infant Survival P.O. Box 3841 Davenport, IA 52808 (Check telephone directory for local guilds or state SIDS Information Counseling Project.)	Consoles families experiencing SIDS by telephone, letter, and home visits; provides the community with information; promotes research.
Sudden Infant Death Syndrome Clearinghouse 1555 Wilson Blvd., Suite 600 Rosslyn, VA 22209 (703-522-0870, ext. 279) Federal SIDS program	Provides information.

DISCUSSION QUESTIONS

1. How would you apply crisis intervention theory and techniques to parents experiencing the sudden death of their infant?
2. How would you apply crisis intervention theory and techniques to siblings experiencing the sudden death of their brother or sister?
3. What are the steps of the grieving process?
4. How does one distinguish between SIDS and child abuse or neglect?
5. Discuss the attitudes of professionals (including yourself) toward child abuse and SIDS. Think about appropriate questions to ask when interviewing a family to determine whether an unexpected infant death is child abuse or SIDS.
6. What factors related to attitudes, beliefs, habits, culture, and socioeconomic and educational levels may or may not influence your approaches to management and intervention of SIDS?
7. Think about your own beliefs and attitudes toward SIDS and how they may assist or be detrimental in working with the families experiencing SIDS.
8. Discuss the attitudes of professionals (including yourself) toward the dying and death of an infant or child.
9. How do you feel about the death of an infant or child as compared with the death of an adult?
10. Do you feel any difference when death is expected as opposed to unexpected?
11. How do you feel about discussing death with a child? At what age is it appropriate? How does one explain SIDS to a sibling?
12. Think about the concept of the "bad" mother who allowed her infant to die. Think about the amount of guilt associated with SIDS.
13. Today, with the increased number of working women, there is an increased use of infant day-care centers. Think about the amount of guilt experienced by the day-care worker involved with SIDS.

Think about the blaming of this person by the parents. Can SIDS also happen in a hospital?

14. Discuss the parental relationship problems resulting from SIDS. What kinds of interventions could be used? Do people grieve similarly?

15. What channels and methods of communication and teaching-learning process will you use with families and referral agencies involved with SIDS?

16. How would you plan for follow-up on referrals?

17. Discuss the latest research in the field of SIDS, including the controversial issue of home apnea monitoring.

18. What are some of the stresses to the family who is monitoring an infant at home?

19. Discuss the effects of apnea monitoring on parental attachment.

20. How would a toddler react to the stresses of the monitoring? How would an adolescent react to the stresses of the monitoring?

21. Do you feel that parents and siblings could benefit from seeing and holding the infant after death?

REFERENCES

1. Aguilera, D., and J. Messick. *Crisis Intervention: Theory and Methodology.* 4th ed. St. Louis: C. V. Mosby, 1982.

2. Arakelian, M. "An Assessment and Nursing Application of the Concept of Locus of Control." *Advances in Nursing Science* 3:25, 1980.

3. Arnon, S. S., et al. "Intestinal Infection and Toxin Production by *Clostridium Botulinum* as One Cause of Sudden Infant Death Syndrome." *Lancet* 1:1273, 1978.

4. Beckwith, J. *The Sudden Infant Death Syndrome.* Rockville, Md.: U.S. Dept. of Health, Education and Welfare, 1978.

5. Cain, A. C., and B. S. Cain. "On Replacing a Child." *Journal of the American Academy of Child Psychiatry* 3:443, 1964.

6. *Good News Bible with Deuterocanonicals/Apocrypha: The Bible in Today's English Version.* New York: American Bible Society, 1978.

7. Guilleminault, C., et al. "Apnea During Sleep in Infants: Possible Relationships with Sudden Infant Death Syndrome." *Science* 190:677, 1975.

8. Helvie, C. *Community Health Nursing, Theory and Process.* Philadelphia: J. B. Lippincott, 1981.

9. Herbst, J., et al. "Gastroesophageal Reflux in the 'Near-Miss' Sudden Infant Death Syndrome." *Journal of Pediatrics* 92:73, 1978.

10. Jackson, E. *Telling a Child About Death.* New York: Hawthorne Books, 1965.

11. Lee, C. A. "On the Thymus Gland, Its Morbid Affections and the Diseases That Arise from its Abnormal Enlargement." *American Journal of Medical Science* 3:135, 1842.

12. Lewak, N., et al. "Sudden Infant Death Syndrome. Risk Factors: Prospective Data Reviewed." *Clinical Pediatrics* 18:404, 1979.

13. Mundinger, M. "Primary Nurse—Role Evolution." *Nursing Outlook* 21:642, 1973.

14. Orem, D. *Nursing: Concepts of Practice.* 2nd ed. New York: McGraw-Hill, 1980.

15. Pachon, P. *Fact Sheet: What Is SIDS?* Rosslyn, Va.: SIDS Clearinghouse.

16. Parad, H. "Preventative Casework: Problems and Implications." In *Crisis Intervention: Selected Readings,* ed. H. Parad. New York: Family Service Association of America, 1965. p. 287.

17. Reisinger, K. "Sudden Infant Death Syndrome: Review and Update." *Pediatric Basics* 27:7, 1980.

18. Schwartz, P. J. "Cardiac Sympathetic Innervation and the Sudden Infant Death Syndrome: A Possible Pathogenetic Link." *American Journal of Medicine* 60:167, 1976.

19. Stark, A., and B. Thach. "Mechanisms of Airway Obstruction Leading to Apnea in Newborn Infants." *Journal Pediatrics* 89:982, 1976.

20. Steinschneider, A. "Prolonged Apnea and the Sudden Infant Death Syndrome: Clinical and Laboratory Observations." *Pediatrics* 50:646, 1972.

21. Steinschneider, A. "Sudden Infant Death Syndrome and Prolongation of the QT Interval." *American Journal of Diseases of Childhood* 132:688, 1978.

22. Sutton, D., et al.: "Prolonged Apnea in Infant Monkeys Resulting from Stimulation of Superior Laryngeal Nerve." *Pediatrics* 61:519, 1978.

23. Swift, P., and J. Emery. "Clinical Observations on Response to Nasal Occlusion in Infancy." *Archives of Diseases of Childhood* 48:947, 1973.

24. Szybist, C. *The Subsequent Child.* New York: National Foundation for Sudden Infant Death Syndrome, 1973.

25. Tonkin, S. "Sudden Infant Death Syndrome: Hypothesis of Causation." *Pediatrics* 55:650, 1975.

26. Valdes–Dapena, M. "Sudden Infant Death Syndrome: A Review of the Medical Literature, 1974–1979." *Pediatrics* 66:597, 1980.

27. Wachowiak, K. "Sudden Infant Death Syndrome: What You Can Do to Help the Family." *RN* 46:49, February 1978.

28. Whaley, L. F., and D. L. Wong. *Nursing Care of Infants and Children.* St. Louis: C. V. Mosby, 1979.

29. Wooley, P. V. "Mechanical Suffocation During Infancy: A Comment on Its Relation to the Total Problem of Sudden Death." *Journal of Pediatrics* 26:572, 1945.

30. Woolsey, S. *Fact Sheet: The Grief of Children.* Rosslyn, Va.: National SIDS Clearinghouse, 1982.

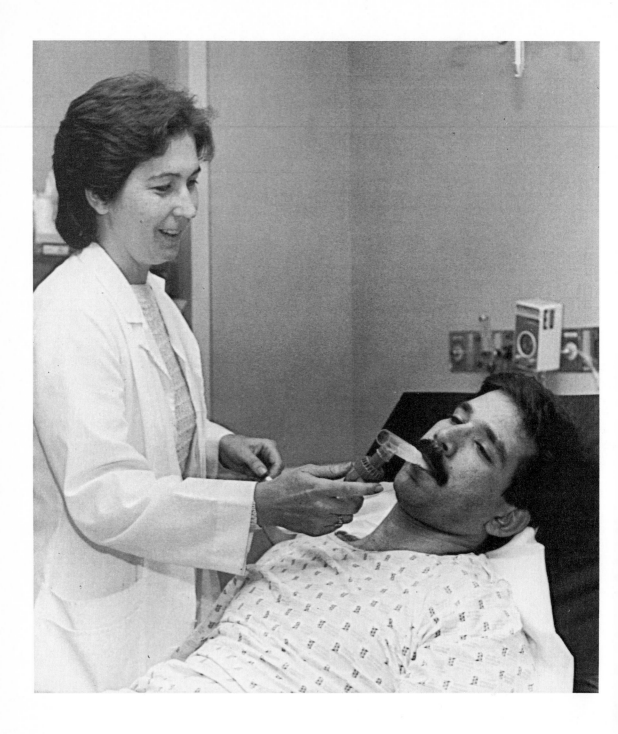

UNIT FIVE

Primary Practice with Young Adults and Adults in Middle Years

The development of the theme of primary nursing throughout the life cycle continues with chapters on problems common to young adults and adults in their middle years. Although the clinical problems chosen could occur in younger people (e.g., diabetes) or could be more prevalent in older people (e.g., coronary artery disease), they do represent major health problems that affect young and middle-aged adults.

The problems discussed in this unit were chosen because they illustrate the scope of primary nursing practice. None of them are simple. Each has the potential for affecting almost every aspect of a person's and family's life. Caring for these clients requires not only the ability to use the nursing process effectively in multiple settings but also a keen awareness of the various roles the nurse assumes in meeting their needs as well as those of their families.

CHAPTER 28

Caring for Adults with Sexually Transmitted Diseases

CLAUDETTE MOBLEY

■

OBJECTIVES

After completing this chapter, the reader will be able to:

☐ Describe the nature and extent of sexually transmitted disease (STD) as a community problem.

☐ Describe or identify the methods of control and treatment used in preventing the transmission of STD.

☐ Define the role of the nurse in primary practice in relation to STD prevention, detection, treatment, counseling, and education.

☐ Determine self-care responsibilities of clients, families, communities in relation to STD.

☐ Identify the legal and ethical issues involved in the prevention of STD.

The number of diseases that can be transmitted sexually is increasing. Once syphilis and gonorrhea were the primary venereal diseases; currently there are at least twenty diseases that can be transmitted through sexual contact. Although syphilis and gonorrhea remain the chief concern of public health officers, diseases like genital herpes and chlamydia are creating serious problems among the population, especially among those of child-bearing age.

This chapter examines the development of sexually transmitted disease (STD) as a major health problem, current treatment methods, and the role of the nurse as primary care giver, health educator, and patient care advocate.

The Magnitude of the Problem

A review of recent statistical information on the incidence of common STDs reveals the magnitude of the problem in the United States and makes clear the dimension of the need for intervention:

7.0 million new or recurrent episodes of genital herpes annually.
3.0 million infections due to chlamydia annually.
3.0 million trichomoniasis cases annually.
2.0 million gonorrhea cases annually.
0.5 million cases of venereal warts annually.
0.1 million new cases of syphilis annually (14)

Changing sexual patterns and increased resistance of organisms to antibiotics are two of the reasons for the statistical increase in the number of cases of STD, but numbers do not begin to relate the tragedy of infertility, damaged infants, psychological trauma, and loss of self-esteem that frequently accompany the diagnosis of STD.

More than half of the estimated 20 million STD victims in 1981 were under age twenty-five; almost one-fourth were victimized before they received their high school diplomas (14). These statistics could be sharply decreased if adequate sex education were provided at early ages. This is discussed in the section relating to community self-care.

In 1980 in New York City there were 10,447 *reported* cases of STD in young people under the age of twenty-one (16). Of that number more than 4,000 cases were found in the eighteen- to nineteen-year-old age-group (16). (The emphasis on *reported* cases indicates that despite the legal requirement to report syphilis and gonorrhea to the Health Department, many cases go unreported or undetected.) Some health care professionals are reluctant to report cases they treat because of the social stigma and embarrassment that might result for their clients.

Statistics themselves do not tell the entire story. In this last quarter of the twentieth century it is frightening that 10,000 young people under the age of twenty-one must confront the harsh reality of having diseases that could have been prevented. It is also frequently frightening to them to have to confront the attitudes of the health professionals who treat them.

Some victims of STD may be reluctant to seek treatment because they fear being categorized "promiscuous," "dirty," "perverted," or any of the other judgmental labels that sometimes are placed on affected people by those with differing value systems or those who do not understand the epidemiology of the disease. They avoid diagnosis and treatment, thereby risking systemic complications, in order to avoid confrontation and judgment. This can be acknowledged to be a non–self-caring behavior on the part of the STD victim, but it is exacerbated by a noncaring attitude on the part of the health care provider. The negative feelings thus generated will not help break the STD cycle; instead they will increase the extent of the community problem.

Overview of STD

There are at least twenty diseases that can currently be considered sexually transmitted. Among these are syphilis, gonorrhea, chancroid, lymphogranuloma venereum, granuloma inguinale, herpes simplex, condylomata acuminata, molluscum contagiosum, pediculosis pubis, scabies, trichomoniasis, candidiasis, and tinea. To this can be added amebiasis, giardiasis, hepatitis B, chlamydia, and moniliasis.

Amebiasis and Giardiasis

Amebiasis and giardiasis are intestinal diseases that are usually found in travelers to foreign countries in which the water supply is contaminated or fresh fruits and vegetables are improperly washed. They have been categorized as STDs after having been discovered in the homosexual community in New York City in 1977 (7). Chlamydia, one of the major public health problems in the United States, causes 40 percent of non-gonococcal urethritis in men, is the predominant cause of mucopurulent cervicitis in women, and is implicated increasingly in pelvic inflammatory disease (PID) (10).

Trichomoniasis

Trichomoniasis is the most widespread STD. The *Trichomonas* protozoa creates the problem and results in a thin, frothy, yellow discharge with itching and foul odor in women and usually no symptoms in men. If it is not treated in both partners concurrently, the disease bounces from partner to partner like a tennis ball. The primary precaution during treatment is that the partners refrain from sexual intercourse, since the disease is communicable for the duration of the infection. Metronidazole (Flagyl) given orally is the treatment of choice for *Trichomonas* infections.

Herpes Simplex

Until 1974–1975 syphilis ranked second to gonorrhea as the most prevalent STD in the United States. Then herpes progenitalis (genital herpes infection) suddenly supplanted syphilis and rivaled gonorrhea in incidence (2).

Herpes simplex is a virus that is classified as type I or type II. Type I is usually found in what is commonly called cold sores, whereas type II is usually cultured from genital lesions; therefore, type II herpes simplex is the causative organism of genital herpes. Although most commonly limited to the genital organs, type II lesions can also occur in the mouth, rectum, and cervix. Herpes has become the most troublesome STD in years. It is chronic, incurable, and rapidly spreading. It is unpredictable in its occurrence and recurrence and is devastating to those who contract it because of its unpredictabil-

ity and chronicity. Nevertheless, it is not yet a reportable disease in the United States. "This is primarily because no control measures are currently available, making it difficult to justify any government surveillance" (1). Because herpes is difficult to detect and cannot be cured, there are no programs for its control, and estimates of those who are affected are just that—estimates.

Herpes is transmitted by skin-to-skin contact with an infected area of the body. The virus, which enters the body either through a break in the skin or through mucous membranes, does not survive on inanimate objects and is not airborne (1). Once inside the body the herpes virus enters the nervous system and remains there indefinitely, lying dormant, until stress, infection, fever, menstruation, or exposure to the sun triggers an outbreak of the disease. The herpes victim never knows when, or if, the outbreak will occur, so he or she constantly lives with fear and uncertainty. Antibiotics are not curative agents for herpes, since the causative organism is a virus. The only treatment to date, acyclovir ointment, shortens the episodes of herpes lesions, but does not cure the disease (1). Acyclovir is applied topically to the lesions (whoever is treating the client should wear gloves) and helps reduce the pain and swelling.

The extent to which herpes is a problem can be summed up in the following quote: "No effective epidemiologic control methods are available; there is no vaccine; transmission is possible without the presence of subjective symptoms or externally visible lesions. Serious sexual problems frequently arise; the perinatal effects on infants can be catastrophic, and herpes is inseparably related to the development of cervical cancer" (9). Research is being conducted to determine why and how this relationship exists.

The lesions of herpes are self-healing. They begin as shallow vesicles and erupt into ulcerations. The ulcer then forms a crust and heals. Pain, itching, tenderness, and edema accompany the formation of the lesions. Dysuria and urinary retention may also occur. Genital herpes has additional implications for young women of childbearing age because of the effects the disease can have on pregnancy and childbirth.

Women who are infected with herpes simplex have a miscarriage rate three times greater than that of the general population. If they reach full term and have active herpes at the time of delivery, there is a better than 40 percent chance that the disease will be transmitted to the newborn baby (2). The mortality rate among such infants is very high, and pregnant women who are actively shedding the herpes virus at the time of labor and delivery must be delivered by cesarean section to prevent transmission to the infant.

Syphilis

In its early primary stage syphilis presents as a chancre on the penis, anus, vagina, rectum, cervix, or, if there has been oral sexual contact, mouth, throat, and pharynx. *Treponema pallidum,* the causative organism of syphilis, invades the body through concealed, moist areas by way of sexual intercourse. The spirochetes enter the lymphatic system almost immediately, multiplying as they go. There are then subsequent multiple sites of infection scattered through the body. The area in which the organism entered the body becomes the site of the characteristic chancre. The chancre is painless, firm, and immovable, and appears from ten to ninety days after exposure. If the victim does not obtain medical attention, the chancre will disappear, often leading the infected person to believe that the disease is cured.

The spirochete continues to multiply, leading to stage II, which is characterized by the appearance of a generalized, dry, nonpruritic body rash, which may also appear on the palms. The rash may be accompanied by a sore throat, hair loss, headaches, and fever and will probably appear about six weeks after the chancre is initially seen. If untreated, the rash will also disappear.

The disease generally enters a latent stage after the rash disappears. Unfortunately the disease process usually continues during the latent stage. Although signs and symptoms may not be evident, the spirochete of syphilis is slowly destroying the heart, brain, and body joints. It will also eventually invade the central nervous system and can be found in the cerebrospinal fluid. Clients have increased difficulty in walking, paresthesia of the lower extremities, and foot ulcers, and experience dulling of pain sensation and the destruction of weight-bearing joints. The disease process can be halted at any point by treatment with penicillin, but the damage done to the heart and brain in the late stages is irreversible. Dilatation and subsequent heart failure are effects of untreated syphilis, as are the previously mentioned neurological effects.

Untreated syphilis can eventually result in blindness, insanity, and death. It can also be passed to an infant in utero. The spirochete crosses the placenta, and the infant is born with congenital syphilis. The mortality rate for such infants is high, if they survive the pregnancy.

Gonorrhea

Gonorrhea, or clap, has reached epidemic proportions in the United States. In 1980 there were 1,004,029 cases reported. The highest rates were in the twenty- to twenty-four-year-old age-group (2). The incubation period is shorter than that of syphilis (three to thirty days versus ten to ninety days), and the initial symptoms are unmistakable. The male victim will have painful urination with a discharge of pus from the urethra. The female victim may or may not have symptoms. If she does, they may include abdominal discomfort, vaginal discharge, and dysuria. Women share with men (particularly homosexual men) a risk of rectal and pharyngeal infection secondary to rectal or oral sexual contact. In addition, there are reported instances of men who test positive for gonorrhea but are asymptomatic. Like women, who are usually the reservoirs of infection, these asymptomatic men become a public health problem.

An infection of the urethra and genital tract, gonorrhea is caused by a gram-negative diplococcus called *Neisseria gonorrhoeae.* It is transmitted through sexual contact. If untreated, it can become life-threatening, and contracting it does not render one immune. Gonorrhea is usually the causative organism in PID, a serious complication in women.

Approximately 10 percent to 17 percent of women with gonorrhea develop PID, infecting such pelvic structures as the endometrial cavity, the fallopian tubes, and the ovaries. Abdominal pain, increased vaginal discharge, dysuria, abnormal uterine bleeding, anorexia, nausea, vomiting, and fever are some of the symptoms associated with PID (11).

Initial episodes of acute PID most commonly occur in single young women, who are in the age-group at highest risk of contracting gonorrhea and other STDs. More than 20 percent of cases result in infertility, and the risk of ectopic pregnancy increases from sixfold to tenfold after PID (5).

Untreated gonorrhea results in sterility in both males and females. In females, infection spreads to the fallopian tubes, which become inflamed and then heal with adhesions that obstruct the tubes and thus prevent fertilization. In the male the gonococcus may cause prostatitis and epididymitis. Epididymitis may lead to sterility. Gonorrhea can also cause arthritis, salpingitis, conjunctivitis, and blindness in infants who are born through a gonococcus-infected vagina. Preventive treatment for gonococcal eye infections in newborns is administered in the form of antibiotic eyedrops in the hospital nursery.

Gonorrhea is the most frequently reported of *all* communicable diseases. It is readily cured by penicillin and probenecid. However, it now takes four times the amount of penicillin to cure gonorrhea as it did ten years ago. And to compound the problem, there are rising numbers of cases of penicillinase-producing *N. gonorrhoeae*, a penicillin-resistant form of gonorrhea. First detected in England and the United States in 1976, these strains spread rapidly, and within four years of the initial report, 1,022 cases had been reported in the United States (4). The evolution of penicillin-resistant organisms will make it increasingly difficult to bring and keep STDs under control, but a concerted effort on the part of all who are concerned with the spread of these diseases will help control them. It must also be understood by all that *every* STD can be repeatedly contracted, and the presence of one does not negate the presence of another. (In other words, it is possible to have more than one STD at the same time.)

Prevention and Screening for Early Intervention

Nurses who are screening for STD must consider several factors in deciding who is a likely candidate. The rule of thumb generally is a young urban male (meaning fifteen to thirty years of age, urban area rather than rural, male more often than female). However, anyone who presents with genital lesions or lesions that have persisted for more than a week should be screened. Those who are in penal institutions, in institutions for the mentally ill or retarded, or in the military should be screened. Prostitutes and male homosexuals also have high incidences of STD, as do sexually active people who frequently change partners. Migrant workers and foreign travelers should also be screened, and anyone with one STD should be screened for others. Sexually transmitted diseases occur worldwide; it cannot be assumed that anyone is immune. Many officials believe that the sexual revolution of the 1960s, the use of oral contraceptives, the mobility of people, liberal use of antibiotics (leading to increased resistance of the STD organisms), and treatment failure are several of the reasons for the increases in reported cases of STD. Attempts have been made to establish programs that would decrease, if not eradicate, certain STDs.

The current methods of control involve the primary and secondary levels of prevention. Although states bear the primary responsibility for venereal disease control activities, the federal government assists the states by providing financial support and personnel through grant programs. Preventing interstate spread is the federal government's responsibility (4). These responsibilities are met in a variety of ways. Public (county and city) clinics, casefinding, contact investigation, and prompt treatment of STD victims and their contacts are examples of secondary prevention.

Primary prevention measures—prenatal and premarital serology tests, education, and consultation—are essential to raising the consciousness of the public and health professionals as well. Sexually transmitted diseases are underreported across the country. Those patients who are cared for by public clinics are always reported to the appropriate government agency, while private doctors and clinics may or may not do the reporting. Thus statistics become skewed, and it is difficult to obtain an accurate picture of trends and incidence.

Youngsters in sex education classes should learn about the consequences of venereal disease. Surprisingly some youngsters still harbor ideas that the illnesses contribute to artistic or creative work or that getting infected is a sign of adulthood (13).

Effective control of STDs is the goal of public education. Media campaigns and hot lines are two of the methods used to accomplish this. The best method, however, is interviewing clients for contacts, followed by location, examination, and treatment of infected contacts (12). Interviewing to locate those contacts is time-consuming and can severely tax the skills of the health professional involved. Helping an STD victim to face the reality of having contracted syphilis, gonorrhea, herpes, or any of the other diseases can be a test of one's ability to be nonjudgmental (the first prerequisite for working with such clients), but the interviewer must still underscore the necessity of immediate treatment for the client, elicit the names of the contacts, stress the confidentiality of the information, and locate and quickly treat the contacts.

Control of STDs depends, to a great extent, on the public perception of them as a problem. Statistics can horrify, but if an attitude of fear or "it only happens to the other guy" prevails, public health officials will continue to see increases each year in the number of STD cases.

Overview of STD Management

The goals of management of STD are to identify actual and potential cases of STD, to intervene as early as possible, to reduce transmission and limit the effects of STD on the client and others, and to foster an optimum level of self-care through education of the client, the client's family, and the public. This section relates to intervention, which aims, primarily through medication, to limit the effects of STD on the individual. An overview of current treatment protocols for STDs is presented in Table 28.1.

Nursing Care

Sexually related problems strike at the most intimate parts of our lives. If sexual intimacy is seen as the epitome of trust and caring, then the diagnosis of STD is devastating, leaving the victim feeling used and worthless. If sexual intimacy is casual, the diagnosis of STD may provoke anger, either at oneself or one or more partners. In either case the intervention of a skilled health professional is necessary to answer questions, clarify misconceptions, defuse anger, elevate self-esteem, promote self-care and healthful attitudes, and have the STD victim and his or her contacts treated. Nurses are in the best position to begin to handle these problems. They cannot effectively handle these problems, however, if they are unsure of their own philosophy and beliefs about sexuality and the expression of it in our society.

The nursing care of a client with STD requires skill, knowledge, sensitivity, and a nonjudgmental attitude. The goals of nursing care are manifold and include cure of disease, prevention of further transmission, treatment of sexual partners, increased knowledge of how these diseases are transmitted, and elimination of many of the myths that surround STD.

Factors Influencing Nursing Care

One human being's ability to care for another depends on a variety of factors: the capacity to care, awareness of limitations, recognition of negative reactions, and the ability to grow despite stress and negativity.

Nurses who must work with STD victims bring their own beliefs and values into that relationship. Intellectually, they may realize that verbal or nonverbal expressions of disgust or revulsion will prevent a caring, curative relationship from developing. Emotionally, they may not be able to avoid reacting. As stated earlier, sexual problems strike at the most intimate parts of our lives. The victims of STD generally feel degraded enough without judgment being passed on their activi-

ties. *Promiscuity* and *permissiveness* are emotion-laden words that are frequently used in conjunction with STDs, and the nurses who allow these or other such emotional words to affect the care they render do a disservice to themselves and their clients. In essence, they set up a noncaring environment and defeat the concept of self-care.

To avoid this atmosphere, several actions are necessary. It is essential for nurses to know their own beliefs and values and how these affect the care they render. If they find that they cannot maintain objectivity and establish a supportive, caring environment, they should remove themselves from the situation. If this is not possible, then they must either send the client to someone else or handle the situation to the best of their ability. Nurses must accept the reality that for various reasons, they will not be able to care for every client they meet. This applies to the client with STD as well. Understanding the reasons for the inability to be caring is a step in the growth process. Admitting the inability to be caring is the first step.

Another factor that influences nursing intervention is the use of oral contraceptives. Many women who use these refuse to consider other methods of contraception. Because oral contraceptives change the pH of the vagina by prolonging the period of alkalinity, they create an atmosphere in which the gonococcus can thrive. Women who use oral contraceptives are more susceptible to gonorrhea. Explanations of the effects of oral contraceptives can and should be given by the nurse, and other methods of contraception should be discussed with the client. For a more detailed description of contraceptives, the reader is referred to chapter 21.

One alternative method of contraception is the condom. The use of condoms has been portrayed humorously in the media through such images as the young man in a small town trying to ask the pharmacist for assistance. The condom is ridiculed today by some, particularly teenagers, who think that their use detracts from the spontaneity of sexual intimacy. But condoms are effective in preventing STDs, especially among the fifteen- to nineteen-year-old group, which is now responsible for 25 percent of all reported cases of gonorrhea, 17.6 percent of all births, approximately 48 percent of all out-of-wedlock births, and 30.4 percent of all abortions (8).

Another factor in nursing intervention is the availability of services. Many clients in public health clinics have to wait a long time to be seen by a health professional. That may mean spending time they can ill afford to be examined. If they cannot take time during the day, there

Table 28.1
STD Treatment Protocols

Disease	Signs and Symptoms	Incubation Period	Common Diagnostic Tests	Treatment
Syphilis Primary	Chancre may appear on genitalia, mouth, anus, breast	Usually appears 3 weeks after exposure	VDRL (blood) Kline	Benzathine penicillin G 2.4 million units I.M. *or* Aqueous procaine penicillin G 600,000 units daily for 8 days
Secondary	Dry, nonpruritic bilaterally symmetrical rash that may appear on palms; malaise, fever, mucous patches in mouth; alopecia, lymphadenopathy	0–10 weeks after chancre appears; usually 6 weeks	Mazzini FTA Darkfield Microscopic	Same as primary
Late	Neurological, cardiac symptoms, gummas—circular or half-moon destructive lesions that can be found on any body organ	5–30 years	Spinal fluid examination (neurosyphilis)	Benzathine penicillin G 6–9 million units I.M. given in 3-million units at 7-day intervals *or* Aqueous procaine penicillin G 6–9 million units given 600,000 units per day
Congenital	Crippling, blindness, facial abnormalities, deafness, stillbirth, nasal discharge, permanent wrinkling and scarring of face, enlarged liver or spleen, anemia, abnormal cry	Acquired in utero after 18th week of pregnancy		Benzathine penicillin G 50,000 units per kilogram of body weight *or* Aqueous procaine penicillin G 100,000 units per kilogram of body weight divided into daily dosage over 10 days
Gonorrhea	Burning sensation in urethra; difficulty or pain on urination; purulent yellow or green discharge; reddened, swollen end of penis; untreated—sterility Female—generally asymptomatic, may have discharge. Untreated PID, ectopic pregnancy, or sterility	3–5 days	Smear of discharge on a gloss slide (male) *or* Culture and sugar fermentation test (female)	Aqueous procaine penicillin G 4.8 million units I.M. in two divided doses *or* Tetracycline 0.5 g P.O. q.i.d. × 5 days *or* Ampicillin 3.5 g with 1 g probenecid

(*continued*)

Table 28.1   *(continued)*

Disease	Signs and Symptoms	Incubation Period	Common Diagnostic Tests	Treatment
Genital herpes	Blisterlike lesions on genitals; sore, burning areas; swollen inguinal nodes; difficult urination; fever, headache, anorexia	Undetermined	Smears *or* Culture of fresh lesions	Symptomatic—no cure known; acyclovir cream is treatment for outbreaks
Trichomoniasis	Frothy white or yellow discharge; unpleasant odor; vaginal itching	1–3 weeks	Smear of discharge	Flagyl 2 g P.O. stat *or* 250 mg P.O. t.i.d. × 7 days; concurrent treatment of sex partner; no alcohol while under treatment
Chlamydia	See LGV			
Amebiasis	Abdominal discomfort, diarrhea containing blood or mucus alternating with periods of constipation or remission	2–4 weeks	Examination of stool specimen	Flagyl *or* Diodoquin
Giardiasis	Diarrhea, abdominal cramps, bloating, frequent loose and smelly stools, fatigue, weight loss	Variable; 6–22 days	Examination of stool specimen	Flagyl *or* Atabrine
Moniliasis	Same as candidiasis, also causes thrush in infants	Same as candidiasis	Gram stain *or* Culture	Same as candidiasis
Pediculosis ("crabs")	Severe pubic itching	7–9 days	Hair under microscope	Kwell shampoo or lotion repeated in 24 hours
Candidiasis	Thick, white discharge resembling cottage cheese; yeastlike odor; white plaques on vagina; severe itching	Variable	Wet mount *or* Culture	Mycostatin suppositories b.i.d. for 7–14 days
Lymphogranuloma venereum (LGV)	Small genital lesion, followed by inguinal bubo, then enlarged inguinal nodes that erupt and drain. *Late S&S:* penile elephantiasis, polypoid growths, anorectal ulcers, strictures	1–3 weeks	Frei skin test	Tetracycline 500 mg P.O. q.i.d. × 2–3 weeks *or* Sulfasoxazole 4 g P.O., followed by 500 mg q.i.d. × 3 weeks
Granuloma inguinale	Painless papule on genitals or thighs, ulceration of papules; granulomatous masses that are friable and red. *Late*	Unknown; estimated to be 50 days	Smear *or* Culture	Streptomycin Tetracycline 500 mg P.O. q.i.d. × 2–3 weeks Erythromycin

Table 28.1 *(continued)*

Disease	Signs and Symptoms	Incubation Period	Common Diagnostic Tests	Treatment
	S&S: scarring, elephantiasis, ulceration of underlying tissue and organs			
Condylomata acuminata (warts)	Soft, red bumps that become pedunculated; appear on glands, foreskin, urinary opening in men; labia, vaginal walls, and perineum in women	1–6 months	Serology (blood test)	Repeated for several weeks: paint warts with podophyllin preparation diluted with alcohol; wash off after 6 hours
Chancroid	Small, red painful papule that appears wherever bacteria entered body; papule becomes pustule that turns into open sore; multiple pustules appear; abscesses and fistulas may develop	3–8 days	Gram stain or smear of drainage	Streptomycin (if sulfa-resistant) 500 mg I.M. b.i.d. × 10–14 days Sulfonamides 1 g P.O. q.i.d. *or* Tetracycline 500 mg × 10–14 days
NGU (non-gonococcal urethritis)	Thin, clear persistent discharge; discomfort when urinating; causative organism in 40 percent of cases—*Chlamydia*	Generally 5–7 days	Smear of discharge	Tetracycline 2 g daily for 7–10 days *or* Tetracycline 1 g daily for 21 days
Scabies	Severe itching between fingers, or on wrists, armpits, breasts, buttocks, thighs, penis, scrotum	Several days to several weeks	Microscopic *or* Clinical	Hot bath, followed by application of Kwell, Evrax, or tetmosol twice a day or emulsion of benzyl benzoate ointment, followed by both the next day
Nonspecific vaginitis	Inflammation of vagina; discharge, itching, or burning	Varies	Smear	Ampicillin 500 mg q.i.d. for 7–10 days *or* Flagyl 250 mg P.O. t.i.d. × 7 days
PPNG	See gonorrhea		Smear culture	Spectinomycin 2 g I.M.
Molluscum contagiosum	Pearly pink to white papules with prominent central pore multiple lesions; appear on the skin	2–7 weeks	Clinical diagnosis	Insertion of phenol into depressed center of lesions
Tinea cruris	Scaly lesions surrounded by small blisters or pustules found in creases of groin or on the thighs		Clinical diagnosis	Antifungicide

are few alternatives, since most clinics do not have evening hours.

Family reactions may also be a factor in nursing intervention. A nurse's plan to treat the exposed wife of an STD victim will not be carried out, despite the need for it, if the husband refuses to tell her. The diagnosis of STD, especially gonorrhea, syphilis, or herpes, has a ripple effect. It affects the STD victim and those with whom he or she has contact. The willingness of the person with STD to assist in locating contacts will affect the ease with which the nurse can intervene in the situation.

Establishing a Nurse-Client Relationship

The first contact with the health care system for a client who suspects that she or he has STD will probably be a nurse. The nurse sets the tone for the initial contact. It will be necessary to obtain certain types of information, such as a sexual history. A sexual history is necessary when clients display any of the classically recognized symptoms of an STD, when they report having previously had STD, if they present intraoral or intrarectal complaints, or if they ask for a VD checkup (8).

Discussion of sexual activities can be painful for both the client and the nurse. The nurse cannot afford to appear judgmental in the conduct of the interview, for goals of treatment and prevention may not be accomplished. Assurances of confidentiality are essential and must be followed through.

As a primary source of care, the nurse is concerned about curing the patient and preventing the spread of the STD. Securing the client's confidence, explaining the procedures to be done and interpreting the results, reinforcing what the physician has explained, and stressing the need to complete treatment as well as to have the sexual partners treated are all part of the nursing care plan for the adult with STD.

Locating the contacts can be a time-consuming process. It is imperative that they be found and treated as quickly as possible. In the role of counselor and educator, the nurse can explain to the STD victim the manner in which these diseases spread, the effects of untreated disease on the individual and others, and the need for complete treatment. The nurse should also be able to determine, through communication with the client, the extent of the blow to self-esteem and the depth of the anger and fear that usually exist in this situation. If they are caring persons in the sense that the nursing theorists describe, nurses will be able to use their knowledge and skill to guide STD victims into better health by helping

them to examine values, beliefs, reasons for actions, and, ultimately, life and life-styles. Nurses will be able to assist the client to set priorities, make well-informed decisions, and be content with those decisions; they will not be disturbed if those decisions are in conflict with their own value systems. For example, if a client's sexual history indicates primarily homosexual contacts, nurses are more helpful when they refrain from attempting to convert the client or to indicate distaste for the client's sexual practices. The nurse must instead try to prevent a recurrence, provide instruction about the client's medication regimen, explain the nature of the disease (how it was contracted and the various methods for determining its presence), emphasize the need for follow-up, and focus on the partners so that they might be notified. As long as clients feel no condemnation or condescension for the way they live, the nurse should be able to promote the growth and caring that is so essential in this situation.

Coordinator Role

A coordinator orchestrates the various efforts involved in resolving a particular problem. As primary care givers, nurses frequently are responsible for contacting other members of the interdisciplinary team and acting as liaisons and advocates. They may refer an STD victim for counseling if indicated. If information on family planning or contraception is needed, nurses can refer clients to appropriate clinics or facilities. As coordinators, nurses should maintain contact with those people to whom clients are referred so that information is shared and care is planned and evaluated.

Assessment

In assessing the client for STD, the nurse must obtain a nursing history, which includes a sexual history. It is vital that the nurse obtain the following information:

- If the client is a female, is she using contraception? Birth control pills and intrauterine devices increase susceptibility to infection.
- Has the client noticed any discharges from vagina or urethra?
- Is there any difficulty or pain on urination?
- Is there any pain on defecation?
- Is there any anal or vulval itching?
- Does the client have a sore throat? Frequency of sore throats?

- Has the client noticed any rashes or lesions on the skin?
- When did any of the problems appear?
- If the client is a female, date of last Pap smear?
- Age of first sexual contact?
- Frequency of intercourse?
- Is there one regular partner? Most recent sexual contact?
- Has there been more than one sexual partner? How many? Most recent sexual contact?
- Has the partner complained of discharges, itching, rashes, or lesions?
- Is sexual contact vaginal, anal, oral, or any combination thereof?
- Are there any allergies, especially to medications?
- What is the client's level of knowledge about STD—its transmission, prevention, and management?
- What health care resources are available to and used by the client?
- What impact—emotionally and socially—has the actual or potential threat of STD made on the client and family?

A physical examination should address the responses to these questions. Blood for testing must be drawn; any lesions must be examined and cultured. Throats must also be examined and cultured. If there are any lesions, are they hard and indurated, or edematous and inflamed? Do they bleed easily? In a female, the nurse must check for abdominal pain and tenderness, fever, headache, lethargy. Are there any enlarged lymph nodes? What type of rash is present? Where is it on the body?

Serology tests for determining the presence of an STD are available only for syphilis. The other diseases are elicited by Pap smears, rectal smears, and cultures. Because cultures take time to grow, suspected gonorrhea, syphilis, or chlamydia should be treated at once rather than risk its being spread to others.

Diagnostic tests commonly used for STDs are listed in Table 28.2. Interpretation of test results can be problematic. Clients have been known to have false-positive and false-negative reactions (Table 28.3). Other physical conditions can evoke such reactions.

Nursing Diagnoses

Establishing nursing diagnoses in a physical, social, and emotional context can help the primary nurse determine the most effective plan of care for the client and family.

The following selected nursing diagnoses are designed to illustrate the application of concepts of primary nursing to common problems of the client with STD.

- Potential transmission of an infection related to such factors as uncertainty about diagnosis and insufficient knowledge about STD
- Potential feelings of rage, disappointment, concern, and confusion related to such factors as the personal meaning of a diagnosis of STD, its social connotations, and its impact on family relationships
- Knowledge deficit related to such factors as misinformation and lack of information
- Potential self-care deficits related to such factors as poor self-image, lack of supportive relationships, and failure to appreciate the importance of individual responsibility

Planning and Implementation

□ **Potential Transmission of an Infection.** Regardless of the method of transmission, infectious diseases must be prevented from spreading. The methods that health professionals have learned—thorough handwashing, proper disposal of soiled articles, isolation or quarantine when necessary, disinfection when necessary—also apply when dealing with STD. There are three goals to be achieved in treating STD: preventing further spread of the infection, achieving good hygiene, and improving individual learning to avoid reinfection and promote general health awareness. Nursing intervention must focus on these areas.

When the client initially presents with physical complaints, the nurse proceeds to determine the source of the problem. The nurse attempts to reassure the client while eliciting the information needed to clarify the complaint. Nursing interventions are based on a combination of the nurse's knowledge, observations, and the answers to these questions.

The nurse will inspect all lesions on the skin and genital and rectal areas. The mouth and the throat will also be inspected, and cultures taken from all open lesions. Blood samples for testing will be drawn, using needle precautions. Care must be taken to prevent infection from entering cuts or other breaks in the skin.

Once all baseline data are obtained, treatment begins. If the STD is reportable, the nurse must file a report. Whether it is reportable or not, teaching must be part of the treatment plan. The nurse must explain the transmission process and emphasize the need to complete the

Table 28.2
Diagnostic Tests for STDs

Disease	Type of Test	How Obtained	Results	Interpretation
Genital herpes	Viral culture	Scrapings from base of fresh lesions	Giant cells with multiple nuclei	Presence of disease. Symptoms resolve in 1–4 weeks.
	Smear	Same as culture	Isolation of virus in 1–3 days	Virus remains in body. Symptoms recur.
Gonorrhea	Culture	Women: cervix, anus, throat, pelvic exam; use cotton swabs to obtain specimen; apply to Thayer–Martin medium in Z-pattern and then streak with loop	Thayer–Martin medium prevents growth of other bacteria. Z-pattern and streaking promote growth of the gonococcus.	Presence of active disease. Warrants antibiotics. Clients must be recultured in 3–7 days while in treatment and 4–6 weeks after completion of treatment. Contacts must be treated within 10 days. Clients should refrain from sexual contact until treatment is complete.
	Smear	Men: penile discharge for exam under microscope	Presence of gram-negative rods means active disease.	
Syphilis Non-treponemal (diagnosis screen asymptomatic people)	VDRL Rapid plasma reagin circle card test	Venipuncture Spinal fluid	Reactive, weakly reactive, nonreactive	Nonreactive = no disease; weakly reactive or positive titers = confirm by treponemal test; begin treatment and retest.
Treponemal (test symptomatic people)	Darkfield microscopic exam	Swab of lesions or aspirated lymph nodes	Spirochete present	Treatment required
	Fluorescent treponemal antibody absorption (FTA-ABS)	Used when client presents with ulcerations; done on blood serum	Negative	Syphilis unlikely
			Borderline	Repeat; if again borderline, syphilis unlikely
			Positive	Past or present infection

course of treatment and avoid sexual contact until treatment is completed. The need for treatment of the sexual partners cannot be overemphasized. Nor can the possibility of the existence of two or more diseases at the same time. As treatment progresses, the nurse can also instruct the male and female clients in proper hygiene and cleanliness to minimize the possibility of reinfection. Vinegar douches and cotton panties or pantyhose can inhibit the growth of bacteria. Using condoms, washing the genitals thoroughly with soap and water before and after sexual intercourse, avoiding vaginal deodorant sprays and tampons will help promote healing

Table 28.3
Patterns of Test Results

Test Result	Reaction
Positive VDRL Reactive FTA-ABS	Can occur with untreated or treated syphilis, congenital syphilis, or other spirochete infections.
Negative VDRL Positive FTA	Indicates adequately treated syphilis, untreated early primary or late infection, or a false-positive FTA. This has been reported in patients with lupus, in drug addicts, and in pregnancy.
Positive VDRL Negative FTA	False positive and may occur with viral infections, malaria, and pregnancy.
Negative VDRL Negative FTA	Occurs in incubating syphilis and when there is no syphilis.

Source: Nelson Gantz and Richard Gleckman. "Serologic Tests for Syphilis." In *Manual of Clinical Problems in Infectious Diseases.* Boston: Little, Brown, 1979, pp. 154–55.

and decrease bacterial growth. It is important that clients understand that there is no immunity against STD. Such diseases can be repeatedly contracted and must be treated each time. The effects of failure to seek treatment can and should be taught as well.

☐ *Potential Feelings of Rage, Disappointment, Concern, and Confusion.* The goals related to this nursing diagnosis are to decrease the emotional level and thus facilitate the learning process. Nursing intervention must calm, reassure, question, interview, and teach. Understanding the concern of the client about the effects of any STD on his or her life is the first step in decreasing the emotional level. At the least, an STD means an inconvenience (curtailing some activities, visits to the doctor's office, cost of medications). At worst, an STD can be life-threatening. Reactions to the diagnosis of STD are as varied as human beings are varied. They can range from little concern to irrationality.

Defusing the concern by listening carefully and asking gentle but probing questions can help the client begin to understand what is happening and help the nurse gather enough information to begin teaching about the need for identifying and treating contacts, the need for the client to begin and continue treatment, and the need to

have follow-up care. The nurse can also begin to discuss risk factors and general hygiene measures.

Socially, the potential exists for withdrawal from others. The goal is to reduce suspicion of others and encourage positive self-images and self-caring behaviors. This is not to say that every person who contracts an STD has a poor self-image. Those who do, however, are at high risk for repeat infections, as are people who have multiple sexual partners.

Part of the nursing intervention in the care of these clients may be referrals to community agencies. If the client seems to need assistance—financial, medical, counseling, substance abuse, family counseling—it is the nurse's responsibility as primary care giver to refer the client to a social worker, a clinic, or outside agencies, all of which may provide some help. Because the diagnosis of gonorrhea, syphilis, or genital herpes can be so devastating, especially when spouses are involved, the nurse may treat the entire family or coordinate services for the entire family. This is not an insignificant job. The larger fabric of society is greatly affected by disease or any other event that results in losses. Because the incidence of STD is at an all-time high in the United States, the number of hours and the amount of productivity lost in the need for treatment and even hospitalization are staggering. Any intervention at any stage can do something to reduce the cost to society.

☐ *Knowledge Deficit.* The client with STD has a tremendous need for both information and acceptance. Even in the last two decades of the twentieth century, there are people who still believe that STDs are transmitted from doorknobs, towels and toilet seats (although there may be some validity to this since the causative organism of trichomoniasis has been found in the dirty water of public toilets). There are also those who have no knowledge of anatomy or how sexually transmitted diseases are contracted. For many victims of STD, seeking treatment may be the first contact with the health care delivery system. For a woman, this might mean her first pelvic examination. For a man, it will likely mean his first penile or rectal exam. How these are handled will frequently determine how willing the STD victim will be to cooperate with the nurse in locating contacts.

☐ *Potential Self-Care Deficits.* The concept of self-care rests heavily on the theory that people want to do what is best for themselves to maintain their health and, given the information and opportunity, will do so. The nurse who is a "caring" person will help promote the self-care potential that each person possesses. In the case of a client with STD, this may be difficult for a nurse to do.

Caring involves developing a trusting relationship that will move a client toward a positive, more aware, healthier state. The classic STD victim is twenty to twenty-four years of age and may have had a number of sexual partners, male and female. Homosexuality, premarital sex, extramarital sex, a variety of partners—all of these phrases mean different things to different people. Because of the nature of these diseases, a nurse may feel uncomfortable with these clients and avoid the caring that may be necessary to help them evaluate their life-styles. Although evaluation may produce no change, it potentially can lead to more discreet selection of partners and to a change in living patterns.

There are self-care responsibilities for everyone concerned with treating and preventing STD, but the initial responsibility lies with the client. People behave in various ways for various reasons; some reasons are known and others are not. People with STD may have a poor self-image or may have never learned to care properly for themselves. In the context of self-care, clients are responsible for recognizing that there are problems, and seeking help, completing necessary treatment, and appearing for follow-up as needed. They are also responsible for helping to locate contacts. Accepting these self-care responsibilities may help the STD victim to improve self-esteem and learn those things that are necessary for better health. For example, if indiscriminate sexual activity is a manifestation of lowered self-esteem, then increasing self-care awareness will help the STD victim become more discriminating and selective in sexual contacts and thus may decrease the number of STD cases.

Other self-care responsibilities include compliance with reasonable recommendations. For instance, if the intervention of a social worker is needed in a particular situation and a referral is made, it is a self-caring person who will follow through on the referral. Self-care demands that clients understand the effects of their actions on themselves and others, and set appropriate priorities. Self-caring people will look closely at their relationships to determine if they are positive and promote health, or if they are negative and destroy health, and what alternatives may be taken.

Self-care responsibilities for those who are named as contacts include being willing to cooperate with the health professionals involved in attempting to stop the spread of STD. They will allow themselves to be treated and name any other people with whom they might have had contact. They may find that the same evaluation process is necessary. The process of learning to be self-caring can be painful for both victim and contact. Complications from untreated disease (e.g., PID, congenital syphilis, herpes in an infant) are a brutal way to learn. Unfortunately too many people ignore the initial signs of infection and thus allow these complications to occur. If changes in life-style do occur, they may well be the result of survival of these complications.

Self-care responsibilities extend to the family. Families can be helped to be more self-caring. A family can be a powerful unit, and the values and beliefs that are taught in the family will influence individuals for the remainder of their lives. Self-care denotes increased responsibility for one's own health and well-being. A family that is devastated by the diagnosis of STD (especially syphilis, gonorrhea, or genital herpes) may not feel capable of making any decisions about treatment, notifying contacts, and following up on care. The decision making involved in treating a three-year-old with STD, a sixteen-year-old with PID from gonorrhea or chlamydia, and a male or female adult with no other problems is going to be different, and the degree of dependence on the health care provider will be different.

One of the family's greatest self-care responsibilities is to provide its members with the information needed to make informed, thoughtful decisions about health. For example, open discussions on sexuality, reproduction, sexual responsibility, and STD are vital to an adolescent's well-being. But waiting until a child is an adolescent to provide this information is not caring, nor does it encourage self-care. The primary nurse can help families become more self-caring by helping them to recognize self-care deficits and to accept appropriate help.

Community self-care responsibility involves various aspects of the STD problem. Because communities are made up of families, a caring atmosphere is essential to promote self-care. Community leaders must ensure that health care and referral agencies are adequate in number and staff to provide care to those victims of STD who require it. Evening clinics staffed by health care professionals who are knowledgeable about STD and its management could be provided by the community. Unfortunately many communities are dependent on governmental funds for the existence of special programs, and cutbacks of these funds can lead to termination of the programs. Self-care responsibilities of the community also include health education, especially for the young, and support for research into STD.

More money is needed for research into STD. This, too, is a self-care responsibility of the community. If the governmental community is unable to meet its obligations to its citizens, smaller communities have the option of seeking funding sources elsewhere. The greatest self-care responsibility of the community is to provide education for its young.

Nurses are not the only health professionals to have self-care responsibilities. Physicians have power that can be used to promote self-care, yet some remain unconvinced of its advantages. Methods of care that do not follow tradition are viewed skeptically in some instances. But consumers are becoming more health conscious and more willing to seek alternatives to established medical practices. There will always be a need for medical care, but self-care is the keystone of primary prevention.

Primary nurses can use their political influence to encourage the establishment of satellite facilities for treatment of STD, to lobby for funds for research, treatment, and staff, and to encourage the establishment of sex education programs, family planning clinics, and counseling groups, as needed.

Evaluation

As nurses, we expect that efforts at intervention will yield positive results. Sometimes we are disappointed to find this does not happen. In the case of STDs, the most common result of nursing intervention related to the medical plan of care will be the cure of the disease. This can be accomplished usually within a week to ten days after diagnosis, provided the client adheres to the medication and treatment regimen. Another expected outcome is the cure of sexual partners. Other outcomes are more difficult to measure and more difficult to place in a time constraint.

Expected nursing outcomes related to nursing diagnoses are (a) control of the spread of STD; (b) more positive feeelings about self and others, leading to reduced feelings of rage, disappointment, concern, and confusion; (c) optimum knowledge of STD—its causes, transmission, prevention, and management—and ongoing self-care behaviors. Small changes may be the only indication a nurse has: a client whose contact with health care professionals has been minimal, nonexistent, or hostile begins to keep appointments and is interested in his or her own progress; another client questions the reasons for treatment as opposed to how someone else with the same disease was treated; another client brings in someone else for treatment. These behavioral changes occur over time, not immediately.

Ethical and Legal Issues

The legal requirement for reporting certain communicable diseases is clearly defined in most states. The fact that there are such statutes emphasizes the need for reporting communicable diseases. If states are going to protect their citizens' health, they must have procedures that ensure the prompt reporting of infectious diseases (16).

Syphilis, gonorrhea, chancroid, and lymphogranuloma venereum are examples of diseases that are reportable by law. Many cases, however, go unreported, obviously in violation of the law. Genital herpes is not a reportable disease, despite the number of new cases that appear each year. Yet some statistics are kept, so that estimates of the number of cases can be made. Locating health care providers who fail to report STD can be difficult, if not impossible. The public has a right to hold health care providers accountable for their actions, or inactions, in halting the spread of STD. Failure to attempt to locate and treat and failure to report the existence of disease are violations of both the law and ethical codes. It is the responsibility of health care providers to protect the health of the public, while respecting, as feasible, the confidentiality of client information. With access to the most intimate and personal information about clients, nurses have both a legal and an ethical duty not to reveal confidential information. Their legal duty arises because the law recognizes a right to privacy. Protecting this right carries a corresponding duty to obey, but the ethical duty is broader and applies at all times (3).

Accountability and ethics are double-edged swords. There are responsibilities on both sides. While professionals are bound legally and ethically to treat STD victims, those victims are equally bound to seek treatment, comply with medical care, avoid any sexual contact until treatment has been completed, and assist in locating contacts. STD victims can be held as accountable for failing to seek treatment as the care provider can be for failing to provide it.

The control of STD is a responsibility of society. Knowledge of methods of prevention should be widespread. Education in sexuality and human reproduction should begin as soon as a child is old enough to ask questions and understand simple answers. Alternative methods of obtaining that education are essential to complement parental teaching. Treatment facilities must be available to all who need them, even if it warrants evening hours. The keystone in any successful program for preventing and treating people with STD is not facilities, but a caring person—a primary nurse—who can relate to them as individuals with diverse problems and needs.

DISCUSSION QUESTIONS

1. You are the primary nurse in a VD clinic and have just informed a male client that his smear was positive for gonococcus. He tells you that his wife is in her first trimester of pregnancy, and has a history of spontaneous abortions. He fears the shock of this diagnosis will cause another miscarriage and insists that she not be told. How will you handle this?

2. A female client is positive for syphilis. She admits to having several sexual partners whom she saw only once or twice. She has no contact with any of them. What are your responsibilities as a care giver? How do you help this client to become more self-caring?

3. A male client has just been diagnosed as having gonorrhea. In the process of interviewing he suddenly stands up, says, "I'll take care of this myself," and refuses to name any contacts. What will you do?

4. A female client, six months pregnant, presents with symptoms that are soon diagnosed as genital herpes. She becomes extremely agitated, blames her husband, and then names someone else as the possible source. She asks you to promise not to inform her husband and then asks, "Will my baby be all right?" How will you respond?

5. A male client comes in with rectal lesions, which test positive for gonococcus and amebiasis. The client flatly denies this and refuses to believe that it is possible. What will you do?

REFERENCES

1. Bettoli, Elena. "Herpes: Facts and Fallacies." *American Journal of Nursing* 82:924–27, June 1982.
2. Campbell, Charles, and R. Jeffrey Herten. "VD to STD:
   Redefining Venereal Disease." *American Journal of Nursing* 81:1629–31, September, 1981.
3. Cazalas, Mary. *Nursing and the Law.* 3rd ed. Germantown, Md.: Aspen System Corp., 1978, 72, 150.
4. Clark, Durean, and Brian MacMahon. "Sexually Transmitted Diseases." In *Preventive and Community Medicine.* 2nd ed., ed. Duncan W. Clark and Brian MacMahon. Boston: Little, Brown, 1981, 415–20.
5. Curras, James. "Economic Consequences of Pelvic Inflammatory Disease in the United States." *American Journal of Obstetrics and Gynecology* 138:848, 1980.
6. Felman, Yehudi. "A Plea for the Condom, Especially for Teenagers." *Journal of the American Medical Association* 241:2517, June 8, 1979.
7. Felman, Yehudi. "Approaches to Sexually Transmitted Amebiasis." *Bulletin of New York Academy of Medicine* 57:201, April 1981.
8. Felman, Yehudi, and James Nikitas. "Obtaining History of Patient's Sexual Activities." *New York State Journal of Medicine* 79:1879, November 1979.
9. Gardner, Herman L. "Herpes Genitalis: Our Most Important Venereal Disease." *American Journal of Obstetrics and Gynecology* 135:554, November 1, 1979.
10. Handsfield, H. Hunter, Walter Stamm, and King K. Holmes. "Sexually Transmitted Diseases." *Journal of the American Venereal Disease Association* 8:85, April/June 1981.
11. Hawkins, Joellen, and Loretta P. Higgins. *Maternity and Gynecological Nursing: Women's Health Care.* Philadelphia: J. B. Lippincott, 1981, 497.
12. Hume, John. "On Reports and Rapport in VD Control." *American Journal of Public Health* 70:946–47, September 1980.
13. Kapel, Saul. "Don't Resist VD Info." *New York Daily News,* January 7, 1982, 54.
14. Kroger, Fred, and Paul J. Wiesner. "STD Education: Challenge for the 80's." *Journal of School Health* 51:242, April 1981.
15. Miele, Alfred, and Edward Edelson. "New York Hit by a VD Epidemic." *New York Daily News,* December 29, 1981, 5.
16. "Reported Cases of Infectious VD from January 1, 1980 to December 31, 1980." New York City Department of Health.

CHAPTER 29

Adults with Tuberculosis

SONYA APPEL

■

OBJECTIVES

After completing this chapter, the reader will be able to:

- Understand the magnitude of tuberculosis as a health problem.
- Identify reasons for persistence of tuberculosis as a major health problem.
- Relate knowledge of the etiology, pathophysiology, and treatment of tuberculosis to nursing assessment and diagnoses.
- Relate knowledge of transmission of tuberculosis to assessment of infectiousness and teaching of appropriate client behaviors.
- Understand the role of the primary nurse in the identification of contacts of tuberculosis clients at risk of new infection.
- Identify nursing care appropriate for selected nursing diagnoses.
- Identify legal and ethical issues related to tuberculosis.

Tuberculosis was the leading cause of death in most of the world in 1882 when Robert Koch announced his discovery of the causative bacillus. Although the death rate from the disease had begun to fall in areas with improved nutrition and standards of living, tuberculosis was still the leading cause of death in the United States in 1906, with more than 200 deaths per 100,000 (18). Clients were then treated with bed rest, good food, and fresh air, preferably in a sanitorium. Isolation of the client from the community was the method of control of transmission of the disease. Many clients stayed years or even decades in sanitoria, which were important parts of tuberculosis control efforts until the middle of this century. As the years progressed, surgery (lobectomy, pneumonectomy, or partial pneumonectomy) or induced pneumothorax was frequently the treatment of choice.

The shift to chemotherapy as the centerpiece of tuberculosis management began after streptomycin, the first drug found to be effective against the tubercle bacillus, was discovered in 1944. As additional drugs were developed in succeeding decades, chemotherapy of tuberculosis became more effective and easier to administer. The setting for client care evolved from the sanitorium to the general hospital to the home. The tuberculosis client today can be treated and cured, in most instances, totally on an outpatient basis, and can be rendered noninfectious in two to three weeks.

Despite these dramatic changes, it is estimated that 10 million cases of tuberculosis still occur each year worldwide, with 4 to 5 million of them being highly infectious, and 2 to 3 million causing death (9). Tuberculosis remains a leading cause of death in many areas of the world and is a problem particularly in the developing countries, where only a fraction of the population has access to health services. In the United States tuberculosis case and death rates have continued to decline overall; the death rate in 1980 was down to approximately 0.8 per 100,000 (10). Nevertheless, more than 20,000 new cases and 1,800 deaths have been reported each year of the first half of the 1980s. The fact that hundreds of cases each year occur in young children demonstrates the continued transmission of the disease

(25, p. 302). Several factors contribute to the continued persistence of tuberculosis in the United States.

It is estimated that 10 to 15 million persons in this country (approximately 6 percent of the population) are already infected with the tubercle bacillus. Even if transmission of new infections were to stop, cases of the disease would develop from this reservoir of infection for many years (13, p. 7).

This infected population is aging, but in many areas of the country it is being replenished to some extent by immigration. In recent decades the geographical pattern of immigration has changed, and the number of entrants has greatly increased. Many immigrants, refugees, and undocumented aliens are coming from areas of the world, including Asia and Latin America, where tuberculosis prevalence is much higher than in the United States (12, p. 11).

New transmission of the disease continues to occur mostly before the cases get into the health care system. Recent immigrants tend to be younger than the native-born infected and may be more likely to be in workplaces and have a greater number of contacts.

Another problem complicating tuberculosis control is the emergence of drug-resistant disease. Resistance is more common among Asians, Africans, and Latin Americans, but it is not limited to the foreign-born (25, p. 307).

Noncompliance with the prescribed regimen on the part of the client is another obstacle to control of the disease. Although therapy is highly effective, it requires months of adherence to the regimen, and many clients are unwilling or unable to comply.

Many health care providers share the perception that tuberculosis is no longer a threat and may therefore be less likely to recognize a potentially infectious case. In part because of this misconception, health departments have lost resources needed to carry out control and prevention measures.

Another factor is a link between the growing numbers of acquired immunodeficiency syndrome (AIDS) cases and tuberculosis incidence. It is thought that the compromised immunity in AIDS cases is resulting in active tuberculosis in those already infected.

Inefficiencies of the tools used against tuberculosis also limit success. Definitive diagnosis and treatment of the disease are both extremely lengthy procedures. Detection of new infections is very resource-consuming, and chemoprophylaxis of those new infections may be as lengthy as treatment of the active disease.

Tuberculosis still occurs in all age-groups and strata of society. However, the greatest risk occurs in urban, male, nonwhite, foreign-born people. The nation's largest cities average more than twice the national case rate. The proportion of foreign-born clients is between 15 percent and 20 percent and may be increasing. The elderly, alcoholic, and malnourished have an increased risk of tuberculosis. These demographic factors contribute to the complexities of the management of the disease (12, p. 11).

The need for medical research to develop a reliable effective vaccine, a rapid diagnostic test, and briefer regimens for treatment and prophylaxis is recognized. Nursing research aimed at enhancing compliant behavior and bringing clients into the health care system earlier would be valuable.

In order to optimize the effectiveness of the tools now available, the nurse working with tuberculosis clients must acquire knowledge of the disease and its treatment and prevention. It is also necessary to recognize and comprehend the complex medical, social, economic, and emotional factors that contribute to the challenges of tuberculosis control. The focus of this chapter is the role of the primary nurse in assessing the needs and implementing the care of the individual client with tuberculosis disease or infection, and in formulating and implementing a plan for minimizing risk to the community. The etiology, transmission, and pathophysiology of the disease are discussed at length, in order to provide the information necessary for assessment, planning, and client education.

The Primary Nurse and Tuberculosis Control—An Overview

The objectives of tuberculosis control have been described in terms of both personal and public health.

The personal health objectives of tuberculosis control are to reduce and eventually eliminate death, disability, illness, emotional trauma, family disruption, and the social stigma still caused by the disease. . . . The public health objectives of

tuberculosis control are to interrupt and to prevent transmission of tubercle bacilli. (4)

Methods for accomplishment of these goals generally fall into the categories of surveillance and containment.

Surveillance is necessary to accumulate epidemiological data on disease frequency and distribution in the community. . . . The successful surveillance activity also assures the availability of diagnostic and treatment services for all patients and initiates containment activities to stop transmission. . . . Containment is concerned with the proper treatment of both the case and the contacts. (4)

The role of the primary nurse is critical in the achievement of the personal and public health objectives through surveillance and containment. There may be no other area of practice in which nursing decisions and interventions will have such far-reaching consequences.

The local health department has the responsibility to assure that clients receive adequate services to contain the disease. The primary nurse may coordinate the services of all the health care team members to achieve that goal. Information may be requested of or transmitted to clerical workers within the health department who maintain a register with updated information about clients under treatment for active tuberculosis as well as those on preventive therapy. Physicians, laboratory personnel, social workers, outreach workers, as well as rehabilitation, vocational, or alcohol abuse counselors may all be involved. Of course, the client and supportive members of his or her family are part of the team. Bringing all of these people together can be a monumental task, and it is frequently the responsibility of the primary nurse to call conferences, gather information, interpret and follow-up on findings, put plans into action, and keep everyone informed about the progress of the client and family.

It is usually the responsibility of the primary nurse to conduct investigations of contacts of infectious cases in the home and in industrial and institutional settings. The crucial nature of this activity in the surveillance and containment of tuberculosis is evidenced by the statistic that 5 percent of newly infected contacts develop disease within one year if not given preventive treatment. The interviewing and teaching skills of the primary nurse will, to a great extent, determine how successfully contacts are identified and brought into the system for testing and treatment when necessary. It is often the judgment of a primary nurse as to which contacts had the kind of exposure to make transmission possible that determines the limits of the investigation.

Public health nurses manage clinics that deliver services to tuberculosis clients, and do much of the teaching and assessment that take place there. The primary nurse maintains the most frequent contact with the client and is the provider in the best position to effect necessary change and ensure the success of the regimen.

It is often a nurse in a hospital or clinic setting who initially instructs the client about the treatment regimen; this first presentation may determine future compliance. Discharge planning by the hospital nurse is also critical. The case of tuberculosis should be reported to public health authorities to permit adequate surveillance and containment activities on their part. An assessment of any particular risks to successful treatment, such as an alcoholic history or inability to afford care, should be conveyed to those authorities. Referrals for medical care and social services, as needed, should be made before discharge. In the case of a client with infectious tuberculosis leaving a hospital with the obvious intent to avoid treatment, public health authorities should be informed immediately so that attempts to initiate treatment can be made, and legal assistance obtained to confine the client if necessary.

Nursing responsibilities for tuberculosis control extend to the nursing home. Recent investigations "show tuberculosis to be a common endemic and even nosocomial infection in nursing homes." The indication is that new tuberculosis infection in elderly residents is more common than previously thought. Measures should be taken for early detection of new cases of disease to prevent transmission; these include surveillance of tuberculin skin tests of employees and sputum studies in cases of unexplained pulmonary infections failing to respond to usual antibiotics (24).

Nurses working with the homeless in shelters should be aware that this is a group at high risk of tuberculosis. Achieving compliance with a treatment regimen may be a particular problem with these people, and administration of medications should be supervised when possible. Clients in drug and alcohol programs and in jails and prisons should also take medications under supervision. Jails and prisons offer particular surveillance and containment challenges because of the high risk of tuberculosis in the population and the increased probability of transmission because of crowded conditions.

Etiology—The Mycobacteria

The causative agent of tuberculosis is *Mycobacterium tuberculosis,* a species of the genus *Mycobacterium* that includes many human pathogens, one of which is *M. leprae,* the organism that causes leprosy. The mycobacteria are bacilli (rods) and are acid-fast. *M. tuberculosis* is a slow-growing, strict aerobe and thrives best in organs with relatively high oxygen tension. It produces niacin; a niacin-positive test is one means of differentiating it from other mycobacteria in the laboratory.

A second species causing tuberculosis in humans is *M. bovis.* Tuberculosis control programs for cattle and pasteurization of milk have been so effective that human infection with *M. bovis* is now rare in developed countries.

A number of other mycobacteria are known to cause human disease; these have often been referred to as "atypical" mycobacteria. Most notable among these are *M. avium-intracellulare* and *M. kansasii.* It is useful for the nurse to have some knowledge of these, particularly as it is often difficult initially to distinguish their disease processes from that of tuberculosis.

M. avium-intracellulare (MAC), or *M. avium* complex, is a grouping of two closely related organisms, *M. avium* and *M. intracellulare.* They can cause pulmonary disease with cavitation closely resembling tuberculosis, lymphadenitis, and disseminated disease. Although the organisms have been isolated from soil, water, and animals, there is little information as to routes of transmission or infection. It is not thought that person-to-person or animal-to-person transmission is likely. Many investigators believe that environmental organisms of MAC are the most important source of infection in humans with pulmonary disease resulting from inhalation of infectious aerosols from water, soil, or dust (19, 26).

MAC pulmonary disease has usually occurred in older white men; geographically the highest incidence has been in the southeastern United States and in the North Central and Pacific regions, with a large proportion of patients from rural areas. Predisposing factors are chronic pulmonary disease, such as chronic obstructive pulmonary disease (COPD), bronchiectasis, previous tuberculosis, or silicosis. Increasingly, disease caused by *M. avium-intracelluare,* particularly disseminated, is being seen in clients with AIDS (19).

Diagnosis of MAC disease requires repeated isolation in the laboratory of multiple colonies of the organism, or isolation of the organism from a closed lesion handled under sterile conditions. Evidence of disease compatible with the diagnosis, which has not been otherwise explained, should also be demonstrated (2, p. 350).

Not all MAC infections progress; some clients improve spontaneously and some reach an equilibrium with the disease. An MAC infection might be the result of a temporary colonization of preexisting cavities and poorly drained areas. Therefore, it is suggested that in a case where immediate treatment is not required, measures to improve pulmonary hygiene be undertaken, after which bacteriologic studies should be repeated. Such measures can include, as appropriate, cessation of smoking, bronchodilator therapy for those with reversible obstruction, antibiotics for those with purulent secretions, and chest physiotherapy. Those with progressive disease are unfortunate, as MAC infections are generally highly resistant to chemotherapy. Treatment regimens used have ranged from triple-drug therapy similar to that used in treatment of tuberculosis, to use of five- or six-drug regimens for clients with advanced or disseminated disease. Resectional surgery is also used in some cases (19, 26).

M. kansasii also causes disease difficult to distinguish from tuberculosis, but it differs from MAC in that it is susceptible to treatment with antituberculosis drugs. M. kansasii is more commonly found in the midwestern and southwestern states. Even in geographical areas with greater prevalence of M. kansasii, it is MAC-caused disease that is being seen in AIDS clients (26).

Transmission

Tuberculosis is transmitted person to person through shared air space. It is not transmitted by hands, dishes, glasses, utensils, or fomites.

When a person with active pulmonary tuberculosis coughs, M. tuberculosis is expelled in tiny droplet nuclei. These droplet nuclei are so small (1 to 10 μm) that air currents keep them airborne and disperse them throughout the room. Tuberculosis clients also shed larger droplets containing numerous bacilli; these play no part in disease transmission. They either fall to the ground or, if inhaled, are caught on the mucociliary blanket and swallowed or expectorated without penetration of the respiratory system. Infection can result when the tiny droplet nuclei are inhaled by a susceptible host and pass beyond the mucociliary protective mechanism to the alveoli.

People who have previously been infected are thought to be largely protected from reinfection by specific immunity mediated by T lymphocytes (18, pp. 701–2).

Tuberculosis is not a highly infectious disease. Clients vary in degree of infectiousness, but for transmission to occur, close, prolonged, or frequent contact is generally necessary.

Pathophysiology

After the tubercle bacilli reach the alveoli, they can multiply with no initial resistance from the host, as they produce no toxins or tissue reaction. The organisms are slowly engulfed by phagocytes but remain viable within them. The bacilli spread through the lymphatic channels to regional lymph nodes and through the bloodstream to other sites. Organisms deposited in areas with high oxygen tension, the apices of the lungs, the kidneys, and bone epiphyses, find an environment favorable to their multiplication. Bacilli reaching the liver or spleen, where oxygen tension is low, seldom affect those organs (18, pp. 701–2).

After several weeks specific immunity mediated by T lymphocytes develops. The characteristic tissue reaction then develops, with epithelioid cell granulomas and caseation necrosis in the pulmonary lesion and in any sites to which the bacteria have spread. This tissue reaction is the result of the cell-mediated response of the host to the living bacilli. Although in a small number of people the initial infection progresses directly to clinical illness, in most instances the acquired immunity limits further multiplication of the bacilli, and the lesions heal by a combination of resolution, fibrosis, and calcification. These lesions may remain dormant for life, or bacilli persisting within them may begin to multiply rapidly and develop progressive disease at any time. The disease is characterized by nodular infiltrations (the tubercles for which it is named), fibrosis, and cavitation (18, pp. 701–2).

The most common site from which active tuberculosis develops is the apical portion of the lung. Cavitation and liquid necrosis, containing abundant bacilli, are produced as the disease progresses in the lungs; these bacilli can then be expelled into the environment to begin the infectious cycle again.

Approximately 15 percent of the tuberculosis cases seen in the United States are extrapulmonary. The incidence of cases of extrapulmonary tuberculosis has not been decreasing as rapidly as that of pulmonary tuberculosis (13, p. 11). In clients with AIDS, extrapulmonary tuberculosis, particularly disseminated, is more common than in other client populations. The most commonly involved areas are the pleurae, lymph nodes, genitourinary tract, and skeletal system; also affected are the central nervous system, the pericardium, and the peritoneum (15). Tuberculosis is not normally infectious from these sites.

Miliary tuberculosis occurs when tubercle bacilli are massively disseminated hematogenously throughout the body and overwhelm defenses to become established in many organs. This manifestation is named for the diffuse, uniform nodules produced, which appear the size of millet seeds on a chest x-ray. The massive dissemination can happen shortly after the initial infection, or years or even decades later from reactivation of a dormant lesion. Even organs that do not have a high oxygen tension become involved, and the prognosis is poor if therapy is not adequate.

Of new tuberculosis infections, 5 percent to 15 percent progress to serious disease within five years if not treated, with the greatest risk occurring the first year after infection. Among those remaining well for five years, a further 3 percent to 5 percent may develop active disease later in life (18, p. 701). A variety of conditions involving compromised immunity are associated with an increased risk of development of active tuberculosis. These include concomitant illness, administration of corticosteroids or cytotoxic agents, alcoholism, and malnutrition. Clients with AIDS, diabetes, or silicosis, or those who have undergone gastrectomy have an increased risk. Children under six years of age also have higher susceptibility.

Assessment and Diagnostic Tests

The onset of tuberculosis can be insidious, and some cases are detected as a result of a routine x-ray. However, most clients with active tuberculosis case-find themselves. Signs and symptoms that may cause a person to seek medical attention include malaise, excessive fatigue, fever, and weight loss. Night sweats, profuse sweating caused by defervescence during sleep, may occur. The client with pulmonary tuberculosis frequently has a cough, which may be productive of green or yellow sputum raised principally in the morning. Hemoptysis may also occur.

Signs and symptoms of extrapulmonary tuberculosis are related to the site of the disease. Genitourinary tuberculosis may present with recurrent urinary tract infections with no growth of common bacterial pathogens, pyuria without bacteriuria, or hematuria. Males may develop epididymitis; females, irregular menses, pelvic inflammatory disease, or infertility (12). Tuberculosis of the cervical or supraclavicular lymph nodes produces an evident enlargement; hilar or mediastinal lymphadenopathy will be detected by x-ray.

Taking a complete history is essential for assessment.

Questions should elicit information as to the client's past medical history, current signs and symptoms, and medical and social factors that might affect the success of a regimen. Clients should be asked about any previous history of tuberculosis, contact with tuberculosis clients, results of tuberculin testing and chest x-rays.

Prior vaccination with BCG (bacillus of Calmette and Guérin) should be noted. BCG vaccine was originally derived from an attenuated strain of M. bovis and first administered to humans in 1921. BCG is recommended for use in the United States in only rare instances, but it is used on a large scale in many other areas of the world, particularly in the developing nations. There are a number of BCG vaccines in use today that vary in effectiveness and degree of tuberculin sensitivity. One study reported in 1979 that followed 115,000 persons in India for seven and a half years showed no evidence of protective effect of the BCG vaccine administered (17). Other trials conducted before 1955 showed protection ranging from 0 percent to 80 percent. As the efficacy of BCG vaccination is uncertain, recommendations call for tuberculin tests to be administered when indicated, despite history of BCG vaccination. As it is not possible to distinguish whether a reaction to a tuberculin test is due to BCG or to tuberculosis infection, and as many persons vaccinated with BCG have come from areas where risk of tuberculosis infection is high, the size of the tuberculin reaction and the need for therapy should be assessed in the usual way (14).

The standard tuberculin skin test for diagnosis of tuberculosis infection is the intradermal Mantoux test. The test is based on the hypersensitivity reaction to injected tuberculin exhibited because of the development of specific immunity after tuberculosis infection. The material injected, purified protein derivative of tuberculin (PPD), is a protein fraction of tubercle bacilli. When PPD is injected intradermally, an induration of the skin owing to edema and accumulation of sensitized lymphocytes occurs and is at its peak in forty-eight to seventy-two hours. The incubation period between infection by the tubercle bacillus and development of the hypersensitivity that is demonstrated by a positive reaction to the tuberculin test is two to ten weeks (2, p. 344).

Several multiple-puncture devices are used in tuberculosis screening. These may use either PPD or Old tuberculin (OT), from which PPD is purified. They all differ from Mantoux tests in that the material injected is not a measured dosage, and results are not as reliable. Positive results from a multiple-puncture test should be confirmed by a Mantoux test, with the exception of a vesiculated reaction. Multiple-puncture tests are not recommended for the diagnosis of tuberculosis infection.

Good technique in administration of a Mantoux test is essential for reliable results. The tuberculin is injected through a plastic syringe with a ¼- to ½-inch, 26- or 27-gauge intradermal needle. The syringe should be filled immediately before the test is to be done to avoid adsorption of the tuberculin into the plastic.

The amount of tuberculin used is 0.1 ml of 5 tuberculin units (TU) PPD; 5 TU is the strength of the solution, which is also referred to as intermediate strength. Sometimes a 250-TU solution is used when a 5 TU fails to produce a reaction that was predicted on clinical evidence. Epinephrine should be available for emergency use.

The site usually used is the volar surface of the left forearm, just below the upper third. The person to be tested should be seated, with the arm resting on a firm, well-lighted surface. The person administering the test should draw the skin of the site taut between the thumb and index finger. The needle should be held bevel upward almost parallel to the skin, and the tip inserted just below the skin surface. Resistance should be felt as the tuberculin is injected, and a tense wheal, 6 to 10 mm in diameter, produced. If a wheal is not produced, the injection was too deep; if a substantial portion of the tuberculin leaks from the site, the injection was too shallow. In either case the test should be immediately repeated at another site at least 5 cm away (21).

The test should be read in forty-eight to seventy-two hours. Only the induration should be measured; the erythema that usually accompanies the reaction has no clinical significance. The margins of the induration should be found by touch, and the transverse diameter of the induration measured and recorded in millimeters. If difficulty locating the margins is encountered, it is often helpful to inspect the reaction in a cross-light.

In most areas of the United States a reaction of 10 mm or more is considered positive or significant; a person with a reading of that size is a reactor. Other species of mycobacteria can cause cross reactions to tuberculin testing. The cut point of 10 mm has been statistically determined to discriminate between tuberculosis infection and cross reactions in most areas of the United States. The larger the size of the reaction, the more likely it is to represent infection with M. tuberculosis.

For tuberculosis suspects (people with clinical evidence of disease) and contacts of clients with sputum-positive tuberculosis, a 5-mm test is considered significant.

It is particularly important to detect newly infected clients, as the greatest risk of breakdown with active disease occurs in the first year or two after infection. A person who has a significant tuberculin skin test for the first time, after having had negative tests in recent years, is a converter and has been infected in the period since the last negative test. A converter is more specifically defined as "a person whose tuberculin reaction changes from less than 10 mm in diameter to 10 mm or more in diameter and increases by at least 6 mm within a period of 2 years" (3).

A phenomenon known as the booster effect can confuse the detection of new infections. Tuberculin hypersensitivity may gradually wane over the years, and a person tested at that point may have a tuberculin reaction read as not significant. However, that test may boost the hypersensitivity so that a subsequent test is significant, producing the illusion that a conversion has occurred. For this reason it is recommended that two-step testing be done initially in a program where periodic tuberculin testing of adults is to be done. If the first test is negative, or not significant, a second test is given a week later. If the second test is not significant, then a significant reaction in the future can be assumed to be due to new infection. If the second test is significant, it is probably due to a boosted reaction from a previous infection.

In some cases the tuberculin test is negative despite the presence of tuberculosis infection. Clients who are seriously ill, including with tuberculosis, may have a suppression of the reaction to tuberculin as well as other hypersensitivity reactions. AIDS, live virus vaccination, neoplastic disease, sarcoidosis, and immunosuppressive therapy may also cause anergy, and therefore a negative tuberculin reaction in an infected person. A tuberculin test should be done as soon as possible on an AIDS suspect, as immunosuppression will develop with progression of the disease. Faulty testing technique may also cause negative reactions in infected clients.

A client with a newly significant tuberculin test should be instructed to have no further tuberculin skin tests done. Although the tuberculin hypersensitivity reaction tends to wane over the years, particularly in the elderly, an infected client may remain PPD positive for life. Additional tuberculin tests would not add further information to an assessment of the client's status.

The determination of whether an infection has progressed to disease will usually be made by x-ray and bacteriologic studies, as well as by signs and symptoms. The next step for a client with a newly significant tuberculin test is a chest x-ray.

Chest X-Ray Examination

Until the 1970s mass community chest x-ray screening was accepted for the detection of tuberculosis. The American Lung Association offered free x-rays to the general population on mobile vans, and health department codes required routine x-ray screenings of various occupational groups. Eventually the yield of active disease from these mass screenings was found to be very low. With increasing concern about radiation exposure, the decreasing prevalence of tuberculosis in the United States, and the reliability of the tuberculin skin test in detecting infection that has not yet progressed to disease, the skin test became the screening method of choice.

However, the chest x-ray remains very important in the diagnosis of tuberculosis. When a person presents with a history or symptoms suggestive of tuberculosis, or a significant tuberculin test, a chest x-ray should be ordered. The abnormality most suggestive of tuberculosis is a multinodular infiltrate with cavitation in one or both of the upper lobes of the lung, although other lobes can be involved. In the client with AIDS, infiltrate may be in any long zone, and cavitation is uncommon. Comparison of current films with others done months or years earlier is particularly valuable, as changes are evidence of the activity of the disease.

Bacteriology

X-ray examination can provide presumptive evidence of tuberculosis, but bacteriologic examination is required for conclusive evidence. The client with a productive cough should be instructed to submit at least three successive early-morning specimens of sputum before treatment of tuberculosis is started. The single morning specimen is preferred to a twenty-four-hour pooled specimen, to avoid overgrowth of contaminants. The client should be encouraged to submit sputum collected after deep coughing and to minimize saliva and nasal secretions. Inhaling steam from a kettle or a bathroom shower might be helpful for some clients who have difficulty raising sputum. Sputum should be collected only in sterile containers and delivered to the laboratory as quickly as possible. Specimens that cannot be delivered immediately should be refrigerated.

If a client does not spontaneously produce sputum, specimens can be obtained by inducing coughing by having the client inhale hypertonic sodium chloride or normal saline solution aerosolized by a nebulizer. Portable ultrasonic nebulizers that can be taken to a client's home are available and are particularly useful when clinic or office facilities do not permit protection of other clients during or after the induction procedure. Specimens produced by induction are watery and should be labeled "induced sputum," to prevent the laboratory's mistaking them for saliva. Sometimes gastric aspiration is used to obtain gastric specimens containing swallowed sputum. This procedure should be done on a fasting stomach before the client has begun to move around in the morning and is usually done for hospitalized clients. Bronchoscopy is done in cases where there are diagnostic problems and specimens may be obtained during the procedure by washing or brushing. Extrapulmonary specimens examined in the bacteriology laboratory include urine, blood, and tissue specimens obtained by biopsy.

The initial procedure used to identify mycobacteria in the specimen is microscopic examination of a stained smear. As mycobacteria are uniquely acid-fast, visualization of acid-fast bacilli under the microscope is evidence of their presence. The various species of mycobacteria cannot be distinguished from one another on a smear; therefore, a definitive diagnosis of tuberculosis cannot be made at this point. However, when findings of acid-fast bacilli on smears are considered with other clinical evidence, a presumptive diagnosis is often made at this point and treatment is started. Conclusive evidence of the presence of *M. tuberculosis* requires growing the organisms in culture and identifying them by differential tests. In addition, specimens containing too few bacilli to be seen on a slide can grow on culture. Conventional methods usually require six to eight weeks before a culture positive for *M. tuberculosis* can be reported; newer methods may permit the report of a positive culture in less than one month. Properties of the culture that are considered for differentiation include growth rate, pigmentation, nitrate reduction, niacin production, and colony morphology. A positive niacin test may be reported by the laboratory with the final reading, as it is such a strong indication of the presence of *M. tuberculosis;* however, certain strains of atypical mycobacteria may also be niacin positive (5).

If a culture is reported as growing mycobacteria other than tuberculosis, certain laboratories can go on to specifically identify which mycobacteria are present. This information can be significant, as some species are more likely to be pathogens and others, to be contaminants.

In extrapulmonary tuberculosis other procedures, such as biopsy and computed tomography scan, may be done. Physical examination alone may not contribute significantly to a diagnosis, but a complete examination is necessary before treatment is begun.

Overview of Management

Treatment of tuberculosis is on an outpatient basis, with hospitalization indicated only for illness too serious to be managed at home, or for diagnostic or medication problems.

The objective of chemotherapy is to kill the bacilli without permitting multiplication of drug-resistant organisms. Even in a population of bacilli susceptible to antituberculosis drugs, a natural mutant that is resistant may occur. To prevent multiplication of these mutants, treatment of tuberculosis is always by at least two drugs. For this reason also, if a regimen is failing, two new drugs rather than one should be added (6).

Drugs should be chosen to which susceptibility is likely. Drug resistance can be primary or acquired. Primary drug resistance occurs in people who have not previously been treated for tuberculosis. Drug-resistant bacilli may have been transmitted and caused disease. Acquired drug resistance occurs in people who have previously been treated, usually because of poor compliance with the medication regimen, or because of a poorly chosen regimen. The incidence of primary drug resistance is relatively low in North Americans, but it is more common in other groups, particularly Asians and Hispanics. Drug resistance should be suspected and susceptibility studies ordered in the laboratory when a client has been previously treated, has been exposed to resistant disease, or is of a group with high prevalence of resistance, or when culture-positive sputum persists after three months of therapy.

The bacteria are thought to exist in the body in several populations that differ in metabolic rates and susceptibility to treatment, the slower growing being more difficult to eradicate. Because of the slow growth rate, and the possibility that some organisms exist in a dormant state, treatment is lengthy and is always for periods that extend past the bacteriologic conversion from positive to negative that can be seen in the laboratory.

Bactericidal drugs are preferred to bacteriostatic. The treatment regimen is shorter when they are used. The regimen selected should be highly effective, with a relapse rate no greater than 5 percent acceptable in the United States, and should have a low risk of toxic effects (23).

When possible, tuberculosis medications should be taken in a single dose before breakfast for maximum effect on the bacilli.

The regimen of antituberculosis chemotherapy recommended by the American Thoracic Society and the Centers for Disease Control as first choice today, for compliant patients with susceptible organisms, consists of two months of isoniazid (INH), rifampin, and pyrazinamide (PZA), followed by four months of INH and rifampin. If INH resistance is suspected, ethambutol may also be given during the first two months. INH and rifampin are both bactericidal and relatively nontoxic; PZA is bactericidal in an acid environment and does not cause a significant increase in toxicity when added to a regimen of INH and rifampin. Ethambutol is bacteriostatic. Recommended drugs for the initial treatment of tuberculosis in children and adults are listed in Table 29.1.

During the first two-month phase of treatment, medications are taken daily. During the second phase the INH and rifampin may be taken daily or twice weekly. This intermittent therapy is recommended particularly when a compliance problem exists and there is a need to supervise the administration of medications.

A nine-month regimen of INH and rifampin is also highly successful and was the standard until the newer six-month regimen. As with the shorter regimen, if INH resistance is suspected, ethambutol should be given along with the INH and rifampin, until drug susceptibility studies are reported. After an initial two months of daily therapy, the medications may be given daily, or twice weekly, if given under supervision.

For clients with AIDS, the first-choice regimen is INH, rifampin, and PZA or ethambutol for two months, followed by a minimum of seven additional months of INH and rifampin, or at least six months after culture conversion to negative.

Isoniazid and rifampin are the treatment of choice for pregnant women with tuberculosis, as the teratogenic potential of PZA has not yet been evaluated (7). A third drug, ethambutol, is added if isoniazid resistance is suspected.

The six-month regimen is thought to be as effective for extrapulmonary tuberculosis as for pulmonary, but as this has not yet been established by clinical trial, longer therapy may be used for lymph node, bone, or joint disease. The nine-month regimen is generally effective for extrapulmonary disease, but in some instances, as in tuberculou meningitis, which is particularly life-threatening, three rather than two drugs are used.

Other medications used for antituberculosis chemotherapy are more limited in usefulness, either because

Table 29.1
Recommended Drugs for the Initial Treatment of Tuberculosis in Children and Adults

Drug	Dosage Forms	Daily Dose*		Maximal Daily Dose in Children and Adults	Twice Weekly Dose		Monthly Cost†		Major Adverse Reactions
		Children	Adults		Children	Adults	Daily	Twice Weekly	
Isoniazid	Tablets: 100 mg, 300 mg‡§; Syrup: 50 mg/5 ml; Vials: 1 g	10 to 20 mg/kg PO or IM	5 mg/kg PO or IM	300 mg	20 to 40 mg/kg Max. 900 mg	15 mg/kg Max. 900 mg	Less than $1	Less than $1	Hepatic enzyme elevation, peripheral neuropathy, hepatitis, hypersensitivity
Rifampin	Capsules: 150 mg, 300 mg‡§; Syrup: formulated from capsules, 10 mg/ml	10 to 20 mg/kg PO	10 mg/kg PO	600 mg	10 to 20 mg/kg Max. 600 mg	10 mg/kg Max. 600 mg	$13 to $21	$4 to $6	Orange discoloration of secretions and urine; nausea, vomiting, hepatitis, febrile reaction, purpura (rare)
Pyrazinamide	Tablets: 500 mg§	15 to 30 mg/kg PO	15 to 30 mg/kg PO	2 g	50 to 70 mg/kg	50 to 70 mg/kg	$19 to $48	$17 to $32	Hepatotoxicity, hyperuricemia, arthralgias, skin rash, gastrointestinal upset
Streptomycin	Vials: 1 g, 4 g	20 to 40 mg/kg IM	15 mg/kg‖ IM	1 g‖	25 to 30 mg/kg IM	25 to 30 mg/kg IM	$23 to $27	$16 to $20	Ototoxicity, nephrotoxicity
Ethambutol	Tablets: 100 mg, 400 mg	15 to 25 mg/kg PO	15 to 25 mg/kg PO	2.5 g	50 mg/kg	50 mg/kg	$27 to $72	$23 to $36	Optic neuritis (decreased red-green color discrimination, decreased visual acuity), skin rash

Note: PO = perorally; IM = intramuscularly.

*Doses based on weight should be adjusted as weight changes.

†Approximate cost to Health Departments for drugs purchased in quantities based on a 70-kg adult. Data from Alabama, Georgia, Wisconsin, and Chicago for 1984 through 1986.

‡Isoniazid and rifampin are available as a combination capsule containing 150 mg of isoniazid and 300 mg of rifampin.

§ A combination of isoniazid, rifampin, and pyrazinamide in a single capsule is being introduced.

‖In persons older than 60 years of age the daily dose of streptomycin should be limited to 10 mg/kg with a maximal dose of 750 mg.

Source: American Thoracic Society and the Centers for Disease Control. "Treatment of Tuberculosis and Tuberculosis Infection in Adults and Children." *American Review of Respiratory Disease* 134:355–63, 1986.

therapy are more limited in usefulness, either because of necessity for parenteral administration or because of higher incidence of toxic effects (see Table 29.2).

The client must be monitored during treatment both for the effectiveness of the medications and for any adverse effects. The effectiveness of the regimen is best monitored by bacteriology studies. One positive culture should be tested for drug susceptibility. Clients should continue to submit sputum regularly at least until two or three successive negative cultures are obtained. For clients who had smears positive for acid-fast bacilli, a more rapid assessment is provided by the count of acid-fast bacilli reported on serial smears. One suggestion is to have clients submit sputum weekly during the initial course of therapy to permit pinpointing of the time of conversion.

Nursing interventions to prevent or identify adverse medication effects are discussed later in the chapter. Major adverse reactions and recommended regular monitoring are summarized in Tables 29.1 and 29.2.

Prevention and Screening for Early Intervention

Transmission of tuberculosis infection requires three elements: (a) a person with sputum containing viable tubercle bacilli who releases those bacilli by coughing; (b) an air space in which the sputum is aerosolized as droplet nuclei and is suspending and diffused; and (c) a susceptible host who inhales the droplet nuclei. Interruption of the cycle of transmission can be accomplished by interventions dealing with each of these elements.

The infectiousness of a source case can be assessed in several ways. Sputum smears are better indicators of

Table 29.2
Second-Line Antituberculosis Drugs*

Drug	Dosage Forms	Daily Dose in Children and Adults†	Maximal Daily Dose in Children and Adults	Major Adverse Reactions	Recommended Regular Monitoring
Capreomycin	Vials: 1 g	15 to 30 mg/kg IM	1 g	Auditory, vestibular, and renal toxicity	Vestibular function, audiometry, blood urea nitrogen, and creatinine
Kanamycin	Vials: 75 mg 500 mg 1 g	15 to 30 mg/kg IM	1 g	Auditory and renal toxicity, rare vestibular toxicity	Vestibular function, audiometry, blood urea nitrogen, and creatinine
Ethionamide	Tablets: 250 mg	15 to 20 mg/kg PO	1 g	Gastrointestinal disturbance, hepatotoxicity, hypersensitivity	Hepatic enzymes
Para-aminosali-cylic acid	Tablets: 500 mg, 1 g Bulk powder	150 mg/kg PO	12 g	Gastrointestinal disturbance, hypersensitivity, hepatotoxicity, sodium load	
Cycloserine	Capsules: 250 mg	15 to 20 mg/kg PO	1 g	Psychosis, convulsions, rash	Assessment of mental status

Note: For definition of abbreviations, see Table 29.1.

*These drugs are more difficult to use than the drugs listed in Table 29.1. They should be used only when necessary and should be given and monitored by health providers experienced in their use.

†Doses based on weight should be adjusted as weight changes.

Source: American Thoracic Society and the Centers for Disease Control. "Treatment of Tuberculosis and Tuberculosis Infection in Adults and Children." *American Review of Respiratory Disease* 134:355–63, 1986.

infectiousness than are cultures. A sputum smear positive for acid-fast bacilli indicates a higher infectious potential than a negative smear, with the potential increasing in proportion to the number of bacilli present. Cavitation seen on a chest x-ray usually indicates high infectiousness. Frequency of cough and high volume of secretions increase the chance of formation of infectious particles. Poor hygienic habits with failure to cover a cough can make transmission more likely.

Chemotherapy is the most effective means of reducing a client's infectiousness. Antituberculosis medications reduce the number of bacilli present, the amount of sputum production, and the coughing owing to tuberculosis. Clients should be taught to cover the nose and mouth with tissues when coughing or sneezing, and to expectorate into tissues or a covered container. Masks are thought to be of limited value, and if used, they must filter out particles as small as 1 μm and fit snugly around the nose and mouth (2, p. 344; 15).

Infectiousness alone is not an indication for hospitalization. If a patient with active pulmonary tuberculosis is hospitalized, a private room with special ventilation should be used, and masks should be worn by health care personnel in the room if the client coughs. A client who started treatment in a hospital can generally be returned to the same household with instructions to not make new contacts until further assessment. Decisions as to when a client can return to work or other community situations must be made on an individual basis. Serial sputum smears should be assessed for declining numbers or absence of bacilli. It is thought that even if there are limited numbers of bacilli in the sputum, the risk of transmission is small when the client is receiving adequate chemotherapy (1). Reduction in cough and other signs and symptoms also indicates response to therapy. Generally, it is thought a client need not be isolated after two to three weeks of therapy (13). The susceptibility of the contacts and the nature of the environment in the situation to which the client would be returning should also be considered. Greater caution would be exercised in returning a nursery school teacher to her classroom than in returning a construction worker to an outdoor site.

The second element required for transmission is an air space shared by a source case and his or her contacts. The volume of shared air is critical, as infection becomes more likely with an increased concentration of infectious particles in the air. A contact in physical proximity to a source case in a small room is at greater risk than a contact situated at a distance in a large area. Ventilation is an important factor, with fresh air being es-

sential to reduce the number of airborne bacteria. Tuberculosis is not spread on fomites, and sterilization or disposal of dishes, utensils, or clothing is not useful.

The third element required for transmission is the susceptible host. Clients who have been infected with tuberculosis in the past have a lower risk from a new exposure to tuberculosis bacilli. The nature of the contact's exposure to the source case is critical, with increased frequency and extent of time in the same air space increasing the risk of transmission.

Prophylactic treatment with INH can intervene to prevent development of disease in the infected. Such preventive therapy is thought to work by decreasing the small bacterial population present. Clinical trials have shown a reduction of the incidence of tuberculosis in clients who have tuberculosis infection by 70 percent to 80 percent during a year of INH. A 50 percent reduction in incidence was shown to extend at least twenty years, with evidence that the level of protection actually exceeded 90 percent for those who took most of the prescribed medication (8, p. 1285).

Most clinical trials of INH have been of twelve months' duration, but good evidence suggests six months of prophylactic therapy gives comparable protection (19, 22). Therefore, current recommendations call for six to twelve months of preventive therapy to decrease the risk of tuberculosis (7).

Clients with new significant tests and negative chest x-rays are offered INH prophylaxis unless contraindicated. The benefits of INH prophylaxis for clients who are not newly infected must be weighed against the risks of INH-related hepatitis. A younger person has the expectation of more years in which tuberculosis can develop. An older person has a greater risk of hepatitis.

Although there has been controversy about INH prophylaxis for reactors under the age of thirty-five who are not newly infected, most medical authorities advise that the benefits outweigh the risks in this situation (8, p. 129S). Reactors over the age of thirty-five who do not have other risk factors, including recent infection, are not generally offered INH. Other clients who will be offered INH prophylaxis are reactors with x-ray evidence of old tuberculosis disease not previously treated, and reactors who have compromised immunity, and HIV reactors of any age. Table 29.3 summarizes indications for preventive therapy.

Nursing Diagnoses

The primary nurse will derive nursing diagnoses particular to an individual client from the data base accumulated by the assessment of the client's physical status and

Table 29.3
Preventive Therapy

Indications

1. Household members and other close associates of newly diagnosed patients
2. Newly infected persons
3. Significant tuberculin skin test reactors with abnormal chest roentgenogram
4. Significant tuberculin skin test reactors with special clinical situations (steroids, diabetes, silicosis, gastrectomy, etc.)
5. Other significant tuberculin skin test reactors up to age 35
6. Other significant tuberculin skin test reactors over age 35 only in special epidemiologic situations

Contraindications

1. Progressive tuberculosis disease (more than one drug needed)
2. Adequate course of INH previously completed
3. Severe adverse reaction to INH previously
4. Previous INH-associated hepatic injury
5. Acute liver disease of any etiology

Special Attention

1. Concurrent use of other medications (possible drug interactions)
2. Daily use of alcohol (possible higher incidence of INH-associated liver injury)
3. Current chronic liver disease (difficulty in evaluating changes in hepatic function)
4. Pregnancy (prudent to defer until post-partum unless contact, new infection, or other urgent indication)

Note: HIV positive clients of any age who are infected with tuberculosis should be offered preventive therapy.

Source: Tuberculosis—What the Physician Should Know. New York: American Lung Association, 1982, Table 4.

the health and social history. Statement of further nursing diagnoses may be necessary as problems evolve during the lengthy treatment period. Nursing diagnoses that will commonly apply to the tuberculosis client are as follows:

· Anxiety related to the possibility of infecting others
· Potential for new infection related to close, prolonged, or frequent contact with a client with active pulmonary tuberculosis

· Potential for injury related to adverse medication effects
· Potential noncompliance with the therapeutic regimen related to:
—knowledge deficit regarding use of medications
—knowledge deficit regarding expected behaviors
—other health problems
—social problems
—lack of access to health care services

Planning and Implementation

This discussion of nursing interventions is related to the nursing diagnoses identified above.

□ *Anxiety Related to Infectiousness.* The distinction between infection and active disease should be explained to all clients with new significant skin tests. Most newly infected clients will be concerned as to whether they can infect others. Such clients should be told that a significant test means only that some tuberculosis bacteria have entered their bodies, or infected them, and that in most cases those bacteria remain dormant for life. Only in the small percentage of people in whom the infection has progressed to active pulmonary disease can infection be transmitted.

The client with active pulmonary disease can be reassured that most clients are noninfectious after two to three weeks of medication. Results of serial sputum cultures showing response to therapy can be shared with the client as additional reassurance.

The route of transmission should be explained, and clients taught to cover the nose or mouth with tissues when coughing or sneezing, and to expectorate into tissues or a covered container. Although the client with active pulmonary disease can also be advised that tuberculosis is generally not a highly infectious disease, and that close, prolonged, or frequent contact usually is necessary for transmission, it is appropriate to tell such a client to not make new contacts during the first two or three weeks of therapy.

□ *Potential for New Infection.* Newly infected clients are identified by a careful investigation of the contacts of an infectious source case. The nurse designing a contact investigation should start by assembling an extensive data base. Information relating to the infectiousness of the source case should be gathered and evaluated. The source case should be interviewed for identification of people with whom he or she had regular contact and to whom infection may have been transmitted. Many clients experience fear and embarrassment at naming contacts, and much reassurance may be required. Contacts listed should not be confined to other household members; work or other community contacts may have spent as much or more time with the source case. It may be necessary to visit a workplace or other community setting to gather data about a shared environment. The assembled data base can then be used to divide contacts into groups with higher and lower probabilities of being infected. All the factors affecting transmission should contribute to this assessment: infectiousness of the source, size and ventilation of the shared environment, and frequency and extent of contact should all be considered. People with the highest risk of infection should then be skin-tested. If evidence of new infections is found, the investigation should be progressively extended through lower-risk contacts until the rate of infection found approximates what is to be normally expected in that community. Clients with compromised immunity, who are at higher risk of developing disease if infected, should also be given high priority for evaluation. Children under six years of age should always be considered to be at increased risk of development of disease and of serious consequences, such as tuberculous meningitis.

Clients found to have positive skin tests should have chest x-rays to exclude the possibility of tuberculosis pulmonary disease. Contacts with any clinical suggestion of tuberculosis should also be given x-rays, as a negative skin test can be due to anergy. All contacts with negative skin tests should be retested ten to fifteen weeks after contact is broken or the source is rendered noninfectious.

All contacts with positive skin tests and negative chest x-rays should be offered INH prophylaxis unless contraindicated. Contacts with a particularly high probability of transmission or of serious consequences of disease, such as children, and people sharing a household with an infectious source, are offered INH even if the initial testing is negative. The INH is continued until the repeat test three months later, at which time it can be discontinued if the test is negative. For clients thought to be infected with INH-resistant organisms, preventive therapy with rifampin can be considered (8, p. 131S).

Present-day chemotherapy can reduce the transmission and incidence of new cases of tuberculosis, but the extent of its effectiveness will depend on the skill with which those for whom medication is indicated are identified, and on the willingness and ability of the clients

to adhere to a regimen with regularity. Identification of those to be treated and their attitude toward a regimen will often depend, to a large degree, on the skill of the primary nurse.

□ **Potential for Injury—Adverse Medication Effects.** The instruction the primary nurse gives to a client about his or her medication regimen is vital to the success of that regimen. The client must understand how to take the medications, as well as be aware of symptoms of adverse effects. The primary nurse should see clients at least monthly, at which time monitoring can be continued and teaching reinforced.

Monitoring for adverse medication effects starts with obtaining baseline data. Blood values, particularly liver function tests, must be determined, as some of the medications can be hepatotoxic. A uric acid baseline is necessary for the client who will be receiving pyrazinamide. Auditory tests should be done if the client is to be given streptomycin; visual tests are necessary for ethambutol administration.

Isoniazid can cause hepatitis and peripheral neuropathy. INH-associated hepatitis is rare in clients under twenty and increases with the age of the client to a frequency of up to 2.3 percent in clients over the age of fifty (6). Because INH-associated hepatitis can be fatal if the drug is continued after it occurs, clients should be given only one month's supply of the medication at a time. Clients should be monitored for signs and symptoms of hepatitis at each monthly visit and should be advised to call immediately if malaise, anorexia, nausea, vomiting, fever, or jaundice occurs. Clients should also be aware that alcohol intake, especially on a daily basis, may increase the risk of hepatitis. If hepatitis is suspected, the medication should be discontinued and blood drawn for liver function tests: serum glutamic oxalacetic transaminase (SGOT), serum glutamic pyruvic transaminase (SGPT), serum bilirubin, and alkaline phosphatase. Although minor elevations can be transient even if INH is continued, use of the drug should be reconsidered if the results of any of the tests are three to five times the normal value.

Peripheral neuropathy during INH administration can occur owing to competition of the INH with pyridoxine, and it is more common in such clients as alcoholics, whose nutrition is impaired. Pyridoxine can be given with INH as prophylaxis.

Rifampin can also be hepatotoxic, and effects should be similarly monitored. The nurse supervising a regimen that includes rifampin should refer to current literature about the many possible drug interactions. Care should be taken to advise clients that rifampin may inhibit the effect of oral contraceptives. Knowing that rifampin colors urine and other body secretions orange, and that contact lenses can be discolored can spare a client needless anxiety.

Pyrazinamide is another potentially hepatotoxic drug and can also result in hyperuricemia. Acute gout is rare.

Streptomycin can cause auditory nerve damage; hearing should be monitored during administration. Ethambutol can cause optic neuritis, which is reversible when the medication is discontinued; color discrimination and visual acuity should be monitored.

□ **Noncompliance.** Noncompliance with the prescribed medical regimen is a particular problem in tuberculosis control, largely because of the extended length of time required for treatment. Clients are asked to take medications for months past the time they feel well again. Failure to complete a regimen for treatment of active disease can result in relapse, necessitating a retreatment regimen that may be more complex and toxic because of drug resistance. Clients who are on a prophylactic regimen are asked to take medications even though they were never ill. Failure to adhere to a prophylactic regimen may not be detected until much later, when a client develops disease.

Responsibility for compliance with a regimen is shared. It is the health care provider's responsibility to give the client the tools necessary to choose appropriate behaviors. The primary nurse working with a client on a tuberculosis regimen should provide information that enables the client to understand what is required of him or her, why it is important, and how to carry out the required behaviors. The client should be helped to feel capable of performing the expected tasks and to identify and deal with obstacles to compliant behavior. Public health officials have the responsibility of assuring that clients with infectious tuberculosis are treated and rendered noninfectious.

The nurse should collect data during the initial history that will enable identification of potential compliance problems. Note should be made of clients with a history of noncompliance. Other health problems, alcohol or drug abuse, and social problems will all affect a client's motivation and ability to comply. Transient or homeless clients present particular problems for delivery of services and in being monitored. Plans to attempt to deal with such preexisting problems should be formulated, and appropriate social service referrals made.

Enhancement of compliance begins with education. Information given to a client must be presented in a way that is appropriate for the individual client's level of comprehension and language. Interpreters of foreign languages should be provided when necessary. Because the amount of information a client will retain at one setting is limited, selectivity of information presented is important. The behaviors required and the benefits to be derived should be identified. The client's comprehension of what is being taught should be periodically assessed. Written material that the client can take home to review verbal instructions is very helpful.

Community resources should be identified for the client. Health department tuberculosis control programs may provide clinic services and medications. Social services may provide transportation or assist in finding more appropriate housing. Clients who are usually outside the health care system, such as undocumented aliens, should have resources for medical care made available to them.

Nurses who manage clinics that deliver services to tuberculosis clients have an opportunity to improve client compliance. Clinic schedules and settings should be planned for easy accessibility for the community. Public transportation should be available. The interval between the time of referral and the appointment, and the waiting time in the clinic should be kept to a minimum. A consistent clinic staff will help to allay the client's anxiety. Availability of translation will improve attendance of those who speak foreign languages. Sending appointment reminders and calling those who did not keep appointments are useful actions.

One indication of compliance is how well appointments are kept. Some tuberculosis programs and clinics have devised creative methods to improve compliance. Contracts to be signed by both provider and client have been used. A reward system, in which the client is actually given a "prize," has been tried. A clinic lottery for which only those who attend are eligible is another suggestion. Certificates of completion of treatment can offer a tangible goal for the client.

Compliance with the medication regimen can be monitored in several ways. The direct method is to measure blood or urine levels of the drugs and their metabolites. A dipstick method to detect INH metabolites in the urine is simple and easy to do in a clinic or home setting.

An assessment of the client's response to therapy gives important information about compliance, but it cannot be relied on alone. A client may take enough medication to convert to sputum-negative cultures but not enough to prevent later relapse. A compliant client may fail to show improvement because of drug resistance. Clients should be asked during interviews, in a nonthreatening way, if they have missed any doses of medication. Pill counts can also be made, either by having the client bring the supply to appointments or during home visits. Public health authorities should be consulted about compliance problems. They have a responsibility to protect the community and may have other resources to draw on.

If consideration of all these factors leads to an assessment of noncompliance, the primary nurse should initiate problem solving. The client should first be invited to state his or her perception of the problem and to participate in seeking a solution. Some problems may be readily resolved. If the client complains of side effects of medications, he or she may be advised to take the drug with meals or to split doses. If lack of transportation is a problem, family members or social services might assist. If misinformation is the problem, teaching and providing written material may be the solution. Home visits can be helpful to elicit problems and solutions, and the increased attention alone may improve a client's motivation. Other team members should also be called on to identify problems and solutions. The support of a family member, the assistance of social services, or an adjustment in the medication regimen by the physician might remove an obstacle to compliance.

Direct supervision of administration of medications may be necessary for some clients. Intermittent administration of medications twice weekly, rather than daily, is more practical in some instances. Some of these clients spend time in settings where nurses are available to supervise, such as drug and alcohol rehabilitation programs, or shelters. Other clients might be required to come to clinics or offices for supervision, or home visits might be made by nurses or outreach workers.

If all strategies fail and an infectious client continues to be noncompliant with a medication regimen, the primary nurse should seek advice from public health and legal authorities regarding confinement of the client for treatment. This is a difficult step to take and is done only as a last resort, but it may be necessary for the protection of the community. The ability to confine a client will vary in different communities, depending on local laws and statutes, the availability of facilities for care, and the willingness to cooperate of court and law officials.

Evaluation

Measures that can be used to evaluate effectiveness of nursing interventions are discussed below.

Anxiety Related to Infectiousness. The client will verbalize understanding of the likelihood of infecting contacts and will demonstrate appropriate hygienic or isolation measures to prevent transmission. Manifestations of anxiety will be decreased.

Potential for New Infection. Newly infected contacts will be identified and offered prophylaxis. Contacts with a particularly high probability of transmission, or of serious consequences of disease, will be offered prophylaxis. The final group of contacts tested will have a rate of infection approximating what is expected in that community.

Potential for Injury—Adverse Medication Effects. The client will verbalize signs and symptoms for which to observe. Signs and symptoms of adverse effects will be identified by the primary nurse, and further complications avoided.

Noncompliance. The client will complete the prescribed course of therapy. Indications that the client is taking the medication may include appropriate measurements of blood and urine levels of drugs and their metabolites, whether appointments with health care providers are kept, the positive assessment of the provider, and the response to therapy.

Ethical and Legal Issues

Reporting cases of tuberculosis is a legal requirement in every state of the United States. Report is made by providers of care, including hospitals, laboratories, and physicians, to the local public health authorities. Very often, reporting is actually implemented by nurses acting as representatives of institutional providers. Compliance with the requirement is necessary for protection of the community in regard to the person being reported, and also for effective planning of surveillance and containment of tuberculosis in the community at large. Other requisites include investigation of contacts and measures to assure that clients receive treatment that renders them noninfectious. Local public health departments coordinate all these surveillance and containment activities and will require periodic sharing of information by providers.

Along with responsibility for the client's best interests, the nurse working with a tuberculosis client has responsibility for the safety of the community and for fulfilling requirements of public health law. At times the interests of the client may appear to conflict with the interests of the community. The nurse may be called on to share with others information that the client would have preferred be kept confidential. An instance is a situation in which the employer of an infectious client must be given enough information for the implementation of an investigation of contacts at the work site. The person being treated for tuberculosis may not want his or her employer to know. The nurse in this situation must be aware of his or her legal obligations and must understand how much information must be shared to permit an effective investigation. Decisions have to be made to best serve individuals, community, and legal interests. Perhaps in this instance a responsible person who could describe the nature of the contact of the other employees could be told who the source case is. The other employees might then be given information about the possibility of transmission, which omits the identity of the source.

Many such situations will occur in which the conventional concept of confidentiality, or the client's perception of his or her own best interests, does not coincide with the nurse's obligation to the community and with what is called for by public health law. The challenge presented is difficult. Effective resolution of these situations begins with a primary nurse who is equipped with adequate knowledge of the disease process and of legal obligations. Skillful and compassionate application of nursing skills and ethical sense can produce solutions that best serve all interests.

CASE STUDY

Mrs. Carter, a twenty-six-year-old mother of two children, ages four and seven, works part-time as a waitress in a local diner. Three weeks ago she began to have a fever accompanied by a persistent cough. She lost five pounds during this time.

Her twenty-eight-year-old husband, John, insisted that she seek help, despite her belief that aspirin, cough syrup, and rest would cure her problem.

When Mrs. Carter was seen by the primary nurse and the physician, a Mantoux tuberculin test was done and a chest x-ray was taken. The result was an 18-mm area of induration. The chest x-ray showed a subapical infiltrate of the left lung.

An interview with Mrs. Carter revealed that she had coffee with two neighbors each morning after the children had gone to school. The only other people with whom she regularly came into contact were two other waitresses and the cook at the diner.

1. Describe your role as the primary nurse in controlling the spread of tuberculosis in this situation.
2. What ethical and legal issues are associated with intervention designed to control the spread of tuberculosis?
3. Noncompliance with the therapeutic regimen is a potential problem for Mrs. Carter. How might you intervene early to prevent noncompliance?

REFERENCES

1. American Thoracic Society. "Guidelines for Work for Patients with Tuberculosis." *American Review of Respiratory Disease* 108:160–61, 1973.
2. American Thoracic Society. "Diagnostic Standards and Classification of Tuberculosis and Other Mycobacterial Diseases." *American Review of Respiratory Disease* 123:350, March 1981.
3. American Thoracic Society. *The Tuberculin Skin Test—1981.* Washington, D.C.: Public Health Service, March 1981, 7.
4. American Thoracic Society. *Tuberculosis, What the Physician Should Know.* Washington, D.C.: Public Health Service, 1982, 14.
5. American Thoracic Society. "Levels of Laboratory Services for Mycobacterial Diseases." *American Review of Respiratory Disease* 28:5, July 1983.
6. American Thoracic Society. *Treatment of Tuberculosis and Other Mycobacterial Diseases, American Review of Respiratory Disease* 127(6):790, 1983.
7. American Thoracic Society and Centers for Disease Control. "Treatment of Tuberculosis and Tuberculosis Infection in Adults and Children." *American Review of Respiratory Disease* 134:355–63, 1986.
8. Bailey, William, Richard Byrd, Jeffrey Glassroth, Philip Hopewell, and Lee Reichman. "Preventive Treatment of Tuberculosis." *Chest* 87:128S, February 1985.
9. "Centennial: Koch's Discovery of the Tubercle Bacillus." *American Review of Respiratory Disease* 125 (supplement):123, 1982.

10. Centers for Disease Control. "Guidelines for Short-Course Tuberculosis Chemotherapy." *MMWR* 29:97–105, 1980.

11. Centers for Disease Control. *Tuberculosis in the United States, 1980.* Atlanta, Ga.: Public Health Service, 1983, 2.

12. Farer, Laurence S. "Incidence and Epidemiology of Tuberculosis in the 1980s." In *Guidelines for the Diagnosis of Tuberculosis Infections,* ed. L. Reichman et al. New York: Audio Visual Medical Marketing, 1984.

13. Farer, Laurence S. "Infectiousness of Tuberculosis Patients." *American Review of Respiratory Disease* 108:152, July 1973.

14. Farer, Laurence S. "Prior BCG Vaccination and PPD Skin Test." *Journal of the American Medical Association* 250:3105, December 9, 1983.

15. Felton, Charles P. "Extrapulmonary Tuberculosis." Presented at *Tuberculosis Update—1985,* a Symposium for Health Care Professionals sponsored by the New York Lung Association, October 22, 1985.

16. Guyton, H. Gerald, and Herbert M. Decker. "Respiratory Protection Provided by Five New Contagion Masks." *Applied Microbiology* 11:66–68, January 1963.

17. Indian Council of Medical Research. "Trial of BCG Vaccines in South India for Tuberculosis Prevention: First Report." *Bulletin of the World Health Organization* 57:819–27, 1979.

18. Iselbacher, Kurt, Raymond Adams, Eugene Braunwald, Robert Petersdorf, and Jean Wilson, eds. *Harrison's Principles of Internal Medicine.* 9th ed. New York: McGraw-Hill, 1978.

19. Iseman, Michael, Raymond Corpe, Richard O'Brien, David Rosenzweig, and Emanuel Wolinsky. "Disease Due to *Mycobacterium avium-intracellulare.*" *Chest* 87:139S–42S, February 1985.

20. IUAT. "Efficacy of Various Durations of Isoniazid Preventive Therapy for Tuberculosis." *Bulletin of the World Health Organization,* 60:555, 1982.

21. Lunn, John A. "Administering and Reading the Mantoux Test." *Guidelines for the Diagnosis of Tuberculosis Infection,* Morris Plains, N.J.: Parke Davis, 1984, 20–21.

22. Snider, Dixie, David Cohn, Paul Davidson, Earl Hershfield, Margaret Smith, and Frank Sulton. "Standard Therapy for Tuberculosis." *Chest* 87:118S, February 1985.

23. Snider, D. E., G. J. Caras, and J. P. Koplan. "Preventive Therapy with Isoniazid." *Journal of the American Medical Association* 255:1579, 1982.

24. Stead, William, et al. "Tuberculosis as an Endemic and Nosocomial Infection Among the Elderly in Nursing Homes." *New England Journal of Medicine* 312:1483–87, June 6, 1985.

25. "Tuberculosis—United States, 1984." *MMWR* 34:302, May 31, 1985.

26. Wolinsky, Emanuel. "Other Mycobacterial Infections—A Problem of Growing Concern." Presented at *Tuberculosis Update—1986,* a Symposium for Health Care Professionals sponsored at the New York Lung Association, October 22, 1986.

CHAPTER 30

Adults with Hypertension

ROSEMARY COLLINS

■

OBJECTIVES

After completing this chapter, the reader will be able to:

- Define hypertension according to current standards.
- State and discuss the major risk factors related to hypertension.
- Identify and describe the types and classifications of hypertension.
- Discuss the physiologic mechanisms that control blood pressure in normotensive and hypertensive clients.
- Describe the clinical manifestations of mild, moderate, and severe hypertension.
- Identify nursing's role in hypertension prevention and screening.
- Apply the nursing process to clients with any stage of essential hypertension.
- Describe strategies and approaches to promote self-care and decision making for lifelong hypertension control.
- Identify and discuss major ethical issues as they relate to care of clients with hypertension.

Hypertension is most simply defined as high blood pressure. The condition is suspected when the blood pressure measurement exceeds the normotensive level for people within defined age-groups. In adults, blood pressures exceeding 140/90 mm Hg are considered abnormal. Hypertension can be classified into three groups: systolic, diastolic, or systemic. In systolic and diastolic hypertension an elevation of only one respective pressure level occurs, either the systolic greater than 140 mm Hg, or the diastolic greater than 90 mm Hg. Table 30.1 presents the recommended scheme for classifying systolic and diastolic hypertension according to blood pressure levels. Systemic hypertension is established when both the systolic and the diastolic measurements are elevated, greater than 140/90 mm Hg.

Because the variability of blood pressure is well known, a single reading is insufficient basis for a diagnosis. In the early stage of development, hypertension may be a *labile* or intermittent process, until it gradually becomes *sustained*. Sustained or definite hypertension is determined when pressure measurements are consistently above 95 mm Hg diastolic or 160 mm Hg systolic. Lesser pressure elevations are described as *borderline* or prehypertension condition.

Detection and control of hypertension is an individual and a public health concern. Elevated blood pressure is clearly recognized as a high cardiovascular risk (38). In particular, hypertensive clients are predisposed to early death from stroke, cardiac disease, or renal failure. This attributable risk increases proportionately as systolic and diastolic pressures rise. Clients with diastolic pressures in excess of 105 mm Hg are regarded to have three times greater mortality (34).

Since the 1960s a dramatic decline has been noted in the cardiovascular mortality rate related to hypertension (53). Other favorable indicators have been an increase in public knowledge about and attitudes toward blood pressure control, and an increase in patient visits to physicians for treatment of high blood pressure and hypertensive heart diasease (18). Much still remains to be accomplished. Hypertension has to be further publicized as a serious disease, not accepted as a condition of the times. Active screening and education remain a concern among high-risk groups and people with limited access to health care.

For clients identified to be hypertensive, blood pressure control involves a lifetime regimen. Resources are needed to support such clients in their decisions to control hypertension by prescribed pharmacological and nonpharmacological therapies. Attitudes of family, friends, and health care professionals can become strong motivators. Hypertension's attributable risks warrant continuing efforts to reduce blood pressure in as many people as possible.

Hypertension is a prevalent ambulatory illness, reported to affect 20 percent of the U.S. adult population. Among groups within the general population, this prevalence may greatly vary. Familial history, involving both parents or a sibling, is one of the best predictors of hypertension. People between twenty-five and fifty-five

Table 30.1
Classification of Hypertension

	Classification
Diastolic Blood Pressure (mm Hg)	
< 85	Normal blood pressure
85–89	High normal blood pressure
90–104	Mild hypertension
105–114	Moderate hypertension
≥115	Severe hypertension
Systolic Blood Pressure (mm Hg)*	
< 140	Normal blood pressure
140–159	Borderline isolated systolic hypertension
≥160	Isolated systolic hypertension

*When the diastolic blood pressure is less than 90 mm Hg.

Source: From The 1984 Report of the Joint National Committee on Detection, Evaluation, and Treatment of High Blood Pressure. U.S. Department of Health and Human Services. NIH Pub. No. 84-1088, June 1984.

years of age usually develop diastolic hypertension, while isolated systolic hypertension is seen most often in people over sixty-five years of age. Generally the incidence of hypertension directly correlates with advancing age and related atherosclerotic vessel changes. Table 30.2 presents other associated sociodemographic factors related to sex, race, age, income, and education. Research still needs to examine the interrelationships between several of these factors. Vigorous detection, counseling, referral, and hypertension follow-up measures are clearly needed within the black population, which has a prevalence and disproportionate severity of hypertension.

More than 90 percent of hypertensive adults have *essential,* or primary, hypertension, which has no discernible cause. *Secondary* hypertension accounts for less than 10 percent of all hypertensive conditions. This form of high blood pressure is induced by specific etiology and is resolved by treatment of the underlying condition. The term benign is used to describe a very slow course of development; it should not be falsely associated with low morbidity. Malignant hypertension develops abruptly and severely, but given prompt medical treatment, its accelerated course can be reversed. Approximately 1 percent to 5 percent of diagnosed hypertensives develop the malignant form.

Overview of Hypertension

Blood pressure is a product of cardiac function, blood vessel diameter, and intravascular volume or viscosity

Table 30.2
Prevalence of Hypertension
by Major Sociodemographic Factors

Factor	Prevalence
Familial history	Increased by familial predisposition, especially if both parents of a sibling are/were hypertensive
Sex	Increased in males, with female rate inclining
Age	Nearly positive linear relationship between increasing age and incidence
Race	Twice as prevalent within black population as among whites. Severity also greater among blacks.
Income	Increased within low-income groups
Education	Increase related to low education level

(Figure 30.1). Several interrelated physiologic mechanisms operate to maintain normotensive blood pressure. These same factors tend to perpetuate hypertensive states. These mechanisms involve (a) the sympathetic nervous system, (b) autoregulation of intravascular volume, and (c) humoral control.

Sympathetic Nervous System. Stimulation of the vasomotor center in the medulla of the brain sets into motion the sympathetic nervous system. Release of norepinephrine at the postganglionic nerve fibers effects short-term vasoconstriction. The adrenal gland also responds to stressors by release of another vasoconstrictor, epinephrine. Internal reflexes are designed to trigger this activity in response to specific physiologic demand. In the presence of elevated blood pressure, factors that may account for an increased sympathetic response must be investigated.

Autoregulation of Intravascular Volume. Any renal condition associated with sodium and fluid retention can produce blood pressure elevation. Conversely, the kidneys exert an antihypertensive action called autoregulation. This compensatory mechanism acts to reduce blood volume by increasing urinary output.

Humoral Control. The kidneys produce and release the enzyme renin under conditions of (a) sodium depletion, (b) decreased renal perfusion, or (c) sympathetic stimulation. Figure 30.2 shows the physiologic conversion of renin to angiotensin I and then to angiotensin II. In turn the adrenal cortex is stimulated to release the hormone aldosterone. As a result, blood pressure will increase owing to vasoconstriction and sodium and water retention. The release of renin will normally cease in high-pressure states. However, conditions that produce renal ischemia will stimulate renin secretion (39).

Secondary Hypertension

The major pathological conditions associated with the development of secondary hypertension include the following:

- Endocrine disorders: primary aldosteronism, Cushing's syndrome, pheochromocytoma, hypothyroidism, hyperparathyroidism
- Renal disease: acute or chronic renal failure, glomerulonephritis, polycystic disease, scleroderma, renovascular hypertension, renin-secreting tumors

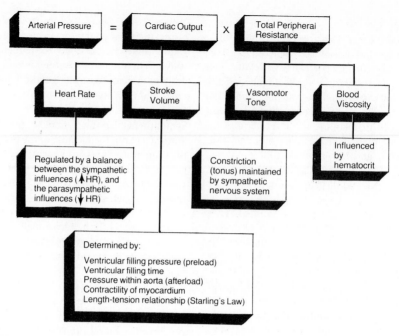

Figure 30.1. Determinants of Arterial Pressure

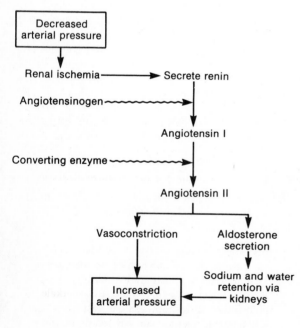

Figure 30.2. Renin-Angiotensin-Aldosterone System

- Coarctation of aorta
- Neurological disorders: increased intracranial pressure, excess catecholamine secretion or stimulation secondary to tumors
- Toxemia of pregnancy

Hypertension can also develop secondary to the ingestion of certain exogenous compounds contained in foods or drugs. Table 30.3 lists common sources of these compounds, which have been implicated as factors in vasoconstriction, sodium and fluid retention, and the elevation of angiotensin II levels. In some of these instances the exact mechanism is not completely understood. Licorice, tobacco, and some liquors, however, are known to contain an aldosteronelike compound (glycyrrhizin) that acts as a pressor agent if ingested in large amounts.

Essential Hypertension

Essential, or primary, hypertension defies explanation; no certain causation has been found. Many theories have been postulated and investigated. Most of these have focused on one or more factors that could create a disturbance in the blood pressure equation: heart rate (HR) × stroke volume (SV) × peripheral vascular resistance (PVR) = blood pressure (BP). Although increased fluid volume or rapid heart rate may be the ini-

Table 30.3
Food and Drugs Implicated in Hypertension

Nicotine	
Caffeine	
Tyramine-containing foods	Chicken liver
	Pickled herring
	Yeast extract
	Beer
	Wines (especially Chianti)
	Matured cheeses (especially cheddar, Brie)
	Broad beans
Over-the-counter sympatho-mimetics	Allergy, cold, and decongestant products
	Alka Seltzer Plus
	Allerest
	Afrin Nasal Spray
	Chlor-Trimeton D
	Coricidin
	Contact
	Dristan
	Sine-Off
	Sinutab
	Sudafed
	Formula 44 D
	Headway Capsules
	Novahistine
	Nyquil
	Triminic
	Vicks Sinex
	Asthma products
	Bronkaid
	Phedral
	Primatine
	Tedral
Prescribed sympatho-mimetics	Epinephrine (Adrenaline)
	Ephedrine
	Isoproterenol
	Phenylephrine (Neo-synephrine)
	Actifed
	Dexedrin (dextroamphetamine)
	Otrivin (xylometazoline)

tial disturbance, sustained pressure elevations are believed to involve increased peripheral vascular resistance. So far there is no common profile for essential hypertension; a mosaic of several interacting factors is most commonly regarded.

Role of Atherosclerosis. The role of atherosclerosis as a cause or result of hypertension remains controversial. Reduction of arterial caliber is associated with atheromatous plaque formation, and this change is evidenced to be underway as early as the second decade of life (48). Yet other studies consistently demonstrate that plaque formation increases in relation to the persistence of hypertension (73). Andrea and others reported structural vascular changes and hypertrophy of smooth muscle in animals exposed to chronic noise (3). This effect has yet to be studied in humans. Other data suggest a hereditary defect in sodium transport and the normal pressure naturesis relationship, such that the kidneys retain sodium and water despite elevated pressures (79). A study by Palfrey indicated that prolonged retention of sodium was induced by isometric exercise in people with mild hypertension, thus potentiating their hypertensive process. Extension of the study to young normotensive males showed no differences in sodium retention or hemodynamic changes, regardless of any familial history of essential hypertension. These data suggest that sodium excretion rates are somehow related to the hypertensive process (57).

Vasomotor Control. Vasomotor control over peripheral vascular resistance is influenced by baroreceptor response to pressure changes sensed within the aortic arch and the carotid sinuses. It is postulated that some hypertensive people experience an upward setting of these baroreceptor set points, which accounts for inappropriate vasoconstriction and sympathetic vasomotor outflow in the presence of elevated blood pressures. Increased vascular resistance may also be the result of vasopressor response.

Plasma Renin. Plasma renin activity assay can be helpful in classifying essential hypertension and selection of appropriate therapy (35, 83). Most people (70 percent) with essential hypertension have normal renin levels. This in fact is considered a true indicator of the condition. Elevated renin levels are usually associated with distinct renovascular pathology, although the increase may also be caused by salt intake, diuretics, oral contraceptives, antihypertensives, severe blood loss, vasodilators, licorice ingestion, or pregnancy. High-renin essential hypertension is uncommon (5 percent to 10 percent), and it is characterized by vasoconstriction with related cardiovascular-renal risks. Clients with primary aldosteronism or Cushing's syndrome typically have low renin profiles. It is also evident in hypervolemia, catecholamine deficiency, and hyperkalemia. Low-renin essential hypertension is found in approximately 25 percent of cases, and it is associated with sodium retention. Classification of essential hypertension according to renin activity in the absence of secondary pathology may give rise to clearer understanding of the etiology.

Catecholamine Effect. Increased levels of norepinephrine in essential hypertension suggest sympathetic overactivity or defective norepinephrine uptake (25). Approximately 5 percent to 10 percent of essential hypertensives have borderline catecholamine levels, without any evidence of pheochromocytoma (10).

Arterial Wall Changes. Early in the course of hypertension there may be no pathological changes. However, multiple changes will probably result from sustained hypertension, usually of more than three months. Large and small arterial structural changes are associated with sustained increase in either systolic or diastolic arterial pressure. Hypertropic changes in the middle arterial layer usually result from systolic hypertension. Damage to the inner lining of the arterioles and edema of the vascular wall is seen in diastolic hypertension. From these similar but characteristic changes atherosclerosis and arteriosclerosis develop. Within the small vessels disruption of the intima results in fibrin accumulation, edema, and intravascular clotting. In larger vessels, especially in areas of high pressure, elastic tissue is replaced by fibrous collagen tissue. The thickened arterial wall becomes less distensible and increases the resistance to blood flow.

The functional effects resulting from arterial wall changes may result in decreased blood supply to the heart, brain, and kidneys. The risk of coronary artery narrowing is greatly increased when moderate or severe hypertension is present in conjunction with diabetes or hypercholesterolemia. When thickening occurs in the major arteries, especially in the upper aorta, greater myocardial work effort is required to overcome the increased resistance to blood flow out of the heart (called increased afterload). Initially the left ventricle will compensate by exerting greater force of ejection. Over time the cardiac muscle fibers will stretch in an attempt to increase the strength of contraction, resulting in left ventricular hypertrophy. This hypertrophy is usually associated with hypertensive heart disease. These changes reflect Starling's law, which states that the more the cardiac muscle is stretched in diastole, the greater the heart will contract in systole. There is, however, a point at which the arterial pressure will surpass the ability of the heart to stretch and effectively contract. When this occurs, cardiac decompensation or congestive heart failure develops.

The kidneys are especially susceptible to damage from vascular hypertrophy and decreased perfusion. As the glomerulus is deprived of renal blood supply, inability to concentrate urine and increased tubular permeability develop and may later progress to renal failure. Sustained rise in arterial pressure may also produce cerebral hypertension. In severe instances necrotizing changes in the small arteries, and aneurysms may result, and the risk may proceed to a massive cerebral infarction.

Retinal changes are an important and reliable index to the severity and prognosis of hypertension. Within the retina pressure-related structural changes in the arteries can be visualized. Minimal or no sclerosis of the retinal arterioles usually implies that the hypertensive condition is either labile or of recent origin. Retinal changes indicative of major organ damage include hemorrhages, exudates, narrowing, and, in severest cases, papilledema.

Clinical Manifestations of Hypertension. Hypertension has been appropriately called the "silent killer," since almost one half of all hypertensive people remain asymptomatic and unaware of their condition.

Occipital headache, apparent on awakening, is often reported as the earliest symptom of hypertensive states. As transient cerebral ischemia develops, complaints of dizziness, light-headedness, tinnitus, and visual changes may be presented. Personality changes, irritability, and memory changes may be indicative of cerebral microinfarctions. Large lesions will produce major strokes.

A high incidence of coronary artery disease is evident within the hypertensive population. Anginal syndrome and palpitations may develop as coronary artery perfusion is diminished. The cardiovascular consequences of severe, sustained hypertension may also include myocardial infarction and aneurysm development within the aorta. As previously described, ventricular hypertrophy develops to compensate for persistently high arterial pressures. As the myocardial strain and oxygen consumption rise, cardiac arrhythmias and early symptoms of congestive failure are seen.

In renal hypertension, increased tubular permeability, hypertrophy, and local edema account for (a) diminished renal perfusion, (b) renal artery stenosis, and (c) tubular dysfunction. These developments are reflected by nocturia and elevated plasma levels of urea and creatinine.

In secondary hypertension, specific clinical manifestations depend on the underlying causative disorder. For example, clients suffering hypertension secondary to pheochromocytoma experience symptoms related to excess circulating catecholamines (chest pain, palpitations, diaphoresis, dilated pupils, weakness, tremors, anxiety).

Complications

Vascular damage is associated with severe hypertension that is poorly controlled and with abrupt discontinuance of medication. If severe, uncontrolled hypertension (diastolic greater than 120 mm Hg) progresses to the accelerated or malignant phase (diastolic greater than 130 mm Hg), fibrinoid necrosing arteriolitis can rapidly lead to organ failure. The target organs for this major hypertensive complication are the brain, retina, heart, aorta, and kidneys. Usually the degree of organ damage correlates well with the level of the pressure. Some clients, however, may tolerate severe pressure elevations without immediate ill effects, whereas others who were previously normotensive may suffer damage from rapid pressure elevations that are only in the moderate hypertension range (12). Generally a diastolic pressure of more than 120 mm Hg is associated with increased risk of imminent organ damage.

Cerebral Effects. Even mildly hypertensive clients have four times the risk of cerebrovascular disease that normotensive clients have. The detrimental cerebral effects of acute hypertension include cerebral infarction, microaneurysms, intracranial hemorrhage, and encephalopathy. The earliest symptom of cerebral damage is occipital morning headaches. As hypertension progresses other signs and symptoms may include fatigue, irritability or agitation, forgetfulness, confusion, numbness or tingling in arms or legs, seizures, and, finally, coma.

Renal Effects. Sudden, extreme blood pressure elevations can also cause severe vasoconstriction of the kidneys' arterioles. The resulting impairment of renal circulation accounts for symptoms of nocturia, proteinuria, azotemia, hematuria, and, eventually, renal failure, if untreated.

Cardiac Effects. Hypertension also increases myocardial oxygen consumption and workload. The chronic result may be left ventricular hypertrophy, with even greater oxygen need demands; heart failure eventually develops. Common symptoms involve dyspnea, cough, diaphoresis, anxiety, and diminished exercise tolerance.

Symptoms indicative of progression to the stages of pulmonary edema are cyanosis, wheezing, moist rales, blood-tinged frothy sputum, and the presence of third and fourth heart sounds. Other cardiovascular sequelae of hypertension are coronary artery disease and the formation of aortic aneurysms.

Retinal Effects. Examination of the client's retinal arteries can provide a reliable index of the severity and prognosis of hypertension. Using the Keith-Wagner-Barker scale, retinal findings are classified into one of five grades. Soft cotton-wool exudates and hemorrhage, in addition to retinal edema and arteriolar narrowing, are present in grade III, hypertensive retinopathy. It is indicative of severe chronic hypertension. The finding of papilledema signals the onset of severe retinopathy (grade IV) and is diagnostic of malignant hypertension.

Acute complications owing to severe blood pressure elevations constitute a clinical emergency, requiring aggressive treatment. Manifestation of hypertensive encephalopathy, intracranial hemorrhage, or heart failure is most critical. The first treatment priority is immediate reduction of the blood pressure. Even potent diuretics often have little effect, since most hypertensive emergencies are vasoconstrictive states. Sodium nitropusside (Nitrostat) is considered the drug of choice, since it lowers the pressure within seconds, regardless of the cause. Its administration requires special preparation and careful monitoring for smooth blood pressure reduction to the desired level. Other rapid-acting agents are available, including diazoxide (Hyperstat), hydralazine (Apresoline), trimethaphane (Arfonad), labetalol (Normodyne, Trandate), clonidine (Catapres), propranolol (Inderal), phenoxybenzamine (Dibenzyline), and, most recently, nifedipine (Procardia). The effectiveness of each of these medications is limited to certain hypertensive emergency situations.

Risk Factors

Life-style factors, such as high dietary sodium, physical inactivity, obesity, excess alcohol intake, emotional stress, and elevated serum cholesterol, must be considered in hypertension risk. Several population studies relate high salt intake to a high incidence of hypertension (19, 56). This hypertensive effect has been associated with increased vascular sensitivity to pressor agents, increased cellular concentration of ionized calcium, and expansion of extracellular fluid volume (9). Other researchers have identified salt-sensitive hypertensive clients, who demonstrate inappropriately high plasma norepinephrine levels for their level of salt intake (15). Contrasting views have been based on evidence that mild to moderate hypertension often does not respond to sodium restriction (46).

Obesity. Defined as 20 percent above the body mass index (weight/height), obesity is clearly related to hypertension risk. Sedentary life-style and physical inactivity have a marked chronic effect on the tendency toward obesity. This condition is associated with a four to eight times greater risk of developing hypertension (81). Programs of weight reduction can be particularly successful, since weight loss may also be accompanied by a decline in plasma renin and aldosterone (80). Studies have also noted that weight control can reduce the incidence of hypertension by as much as 41 percent (81).

Alcohol Consumption. Habitual alcohol intake is another hypertension risk factor (17). An intake of two beers a day (30 ml ethanol) is reported to produce a consistent blood pressure increment between 2 and 6 mm Hg (65). Higher plasma renin concentrations have also been related to high alcohol consumption.

Stress. A linkage between stressful events and the development of hypertension has also been identified. These stimuli include unpleasant working conditions, competition, and low economic conditions. People with hypertension demonstrate greater anger and hostility than the normotensive population (76).

The diagnosis of hypertension has itself been implicated as a source of high anxiety (70). It is, however, thought that underlying personality traits actually determine which situations are stressful and the response of individuals to the situation.

Personality Profile. While no clear-cut personality profile has been formulated, it has been identified that adeptness in social skills, adaptability, and flexibility are important to the maintenance of normotension (71). Failure in appropriate use of these skills and coping mechanisms in highly competitive or stressful situations strongly correlates with the development of hypertension. Data also note that some people display a high degree of "engagement," that is, investment or involvement in social transaction (4). The process of engagement can produce either negative or positive effects and emotions. Those who are chronically engaged in predominantly negative transactions generally demonstrate hypertension (4).

Diet and Serum Lipids. It is a popular contention that atherosclerosis constitutes the primary cause of hypertension. At this time there is sufficient evidence to incriminate metabolic processes associated with excess body fats (lipids) as a prominent factor in atherosclerosis development. In major international studies typical American diets ranked second highest in the total consumption of saturated fats (19 percent), producing among the highest levels of blood cholesterol (range 220 to 280 mg/dl) (8).

There is evidence that among the blood's fat protein molecules, low-density lipoproteins and very low density lipoproteins contain the largest portion of cholesterol and triglycerides. Subsequently, elevated low-density lipoproteins increase the risk of hypertension from fatty artery disease.

There is much more to be learned about the optimal levels of cholesterol, low-density lipoproteins, and triglycerides. Although clinical evidence bearing on atherosclerosis is far from complete, elevated triglyceride levels have been associated with diabetes mellitus, high sugar diets, excess alcohol consumption, obesity, and birth control pills. As a risk factor, high blood cholesterol levels can be avoided, controlled, or corrected by diet and, in extreme cases, by drugs. The benefit of physical exercise includes a reduction in serum lipid levels.

Caffeine Consumption. Excess caffeine intake is suggested as a possible risk factor on the basis that it stimulates catecholamine release, which is incidental to vasoconstriction and cardiac excitation. The components of tobacco smoke have also been linked with arterial damage and possibly the development of atherosclerosis. This risk is particularly manifested in chain smokers.

Prevention and Screening for Early Intervention

Nurses, as members of the largest health profession, have many opportunities to conduct hypertension case finding, education, and referral. It is a recognized area of independent nursing practice. Any basis for health care, regardless of the phase or subspecialty, should present an opportunity for blood pressure assessment (78). Nurses may conduct this activity in a myriad of practice settings, including, but not limited to, industrial and corporate organizations, correctional facilities, senior citizen centers and residences, church-sponsored group meetings, and, of course, within their own families and social circles. Nurses' expertise is also needed in the planning, development, and implementation of primary programs. One such program was particularly successful with the involvement of nurses indigenous to the community's culture and operating on a pay-as-you-can fee schedule (11).

To maximize nursing's potential, hypertension must be given special emphasis in basic nursing curricula and continuing education. One of the most important resources for professional information and educational program guidelines is the National High Blood Pressure Program, based in Washington, D.C. (54). Effective participation in primary hypertension care requires (a) basic interpersonal skills, (b) knowledge of predisposing hypertension risk factors, (c) accurate skill in blood pressure measurement, and (d) understanding of the current guidelines for hypertension screening and referral.

Factors That Affect Blood Pressure Measurement. Accurate blood pressure screening begins with the identification and control of any stimuli that may be incidental to pressure elevation. Table 30.4 presents common factors that should be avoided. Environmental location, verbal conversation, and even the presence of medical professionals can produce alterations. Emotional response attributed to a clinic setting or the arrival of the physician has been associated with the occurrence of "office hypertension." Blood pressures taken under usual living conditions by a nurse or a trained family member may be more indicative of the norm. Because verbal activity and the client's emotions can underlie significant pressure elevations, the measurement of blood pressure should precede any efforts to encourage the client to "ventilate" feelings and concerns (47).

Measurement Technique. Reliable pressure measurement requires use of correct and consistent technique. Either an aneroid or mercury sphygmomanometer can be used. The instrument should be well maintained and properly calibrated (aneroid) at least once a year. Table 30.5 presents important criteria for cuff selection. Too small a cuff may result in the classification of normotensives as hypertensives (cuff hypertension), and conversely, using too large a cuff may cause hypertensives to appear normotensive. It is also important to keep the client's forearm positioned at the level of the heart and extended slightly. False low readings occur when the arm is raised above the heart level, and false high readings when the arm is dropped below. In all situations upper arm constriction, by rolled sleeves or a too-tight cuff, should be avoided.

Position the bottom edge of the cuff one inch above the antecubital area, with the bladder over the brachial artery. The cuff should be inflated to a pressure 30 mm Hg above the level at which the radial pulse disappears and then slow deflation begun at a rate of 2 mm Hg per second. The stethoscope head should be applied firmly, but with as little pressure as possible, to the antecubital space over the palpated brachial artery. As seen in Figure 30.3, there are five phases to the Korotkoff sounds.

Systolic pressure should be read at the first regular tapping sound (phase one). An auscultatory gap in phase two may lead to the error of reading a false systolic pres-

Table 30.4
Factors That Influence Blood Pressure Elevation

Apprehension
Cold
Smoking
Pain
Recent large meal
Full bladder
Caffeine
Crossed legs

Table 30.5
Recommendations for Blood Pressure Cuff Selection

Arm Circumference at Midpoint (cm)*	Cuff Size	Bladder	
		Width (cm)	Length (cm)
17–26	Small adult	11	17
24–32	Adult	13	24
32–42	Large adult	17	32
42–50+	Thigh	20	42

*Midpoint of the arm is defined as half the distance from the acromion to the olecranon.

Source: From Recommendations for Human Blood Pressure Determination by Sphygmomanometers. American Heart Association, 1980. Publication 70-019-B, 12-80-100M.

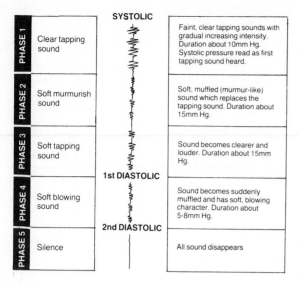

		SYSTOLIC	
PHASE 1	Clear tapping sound		Faint, clear tapping sounds with gradual increasing intensity. Duration about 10mm Hg. Systolic pressure read as first tapping sound heard.
PHASE 2	Soft murmurish sound		Soft, muffled (murmur-like) sound which replaces the tapping sound. Duration about 15mm Hg.
PHASE 3	Soft tapping sound	1st DIASTOLIC	Sound becomes clearer and louder. Duration about 15mm Hg.
PHASE 4	Soft blowing sound	2nd DIASTOLIC	Sound becomes suddenly muffled and has soft, blowing character. Duration about 5-8mm Hg.
PHASE 5	Silence		All sound disappears

Figure 30.3.   Phases of Korotkoff Sounds

sure, perhaps 10 to 30 mm Hg below the true systolic level. Caution being advised, the pressure can be first taken by palpation to identify the true level of the systolic pressure.

Two different numerical points can also be designated as the diastolic pressure. The onset of muffling (fourth phase) should be used as the best index of diastolic pressure in states such as hyperthyroidism or aortic insufficiency or after exercise. Otherwise, the fifth phase, which occurs when sounds become inaudible, should be regarded as the best index of adults' diastolic blood pressure.

If the cuff is not totally deflated between successive measurements, venous congestion will likely produce false elevation of the later measurement. Baseline blood pressure should be the average of two or more measurements. Multiple measurements are recommended when a client demonstrates a high level of engagement (reaction to persons and circumstances) (69). If a significant discrepancy (10 mm Hg or more) is noted between arms, further evaluation should be based on the pressures taken in the arm with the higher reading.

Interpreting Blood Pressure to the Client.   Almost anyone can be trained to take an accurate blood pressure measurement by the manual method. In addition, coin-operated computerized sphygmomanometers and compact electronic blood pressure kits have also been pop-

ularized. Blood pressure measurements taken by nonprofessionals or by electronic devices are a matter of concern for several reasons. These situations may lack necessary explanation and health counseling, be a substitute for important health care visits, or promote client overreaction or overconsciousness about insignificant blood pressure fluctuations (27).

Nurse professionals are recognized to be one of the client's most helpful sources of health information (18). On the occasion of blood pressure measurement, counseling and instruction should include (a) the meaning of the blood pressure's numerical value, (b) recommended follow-up based on the current measurement, (c) desirability of normotensive state to avoid health risks, and (d) identification of controllable risk factors. Follow-up criteria, established by the National High Blood Pressure Program for initial and secondary blood pressure assessment are presented in Table 30.6.

Blood pressure screening does not present as great a problem as the client's need for motivation to carry out subsequent recommendations for follow-up and control. The independent adult must assume an active role if the desired goals for well-being are to be realized. The nurse's interpersonal skills are used to explore the client's understanding of hypertension and its consequences, typical health promotion behaviors and stressors, personal priorities, openness to teaching and counseling, and coping resources. This assessment should include familial and other significant relationships. These people may provide vital forms of social support, including encouragement, companionship, real concern, needed reminders, and practical assistance (transportation to health care site).

Because there is no conclusive causation, there are no guaranteed measures for prevention of essential hypertension. Risk factors relevant to each individual client will become the foundation for preventative intervention. The best overall result may be produced by a family-centered approach, especially if high risks prevail.

General client/family recommendations should include dietary change, regular exercise, weight reduction, and reduction of alcohol intake and cigarette smoking. The nurse should suggest progressive modifications and advise against drastic efforts, which can have recognized dangers and long-term ineffectiveness. As a final observation, nurses should give attention to their own personal behaviors (smoking, obesity, excess caffeine consumption), which may transmit contradictory messages to the client.

Table 30.6
Follow-up Criteria for First- and Second-Occasion Blood Pressure Measurement

Diastolic (mm Hg)	Follow-up	Systolic* (mm Hg)	Follow-up
First-Occasion Measurement			
< 85	Recheck within 2 years	< 140	Recheck within 2 years
85–89	Recheck within 1 year	140–199	Confirm promptly (within 2 months)
90–104	Confirm promptly (within 2 months)	≥ 200	Evaluate or refer promptly (within 2 weeks)
105–114	Evaluate or refer promptly (within 2 weeks)		
≥ 115	Evaluate or refer immediately		
Second-Occasion Measurement			
< 85	Recheck within 2 years	< 140	Recheck within 1 year
85–89	Recheck within 1 year	≥ 140	Evaluate or refer promptly for care
≥ 90	Evaluate or refer for care		

*When diastolic blood pressure is less than 90 mm Hg.

Source: From The 1984 Report of the Joint National Committee on Detection, Evaluation, and Treatment of High Blood Pressure. U.S. Department of Health and Human Services. NIH Pub. No. 84-1088, June 1984.

Nursing Care

Mild to moderate hypertension has a significantly greater prevalence than severe hypertension. Regardless of its stage, essential hypertension presents a chronic health problem; effective interventions promise only control, not a cure. It is a unique opportunity for nurses to demonstrate the fullest scope of professional practice. The goals and objectives for nursing care of hypertensive clients focus on the following:

- Follow-up all clients at recommended intervals.
- Identify, with the client, those controllable factors that contribute to hypertension, and mutually plan toward their modification.
- Assist clients and family to accept diagnosis of hypertension and a lifelong regimen for control.
- Promote self-care patterns in accordance with any prescribed medical treatment.
- Refer the client to available community resources for health management assistance.

- Assess the client's response to specific and overall elements of the therapeutic plan.
- Promptly refer the client for medical treatment of severe or acute blood pressure elevations.

Assessment

In the collection of a data base, the nurse generally focuses on data known to be pertinent to hypertension. However, active listening, sensitivity to client responses, and exploration of cues are more important than any specific format. The major areas of assessment are the health history, physical examination, findings of relevant diagnostic tests, and psychosocial assessment.

Health History. In the health history the client is questioned regarding

- recent or chronic illnesses;
- familial incidence of hypertension or other cardiovascular disease;
- physical complaints, especially morning headache,

dizziness, palpitations, blurred vision, epistaxis, nocturia, or hematuria;

- current weight/height and any recent weight loss or gain;
- known food, drug, or environmental allergies;
- use of current medications, both prescribed and over-the-counter;
- cigarette smoking and efforts to stop;
- daily exercise, either for recreation or work-related, and usual amount of sleep and rest; and
- usual dietary consumption of red meats, cheese, sausage, organ meats, eggs (cholesterol); ham, bacon, luncheon meats, condiments, bakery goods, prepared processed meals, snack foods, or added salt in cooking or seasoning (sodium); and alcohol in any form (wine, beer, mixed drinks).

Physical Examination. Besides blood pressure measurement, the severity of hypertension is evaluated by physical examination. Significant changes or evidence of vascular damage that may be observed, include the following:

- Ophthalmoscopic examination: increased light reflex, narrowed arteries, hemorrhages, exudates, or papilledema
- Neurologic examination: Babinski reflex, hyperreflexia, hemiparesis, or hemiplegia
- Abdominal examination: unilateral mass or abdominal bruit
- Cardiovascular examination: third or fourth heart sounds; carotid, femoral, or radial pulse changes indicative of occlusive disease; tachycardia

The heart and aorta are also examined by means of electrocardiography and chest x-ray.

Pertinent laboratory tests include blood tests (complete blood count; serum levels of potassium, calcium, creatinine, cholesterol, triglycerides, urea nitrogen; and renin–sodium profile) and urinalysis.

When indicated, more specific tests for pheochromocytoma, primary aldosteronism, Cushing's syndrome, or renal disease may be ordered to rule out secondary hypertension.

Psychosocial Assessment. This assessment also provides most important information about the presence and management of stress. The fallacy still prevails, characterizing hypertensive clients as visibly high-strung, tense, and nervous people. But in fact, hypertensive clients may appear calm, relaxed, and placid. Research has shown that increased blood pressure,

tachycardia, and hyperpnea are entirely appropriate responses to stress. At times stress and its accompanying physical changes can make the body perform better. But the same cannot be said of prolonged stress, which contributes to hypertension development. The client's personality plays an important role in reaction to stressful events. Chronic anger is also regarded as predisposing to high blood pressure.

Assessment should include pertinent psychosocial information: (a) relationships with family, friends, and significant others; (b) interrelationships with co-workers, superiors, and the like; (c) nature and degree of domestic, occupational, and social stress; (d) usual reactions to upsetting events and situations; and (e) any recent life crisis. The various reactions of clients to illness and the impact of these reactions must be recognized. Depression, denial, anxiety, or anger may arise on diagnosis of hypertension. Clients' lives are guided by a set of personal norms and values, which includes the meaning of illness and its consequences. The primary nurse needs to gain an appreciation of the clients' life situations and then identify and nonjudgmentally accept their beliefs, perspectives, priorities, and social interests.

Nursing Diagnoses

Hypertension presents many problems, most centering on the client's lack of knowledge or poor adherence to treatment regimens. By synthesis of gathered data, the problems unique to the individual client can be derived. Clinical problems and nursing diagnoses should be differentiated, since primary nurses have varying degrees of authority in their management (13). Within the nursing role the nurse may identify *clinical problems* that require medical collaboration and prescriptive authority, as well as *nursing diagnoses*, for which the nurse can assume direct responsibility.

Examples of clinical problems include (a) mild blood pressure elevation unresponsive to nonpharmacologic interventions, (b) dietary modification for an obese hypertensive client on a diabetic insulin regimen, (c) adverse side effects of antihypertensive drugs, (d) acute pressure elevations or other manifestations requiring urgent treatment and possible hospitalization, (e) exercise limitations in hypertension, complicated by angina or other cardiac pathology.

In the care of hypertensive clients, nursing diagnoses commonly relate to either knowledge deficits or noncompliance (specific). Relating each diagnosis to its causative or contributing factors will give direction to individualized intervention, as presented in Table 30.7.

Priorities of care must be established for clients who have multiple problems. More accurately, priorities of care should address client goals rather than the diagnostic problem statements. Client validation is important in establishing the accuracy of the nursing diagnoses and for mutual goal setting for long-term cooperation. This interactive process responds to clients' individual needs, but some clients may not be willing or able to participate. When a familial predisposition to hypertension is assessed, realistic reduction of controllable risk factors is of major importance.

Planning and Implementation

Nursing care in hypertension is directed toward the control of blood pressure levels by the promotion and maintenance of appropriate client behaviors. Nursing interventions focus on educating, counseling, and supporting clients and their families in the implementation of prescribed regimens for blood pressure control. The intervention for selected nursing diagnoses is presented here.

□ **Knowledge Deficit and General Aspects of Self-Care.** Health education is an intrinsic part of every nurse-client encounter, but still a framework should be

Table 30.7
Nursing Diagnoses in Hypertension

Knowledge deficit related to:

1. Hypertension risk factor(s)
2. Effect/consequences of high blood pressure
3. Weight control
4. Low/moderate sodium diet
5. Low cholesterol diet
6. Stress management and relaxation techniques
7. Self-monitoring of blood pressure
8. Newly prescribed antihypertensive drug(s)
9. Reportable complications

Noncompliance related to:

1. Unpleasant side effects of prescribed drug(s)
2. Complex, prolonged antihypertensive therapy
3. Disbelief that treatment for hypertension is needed
4. Unsuccessful experience with blood pressure control regimen
5. Expense of antihypertensive medication within limited income
6. Nonsupportive family relationships

used to make it a conscious, organized effort. Its effectiveness depends on the relevancy and comprehensibility of the presentation and on the readiness of the client to learn. Teaching methods, both formal and informal, should reflect principles of adult education, with emphasis on the clients' control over their behavior (77). It is helpful to follow prepared guidelines of educational content useful to most hypertensive clients. The nurse must remember, however, that not every client needs, wants, or is capable of learning everything about hypertension. The educational plan must have priorities based on mutually identified needs. A simple questionnaire can be used to identify what the client and family want to know (5).

The reality of self-care is contingent on the client's understanding of what needs to be done. Terminology and educational materials should be suited to the client's level of comprehension. Medical jargon is best avoided, unless the terms can be clearly defined by analogies. A particular educational challenge is presented by the approximately 23 million American adults who are labeled as functionally illiterate (23). The content, presentation method, and the literacy demand of verbal and written instructions must be appropriate if the client is to achieve a reasonable level of self-care. Strategies that meet the client's language, logic, and experience can improve comprehension.

The client's usual sources of health information should be discussed—for example, magazines, newspapers, television programs, families, and acquaintances. Support accurate knowledge and understanding, and correct misinformation. Reinforce learning and promote information sharing with others by the use of printed information and instruction sheets. Materials for specific client needs should be developed. The educational program is aimed at both the client and significant others who are part of the support system.

All pertinent information should not be presented in one session. Effective education requires more than the giving of information. Interpersonal skills are needed to promote an active process on the part of the learner. Learning activities should be designed to assist the client in the application of information for decision making and problem solving (26).

Social support can be a strong positive force in encouraging the client's well-being and her or his acceptance of necessary life-style change. Self-help groups can be especially important when family members are not available or are nonsupportive. Like diabetics and heart attack survivors, people with hypertension can benefit from support groups based on their disease commonality. Some clients may need to be directed to more established groups for specific assistance with alcoholism, overeating, or domestic problems. The National Self-Help Clearinghouse should be contacted for information about local groups or suggestions about how to start new self-help groups.

Knowledge about illness and its treatment does not necessarily lead to positive health behavior. Three premises for client achievement and maintenance of long-term hypertension control are as follows (49):

1. Active client participation favors successful management of high blood pressure.
2. Clients are ultimately in charge, and the responsibility of the professional as health adviser is to assist clients in assuming this role in the decision-making process.
3. Interaction between the professional and client is a critical factor in achieving blood pressure control over a period of time.

The basis for this participation requires that the client and family clearly understand the condition of hypertension and accept responsibility for self-care activities. These self-care activities must be mutually identified as being within the client's physical and psychological ability.

The degree to which clients are willing to follow recommendations is related somewhat to the personal cost associated with them, in terms of depriving self. Treatment of hypertension may interfere with clients' other priorities. It is necessary to use an approach that encourages the client to express concerns and perceptions that may interfere with blood pressure control recommendations. Whenever possible, treatment plans should allow the client as normal a life-style as possible. To be instrumental, nurses must explore ways in which the client can effectively and realistically incorporate recommended activities into daily schedules. While several drastic life-style modifications might be desirable, such a complete change in a person is unrealistic. A priority list for self-care modifications may be recommended by the nurse, but ultimately it will be the client's decision. Ways must be sought to facilitate the client's decision making. For example, the nurse can tactfully assist the client in acknowledging a tendency to make excuses or to rationalize.

The health belief model supports an educational process for blood pressure control. It proposes that a major motivation for undertaking change in health behavior and gaining necessary knowledge is the desire to avoid the perceived threat of disease (6). The nurse should not be an unnecessary alarmist, but he or she should communicate the seriousness of the condition and the importance of following the regimen. Caution must be exercised in this approach. If a fatalistic view is communicated, some clients may believe that there is little they can do to prevent the inevitable (45).

Long-term goals may seem nebulous to the client. Furthermore, the client's effort may not have immediate results that are reinforcing enough to maintain motivation. It is often helpful to formulate a mutual contract that establishes outcomes that are less vague, more observable, and more easily measured. Realistic short-term goals can eventually reach long-term goals, whereas overly ambitious goals may sabotage the possibility of success.

Contingency contracting can support client changes in self-care behaviors. This method uses both goal setting and a system of incentives and rewards to achieve goals. In addition to increased attention from the nurse and social support, many other possible rewards or incentives can be identified. By talking and listening to clients the nurse can find out what is important to them.

☐ *Knowledge Deficit of Proper Diet.* Reduction in dietary sodium is a therapeutic recommendation for most hypertensive clients. In general our society has acquired a taste for sodium, and most adults consume several times the recommended daily intake of sodium (2 g). For this reason the same advice would probably benefit all people, regardless of age, in the prevention of hypertension.

Dietary counseling should be flexible, aimed toward the client's developing sodium control in a diet that still allows eating enjoyment. Long-standing food preparation and eating habits may need to be altered. The client's motivation may be influenced by cultural pattern, attitudes toward meals, and family expectations. Rigid sodium restriction (500 mg/day) is often impractical and unnecessary. Mild to moderate sodium reduction can usually be achieved by reducing intake of processed foods (canned or frozen), cold cuts, milk and milk products, most cheeses, and pretzels, nuts, and other snack foods. Clients are reminded that the sodium content of foods should not be judged by the presence or absence of "salty" taste. Much depends on their ability and willingness to read the sodium content on the package label. Any food containing 1.25 g or more of sodium per serving should be avoided.

Clients can benefit from instruction about preparing economical, palatable foods that are low in sodium content. Numerous cookbooks containing low-sodium recipes are available in bookstores and from public libraries. Client group meetings can include recipe trading, "cooks only" meetings, or potluck low-sodium buffets. Copies of low- and high-sodium food and beverage lists should be available for both clients and family members. Emphasis needs to be placed on the elimination of added salt and the substitution of alternative seasonings, such as onion and garlic. Clients who do not have a history of renal disease and who are not taking either potassium supplements or potassium-sparing diuretics may use salt substitutes, most of which contain potassium.

Adoption of a low-fat diet is also prudently recommended for the general U.S. population. Clients should be advised to consume dairy products in moderation and to substitute fish, poultry, or veal for more fatty meats (beef, pork). If the client's cholesterol or triglyceride levels are elevated, more specific dietary counseling and a calorie-controlled plan are necessary.

☐ *Knowledge Deficit of Weight Reduction Methods.* For some people, weight reduction is the only measure needed to reduce blood pressure. One of the first steps that nurses can take in providing quality care is an assessment of any client's weight. Once the data indicate a need for reduction, a dietary plan is calculated and an exercise regimen prescribed. The long-range goal should be a gradual but steady weight loss until the optimum weight is reached.

As cardiac status and general health permit, clients should be encouraged to engage in one to one and a half hours of mild exercise daily. This not only aids in weight reduction but also helps to release pent-up stress. Suggested activities include walking, golf, bowling, and swimming. For some clients, enrolling in a physical fitness program is desirable.

Some clients are able to diet alone; others benefit from groups. Popular diet programs that emphasize group support are Weight Watchers, TOPS, TRIMS, and Overeaters Anonymous. Total family involvement in fitness and weight control programs can be supportive for the client. Weight reduction may be extremely difficult if the basis for obesity is emotional; psychotherapy may be needed.

☐ *Knowledge Deficit of Stress Management.* Elevated blood pressure is associated with stress. Clients whose jobs involve high psychological demands and little opportunity for personal control and clients with type A behavior are especially subject to stress. Stressful family relationships may contribute significantly to raising a client's blood pressure. Often clients can readily identify their tension-creating situations, but they do not realize that they have any control over the situation.

For general health, clients should be encouraged to realize the greatest possible relaxation from periodic rest periods, after-work recreation, holidays, and vacations. According to clients' individual interests, hobbies or club memberships can be suggested. The importance of a relaxed home environment should be emphasized. Intimacy and agreeable companionship, even the presence of lovable pets, can play a significant role in blood pressure control.

Removing oneself from stressful situations (e.g., changing jobs) may seem to be a reasonable choice of actions, yet some clients find this unacceptable. Such choices might not be necessary if clients learned to handle stress differently. Therapeutic relaxation techniques, practiced ten to twenty minutes once or twice a day, can mitigate stress when avoidance is not possible. Biofeedback, self-hypnosis, rhythmic breathing, and exercise can also produce lasting reduction in blood pressure (24, 82). There is some indication, however, that relaxation techniques are more time-consuming, produce less uniform response, and are not as effective as antihypertensive therapy (16). Tranquilizers may be helpful, but preferably their use should be limited to clients who have extreme anxiety or whose ability to cope is exhausted. Some clients need professional psychological referral. Hospital-sponsored clinics and corporate-based stress management programs have boomed in recent years. Nurses are reminded that clients who face the relentless stress of low income and crowded living conditions may not be able to take advantage of formal stress management programs.

In coping with specific stressors, referral to peer or self-help support groups can be an effective intervention. As presented in Table 30.8, available self-help/peer support groups are as diversified as the human problems that create personal or family stress.

☐ *Knowledge Deficit of Blood Pressure Self-Monitoring.* It has been noted that clients' active involvement in their care improves adherence to therapy (66). Self-monitoring of blood pressure can serve as an adjunct to hypertension therapy. It may help clients to (a) identify factors that affect blood pressure levels, (b) observe the positive effects of therapy, and (c) realize convenience and economic savings from fewer health care appointments. Their periodic reporting of self-monitored blood pressure recordings to the health professional must be part of this program.

Table 30.8
*Self-Help and Support Groups Dealing
with Stressful Life Behaviors or Circumstances*

Stressor	Self-Help/Support Groups
Substance abuse	Alcoholics Anonymous
	For the Alcoholic
	Al-Anon
	Friends and Parents of Renaissance Project
	Pil-Anon Family Program
Dependent family	Project Time Out
	Spouse Support Group
Parenting	Parents Anonymous
	Single Parents: Learning and Sharing
	Families Anonymous
	Tough Love
	Kindred Spirits
Bereavement	Bereaved Parents
	Widowed to Widowed Network
	Families of Homicide Victims Support Group
	Friends and Relatives of Victims of Suicide
	Senior Support Group: Coping with Loss
Miscellaneous	Wellness Support Group

Note: Regional information on self-help and mutual support groups can be obtained from National Self-Help Clearinghouse, Graduate School and University Center/CUNY, 33 West 42nd Street, Room 1206A, New York, New York 10036.

Source: From Westchester Self-Help Clearinghouse. Directory of Self-Help Groups in Westchester County. 1985 Guide to Mutual Support Groups. Valhalla, New York.

Accurate at-home blood pressure recording can be an excellent means of monitoring blood pressure, since it usually provides more representative pressures. Self-monitoring, however, does not always lead to other behaviors designed to control blood pressure (33). Obviously self-monitoring is not acceptable or appropriate for all clients or their families. It may be difficult to convince some clients that variable pressure levels are normal. There is also a possibility that some clients may be inclined to make unprescribed dosage adjustments or discontinue their antihypertensive medications. Although blood pressure measurement is an easily taught skill, treatment decisions regarding self-monitoring require professional examination of the individual client's ability and motivation and the anticipated benefits.

Achievement of long-term blood pressure control ne-

cessitates the continuation of an effective treatment program. Subsequent nurse–client encounters are important to track progress toward hypertension control and to evaluate information retention and behavioral change. Follow-up visits should emphasize the controllable rather than the curable nature of hypertension. Frequency of follow-up visits is guided by the progress toward blood pressure control and the client's need for reinforcement.

☐ *Knowledge Deficit of Antihypertensive Drug Therapy.* There is convincing evidence that antihypertensive drug therapy effectively controls blood pressure. Ideally the result is accomplished without toxic or unacceptable side effects, major disruption of life-style, or great financial expense. Nonpharmacological therapies and surveillance are usually prescribed for mild hypertension, in the absence of multiple risk factors (31). If this approach is ineffective after a limited period of time, antihypertensive drug therapy is then initiated. Generally no one drug or combination of drugs works successfully for all clients. When a choice is available, the drug with fewest side effects, least client inconvenience, least required frequency, and lowest cost is preferred.

Nurses must be knowledgeable about the antihypertensive drugs prescribed for their clients if they are to significantly contribute to the success of the pharmacological regimen. Drug education for clients and their families is essential if their cooperation is to be enlisted. Figure 30.4 presents the recommended stepped-care drug therapy program for hypertension control. This progressive regimen involves initial use of diuretics in increasing therapeutic doses and then the addition of other agents as needed until control is achieved. The drugs that may be used include the following:

- Diuretics: thiazide derivatives, loop diuretics, potassium-sparing agents
- Adrenergic inhibiting agents: beta-adrenergic blockers, central-acting adrenergic inhibitors, peripheral-acting adrenergic inhibitors, alpha-1-adrenergic blockers, combined alpha- and beta-adrenergic blockers
- Vasodilators
- Angiotensin-converting enzymes

Slow-channel calcium entry blockers may be acceptable as step 2 or 3 drugs (78).

The extent of client education about prescribed medications is best guided by assessment of their interest, comprehension, and need to know in the context of what is necessary for safe, effective treatment. The two

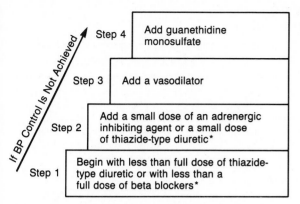

Figure 30.4. Stepped-Care Drug Therapy Program for Hypertension

*Proceed to full dose if necessary and desirable.

Source: Adapted from The 1984 Report of the Joint National Committee on Detection, Evaluation, and Treatment of High Blood Pressure. U.S. Department of Health and Human Services. NIH Pub. No. 84-1088, June 1984.

most important aspects of the drug education program are the prescribed medication schedule and the adverse side effects. Client cooperation is necessary in devising an acceptable medication schedule. Above all other treatment aspects, the continuation of a prescribed medication schedule for as long as ordered should be stressed. Antihypertensive drugs are safe and effective for long-term use.

Drug-induced side effects can occur among any age-group, but they seemingly occur with greatest incidence among clients in their fifties. Most side effects are minor or will disappear as clients adjust to the medication. They can therefore be termed acceptable, since they do not interfere greatly with life-style, a factor that enhances compliance with continued drug therapy.

Clients should always be informed of any common drug side effects that may interfere with work performance, safety, or leisure plans. Side effects associated with antihypertensive drug therapy include decreased mental acuity, weakness, depression, exercise intolerance, nausea, vomiting, and other discomforts (leg cramps, calf pain). Table 30.9 presents side effects of and comments on specific antihypertensive agents.

Client and family education should include the identification of major side effects, actions to minimize any distress, and instructions for contacting the primary care professional. Clients should be clearly advised not to stop their medication without first contacting the physician or nurse.

Some clients may develop acute hypotensive reactions during antihypertensive drug therapy. Clients and their concerned family members should be taught how to prevent these reactions, as well as what to do if they occur. Precautions include the following:

- Avoid standing motionless for prolonged periods of time, since this may cause pooling of blood in the lower extremities. Periodic muscle activity can decrease this effect.
- If faintness, weakness, or nausea occurs, sit or lie down immediately. When lying down, elevate the feet higher than the head and flex thigh muscles and toes to promote cerebral blood flow.
- Always rise slowly from a lying to a sitting position and then from a sitting to a standing position to allow time for the vascular system to adjust to the changes.
- Avoid extremely hot baths, excessive amounts of alcohol, and immobility after exercise, since these conditions may promote blood vessel dilation.
- Avoid constipation, since it may cause either an increased or irregular absorption of the medication.
- Report frequent episodes of postural hypotension. Ace bandages or elastic support stockings may need to be worn to promote blood return from the lower extremities.

Treatment of winter colds and coughs presents a special problem for hypertensive clients. Although labels on cough and cold remedies advise against taking without consulting a physician, clients may not heed this. Preparations containing norephedrine, pseudoephedrine, and antihistamines interact with antihypertensive medications and should not be taken without physician approval (85).

☐ **Noncompliance.** The terms *adherence* and *compliance* are often used to describe clients' maintenance of prescribed regimens. Problems of noncompliance may be characterized by missing scheduled appointments, failure to take medications according to schedule or dosage, failure to report adverse side effects of medication, and lack of effort toward life-style modification. It is reported that approximately half of all clients treated for hypertension do not adhere to the prescribed treatment plan (75). Established educational programs may have no long-term effect on some clients' adherence behavior (64). Smoking and weight reduction are behaviors recognized to be most resistant to change (86).

It is important to distinguish between compliance and the outcome of compliance. Sustained or progressively elevated blood pressures should not be solely interpreted as a measure of nonadherence until validated. For ex-

Table 30.9
Antihypertensive Agents

Agent	Side Effects	Comments

Diuretics
Thiazides and Related Sulfonamides
  Bendroflumethiazide (Naturetin)
  Benzthiazide (Hydrex)
  Chlorothiazide sodium (Diuril)
  Chlorthalidone (Hygroton)
  Cyclothiazide (Fluidil, Anhydron)
  Hydrochlorothiazide (Esidrex, HydroDiuril)
  Hydroflumethiazide (Diucardin, Saluron)
  Indapamide (Lozol)
  Metolazone (Diulo)
  Methyclothiazide (Enduron)
  Polythiazide (Renese)
  Quinethazone (Hydromox)
  Trichlormethiazide (Diurese, Naqua)
	Dry mouth, thirst, weakness, drowsiness, lethargy, muscle aches, fatigue, GI disturbance
	
	Orthostatic hypotension may be potentiated by alcohol, sedatives, or narcotics.
	
	Hypokalemia, hyperuricemia, glucose intolerance, elevated cholesterol and triglycerides
		May be ineffective in renal failure. Hypokalemia increases digitalis toxicity. Hyperuricemia may precipitate acute gout.
		
		Contraindicated in known sensitivity to sulfonamide-derived drugs.

Loop Diuretics
  Bumetanide (Bumex)
  Ethacrynic acid (Edecrin)
  Furosemide (Lasix)
		Effective in chronic renal failure. Caution regarding hypokalemia and hyperuricemia. Hyponatremia may occur in the elderly.

Potassium-sparing Agents
  Amiloride hydrochloride (Midamor)
  Spironolactone (Aldactone)
  Triamterene (Dyrenium)
	Hyperkalemia, skin eruptions, urticaria, sexual dysfunction, mental confusion, gynecomastia (amiloride and spironolactone), ataxia	Danger of hyperkalemia in patients with renal failure.
		
		Decrease dosage if drowsiness, lethargy, confusion, or ataxia occurs.
		
		Give drug after meals to avoid diarrhea and other GI symptoms.

Adrenergic Inhibitors
Beta-Adrenergic Blockers
  Atenolol (Tenormin)
  Metoprolol tartrate (Lopressor)
  Nadolol (Corgard)
  Oxprenolol hydrochloride (Iset, Trasicor)
  Pindolol (Visken)
  Propranolol hydrochloride (Inderal)
  Propranolol long-acting (Inderal LA)
  Timolol maleate (Blocadren)
	Bradycardia, fatigue, insomnia, bizarre dreams, sexual dysfunction, elevated triglycerides, lightheadedness	Contraindicated in clients with asthma, chronic obstructive lung disease, congestive heart failure, heart block, and sick sinus syndrome.
		
		Use with caution in diabetes mellitus and peripheral vascular disease.
		
		Clonidine and guanabenz: rebound hypertension may occur with abrupt stoppage.

Central Adrenergic Inhibitors
  Clonidine hydrochloride (Catapres)
  Guanabenz acetate (Wytensin)
  Methyldopa (Aldomet)
	Orthostatic hypotension, drowsiness, fever, liver damage, anemia, impotence	Methyldopa: may cause liver damage.
		(continued)

Table 30.9 (continued)

Agent	Side Effects	Comments

Adrenergic Inhibitors
Peripheral Adrenergic Antagonists
   Guanadrel sulfate (Hylorel)
   Guanethidine monosulfate (Ismelin)
	Orthostatic hypotension (very common), diarrhea, impotence, loss of ejaculation	Use with caution in elderly because of orthostatic hypotension.

Rauwolfia Alkaloids
   Rauwolfia (whole root)
   Reserpine (Serpasil)
	Drowsiness, lethargy, nasal congestion, bradycardia, depression, gastric hyperacidity	Contraindicated in clients with history of depression, psychosis, obesity, chronic sinusitis, peptic ulcer.

Alpha$_1$-Adrenergic Blocker Prazosin hydrochloride (Minipress)	"First dose" syncope, orthostatic hypotension, weakness, palpitations	Use with caution in elderly because of orthostatic hypotension.
Combined Alpha- and Beta-adrenergic Blocker Labetalol hydrochloride (Trandate, Normodyne)	Nausea, fatigue, dizziness, asthma, headache (rare)	Contraindicated in sick sinus syndrome, heart block. Use with caution in heart failure, asthma, chronic obstructive lung disease, diabetes mellitus.

Vasodilators
   Hydralazine hydrochloride (Apresoline)
   Minoxidil (Liniten)
	Headache, tachycardia, fluid retention	May precipitate angina in patients with coronary artery disease.
		Hydralazine: large doses may produce lupus syndrome.
		Minoxidil: may cause or aggravate pleural or pericardial effusions.

Angiotensin-Converting Enzyme Inhibitors Captopril (Capoten)	Rash, proteinuria, leukopenia, taste change	Can cause reversible, acute renal failure in clients with bilateral renal arterial stenosis.

ample, some clients demonstrating 100 percent adherence to their prescribed medication schedule do not achieve blood pressure control because either the drug choice was ineffective or drug tolerance developed. An 80 percent adherence rate to effective medications was found in one study to be sufficient to achieve the therapeutic goals for the majority of hypertensive subjects. For most people, however, frequent medication times are problematic (33).

Every reasonable effort should be made to determine the cause of noncompliance. The nurse should always convey a nonjudgmental attitude and avoid making assumptions or prejudgments. Some clients may lack consistency of motivation, be angry because of unsatisfied expectations, or be in disagreement with the treatment plan. The quality of the nurse–client interaction may have an effect on adherence. Empathy is essential to the interpersonal relationship. The nurse must sense the client's world and use this perception in a therapeutic manner. Authoritarianism can inhibit this process (29). The therapeutic relationship is a partnership, so decision making and responsibility for outcomes are actually (although disproportionately) shared. Most important of all, clients, even noncompliant ones, must be assured of continued care and support.

Strategies to facilitate compliance appropriately address the cause of the problem. Appointments should be scheduled to accommodate job and family obligations (and conflicts). Date and time of appointments should be verified in writing. On the scheduled day the waiting time should be minimal, if not avoided, and a primary nurse should be available to the client. Outreach programs, involving postcards, phone calls, and, if feasible, home visits, are costly, but they may be needed to reach clients who miss appointments. Adherence to medication schedules can be supported by medication calendars, pill trays, or the association of medication time with routine daily activities. The occurrence of unpleasant side effects is often the basis of noncompliance.

Evaluation

As an initial outcome of the hypertension teaching plan, clients should be able to verbalize (in their own words) an accurate understanding of their condition and the recommended blood pressure goals. These cognitive outcomes will be more readily achieved than the following, which relate to expected change in client behavior:

- Lose weight as prescribed.
- Adhere to a prescribed diet for sodium, cholesterol, or caloric reduction.
- Reduce caffeine intake.
- Participate in a regular program of exercise.
- Reduce (or eliminate) the number of cigarettes smoked.
- Take medication according to the prescribed schedule and dose.
- Eliminate major environmental stressors.
- Incorporate rest and relaxation into daily routines.
- Demonstrate the ability to accurately take one's own blood pressure, if applicable.
- Formulate plans for regular, lifelong follow-up.

Clients who understand the seriousness of their condition or those who are symptomatic will probably be more motivated—or resigned—to these immediate and lifelong expectations. Too many changes should not be approached at once; priorities must be set mutually. To make progress visible, attainable goals should be established and evaluated at each visit. The nurse should convey enthusiasm and commitment about progress toward goal achievement.

The ultimate goal of programs for blood pressure control is to achieve and maintain diastolic pressure at or below 90 mm Hg. A more limited goal may be acceptable for some clients, since the result must be consistent with safety and tolerance. Usually the beneficial effects of antihypertensive drug therapy are not apparent for two weeks or longer. Intervals of two to three months may be allowed before "stepping up" to the next medication level. This approach allows individualization and flexibility; normotensive levels are achieved in more than 80 percent of the client population (78).

The occurrence of minimal, if any, side effects is desired and may be achieved through more effective problem solving. Clients are expected to report their symptoms before altering or discontinuing their medication schedule. When evaluation indicates that the pharmacological regimen is ineffective, further collaboration between the primary nurse and the physician is indicated.

Ethical and Legal Issues

At some point in the care of hypertensive clients, most nurses will ask the frustrating question, "Why won't clients do what is best for them?" (87). This question, with potential underlying authoritarianism, characterizes an ethical dilemma. Past health planning and delivery was largely based on the premise that the health care professional was "in charge" and that the client (then known as the patient) assumed a passive, recipient role. Today there are instead health care consumers, clients, and partners in care. The media and other information sources have educated the adult population about illness and disease, available treatments, and their rights within health care relationships. It has been stated that faith in the health care professional as an authority is also diminished (26).

While nurses seek to offer advice that they regard to be professionally appropriate, clients seek to reach goals that are consistent with their own expectations and priorities. Perspectives differ and recommendations that the nurse regards as being necessary and reasonable may be viewed differently by the client. The values of the nurse may be reflected in the instructions and alternatives that are stressed. Clients' beliefs, values, and social influences may impact significantly on their willingness to follow any recommended treatment or behavior change.

Most clients will balance the consequences of following or not following the recommended treatment. Nurses may be tempted to coerce by arousing fear, threatening rejection, or using force when clients do not accept their recommendations. But such behavior is unethical. Likewise, some clients may try to coerce the nurse.

Negotiation is an ethical and necessary process in the nurse–client partnership for hypertension control. It is a model of mutual participation in which areas of agreement and disagreement are identified and discussed and compromises acceptable to both client and nurse are rewarded. It is characterized by the nurse's high degree of empathy and recognition of the client's individual needs. It encompasses the realization that the nurse does not always know what is best for clients and comprehend the many problems clients face in following the treatment recommendations. Negotiation is a framework that can facilitate conclusion of a satisfactory plan that more closely approximates both the client's and the nurse's goals.

CASE STUDY

Assume that you are the primary nurse in a health center and that you are assessing Mr. Jackson, a 55-year-old owner of a small business in a suburban town. His blood pressure is 146/92, and he is twenty pounds overweight. He tells you that he has had many problems with his business in the past six months, requiring him to work twelve to fifteen hours a day. He is also having problems with his marriage of twenty years. You also learn that he does not exercise regularly and eats often at quick food restaurants. Foods most often consumed include cheese, beef, fried potatoes, ice cream, and beer.

1. How should you respond to Mr. Jackson's blood pressure reading?
2. How does Mr. Jackson's diet compare with current recommendations for a healthy diet? What should Mr. Jackson be taught about the kinds of foods he eats?
3. What are some probable stressors in Mr. Jackson's life? How could you as a primary nurse help him to handle stress effectively?
4. What information should you share with Mr. Jackson about risk factors in hypertension?
5. What is an appropriate response on your part to Mr. Jackson's weight?
6. What can you as the primary nurse do to protect Mr. Jackson's right to autonomy in managing his own health?

REFERENCES

1. Admire, J. B., et al. "Hypertension Control—Meeting the 1990 Objectives for the Nation." *Public Health Reports* 99:300, 1984.
2. American Medical Association, U.S. Department of Environmental, Public, and Occupational Health. *Stress, Work and Health.* Chicago: November 1980.
3. Andrea, L., et al. "Mechanism of the Hypertensive Effect of Noise." *Clinical Science* 61:895, 1981.
4. Baer, P. E., et al. "Assessing Personality Factors in Essential Hypertension with Brief Self Report Instrument." *Psychosomatic Medicine* 41:321, 1979.
5. Barrett, N., et al. "What Patients Really Want to Know." *American Journal of Nursing* 81:1642, 1981.
6. Becker, M. H., ed. *The Health Belief Model and Personal Health Behavior.* Thorofare, N.J.: Charles B. Slack Co., 1974.
7. Black, H. R. "Hypertension Therapy—Prescribe for Compliance: Simplify the Regimen." *Consultant* 24:333, 1984.
8. Blackburn, H. "Risk Factors in Cardiovascular Disease." In *The American Heart Association Heart Book,* ed. R. Hurley. New York: E. P. Dutton, 1980.
9. Blaustein, M. P. "Sodium Ions, Calcium Ions, Blood Pressure Regulation and Hypertension." *American Journal of Physiology* 232:165, 1977.
10. Bravo, E. L., et al. "Clonidine Suppression Test: A Useful Aid in the Diagnosis of Pheochromocytoma." *New England Journal of Medicine* 305:623, 1981.
11. Brown, A. L., et al. "Elevated Blood Pressure Among Harlem Residents." *Nurse Practitioner* 7:27, 1982.
12. Burris, J. F. "Hypertensive Emergencies." *American Family Physician* 32:97, 1985.
13. Carpenito, L. J. *Nursing Diagnosis—Application to Clinical Practice.* Philadelphia: J. B. Lippincott, 1983.
14. Chobian, A. V. "Hypertension—Diagnosis, Complications, Therapy." *Clinical Symposia* 34:3, 1982.
15. Compezi, V. M. "Abnormal Relationship Between Sodium Intake and Sympathetic Nervous System Activity in Salt Sensitive Patients with Essential Hypertension." *Kidney International* 21:371, 1982.
16. Cottier, C., et al. "Treatment of Mild Hypertension with Progressive Muscular Relaxation: Predictive Value of Indexes of Sympathetic Tone." *Archives of Internal Medicine* 144:1954, 1984.
17. Crique, M. H., et al. "Alcohol Consumption and Blood Pressure: The Lipid Research Prevalence Study." *Hypertension* 3:557, 1981.
18. Cunningham, S., et al. "Current Status of Blood Pressure Control." *Nurse Practitioner* 7:37, 1982.
19. Dahl, L. K., et al. "Etiologic Role of Sodium Intake in Essential Hypertension in Humans." *Journal of Experimental Medicine* 118:607, 1963.
20. Daniels, L. M., et al. "Monitoring and Facilitating Adherence to Hypertension Therapeutic Regimens." *Cardiovascular Nursing* 16:2, 1980.

21. Devon, H. A., et al. "Health Beliefs, Adjustment to Illness, and Control of Hypertension." *Research in Nursing and Health* 7:10, 1984.

22. Dickson, E., et al. "A Hypertension Follow-up Program . . . Nurses Can Dramatically Increase Patient Cooperation and Compliance." *Nursing Health Care* 4:508, 1983.

23. Doak, E., L. G. Doak, and J. H. Root. *Teaching Patients with Low Literacy Skills.* Philadelphia: J. B. Lippincott, 1985.

24. Dowdall, S. A. "Breathing Techniques That Help Reduce Hypertension." *RN* 40:73, 1977.

25. Esler, M., et al. "Norepinephrine Kinetics in Essential Hypertension: Defective Neuronal Uptake in Some Patients." *Hypertension* 3:149, 1981.

26. Falvo, D. R. *Effective Patient Education: A Guide to Increased Compliance.* Rockville, Md.: Aspen Systems, 1985.

27. Flynn, J. B., et al. "Coin-operated Sphygmomanometers." *American Journal of Nursing* 81:533, 1981.

28. Forsyth, G. L. "Exploration of Empathy in the Nurse-Client Interaction." *Advances in Nursing Science* 2:53, 1979.

29. Forsyth, R. A. "Hypertension—Criteria for Diagnosis and for Initiating Therapy." *Consultant* 24:306, 1984.

30. Foster, S. B., et al. "Influence of Side Effects of Antihypertensive Medications on Patient Behavior." *Cardiovascular Nursing* 14:2, 1978.

31. Freis, E. D. "Should Mild Hypertension Be Treated?" *New England Journal of Medicine* 307:306, 1982.

32. Gelfont, B. "Hypertension Protocol." *Nurse Practitioner* 8:25, 1983.

33. Haynes, R. B., D. Taylor, and D. Sackett, eds. *Compliance in Health Care.* Baltimore: Johns Hopkins University Press, 1979.

34. Helgeland, A. "Treatment of Mild Hypertension—The Five Year Study." *American Journal of Medicine* 69:725, 1980.

35. Hollifield, J. W. "Essential Hypertension—Renin Levels as Guides for Therapy." *Consultant* 18:147, 1978.

36. Houston, M. C. "Hypertension—Examining Dietary Sodium as Cause and Therapy." *Consultant* 25:235, 1985.

37. Janz, N. K. "Contingency Contracting to Enhance Patient Compliance: A Review." *Patient Education and Counseling* 5:165, 1984.

38. Kannel, W. B. "Some Lessons in Cardiovascular Epidemiology from Framingham." *American Journal of Cardiology* 37:269, 1976.

39. Kaplan, N. M. "Mechanism and Pathophysiology of Essential Hypertension." In *Current Update: Aldomet in the Management of Hypertension,* ed. M. H. Maxwell. West Point, Pa.: Merck, Sharp & Dohme, 1978.

40. Kasanoff, D. "Mild Hypertension: Treat All Patients?" *Patient Care* 17:171, 1983.

41. Kerr, J. A. "Adherence and Self Care . . . Patients Treated for Hypertension." *Heart & Lung* 14:24, 1985.

42. Langford, H. G. "Drug and Dietary Interaction in Hypertension." *Hypertension* 4:166, 1982.

43. Lee, K. A. "High Blood Pressure." In *Cardiac Nursing,* ed. S. L. Underwood et al. Philadelphia: J. B. Lippincott, 1982.

44. Lenfant, C., et al. "Trends in Hypertension Control in the U.S." *Chest* 86:459, 1984.

45. Levine, D. M., et al. "Health Education for Hypertensive Patients." *Journal of the American Medical Association* 241:1700, 1979.

46. Ljung, H., et al. "Sodium Excretion and Blood Pressure." *Hypertension* 3:138, 1981.

47. Lynch, J. J., et al. "The Effects of Talking on Blood Pressure and Normotensive Individuals." *Psychosomatic Medicine* 43:25, 1981.

48. McCombs, J., et al. "Critical Patient Behaviors in High Blood Pressure Control." *Cardiovascular Nursing* 16:4, 1980.

49. McGurn, W. C. *Hypertension in People with Cardiac Problems: Nursing Concepts.* Philadelphia: J. B. Lippincott, 1981.

50. McNamara, J., et al. "Coronary Artery Disease in Vietnam Casualties." *Journal of the American Medical Association* 216:1185, 1971.

51. Maloney, R. J. "Hypertension Update!" *Critical Care Update* 9:7, 1982.

52. Morisky, D. E., et al. "Five Year Blood Pressure Control and Mortality Following Health Education for Hypertensive Patients." *American Journal of Public Health* 73:152, 1983.

53. National Heart, Lung, and Blood Institute, based on data from National Center for Health Statistics, Vital Statistics Bureau, U.S. Department of Health, Education and Welfare.

54. National High Blood Pressure Education Program. *Guidelines for Educating Nurses in High Blood Pressure Control.* Washington, D.C.: National Heart, Lung, and Blood Institute, March 1980. NIH Pub. No. 80-1241.

55. Page, I. H. "Hypertension—The Fledgling of Modern Medical Practice." *Postgraduate Medicine* 61:203, 1977.

56. Page, L. B., et al. "Antecedents of Cardiovascular Disease in Six Solomon Island Societies." *Circulation* 49:1132, 1974.

57. Palfrey, M., et al. "Prolonged Isometric Exercise." *Hypertension* 3:182, 1981.

58. Pascual, A. V. "Hypertensive Crisis: Diagnosis and Strategies in Treatment." *Hospital Medicine* 17:43, 1981.

59. Pender, N. J. "Physiologic Responses of Clients with Essential Hypertension to Progressive Muscle Relaxation Training." *Research in Nursing and Health* 7:197, 1984.

60. Powers, M. J., et al. "Factors Influencing Knowledge, Attitudes, and Compliance of Hypertensive Patients . . . Four Aspects of an Educational Program." *Research in Nursing and Health* 5:171, 1982.

61. Report of Subcommittee of the Postgraduate Education Committee. *Recommendations for Human Blood Pressure*

Determination by Sphygmomanometers. American Heart Association, 1980. Pub. No. 70-019B. 12-80-100M.

62. Rocella, E. J. "Progress and Lessons Learned from the National High Blood Pressure Education Program." *Patient Education Counseling* 6:103, 1984.

63. Rosch, P. "Stress and Cardiovascular Disease." *Comprehensive Therapy* 9:6, 1983.

64. Sackett, D. L., et al. "Patient Compliance with Antihypertensive Regimens." *Patient Counseling and Health Education,* 1978, 18.

65. Saunders, J. B., et al. "Alcohol Induced Hypertension." *Lancet* 1:653, 1981.

66. Schulman, B. A. "Active Patient Orientation Outcomes in Hypertension Treatment: Application of a Socio-organizational Perspective." *Medical Care* 17:267, 1979.

67. "Self-monitoring of Blood Pressure Improves Treatment of Hypertension During Pregnancy." *Nurses Drug Alert* 8:88, 1984.

68. Singer, M. T. "Engagement Involvement: A Central Phenomenon in Psychophysiological Research." *Psychosomatic Medicine* 36:1, 1974.

69. Smyth, K., et al. "Engagement Involvement and Blood Pressure Change: A Methodological Inquiry." *Nursing Research* 29:270, 1980.

70. Soghikian, K., et al. "Psychological Variables and High Blood Pressure." *Preventive Medicine* 8:223, 1979.

71. Sparacino, J. "Blood Pressure, Stress, and Mental Health." *Nursing Research* 31:89, 1982.

72. Stahl, S. M., et al. "Effects of Home Blood Pressure Measurement on Long-term Blood Pressure Control." *American Journal of Public Health* 74:704, 1984.

73. Stamler, J., R. Stamler, and T. N. Pullman, eds. *The Epidemiology of Hypertension.* New York: Grune & Stratton, 1967.

74. Steckel, S. B. "Hypertension Compliance: When Patient Will Power Fails a Written Contract May Succeed." *Consultant* 22:129, 1982.

75. Stone, C. C. Patient Compliance and the Role of the Expert. *Journal of Social Issues* 35:34, 1979.

76. Sullivan, P., et al. "Anxiety, Anger and Neurogenic Tone in Hypertensives." *Hypertension* 11:119, 1981.

77. Swain, M. S., et al. "Influencing Adherence Among Hypertensives." *Research in Nursing and Health* 4:213, 1981.

78. The 1984 Report of the Joint National Committee on Detection, Evaluation, and Treatment of High Blood Pressure. U.S. Department of Health and Human Services, June 1984. NIH Pub. No. 84-1088.

79. Tobian, L., et al. "Effect of Perfusion Pressures in the Output of Sodium and Renin and the Vascular Resistance in Kidneys of Rats with 'Post Salt' Hypertension." *Archives of Research* 36:162, 1975.

80. Tuck, M. L., et al. "The Effect of Weight Reduction on Blood Pressure, Plasma Renin Activity, and Plasma Aldosterone Levels in Obese Patients." *New England Journal of Medicine* 304:930, 1981.

81. Tyroler, H. A., D. Heyden, and C. Homes. "Weight and Hypertension: Evans County Studies of Blacks and Whites." In *Epidemiology and Control of Hypertension,* ed. O. Paul. New York: Stratton International Medical Book Co., 1975.

82. Wallis, C. "Stress—Can We Cope?" *Time,* June 9, 1983, 48.

83. Weber, M. A., and J. H. Laragh. "Hypertension." In *Current Therapy,* ed. H. F. Conn. Philadelphia: W. B. Saunders, 1978.

84. "When Is Hypertension Hypertension? Blood Pressure Must Be Measured More Than Once." *Nurses Drug Alert* 7:52, 1983.

85. White, W. B., et al. "Drugs for Cough and Cold Symptoms in Hypertensive Patients." *American Family Physician* 31:183, 1985.

86. Wyka–Fitzgerald, C., et al. "Long-term Evaluation of Group Education for High Blood Pressure Control." *Cardiovascular Nursing* 20:13, 1984.

87. Yoos, L. "Compliance: Philosophical and Ethical Considerations." *Nurse Practitioner* 6:27, 1981.

CHAPTER 31

Adults with Chronic Renal Failure and End-Stage Renal Disease

MARJATTA HERRANEN

■

OBJECTIVES

After completing this chapter, the reader will be able to:

- Define the terms chronic renal failure (CRF) and end-stage renal disease (ESRD).
- Describe the magnitude of CRF and ESRD as health problems in the United States.
- Describe the pathophysiology of CRF.
- Identify factors that contribute to the onset and progression of CRF.
- Identify nursing measures that can be used to prevent and screen for early intervention in CRF.
- Relate the nursing assessment of the client with CRF to nursing diagnoses.
- Discuss nursing intervention and evaluation related to selected nursing diagnoses.
- Identify ethical issues related to CRF.

Chronic renal failure (CRF) is a complex clinical condition characterized by the gradual and inexorable deterioration of kidney function. The constellation of signs, symptoms, and physiochemical manifestations associated with decreased renal function is known as uremia or uremic syndrome. The term end-stage renal disease (ESRD) is used to denote the progression of renal failure to a stage at which a definitive replacement therapy, such as peritoneal dialysis, hemodialyis, or renal transplantation, is necessary for survival (13).

ESRD is a relatively recent entry among the treatable chronic diseases. The major advances in therapy—dialysis and renal transplantation—were made in the 1960s and became widely available after 1972, when Public Law 92-603 extended the entitlement for Medicare insurance benefits to almost anyone who required chronic replacement therapy. An estimated 92 percent to 95 percent of all clients with ESRD are currently eligible for either Medicare or Medicaid (18).

Since the beginning of the federal reimbursement program, the number of clients who receive replacement therapy has increased yearly. In 1984, 27,000 new clients began receiving replacement therapy. The total number of clients now being treated is approximately 90,000. Current projections indicate a leveling off in the number of new clients each year through the mid-1990s.

The total incidence of chronic renal disease is unknown; reported estimates are 150 to 200 per million persons, only 15 percent to 20 percent of whom will eventually reach ESRD. The vast majority of these people will be treated conservatively (3).

The current costs to Medicare for treating ESRD now exceed $2.8 billion per year. This figure does not reflect the costs accrued before reaching ESRD; nor does it include the losses in productivity during the progression of renal failure and when rehabilitation during replacement therapy is only partially successful. Because hemodialysis and peritoneal dialysis are increasingly performed at home, there may be other, hidden costs that are difficult to assess.

The Nature of the Problem

The kidneys play a vital role in the maintenance of the body's internal environment through complex excretory, metabolic, and endocrine functions. The approximately 1 million nephrons in each kidney regulate the volume, composition, and pH of body fluids. Each minute one-quarter of the circulating blood volume passes through the glomerular capillaries, filtering approximately 130 ml of plasma. Between 1,000 and 2,000 ml of urine is formed for excretion in 24 hours.

The kidneys perform such functions as the following:

- Maintenance of fluid and electrolyte composition of the body fluids through the retention or excretion of water, sodium, potassium, and chlorides
- Maintenance of acid–base balance through conservation of bicarbonate and excretion of excess hydrogen ions
- Excretion of metabolic waste products, such as urea, uric acid, and creatinine
- Regulation of extracellular fluid volume and blood pressure through the renin–angiotensin system, renal prostaglandins, and renal kallikrein–kinin system
- Control of the red blood cell mass through erythropoietin
- Maintenance of calcium and phosphate balance and production of an active metabolite of vitamin D, all of which affect the integrity of the skeletal system
- Degradation and catabolism of hormones such as insulin glucagon, calcitonin, and parathyroid hormone
- Detoxification and elimination of toxins and drugs

As shown in Table 31.1, significant impairment of renal function and therapies used in the management of renal disease can affect many body systems, leading to a variety of clinical manifestations.

Table 31.1
Effects of Renal Failure on the Body

System	Contributing Factors	Effect
Cardiovascular	Volume overload, increased activity of renin–angiotensin system, increased peripheral vascular resistance, anemia, uremic toxins, acidosis, atherosclerosis, anticoagulant administration, underdialysis	Hypertension, decreased exercise tolerance, dyspnea, orthopnea, gallop, congestive heart failure, peripheral edema, angina, pericarditis, effusion, tamponade
Pulmonary	Uremic toxins, volume overload, congestive heart failure, increased susceptibility to infections	Pulmonary congestion, pleural effusion, pleuritis, interstitial pneumonias
Hematologic (anemia, usually normocytic normochromic)	Decreased erythropoietin, decreased erythrocyte production and life span, iron and folate deficiency, blood loss owing to extracorporeal dialysis and laboratory sampling, decreased platelet adhesiveness	General weakness, fatigue, tachycardia, congestive heart failure, feeling cold, prolonged bleeding time
Gastrointestinal	Accumulation of waste products, acidosis, elevated parathyroid hormone levels, prolonged bleeding time, aluminum hydroxide ingestion	Uremic breath odor, metallic taste, stomatitis, thirst, epigastric discomfort, anorexia, nausea, vomiting, hematemesis, colitis, constipation
Metabolic/endocrine		
Carbohydrate intolerance	Altered insulin release, peripheral insulin antagonism, delayed renal degradation of insulin, abnormal growth hormone, abnormal glucagon, abnormal parathyroid hormone levels	Fasting euglycemia, spontaneous hypoglycemia, diminished insulin requirement in diabetics
Hyperlipidemia	Increased synthesis, impaired catabolism	Hypertriglyceridemia, increased incidence of cardiovascular complications
Reproductive	Uremic toxins, hormonal disturbances, stress of chronic illness, autonomic neuropathy	Decreased libido Female: menstrual irregularity, nonovulatory cycles, amenorrhea, cystic ovarian disease Male: oligospermia or azoospermia, impotence

(continued)

Four stages in the progression of CRF are commonly identified.

Diminished Renal Reserve. At this stage all of the excretory and regulatory functions are well preserved. Laboratory findings show normal serum urea, creatinine, and creatinine clearance. The client is asymptomatic unless stressed by a severe systemic event, such as major surgery, trauma, or heart attack, at which time diminished renal reserve becomes evident.

Renal Insufficiency. At this stage laboratory findings include mild azotemia, elevations of urea and creatinine, and reduced creatinine clearance. The client may experience fatigue, nocturia, itching, and difficulty in concentrating.

Frank Renal Failure. At this stage more than 80 percent of renal function is lost and uremic manifestations increase both in number and in intensity. Laboratory tests show markedly increased serum urea and creatinine, hypocalcemia, hyperphosphatemia, metabolic acidosis, and isosthenuria.

End-Stage Renal Disease. All of the consequences of renal failure begin to appear and replacement therapy is mandatory to maintain life (7).

Table 31.1 (continued)

System	Contributing Factors	Effect

Neurological
  Central
  Dialysis encephalopathy
  Peripheral
  Carpal tunnel syndrome
  Autonomic
  Dialysis disequilibrium
	Uremic toxins, electrolyte imbalance, elevated parathyroid hormone levels, aluminum ingestion, exposure in dialysis, anemia chronic illness state, abnormal plasma catecholamines, rapid removal of urea	Insomnia, shortened memory and attention span, confusion, irritability, halting speech, seizures, depression, numbness, burning and restless feet, decreased nerve conduction velocities, tingling, weakness of fingers and hands, pain, orthostatic hypotension, decreased sweat gland function, headache, nausea, vomiting, tremors, seizures after hemodialysis

Skeletal (renal osteodystrophy)	Absence of active vitamin D metabolites, decreased absorption of calcium, secondary hyperparathyroidism, accumulation of phosphates, acidosis, malnutrition	Muscle weakness, bone pain, fractures, delayed healing of fractures, pruritus
Integumentary	Decreased activity of sebaceous and sweat glands, anemia, retained urochrome, multiple transfusions, prolonged bleeding time, increased capillary fragility, pruritus, malnutrition, acidosis	Dry and scaly skin, diminished perspiration, pallor, yellow-brown or grayish-bronze color, purpura, ecchymosis, petechiae, poor wound healing

Source: G. Eknoyan and J. P. Knochel. *The Systemic Consequences of Renal Failure.* Orlando, Fla.: Grune & Stratton, 1984; D. P. Earle. *Manual of Clinical Nephrology.* Philadelphia: W. B. Saunders, 1982; W. Flamenbaum and R. J. Hamburger. *Nephrology: An Approach to the Patient with Renal Disease.* Philadelphia: J. B. Lippincott, 1982.

Complications

Anemia. The primary cause of anemia in CRF is decreased production of erythropoietin by diseased kidneys, although hemodialysis and repeated blood sampling also contribute.

Anemic clients, particularly the elderly, are regularly assessed for cardiovascular symptoms—tachycardia, dyspnea, palpitations, and angina. When cardiovascular symptoms interfere with activities of daily living, blood transfusions are usually indicated.

Oral iron supplements are given when iron deficiency anemia is present. Ferrous sulfate, 300 mg, is given one to three times daily either one hour before or two hours after meals, to reduce gastric irritation. Phosphate binders, such as aluminum hydroxide gel, help to reduce gastric irritation. Because ferrous sulfate and phosphate binders are constipating, stool softeners and bulk laxatives may be given. Dietary fiber may also be increased. When bulk laxatives are ineffective, stimulant laxatives and enemas, such as Fleet's oil-retention enemas, may be used to relieve constipation. Commonly used hematinic agents and laxatives are listed in Table 31.4.

Both anemia and constipation often respond positively to increased physical exercise. Clients are encouraged to increase their physical activity within tolerable levels. Walking interspersed with rest periods is suitable for most clients.

Two other measures used to manage anemia are folic acid and androgen therapy (see Table 31.4). Sometimes nandrolone decanoate for women and testosterone for men are given over an extended period.

Pericarditis. Pericarditis, inflammation of the parietal and visceral membranes surrounding the heart and the accumulation of serosanguineous exudate in the pericardial sac, is frequently seen in clients who are entering replacement therapy and who are being dialyzed. The cause of this problem is uncertain, although the presence of uremic toxins and persistent volume overload may contribute to it.

Manifestations of pericarditis include increasing fatigue, malaise, weight loss, and low-grade fever. Chest pain that improves when the client sits upright and that is accompanied by hypotension, narrow pulse pressure, and pericardial friction rub is highly suggestive of pericarditis (7). Arrhythmias may be observed.

Medical management includes increasing the frequency of dialysis from three times a week to daily until improvement is observed. If the client fails to respond to conservative measures, the pericardium may be drained surgically (7).

Nursing assessment of vital signs, interpretation of findings, and reporting of observations help to control this serious complication. Explanation of events and encouraging the client to limit weight gain during the interdialytic period help to speed recovery.

Aluminum Encephalopathy. A complication that may be attributed to replacement therapy is aluminum encephalopathy—deposition of aluminum in the bone and gray matter of the brain, resulting in a complex neurological syndrome characterized by stuttering, hesitant, and dysphasic speech, myoclonus, dementia, and seizures (14).

Peripheral Neuropathy. Slowing of both motor and sensory nerve conduction velocity and concomitant muscle weakness are common in CRF. Manifestations include painful paresthesias of the extremities, "restless leg" syndrome, muscle weakness, and loss of deep tendon reflexes. It is more commonly seen in the lower than in the upper extremities. Its cause in most clients is unknown, although clients on peritoneal dialysis seem to be affected less often than clients on hemodialysis. Prolonging dialysis time may relieve symptoms.

Risk Factors

As shown in Table 31.2, the major risk factors associated with ESRD are hypertension, diabetes mellitus, and primary renal disease (glomerulonephritis, nephrosis, and nephrotic syndrome). These three risk factors accounted for two-thirds of the newly diagnosed ESRD patients who received Medicare in 1983.

The incidence of ESRD increases with age. In 1983 almost one-half of the patients (45 percent) were sixty years of age or older. This is due in part to the progressive loss of functioning nephrons that begins in the fifth decade, caused by normal aging (19).

ESRD is more common in men than in women, and

Table 31.2
Newly Diagnosed Medicare ESRD Clients by Primary Diagnosis (Network 25)—1983

Primary Diagnosis	Percentage
Hypertension with cardiac and renal complications	22
Diabetes mellitus with other complications	22
Glomerulonephritis, nephrotic syndrome, and nephroses	21
Congenital anomalies	5
Urinary system diseases	4
All others	10
Unreported	15

Source: Office of Statistics and Data Management. *End-Stage Renal Disease Patient Profile Tables.* Washington, D.C.: DHHS, June 5, 1985.

whites are affected more than twice as frequently as blacks (19).

Table 31.3 lists some of the causes of CRF. The list is not exhaustive, but it does include some of the more common causes.

Prevention and Screening for Early Intervention

Active identification of the population at risk is of primary importance in preventing the onset and progression of CRF (6). Diverse strategies are needed. Screening of renal function among the risk groups should be done frequently with the aim of modifying behaviors that increase risk.

Programs for the detection of hypertension are offered by numerous groups—the American Heart Association, private industry, private and public health care institutions, and the mass media. These programs, in addition to detecting unsuspected hypertension, aim to enhance public awareness of the health hazards of hypertension. Of particular importance is increasing client compliance with hypertension treatment programs. Clients are usually asymptomatic and lack understanding of the potential risks involved in improper medical management. The medications they take have side effects, and the rewards for taking them are not easily visible (10).

Table 31.3
Origins of Chronic Renal Failure

Congenital/Hereditary
  Hypoplasia
  Dysplasia
  Obstructive oropathy
  Cystinosis
  Oxalosis
  Allport's syndrome
  Fabry's syndrome
  Fanconi's syndrome
  Polycystic (infant and adult forms)
  Sickle cell disease
Primary Renal Diseases
  Glomerulonephritis (acute, rapidly progressive, chronic)
  Renal tubular acidosis
  Pyelonephritis
  Neoplasms, nephrolithiasis
Systemic Causes
  Diabetes mellitus
  Hypertension
  Systemic lupus erythematosus
  Vasculitis
  Multiple myeloma
  Amyloidosis
  Scleroderma
  Gout
  Tuberculosis
Other Factors
  Analgesic abuse
  Heroin abuse
  Metals: silver, gold, bismuth
  Hydrocarbons
  Malignancies

Maintenance of euglycemia—blood glucose between 70 and 150 mg/dl—in the diabetic can impact on the development of renal disease. General health measures such as maintenance of ideal body weight and moderate protein and salt ingestion are beneficial in the prevention and control of both hypertension and diabetes.

Treatment of urinary tract infections can be accomplished by several methods: (a) using aseptic technique when instrumentation of the urinary tract is unavoidable (6); (b) minimizing the use of indwelling catheters by teaching clients how to catheterize themselves and use other forms of bladder training (16); and (c) screening for bacteriuria, even when asymptomatic, in such high-risk groups as diabetics and pregnant women in their third trimester. When infections are discovered, adequate treatment with follow-up examination at the end of the prescribed therapy is advocated (6). Treatment of all streptococcal infections is particularly important.

Reducing the exposure of people to nephrotoxic substances can also help prevent CRF. Risk reduction measures include an appreciation of the importance of knowing whether or not a substance is nephrotoxic before using it (particularly important in those with known renal damage), control of over-the-counter consumption of nonnarcotic analgesics, and safe handling of industrial chemicals known to be nephrotoxic.

Management of Chronic Renal Failure and End-Stage Renal Disease

There are currently three replacement therapies available to clients. Each of these is discussed briefly.

Renal Transplantation

The best chance of return to normal life is offered by transplantation of a healthy kidney, from either a living donor or a cadaveric donor. In the past, kidney rejection and the side effects of drugs used to reduce rejection significantly limited transplantation. New immunosuppressive agents, such as cyclosporine A, and monoclonal antibodies used either in conjunction with or instead of traditional agents such as steroids and azathioprine, and the growing understanding of host-versus-graft reactions continue to improve graft survival and reduce complications.

Not all clients are suitable candidates for transplantation. Advanced age and the presence of multiple medical, social, or psychological problems exclude many clients.

The scarcity of kidneys available for transplantation limits the number of people who can benefit from this treatment option. Several states recently began to address the problem by enacting laws that facilitate requesting organs for transplantation on death of the donor. New York State: Required Request Law 4925-C is an example. Organ donor cards that can be carried in one's wallet and driver's licenses on which one can give permission for organ donation are instrumental in raising the number of organs that become available for transplantation.

Hemodialysis

Hemodialysis, an extra-corporeal process of blood purification, requires repeated access to the circulatory system, a semipermeable membrane (dialyzer), and a machine that enables blood and dialyzate solution to be brought into contact with each other so that diffusion of accumulated waste products and removal of excess water can occur. Systemic anticoagulation with heparin is necessary in most cases as well as continuous monitoring to prevent complications (8).

This treatment modality can be performed in different settings, depending on the client's medical condition and desire, and the availability of a partner. The majority of clients (83 percent) are dialyzed in either hospital or independent satellite dialysis units. Only a small number are dialyzed at home by either family members or trained assistants (17).

Although the level of waste products and body water, and metabolic acidosis can be controlled by performing hemodialysis three times weekly, many systemic manifestations of ESRD remain.

Hemodialysis requires permanent access to the circulatory system. Fistulas and grafts, usually located in the arms, offer the best long-term access. Both are created surgically and are not used until healing is complete. A disadvantage of fistulas and grafts is repeated access by way of needles. Transcutaneous buttons (i.e., hemasites), usually implanted in the upper arm fistula or graft, permit repeated access to circulation without needle puncture (20). Clients are taught to assess the patency of fistulas and grafts by palpating them daily for thrills or by listening for bruits (extracardiac murmurs). They are also instructed to avoid wearing restrictive clothing or applying pressure to the sites. Potential complications include infections, clotting, and aneurysms, all of which require immediate corrective action.

Temporary access for hemodialysis can be achieved by means of shunts or right atrial catheters (i.e., Hickman catheters). Both can be used immediately after implantation. They are, however, prone to infections, clotting, and dislodgment, and they seldom last longer than a few months. Use of the affected limb is limited, and showers are prohibited unless the site is well protected. The client and family are taught emergency procedures that may be needed to handle life-threatening situations.

Peritoneal Dialysis

Peritoneal dialysis, intracorporeal blood purification, uses the visceral and parietal peritoneal membranes as semipermeable membranes. Dialysate is instilled into the abdominal cavity through either a temporary or a permanent catheter (8). The dialysate remains in the abdominal cavity for a predetermined period before it is drained and fresh dialysate is instilled.

The most common form of peritoneal dialysis is continuous ambulatory peritoneal dialysis (CAPD). Dialysate is exchanged without a machine four to five times a day, usually by the client, although a disabled person may use a partner. Use of a cycling machine at night gives the client dialysis-free time during the day. Advantages of CAPD include freedom from machines, cannulations, and treatment center schedules and less rapid changes in the volume and composition of body fluids. Less restricted diet and simplicity of technique make this form of dialysis suitable for many clients. Success of CAPD depends on the client's ability and motivation for self-care. Disadvantages include inevitable losses of protein, which must be compensated for by increased protein intake, and the increased risk for infections either at the catheter exit site or in the peritoneal cavity. Repeated infections diminish the ability of the peritoneal membrane to dialyze. It is not uncommon for a client to go from one treatment modality to another.

Medications commonly used in the management of clients with CRF are listed in Table 31.4.

Nursing Care

Nursing care of clients with CRF poses a constant challenge. The main goal of nursing intervention is the maintenance of the client's independence while coping with a chronic health problem. When planning care, the primary nurse considers the progressive nature of renal failure, the individual differences among clients and their families, and the overriding principle of the client's right to self-determination. Care includes client and family teaching, counseling, and support while continuously evaluating and modifying care as new situations arise.

Assessment

Assessment of the client with either known or suspected renal impairment includes a thorough physical examination, a health history, and a series of laboratory and radiological studies designed to delineate the type and degree of renal involvement. The health history should include a history of renal and systemic diseases (e.g.,

Table 31.4
Pharmacological Treatment of Chronic Renal Failure

Category/Indications	Drug	Nursing Management
Antihypertensives		
Adrenergic inhibitors		
Peripheral	guanethidine monosulfate (Ismelin)	Evaluate for orthostatic hypotension by measuring blood pressure while supine, standing, and sitting; evaluate for impotence; advise to avoid strenuous exercise.
Central	methyldopa (Aldomet)	Evaluate for orthostatic hypotension, edema, weight gain, dry mouth.
Alpha blockers	prazosin hydrochloride (Minipress)	Evaluate for palpitations, orthostatic hypotension, dry mouth.
Beta blockers	propranolol hydrochloride (Inderal)	Evaluate for masking of hypoglycemia in diabetic, discontinue gradually to avoid angina and increased risk of myocardial infarction.
	nadolol (Cogard) timolol maleate (Timoptic) pindolol (Visken) metroprolol tartrate (Lopressor) atenolol (Tenormin)	Evaluate for bradycardia, congestive heart failure; administer before meals to enhance absorption; discontinue gradually.
Alpha and beta blockers	labetalol hydrochloride (Normodyne)	
Converting enzyme inhibitors	captopril (Capoten)	Evaluate for leukopenia, particularly in the presence of immunosuppressive therapy; loss of taste; skin rash; decreased renal function; proteinuria.
Vasodilators	hydralazine hydrochloride (Apresoline) minoxidil (Loniten)	Evaluate for tachycardia, skin rash, lupuslike symptoms; administer with meals; evaluate for tachycardia, edema, congestive heart failure, hypertrichosis.
Vitamins		
Vitamin D	calcitriol (Rocaltrol) dihydrotachysterol (DHT)	Evaluate for signs of hypercalcemia, nausea, vomiting, weakness, headache, somnolence; monitor serum calcium and phosphorus levels.
Vitamin B_9	folic acid (Folacin)	Instruct client to take after dialysis treatment.
Hematinics	ferrous sulfate (Feosol)	Instruct client to take 1 hour before meals, *not* with antacids; instruct to observe for constipation.
	iron dextran (Imferon)	Administer test dose; inject deeply using Z track; observe for potential shock.
Androgenic agents	nandrolone decanoate (Deca-Durabolin) fluoxymesterone (Halotestin)	Evaluate for acne, hirsutism; evaluate hemoglobin, hematocrit.
Antipruritics (Antihistamines)	cyproheptadine (Cyprodine) trimeprazine tartrate (Temaril)	Evaluate for drowsiness, dry mouth; instruct client to avoid activity requiring mental alertness; instruct client to avoid alcohol.
Stool softeners and laxatives		
Emollients, lubricants	docusate sodium (Colace)	Instruct client to take regularly to prevent constipation.
Mineral oil		Limit use to avoid loss of fat-soluble vitamins.

(continued)

Table 31.4 (continued)

Category/Indications	Drug	Nursing Management
Stool softeners and laxatives		
Bulk laxatives	psyllium hydrophilic muciloid (Metamucil)	Effectiveness depends on fluid intake.
Stimulants	castor oil, senna (Senokot) bisacodyl (Dulcolax)	Use only to relieve acute constipation; can be habit-forming.
Miscellaneous		
Resin exchange	sodium polystyrene sulfonate (Kayexalate)	Monitor for signs of hypokalemia, diarrhea, or impaction.
Phosphate binding agents	aluminum hydroxide (Amphojel) aluminum carbonate gel (Basaljel)	Avoid taking with iron, constipating.
	calcium carbonate (Os-cal)	Monitor serum calcium and phosphate levels.

include a history of renal and systemic diseases (e.g., hypertension and diabetes), a pharmacological history, work and leisure activities, and symptoms associated with CRF (see Table 31.1). The nursing assessment includes the client's perceptions of the illness experience and its meaning to the client and family, and previous coping mechanisms.

Diagnostic and laboratory tests commonly used and the findings associated with CRF may be found in Tables 31.5 and 31.6.

Nursing Diagnoses

The following list of nursing diagnoses is designed to guide the primary nurse in planning nursing care for the client with CRF, particularly those with ESRD. It is not exhaustive, since each client will have unique needs, but it does include major areas of common concern.

- Fluid volume alteration (excess and deficit) related to impaired regulatory function
- Alteration in electrolyte balance related to impaired regulatory function
- Alteration in nutrition (deficit) related to such factors as nausea, vomiting, anorexia, and depression
- Alteration in bowel elimination (constipation) related to such factors as altered dietary and fluid intake
- Potential impairment of skin integrity related to such factors as accumulation of toxic waste products and pruritus
- Activity intolerance related to such factors as fatigue

Table 31.5
Diagnostic Studies and Usual Findings in CRF

Test	Findings
Kidney–ureter–bladder plain roentgenogram	Location, size, and shape of kidneys, ureters, bladder; presence of calculi; nephrocalcinosis
Sonography (noninvasive sound wave imaging)	Alterations in size and shape of kidneys, collecting system; presence of cysts, calculi, collections of blood, pus, urine, lymph
Scanning (radio isotope uptake)	Alterations in renal perfusion and function
Intravenous urography (contrast-mediated x-ray)	Serial views of kidneys and lower urinary tract; fine resolution of structural abnormalities
Biopsy—percutaneous or open; light, electron, immunofluorescence microscopic techniques	Identify affected intrarenal structures, glomeruli, interstitium, define degree

- Depression related to such factors as stress of therapy and multiple losses
- Fear and anxiety related to such factors as pain, the nature of therapy, and the death of fellow clients

Planning and Implementation

□ **Alteration in Body Fluid Volume.** As the regulatory mechanisms of the kidney begin to fail, both excess and

Table 31.6
Comparison of Normal and CRF Values

Test	Normal Adult Value	CRF Value
Hematology		
Hemoglobin	12–18 g/dl (male); 12–16 g/dl (female)	6–11 g/dl
Hematocrit	42–54% (male); 38–46% (female)	15–30%
Platelets	130,000–370,000/mm³	Qualitatively different
Coagulation—bleeding time	1–9 min	Prolonged
Electrolytes		
Serum Potassium	3.5–5.0 mEq/liter	5.0–6.0 mEq/liter or above
Total carbon dioxide content	22–34 mEq/liter	12–20 mEq/liter
Serum Calcium	4.5–5.5 mEq/liter	Usually lower in the absence of vitamin D and calcium supplements, and phosphate control
Serum Magnesium	1.5–2.5 mEq/liter	Elevated without intake control
Immune Response		
Antistreptolysin titer (ASO)	less than 85 Todd units/ml	200–3,000 Todd units
Hepatitis B		
Surface antigen	Negative	Positive in small percentage
Surface antibody	Negative	Positive post-recovery or vaccination
Other		
Blood urea nitrogen	8–20 mg/dl	50–100 mg/dl
Serum creatinine	0.2–0.6 mg/dl in males; 0.6–1 mg/dl in females	8–20 mg/dl
Serum phosphate	2.5–4.5 mg/dl	Elevated in the absence of phosphate binders
Calcium phosphorus product	30–40	Above 40
Alkaline phosphate	Values vary with laboratory method used	Elevated
Triglycerides	10–190 mg/dl (varies with age)	Often elevated
Parathyroid		
Hormone		
C-terminal fraction		Elevated
N-terminal fraction		Elevated
Creatinine clearance	74–125 ml/miné (calculated on basis of body surface)	0–20 ml/miné

Source: Diagnostics. 2nd Edition. Springhouse, Pa.: Springhouse Corporation Book Division, 1986.

deficit in the volume of body water may occur. By far the more common is volume overload resulting from accumulation of sodium and water. Its manifestations range from mild to severe and include weight gain, edema, lowering of hematocrit, and signs of circulatory overload: hypertension, bounding pulse, dyspnea, orthopnea, distended neck veins, and, if overload is extreme, frank pulmonary edema. Dependent edema without the manifestations of circulatory overload occurs when hypervolemia coexists with low plasma protein levels, as seen in protein malnutrition and severe proteinuria. Hypovolemia is seen as a consequence of salt-wasting polyuria or when the client is unable to ingest adequate amounts of fluids to compensate for daily losses.

In planning nursing interventions addressing potential

and real problems in fluid homeostasis, accuracy in data collection cannot be overemphasized. Fluid intake is correlated by assessment of losses. This includes periodically measuring urine output, as the amount is likely to change during disease progression and alterations in medical management. The daily insensible losses through the skin, by breathing, and in stool are estimated and the optimum intake level is determined. Safe interdialytic weight gain in hemodialysis ranges from 3 to 5 pounds, depending on the client's body size and the presence or absence of other contributory factors. Because most clients have to restrict their intake, the following is a discussion of nursing strategies in assisting clients to maintain optimum fluid levels. Measuring both intake and output and keeping records are useful for establishing accurate guidelines and verifying results; underestimation of intake and overestimation of output are common. The client should be weighed each day, preferably at the same time, using the same scale, and while wearing the same amount of clothing, thus minimizing the error in results. If thirst is present, separating fluid intake from mealtimes and dividing the total allowed amount into several small portions, to be ingested throughout the day, can alleviate this symptom. Maintaining moist mucous membranes by sucking on hard candy can be useful for some clients, as can frequent rinsing with mild mouthwash, particularly when an unpleasant, metallic taste is present. The client is taught how to recognize signs and symptoms of hypovolemia and hypervolemia. In hypovolemia the client may experience lower than normal blood pressure, tachycardia, dizziness, weakness, and fainting when changing position from supine to vertical. Hypovolemia is likely on peritoneal dialysis when the inevitable water losses resulting from the hypertonicity of dialyzate cannot be replaced by intake.

□ *Alteration in Electrolyte Balance.* By the time creatinine clearance has decreased to 5 ml/min, potassium homeostasis needs constant attention. Potential for hyperkalemia is ever present; contributory factors include excessive ingestion—the limit usually prescribed is 2,000 mg daily—persistent metabolic acidosis, bleeding, and administration of transfusions. Although dialysis clients appear to tolerate potassium levels that are significantly higher than normal with minimal side effects, levels that exceed 6 mEq/liter can cause cardiac arrhythmias, bradycardia, and death. Electrocardiographic manifestations include prolongation of P-R interval, widened QRS complex, and elevated T waves. Primary treatment in acute life-threatening hyperkalemia is hemodialysis, since rapid excess potassium re-

moval can be accomplished. Other options are oral or rectal administration of sodium polystyrene sulfonate (Kayexalate), diluted in water or sorbitol. This exchange resin removes potassium by 1:1 exchange with sodium; a client with concomitant hypervolemia must be carefully observed for potential worsening of manifestations. Temporary lowering of serum potassium levels can be achieved with the administration of 50 percent glucose with regular insulin. Sodium bicarbonate is used as well when the amount of sodium poses no threat to the client.

Potential for hypokalemia exists for the client on peritoneal dialysis. As the dialyzate used does not contain potassium, gradual and constant removal takes place. Manifestations include rapid, irregular pulse and ventricular fibrillation if the potassium level drops significantly. Hypokalemia is particularly dangerous for the digitalized client potentiating arrhythmias and signs of digitalis toxicity. Ascertaining adequate daily intake is the best strategy. Usually this poses no problems to the client, since adding potassium-containing foods to the diet increases food choices and enhances palatability; only clients who, during their course of replacement therapy, change from hemodialysis to peritoneal dialysis may experience this new freedom as frightening.

Another persistent alteration in the composition of body fluids is metabolic acidosis. Conservation of bicarbonate and excretion of excess hydrogen ions cannot take place in the diseased kidney. Manifestations include compensatory Kussmaul-like breathing, low total carbon dioxide level, and elevations in uric acid, phosphates, urea, and creatinine. Dialyzate containing bicarbonate, lactate, or acetate is used in the dialytic process, allowing some replenishment of bicarbonate stores. In severe acidosis, additional bicarbonate may be administered orally.

Alterations in calcium phosphorus homeostasis occur in CRF. Increases in the levels of serum phosphates result when excretion through the kidney becomes impaired. Calcium absorption from the gut, on the other hand, necessitates the presence of the active form of vitamin D, which in turn is manufactured by the healthy kidney. As serum calcium levels fall and phosphate levels rise, parathyroid hormone is manufactured in response, in an attempt to maintain stable circulating calcium levels. As the calcium is obtained from the bone, renal osteodystrophy develops, characterized by bone reabsorption, osteoporosis, osteomalacia, or osteitis fibrosa. Observable manifestations of renal osteodystrophy include slowing or complete cessation of growth in children, pathological fractures, bone pain, muscle weakness interfering with ambulation (23).

As dietary restriction of phosphates is not feasible without simultaneously seriously restricting protein intake, antacids are used as phosphate binders in the gut, thus facilitating the excretion of phosphates in the stool. Aluminum hydroxide-containing liquid or tablets are most commonly used for this purpose. The client is instructed to take 1 to 2 oz or one or two tablets one-half hour after each meal. As aluminum hydroxide can bind other substances, such as iron, it is important to separate these. Another side effect of antacids is constipation, and many clients fail to ingest the prescribed amount because of this complication. Preventive interventions will be discussed in the section on nutrition and elimination. The use of calcium supplements, in the form of calcium carbonate, is increasing; caution must remain in the use of calcium, if the serum phosphate level is not within normal limits, deposits of calcium in the soft tissues (i.e., blood vessels) can follow.

Two active forms of vitamin D are currently available: calcitriol and dihydrotachysterol. Both are used as a daily supplement to enhance calcium absorption from the gut. As hypercalcemia may occur as the consequence, serum calcium levels are to be evaluated regularly. Signs and symptoms of hypercalcemia include weakness, somnolence, nausea, and vomiting.

Serum parathyroid hormone levels are monitored regularly to ascertain response to this combined therapy.

□ *Alteration in Nutrition.*   Nausea, anorexia, and vomiting are frequently the symptoms of uremia that propel the beginning of dialytic replacement therapy. Although amelioration of these symptoms is achieved by dialysis, they may continue to interfere with the consumption of adequate nutrition and pose a difficult challenge for both the client and the staff working with him or her. The cause of anorexia is multifactorial. It may be due to depression, rapid fluctuations of fluid and electrolyte balance occurring as a consequence of hemodialysis, or inadequate removal of waste products during dialysis. The client is constantly threatened with the vicious cycle of inadequate nutrient intake, followed by increased tissue catabolism and rising urea and creatinine levels, which in turn may worsen the already existing anorexia (24). Other factors that influence appetite are the presence of concurrent illness, medications, and anemia (12). The sedentary life-style assumed by many clients can also contribute to loss of appetite. Deficiency of zinc has been reported to alter the taste sensation (12), and fluid and salt restrictions that are often necessary further diminish the desire to eat. The gastrointestinal tract is often irritable, seemingly without a cause; the diabetic client is particularly prone to gastroparesis and delayed emptying. Ulcerations of the mouth and gastrointestinal tract, and constipation or diarrhea also impede the consumption of adequate nutrients.

Although variations do exist, depending on the client's particular circumstance, the daily requirements for nutrients and vitamins closely parallel those recommended to healthy people. As some vitamin and amino acid losses result from the dialytic therapy, water-soluble vitamins are recommended as supplements, as is folic acid, 1 mg daily, taken after dialysis. Protein consumption should reach 0.8 to 1 mg/kg of body weight. As mentioned previously, protein losses increase during peritoneal dialysis; thus the need for increased protein intake is necessary to prevent malnutrition and wasting. Protein intake should consist of high biological-value protein, for example, eggs, meat, and fish. Milk as a source of protein must be limited when phosphate accumulation is noted. Forty to sixty grams protein restriction is used during the predialytic phase before replacement therapy to minimize uremic symptoms. Sometimes essential amino acid supplements are recommended in order to spare proteins. Carbohydrates and fats must be consumed in adequate quantities, since the end products of their metabolism, carbon dioxide and water, do not significantly burden the kidney. Because this dietary regimen may be prolonged, the client is frequently assessed for signs of progressive wasting—decreased body weight, body fat, and lean body mass, as well as altered plasma proteins.

The client is assisted by the primary nurse in making realistic plans for a diet. This includes taking into account a multitude of factors that influence a person's eating habits; economic, cultural, and demographic influences should be taken into account, as well as the client's understanding of his disease and perception of his role in controlling it. By making realistic plans with the client, the primary nurse can influence client compliance.

Maintaining long-term protein restrictions may prove to be a difficult challenge for many clients. For many years the diet in the Western societies has been high in protein; popular weight reduction regimens advertised and promoted among the public use as the basis of weight reduction limitation of carbohydrates and fats and encourage high protein intake. By educating the public on proper nutrition, nursing can enhance the impact of people's current growing interest in health.

General measures that may enhance eating include good oral hygiene, alleviation of thirst by dividing allowed fluid intake into several small portions to be taken during the day and by sucking on hard candy, and ingesting several small meals instead of a few large ones. Many clients may also be responsive to learning new ways of food preparation by adding herbs and spices, as well as including food items unfamiliar to them. Sharing in the success of other clients, sharing recipes, and striving for a positive outlook can diminish the sense of deprivation often experienced by clients. The impact of the family constellation cannot be overestimated; explaining the diet to household members often leads to improved compliance and improved health.

□ *Alteration in Bowel Elimination—Constipation.* Management and prevention of constipation require constant attention. Because many of the contributory factors cannot be eliminated, use of stool softeners (docusate sodium) or bulk-producing laxatives may be necessary as an ongoing preventive measure. Increasing fiber intake is also recommended, but many clients resist this intervention. Stimulant laxatives or small oil-retention enemas, such as Fleet's oil-retention enemas, can relieve acute constipation. Constipation may also improve with increased physical activity; the client should be encouraged to be as active as possible.

□ *Potential Impairment of Skin Integrity.* Manifestations of renal disease in the integumentary system are numerous and often troublesome to the client. Moderate to severe pruritus is reported to occur in 60 percent to 85 percent of all clients undergoing maintenance replacement therapy, and common to all is the poor response to the traditional interventions with antihistamines and the like (1, 9). The cause of uremic pruritus is not fully understood; potential contributing factors are the accumulation of toxic waste products and elevations of parathyroid hormone, phosphates, and calcium. Another contributing factor is the excessive dryness of the skin; this in turn is thought to be due to the diminished function of the sebaceous glands.

Ultraviolet light treatments, when performed under close medical supervision, have been beneficial (19). Some alleviation of itching can be achieved by using lanolin-based soaps and creams, by avoiding prolonged hot showers and baths, and by wearing loose-fitting clothing in layers so that adjustment to the changes in the ambient temperature can be easily accomplished. Another aspect of uncontrollable itching is the inevitable scratching of the skin, leading to excoriations and increased potential for bacterial entry to the system, and thus infections. Fatigue resulting from lack of sleep makes caring for personal hygiene difficult and the client finds himself on the vicious cycle of becoming in-

creasingly tired and less and less capable of taking care of personal needs.

The sallowness and grayness of uremic skin, thought to be due to waste accumulation and hyperpigmentation, also sets the client apart from healthy people and reinforces the acceptance of the sick role. Ecchymosis, caused by platelet dysfunction, also contributes to viewing oneself as being different from others. Nursing strategies include positive reinforcement and encouragement of the client, monitoring of laboratory values for adequacy of dialysis, and periodic review of medications in order to enhance the client's compliance with the therapeutic regimen.

□ *Activity Intolerance.* The reasons for the persistence of activity intolerance are numerous and interwoven. The demands of the therapy itself—particularly hemodialysis—are considerable. The repetitive phenomena of fatigue and lethargy owing to the accumulation of water and waste products in the body, followed by the physical consequences of the rapid removal of the same, contribute to the fatigue and lack of energy. Although some habituation to these fluctuations occurs over time, no client is unaffected. Anemia and impaired nutritional status diminish the general level of wellness experienced, and thus contribute to the fatigue. A total or partial reversal of sleep pattern—inability to fall asleep for more than short periods during the night—occurs frequently in CRF. In addition, the spectrum of psychosocial stresses discussed elsewhere in this chapter influences the client's perception of wellness, his ability to fall asleep and maintain sleep, and his tolerance for the lack of sleep.

The nurse assists the client in analyzing and explaining his particular causes for fatigue and helps him to modify his activity in order to maximize rest. Several short rest periods during the day are preferable to the use of sedatives; physical activity, when tolerated, enhances the client's ability to fall asleep.

□ *Depression.* Depression or depressive effect is experienced by most clients with CRF at least some time during their use of the different replacement therapies. The cause of depression is complex and multifaceted but centers around the multiple losses suffered by the client and the stresses inflicted by the various forms of therapy. Every aspect of life is affected; never again feeling as well as before therapy was begun is a frequently heard comment in dialysis units. Loss of a vital body function is combined with losses or alterations in usual roles, be they family, sexual, work, or society. Stresses resulting from the need to follow dietary and medication regimens and dialysis schedules that usually better accommodate the needs of the center rather than the client's all serve to negatively influence the client's self-concept and self-esteem. Shame and anger at being ill and different from others contribute to the sense of worthlessness and result in lowered toleration for frustration. Behaviors that the nurse may observe include seemingly inappropriate bursts of anger, excessive demands, manipulative and irritable patterns of interacting with family and health care personnel. Withdrawal from social interaction, increased somatic complaints, requests for pain medication are also potential manifestations of depression. Problems of elimination, sleep, and appetite that can arise from other, nonrelated sources as well can exacerbate the client's emotional status.

The client expresses feelings of giving up as life, as it is currently experienced by him, offers no joy or satisfaction. Planning for the future may cease. Often the client does not want to assume even a minor part in his care, claiming incapability to do so; the secondary gains of the sick role may bring temporary solace and satisfy some unconscious, basic needs. Fears of becoming abandoned by family or professional staff become evident by the growing number of somatic symptoms that require constant attention. Previous coping capabilities are often denied or minimized; the message is "Take care of me, stay with me, do not abandon me."

Nursing interventions are based on the recognition and acceptance of the client's feelings. The sources of stress that are real are identified and discussed, positive aspects of self are discovered and explored jointly with the client and his family. Previously successful coping strategies can be identified, and new ones are discovered either by sharing with fellow clients or by nursing interventions. The primary nurse can provide constancy and continuity in the relationship with the client. Allowing the client time to grieve for the losses, real or imaginary, will create new opportunities for regaining mastery over some aspect of life. Moving toward the stage of acceptance involves a new and more realistic view of self. The nurse facilitates this process by teaching the client about the nature of his illness, correcting misconceptions and fantasies. Teaching should be individualized, taking into account the client's readiness for learning, the manner in which integration of new material is maximal, and the time required to achieve the jointly established goals.

Inclusion of family members in care can affect the client's sense of isolation and powerlessness and enhance sharing of feelings between the client and his significant others. Use of a peer group as a source of support and information can stem the sense of isolation and separateness experienced by the client.

□ *Fear and Anxiety.* Fear and anxiety are common phenomena. The client fears pain, mutilation, and death. Death of a fellow client who sat close by in the treatment center affects the already fragile sense of self and increases the sense of vulnerability. Openness and acceptance of feelings, exploration of the meaning of life and death in a supportive environment can help the client to move toward the discovery of new meaning in life, to accept the differences imposed by the illness while maintaining a sense of dignity and worth.

Evaluation

The following behaviors exemplify some of those that may be used to measure the outcomes of nursing intervention.

Fluid Volume Alteration. The client maintains appropriate interdialytic weight gain. Signs of volume overload (e.g., shortness of breath, hypertension, and edema) are absent.

Alteration in Electrolyte Balance. Serum potassium, calcium, and phosphorus levels are within normal limits.

Alteration in Nutrition. The client will maintain a low-protein diet with sufficient calories from carbohydrates and fats to maintain body mass.

Alteration in Bowel Elimination. The client returns to a normal bowel pattern. He eats a diet high in fiber and exercises regularly, as tolerated.

Potential Impairment of Skin Integrity. The client's skin remains clean and intact. Uncontrolled pruritus is absent.

Activity Intolerance. The client verbalizes an understanding of the importance of and a willingness to engage in regular physical activity. Client and nurse collaboratively plan an exercise program that the client consistently follows. The client includes sufficient rest periods in daily routine to prevent excessive fatigue.

Depression. The client participates in planning care and assumes self-care at a level deemed appropriate to his or her physical status. The client makes flexible short- and long-term plans and deals realistically with fluctuations in the level of health. The client maintains satisfying social interactions with peers, friends, and colleagues.

Fear and Anxiety. The client correctly identifies sources of stress and takes corrective action. The client demonstrates a variety of effective coping mechanisms when undergoing stressful events. The client prepares for eventual death.

Ethical Issues

When the federal government became involved in caring for clients with ESRD, all previous social, psychological, and biochemical criteria that affect access to chronic replacement therapy were eliminated. It was initially estimated that 70 percent of the clients would receive kidney transplants, and that 50 percent of those treated with dialysis would be treated at home. Despite legislative efforts to increase the availability of cadaveric organs, the number of kidney transplants has not increased as anticipated. Initial reimbursement structures discouraged home dialysis, thus contributing to the spiraling costs of ESRD programs.

The unanticipated growth in costs of maintaining ESRD programs has led to questions about the allocation of public resources. Is it fair to single out one group of clients for public support when other catastrophic illnesses lack such support?

Other ethical questions raised by the technology of replacement therapy are these: Has universal benefit led to too much treatment? Are there clients who ought to be denied dialysis? Should dialysis be discontinued for clients who show no hope of rehabilitation (15)? What roles should the client, the client's family, care givers, and the government assume in making decisions about care, including whether or not and when to terminate care?

Quality of life issues versus quantity of life issues are not unique to renal care, yet the decisions made and the ways they are implemented will have an important impact on the entire health field. The primary nurse's role as client advocate mandates participation in these difficult and complex deliberations.

Caring for clients with CRF poses a difficult challenge for primary nurses who spend extensive amounts of time with such clients while anticipating and observing their deterioration and, eventually, death. Nurses bear the brunt of clients' attempts to cope with illness—anger, frustration, acting out, depression, and withdrawal. When confronted with the many demands of these clients, primary nurses often feel inadequate. In an effort to deal with this inadequacy, they may set unrealistically high expectations for their performance as well as that of their clients. They may not allow clients to participate in planning and implementing care. It is most important for primary nurses to understand how caring for chronically and terminally ill clients affects them and how their needs, in turn, affect care. Using colleagues for support and seeking counsel from clinical nurse specialists, both psychiatric and renal, can help them to deal constructively with their stresses.

REFERENCES

1. Blachley, J. D. "Uremic Pruritus: Skin Divalent Ion Content and the Response to Ultraviolet Phototherapy." *American Journal of Kidney Diseases* 5:237–41, 1984.
2. Brenner, B. M., et al. "Dietary Protein Intake and the Progressive Nature of Kidney Disease." *New England Journal of Medicine* 30:652–58, 1982.
3. Burton, B. T. "Current Concepts of Nutritional Therapy in Chronic Renal Failure." *Journal of American Dietetic Association* 82:359–63, 1983.
4. Chyatte–Underwood, H., et al. "Effects of Low-risk Exercise Therapy for Chronic Dialysis Patients." *Dialysis and Transplantation* 14:688–95, 1985.
5. Davidson, M. B. *Diabetes Mellitus: Diagnosis and Treatment.* New York: John Wiley & Sons, 1981.
6. Dodge, W. F. *Evaluation of Screening and Health Maintenance.* NIH Publication No. 78–855. Washington, D.C.: National Institutes of Health, 1978, 1–15.
7. Eknoyan, G., and J. P. Knochel. *The Systemic Consequences of Renal Failure.* Orlando, Fla.: Grune & Stratton, 1984.
8. Flamenbaum, W., and R. J. Hamburger. *Nephrology: An Approach to the Patient with Renal Disease.* Philadelphia: J. B. Lippincott, 1982, 561–69.
9. Gilchrest, B. A., et al. "Relief of Uremic Pruritus with Ultraviolet Therapy." *New England Journal of Medicine* 297:136–38, 1978.
10. Hartmut, H., et al. "The Use of Deferoxamine in the Management of Aluminum Accumulation in Bone in Patients with Renal Failure." *New England Journal of Medicine* 311:140–44, 1984.
11. Kaplan, N. M. "Management Strategies in Hypertension." In *Hypertension,* ed. B. M. Brenner and H. Jay. New York: Churchill Livingstone, 1981, 355–56.
12. Kensit, M. "Appetite Disturbances in Dialysis Patients." *Journal of the American Association of Nephrology Nurses and Technicians* 6:194–99, 1979.

13. Lancaster, L. E. "End-Stage Renal Disease: Pathophysiology, Assessment, and Intervention." In *The Patient with End-Stage Renal Disease,* ed. L. E. Lancaster. New York: John Wiley & Sons, 1984, 2.

14. Lederman, R. J., and C. E. Henry. "Progressive Dialysis Encephalopathy." *Annals of Neurology* 4:199–204, 1983.

15. Levy, N. *Psychonephrology.* New York: Plenum, 1981.

16. Michigan Nurses Association. Curn Project. *Clean, Intermittent Catheterization.* Orlando, Fla.: Grune & Stratton, 1982.

17. National Kidney Foundation. *Health Care Financing Administration End-Stage Renal Disease Program Highlights 1984.* Available from National Kidney Foundation, Inc., 2 Park Ave., New York, N.Y., 10016, 1984.

18. Nogueira, H., et al. "Anemia in Chronic Renal Failure." *Dialysis and Transplantation* 14:483–89, 1985.

19. Office of Statistics and Data Management. *End-Stage Renal Disease Patient Profile Tables.* Washington, D.C.: DHHS, June 5, 1985.

20. Orr, M. L. "Public Policy Issues in ESRD Care." In *The Patient with End-Stage Renal Disease,* ed. L. E. Lancaster. New York: John Wiley & Sons, 1984, 336.

21. Orr, M. L. "Drugs and Renal Disease." *American Journal of Nursing* 81:969–71, 1981.

22. Reed, G. "Potassium the Chief Electrolyte." In *Monitoring Fluid and Electrolytes Precisely.* Horsham, Pa.: Intermed Communications, 1978, 79–88.

23. *Renal Osteodystrophy.* Pitman, N.J.: American Association of Nephrology Nurses and Technicians, 1981.

24. Simmons, R., et al. *Manual of Vascular Access, Organ Donation and Transplantation.* New York: Springer–Verlag, 1984.

25. Underwood, H. C., D. D. Gardenas, and N. G. Kutner. "Effects of Low-risk Exercise Therapy for Chronic Dialysis Patients." *Dialysis and Transplantation* 14:688–95, 1985.

26. Walser, M. "Nutritional Management of Chronic Renal Failure." *American Journal of Kidney Diseases* 1:261–75, 1982.

C H A P T E R   3 2

Adults with Coronary Artery Disease

GLORIA CALIANDRO

■

OBJECTIVES

After completing this chapter, the reader will be able to:

- Identify the magnitude of coronary artery disease (CAD) in the United States.
- Relate the pathophysiology and complications of CAD and myocardial infarction to client problems requiring nursing intervention.
- Identify factors that contribute to the onset and progression of CAD.
- Identify measures that can be used in the prevention of and screening for early intervention in CAD.
- Identify the role of the primary nurse in the prevention of and screening for early intervention in CAD.
- Relate the nursing assessment of the client with CAD to nursing diagnoses.
- Discuss nursing intervention and evaluation related to selected nursing diagnoses for the client with CAD.
- Recall ethical and legal issues related to CAD.

Cardiovascular disease (CVD) is the number one health problem in the United States today. Each year millions of Americans are affected, causing physical and emotional pain and suffering as well as social disruption. For the nurse, CVD represents a challenge and an opportunity to implement concepts of primary nursing care.

The focus of this chapter is the role of the primary nurse in preventing coronary artery disease (CAD), in identifying and reducing risk factors associated with CAD, in functioning as a member of a multidisciplinary health team, and in planning and implementing a plan of nursing care designed to ameliorate selected client problems. Caring for the acutely ill client who may be hospitalized in a coronary care unit is beyond the scope of this text, and the reader is referred to appropriate texts on coronary care nursing.

Overview of Coronary Artery Disease

Incidence

According to estimates supplied by the American Heart Association, 43.5 million Americans had some form of CVD in 1982; 4.67 million of these persons had CAD. Approximately 1.5 million Americans had heart attacks (the major complication of CAD) in 1982, an average of 4,109 heart attacks per day, or three per minute (20).

Diseases of the heart and blood vessels are also the major cause of death among Americans. Almost one-half (49.6 percent) of all deaths in the United States during 1982 were due to CVD. More than twice as many people died of CVD as died of cancer, the second leading cause of death in the United States. Heart attack is the single greatest cause of death, claiming 554,900 lives in 1982 (20). Although the death rate from CVD increases with age, these diseases continue to claim a large number of lives of people under sixty-five years of age. In 1980, 41.6 percent of the people between the ages of forty-five and sixty-four and 17.3 percent of the people between the ages of twenty-five and forty-four died of CVD (30).

Although heart disease remains a major health problem, the mortality rate from coronary heart disease is decreasing. As shown in Table 32.1, the age-adjusted death rate per 100,000 population peaked in 1960, when it was 238.5. By 1980 the rate had declined to 149.4.

Added insight into the problem is revealed in the trends in morbidity and mortality rates for myocardial infarction. In a study of 6,436 employees of the DuPont Company over a twenty-six-year period, from 1957 through 1983, investigators found a steady decline in morbidity and mortality rates, especially among white-collar salaried employees (42). In a second study, the Minnesota Heart Survey, men and women between the ages of thirty and seventy-four in the Minneapolis–St. Paul area were studied for a ten-year period, from 1970 through 1980, during which time investigators also observed a decline both in admissions to the hospital for myocardial infarction and in death rate before arrival at

Table 32.1
Age-Adjusted Death Rates for Coronary Heart Disease, United States, 1940–1980

Year	Death Rate
1940	207.2
1945	208.2
1950	226.4
1955	226.0
1960	238.5
1965	237.7
1970	228.1
1975	172.2
1980	149.4

Note: Rate per 100,000 population, age adjusted to U.S. population, 1940.

Source: R. L. Levy "Prevalence and Epidemiology of Cardiovascular Disease." In *Cecil Textbook of Medicine*, ed. J. B. Wyngaarden and L. H. Smith. 17th ed. Philadelphia: W. B. Saunders, 1985, p. 156.

hospitals and in the emergency rooms (16). In both studies the investigators concluded that the decline in mortality rates was probably due to improved medical care. The decline in morbidity was attributed in the latter study to probable changes in risk factors.

The overall death rate for people under sixty-five has been declining in the United States. Decreased mortality from CVD was cited by the surgeon general of the United States as a major cause. The decline in mortality from CVD coincides with the reduction in several important risk factors specifically related to CAD—cigarette smoking by men, consumption of high-fat diets, average serum cholesterol levels, and the number of people with untreated hypertension (19).

Morbidity and mortality rates present only two aspects of the problem associated with CVD. The American Heart Association estimated that in 1985 CVD cost Americans $72.1 billion. The major portion, $43.7 billion, went for hospital and nursing home services, but lost output owing to disability cost Americans $13 billion. CVD is second only to respiratory disease in terms of days of disability.

Pathophysiology

The underlying problem in most cases of CAD is atherosclerosis of the coronary arteries. Atherosclerosis is defined as a disease primarily of medium and large arteries in which there is the development of raised, fibrofatty plaques called atheromas on the intima of the arteries. Any portion of the artery may be affected, especially points of bifurcation, and multiple lesions are typical.

In childhood there is concentric fibromuscular thickening of the arteries and by age ten, fatty streaks may be found on the intima of apparently healthy children. Whether or not this represents the early stages of atherosclerosis is debatable, but in the person predisposed to atherosclerosis, atheromas are imposed on these changes. Atheromas in the early stages are fibrofatty plaques appearing as soft, yellow raised lesions. They are mainly composed of cholesterol and cholesterol ester. These plaques gradually progress to fibrous lesions in which calcium salts may be deposited. When damaged, atheromas may ulcerate and hemorrhage. The end results of atheroma development are occlusion of the arterial lumen and loss of normal elasticity and integrity of the arterial wall. Symptoms occur when occlusion reduces the blood flow to tissues distal to the plaques enough to produce ischemia.

Atherosclerosis is a generalized phenomenon that tends to affect arteries throughout the body. Therefore, a person who presents with CAD may also have involvement of other arteries, such as those in the periphery, neck, and brain.

Angina pectoris is a clinical syndrome characterized by chest pain resulting from ischemia of the heart muscle. It occurs when the demand for oxygen exceeds the supply, most often as a result of atherosclerosis. When the lumen of the coronary artery is narrowed by at least 50 percent, symptoms of angina may occur with physical exertion. Symptoms at rest tend to occur when the degree of narrowing reaches 70 percent or more. Factors that can precipitate an attack of angina include coronary artery spasm, platelet aggregation, exercise, eating, exposure to cold, and emotional stress.

The typical person with an attack of angina pectoris complains of chest discomfort that is described as either substernal or left precordial pain, tightness, heaviness, or pressure. Occasionally the discomfort may occur in the back, forearm, or jaw. It is relieved by rest or a vasodilator such as nitroglycerin. Some people may have ischemia without discomfort. This is known as silent angina.

Angina pectoris is classified according to types as shown in Table 32.2. The significance of the types varies.

Complications

Myocardial Infarction. The major complication of CAD is myocardial infarction: necrosis of the myocardium secondary to ischemia. The most common cause of myocardial ischemia is atherosclerosis of the coronary arteries. Coronary artery thrombosis is present in almost all instances of myocardial infarction, but

Table 32.2
Types of Angina Pectoris and Their Significance

Stable Angina: Occurs with exercise or effort; onset and course are predictable; usually relieved promptly by nitroglycerin

Unstable Angina: Occurs with increasing frequency and with less effort; may occur at rest; lasts for longer periods; does not respond as well to nitroglycerin; warrants prompt medical attention as may be an indicator of myocardial infarction

Prinzmetal's Angina: Occurs at rest; is associated with coronary artery spasm; usually responds to vasodilators and calcium antagonists

---

whether thrombosis precedes or follows myocardial infarction is uncertain. The majority of infarctions occur in the left ventricle. The degree of cardiac impairment depends on the site and extent of infarction.

A person having a myocardial infarction typically presents with severe chest pain that may be either substernal or precordial. Some people, however, describe the experience as a heaviness or tightness of or a weight on the chest. It may radiate to other areas of the body (e.g., the back, jaw, neck, or left arm). Regardless of the location of discomfort, it usually lasts for more than thirty minutes and may be associated with diaphoresis and nausea. Some people have none of the above. Their infarctions are labeled silent infarctions. All people suspected of having a myocardial infarction should receive prompt medical care.

Dysrhythmias. Dysrhythmias may complicate CAD, especially when the client has had a myocardial infarction. More than 90 percent of the clients with acute myocardial infarction develop ventricular premature beats in the first seventy-two hours after infarction (58). These may persist into the recovery phase. Antiarrhythmic drugs may be used to treat dysrhythmias, and if heart block is present, either a temporary or a permanent pacemaker may be necessary.

Congestive Heart Failure. The precursors to congestive heart failure in almost 90 percent of the clients with it are either hypertension or CAD or both (14). Clinical manifestations of heart failure include dyspnea, orthopnea, paroxysmal nocturnal dyspnea, systemic venous congestion, weight gain, dependent edema, and engorged liver. Coughing, wheezing, breathlessness, rales, and cyanosis are associated with acute left ventricular failure.

Management of congestive heart failure includes bed rest to reduce the demands on the heart, diuretics and decreased sodium intake to reduce circulating blood volume, and vasodilators to reduce the afterload on the failing heart. The use of digitalis in treating congestive heart failure is controversial.

Risk Factors

The American Heart Association has identified a number of risk factors in CAD. These are categorized as major risk factors that can be changed, major risk factors that cannot be changed, and contributing factors. *Major risk factors that can be changed* include those discussed in the following paragraphs.

Cigarette Smoking. The surgeon general of the United States, in assessing the significance of cigarette smoking to the development of CAD, wrote: "Cigarette smoking should be considered the most important of the known modifiable risk factors for coronary heart disease" (54). Data from the Framingham Heart Study indicate that the probability of developing CAD is consistently greater in both sexes even when other risk factors—elevated blood pressure, elevated serum cholesterol, and glucose intolerance—are taken into account (7).

People who smoke have a much greater risk of having a heart attack than do nonsmokers, and the risk increases with the number of cigarettes smoked daily. It has been suggested that 30 percent to 40 percent of the annual deaths from heart attacks can be attributed to smoking. The risk of having a fatal heart attack increases with early initiation of cigarette smoking, long total exposure to smoking, and deep smoke inhalation. People can reduce their risk of death from heart attack caused by smoking by smoking cessation, but a decade may be required before their risk approximates that of the nonsmoker.

High Blood Pressure. Hypertension has long been associated with the development of CAD. There is some evidence that the risk of developing atherosclerosis and CAD increases when the blood pressure exceeds 140/90. Data from the Framingham Heart Study indicate that the risk of developing CAD is consistently higher in men and women as their blood pressure increases (7).

Elevated Serum Cholesterol. Fifty percent of middle-aged Americans have a serum cholesterol in excess of 200 mg/dl. Epidemiological studies have shown that in populations in which the average serum cholesterol level is below 150 mg/dl (e.g., in the Orient), the risk of developing atherosclerosis is low. The risk increases as the average serum cholesterol levels increase (18).

Heart attacks are more frequent in people with elevated serum cholesterol. Men and women aged thirty-five to forty-four who have serum cholesterol levels in excess of 265 mg/dl have five times the number of heart attacks as people with levels below 220 mg/dl (19).

A number of studies have been done on the relationship of lipoproteins, carriers of cholesterol in the body, to the development of atherosclerosis and CAD. High-density lipoprotein (HDL) is responsible for transporting cholesterol from peripheral tissues (e.g., the arteries) to the liver, where it is catabolized. It is *inversely* related to the incidence of atherosclerosis and CAD. As the level of HDL rises, the incidence of CAD decreases.

Low-density lipoprotein (LDL) and very low density

lipoprotein (VLDL) are both linked to the onset and progression of atherosclerosis. As the levels of LDL and VLDL rise, the incidence of atherosclerosis increases (18, 25, 43).

Certain factors are known to affect cholesterol and lipoprotein levels. Serum cholesterol levels are higher in people who consume diets high in saturated fatty acids, cholesterol, and total calories; in diabetics; in obese people; in sedentary people; and in people with familial hyperlipidemia.

The role that plasma triglycerides play in the development of atherosclerosis is not as clear as that of cholesterol, LDL, and HDL. There is evidence, however, that an elevation of triglycerides occurs in some people with atherosclerosis and CAD (55, 56).

Diabetes.   Cardiovascular disease is a major cause of death among diabetics and is far more prevalent in diabetics than in nondiabetics because of accelerated atherogenesis. Diabetics have higher serum cholesterol and triglyceride levels than do nondiabetics. Most forms of hyperlipoproteinemia are more common in diabetics than in nondiabetics. HDL levels tend to be decreased in uncontrolled diabetes.

Major risk factors that cannot be changed include the following.

Heredity.   The incidence of atherosclerosis and CAD is higher in people with a family history of atherosclerosis, coronary disease, diabetes, hypertension, and familial hypercholesterolemia. There is some evidence that blood pressure is heritable.

Sex.   Morbidity and mortality rates from CAD are higher in men than in women, even after menopause, when the rate begins to increase in women. Data from the Framingham Heart Study illustrate this point. A fifty-year-old man who does not smoke and has a systolic blood pressure of 135 and a serum cholesterol level of 185 (considered low-risk) has a probability of developing CAD in six years of 3.6 per 100. A fifty-year-old woman (the usual age of menopause) matched for risk factors (smoking, blood pressure, and serum cholesterol) has a probability of 1.2 (7).

Race.   Based on American Heart Association estimates for 1982, black men and women over the age of eighteen in the United States have almost one and one-half times the number of cases for hypertension as white men and women. The increased risk of CAD is probably related to the increased incidence of this risk factor.

Age.   The incidence of CAD increases with age for men and women. Risk factors associated with CAD (e.g., diabetes and hypertension) also increase with age.

Contributing factors to CAD include the following.

Obesity.   There is evidence that diabetes, hypercholesterolemia, hypertriglyceridemia, low HDL levels, increased LDL levels, and hypertension are associated with obesity. These may account for the increased risk of CAD with obesity.

Lack of Exercise.   Research has shown that there is an *inverse* relationship between CAD and physical activity. Studies have shown that people who exercise regularly tend to have higher HDL levels (23), smoke less (6), and are able to control hypertension more effectively (39). Their overall CAD risk is lower than it is for those who are inactive (28).

Stress.   The relationship of stress to CAD is less certain than other risk factors, such as hypertension and serum cholesterol levels, despite the number of studies done. In their classic book, *Type A Behavior and Your Heart,* Friedman and Rosenman linked heart disease to the type A personality—a hard-driving, aggressive, achieving person (15). Data from the Framingham Heart Study also support this linkage (7). In a more recent investigation, however, no relationship between type A behavior and the long-term outcome of acute myocardial infarction was found (5).

As indicated thus far in the discussion of risk factors, there is a significant increase in the risk of CAD when two or more risk factors are present. According to information supplied by the American Heart Association, the risk of having a heart attack is more than three times greater for a person who smokes cigarettes and has an elevated serum cholesterol level and hypertension than it is for a person whose risk is limited to cigarette smoking (20).

Prevention and Screening for Early Intervention

Primary prevention is directed toward modifying risk factors in the general population and specifically in high-risk people who do not exhibit clinical manifestations of CAD. Ideally it begins in early childhood, when children are taught at home and in the classroom the essentials of healthy living to prevent CAD—no smoking, proper nutrition, proper exercise, maintenance of optimum body weight, stress control, and regular health assessments to detect and permit early intervention for risk factors. Intervention aimed at primary prevention of specific risk factors is described in succeeding paragraphs.

The primary nurse's role in preventing CAD includes teaching and counseling to reduce risk factors as early as possible. In the overview of CAD it was indicated that some evidence of fatty changes in arteries are seen in children. When a child has a parent with CAD it is especially important to intervene early. Mothers of high-risk children need to be taught how to help their children lead healthy lives. The primary nurse may also be a resource for health education in schools.

Smoking. The increased risk of CAD associated with smoking is due not only to the number of cigarettes smoked for any specific time period, but also to total lifetime consumption (57). Ideally, smoking should be stopped before it begins, which means directing efforts toward children in grades five through nine, a period when children commonly adopt the habit. Content related to the hazards of cigarette smoking can be included in school curricula. The impact of the instruction is limited, however, unless the child is exposed to nonsmoking role models, including nurses. Some schools use nonsmoking members of the peer group to implement their smoking education programs. But this exposure must be extended to the home. It is difficult for children to internalize the need to not smoke when they observe their parents smoking. Adults may be referred to programs designed to help them quit smoking.

The American Heart Association, in its booklet entitled *Calling It Quits,* lists some useful tips and hints to help people stop smoking (1).

- List your reasons for quitting.
- Positively decide that you want to stop smoking.
- Set a target date for quitting and stick to it.
- Involve a friend or spouse in your effort.
- Switch brands and cut down on the number of cigarettes you smoke each day.
- On the day you quit, throw away all of your matches and cigarettes.
- Change your habits, especially those you associate with smoking.
- Celebrate each anniversary you remain an ex-smoker.

Other measures designed to reduce cigarette smoking include limiting smoking to designated areas in work and public places, establishing industrial policies and programs to discourage smoking, offering premium discounts on life insurance to people who have never smoked, and increasing the cost of cigarettes through reduction of the tobacco subsidy and higher cigarette taxation. Primary nurses can use their influence as health professionals to help accomplish these.

Nutrition. Since 1977 at least ten major reports dealing with nutrition of American people have been published by federal, professional, and health organizations (3). Although they vary in specific recommendations, all agree that there is a relationship between health and dietary intake. The aims of dietary intervention to prevent and control CAD are to reduce risk factors—dyslipidemia, obesity, hypertension, and diabetes.

In December 1984 the National Heart, Lung and Blood Institute of the National Institutes of Health issued a consensus statement that recommended the following dietary changes for all Americans over two years of age as one means of lowering blood cholesterol and preventing heart disease (31):

- Reduce calories from fat from the present average 40 percent level to 30 percent.
- Reduce intake of saturated fats to 10 percent or less of total calories.
- Reduce dietary cholesterol to no more than 250 to 300 mg daily.
- Increase, but do not exceed, intake of polyunsaturated fats to 10 percent of total calories.
- Reduce intake of total calories, if necessary, to correct obesity and maintain ideal body weight.
- Give special attention to managing other risk factors (e.g., cigarette smoking, diabetes, and physical inactivity) in people with elevated blood cholesterol.

In general, a diet consistent with the above guidelines would contain more grains, legumes, cereals, fruits, vegetables, fish, and poultry (served without skin). Current research indicates that as little as two fish dishes per week may help prevent CAD (26). The consumption of fish oils also may be effective (44). Such a diet would contain less meat, eggs, cheese, oils, and milk. Foods would preferably be cooked without frying. Skim milk and margarine would replace whole milk and butter. When eaten, meat would be lean and in smaller portions. There would be less salt and sugar, and total calories would be limited to those required to maintain optimum weight.

Dietary compliance can be a problem, two of the major reasons being the nature of the diet and the meaning of dietary change to a person. A low-fat, low-cholesterol diet can be unpalatable, although it does not have to be, and unless one prepares the diet from basic ingredients, following it can be a problem. Restaurants and food processors cater to the general public, whose eating habits tend toward foods that are high in fat and cholesterol. In many restaurants, however, it is possible to ask for and get low-fat, low-cholesterol meals, and if one shops diligently enough, it is possible to find prepared foods in the supermarkets that conform to dietary demands.

Generally, changing one's dietary habits is not an easy task. Our motivation for eating is complex. People eat not only because they are hungry and need body energy, but also to meet emotional and social needs. Changing one's eating habits is, in essence, changing a big part of one's life-style. Essential to successful long-term change in dietary practices is personal commitment to change, adequate support from family and significant others, and consideration of such essential factors as availability of food and ability to select and properly prepare the recommended diet. Preferably the entire family is involved in dietary change—the children, who are at higher risk because of heredity, and the spouse, who is usually involved in food preparation.

Other factors that may influence compliance are low level of education, low socioeconomic status, lack of understanding of the illness by the client, and inadequate communication. The initial motivation to comply has less effect on compliance than these do.

A teaching program designed to assist clients to change their dietary practices generally includes a discussion of the relationship between heart disease and diet, choosing and preparing foods, food shopping (including how to read labels), and how to incorporate dietary changes into one's life-style. Preferably classes should extend over several weeks to allow the client to implement what has been learned, to identify individual problems, and to provide feedback and support. The client should be either given recipes or referred to cookbooks, and the spouse should, if at all possible, attend all classes. Each is given a dietary prescription and a complete explanation of it. In some settings dietary teaching and counseling are done by a nutritionist; in other settings it may be the responsibility of the primary nurse.

Exercise. A program of regular vigorous physical activity, such as brisk walking, running, jogging, swimming, and cycling, that begins in childhood and continues through old age may protect against CAD.

People over age forty and anyone with symptoms suggestive of CAD or risk factors such as elevated serum cholesterol or hypertension should have a thorough cardiovascular assessment before embarking on an exercise program. Exercise programs should begin slowly and increase over a period of weeks to months. Engaging in exercise that is enjoyable and fits easily into one's life-style helps to promote long-term adherence.

Stress. Stress is a term that relates to a multitude of problems. Many factors produce stress, some of the more common being personality type, jobs, family relationships, socioeconomic status, and health status. A program that is effective in reducing stress begins with the identification of specific stressors that affect individuals and families. Stress reduction can be achieved to some degree when (a) stressors are correctly identified, (b) the individual and family admit that the stressors affect them adversely, (c) the individual and family are open and committed to change, and (d) appropriate resources, such as the primary nurse, for facilitating change are available and used.

Heredity. Because children of parents with CAD, hypertension, diabetes, and familial hyperlipidemia are at higher risk for developing CAD than are children of unaffected parents, screening for CAD appropriately begins early for such children. One program that can be used for screening and early intervention is presented in Table 32.3.

Today the American public is aware of the risk factors associated with CAD and of ways of changing their life-styles to reduce them. This awareness is due not only to the vast amount of research that has increased our knowledge of CAD, but also to the amount of exposure given through the media. Industry has joined by increasing employee health programs specifically aimed at reducing CAD.

The importance of primary nurses keeping up-to-date on research and reports issued by groups such as the American Heart Association and the National Institutes of Health and of adopting a healthy life-style themselves cannot be overemphasized. Nurses are role models, and their clients are influenced by their actions. Imagine the impact a nurse who smokes will make while counseling a client to give up smoking. If we believe that reducing risk factors is important to preventing CAD, nurses must be willing to reduce such factors in their own life-styles.

Management of Coronary Artery Disease

The major goals of management in CAD are to prevent extension of the atherosclerotic process; to prevent

Table 32.3
A Program for Pediatric Prevention
of Coronary Heart Disease

Age	Recommendations
Birth–1 yr	Family history; early (less than 55 years old) myocardial infarction or cerebrovascular accident in close relatives; parental hypertension, hypercholesterolemia, obesity, diabetes, smoking Follow growth* Nutritional counseling: breast-feeding, formula versus whole milk, dietary fat, sodium, sugar, weaning to solid food
2–5 yr	If family history is positive, screen for cholesterol; follow blood pressure and weight; counsel regarding dietary fat and sodium
5–12 yr	Observe growth and blood pressure; nutritional referral if obese Check parental smoking, and family and school exercise activity
12–18 yr	Follow blood pressure, weight; check cholesterol if obese or if family history is positive Counsel regarding smoking, alcohol, exercise, and diet

*At each age level if abnormal growth, hypertension, or elevated cholesterol is detected, careful study is warranted to rule out secondary causes or contributory illness.

Source: A. McKinnon. "Prevention of Heart Disease in Children." In *Cardiology Clinics,* ed. G. D. Curfman and A. Leaf. 3:289, 1985.

myocardial infarction, or reinfarction if the person has already sustained one; and to help the client live a productive and satisfying life. In accomplishing these goals, nurses are viewed as occupying a pivotal position. Through their expertise as teachers, counselors, and managers of client care they have the capacity to help set specific goals for individual clients, design and implement appropriate strategies for meeting these goals, and monitor the degree of goal attainment. Nurses who are knowledgeable about comprehensive cardiac care are aware of resources that clients and their families need, how to secure these resources through referral, and how to coordinate care so that resources are used appropriately.

Care begins as soon as the client is diagnosed as hav-

ing a problem. For the client who has been hospitalized with a myocardial infarction, this may be in the coronary care unit. It continues until the client has adapted his or her life-style to include the essentials of the program.

Some of the principles of effective care are as follows:

- Care should be comprehensive, addressing the physical, psychological, social, and spiritual needs of the client and family.
- Care is a multidisciplinary effort in which the nurse has a unique role.
- Care should be a collaborative effort between the client, the client's family, and health care professionals.
- Care should include teaching and counseling directed at specific needs and monitoring client and family responses to it.
- When selecting strategies for implementing care, those strategies that offer the greatest potential for long-term adherence should be considered.
- Ideally, the client and family should relate to the same health care professionals over an extended period of time. If at all possible, there should be a primary nurse who assumes responsibility for the client's care and is the primary contact for nursing intervention.

Nursing Care

Nursing care of the client with CAD adheres to the principles of effective care described above. It begins with a comprehensive assessment of the client and concludes with evaluation of the effectiveness of nursing strategies in reaching problem resolution.

Assessment

Assessment of the client with CAD includes a complete health history, physical examination, and findings of laboratory and diagnostic tests to determine the extent of pathology and the risk of developing complications, such as myocardial infarction. Nursing diagnoses derive from this data base and the nurse's knowledge of generally accepted preventive care. The nursing care plan is based on the nursing diagnoses.

Health History. Information specific to CAD elicited in the health history includes the following:

- Personal history of common cardiovascular symptoms: chest pain (onset, quality, duration, location, referral, degree of severity, precipitating

factors, means of alleviating, and associated symptoms, e.g., weakness, faintness, sweating, and nausea), cyanosis, palpitations, shortness of breath, dyspnea (on exertion and paroxysmal nocturnal), orthopnea (indicate number of pillows needed to relieve it), hemoptysis, edema, high blood pressure, headaches, dizziness, loss of consciousness, and changes in visual fields (e.g., blind spots)
- Past diagnosis of heart disease, hypertension, diabetes, retinal hemorrhage, dyslipidemia, stroke, and peripheral vascular disease
- Family history of heart disease, hypertension, diabetes, dyslipidemia, stroke, and peripheral vascular disease
- Relationships with family and significant others
- Occupation, working environment, relationships with co-workers, and satisfaction with employment
- Rest and leisure activities
- Exercise (type and amount)
- Diet (kinds and quantity of foods eaten; use of fats, salt, and sugar)
- Knowledge of CAD, its prevention and management
- Self-care ability and utilization of health care resources
- Response to health and illness, including perceived impact of CVD on the individual and family, motivation to change life-style as needed, and coping mechanisms

Physical Examination.   Information specific to CAD that is collected during the physical examination is found in Table 32.4. Some clients with CAD have no abnormal findings on physical examination. The nature and extent of findings depend on the degree of pathology and how much cardiac function is impaired.

Diagnostic Tests.   Selected tests that are commonly done to help diagnose the presence and determine the extent of CAD are found in Table 32.5.

Nursing Diagnoses

Although nursing diagnoses are individualized for each client, the following diagnoses are typical of those used in planning care:

- Potential noncompliance with overall care related to such factors as lack of knowledge and inadequate support
- Alteration in comfort: chest pain related to myocardial ischemia
- Exercise deficits related to such factors as lack of knowledge about optimum exercise and failure to select activities compatible with one's life-style
- Sexual dysfunction related to such factors as loss of libido, and fear
- Fear, anxiety, and depression related to such factors as the perceived threat of death and the impact of CAD on the client and family.

Nursing diagnoses related to smoking and nutrition are not included in this section because they are discussed in detail in the section on prevention.

Planning and Implementation

The following discussion of nursing intervention is directed to selected problems experienced by clients with CAD, with or without myocardial infarction, and is derived from the nursing diagnoses above.

☐ **Noncompliance.**   Coronary artery disease is a multifactorial problem. An effective approach to the problem is one that helps the client and family understand the nature of the problem and aims to reduce as many of the risk factors as possible, especially those that can be modified. Much of the discussion of primary prevention presented earlier is applicable here, but the emphasis in this section will be on what constitutes a comprehensive cardiac care program and how nurses can assist clients and their families to comply with the program over an extended period.

Essential elements of a comprehensive cardiac care program are as follows:

A program for monitoring the client's status
A teaching program that focuses on the following:

- The nature of the problem—normal cardiac functioning, development of atherosclerotic lesions and how they affect the body. If the client has had a myocardial infarction, content related to changes in the heart that occur with infarction and the healing process are included.
- Risk factors associated with CAD and how to reduce them
- Activity—kinds and amounts permitted (including leisure activity), kinds to avoid, and how to monitor responses to physical activity

Table 32.4
Assessment of the Heart and Vessels in Coronary Artery Disease

Assessment	Normal Findings	Comments
Blood pressure	120/80, varies with age	Should be measured in both arms and while standing and reclining. There should be little difference between the various readings. Elevated blood pressure is a common finding. When elevation is found, blood pressure should be retaken after the client relaxes. A single elevation does not indicate hypertension.
Radial pulse	Rate between 50 and 100 beats per minute, full volume, regular rhythm	Dysrhythmias, especially ventricular premature contractions, are common after myocardial infarction. Bradycardia and tachycardia may be associated with myocardial infarction.
Heart sounds	First (S_1) and second (S_2) heart sounds are clearly audible. Third (S_3) and fourth (S_4) are not heard. No murmurs, clicks, or gallops. Rhythm regular. Rate between 50 and 100 beats per minute.	In myocardial infarction there may be paradoxical splitting of S_2. S_3 may be heard. S_4 usually heard. Murmurs may be present.
Apical impulse	Faint pulsation less than 2 cm in diameter located in either 4th or 5th intercostal space just medial to left midclavicular line	More forceful in hypertension.
Carotid artery pulsations	Consists of single positive wave that is full, regular in rhythm, and equal bilaterally. No bruits.	Unequal carotid pulses may be seen in atherosclerosis of the carotid arteries. Amplitude of pulse decreased when left ventricular output is impaired. Auscultation of carotid arteries frequently reveals bruits when atherosclerotic narrowing is present.
Jugular venous pulsations	Undulating pulse with three positive waves visible when pulse rate is slow. Veins distend when client is reclining. At 45° angle, veins are barely distended above clavicle.	Venous distension persists in upright positions in right ventricular failure.

- Diet—kinds and quantity of foods to eat, foods to avoid
- Smoking—the importance of not smoking and resources to assist with breaking the smoking habit
- Sex—when to resume and handling problems related to sex for the client who has had a myocardial infarction
- Work—when to return and at what level, and planning rest periods at work for the client who has had a myocardial infarction
- Stress—common stressors, recognizing responses to stress, and general strategies for dealing with stress
- Medications—what they are, effects, dosages, administration, adverse effects and what to do when they occur, and precautions to observe (e.g., interaction of medication with other substances and storage of medication)
- Community resources available to the client and family
- Specific details of the plan of care for the individual client, planned tests or procedures, time and place of return visits, who to contact for

Table 32.5
Tests Used to Diagnose Coronary Artery Disease

Test	Rationale for Using	Comments
Chest x-ray	Assess size and position of heart, condition of great vessels, and pulmonary circulation	Arterial calcification may be seen in atherosclerosis. Pulmonary vascular engorgement and fluid accumulation in interstitial tissues of lung may be seen with left ventricular failure
Electrocardiogram	Most widely used noninvasive test of cardiac status and function. Used to identify areas of myocardial ischemia and infarction and to determine conduction defects	S-T segment deviation seen in myocardial ischemia. Q waves seen in myocardial infarction. Conduction defects (e.g., ventricular premature beats and heart block) may be associated with myocardial infarction
Cardiac catheterization and coronary angiography	Assess the ability of heart muscle to contract and visualize the condition of coronary arteries. Help in identifying candidates for coronary artery bypass surgery	Location and extent of atherosclerotic lesions can be determined
Thallium-201 and technetium-99m	Measure regional myocardial perfusion	Regional myocardial perfusion is decreased in coronary artery occlusion and infarction
Creatine kinase-MB (CK-MB)	Detect myocardial damage	CK-MB is found in myocardial cells and released with cellular damage. Normally less than 3 IU/liter; increased levels may be detected in the serum two hours after myocardial infarction. It peaks in 10 to 12 hours and returns to normal in twenty-four hours
Serum lipid profile (cholesterol, HDL:LDL, triglycerides)	Detect hyperlipidemia	Cholesterol and triglycerides are commonly increased in coronary artery disease. HDL is commonly decreased in proportion to LDL
Fasting serum glucose	Detect glucose intolerance and diabetes	Levels in excess of 120 mg/dl indicate possible diabetes
Stress test	Determine response of coronary circulation to increased demand	S-T segment deviation, indicating myocardial ischemia, seen when demand exceeds supply in coronary circulation. Helps to determine activity level in rehabilitation

information about care, and what to do in case of emergency

An exercise program that may be either supervised or unsupervised
Nutritional counseling
Psychological counseling
Spiritual counseling

Both group and individual sessions may be used to implement care. Nurses may lead any or all of the sessions, depending on their level of expertise in the content and in group work. Self-help groups, such as those sponsored by the American Heart Association, can effectively augment the professional programs. These groups give clients and their families an opportunity to share common concerns and ways to cope with them.

They also help reduce social isolation and provide emotional support that may be lacking elsewhere (45).

A variety of factors can influence compliance. These can roughly be divided into four groups—the client, facilities and services, health care personnel, and client support. Within the client are such factors as perception of illness, understanding of the program, perception of the value of care, and such psychological problems as fear, anxiety, depression, and denial. Factors related to facilities and services include cost, accessibility, and time commitment. Examples of factors related to health care personnel that influence compliance are attitudes toward the client and family, the quality of relationship they establish, and the kind of feedback they give. Primary supports for the client are the spouse, the physician, the primary nurse, friends, and relatives. In terms of compliance, the spouse can have a significant influence (22, 33, 35).

Dealing with the problem of noncompliance begins with uncovering the reasons for noncompliance. This can be done initially with the client in an individual counseling session, followed by a joint session with the spouse. Once the underlying problems are determined, appropriate strategies for solving them can be selected. For example, a client may not be complying with an exercise program because his wife is afraid he might have a heart attack and die while exercising. She constantly discourages him from exercising. One strategy that may alleviate this problem is to have the wife observe the exercise test on her husband and perhaps get on the bicycle or treadmill herself so she will know what it is like. Research has shown that this approach increases both the client's and the spouse's perception of the client's self-efficacy (53). Increased self-efficacy is linked to increased compliance (38).

□ **Chest Pain.** The chest pain of CAD and myocardial infarction is due to ischemia of the myocardium; therefore, efforts to relieve this problem are directed toward increasing the supply of blood to the myocardium and decreasing myocardial demand for oxygen. The most widely used method of increasing blood supply is the administration of coronary artery vasodilators. Some commonly used drugs are listed in Table 32.6.

Teaching clients how to use these drugs effectively enhances pain relief. For example, to prevent angina, clients are taught to take nitroglycerin sublingually before engaging in strenuous physical activities, emotionally stressful situations, and sexual intercourse. If angina does occur, the client should take nitroglycerin sublingually as soon as possible and stop doing whatever precipitated the pain. Either sitting or lying down helps relieve the pain by decreasing myocardial oxygen demand. Other measures that may be used include deep muscle relaxation, imagery, and thought control. Thoughts that attempt to fight chest pain tend to increase anxiety and pain, whereas thoughts that acknowledge the pain and focus on the idea that it will pass do not (49). If the pain is unusually severe or persists after taking two or three nitroglycerin tablets, the client should promptly seek medical attention. For clients who have recurring angina, long-acting nitrates, beta-adrenergic blocking drugs, and calcium antagonists may be used.

In order to allay fear and help clients to make intelligent decisions about when to promptly seek medical attention, clients are taught to identify precipitators of angina in themselves, to recognize when they are at their limit for physical and emotional stress, and to know how their angina feels. They are also encouraged to think of angina as a warning that needs to be heeded, rather than as a sign of an impending catastrophe. In most instances clients can relieve their angina by appropriate intervention and prevent more serious consequences; however, when angina exceeds what the client usually experiences, it is time to seek medical help.

Smoking cessation and exercise can also help to relieve angina. Some of the untoward effects of cigarette smoking are increased pulse rate and vasoconstriction associated with nicotine and a reduction of oxygen available to tissues associated with the inhaled carbon monoxide. As a client becomes more physically fit through exercise, the heart rate and blood pressure levels tend to decrease, lowering myocardial oxygen demand.

□ **Exercise Deficits.** The exercise component of the cardiac care program begins at the earliest feasible time. For the client with CAD who has not had a heart attack, this is as soon as the diagnosis is made and exercise tolerance is assessed.

After myocardial infarction and before discharge from the hospital, the intensity and duration of physical activity are gradually increased until the client is able to perform at a level comparable to that expected on return home. This prepares the client both physically and psychologically to resume activities of daily living and increases self-efficacy.

On discharge from the hospital the client may be referred to a supervised exercise program associated with a health care facility, a medically supervised home exercise program, or an unsupervised home program. Some community agencies, such as the Young Men's Christian

Table 32.6
Selected Drugs Used in the Treatment of Angina Pectoris

Category/Drug	Indications for Use	Comments and Nursing Management
Nitrates		
Nitroglycerin sublingual (Nitro-stat)	Coronary artery dilator; for acute angina attacks	If angina persists longer than 15 minutes or requires more than three tablets, notify physician. May be used 5 to 10 minutes before engaging in activities associated with angina. Tolerance may develop. Do not drink alcohol or use tobacco while using. May potentiate hypotensive effects of other concurrent cardiovascular drugs.
Nitroglycerin ointment 2% (Nitrostat)	Coronary artery dilator; used in the prophylaxis of angina	Apply to skin (usually chest, but other areas may be used) using dose-measuring applicator supplied with medication. Cover applicator and tape in place.
Isosorbide dinitrate (Isordil)	Coronary artery dilator; used in the prophylaxis of angina	Tolerance may occur.
Calcium Antagonists		
Nifedipine (Procardia)	Relief of coronary artery spasm	May interact with nitrates and beta blockers, leading to hypotension. Check drug interaction literature. Assess for hypotension during titration.
Verapamil hydrochloride (Isoptin, Calan)	Relief of coronary artery spasm	May have additive effect when used with other vasodilators. Use cautiously in clients with hepatic or renal damage. Contraindicated in severe left ventricular dysfunction and 2d or 3d degree heart block.
Beta-adrenergic Blockers		
Propranolol hydrochloride (Inderal)	Relieves angina by reducing heart rate and systolic blood pressure; for long-term management	Interacts with a number of drugs. Check drug interaction literature. Do not discontinue abruptly, as may exacerbate angina and precipitate myocardial infarction. Administer on empty stomach. Do not drink alcohol while using. Contraindicated in sinus bradycardia, 2d or 3d degree heart block, and congestive heart failure.
Dipyridamole (Persantine)	Coronary artery dilator for long-term management	Take at least 1 hour before meals. Not effective for acute angina attacks. Response to drug may be delayed 2 to 3 months.

Association, also have cardiac rehabilitation programs. If the program is supervised, it should comply with the standards for cardiac rehabilitation programs set by the American Heart Association (11). These standards assure that the proper personnel and facilities are available and used, that the client is appropriately assessed at various points in the program, and that provisions are made for handling emergencies. Before engaging in an exercise program, the client ideally should be tested for exercise tolerance.

The basic exercise program is the same for all clients, the difference being the intensity and duration of exercise based on exercise testing. It consists of a five- to ten-minute warmup phase, followed by a fifteen- to thirty-minute dynamic phase. The dynamic phase may consist of treadmill walking, riding the bicycle ergometer, or upper extremity exercises, or a combination of these. After the dynamic phase there is a five- to ten-minute cool-down phase that consists of walking or stretching exercises. This phase allows the heart rate to return to the baseline more gradually and helps to maintain cardiovascular stability. Exercise sessions are held three times weekly, preferably not on consecutive days, at an intensity sufficient to achieve 70 percent to 85 percent of the peak heart rate achieved in a symptom-limited exercise test.

For clients who are not enrolled in programs as described, two to three miles of walk-run activity three times a week is sufficient to maintain a cardiovascular training level. Alternatives to walk-run activity include swimming and rope jumping (11). Whatever the type of exercise, regularity and continuity throughout the year are essential.

Long-term compliance is necessary to benefit from exercise, yet compliance with cardiac exercise programs is low. Some of the factors associated with noncompliance reported in studies include program inconvenience, transportation difficulties, psychosocial problems, and medical problems, such as deteriorating cardiovascular status. Noncompliers also tend to be smokers, to be inactive in their leisure time, and to have spouses who are either neutral or negative to their participation in the program (37).

□ **Sexual Dysfunction.** Studies indicate that a number of clients have sexual dysfunction after myocardial infarction (4, 21, 40, 41). In one study of 100 couples 49 percent decreased the frequency of sexual intercourse and 24 percent did not resume sexual intercourse after myocardial infarction (41). In another study that examined sexual patterns over a period of time, investigators found that by six weeks postinfarction, 62 percent had resumed sexual intercourse and by six months, 93.9 percent had resumed sexual intercourse (52). Studies also indicate that clients who resume sexual activity have sexual intercourse less frequently, even after they resume a normal life-style (4, 21).

Reasons given for the decrease in or failure to resume sexual activity are, in decreasing order of frequency, loss of libido, client's and partner's fears, and depression. Some of the fears expressed were chest pain, heart at-

tack, inability to perform sexually, and sudden death (40). Rarely use of beta blockers may decrease sex drive and performance. Although 41.9 percent of the clients in one study had tachycardia or angina during intercourse, physical symptoms do not seem to be the major reason clients do not resume their preinfarction level of sexual activity. Emotional reasons seem to be the primary cause (21).

Asymptomatic clients can usually resume sexual activity approximately four weeks after returning home or when other usual activities of daily living are resumed (58, 59). The physiological demand of sexual intercourse is equivalent to walking briskly on a street or climbing one or two flights of stairs. Clients who experience angina during intercourse may take nitroglycerin sublingually beforehand to prevent it.

Before discharge from the hospital, clients who have had a myocardial infarction and their partners should receive complete instruction about resuming sexual activity and be given an opportunity to explore their feelings related to it. Although it is customary to give instruction to the client, partners are often omitted. In one study 55 percent of the wives of clients received no instruction before their husbands' discharge (41). Instruction ideally should include the physiological demands of sex, safety, alternative positions for intercourse, and the importance of discussing their fears and problems. Clients are also encouraged to exercise regularly, as physical fitness is associated with increased sexual activity.

Coronary artery disease and myocardial infarction may lead to marital conflict in some couples. The degree of conflict is related to a number of factors, including ability of the couple to communicate satisfactorily before the illness, emotional characteristics and problems of each partner before the illness, the impact the illness has on socioeconomic status, the couple's response to the illness, and the impact of illness on roles. Psychological counseling, both individual and couple, can be an effective means of dealing with this.

□ **Fear, Anxiety, and Depression.** Fear, anxiety, and depression are common responses to CAD, especially myocardial infarction. Studies indicate that anxiety and depression are the most prevalent maladaptive responses to heart illness (46, 49). These feelings may impact on almost any aspect of a person's life—marital relationships, family relationships, work, recreation, and self-concept. Likewise, many aspects of a person's life can affect the level of fear, anxiety, and depression experienced. Any attempt to relieve these feelings warrants a holistic approach to the client, considering not only the present illness, its meaning and impact, but also other factors from the client's past and present life, including support systems.

Fear is a response to something or some event that can be identified and that threatens the person. Throughout the ages we have identified in our literature the close connection in our thinking and feeling between the heart and life. Perhaps Virgil said it best in the *Aeneid* when he wrote: "Here are the tears of things; mortality touches the heart." It is not surprising, then, that the fear most consistently associated with heart disease is death. Having a heart attack can be a sobering event, for it forces one to face the fact that we are all mortal, life is limited, and, for this person, life may be short. When faced with this thought, anxiety and depression may ensue. Fear of death is only one fear common to cardiacs. Other fears expressed include limitations that heart disease will impose physically, economically, and socially.

Anxiety is a generalized response to something that is not identifiable. According to the *Diagnostic and Statistical Manual of Mental Disorders* (10, pp. 214, 233), a person is said to be anxious when exhibiting the following symptoms: motor tension (e.g., shakiness, restlessness), autonomic hyperactivity (e.g., sweating, tachycardia), apprehensive expectation (e.g., worry, anticipation of some misfortune), and vigilance and scanning (e.g., increased distractibility, insomnia).

As one examines these symptoms it becomes apparent that they are also common manifestations of physical illness. Therefore, it may be difficult to recognize anxiety in some clients unless the nurse spends time talking with the client and exploring feelings. This may be overlooked when the emphasis is placed on restoration and maintenance of physical functioning.

Depression is a dysphoric mood characterized by such symptoms as feelings of sadness, hopelessness, and worthlessness, loss of interest in usual activities, decreased appetite, insomnia, loss of energy, and difficulty thinking and concentrating (10). It is a common concomitant of crises, of which a major illness is an example, but it may be associated with other factors, for instance, neurochemical changes (decreased serotonin in the brain) and medications (antihypertensives being an example). The depression observed in a client after a myocardial infarction may also be part of a problem that existed before the illness.

If there is doubt about whether or not the client is depressed and the degree of depression, or about how to intervene, a psychiatric nurse clinician or psychiatrist may be consulted. It is particularly important to correctly assess the severity of depression, as suicide does occur in depressed people. Clients who have suicidal ideation, such as thoughts of "I wish I were dead" or "There's no reason for me to go on living," and clients who make suicidal gestures or attempts should be immediately referred for evaluation and care.

If the client has been hospitalized, the nurse should recognize that the incidence of both anxiety and depression tends to peak in the posthospital period and to be greater than what clients anticipated (46). Therefore, it is important in the first few months after hospitalization to spend some time with the client during each contact, exploring feelings and adjustment to the recovery phase. This is also a time for helping the client to acquire a positive philosophy of illness and recognize that being confronted with a serious problem can be an opportunity for personal growth. It can be a stimulus for rethinking life's priorities and focusing on what is truly important. Paradoxical as it may seem, having a serious illness can lead to greater meaning in life when clients and their families are helped to deal constructively with it.

When planning care for the anxious or depressed client, the family is appropriately included. Studies indicate that clients with CAD seek and receive most of their social support from relatives, friends, and their doctors instead of from professional services (46). Intervention is on different levels. For the nurse without advanced preparation in psychiatric nursing, intervention may predominantly consist of therapeutic listening to the client and family and referral to appropriate resources as necessary. The psychiatric nurse clinician, however, can help the client and family explore their problems in greater depth, including the social and physical manifestations of their problems, and develop more effective coping skills (32). The severely anxious and depressed and those requiring psychotropic drugs are appropriately under the care of a psychiatrist. To be most effective, intervention must be early and continue for a long enough period of time to allow the client and family to work through their problems and acquire adequate coping skills.

Evaluation

The following behaviors exemplify some that may be used to measure the outcomes of the nursing intervention.

Noncompliance. The client and his or her family will demonstrate an understanding of CAD and its prevention and management. The client will keep scheduled appointments and engage in prescribed activities.

Chest Pain. The client will use vasodilators and other methods of pain control, as prescribed. The client will modify activities and stress level to minimize chest pain. Her or his chest pain will not increase in frequency or severity.

Exercise Deficits. The client and his or her family will verbalize knowledge of optimum exercise. The client will demonstrate compliance with the exercise program.

Sexual Dysfunction. The client and his or her partner will discuss between themselves and with professional staff sexual problems as they arise. The client and partner will verbalize satisfaction with sexual activity.

Fear, Anxiety, and Depression. The client and his or her family will recognize manifestations of fear, anxiety, and depression. The client and family will seek care from the primary nurse and other health professionals. The client and family will exhibit fewer or no manifestations of fear, anxiety, and depression.

Ethical and Legal Issues

Ethical and legal issues related to CAD are diverse and broad in scope, ranging from the issue of client autonomy in making daily decisions about compliance with care to the complex issues of heart transplantation and the right to die unimpeded by mechanical life-support systems. A thorough discussion of ethical and legal issues may be found in chapters 5 and 6. A few of the questions that primary nurses may face are as follows.

What are the limits to client autonomy in planning and implementing care? How much can the primary nurse and other health care professionals intervene on behalf of the client?

When is informed consent truly informed? This is particularly relevant when new forms of treatment are being tried, or the client is part of an investigation.

Where should the emphasis on expenditure of funds be placed? On prevention of CAD? On care of acutely ill clients? On research and development into secondary prevention of CAD? On rehabilitation?

How can a primary nurse respond to a client's wish to die unimpeded by mechanical life-support systems while remaining within acceptable ethical and legal boundaries?

CASE STUDY

David Silverstein, a fifty-five-year-old self-employed stockbroker, is being discharged from the hospital after an uncomplicated myocardial infarction sustained two weeks ago.

He is 5 feet 10 inches tall and weighs 190 pounds. His average blood pressure is 150/90; his pulse averages eighty-eight and is regular. The most recent electrocardiogram shows a small infarction in the anterior wall of the left ventricle. There are no dysrhythmias or heart block.

Mr. Silverstein's serum cholesterol is 260 mg/dl, with HDL being 55 and LDL being 168. These values place him in the 90 percent risk category for CAD. His triglyceride level is 85 mg/dl, indicating that he does not have hypertriglyceridemia. He is being discharged on a 1,500-calorie, low-fat, low-cholesterol diet and is enrolled in a six-week nutrition program conducted by the nutritionist associated with the rehabilitation program. The nutritionist gave him a copy of his dietary guidelines and initiated diet teaching two days ago.

After discharge Mr. Silverstein will have his exercise test, following which an exercise prescription will be written. He is already enrolled in the two-month exercise program that is part of the rehabilitation program. It meets for one hour three times a week, with unsupervised exercise on remaining days.

You are the primary nurse and have responsibility for managing Mr. Silverstein's rehabilitation and for teaching, with the exception of diet teaching.

Mr. Silverstein is married and has two sons, aged twenty-five and twenty-three. He is financially secure and has comprehensive medical insurance that covers most expenses.

1. Describe your role as the primary nurse in this situation.
2. Outline a plan of teaching for Mr. Silverstein and his wife.
3. What is an appropriate approach to handling his sons' increased risk for CAD?

REFERENCES

1. American Heart Association. *How to Quit: A Guide to Help You Stop Smoking.* Dallas: American Heart Association, 1984.
2. Arntzenius, A. C., et al. "Diet, Lipoproteins, and the Progression of Coronary Atherosclerosis." *New England Journal of Medicine* 312:805, 1985.
3. Behlen, P. M., and F. J. Cronin. "Dietary Recommendations for Healthy Americans Summarized." *Family Economics Review* 3:17, 1985.
4. Block, A., J. P. Maeder, and J. C. Haissly. "Sexual Problems After Myocardial Infarction." *American Heart Journal* 90:536, 1975.
5. Case, R. B., et al. "Type A Behavior and Survival After Acute Myocardial Infarction." *New England Journal of Medicine* 312:737, 1985.
6. Cooper, K., et al. "Physical Fitness Levels vs. Selected Cor-

onary Risk Factors: A Cross-Sectional Study." *Journal of the American Medical Association* 236:166, 1976.

7. *Coronary Risk Handbook—Estimating Risk of Coronary Heart Disease in Daily Practice.* Dallas: American Heart Association, 1973.

8. DeBush, R. F., et al. "Medically Directed At-Home Rehabilitation Soon After Clinically Uncomplicated Acute Myocardial Infarction: A New Model for Patient Care." *American Journal of Cardiology* 55:251, 1985.

9. DeVries, W. C., et al. "Clinical Use of the Total Artificial Heart." *New England Journal of Medicine* 310:273, 1984.

10. *Diagnostic and Statistical Manual of Mental Disorders.* 3d ed. Washington, D.C.: American Psychiatric Association, 1980.

11. Erb, B. D., et al. "Standards for Supervised Cardiovascular Exercise Maintenance Programs." *Circulation* 62:669A, 1980.

12. Fielding, J. E. "Smoking: Health Effects and Control," Pt. 1. *New England Journal of Medicine* 313:491, 1985.

13. Fielding, J. E. "Smoking: Health Effects and Control," Pt. 2. *New England Journal of Medicine* 313:555, 1985.

14. Firth, B. G. "Southwestern Internal Medicine Conference: Chronic Congestive Heart Failure—The Nature of the Problem and Its Management in 1984." *American Journal of the Medical Sciences* 288:178, 1984.

15. Friedman, M. and R. H. Rosenman. *Type A Behavior and Your Heart.* New York: Fawcett, 1981.

16. Gillum, R. F., et al. "Sudden Death and Acute Myocardial Infarction in a Metropolitan Area, 1970–1980." *New England Journal of Medicine* 309:1353, 1983.

17. Goldberg, L., and D. L. Elliot. "The Effect of Physical Activity on Lipid and Lipoprotein Levels." *Medical Clinics of North America* 69:41, 1985.

18. Gotto, A. M., et al. "Recommendations for Treatment of Hyperlipidemia in Adults—A Joint Statement of the Nutrition Committee and The Council on Arteriosclerosis." *Circulation* 69:1065A, 1984.

19. *Healthy People—The Surgeon General's Report on Health Promotion and Disease Prevention.* Washington, D.C.: U.S. Department of Health, Education and Welfare, Public Health Service, 1979.

20. *Heart Facts 1985.* Dallas: American Heart Association, 1985.

21. Hellerstein, H. K., and E. H. Friedman. "Sexual Activity and the Postcoronary Patient." *Archives of Internal Medicine* 125:987, 1970.

22. Hubbard, P., A. F. Muhlenkamp, and N. Brown. "The Relationship Between Social Support and Self-care Practices." *Nursing Research* 33:266, 1984.

23. Hutten, J. K., et al. "Effect of Moderate Physical Exercise on Serum Lipoproteins." *Circulation* 60:1220, 1979.

24. Knox, R. A. "Heart Transplants: To Pay or Not to Pay." In *Medical Ethics,* ed. N. Abrams and M. D. Buckner. Cambridge, Mass.: MIT Press, 1983, ch. 109.

25. Kromhout, D., A. Arntzenius, and E. Van der Velde.

"Diet, Total/HDL-Cholesterol and Coronary Lesion Growth." *Circulation* 70: II–1, 1984.

26. Kromhout, D., E. D. Bosschieter, and C. L. Coulander. "The Inverse Relation Between Fish Consumption and 20-Year Mortality from Coronary Heart Disease." *New England Journal of Medicine* 312:1205, 1985.

27. Leaf, A. "MGH Trustees Say No to Heart Transplants" (I). In *Medical Ethics,* ed. N. Abrams and M. D. Buckner. Cambridge, Mass.: MIT Press, 1983, ch. 110.

28. Leon, A. S. "Physical Activity Levels and Coronary Heart Disease." *Medical Clinics of North America* 69:3, 1985.

29. Leon, A. S., et al. "Relation of Leisure Time Physical Activity to Mortality in the Multiple Risk Factor Intervention Trial (MRFIT)." *Circulation* 70:II–64, 1984.

30. Levy, R. I. "Prevalence and Epidemiology of Cardiovascular Disease." In *Cecil Textbook of Medicine,* ed. J. B. Wyngaarden and L. H. Smith. 17th ed. Philadelphia: W. B. Saunders, 1985, ch. 39.

31. *Lowering Blood Cholesterol to Prevent Heart Disease.* Bethesda, Md.: National Heart, Lung, and Blood Institute, National Institutes of Health, 1985.

32. Lynch, P., and M. N. Stevens. "Depression and the Physically Ill." In *Nursing Intervention in Depression,* ed. C. A. Rogers and J. Ulsafer–Van Lanen. Orlando, Fla.: Grune & Stratton, 1985, ch. 4.

33. McKool, K., and K. Nelson. "A Practice of Cardiac Rehabilitation." *Cardiology Clinics* 3:269, 1985.

34. McMahon, M., and R. M. Palmer. *"Exercise and Hypertension." Medical Clinics of North America* 69:57, 1985.

35. Mayou, R., A. Foster, and B. Williamson. "The Psychological and Social Effects of Myocardial Infarction on Wives." *British Medical Journal* 1:699, 1978.

36. Miller, P. L., et al. "MGH Trustees Say No to Heart Transplants" (II). In *Medical Ethics,* ed. N. Abrams and M. D. Buckner. Cambridge, Mass.: MIT Press, 1983, ch. 111.

37. Oldridge, N. B. "Compliance and Exercise in Primary and Secondary Prevention of Coronary Heart Disease: A Review." *Preventive Medicine* 11:56, 1982.

38. O'Leary, A. "Self-efficacy and Health." *Behaviour Research and Therapy* 23:437, 1985.

39. Paffenbarger, R. S., Jr., et al. "Chronic Disease in Former College Students. XX. Physical Activity and Incidence of Hypertension in College Alumni." *American Journal of Epidemiology* 117:245, 1983.

40. Papadopoulos, C., et al. "Myocardial Infarction and Sexual Activity of the Female Patient." *Archives of Internal Medicine* 143:1528, 1983.

41. Papadopoulos, C., et al. "Sexual Concerns and Needs of Post-coronary Patient's Wife." *Archives of Internal Medicine* 140:38, 1980.

42. Pell, S., and W. Fayerweather. "Trends in the Incidence of Myocardial Infarction and in Associated Mortality and Morbidity in a Large Employed Population, 1957–1983." *New England Journal of Medicine* 312:1005, 1985.

43. Peters, W. L., D. M. Hegsted, and A. Leaf. "Lipids, Nutrition, and Coronary Heart Disease." *Cardiology Clinics* 3:179, 1985.

44. Phillipson, B. E., et al. "Reduction of Plasma Lipids, Lipoproteins, and Apoproteins by Dietary Fish Oils in Patients with Hypertriglyceridemia." *New England Journal of Medicine* 312:1210, 1985.

45. Pinneo, R. "Living with Coronary Artery Disease." *Nursing Clinics of North America* 19:459, 1984.

46. Razin, A. M. "Psychological Intervention in Coronary Artery Disease: A Review." *Psychosomatic Medicine* 44:363, 1982.

47. Reid, V., et al. "Factors Affecting Dietary Compliance in Coronary Patients Included in a Secondary Prevention Programme." *Human Nutrition: Applied Nutrition* 38A:279, 1984.

48. Robbins, S., M. Angell, and V. Kumar. *Basic Pathology.* 3d ed. Philadelphia: W. B. Saunders, 1981.

49. Rovario, S., D. S. Holmes, and R. D. Holmsten. "Influence of a Cardiac Rehabilitation Program on the Cardiovascular, Psychological, and Social Functioning of Cardiac Patients." *Journal of Behavioral Medicine* 7:61, 1984.

50. Runions, J. "A Program for Psychological and Social Enhancement During Rehabilitation After Myocardial Infarction." *Heart & Lung* 14:117, 1985.

51. Shekelle, R. B., et al. "Diet, Serum Cholesterol, and Death from Coronary Heart Disease." *New England Journal of Medicine* 304:65, 1981.

52. Stern, M. J., L. Pascale, and A. Ackerman. "Life Adjustment Postmyocardial Infarction." *Archives of Internal Medicine* 137:1680, 1977.

53. Taylor, C. B., et al. "Exercise Testing to Enhance Wives' Confidence in Their Husbands' Cardiac Capability Soon After Clinically Uncomplicated Acute Myocardial Infarction." *American Journal of Cardiology* 55:635, 1985.

54. *The Health Consequence of Smoking: Cardiovascular Disease. A Report of the Surgeon General.* Rockville, Md.: Department of Health and Human Services, 1983.

55. "The Lipid Research Clinics Coronary Primary Prevention Trial Results: I. Reduction in Incidence of Coronary Heart Disease." *Journal of the American Medical Association* 251:351, 1984.

56. "The Lipid Research Clinics Coronary Primary Prevention Trial Results: II. The Relationship of Reduction in Incidence of Coronary Heart Disease to Cholesterol Lowering." *Journal of the American Medical Association* 251:365, 1984.

57. Weintraub, W. S., et al. "Importance of Total Life Consumption of Cigarettes as a Risk Factor for Coronary Artery Disease." *American Journal of Cardiology* 55:669, 1985.

58. Wenger, N. "Rehabilitation After Myocardial Infarction." *Comprehensive Therapy* 11:68, 1985.

59. Willerson, J. T. "Acute Myocardial Infarction." In *Cecil Textbook of Medicine,* ed. J. B. Wyngaarden and L. H. Smith. 17th ed. Philadelphia: W. B. Saunders, 1985, ch. 49.2.

60. Woolley, F. R. "Ethical Issues in the Implantation of the Total Artificial Heart." *New England Journal of Medicine* 310:292, 1984.

CHAPTER 33

Adults with Diabetes

CAROLYN AUERHAHN

■

OBJECTIVES

After completing this chapter, the reader will be able to:

☐ Differentiate between insulin-dependent and non-insulin-dependent diabetes mellitus with regard to pathophysiology, characteristics, cause, and management.

☐ Discuss the complications of diabetes with regard to their impact on the client.

☐ Discuss the implications for the nurse of the psychosocial aspects of diabetes.

☐ Describe the components of the management regimen.

☐ Discuss the client's role in the management of diabetes.

☐ Describe each of the components of the nursing process as it relates to the diabetic client.

☐ List three potential problems that may be encountered in the implementation of the nursing care plan.

☐ List three ethical/legal issues related to diabetes.

Diabetes is one of the most common chronic diseases in the United States. It is estimated to affect at least 6 percent of the forty- to fifty-nine-year age-group and 13 percent of those aged sixty to seventy-four (7). The incidence has increased in recent years and will continue to increase, owing to a variety of factors such as increased life expectancy, increased prevalence of obesity, and decreased death rate among diabetics. Diabetes is one of the leading causes of heart disease, blindness, and kidney disease, as well as the leading cause of amputation, in the United States and in many other developed countries.

Diabetes can be managed. It is as individual in its responses to treatment as the people it affects. Therein lies the key to its management—the individual. There are few, if any, other chronic diseases in which clients play as major a role in disease management as they do in diabetes. The very nature of the disease demands their active participation on a daily basis. It is the role of the nurse, as part of the health care team, to assist them in this endeavor. The purpose of this chapter is to provide the primary nurse with the knowledge and tools needed to fulfill this role.

Overview of Diabetes Mellitus

Classification and Diagnosis

Before the 1970s diabetes was viewed as one disease with varying degrees of severity. Terminology reflected the age of onset or difficulties encountered in management, and was not uniformly applied. Research during the 1960s and 1970s indicated that diabetes was in fact a heterogeneous syndrome, and the need for a revision in nomenclature became evident.

The 1979 the National Diabetes Data Group (NDDG) developed the classification system in current use today (see Table 33.1). This nomenclature reflects the inherent defect in glucose metabolism and provides for uniformity in classification. This chapter deals in depth with insulin-dependent and non-insulin-dependent diabetes mellitus.

Table 33.1
Classification of Glucose Intolerance

Class	Former Terms
Diabetes mellitus Insulin-dependent, type I	Juvenile-onset diabetes, ketosis-prone diabetes, brittle diabetes
Non-insulin-dependent, type II 1. Nonobese 2. Obese	Adult-onset diabetes, maturity-onset diabetes, ketosis-resistant diabetes stable diabetes
Impaired glucose tolerance (IGT)	Asymptomatic diabetes, chemical diabetes, borderline diabetes
Gestational diabetes	Gestational diabetes
Previous abnormality of glucose tolerance (Prev AGT)	Prediabetes, potential diabetes
Potential abnormality of glucose tolerance (Pot AGT)	Prediabetes, potential diabetes

Source: Classification and Diagnosis of Diabetes Mellitus and Other Categories of Glucose Tolerance. National Diabetes Data Group, National Institutes of Health, Bethesda, Md., 1979.

As with the earlier terminology, the criteria for diagnosis were inconsistent. Considering the impact of the diagnosis of diabetes on the patient, it is essential that there be consistency in diagnostic criteria.

Current diagnostic criteria, as developed by the NDDG (31), are as follows: Normal glucose levels are defined as fasting plasma glucose less than or equal to 115 mg/dl and two-hour oral glucose tolerance test (OGTT) values less than or equal to 140 mg/dl. A diagnosis of diabetes mellitus in the nonpregnant adult can be made if any one of the following is found:

a. Classic symptoms of diabetes, such as polyuria, polydipsia, ketonuria, and rapid weight loss, with an unequivocal elevation (≥ 200 mg/dl) of plasma glucose
b. Elevated fasting plasma glucose greater than or equal to 140 mg/dl on more than one occasion
c. Elevations during OGTT of plasma glucose

greater than or equal to 200 mg/dl at two hours *and* some other point between fasting and two hours on more than one occasion

The diagnosis of diabetes mellitus in the nonpregnant adult is usually made based on (a) or (b). The OGTT is being used with less frequency as a method of diagnosis in the nonpregnant population.

Insulin-Dependent Diabetes Mellitus (IDDM), Type I. IDDM, or type I diabetes, is characterized by sudden onset. The client presents with a history of polyuria, polydipsia, nausea, vomiting, ketonuria, weight loss, and fatigue. Rapid, deep respirations (Kussmaul's breathing) and acetone on the breath may be present and are classic symptoms of diabetic ketoacidosis. Hospitalization is frequently required at the time of diagnosis. Clients with IDDM are insulinopenic and ketosis-prone, requiring insulin by injection to sustain life. Onset is generally in childhood but can occur at any age (31). IDDM accounts for only a small percentage of the total diabetic population. Causative factors are both genetic and environmental.

Studies involving identical twins indicate a powerful genetic influence in the cause of IDDM. However, because IDDM was found to occur in only 50 percent of co-twins of affected clients, environmental factors have been implicated as playing a major role in the development of IDDM in genetically susceptible clients (27). Environmental factors appear to be both viral and chemical (17). Indications are that the process by which the disease occurs is autoimmune. Pancreatic islet cell antibodies have been identified at the time of diagnosis in clients with IDDM (27).

The physiological defect in IDDM is insulin deficiency. Insulin's role in glucose utilization is to facilitate the transport of glucose from the bloodstream into the cells (28). It is only within the cells that glucose can be used as an energy source. In addition, it is the presence or absence of insulin that determines whether the body is in a "fed" state or a starvation state (28). In IDDM there is little, if any, endogenous insulin production by the beta cells of the pancreas, and unless an adequate supply of exogenous insulin (by injection) is provided, the following will occur: Glucose will build up in the bloodstream, resulting in the symptoms associated with hyperglycemia—polyuria, polydipsia, polyphagia, fatigue, and weight loss. In addition, in a starvation state the body attempts to supply the cells with needed energy by manufacturing fuels such as glucose and free fatty acids. Glucose will be produced from glycogen stores in the liver and skeletal muscles (gly-

colysis) and by the hepatic conversion of amino acids to glucose (gluconeogenesis) (28). In IDDM this attempt at compensation only results in increased hyperglycemia. Free fatty acids will be formed by the breakdown of adipose tissue and can result in the life-threatening complication of diabetic ketoacidosis.

The treatment of IDDM consists of a combination of insulin by injection, diet, and exercise. The use of oral hypoglycemic agents is contraindicated in IDDM.

Non-Insulin-Dependent Diabetes Mellitus (NIDDM), Type II. NIDDM, or type II diabetes, is characterized by an insidious onset, frequently presenting with minimal or no symptoms of hyperglycemia. The disease may be present for years before the diagnosis is made. In many cases the diagnosis is initially suspected and later confirmed after an abnormal serum glucose level is obtained in the course of a routine physical examination. The onset generally occurs after the age of forty, but it can present at an earlier age. There are two distinct subclasses of NIDDM: obese (60 percent to 90 percent) and nonobese (10 percent to 40 percent). These clients are not ketosis-prone and may have insulin levels that are mildly decreased, normal, or elevated. They are not dependent on insulin to sustain life but may require it to control persistent symptoms or excessive hyperglycemia (31). NIDDM accounts for the majority of the total diabetic population. Both genetic and environmental factors are implicated in the cause of NIDDM.

Genetics plays a major role in the cause of NIDDM. Studies involving identical twins indicate a concordance rate of 95 percent with regard to the presence of NIDDM. In addition, the co-twins in the remaining 5 percent exhibited abnormal glucose tolerance (27). In a disease occurring, for the most part, after the age of forty the data point strongly to the inherited nature of NIDDM. The exact nature of the genetics of NIDDM is yet to be determined (17). The environmental factors implicated are lack of exercise, quantitative and qualitative food intake, obesity, and psychosocial stress (37). Obesity is the major precipitating environmental factor in the development of NIDDM in a genetically predisposed client (11).

The physiological defect in NIDDM is insulin resistance. Insulin resistance may be caused by numerous factors, such as the secretion of abnormal or ineffective insulin by the pancreas, circulating insulin antagonists (e.g., anti-insulin antibodies), or target tissue defects (either insulin receptor defects or postreceptor defects) (32). Insufficient glucose transport occurs and hyperglycemia results. Diabetic ketoacidosis does not generally occur because circulating insulin levels are sufficient to prevent it (see IDDM).

The treatment of NIDDM consists of diet alone, diet and an oral hypoglycemic agent, or diet and insulin. Exercise has been suggested as an adjunct to any of these regimens (8).

Complications

The complications of diabetes are both acute and chronic (see Table 33.2). Acute complications are episodic and life-threatening if untreated. Chronic complications involve the nervous and circulatory systems and can result in severe disability or death.

Acute complications are caused by acute aberrations in blood glucose levels. There are numerous precipitating factors, such as infection, stress, drug interactions, and noncompliance with management regimens. Response to treatment is generally good.

The devastating long-term effects of the chronic complications of diabetes have led to a tremendous research effort in the areas of cause, treatment, and prevention. The exact mechanism(s) for the development of these complications remains unclear, and research is ongoing.

Table 33.2
Complications of Diabetes Mellitus

Complication	Symptoms	Treatment	Impact on Patient
Acute			
Diabetic ketoacidosis	Polydipsia, polyuria, polyphagia, nausea, vomiting, altered level of consciousness, weakness, weight loss, Kussmaul's breathing, acetone breath	Hospitalization for stabilization with I.V. fluids, insulin, and supportive measures	If untreated, can progress to coma and death.
Hyperosmolar hyperglycemic nonketotic coma	Dehydration, decreased level of consciousness, polydipsia, polyuria, polyphagia, nausea, vomiting, hypotension, hyperthermia, tachypnea, focal seizures	Hospitalization for stabilization with I.V. fluids and insulin	If untreated, can progress to coma and death.
Hypoglycemia (insulin reaction)	Hunger, sweating, tachycardia, tremors, light-headedness, altered level of consciousness, grand mal seizures	Glucose, if able to swallow orally, in form of food; glucagon or I.V. dextrose if unconscious	If untreated, can progress to coma and death.
Chronic			
Neuropathies			
Peripheral	Numbness, burning, tingling, pain, loss of sensation—usually lower extremities but can affect upper extremities as well	Dilantin, Tegretol, Elavil usually ineffective. Aldose reductase inhibitors under investigation	Pain, reduction in activities of daily living, increased risk of amputation
Autonomic gastroparesis	Feeling of fullness, early satiety, vomiting undigested food hours after consumed	Reglan usually effective	Increased risk of hypoglycemia
Diabetic diarrhea	Nocturnal, explosive diarrhea	Usually refractory to antidiarrheals	Extreme embarrassment. Potential for dehydration
Cardiac	Orthostatic hypotension usually severe; fixed heart rate	If orthostatic changes are significant, Florinef is tried.	Increased risk of injury secondary to "fainting"
Neurogenic bladder	Incomplete emptying of bladder	Urecholine, intermittent self-catheterization. Long-term antibiotic therapy may be necessary.	Increased incidence of urinary tract infections

(continued)

Table 33.2 (continued)

Complication	Symptoms	Treatment	Impact on Patient
Chronic			
Neuropathies			
Impotence	Inability to maintain or sustain an erection. Complete workup to rule out other causes is essential.	Penile implant, counseling	Decreased quality of life. Psychological difficulties
Microvascular			
Nephropathy	Proteinuria, nephrotic syndrome, azotemia. Can progress to hypertension, edema, congestive heart failure, and encephalopathy.	Aldose reductase inhibitors under investigation. Dialysis and renal transplant in end-stage disease.	As renal function decreases, increased risk for hypoglycemia. Can progress to death.
Retinopathy	Asymptomatic—usually detected on routine eye exam. Severe proliferative changes can lead to hemorrhage of retinal vessels.	Follow-up essential. Laser photo-coagulation, vitrectomy. Aldose reductase inhibitors under investigation	Major cause of blindness
Macrovascular			
Atherosclerotic coronary artery disease	Angina pectoris or no symptoms	Symptomatic treatment of angina, coronary artery bypass surgery, anticoagulants	Myocardial infarctions—"silent" and acute; sudden death
Atherosclerotic cerebrovascular disease	Carotid bruits, transient ischemic attacks, or no symptoms	Anticoagulants, carotid angioplasty	Cerebrovascular infarction, sudden death
Peripheral vascular disease	Intermittent claudication	Increased walking, vascular surgery	Increased risk of amputation; if coexisting peripheral neuropathy, risk is tremendous.

Various treatment modalities are also the subject of numerous clinical studies. Chronic complications account for the reduction of the average life expectancy of diabetic clients to one-third less than that of the general population (10). Therefore, the prevention of complications becomes a priority. A relationship between the control of the disease and the occurrence of complications is alluded to in the literature (5, 34). Research continues in an effort to more clearly define this relationship. Response to current treatment modalities is generally suboptimal.

Psychosocial Aspects

An understanding of the psychosocial aspects of diabetes is essential when caring for the diabetic client. The diagnosis of diabetes carries with it the threat of severe, disabling, and life-threatening complications. The client will be required to assume the primary responsibility for a management regimen, which at times may be complex, on a daily basis. In addition, the diabetic client will have to work through the stages of adaptation associated with the diagnosis of any chronic illness.

The stages of adaptation to chronic illness, as identified by Crate (14), are shown in Table 33.3. The adjustment process can be viewed as a continuum. The client's progress along this continuum toward successful adaptation is an orderly process—one stage at a time in sequence. Fear, anxiety, and confusion can interfere with the client's adjustment. Regression along this continuum can occur in the event of a crisis (e.g., the development of a complication such as retinopathy). Depression is a common manifestation of unsuccessful adaptation.

Poor adjustment patterns may be demonstrated by the following behaviors:

1. Inactivity and over-dependence on other family members and/or health professionals

Table 33.3
*Adaptation to Chronic Disease
and Associated Client Behavior*

Stage	Behavior
Disbelief (denial)	Denies disease; disregards management regimen; ignores attempts at educational interventions.
Developing awareness	Blames self or others for the disease; displays anger.
Reorganization	Begins to seek information about disease; avoids discussion of disease with family and friends.
Resolution and identity change	Seeks out others with same condition; actively seeks information; openly displays emotions about diagnosis; strives for greater level of independence.
Successful adaptation	Actively involved in planning care; makes decisions about implementation of management regimen.

Source: Adapted from D. A. Billie, ed. *Practical Approaches to Patient Teaching.* Boston: Little, Brown, 1981.

2. Over-independence and denial of realistic dangers with increased participation in risk-taking activities
3. Withdrawal and resentment, especially if "mutilated" by complications of the disease
4. Denial of the disease or complication to the point of refusing to follow a medical program
5. Manipulation by taking advantage of the disease or complication to gain more attention and avoid restrictive treatment. (20)

Management of Diabetes Mellitus

The long-term goal of the management of diabetes mellitus is the prevention of complications. Short-term goals are to achieve and maintain blood glucose levels as close to normal as possible, to teach and encourage self-care, and to foster independence in the diabetic client. The components of the management regimen are diet, medications, exercise, home monitoring, and patient education.

In order to attain the overall goals of management, a team approach is essential. The team should consist of a physician, a primary nurse, a dietitian, *and the client.* Client noncompliance is a major problem in diabetes management. Therefore, the client should be an active participant in planning the management regimen, as the implementation of this regimen on a daily basis will be primarily his or her responsibility. Mutually agreed on goals need to be established, as do the methods to be used to attain them. An individualized, realistic management regimen must be designed that will encourage compliance. Although it may be suboptimal initially, over time the goals may be expanded to more closely approach the overall goals of diabetes management. Diabetes is difficult to manage, and time and patience on the part of the health care team are essential to ensure a successful outcome.

Components

The components of management include diet, medications, exercise, home monitoring, and patient teaching.

Diet. Diet plays an important role in the management of diabetes. For the insulin-dependent patient it is used in combination with insulin and exercise to achieve blood glucose levels as close to normal as possible. For the non-insulin-dependent client its primary objective is weight reduction (36).

Dietary strategies differ for the insulin-dependent client and the non-insulin-dependent client. Consistency in meal scheduling, caloric and nutrient distribution, and the addition of snacks are essential in IDDM, whereas a decrease in calories may be the only strategy needed in NIDDM (1). Compliance with diet is usually the most difficult component of the management regimen for the client. Education, counseling, and tailoring the diet to personal or ethnic preferences increases compliance (1, 29).

The diet prescription is based on the client's caloric requirements and nutritional needs. It is generally composed of 50 percent to 60 percent carbohydrate, 12 percent to 20 percent protein, and 30 percent to 35 percent fat (1), but the nutrient composition may be altered if coexisting medical problems dictate. The diet prescription is translated into a meal pattern, using the exchange system.

The exchange system is based on the principle of grouping foods of similar nutrient composition (1). This system enables the client to plan meals by selecting the appropriate number of foods from each group. Using this system requires careful attention to portion sizes.

Medications.   The primary medications used in the treatment of diabetes are oral hypoglycemic agents and insulin.

Oral Hypoglycemic Agents (Oral Sulfonylureas). Oral hypoglycemic agents (OHAs) are indicated in the treatment of NIDDM. There are two subgroups of OHAs: first-generation and second-generation (Table 33.4). OHAs are effective in improving glucose metabolism by ameliorating the insulin resistance associated with this type of diabetes (26). Although still somewhat controversial, the actions of OHAs are believed to be increased secretion of insulin by the beta cells of the pancreas and increased peripheral sensitivity to the action of insulin at both receptor and postreceptor sites (23, 26).

Adverse effects are hypoglycemia, gastrointestinal disturbances, hematological effects, skin reactions, and miscellaneous side effects such as water retention and hyponatremia (23). The incidence of these effects is low. They occur more frequently in the elderly population and are reversible when the drug is discontinued. Hypoglycemia is the most common serious side effect and may be prolonged. Drug interactions also are common and consist of either increased or decreased hypoglycemic effect. They most frequently occur with thiazides, glucocorticosteroids, beta-blockers, salicylates, coumarin derivatives, and alcohol (23).

Insulin.   Insulin therapy is mandatory in IDDM to sustain life and may be useful in NIDDM to control persistent symptomatic hyperglycemia. Table 33.5 describes the various types of insulin available.

The goal of insulin therapy is to normalize blood glucose levels over a twenty-four-hour period. This is best accomplished by a regimen of multiple daily injections or the use of a continuous subcutaneous insulin infusion pump. Multiple daily injection regimens consist of a combination of short-acting and intermediate- or long-acting insulins. Short-acting insulin is used exclusively in insulin pump therapy. Both approaches are aimed at simulating the insulin secretion patterns found in the nondiabetic. Similar results can be obtained with either approach.

Adverse effects of insulin therapy are hypoglycemia, insulin allergy, and lipodystrophy. Hypoglycemia is the most frequent and most serious side effect. Insulin allergy is uncommon and can be local or systemic. Local allergy is usually self-limiting. Desensitization kits are available for the treatment of systemic allergy. Lipodystrophy is uncommon and presents as either lipoatrophy or lipohypertrophy. The causes are unknown and the only ill effects are cosmetic (15). Drug interactions can occur and parallel those seen with oral hypoglycemic agents (23).

Exercise.   Exercise is indicated in both IDDM and NIDDM. The effect on blood glucose control is variable. For the well-controlled insulin-dependent diabetic client exercise lowers blood glucose levels and is an important part of daily management. In the presence of hyperglycemia (≥ 300 mg/dl), however, exercise may worsen control and actually precipitate ketoacidosis (22). For the non-insulin-dependent diabetic client the effects of exercise on blood glucose values are less clear; however, it should prove a useful adjunct to diet to achieve weight loss (8).

Exercise for the diabetic client is not without risks. Profound symptomatic hypoglycemia can occur and may be related to injection sites, peak activity of insulin, and timing of meals. Complications such as neuropathy and retinopathy may be worsened, and if coronary artery disease is present, arrhythmias, ischemia, or infarction can occur. Before an exercise program is initiated, medical clearance should be obtained (8).

Home Monitoring.   In order for management goals to be attained it is necessary to have as much data about blood glucose control as possible. A random blood glucose or glycosylated hemoglobin value obtained during an office visit is insufficient data on which to base management decisions. Therefore, it is necessary for the client to monitor blood glucose control on a daily basis, keeping records of results and supplying the physician with these records. Home monitoring may consist of

---

Table 33.4
Oral Hypoglycemic Agents

All sulfonylureas must be given before a meal. Observe the client for adverse effects. Use is contraindicated in insulin-dependent diabetes mellitus and pregnancy, and in clients who have a history of sulfa drug allergy.

First-generation sulfonylureas
   Tolbutamide (Orinase)
   Tolazamide (Tolinase)
   Acetohexamide (Dymelor)
   Chlorpropamide (Diabinese)
Second-generation sulfonylureas
   Glipizide (Glucotrol)
   Glyburide (Micronase, Diabeta)

Table 33.5
Insulin Preparations in Current Use

Type	Appearance	Onset of Action	Peak Activity (h)	Duration (h)
Regular	Clear	Rapid	2–4	6–8
Semilente	Cloudy	Rapid	3–8	10–16
NPH	Cloudy	Intermediate	6–12	18–26
Lente	Cloudy	Intermediate	6–12	18–26
Ultralente	Cloudy	Prolonged	14–24	28–36
Protamine zinc	Cloudy	Prolonged	14–24	26–36

Source: Eli Lilly Industries, Inc., Eli Lilly & Co., Indianapolis, IN 46285.

either urine testing or capillary blood glucose monitoring. Capillary blood glucose monitoring is the preferred method, owing to limitations in the use of urine testing as a method of assessing diabetes control (9, 19).

The client pricks his or her finger with an automatic lancet device, places a drop of blood on a reagent strip, waits a specified length of time, wipes the strip dry, and then either reads the strip visually by comparing it with color blocks on the bottle, or inserts it into a glucose reflectance meter and receives a digital readout. The accuracy of this form of monitoring is excellent, provided that there is adherence to all aspects of the procedure (19). The frequency of monitoring will depend on individual management regimens.

Capillary blood glucose monitoring is virtually without risk to the client, and the data obtained are invaluable. Although this form of monitoring is more expensive than urine testing, the benefits to the client are without question. In addition, third-party reimbursement is available in many instances.

Client Education. The success of any diabetes management plan depends on all its components, being adhered to on a daily basis. The primary responsibility for this rests with the client. The importance of client education in the management of diabetes cannot be overemphasized. Unless the client knows why and how to take care of the disease, the management plan will not be successful. Although all members of the health care team share the responsibility for client education, it is usually the nurse who assumes the role of diabetes educator. Not only is this an appropriate role for the nurse, but it is also the primary component of nursing management of the diabetic client.

Prevention and Screening for Early Intervention

Prevention

The prevention of a disease or its complications is based on the identification and reduction of risk factors. A risk factor is a variable that increases the likelihood of developing a specific disease or complication. There are basically two types: those that can be modified and those that cannot. For example, age, sex, and family history cannot be changed. Weight, cigarette smoking, and a sedentary life-style can be modified. The more risk factors present, the greater the likelihood of developing the disease, and vice versa.

Known risk factors for the development of diabetes mellitus are age, positive family history, history of gestational diabetes, and obesity. Of these, the only modifiable factor is obesity. As mentioned earlier, certain life-style components are implicated in the cause of diabetes mellitus. Life-style components are also a factor in the development of some of the complications of diabetes, such as coronary artery disease (2). An assessment of life-style components, such as diet, activity level, tobacco use, and stress, is essential to identify those that pose the greatest risk for the development of complications.

Efforts toward preventing diabetes in a person at risk should be directed at the prevention or reduction of obesity. To reduce the client's risk of complications, modifiable risk factors must be identified and a plan of attack to reduce or eliminate them must be formulated.

The diabetic client plays a major role in the prevention of complications. In addition to making necessary life-style changes, the client must carry out daily health maintenance measures. These include foot care, skin care, dental hygiene, general hygiene, and compliance with the management regimen (2). The nurse's primary role in the prevention of complications is to assist diabetic clients in carrying out their responsibilities. Education, counseling, support, and referral to community resources are essential.

Screening

In addition to known risk factors, the following have been identified (21) as indications for testing for diabetes:

- Elevated blood glucose
- Glycosuria
- Unusual, unexplained weight loss
- Polyuria, polydipsia, polyphagia
- Recurrent infections
- Presence of metabolic conditions frequently associated with diabetes (e.g., elevated triglyceride, cholesterol, or uric acid levels)
- Unexplained presence of neuropathy, retinopathy, peripheral vascular disease, or coronary artery disease
- Pregnancy (for gestational diabetes)
- Giving birth to a baby weighing nine pounds or greater
- History of multiple spontaneous abortions or birth defects

If any of these are present, referral to a physician for diagnostic workup is essential for early intervention.

Nursing Care

Assessment

A comprehensive nursing history, physical assessment, and diagnostic test results constitute the data base essential for developing the nursing care plan.

The components of the nursing history that are relevant to the diabetic client are as follows.

Age at Onset/Duration. This provides data regarding the client's risk for complications, adaptation stage, or adjustment difficulties.

Treatment Before Admission. Both prescribed and actual treatment should be ascertained. They may differ. Reasons for differences will require further assessment. For example, the prescribed treatment may include capillary blood glucose monitoring before meals and at bedtime. However, clients may not be complying because they cannot afford the supplies.

Control: Signs and Symptoms. When asked, "How good is your blood glucose control?" most clients will respond "pretty good" or "okay." To obtain more accurate information about control, question the client regarding the presence and frequency of symptoms of both hyperglycemia and hypoglycemia. Nocturia is a good indication of hyperglycemia, especially if the client is taking diuretics for coexistent hypertension. Frequent hypoglycemic episodes in a client with normal blood glucose levels will require further assessment regarding meal and exercise patterns.

Presence of Complications. It is essential to ascertain the presence of complications. For example, the client with peripheral neuropathy will need a strong emphasis on foot care to help reduce the risk of amputation. The client with retinopathy may have visual impairments that interfere with aspects of insulin administration or home monitoring.

Compliance. The admission of a client with a diagnosis of uncontrolled diabetes mellitus does not necessarily indicate noncompliance. Stress or infection may have precipitated the loss of control. An assessment of the degree of compliance, as well as the reasons for noncompliance, will be derived from other components of the history and other assessment parameters.

Knowledge Base. Never assume that because a client has had diabetes for many years, that he or she understands the disease or has been taught to manage it. Even clients who have attended formal diabetes education programs may have knowledge deficits that interfere with the management of their disease. The educational intervention may have occurred at the wrong time, or other barriers to learning may have been present. Assessment of the client's knowledge of diabetes is an important aspect of the nursing history. Knowledge deficits are a frequent cause of noncompliance.

Self-Care Measures. Question the client regarding home monitoring, health maintenance measures, and life-style components.

Psychosocial Aspects. An assessment of the client's adjustment to the disease is essential in order to develop a care plan. Also collect data regarding the client's health care beliefs, home situation, work schedule, and financial status. These may impact on the daily management of the disease.

Aspects of the physical assessment especially relevant to the diabetic client are as follows.

Vital Signs. Cardiovascular complications are common in diabetics, especially after the age of forty. There is also a high frequency of coexisting hypertension in this group.

Skin. Observe for excessive dryness, rashes, and the presence of skin infections. Staphylococcal and monilial infections are common in clients with poor control. Infections caused by *Staphylococcus aureus* may be found anywhere on the body. Monilial infections are found in warm, moist areas, such as body creases, the inguinal area, and under the breasts, especially in obese patients. Observe injection sites for areas of redness or induration (local allergy), depressions (lipoatrophy), or excessive fatty deposits (lipohypertrophy).

Mouth. Observe for dryness of mucous membranes, evidence of monilial infection, and condition of teeth and gums. A diabetic client who is poorly controlled for a prolonged period may become dehydrated. Fissures or cracks at the angles of the mouth (cheilosis) or white curdy patches on the palate or tongue are indications of monilial stomatitis. Diabetic clients are especially prone to gum disease and an increased incidence of dental caries.

Lower Extremities. A thorough assessment of the legs and feet is essential when caring for the diabetic client. Observe for evidence of peripheral vascular disease: absent or decreased pulses; changes in skin color, temperature, appearance, or hair distribution. Observe for areas of redness or swelling and the presence of leg or foot ulcers. In chronic arterial insufficiency, ulcers are generally found on the toes or in areas of pressure (as from ill-fitting shoes). Ulcers resulting from chronic venous insufficiency are found at the ankle or above. Assess clients also for loss of sensation secondary to either peripheral neuropathy or peripheral vascular disease.

Diagnostic Tests. The focus of diagnostic tests ordered for the diabetic client will be to assess the level of diabetic control and to detect or monitor complications.

The role of the nurse will be to explain the procedure and the reasons for the test and to provide support for the client if needed. It is not the role of the nurse to report test results to the client. Normal values for laboratory tests will vary from one setting to the next. The normal range is generally included on the printed report or can be obtained from the laboratory. Common tests ordered include the following:

- *Chemistry profile*—to determine blood glucose level, assess renal function (BUN, creatinine, K^+, or PO_4), and detect the presence of other metabolic abnormalities associated with diabetes (elevated triglycerides, cholesterol, or uric acid)
- *Urinalysis*—to detect glycosuria, ketonuria, proteinuria, or the possibility of urinary tract infection
- *Twenty-four-hour urine collection*—to assess renal function (creatinine clearance) and determine the extent of proteinuria or glycosuria
- *Glycosylated hemoglobin* (may be ordered as $HgbA_{1c}$ or $HgbA_1$). This refers to a permanent attachment of glucose molecules to hemoglobin A. At high blood glucose levels more hemoglobin is bound to glucose. Glycosylation of hemoglobin is a slow, irreversible process that occurs throughout the life span of the red blood cell. Because the half-life of the red blood cell is sixty days, the measurement of glycosylated hemoglobin can reflect average blood glucose concentration over the preceding two months. It is unaffected by recent food intake, exercise, or stress levels [24]. It is a good indication of chronic blood glucose control.
- *Electrocardiogram*—to detect or monitor the presence of cardiovascular complications (e.g., coronary artery disease, "silent" myocardial infarction)
- *Nerve conduction velocity studies.* In this electrophysiological method of determining peripheral nerve function, electrodes are placed at points along the major nerves in the upper and lower extremities. The rate at which electrical impulses travel along the nerves is measured. In the presence of neuropathy there will be a slowing in the rate. During the test the client will experience sensations ranging from minor discomfort to "severe" pain.
- *Ophthalmology consult*—to detect or monitor retinopathy. A routine fundoscopic examination is done. Fluorescein angiography may be ordered if

retinopathy is present. A radiopaque dye is injected intravenously, and photographs of the retinal vessels are taken. The client may experience some discomfort from the dye, but this test carries a relatively low risk.

Nursing Diagnoses

After compiling the data base the nurse completes the assessment by formulating nursing diagnoses. Carpenito (12) has identified the following nursing diagnoses as relevant to the diabetic patient.

- Potential impairment of skin integrity related to increased susceptibility to fungal infection, pruritus secondary to vascular condition, and increased blood sugar
- Potential sexual dysfunction (male) related to erectile problems secondary to peripheral neuropathy
- Potential alterations in tactile sensory perception related to paresthesia secondary to peripheral neuropathies
- Potential alterations in visual sensory perception related to retinopathy
- Potential for injury related to decreased tactile sensation and diminished visual acuity
- Alteration in peripheral tissue perfusion related to decreased neurovascular function secondary to peripheral neuropathies
- Potential for infection related to depleted host defenses and depressed leukocytic phagocytosis secondary to hyperglycemia
- Alteration in nutrition—greater than body requirements—related to intake in excess of activity expenditures
- Alteration in nutrition—less than body requirements—related to insufficient fulfillment of caloric requirements to maintain growth and development
- Potential noncompliance related to the complexity of adhering to the prescribed regimen
- Powerlessness related to the uncertainty of the disease and the development of complications
- Knowledge deficit of, for example, the disease itself, nutrition (meal planning), weight control, exercise program, medications, foot care, signs and symptoms of complications, record keeping, blood and urine testing, hypoglycemia and hyperglycemia, and community services (support groups).

This list represents only some of the possible nursing diagnoses. Additional problems that may be encountered are as follows:

- Alterations in comfort—pain related to peripheral neuropathy
- Ineffective individual coping related to significant life changes—new diagnosis diabetes mellitus
- Disturbance in self-image related to amputation secondary to peripheral vascular disease
- Alterations in patterns of urinary elimination (polyuria, nocturia) related to hyperglycemia
- Fear related to possibility of complications

The lists above are intended to be used only as examples of possible nursing diagnoses for the diabetic client. When formulating nursing diagnoses for an individual client it is essential that the diagnosis be derived from an in-depth analysis of the data base for that particular person. By identifying not only the individual problem, but also the individual cause, the nurse will be able to clearly define patient goals as well as nursing interventions needed to effect change (35).

Planning and Implementation

The first step in developing the nursing care plan is to rate the nursing diagnoses with regard to the impact of each on the client. Maslow's hierarchy (30) and Crate's stages of adaptation (14) are excellent tools on which to base this priority rating.

Maslow identified five levels of needs: physiological, safety, belonging and love, esteem (of self and of others), and self-actualization. Needs at the first level (physiological) must be met before those of the second and so forth. Applying Maslow's theory to care planning, the nursing diagnoses that reflect, for example, acute physiological or safety needs receive a higher priority than those dealing with the need for self-actualization.

Crate's stages of adaptation are important when determining educational aspects of patient care. Educational interventions according to stage of adaptation are as follows (2):

Denial/Disbelief	Teach only survival skills
Developing Awareness	Teach survival skills
Reorganization	Teaching of mutually agreed on goals may be started
Resolution/Identity	Teach mutually agreed on goals
Change	Client strives for self-sufficiency

After rating the nursing diagnoses, a care plan for each is developed. Nursing actions and short-term and long-term goals are established. As discussed earlier at length, it is essential that the diabetic client be involved in goal setting whenever possible.

It is beyond the scope of this text to develop care plans for each of the possible nursing diagnoses for the diabetic client. Several examples of detailed care plans are found elsewhere in the literature (16, 25), and I urge the reader to use these references. This text focuses on two of the many possible nursing diagnoses—knowledge deficit related to such factors as inadequate content presented in a manner that the client can comprehend and apply, and noncompliance related to such factors as lack of motivation and resistance to change.

□ *Knowledge Deficits.* As discussed earlier, the primary nursing responsibility when caring for the diabetic client is patient education. Developing an individualized teaching plan is essential when planning care.

Knowledge deficits have been identified during the assessment phase. A teaching plan directed at correcting these deficits is based on the client's current level of understanding, ability to comprehend, physical limitations, level of acceptance of illness and prescribed treatment, home situation, financial status, and ability to cope with illness, physical limitations, and other life responsibilities (3). The teaching plan will allow for the client's health status, procedures and treatments to be performed, medications, diet, activity level, and other aspects of the treatment regimen (3).

Figures 33.1 and 33.2 are examples of teaching plans for the diabetic client. They are designed to meet basic patient education requirements.

The content delivered for each learner objective will depend on numerous factors, such as educational level, adaptation stage, and readiness to learn. Teaching can be accomplished in one-to-one sessions or group classes or by self-learning through handouts. The educational process is ongoing and does not necessarily require formal sessions. Procedures such as insulin administration, monitoring, and foot care can be taught while the nurse is performing them. Return demonstrations are essential when teaching a procedure. Other areas of content can be addressed when explaining procedures or diagnostic tests or when answering clients' questions. Documentation on the teaching plan of nursing actions as well as clients' responses and comprehension is an integral part of the teaching process.

Three potential problems may be encountered when caring for the diabetic client. Barriers may be present that interfere with learning. Clients may not be motivated to accept the responsibilities of their care. They may resist change.

Barriers to learning may be physical, cultural, intellectual, or psychological.

Physical Barriers. Many diabetic clients have visual impairments or fluctuations in visual acuity. Older clients may have hearing deficits or problems with fine hand coordination. Physical barriers may interfere with procedures, and another person may need to assume the responsibility for those aspects of care. Another approach is the use of an ever-growing number of aids for visually impaired diabetic clients (13).

Cultural Barriers. The clients' health care beliefs will impact on their responses to health and illness. For effective learning to occur it is essential to understand and approach the teaching process from the clients' perspective. Language barriers may be present. An interpreter may be necessary, but be aware that the message may be filtered when you use a translator. Some educational materials are available in languages other than English.

Intellectual Barriers. Slow learners and nonreaders usually do not benefit from written materials. Demonstration and audiovisual aids are helpful for such clients.

Psychological Barriers. Most diabetic clients will know others with the disease. They may have preconceived ideas about diabetes that are inaccurate, or have had previous experiences with others that may have frightened them. As described earlier, the stage of adaptation will also impact on learning (2).

□ *Noncompliance.* Lack of motivation is perhaps the most difficult problem encountered when caring for diabetic clients. The client's cooperation and compliance are mandatory in order to attain the overall goals of the management plan. Unmotivated clients are usually noncompliant. The reasons for lack of motivation are multitudinous, as are the remedies. The educational process can be an effective way to motivate clients and thus enhance compliance. The following suggestions are from a "non-compliant diabetic and professor" (33):

1. treat the patient as a person first and a diabetic second
2. let people with diabetes know they are not alone
3. present the education and treatment as a positive act for wellness that offers the diabetic options from which to choose
4. remind the patient that diabetes educators are human

PURPOSE: Provide basic knowledge to assist the patient in controlling her/his diabetes.

LEARNER OBJECTIVE: Patient and/or significant other demonstrates a knowledge of:	Content Delivered	Learner Objectives Met	Comments— Use NA if not applicable
	Date and Initials	Date and Initials	Date and Initials
I. Diabetes and what it means			
II. Type of insulin, dosage, and time to administer			
III. Insulin administration			
IV. Symptoms of hypoglycemia and action to take			
V. Symptoms of hyperglycemia and action to take			
VI. Urine/Capillary blood glucose monitoring			
VII. Diabetic exchange diet, including number of calories in individualized meal plan			
VIII. Role of exercise in treatment plan			
IX. Follow-up care (i.e. appointment(s) with MD/clinic/dietitian)			
X. General hygiene measure			
XI. When and where to call if problems arise			
XII. The importance of wearing Medic-Alert identification			

EVALUATION/SUMMARY:

Figure 33.1.   Basic Patient/Family Teaching Plan for IDDM

Source: Westchester County Medical Center, Department of Nursing, Valhalla, N.Y.

5. try to prevent the patient from becoming dependent upon the diabetes educator for treatment, motivation and support
6. try to get the patient to establish a dispassionate, objective attitude towards treatment
7. remember that diabetes is an expensive disease
8. be accessible

Resistance to change is a major problem when caring for the diabetic client. Compliance with the management plan will involve numerous changes in the client's life-style. Each client will respond differently to the concept of change. Three types of resistance have been identified (4): resistance to the consequence of change, resistance to the change when it threatens the client's integrity, and resistance directed at the change agent. Resistance is usually manifested as a combination of the three types. The nurse's role as a change agent is that of facilitator and logician. Teaching new concepts and

skills and supporting the integration of these into the client's life-style are essential (4). Effecting positive change is lengthy and time-consuming. Identification and utilization of appropriate resources are necessary. Family members or a close friend may prove to be an invaluable resource. Community resources include the local chapter of the American Diabetes Association, which provides such services as education and peer support. Referral to other health care professionals, such as registered dietitians and podiatrists, is also indicated. With the proper guidance and support, resistance to change can be reduced and perhaps conquered.

Evaluation

Evaluation of the client's response to nursing intervention depends on the nursing diagnosis and intervention. The following evaluation criteria are typical for

PURPOSE: Provide basic knowledge to assist the patient in controlling her/his diabetes.

LEARNER OBJECTIVE: Patient and/or significant other demonstrates a knowledge of:	Content Delivered	Learner Objectives Met	Comments— Use NA if not applicable
	Date and Initials	Date and Initials	Date and Initials
I. Diabetes and what it means			
II. Diet (a) relationship of body, weight and glucose tolerance			
(b) diabetic exchange diet, including number of calories in individualized meal plan			
III. Role of exercise in treatment plan			
IV. Oral hypoglycemic agents; name, dose, time, and side effects			
V. Symptoms of hypoglycemia and action to take			
VI. Symptoms of hyperglycemia and action to take			
VII. Urine/Capillary blood glucose monitoring			
VIII. Follow-up care (i.e. appointment(s) with MD/clinic/dietitian)			
IX. General hygiene measures			
X. When and where to call if problems arise			
XI. Importance of wearing Medic-Alert identification			

EVALUATION/SUMMARY:

Figure 33.2. Basic Patient/Family Teaching Plan for NIDDM

Source: Westchester County Medical Center, Department of Nursing, Valhalla, N.Y.

a nursing diagnosis of knowledge deficit with teaching as the intervention. The minimum criteria that must be met for each learner objective in the sample teaching plans are as follows.

Diabetes and What It Means. The client should verbalize that he or she has diabetes and that this is a life-long condition that requires medical follow-up. The client should also verbalize that he or she needs to follow a diet plan (and take prescribed medicine).

Diet. The client should demonstrate a knowledge of the diabetic exchange diet, including the number of calories in an individual meal plan. Proper portion size within each exchange and selection of appropriate foods are basic requirements. The client should verbalize the importance of attaining and maintaining desirable weight.

Medications. *Oral Hypoglycemic Agents:* The client should verbalize the name of the drug, the dose, and the time of ingestion (before meals). He or she should verbalize that the medication is not insulin, but that it helps the body's insulin to work more effectively. The client should verbalize possible side effects of the drug. *Insulin:* The client identifies the type of insulin, the dose, and the time of administration. The client demonstrates correct administration of insulin, including site selection and rotation.

Exercise. *Non-Insulin-Dependent:* The client verbalizes the benefits of exercise: when used in conjunction with a diet, it results in greater weight loss, improves cardiovascular status, enhances one's sense of well-being. The client verbalizes that a planned progressive program should be established, with a full cardiac evaluation before the program is initiated. *Insulin-Dependent:* The client verbalizes the following concepts: if blood sugar is well controlled (under 300), including exercise in the daily routine can help to maintain good control; if blood sugar is poorly controlled, or the client is ill, exercise should not be engaged in until control is regained.

Hypoglycemia. The client should be able to state at least three or more of the following symptoms: nervousness, irritability, weakness, sweating, headache, hunger, trembling, impaired vision, change of behavior, tingling sensation in upper lip, and convulsion. The client should verbalize action to take: 4 oz orange juice, 8 oz milk, 2 packages of sugar, cake-decorating gel, commercially prepared glucose preparation. Repeat in fifteen minutes if necessary; if no response, seek medical attention at once.

Hyperglycemia. The client should be able to state at least three or more of the following symptoms: increased thirst, dry mouth, excessive urination, nausea and vomiting, drowsiness, decreased appetite, weakness, dizziness, rapid breathing, and coma. The client should verbalize action to take: test blood or urine sugar and urine for acetone; call the physician, clinic, or emergency department as indicated.

Monitoring. The client verbalizes the rationale for the type of monitoring (capillary blood glucose or urine). The client demonstrates the procedure, including the recording of results.

General Hygiene Measures. The client verbalizes the importance of daily foot care, skin care, and dental care. The client demonstrates procedures as indicated.

Follow-up Care. The client verbalizes knowledge of follow-up care, for example, appointments with physician, clinic, dietitian.

When and Where to Call. The client describes the circumstances that warrant seeking medical attention and where to go to obtain care.

Medic Alert ID. The client verbalizes the rationale for identification and how to obtain a Medic Alert identification bracelet or necklace.

Nursing intervention related to compliance is evaluated in terms of such behaviors as the client's ability to identify reasons for noncompliance, to identify and accept needed behavioral changes, and to demonstrate behaviors consistent with the plan of care.

Ethical and Legal Issues

One of the major issues confronting the diabetic client is the economic impact of diabetes. Diabetes is an expensive disease. The cost of medical care, medications, supplies, and ancillary services continues to escalate. Diabetes affects the client's eligibility for and coverage by health insurance, adding to the cost borne directly by the client. It can affect the client's employability, work performance, and longevity (18).

Galloway and associates (18) have identified eight strategies that the diabetic client may find useful to reduce the economic impact:

1. Adopt a life-style that promotes good health.
2. High-risk clients should purchase life insurance with additional purchase benefits (rider with guaranteed issue).
3. Obtain career counseling.
4. Maintain group health insurance.
5. Obtain medical care from diabetes specialists who have access to patient education services (nurses, dietitians).
6. Become well educated in the management of the disease.
7. Promptly seek medical attention for all health problems, including those both related and unrelated to diabetes.
8. If a change in employment is considered, anticipate the effect of diabetes on obtaining health insurance.

Reducing the economic impact is not solely the responsibility of the diabetic client. Society as a whole also has an obligation in this area. Although the client directly bears much of the cost of health care, the costs to society are reflected in increased life and health insurance premiums, increased health care costs, and increased social welfare costs secondary to the long-term complications of the disease. Availability of insurance for the diabetic client varies from state to state and is, for the most part, suboptimal. Third-party reimbursement for client education services is virtually nonexistent. By increasing the availability of low-cost health insurance and by providing reimbursement for client education, the economic impact of diabetes for both the client and society may be substantially reduced.

Another issue that needs to be addressed is that of compliance. Compliance is defined as "1. act of complying. 2. a disposition to yield to others" (6). When this definition is analyzed within the context of the goals of diabetes management, the conflict between the two becomes apparent. Another aspect of this issue is that in most instances, compliance becomes synonymous with good and noncompliance, with bad. Many times health care providers "abandon" noncompliant clients in favor of compliant ones. What is the primary nurse's role in the area of compliance? Is it our responsibility to make clients comply no matter what method is required—use of fear, threats of or the actual withdrawing of care, or expressing our disappointment, and thereby eliciting guilt? Is it not instead our role to foster independence and self-care? To educate clients so that they can make well-informed decisions? To support their right to make decisions regarding the promotion, maintenance, and restoration of their health? To redefine the term compliance so that it is in keeping with the philosophy of nursing? Unfortunately there are no simple answers to any of these questions. Perhaps nursing's role is to develop a term more in keeping with the goals of client care and to educate the public in the use of this term.

The last issue to be addressed is client education, an essential aspect of the care of the diabetic client. To the overworked, harried nurse who is caring for several acutely ill clients, client education may become a luxury, and therefore receive a low priority. Given the staffing situation in most acute care facilities, this becomes a very real issue. However, the primary nurse has both ethical and legal responsibility to provide client education. The nurse practice act in most states mandates client education as part of nursing practice. In addition, the care of the diabetic client mandates client education as an ethical responsibility. Many times that which is ideal and that which is realistic are far apart. The key to the solution of the problem of the distance between ideal and realistic lies in the word "provide." Provision of education may be the actual act of teaching. It may also be the referral to a diabetes educator within the institution or, on discharge, in the community. Nurses must be as resourceful in the provision of client educa-

tion as they are in the provision of other aspects of care.

CASE STUDY 1

M. J., a twenty-seven-year-old white female, is admitted with a diagnosis of uncontrolled diabetes mellitus. She has had diabetes since age three and is insulin-dependent. Before admission she was taking NPH insulin, 46 units daily. She was given a 1,500-calorie ADA exchange diet to follow but admits to being unable to do so because "it costs too much" and she "can't be bothered with it." She has a history of diabetic retinopathy and is followed in a retina clinic, where she has been treated with laser photo-coagulation several times over the past five years.

M. J. is married but has no children. She was pregnant two years ago and delivered a stillborn infant. She has had difficulty dealing with this and is being followed by a psychiatrist. Her husband is also an insulin-dependent diabetic who is not well controlled. They are both anxious to have a normal, healthy child.

M. J. is a high school graduate and is employed full time as a shipping clerk. She denies any financial problems.

On admission M. J. states that she generally feels well but admits to polyuria, polydipsia, polyphagia, and nocturia. She tests her urine infrequently; when she does urine tests, they are usually 2 percent or greater. She denies ketonuria. Her blood glucose on admission is 563, acetone negative. Her height is 5 feet 3 inches, and her weight is 145 lbs.

For this case study:

1. Discuss the psychosocial aspects and their implications for care planning.
2. Identify potential problems and discuss possible solutions.
3. List four major nursing diagnoses.
4. Develop a care plan for one of the nursing diagnoses.

CASE STUDY 2

H. F., a sixty-two-year-old white male with newly diagnosed non-insulin-dependent diabetes mellitus, reports symptoms of polyuria, polydipsia, polyphagia, fatigue, and a weight loss of 40 lbs over a six-month period. He admits to having refused to "see a doctor" despite repeated requests made by his wife to have him seek medical attention. He attended a health fair at his wife's insistence and was found to have a blood glucose of over 400. He was admitted the next day for evaluation and control of his blood glucose. On admission his blood glucose was 524, acetone negative, height 5 feet 7 inches, and weight 140 lbs.

H. F.'s past medical history is negative for other chronic diseases or major illnesses. His family history is positive for diabetes. His mother had diabetes for many years, was a bilateral above-the-knee amputee, and had lost most of her vision because of diabetic retinopathy. She had lived with H. F. and his wife for five years before her death last year after a massive stroke.

H. F. lives with his wife, who is a medical secretary, and has three grown children. He is retired, having recently turned over his plumbing business to his son so that he "could enjoy his remaining years." His hobbies include carpentry and gardening.

During the nursing interview H. F. is pleasant and verbalizes well but appears anxious when discussing his diagnosis. He terminates the interview abruptly because he is "tired and needs his rest."

For this case study:

1. Identify H. F.'s stage of adaptation, according to Crate, and its implications for developing a management plan.
2. List the components of the management plan.
3. List three major nursing diagnoses.
4. Develop an individualized teaching plan to be implemented during the hospital admission.
5. Discuss discharge planning for H. F.

REFERENCES

1. Aaron–Young, C., and N. Del Savio. "Diet and Diabetes." In *Principles of Diabetes Management,* ed. M. Bergman. New York: Medical Examination Publishing Co., 1987.
2. Auerhahn, C., and J. Morgan. "Health Maintenance of the Diabetic Patient." In *Principles of Diabetes Management,* ed. M. Bergman. New York: Medical Examination Publishing Co., 1987.
3. Auerhahn, C., and R. Wehrhagen. *Standards of Nursing Practice: Outpatient Department.* Valhalla, N.Y.: Westchester County Medical Center, 1985.
4. Bailey, B. J. "Using Change Theory to Help the Diabetic." *The Diabetic Educator* 9:37–39, 56, Fall 1983.
5. Barbosa, J. "Diabetes: The Science and the Art, Hypoglycemia v. Complications" (editorial). *Archives of Internal Medicine* 143:118–19, 1983.
6. Barnhart, C. L., and J. Stein, eds. *The American College Dictionary.* New York: Random House, 1966, 247.
7. Bennett, P. H. "The Epidemiology of Diabetes Mellitus." In *Diabetes Mellitus and Obesity,* ed. B. N. Brodoff and S. Bleicher. Baltimore: Williams & Wilkins, 1982.
8. Bergman, M., and C. Auerhahn. "A Perspective on Exercise and Diabetes." *American Family Physician* 32:105–11, 1985.
9. Bergman, M., and P. Felig. "Self-monitoring of Blood Glucose Levels in Diabetes, Principles and Practice." *Archives of Internal Medicine* 144:2029–34, October 1984.
10. Brownlee, M. "Diabetic Complications: An Overview." In

Diabetes Mellitus and Obesity, ed. B. N. Brodoff and S. Bleicher. Baltimore: Williams & Wilkins, 1982.
11. Cahill, G. F. "Obesity." In *Diabetes Mellitus and Obesity,* ed. B. N. Brodoff and S. Bleicher. Baltimore: Williams & Wilkins, 1982.
12. Carpenito, L. *Nursing Diagnosis: Application to Clinical Practice.* Philadelphia: J. B. Lippincott, 1983, 97–98.
13. Cleary, M. E. "Aiding the Person Who Is Visually Impaired from Diabetes." *The Diabetes Educator* 10:12–23, Winter 1985.
14. Crate, M. A. "Nursing Functions in Adaptation to Chronic Illness." *American Journal of Nursing* 65:72–76, 1985.
15. Danowski, T. S. "Usage of Insulin in Type I and Type II Diabetes." In *Diabetes Mellitus and Obesity,* ed. B. N. Brodoff and S. Bleicher. Baltimore: Williams & Wilkins, 1982.
16. Doenges, M. E., M. F. Jeffries, and M. F. Moorehouse. *Nursing Care Plans: Nursing Diagnoses in Planning Patient Care.* Philadelphia: F. A. Davis, 1985, 482–99.
17. Frankel, N. "On the Etiology of Diabetes Mellitus." In *Diabetes Mellitus,* vol. 5, ed. H. Rifkin and P. Raskin. Bowie, Md.: Robert J. Brady Co., 1981.
18. Galloway, J. A., P. Sinnock, and J. A. Davidson. "Economic Impact of Diabetes Mellitus." In *Diabetes Mellitus: Management and Complications,* ed. J. M. Olefsky and R. S. Sherwin. New York: Churchill Livingstone, 1985.
19. Gonder-Frederick, L., et al. "Patient Blood Glucose Monitoring: Use, Accuracy, Adherence, and Impact." *Behavioral Medical Update* 6:12–16, 1984.
20. Guthrie, D. W. "Psychosocial Side of Diabetes and Its Complications." *The Diabetes Educator* 8:24–28, Summer 1982.
21. Harris, M. "Classification and Diagnosis of Diabetes Mellitus." In *Diabetes Mellitus: Problems in Management,* ed. D. Schnatz. Menlo Park, Calif.: Addison-Wesley, 1982.
22. Horton, E. S. "Exercise as a Therapeutic Tool in the Treatment of Diabetes Mellitus." *31st Postgraduate Course: Changing Strategies in the Management of Diabetes.* American Diabetes Association, 1984.
23. Jackson, J. E., and R. Bressler. "Oral Hypoglycemics and Drug Interactions with Them and Insulin." In *Diabetes Mellitus and Obesity,* ed. B. N. Brodoff and S. Bleicher. Baltimore: Williams & Wilkins, 1982.
24. Johny, A. "Glycosylated Hemoglobin Test as an Educational and Motivational Tool." *The Diabetes Educator* 10:37, 62, Fall 1984.
25. Kim, M. J., G. K. McFarland, and A. M. McLane. *Pocket Guide to Nursing Diagnosis.* St. Louis: C. V. Mosby, 1984, 83–89.
26. Lebovitz, H. E. "Oral Hypoglycemic Agents." In *The Diabetes Annual/1,* ed. Alberti and Krall. Amsterdam: Elsevier, 1985.
27. Leslie, R. D. G., and D. A. Pyke. "Genetics of Diabetes." In *The Diabetes Annual/1,* ed. Alberti and Krall. Amsterdam: Elsevier, 1985.

28. Levine, R. "Insulin Action: Physiological and Biochemical Aspects." In *Diabetes Mellitus and Obesity,* ed. B. N. Brodoff and S. Bleicher. Baltimore: Williams & Wilkins, 1982.

29. Maras, M. L., and C. L. Adolphi. "Ethnic Tailoring Improves Dietary Compliance." *The Diabetes Educator* 10:47–50, Winter 1985.

30. Maslow, A. *Motivation and Personality.* New York: Harper & Row, 1970.

31. National Diabetes Data Group. "Classification and Diagnosis of Diabetes Mellitus and Other Categories of Glucose Intolerance." *Diabetes* 28:1039–57, December 1979.

32. Olefsky, J. M. "Insulin Resistance and Insulin Action in Obesity and Non-Insulin-Dependent (Type II) Diabetes Mellitus." In *Diabetes Mellitus and Obesity,* ed. B. N. Brodoff and S. Bleicher. Baltimore: Williams & Wilkins, 1982.

33. Raymond, M. W. "Teaching Toward Compliance: A Patient's Perspective." *The Diabetes Educator* 10:42–44, Fall 1984.

34. Tamborlane, W. V., and R. S. Sherwin. "Diabetes Control and Complications: New Strategies and Insights." *Pediatrics* 102:805–13, June 1983.

35. Tartaglia, M. J. "Nursing Diagnosis: Keystone of Your Care Plan." *Nursing85* 15:34–37, March 1985.

36. Wing, R. R., L. H. Epstein, and M. P. Norwalk. "Dietary Adherence in Patients with Diabetes." *Behavioral Medical Update* 6:17–21, 1984.

37. Zimmet, P., and H. King. "The Epidemiology of Diabetes Mellitus: Recent Developments." In *The Diabetes Annual/1,* ed. Alberti and Krall. Amsterdam: Elsevier, 1985.

C H A P T E R   3 4

Adults with Human Immunodeficiency Virus Infection and Acquired Immunodeficiency Syndrome

JO ANNE BENNETT

·

OBJECTIVES

After completing this chapter, the reader will be able to:

- Explain current understanding of the cause of acquired immunodeficiency syndrome (AIDS), including the possible role of cofactors in addition to a specific viral agent.
- Differentiate between lymphadenopathy syndome, AIDS-related complex, and AIDS, including symptoms, diagnosis, and prognosis.
- Explain the pathogenesis of opportunistic diseases associated with human immunodeficiency virus (HIV) infection.
- Compare the chains of infection of human immunodeficiency virus (HIV) and the opportunistic organisms.
- Identify appropriate isolation precautions for AIDS and related infections, and indicate when they are necessary.

- Explain how the risk of HIV transmission can be reduced or eliminated.
- Discuss medical interventions currently available or being investigated in the management of AIDS and related conditions.
- Describe physical, psychological, social, and spiritual needs and problems that are often associated with HIV disease.
- Discuss acute and long-term nursing interventions in the context of a multidisciplinary approach to supporting the person with HIV disease and his or her family.
- Analyze ethical and legal implications of HIV risk, infection, screening, treatment, and research.

Since it was first recognized as a distinct disorder in 1981, acquired immunodeficiency syndrome (AIDS) has presented a unique public health challenge that has been met with varying degrees of responsiveness by governments at all levels and the health care system (30, 52, 57). In the spring of 1983 Margaret Heckler, then secretary of health and human services, declared AIDS to be the nation's number one health problem. At that time fewer then 1,500 persons had been diagnosed.

Initially health care providers and the community at large were not so prepared to respond adequately—with or without governmental assistance—to social problems related to AIDS. Volunteers provided such services as crisis intervention, support for individuals and families, legal aid, financial advocacy, and bereavement counseling. Fortunately advances in immunology, virology, and molecular biology in the 1970s had prepared a ready stage on which scientists could examine issues pertinent to the cause, prevention, and cure of AIDS (1, 8).

Productive research was immediate and continues. Although many questions remain unanswered, the knowledge we have gained in a relatively short period of time should help stem the rising incidence of infection, allay public fear, and provide the basis for planning and delivering therapeutic and supportive care.

No one knows what the long-term effects of AIDS will be. Rational planning for current and evolving needs and problems of a growing number of clients is essential. The purpose of this chapter is to help nurses better understand AIDS, the problems associated with it, and the nurse's role in providing primary care to individuals, families, and communities.

Overview of AIDS

To understand the significance of the problem, one must consider some of the facts about AIDS. This disease primarily affects young people. Seventy percent of those affected are forty years of age or younger; 22 percent are under thirty (50). Before they are diagnosed with human immunodeficiency virus (HIV)-related problems, people with AIDS are generally healthy (50).

Among never-married males fifteen years of age and older, the incidence rate of AIDS was 14.3 per 100,000 in 1984—about half the incidence rate of polio at the peak of the polio epidemic of 1952 and considerably lower than the current incidence of chicken pox among five- to nine-year-old children. The incidence rates in some areas, however, are higher. In New York City and San Francisco the rates are eighteen and twenty-three times higher, respectively, than elsewhere in the United States (20).

The national death rate for AIDS in 1984 was 0.5 per 100,000. Among males between the ages of thirty and thirty-nine in New York City (where 42 percent of AIDS deaths had occurred) it was 88 per 100,000, higher than the rates for homicide and liver disease, the second- and third-ranking causes of death for men in that age-group. AIDS was the second leading cause of death in New York City for women thirty to thirty-four years old and fourth for twenty-five- to twenty-nine-year olds (20).

Mortality from AIDS varies depending on sex, race, age, and disease manifestations. White women and black and Hispanic men and women have poorer prognoses than white men (40). Overall, about 15 percent survive five years after being diagnosed with AIDS. Survival after *Pneumocystis* pneumonia is improving, probably because of earlier diagnosis and better treatment. Most attention has been given to AIDS as a life-threatening infectious disease. But AIDS is also a chronic disease that has an impact on every aspect of a person's daily life.

Immunosuppression

AIDS is the most severe end (observed to date) of a continuum of illness related to HIV infection. Previously used terms for HIV are HTLV-III (human T-lymphotrophic virus, type III), LAV (lymphadenopathy-associated virus), ARV (AIDS-related retrovirus), and IDAV (immunodeficiency-associated virus).

HIV preferentially infects the T_4 cell. Viral replication involves transforming the genetic makeup of an infected

T_4 cell so that when the T_4 cell is stimulated by infectious or other foreign antigen(s), it reproduces HIV instead of itself. New virions then infect other T_4 cells, thus reducing the number of functional T_4 cells. Monocytes that have T_4 receptors can also be infected by HIV. Without adequate defense by monocytes and T_4 cells, flora that usually do not cause disease have the opportunity to invade and overwhelm. B lymphocytes are also affected by HIV, although the process is not fully understood. The result is diminished humoral immunity.

Effect on Nervous System

HIV also attacks nervous tissue, brain cells that contain the surface protein Leu-3, the same protein that serves as the HIV receptor on the T_4 cell. Even under normal circumstances the central nervous system (CNS) is not fully exposed to the immune system so it is less able than other organ systems to resist organisms that cross the blood-brain barrier. In immunosuppressed clients the cellular immune response is even weaker. It is not surprising then that as many as 60 percent or more of people with HIV infection may develop neurological dysfunction (2, 14). About 10 percent to 20 percent exhibit progressive dementia without apparent focal lesions and no other identifiable pathogen, suggesting that the symptoms are directly caused by HIV infection of the brain, not other opportunistic infections (24). Neurological problems—encephalopathy, encephalitis, myelopathy, dementia, and peripheral neuropathy—often precede the symptoms of immunological defects (7, 37–39).

Transmission

HIV is transmitted by sexual contact, by direct inoculation with contaminated blood or blood products, from parent to newborn in utero or during childbirth, and in breast milk. The reservoir of HIV is the human organism (T_4 cells and brain tissue). The virus is passed directly from person to person. A person's risk (i.e., probability) of becoming infected depends on risk of *exposure* to the causative virus (HIV). Exposure involves intimate (mucosal) contact with an infected person's concentrated body fluids (semen and blood), which allows fluids containing infected lymphocytes to enter the circulation of the uninfected person. Intimate contact occurs during sexual activities, heterosexual and homosexual, especially when there is exchange of semen (32). Direct inoculation can occur when contaminated blood is injected from a used syringe or needle.

Homosexual men and intravenous drug abusers have a greater likelihood of exposure to the blood or semen of someone who is already infected. Risk reflects prevalence of infection among potential partners. Prevalence of infection is not so high among heterosexuals who do not abuse intravenous drugs because they have had less frequent exposure (i.e., intimate contact) to those who are infected. Homosexual men and intravenous drug abusers in the United States compose relatively isolated reservoirs of infection. In other countries, where there are not large separate communities of gay men or intravenous drug abusers, the original pattern of distribution of infection appeared quite differently. For example the prevalence of infection among women and men in African countries was apparently evenly distributed.

Limiting the number of one's sexual partners alone does not eliminate risk of exposure. When AIDS was first recognized, those who were diagnosed often reported having had many sexual partners. That experience reflected the size of the reservoir (i.e., how many people are infected) at that time. But infection does not require several partners. As prevalence of infection mounts, more potential partners are infected, thus increasing the probability of exposure in any single encounter.

Less than 2 percent of AIDS cases have been related to infection from transfusion. One-third of these cases involved factor VIII transfusions to hemophiliacs (50). Only blood donations made before March 1983 have been involved. At that time the Public Health Service asked people in identified risk groups to refrain from donating blood (53).

Fortunately the nation's blood supply is no longer part of the reservoir of HIV infection. Since March 1985 the U.S. Food and Drug Administration has required all blood to be screened for antibody to HIV. The ELISA (enzyme-linked immunosorbent assay) antibody screening tests, although nonspecific, are highly sensitive and reliable (49, 51). HIV cannot withstand heat greater than 56°C. Clotting factor concentrates now undergo a special heat treatment (lyophilization) to eliminate the virus.

HIV is less contagious and less virulent than other viruses, such as hepatitis B and influenza. Infection requires a relatively large quantity (dose) of virus. The quantity of virus that is transmitted can vary from one type of exposure to another. Inadequate dose explains why health care workers whose blood or mucous membranes have been accidentally exposed to blood from infected persons through needlesticks, spills into broken skin, and splashes into eyes rarely develop antibody to the virus. The risk of infection following such exposure is less than 0.03 percent. Even a relatively large quantity of infected blood or semen may not contain a large concentration of virus. The concentration of HIV in blood and semen may depend on an infected person's relative disease state. Soon after infection, virus replication may not yet be great enough for an adequate dose even with transfer of large amounts of blood or semen. There may also be little or no viremia in late-stage AIDS, after significant T_4 cell destruction has taken place.

Natural History

Not all infection inevitably progresses to AIDS, the most severe manifestations of HIV infection. The pathology of HIV disease is shown in Figure 34.1. As yet we cannot make prognoses for infected individuals. Perhaps as many as one-third will not develop AIDS. Some even remain completely asymptomatic, with or without immune abnormalities detectable by laboratory tests.

It is believed that various cofactors may contribute to different patterns of disease development. Hence, people with different risk factors have different rates of incidence of various opportunistic diseases. For example, Kaposi's sarcoma has been frequent among gay men with AIDS, but infrequent among hemophiliacs or intravenous drug abusers with AIDS. Tuberculosis frequently occurs among intravenous drug abusers, but not among the other groups.

The Centers for Disease Control in Atlanta have classified HIV manifestations into four categories: I, acute, transient flulike symptoms that occur following primary infection; II, asymptomatic infection; III, PGL; IV, other symptoms, alone or in combination. ARC and AIDS fall into category IV (44, 48).

Complications

Persistent generalized lymphadenopathy (PGL). PGL is a common sign. Often it occurs in combination with other symptoms, including non-life-threatening opportunistic diseases such as herpes simplex and oral candidiasis. About one-third of people with PGL (according to one longitudinal study) develop AIDS within four and one-half years. For many these symptoms may be a chronic manifestation of HIV infection. ARC (AIDS-related complex) refers to any combination of two symptoms *plus* two laboratory abnormalities (see Assessment section).

***Pneumocystis Carinii* Pneumonia (PCP).** This is the most common disease seen in clients when AIDS is diag-

nosed. More than 50 percent present with this infection; many more develop it later. Pneumocystis pneumonia has a subtler onset, a slower progression, and a longer duration in people with AIDS than it has in other immunosuppressed populations. It also requires a longer course of antibiotic therapy (up to one month). Without continued antibiotic therapy, over one-third of clients develop recurrent PCP.

Other Infections. Almost every organism that affects people with HIV can infect the CNS: toxoplasma, cryptococcus, cytomegalovirus (CMV), herpes, mycobacteria.

Opportunistic organisms include endogenous parasites that are not new to the immunodeficient host (31, 34). Virtually all AIDS clients may have CMV infection, although they may not manifest a CMV-related illness. Disorders caused by CMV include diffuse pneumonia (usually complicated by multiple organisms), gastrointestinal ulcerations, adrenal gland necrosis, and chorioretinitis progressing to blindness.

Tuberculosis, pulmonary or extrapulmonary, may be an early sign of AIDS in the economically disadvantaged or those who use intravenous drugs (26).

Kaposi's Sarcoma (KS). This rare multifocal vascular tumor of the skin, mucous membranes, lymph nodes, and visceral organs classically occurs in the middle years to later in life, usually in men of Mediterranean or Jewish extraction. It typically follows an indolent clinical course and is not life-threatening, but in those receiving immunosuppressive drugs and those with AIDS, it is more aggressive. The incidence of KS in gay men with AIDS has dropped markedly, from over 90 percent through 1985 to only 9 percent in 1987 (50).

Other Tumors. Several types of primary CNS lymphoma, usually of the large-cell type, occur with AIDS. Systemic lymphoma with CNS infiltration is also common.

Prevention and Screening

Guidelines for Safe Sex. Sex is the primary way HIV is spread. It is often not possible to know if a potential sexual partner is infected, but risk can be reduced if body fluids are not exchanged during sexual activity. Specifically, a man should not ejaculate inside his partner (male or female) unless he is wearing a condom. This precaution is recommended for vaginal, rectal, and oral intercourse. The condom's efficacy as a barrier to

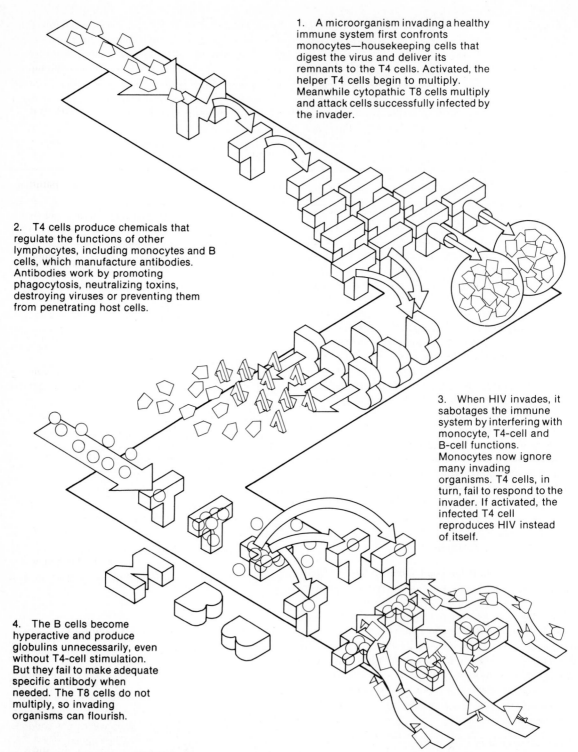

1.   A microorganism invading a healthy immune system first confronts monocytes—housekeeping cells that digest the virus and deliver its remnants to the T4 cells. Activated, the helper T4 cells begin to multiply. Meanwhile cytopathic T8 cells multiply and attack cells successfully infected by the invader.

2.   T4 cells produce chemicals that regulate the functions of other lymphocytes, including monocytes and B cells, which manufacture antibodies. Antibodies work by promoting phagocytosis, neutralizing toxins, destroying viruses or preventing them from penetrating host cells.

3.   When HIV invades, it sabotages the immune system by interfering with monocyte, T4-cell and B-cell functions. Monocytes now ignore many invading organisms. T4 cells, in turn, fail to respond to the invader. If activated, the infected T4 cell reproduces HIV instead of itself.

4.   The B cells become hyperactive and produce globulins unnecessarily, even without T4-cell stimulation. But they fail to make adequate specific antibody when needed. The T8 cells do not multiply, so invading organisms can flourish.

Figure 34.1.   The Effect of HIV Infection

Source: Copyright 1986 American Journal of Nursing Company. Reprinted with permission from the *American Journal of Nursing* 86:1019.

HIV has been demonstrated, but it must be *used all the time* to ensure safety. A diaphragm is *not* an effective barrier. Activities that can injure mucous membranes or impair skin integrity are also risky. Sexual activities that do not involve the exchange or passing of any body fluids between partners (e.g., cuddling, massaging, body rubbing, kissing a partner's skin, and mutual masturbation) are considered safe.

The key to safety is recognizing potential risk. "Know your partner" is a cardinal rule: anonymous sex and one-night stands are risky. How well each partner knows his or her previous partners' sexual and drug use history suggests how reliably potential risk can be assessed. Since there is always the possibility of previous exposure, specific precautions must always be taken.

Teach clients (whether risk is apparent or not) how to use condoms and not to allow semen, urine, or other excretions from one partner to enter the other (by vagina, rectum, or mouth).

Nonsexual Exposure to HIV. Parenteral drug use poses a variety of dangers to health, not least of which is HIV infection. Substance abuse has never been more dangerous. Nurses should advise people who inject drugs to seek help with detoxification and to enroll in rehabilitation programs. If they continue to inject drugs, the nurse should urge them to reduce the risk of AIDS by taking the following precautions: use one's own equipment and do not share it with anyone else; sterilize equipment by boiling it in water for fifteen minutes or by cleaning it with alcohol or bleach after each use and then soaking it in alcohol or bleach until the next use; and clean the skin with alcohol before injecting drugs. Drug users should also be counseled to practice safe sex *even after they have stopped using drugs.*

Personnel in hospitals and other health care institutions should treat all body products—secretions, excretions, and blood—as potentially infectious, regardless of whether or not a client has any diagnosed infection (19). Diagnosis of an infection may not be made until after a client has been treated. Many infections remain undiagnosed.

Exposure to HIV can be prevented by blood and body fluid precautions (42, 43, 46). The specific purpose of blood and body fluid precautions with HIV is to prevent contaminated fluids, especially blood and semen, from getting into an uninfected person's bloodstream. Since the skin is an effective barrier, the concern is for invasive procedures and situations in which the skin is not intact. The use of sterile instruments and aseptic technique is indicated for invasive procedures. Handwashing remains a most important measure to prevent contaminated material from being carried to potential portals of entry, such as open wounds and venipuncture sites. Safe handling of contaminated materials, especially sharp instruments that may puncture one's own skin and liquids that may splash onto exposed mucous membranes, is also imperative.

Compared with many other infections, HIV is difficult to transmit. It probably does not survive for longer than twenty minutes outside the human body, even when mixed in serum proteins. It is not transmitted by sneezing, coughing, or spitting; by handshakes or other nonsexual physical contact; by toilet seats, bathtubs, showers, or swimming pools used by infected people; by utensils, dishes, or linens used by an infected person; by food prepared or served by an infected person; by articles handled or worn by an infected person; or by being around an infected person, even on a daily basis over a long period of time. Caring for AIDS clients, even when there is intensive exposure to contaminated secretions, is *not* a high-risk activity (13, 25, 35, 47).

Disinfection. Alcohol, hypochlorite (bleach), hydrogen peroxide, phenolics (e.g., Lysol), and paraformaldehyde effectively inactivate HIV at relatively low concentrations. Contaminated surfaces should be cleaned and then disinfected with 0.5 percent sodium hypochlorite (NaOCl), which is a 10 percent solution of household bleach (one part bottled bleach *freshly* diluted in nine parts water). An effective alternative to those solutions is heating to 56°C. for ten minutes (27, 42, 43). Normal sanitary practices in any household will prevent the growth of fungi and bacteria that may potentially cause illness to both immunocompromised and immunocompetent people. Special precautions with clients' laundry and eating utensils are *not* necessary. Bathroom facilities and kitchen utensils may be shared with others. Sponges used to clean counters in the kitchen where food is prepared should *not* be the same sponges used to clean toilets or bathroom-type spills (25).

Community Education. An important primary nursing role, community education to prevent AIDS and AIDS hysteria must address not only those who seek information, but also those who think they have nothing to fear. Of equal importance, attention must also be given to reassuring those who are not likely to be exposed to infection.

Although the American public has a growing health consciousness and scientific sophistication, there is nevertheless considerable misunderstanding of basic concepts of contagion and principles of infection control related to AIDS. Discussions of immunity and the body's defenses are rife with dated half-truths, misleading statements, and factual errors. As teachers, primary nurses must be careful to explain issues and relationships accurately. This means reviewing principles of immunology, virology, and nutrition more extensively themselves and being alert to their own misconceptions, as well as those of others.

The language used to communicate about AIDS may be confusing and misleading. For example, saying that the virus is not spread by casual contact often arouses, instead of allaying, the fears of many who perceive their contact with potential AIDS patients as far more than casual. What epidemiologists mean by the term casual is nonsexual interpersonal contact. Explaining terms carefully and ascertaining the listener's level and accuracy of comprehension can help to overcome this problem.

Teenagers and young adults are at greatest risk for HIV and other sexually transmitted diseases. Information about AIDS should be an integral part of high-school sex-education programs and classes about drug abuse. Curricula must include these programs early so that adolescents are informed *before* they begin to experiment. Explanation about exposure must be clear and specific. Euphemisms do not inform; often they confuse. Likewise, clinical language is not always helpful. Sexually explicit language, including street slang, although offensive to many, may in fact be the key to communicating accurately. Printed materials must be geared to the understanding and reading ability of the intended audience. Thus, visual aids, including cartoons, may be necessary. Research is needed to determine what teaching frameworks are most effective in achieving compliance with "safe" behaviors.

Many concerns about AIDS may reflect homophobia and lack of empathy for particular groups affected by the disease. Thus education programs may have to address topics other than epidemiology and infection control.

Immunization. Vaccination would probably be the most reliable way to prevent further disease spread (12). Vaccine-induced antibodies could be directed toward the structural proteins of the virus. Researchers are concentrating on the envelope proteins because they seem to evoke the most powerful immune response.

Recombinant DNA technology has already successfully incorporated HIV genes into bacteria, yeast, and mammalian cells. However, it is not known if such products provide adequate amounts of appropriate anti-

gens. If they do, an advantage of this technology is that the vaccine would not contain any infective material because only a small portion of the viral genome is used. Another advantage is that high-yield production is possible. Although testing of the vaccine's safety in humans began in 1987, availability of a vaccine is years away. The single best defense against AIDS is an educated public.

HIV Antibody Screening. Effective screening of blood to prevent contaminated transfusions is accomplished by detecting antibody to the structural proteins of the virus (49, 53). The presence of antibody demonstrates that a person has been infected and suggests that virus is probably present. It does not indicate a person's prognosis. A negative test indicates that a person either has not been infected or has only recently been exposed but has not yet developed antibody. An infected person may take up to three months to develop antibody. During this time an antibody test is negative. For this reason people who may have been exposed to HIV must not donate blood.

It is important to remember that a negative result is not a constant. A negative result is meaningful only until the next potential exposure.

Prechildbearing screening is recommended both to prevent perinatal viral tranmission *and* to protect the mother (46). The incidence of infection in infants born to infected mothers is about 40 percent. Women who are infected with HIV are likely to develop AIDS complications either during or after pregnancy; they also suffer a higher mortality than those who do not become pregnant. The incidence of pregnancy complications in such women is higher than in uninfected women (4).

Pregnant women who may have been exposed but test negative should repeat the test after six months. A pregnant woman who is seropositive may not want to complete the pregnancy. If an infected woman does give birth, the infant should be followed carefully and tested for antibody *after* reaching fifteen months of age.

Overview of Management

A positive antibody test does not mean a person has AIDS or will definitely develop AIDS. After a positive antibody test, a complete physical examination, including an immunological profile, provides a basis for continuing assessment. Most people will probably remain infected for life and should be followed regularly. The goals of management of the person with HIV infection are to (a) reduce foreign antigen stimulation of T$_4$ cells, (b) limit replication of HIV, (c) prevent and treat opportunistic infections, and (d) restore immune function (9, 18).

Although one cannot offer assurances, sound advice to the seropositive (i.e, already infected) person can be based on what is known about the immune system, HIV replication, and T$_4$-cell cytopathology.

The most obvious—and most important—advice is to beware of foreign antigen stimulation. *Safe sex guidelines are as important for the person who is already infected with the virus as for those who are trying to avoid infection.* The virus can be latent for long periods. It relies on immune activation and T$_4$-cell production for its own replication. Without a supply of T$_4$ cells to invade, its opportunity to multiply within the infected host will be limited. People with HIV infection, whether or not they are manifesting AIDS, ARC, or any symptoms, should avoid exposure to other viruses and sexually transmitted organisms and to reinfection by HIV.

Clients are counseled to avoid exposure to people with viral infections, to be cautious around excreta of pets, especially that of birds and cats, to practice safe-sex precautions, to avoid sharing articles such as razors, and to care for wounds promptly and properly. Wounds should be cleaned promptly with soap and water and covered to prevent entry of organisms. Wounds that do not heal should be reported to a physician. Because intestinal parasites are frequent causes of infection in people with HIV disease, clients must observe precautions when preparing foods. Fruits and vegetables should be peeled, since disease-causing organisms may be present on their surfaces. Cook meats well, as they may contain harmful organisms. Wash hands with soap and water after handling raw meat. Clean kitchen counters with scouring powder to remove food particles.

Clients are counseled to advise physicians about their immunodeficiency before taking any vaccines. Many vaccines contain altered living—"attenuated"—viruses that will not harm those who have normal immunologic capabilities, but might be a problem for those with immunodeficiency. Household members should also not receive live-virus vaccines. Flu vaccines contain *killed* virus. People with immunodeficiencies, including AIDS, ARC, or other HIV symptoms, should be vaccinated each year against flu. Care givers and household members should also be vaccinated.

A number of viral agents are being tested for effectiveness in either killing HIV or stopping its replication (17,

18). So far, zidovudine (Retrovir)—still called by many azidothymidine (AZT)—and ribavirin (Virazole) seem the most promising because they both can be taken orally, cross the blood-brain barrier, and have not caused serious side effects. The latter is an important criterion because it is likely that antiviral therapy will have to be continued for life. Zidovudine was approved for treatment of AIDS and ARC in adults in early 1987. Hematologic side effects have limited its use in some people with severe disease. Its long-term effectiveness and usefulness in treating patients with asymptomatic HIV infection, neurologic symptoms, or KS is still being assessed. Other antiviral drugs being tested include ansamycin, phosphonoformate, ampligen, and dideoxycytidine. The ultimate goal is to intervene as early in infection as possible, before the virus can do major damage to the immune or neurological system. Antiviral combinations are being tried with the hope of not only improving effectiveness but also improving tolerance by reducing adverse effects.

Attempts at restoring immune function are complicated because AIDS does not reflect a single physiological status. Each client responds differently. Although drugs known to boost the immune system, such as isoprinosine, thymopectin, alpha interferon, gamma interferon, and interleukin 2, have been tried with little or no success in AIDS clients, the hope is that their effect will be seen when used in combination with antiviral agents. Bone marrow transplantation has been tried and is being repeated with adjunctive antiviral treatment. Plasmapheresis, which removes circulating immune complexes and suppressive factors, is also being tried. Immunoglobulin therapy is being used with success in children with AIDS.

When opportunistic infections occur they are treated vigorously with appropriate antimicrobials. Often a longer course of treatment is necessary than in treating immunocompetent clients. Recurrence of infection after treatment stops is frequent. Antimicrobials are routinely prescribed prophylactically to prevent recurrence of PCP, herpes, and candidiasis. Clinical trials are under way to compare the prophylactic regimens used against PCP: pentamidine inhaled (at various dosages), dapsone, trimethoprim-sulfamethoxazole, and sulfadoxine-pyrimethamine (9). Caution clients not to take drugs that have not been prescribed because of potential interactions with prescribed drugs and potential impact on immunity. Ribavirin, for example, impairs zidovudine absorption.

Adequate nutrition is important in maintaining the integrity of the immune system. Malnutrition impairs skin integrity and alters antibody formation, phagocytic function, intestinal flora, and body fluid composition. The impact of malnutrition on infectious disease severity has been documented many times over.

Nursing Care

The nurse may encounter a person with HIV infection in a variety of situations. The setting may be the home, the worksite or school, a community social service or health care agency, a drug detoxification or rehabilitation program, a shelter for the homeless, or a hospice. The person may be seen in oncology, dermatology, pediatrics, prenatal, allergy, neurology, ophthalmology, and mental health clinics. In some states AIDS is also a major concern in prisons.

Clients with HIV infection experience different disease courses. Moreover, a person's situation is likely to be in frequent, if not constant, flux. The HIV-infected person who has not experienced an opportunistic disease can also be overwhelmed. Symptomatic relief is not always readily available. Frequent reassessment and reordering of needs and goals are essential.

Assessment

A comprehensive health history, a physical assessment, and data from laboratory tests are the basis for developing the nursing care plan.

Health History. A comprehensive health history for the client with HIV infection would include the following information:

- Chronic problems related to HIV infection, such as:
  —unexplained tiredness, combined with headache, dizziness, or light-headedness;
  —continued (intermittent) temperature of 38° C. (100.5° F.) or greater for longer than two months;
  —profuse, sometimes drenching, night sweats;
  —weight loss of more than 15 lb or more than 10 percent within one to two months that is not due to diminished caloric intake or increased physical activity;
  —swollen glands in the neck, armpits, or groin (greater than 1 cm) that persist longer than two or three months;
  —heavy, dry cough that is not from smoking and has lasted for too long to be a cold or flu;
  —thrush (a thick white coating of the tongue or throat) which may be accompanied by a sore throat;
  —shortness of breath;
  —bruising more easily than normal;
  —purple or discolored growth (patches) on skin, possibly first seen on the ankles and legs or the mucous membranes inside the mouth;
  —unexplained bleeding from any body opening or from growths on the skin or mucous membranes.
- Treatment for symptoms before the present entrance into the health care system. Knowing the dates, types, and providers of treatment helps the nurse to understand the current episode in the context of previous care.
- Self-care measures. The types and effectiveness of self-care measures in alleviating symptoms should be determined.
- Impact of the illness on the person, socially and emotionally. Isolation; loss of job, friends, and partners; depression; and ineffective coping skills are some areas that require exploration.
- Support network. People who may assist in caring for the client should be identified and their relationship with the client explored. Community resources, their availability, and the client's eligibility and willingness to use them should be investigated.
- Knowledge of HIV disease. Knowing the extent and accuracy of the client's knowledge of HIV infection and related disorders is essential to appropriate teaching, relieving emotional distress, enhancing compliance with medical regimens, and promoting effective self-care.

Physical Examination. Aspects of the physical examination that warrant attention include the following:

- Vital signs. Intermittent fever is common.
- Body weight. Loss of weight and severe wasting are common, especially when such problems as oral and esophageal lesions make eating difficult, when diarrhea inhibits absorption, when appetite is depressed, and when fatigue or other symptoms limit the person's ability to shop and prepare meals.
- Mucous-membrane and skin integrity. As indicated earlier, thrush is common. Kaposi's

sarcoma and herpes lesions can affect the mouth, rectum, gastrointestinal tract, and soles of the feet. Rashes and seborrhea are common.

- Lymph nodes. Persistent lymphadenopathy, may be a physiological response to the viral infection. A sudden reduction in lymph node number or size is an ominous sign.
- Abnormal bleeding. Thrombocytopenic purpura is a common manifestation of HIV infection.
- Neurological function. Confusion, disorientation, memory lapses, musculoskeletal weakness, tremors, cramps, and mood swings may indicate opportunistic infections or tumors, drug toxicities, electrolyte or nutrient imbalance, depression, or cerebral hypoxia.

The immunological defects related to HIV infection are diverse and involve *both* cellular and humoral immunity. Laboratory findings are neither diagnostic nor specific. There is an absolute decline in the number of circulating T_4 cells ($400/mm^3$) and a reduced $T_4:T_8$ ratio ($1:0$). Cutaneous anergy and elevated serum globulin levels are noted in most clients. Thrombocytopenia and anemia also are common.

Other laboratory tests that are being used in research settings include lymphocyte transformation studies, which measure some of the functional abilities of lymphocytes to respond to or be stimulated by foreign substances called antigens or mitogens, and elevations of the erythrocyte sedimentation rate or circulating immune complexes (CIC), anti–T cell autoantibodies, $alpha_1$-thymosin levels, $beta_2$-microglobulins, and an acid-labile form of alpha interferon (10, 28).

Clear distinctions between AIDS and ARC, and other HIV-related conditions are not possible from a biological point of view. However, severe laboratory abnormalities are associated with more severe symptoms and a poorer prognosis.

Nursing Diagnoses

The following nursing diagnoses represent those that could be encountered by the primary nurse caring for a person with HIV-related disease and are the point of reference for developing the nursing care in this chapter:

- Fear and anxiety related to such factors as concern about future disease development and ability to cope with potential problems
- Discomfort related to the broad range of symptoms and treatment
- Altered roles and interpersonal relationships

related to the impact of symptoms on work and social routines and the requirements of managing own health care
- Ineffective family coping related to the stigma associated with AIDS, homosexuality, substance abuse and the realities of the disease and its prognosis
- Grief related to loss of job, status, and other important activities
- Impaired nutrition related to the infectious process, which increases caloric requirements, reduced intake, the use of nutrient nostrums, specific nutrient deficits and loss of appetite
- Alterations in elimination such as diarrhea and constipation associated with altered diet, fluid intake, drug therapies and GI disorders
- Alterations in sleep-rest-activity patterns related to fatigue and depression
- Alterations in perception and cognition related to depressive disorders, disrupted daily habits, CMV retinitis and neurologic disorders
- Knowledge deficit about HIV and associated opportunistic problems related to misunderstanding and misinformation about contagion, disease symptoms, and treatment

Planning and Implementation

The person with AIDS or ARC requires more than treatment for the disease itself. The primary nurse must focus on a complex range of emotional and physiological effects. Emotional support and physical comfort measures are nursing priorities. Symptoms depend on the opportunistic diseases that are present.

People with AIDS usually have multiple admissions to the hospital; therefore, good communication between in-hospital nursing staff and those assisting clients at home is essential to ensure that emotional and physical needs are met. A client who is living at home may need social assistance if family and friends cannot provide adequate support and physical care. Home care attendants, sometimes around the clock, may be needed. Regardless of the needs, clients should be encouraged to take an active role in decision making and treatment.

☐ *Fear and Anxiety.* People with symptomatic HIV infection are doubtlessly extremely worried about future disease development. How well they are able to manage physically often depends on how constructively they can cope with their worry and anxiety. Some become extremely health conscious, seeking advice about health-promoting behaviors and ways to avoid infection. Others deny their risk and may actually behave contrarily, pursuing risky activities (unsafe sex or parenteral drug use) and physically overtaxing their bodies.

Some people with symptoms may deny the implications of their symptoms, telling themselves and others that their problems are related to other causes, such as working and playing too hard or not getting enough sleep to explain fatigue; not eating right to explain weight loss or altered bowel function; the flu, allergies, and so on to explain persistent or intermittent cough, anorexia, fevers, rashes, and other symptoms. Poor compliance with medical advice and specific treatment programs can be a sign of denial.

Denial often does not occur until after diagnosis of an opportunistic disease, when AIDS itself is a reality. However, confirmation of AIDS may at first bring a sense of relief from waiting, wondering, and dreading the possibility. When diagnosed, a person can begin to deal with a reality. For those whose earlier symptoms could not be related to any specific disease or syndrome, a firm diagnosis—even one as serious as AIDS—permits the person not to feel like a hypochondriac. Clients often comment that they had begun to think they were imagining symptoms or suffering psychogenic problems, or that their friends thought they were being unduly anxious. They also hope that with the diagnosis may come the possibility of treatment that will bring, if not cure, some relief from symptoms.

Denial is a useful defense mechanism. It often helps a person maintain a positive outlook, reduces stress, and enables the person to cope (56). Challenge a client's denial only when it compromises health.

Just as the course of illness differs for each person, so, too, different people will perceive and respond to the diagnosis differently. Perceptions are influenced by previous knowledge and experience with the disease. Many people know about HIV contagion, prevalence, and mortality. Although less is publicized about the chronicity of the disease and its daily impact, many (if not most) gay men, especially in larger cities, probably have known several people who have had the disease. Thus they're likely to have some specific frame of reference that can be both helpful and alarming. Whatever their initial reaction, recognition of the potentially terminal nature of the disease is often subsumed by its chronicity and multiple challenges to living.

□ *Discomfort.*   The range of physical symptoms that accompany HIV-associated disorders is broad. The primary nurse needs to anticipate discomforts, prepare the

client for side effects of treatments, and make relief available, if possible. Comfort regimens may have to be altered frequently. Check for efficacy. Topical analgesics, such as viscous Xylocaine are often indicated for mucous membrane lesions. Antifungal troches may be more easily tolerated if they are iced. Discuss options with the client and allow experimentation to find the most desirable method or combination of methods.

Another cause of discomfort in clients with AIDS or at risk of AIDS is "AIDS anxiety." AIDS anxiety is believing that every cough is pneumocystis pneumonia, looking for Kaposi's sarcoma lesions several times a day, and dreading minor infections as harbingers of life-threatening illness. Although physically asymptomatic, some people who think they're at risk for developing the disease—"the worried well"—are somatically preoccupied and may suffer actual panic attacks in addition to generalized anxiety and hypochondriasis. Obsessional thinking about disease can impair social and occupational functioning. Those who are not free to share their problem with professional colleagues and co-workers are at even greater risk of distress. Stress reduction techniques can reduce anxiety. Sometimes more specific intervention is needed.

People with AIDS suffer a dramatic change in self-esteem, daily habits, and general life-style, more so than patients with other terminal diseases, such as cancer. Drastic changes in their physical appearance may include profound weight loss and muscle wasting, hair loss, Kaposi's sarcoma lesions, and other skin disorders. The altered body image can interfere with personal identity, role performance, sexuality, and the ability to maintain meaningful relationships. Strangers react with fear, shock, or curiosity. The client may develop a negative self-image or may actually grieve for the loss of his or her "old self." Withdrawal from former activities presents an additional loss.

An important nursing goal is to break down social isolation. The nurse can minimize the client's emotional distress by discouraging unnecessary isolation protocols. Remember, the purpose of infection control is to isolate the pathogen, not the client. Activity restrictions should be based on how the client feels, not the diagnosis. Avoid unnecessary restrictions on client activities. Encourage participation in social, recreational, and occupational pursuits. The nurse may need to reassure the client's family and friends so that they don't encourage unnecessary dependence (5). Conversely, the client may need help to accept dependence, to ask for and accept help. And family and friends may need help to recognize the client's needs and to keep from being overwhelmed themselves.

Work and social routines may be considerably affected by HIV infection, even if full-blown AIDS does not evolve. Recurrent respiratory or gastrointestinal illnesses or general malaise may require frequent, and sometimes prolonged, absences from work. Some clients have to give up their occupation because they can no longer meet its physical demands. Symptoms can have an impact on home life and self-sufficiency. Even when physical symptoms are not severe, managing one's health care can practically fill a client's calendar and even require assistance to coordinate clinic appointments, transportation, applications for insurance benefits, and so on.

The primary nurse is in a position to help identify problems early, to help clients recognize their response to various problems, and to help them deal not only with concrete concerns such as symptom relief, basic self-care, and home management, but also with their feelings about what is happening to them. Not all problems can be resolved, but some can be either prevented or ameliorated with timely supportive intervention.

□ *Altered Roles and Interpersonal Relationships.* Relationships invariably undergo major changes. In some cases there is devastating social isolation, sometimes iatrogenic (for example, when unnecessary isolation precautions are implemented or when other activity restrictions are inappropriately recommended). Being treated as a person with a rare disease and being a participant in research can add to one's sense of isolation.

Anger can be directed at the health care provider who cannot offer hope or answer questions, but counsels participation in experimental treatment. Insensitivity by a few staff members, even if others are supportive, can augment a person's sense of isolation.

Changed patterns of social life may be due to physical and psychological problems. Some changes are a result of the person's attempt to cope with the disease. In some instances isolation may be self-imposed to avoid discussing the facts. Withdrawal may be symptomatic of depression.

Some changes occur because friends and family withdraw from the client to cope with their own fear of the disease or anticipatory grief. Isolation is worsened if friends and family have difficulty adjusting to the disease. In some cases parents and wives first learn of the client's homosexuality or intravenous drug use when AIDS is diagnosed. They have to face this surprise at the same time that they may be coping with the severity

of AIDS. Or, having previously coped with the person's struggle to conquer a drug problem, they now face a perhaps even more frightening aftermath.

Clients are encouraged to express their feelings and discuss relationships and activities with others. Clients may indicate that friends resist talking about important topics, like the disease itself or the possibility of death. They may want to discuss changes in relationships.

Reworking previous social relationships may include developing new patterns of sexual expression. Alterations in libido owing to disease or medications can make this task even more difficult. Clients often express a need for intimacy that is not being fulfilled, especially if they have lost a lover. They may need encouragement to try alternate physical expressions and to experiment to find new satisfactions. The need for simple physical contacts—touching, holding hands, an embrace—cannot be overemphasized. Many clients are young and have not established a relationship that involves a deep personal commitment. Some are compulsively sexually active and do not seek intimacy through sex.

Life-style changes can also contribute to the illness cycle as well as to the accompanying stress. Some clients have a lot of support available to them in their personal environment, while the social systems of others may put their health at greater risk. For some the situation is complicated by previous and ongoing health problems. Alcohol and other drug abuse is a serious and not infrequent problem (3).

The stress of illness and its associated emotional and social stressors often present a risk to the client's substance abuse rehabilitation. The availability of adequate counseling is important. Referral, follow-up, and monitoring are necessary adjuncts to the primary nurse's own intervention.

□ *Ineffective Family Coping.* The impact of AIDS reaches beyond those who have been infected and those who think that they may have been. The nurse's client may be a relative, lover, or friend of a person with AIDS. Sometimes they seek help for themselves, but often unless a care giver makes specific inquiry, they do not acknowledge their own needs, much less seek help.

The psychological distress for families and friends may be greater and more complex than with other life-threatening illnesses because AIDS is so stigmatizing and because it has been associated with so much mystery. The social stigma of the diagnosis involves a presumption about the person's life-style that can be a source of stress. The stigma further complicates the family's bereavement, especially if they do not feel free to discuss their grief when the client dies and reminisce about the lost loved one, including the circumstances of illness and death.

For a lover or spouse, knowing that one has had intimate contact with someone who is dying of a sexually transmitted contagious disease can be shattering. When the client is a male homosexual, health care workers are often surprised to see men care for each other so deeply. Often gay clients' lifelong partners encounter discrimination and legal impediments as they try to help their loved ones through illness. Psychological demands pile on top of existing grief and health worries.

Gay men whose friends have AIDS are particularly vulnerable because they can readily identify with their sick friends. They may even overidentify. They may also feel awkward discussing the illness, or have problems working through their own fears. For other friends who may not have known about the person's life-style, the situation may be similarly awkward. They may not know how to be supportive even if they want to. But there is no time for an "out of sight, out of mind" philosophy. If a person believes that he or she has failed a friend when needed most, or until it was too late, overwhelming guilt can add to grief.

The primary nurse must be prepared to help client, family, and friends learn how to face the realities of the disease. Empathy and a nonjudgmental attitude can reduce distress and facilitate discussion of difficult issues and uncomfortable feelings (5). Separate peer support groups for clients and for care partners, including groups for wives and mothers, have been an effective way for them to share problems, discuss possible solutions, and exchange information. The goal of peer counseling is the establishment of an ongoing, accepting, open social relationship in which intense emotions can be shared. Sharing helps to dilute their negative effects (56). The social component is an important feature of this modality. In addition, couples' groups can focus on interpersonal needs and strengthening relationships during most severe stress. Individual and/or family therapy is often helpful, especially for people whose cultural backgrounds do not dispose them to group discussion. This is an important consideration with Latino clients.

□ *Grief.*   A young person who is diagnosed with a debilitating, life-threatening disease experiences many losses: loss of job, status, and, often, other important activities; loss of future, planning and preparing for which may be an integral part of the person's current life and identity; social losses; and loss of physical strength and health. People with HIV infection often have experienced the deaths of several, sometimes many, friends and associates. Bereavement overload can be a significant problem. The person needs to be able to discuss these losses and his or her feelings about them. He or she also needs to be allowed to anticipate losses and to openly discuss this anticipation.

□ *Impaired Nutrition.*   The immunopathology of HIV infection compromises a person's reserves and defenses against disease. Therefore, it is important for the primary nurse to counsel the client about nutrition and to intervene early if nutritional reserves are compromised. The diet should include concentrated sources of calories and protein. The primary nurse may suggest enteral supplements and help plan menus that are high in calories (at least 4,000 kcal/d) and high in protein (150 g protein). Weight and nutritional intake must be consistently monitored from the time of diagnosis of HIV infection or ARC symptoms.

Many factors can contribute to nutritional deficits. The infectious process, neoplastic growth, fever, chills, and profuse sweating all increase caloric requirements. Inadequate nutrition may be related to loss of appetite, malaise, and diarrhea. The person who suffers from diarrhea may avoid eating because of the fear that eating will produce diarrhea. The primary nurse should explain how excess stool losses increase food requirements and help plan menus with foods that are both highly nutritious and easily absorbed.

Life-style alterations can also contribute to the illness cycle. For example, a person whose social life has revolved around work will suffer a significant loss if work is no longer possible. Those who usually ate out rather than cooking at home will have a significant adjustment that may affect the adequacy of their nutrition if they are confined at home. Finances may also adversely affect the situation. If the client is sleeping more, both meals and snacks may be skipped. The primary nurse should explain that sleep is not a substitute source of energy.

When lesions in the mouth or the esophagus are extensive, a moist diet of smooth consistency is appropriate. A combination of blended or pureed foods and liquids is usually preferred over a full liquid diet. Watermelon, grapes, and peeled cucumbers tend to be tolerated better than other fruits and juices. Rinsing the mouth with a local anesthetic, such as viscous xylocaine, fifteen to twenty minutes before meals also helps. Instruct the client to hold the solution in the mouth *for several minutes* before swallowing.

☐ *Altered Elimination.* Profuse secretory diarrhea accompanying Kaposi's sarcoma and gastrointestinal infections may necessitate hospitalization. An acutely ill person may lose as many as 12 to 13 liters of fluid within a twenty-four-hour period. This requires meticulous intake and output monitoring to keep up with needed fluid, electrolyte, mineral, and vitamin replacement. Partial or total peripheral nutrition may be required even when the client returns home. Perianal lesions aggravate the potential for skin breakdown.

Constipation is, somewhat ironically, also a not infrequent problem—usually a result of altered diet and fluid intake or the effect of analgesics. Fluid intake should be at least 3,000 ml/d.

☐ *Altered Sleep-Rest-Activity Patterns.* Activity intolerance may be due to fatigue. For example, the client who is suffering from severe diarrhea, respiratory insufficiency, or inadequate nutrition is easily exhausted. Various physical problems can disturb sleep and rest: clients with respiratory problems frequently have nocturnal dyspnea; drenching sweats may wake the client several times during the night; many experience insomnia. Round the clock drug regimens, such as AZT, also make uninterrupted sleep impossible. Altered sleep-wake patterns may be a symptom of depression.

☐ *Altered Perception and Cognition.* Behavioral changes and communication problems may be manifestations of depressive disorders. Mood swings are not uncommon. Disorganized thinking may be a response to disrupted daily habits or the inability to cope with crisis. At times, thinking may be repetitive and obsessive. Confinement and sleep-rest disruptions may disorient the person. Without customary or adequate diversions, cognition may be altered.

Sensory-perceptual alterations may also reflect neurological disease—HIV infection or an opportunistic tumor or infection—or the adverse effects of drugs. Encephalopathy, also known as AIDS dementia, can also result from profound metabolic disturbances. These symptoms can be particularly difficult for family and friends, especially if the client manifests paranoia. Vision loss is a devastating effect of CMV.

☐ *Knowledge Deficit About HIV and Related Opportunistic Problems, Treatment Options, Care Requirements, and Available Resources.* People with AIDS are vulnerable to misinformation and misinterpretation of information, especially about opportunistic infection risks and appropriate treatment. Many, for example, may be led to believe that the common cold or a small finger cut may bring their doom. In fact, such problems are not likely to activate the disease. The nurse can explain the specificity of the immune defects and the nature of opportunism. Reviewing the purpose of specific isolation precautions and emphasizing what is not necessary can clarify misconceptions.

When clients are receiving experimental therapies, the details of clinical trials should be carefully explained: the client should understand the purpose of the study, the nature of the trial, whether a placebo may be used, the expected duration of involvement, and the possible side effects, including any impact of alternative therapies. Some points have to be reiterated as the trial continues. Health care personnel should refrain from giving false expectations or suggesting a premature interpretation of results.

For the primary nurse, the challenge is threefold: to keep informed, to understand what is known, and to be alert to new developments. Scientific journals, not public media, should be used as sources of information.

Evaluation

The effectiveness of nursing intervention can be measured by progress toward the achievement of the following goals:

- The client will continue productive social involvement in family, community, and occupational activities.
- The client will engage only in sex practices that are safe.
- The client and household members will use only those measures for disinfection that are necessary.
- The client will maintain his or her weight.
- The client will actively participate in planning and decision making about goals for medical, nursing, and rehabilitative care.
- The client will follow prescribed medical regimens.
- The client will know about resources that are available to him or her, including social services, financial benefits, drug trials, and psychological support programs.
- The client will be able to discuss his or her perception of the experience of illness and feelings about prognosis with care givers and with family and friends.
- The client will be physically comfortable.
- The client and family will be able to anticipate

psychophysiological changes that evolve as illness progresses.
- The client will perceive that adequate support is readily available to assist him or her with home maintenance and physical and health needs.
- The client will be able to plan for his or her death and closure of legal and social affairs.
- The client with sensory–perceptual or cognitive impairment will have a safe environment that promotes maximum independent activity.

Ethical and Legal Issues

Ethical issues surrounding AIDS include concerns about distributive justice and the implications of technology that primary nurses confront in numerous other clinical situations: access to care, right to die, termination of life support, confidentiality, informed consent, scarce resources, birth control, and abortion. AIDS brings new questions to these areas of concern. Research questions encompass not only clinical research, but also epidemiologic data collection necessary for protecting public safety.

The key moral responsibility for professionals is to provide nonjudgmental, compassionate, appropriate physical and emotional care without discrimination. Although some instances of nurses refusing to care for clients with AIDS have been reported, the more frequent problem is the unnecessary use of isolation instead of appropriate precautions. This not only unnecessarily isolates the client, but also alarms others and sets an incorrect example for auxiliary staff. Nurses are not expected to be fearless, but they are expected to be knowledgeable and to base their actions on a scientific rationale and an individualized assessment of client needs. Clients frequently say that the worst part of the hospitalization experience is "feeling like a pariah," being in a single room and having staff avoid them.

Attitudes about caring for people with AIDS may be related to factors other than the disease or the fear of developing the disease. We tend to empathize with those whose life situation is most similar to our own (21). The AIDS epidemic may have activated underlying anxieties and fueled negative attitudes about homosexuality and drug abuse (11). Homophobia may not only justify detachment from clients, but could also displace feelings of frustration and helplessness in the face of an illness that has high morbidity and mortality among the young. Racism may also be an issue. Terminality has been found to be an important factor in nurses' avoidance of clients with other illnesses (55).

People with AIDS or at risk for HIV infection may face a variety of legal problems. In some states homosexual activities are against the law, and drug use violates federal and state statutes. Some people with AIDS have been *illegally* dismissed from employment. Almost all states and U.S. territories have fair employment laws that forbid discrimination based on physical disability or handicap. The exceptions are Arizona, Delaware, Puerto Rico, and the Virgin Islands (23). A federal law, the Vocational Rehabilitation Act of 1973, deals with employment discrimination on the basis of physical disability by federal contractors and programs receiving federal assistance. The latter would include most hospitals and social service agencies. Essentially these laws mandate that employees who are physically able to work without presenting *a real and significant danger* to others or themselves must be allowed to do so, even though they have some physical or medical condition that is potentially or actually disabling (15).

Like any client's diagnosis, the HIV or AIDS diagnosis itself is confidential information. Signs on a person's bed, on the door to the room, or affixed to the chart are inappropriate. (Even notices to use blood and body fluid precautions are not necessary because *all* blood and moist body substances should *always* be handled as *potentially infectious*.) Beware of betraying confidence about personal and sexual history. This information should be discussed only by those who need to know it, and then only in the context of planning and providing care. Conversely, beware of making erroneous assumptions about clients' life-styles. A person's situation and history are likely to be very different from any composite presented in a textbook.

Who needs to know what? Answer this question by asking a second question: What will be done with the information? Many people may participate in a client's care, but *few need to know details about his or her sexual life or family relationships.* The information may be important to making a diagnosis (although probably less so now than several years ago, when symptoms were less well known). Such data can be important to the epidemiological record but every nurse does not need to know about how a client became infected. Those who will provide specific counseling about healthier life-style patterning will need to discuss ongoing activities with the client so that together they can decide what adjustments are workable, and how.

Do not assume that friends and family members know the diagnosis, even if they are frequent visitors or even if the person has been diagnosed for some time and his condition has severely deteriorated. Discuss this issue with the client. Allow him or her to elaborate feelings, and assure the client that privacy will be protected. For some, this worry can be a stressor.

The issue of confidentiality is also raised in relation to screening for HIV infection (i.e., antibody testing). In order to answer people's questions accurately, find out what reporting procedures are being followed at your agency. A variety of methods have been proposed to ensure confidentiality of test results. You can assure people more reliably if you have specific information rather than merely suggesting what can be or might be done. Informed consent involves knowing who will have access to information, so be sure you let clients know *before* you obtain the information. How are records of antibody testing kept? Where are test results recorded? Who has access to the information—the personnel department? an employee's supervisor? the company's insurer? the local department of health? other government agencies? Other blood collection centers? These issues are likely to arise frequently in primary care settings, such as schools and the workplace. Some agencies and health departments offer anonymous testing. Anonymous testing means that *no* record of a person's being tested is kept and neither specimens nor test results are labelled with the person's identifying information. Hospital and clinic records are, obviously, never anonymous. Some hospitals have employed routine testing without clients informed consent and without informing them of the results. A client's insurer has general access to his or her medical and hospital records.

REFERENCES

1. Altman, D. *AIDS in the Mind of America*. Garden City, N.Y.: Anchor Press/Doubleday, 1986.
2. Beckhan, M. M., and E. B. Rudy. "Acquired Immunodeficiency Syndrome: Impact and Implication for the Neurological System." *Journal of Neuroscience Nursing*. 18:5, 1986.
3. Belmont, M., et al. *Resource Utilization by AIDS Patients in the Acute Care Hospital*. 1986. Available from The Health Services Improvement Fund, Inc., 622 Third Avenue, New York, N.Y. 10017.
4. Bennett, J. A. "AIDS Epidemiology Update." *American Journal of Nursing* 85:968, 1985.
5. Bennett, J. A. *Caring for the AIDS Patient*. Rev. ed. (Video) Los Angeles: The Hospital Satellite Network, 1986.
6. Bennett, J. A. "HTLV-III AIDS Link." *American Journal of Nursing* 85:1086, 1985.
7. Black, P. H. "HTLV-III, AIDS, and the Brain." *New England Journal of Medicine* 313:1538, 1985.
8. Brandt, E. N. "The Concentric Effects of the Acquired Immunodeficiency Syndrome." *Public Health Report* 99:1, 1984.
9. Collaborative DHPG Treatment Study Group. "Treatment of Serious Cytomegalovirus Infections with 9-(1,3-dihydroxy–2-propoxymethyl) guanine in Patients with AIDS and Other Immunodeficiencies." *New England Journal of Medicine* 114:801, 1986.
10. DeVita, V. T., S. Hellman, and S. A. Rosenberg, eds. *AIDS: Etiology, Diagnosis, Treatment and Prevention*. Philadelphia: J. B. Lippincott, 1985.
11. Douglass, C. J., C. M. Kalman, and T. P. Kalman. "Homophobia Among Physicians and Nurses: An Empirical Study." *Hospital Community Psychiatry* 16:1310, 1985.
12. Francis, D. P., and J. C. Petricciani. "The Prospects for and Pathways Toward a Vaccine for AIDS." *New England Journal of Medicine* 313:1586, 1985.
13. Friedland, G. H., et al. "Lack of Transmission of HTLV-III/LAV Infection to Household Contacts of Patients with AIDS or AIDS-Related Complex with Oral Candidiasis." *New England Journal of Medicine* 314:344, 1986.
14. Gapen, P. "Neurological Complications Now Characterizing Many AIDS Victims." *Journal of the American Medical Association* 248:2941, 1982.
15. Gay Men's Health Crisis Legal Services. *Legal Aspects of AIDS*. New York: Gay Men's Health Crisis Legal Services, 1984.
16. Goedert, J. J., et al. "Three-Year Incidence of AIDS in Five Cohorts of HTLV-III-Infected Risk Group Members." *Science* 231:992, 1986.
17. Gupta, A., D. E. Novick, and A. Rubinstein. "Restoration of Suppressor T-Cell Functions in Children with AIDS Following Intravenous Gamma Globulin Treatment." *American Journal of Diseases of Children* 140:143, 1986.
18. Hirsch, M. S., and J. C. Kaplan. "Prospects for Therapy for Infections with HTLV-III." *Annals of Internal Medicine* 103:750, 1985.
19. Jackson, M. M., and P. Lynch. "Infection Control: Too Much or Too Little?" *American Journal of Nursing* 84:208, 1984.
20. Kaplan, J. E. "A Modern-Day Plague." *Natural History* 95:28, 1986.
21. Katz, R. L. *Empathy: Its Nature and Uses*. New York: Free Press of Glencoe, 1963.
22. Klatzman, D., and L. Montagnier. "Approaches to AIDS Therapy." *Nature* 319:10, 1986.
23. Leonard, A. S. "The Legal Issues." In *AIDS: The Workplace Issues*, ed. D. Bohl. New York: American Management Association, 1985.
24. Levy, R. M., D. E. Bredesen, and M. L. Rosenblum. "Neurological Manifestations of the Acquired Immunodeficiency Syndrome (AIDS): Experience at UCSF and Re-

view of the Literature." *Journal of Neurosurgery* 62:475, 1985.

25. Lusby, G., and H. Schietinger. *Infection Precautions for People with AIDS Living in the Community.* New York: Gay Men's Health Crisis, 1984.

26. Maayan, S., et al. "Acquired Immunodeficiency Syndrome (AIDS) in an Economically Disadvantaged Population." *Archives of Internal Medicine* 145:1607.

27. Martin, L. S., J. S. McDougal, and S. L. Loskoski. "Disinfection and Inactivation of the Human T-Lymphotropic Virus Type III/Lymphadenopathy-Associated Virus." *Journal of Infectious Diseases* 152:400, 1985.

28. Mass, L. *Medical Answers about AIDS.* Rev. ed. New York: Gay Men's Health Crisis, 1985.

29. National Society for the Prevention of Blindness (NSPB). "NSPB's Task Force Report on AIDS and Eye Health Care." *Sightsaving* 54:6, 1986.

30. Norman, C. "Congress Likely to Halt Shrinkage in AIDS Funds." *Science* 231:1364, 1986.

31. Polsky, B., and D. Armstrong. "Infectious Complications of Neoplastic Disease." *American Journal of Infectious Control* 13:199, 1985.

32. Redfield, R. R., et al. "Frequent Transmission of HTLV-III Among Spouses of Patients with AIDS-Related Complex and AIDS." *Journal of the American Medical Association* 253:1571, 1985.

33. Redfield, R., D. C. Wright, and E. C. Tramont. "The Walter Reed Staging Classification for HTLV-III/LAV Infection." *New England Journal of Medicine* 314:131, 1986.

34. Rosenow, E. C., M. D. Wilson, and F. R. Cockerill. "Pulmonary Disease in the Immunocompromised Host." *Mayo Clinical Proceedings* 60:473, 1985.

35. Sande, M. A. "Transmission of AIDS: The Case Against Casual Contagion." *New England Journal of Medicine* 114:380, 1986.

36. Schorr, J. B., et al. "Prevalence of HTLV-III Antibody in American Blood Donors." *New England Journal of Medicine* 313:384, 1985.

37. Shaw, G. M., et al. "HTLV-III Infection in Brains of Children and Adults with AIDS Encephalopathy." *Science* 227:117, 1985.

38. Snider, W. D., et al. "Neurologic Complications of Acquired Immune Deficiency Syndrome." *Annals of Neurology* 14:403, 1983.

39. Stagno, E. "Toxoplasmosis." *American Journal of Nursing* 80:720, 1980.

40. State of New York Department of Health. *AIDS Institute Newsletter,* October 1985, 3.

41. Staver, S. "Insurers Eye Screening for AIDS." *American Medical News,* September 6, 1985, 1.

42. U.S. Centers for Disease Control. "Acquired Immune Deficiency Syndrome (AIDS): Precautions for Clinical and Laboratory Staffs." *Morbidity and Mortality Weekly Report* 31:577, 1982.

43. U.S. Centers for Disease Control. "Acquired Immunodeficiency Syndrome (AIDS): Precautions for Health Care Workers and Allied Professionals." *Morbidity and Mortality Weekly Report* 32:450, 1982.

44. U.S. Centers for Disease Control. "Classification System for Human T-Lymphotropic Virus Type III/Lymphadenopathy-Associated Virus Infections" *Morbidity and Mortality Weekly Report* 35:334–339, 1986.

45. U.S. Centers for Disease Control. "Education and Foster Care of Children Infected with Human T-Lympotropic Virus Type III/Lymphadenopathy-Associated Virus." *Morbidity and Mortality Weekly Report* 34:517, 1985.

46. U.S. Centers for Disease Control. "Prevention of Acquired Immune Deficiency Syndrome (AIDS): Report of Inter-Agency Recommendations." *Morbidity and Mortality Weekly Report* 32:101, 1983.

47. U.S. Centers for Disease Control. "Recommendations for Assisting in the Prevention of Perinatal Transmission of Human T-Lympotropic Virus Type III/Lymphadenopathy-Associated Virus and AIDS." *Morbidity and Mortality Weekly Report* 34:721, 1985.

48. U.S. Centers for Disease Control. "Revision of the CDC Surveillance Case Definition of Acquired Immunodeficiency Syndrome" *Morbidity and Mortality Weekly Report* 36(suppl no. 15):35–95, 1987.

49. U.S. Centers for Disease Control. "Update: Public Health Service Workshop on Human T-Lymphotropic Virus Type III Antibody Testing—United States." *Morbidity and Mortality Weekly Report* 34:477, 1985.

50. U.S. Centers for Disease Control. Center for Infectious Disease. *Acquired Immune Deficiency Syndrome (AIDS) Weekly Surveillance Report.* December 14, 1987.

51. U.S. Centers for Disease Control, et al. "Provisional Public Health Service Inter-Agency Recommendations for Screening Donated Blood and Plasma for Antibody to the Virus Causing Acquired Immunodeficiency Syndrome." *Morbidity and Mortality Weekly Report* 34:1, 1985.

52. U.S. Congress, Office of Technology Assessment. *Review of the Public Health Service's Response to AIDS* (OTS-TM-H–24). Washington, D.C.: U.S. Government Printing Office, 1985.

53. U.S. Food and Drug Administration. "Progress on AIDS." *FDA Drug Bulletin* 15:27, 1985.

54. Valle, S. L., et al. "Diversity of Clinical Spectrum of HTLV-III Infection." *Lancet* 1(8424):301, 1985.

55. Wegmann, J. "Avoidance Behaviors of Nurses as Related to Cancer Diagnosis and/or Terminality." *Oncology Nursing Forum* 6:8, 1979.

56. Wein, K., and D. Lopez. *Overview of Psychological Issues Concerning AIDS.* New York: Gay Men's Health Crisis, 1983.

57. World Health Organization Collaborating Centre on AIDS. *AIDS Surveillance in Europe* (Report No. 8). Paris: WHO, 1985.

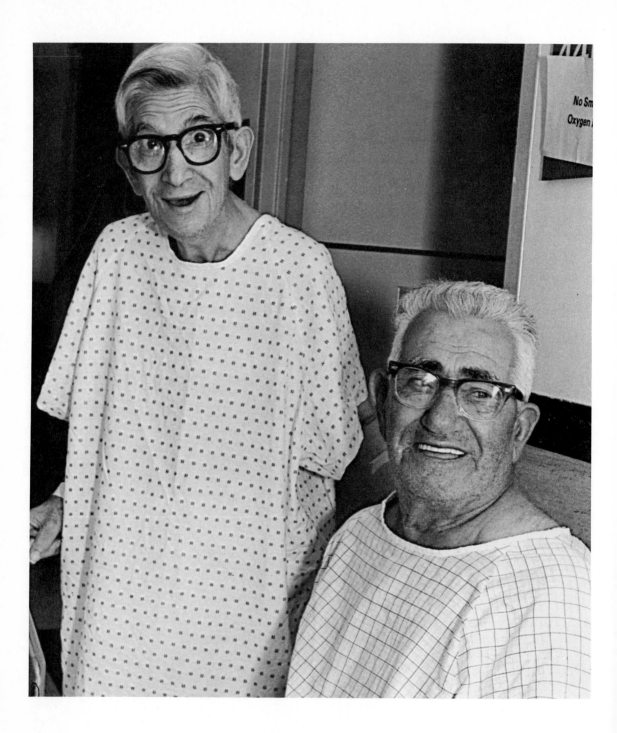

UNIT SIX

Primary Practice with Older Adults

■

Unit Six begins with an introduction to the older adult and provides a point of reference for understanding the chapters on health problems primarily associated with the older adult. In chapter 35 the reader learns about the scope of physical, socioeconomic, and emotional problems of the increasing number of elderly people in American society and how they and their families will require more services from nurses prepared to deliver comprehensive, continuous care than ever before. The discussion of common geriatric problems prepares the reader for the subsequent chapters, which deal with problems of the older adult compounded by selected diseases.

Unit Six includes chapters on chronic obstructive pulmonary disease, stroke, arthritis, and degenerative neuromuscular disease (multiple sclerosis, Parkinson's disease, and Alzheimer's disease). These disease conditions were selected because they occur more often with advancing age and they illustrate application of the concepts of primary nursing care to long-term, complex problems involving multiple body systems and having significant multidimensional effects on the client and family.

CHAPTER 35

The Older Adult

TERRY T. FULMER

■

OBJECTIVES

After completing this chapter, the reader will be able to:

☐ Describe demographic trends in America's older adults and discuss their relevance to nursing care needs.

☐ Discuss nursing resources available for the promotion of gerontological nursing.

☐ Develop an appreciation for the ethical dilemmas involved in caring for the older adult.

☐ Delineate areas of nursing practice for the older adult that need advanced research.

☐ Identify priorities in the nursing assessment of older adults.

☐ Evaluate common clinical syndromes of the older adult.

Demographics of Aging

Nursing care of the older adult is rapidly becoming a specialty area that can no longer be thought of as an extension of medical-surgical nursing. Although maximum life expectancy has not changed, there has been a dramatic increase in average life expectancy that has changed the demographic profile of the United States. In 1900 only 4 percent of the population lived beyond sixty-five years of age. In 1980 fully 11 percent of the population survived beyond age sixty-five, and it is projected that by the year 2040, 21 percent of the population will live beyond age sixty-five. This will mean 66 million older adults will potentially need nursing care (28). It is also important to note that of these people, the "old-old" are the fastest growing segment of the aging population. Americans over seventy-five years of age will increase from 35 percent to 45 percent of the elderly population, and those eighty-five years of age and older will increase threefold, from 2 million to 6 million persons, in the next fifty years (17).

Not only are Americans living longer, but they are living better. Most older people are perfectly capable of living independently and fully 95 percent do so. Innovative programs that lend support to older adults are making it possible for them to live in their own homes or residential communities until they die. The trend toward health maintenance programs and actions directed toward the prevention of health problems are clearly making a difference. Nursing care that emphasizes healthy living is an important component to the total health care of America's elderly. Ideally, healthy aging begins at birth. Children today need to be taught successful health practices in their formative years that will carry them through to a long and healthy life.

Utilization of Health Care Resources

Utilization of health care by older adults is also shifting and reflects the increased use owing to disability and disease, which rise sharply with age. Rowe and Besdine state that "these demands will continue to escalate, and the strain on the health care system will increase disproportionately since the elderly, having more illnesses, use more services" (24). According to Gibson and Fisher, elders over sixty-five years of age use 40 percent of all "acute" hospital bed days, buy one-quarter of all prescription drugs, spend 30 percent of the national health care budget, and occupy 1.1 million nursing home beds (16).

Long-Term Care

Long-term care has become a big business in the United States and 5 percent to 7 percent of all elderly are in nursing homes at any given time. The "typical" nursing home resident is very old; the average age is eighty-two and more than 85 percent are over the age of seventy-five. Most are women. Minorities are under-represented at this time, and most residents have serious health problems, with an average of 3.5 chronic disorders per person. Less than half the residents are independently ambulatory and nearly one-third need assistance in eating, while another two-thirds need help with other activities of daily living (29). Clearly, the demand for nursing care is extraordinary in this age-group and will only increase in the coming decades.

Nursing Resources

Specialty Preparation/Education

Given the demand for nursing care services by our aging population, what resources are available in terms of nurses with advanced preparation in the field of gerontological nursing? The American Nurses' Association (ANA) reports that there are currently twenty-three programs that offer a master's degree with specialization in gerontological nursing (3). As of 1978 there were 150 nurses graduated from these programs. One of the major problems of these programs cited by Ida Martinson is that of adequately prepared faculty (20). The majority of faculty in these programs have obtained their knowledge through self-study. This may be changing, however, as there are now sixteen doctorally prepared nurses with specialization in the area. However, of the 1.9 million nurses in this country, only 7 percent have master's and doctoral degrees. Furthermore, only 0.2 percent of nurses functioning in the expanded role as defined by the ANA are in gerontological nursing practice (5). These numbers suggest that innovations in the care of the gerontological client will be slow until there are more nurse educators prepared in the specialty who can produce nurses qualified to meet the client demand. This is not to suggest that only those nurses who receive an advanced degree are qualified to provide geriatric care! The onus will most certainly be on the new graduate, fresh from college, who will, it is hoped, have had a scientific, as well as an enthusiastic, introduction to the nursing care needs of the elderly.

Long-Term Care

The nursing care needs of America's elderly in long-term care are not being met by professional nurses. Aiken states that, on the average, there are only 1.5 licensed nursing providers (registered nurses and licensed practical nurses) for each 100 nursing home residents (2). Further, even in skilled nursing facilities, only 40 percent of the homes have, at best, one nurse present throughout a twenty-four-hour period. (Only 17 percent of American physicians make nursing home visits.)

The good news is that the number of nurses working in long-term care is rapidly increasing. During the period from 1972 to 1979 there was a 42 percent increase in the number of nurses working in long-term care, and a 20 percent increase in the number of nurses employed by home health agencies (25). It still remains dubious that there will be an adequate supply of professional nurses to meet the demands for long-term care in the future. Factors that contribute to the undersupply include:

- the growth of the elderly population,
- noncompetitive salaries,
- limited opportunities for career advancement,
- unfavorable work conditions,
- a decrease in applicants to and graduates of nursing schools,
- a paucity of gerontological nurse training, and
- low status.

The challenge of nursing during the next decade may well be the reversal of these factors in order to enhance the likelihood of long-term care as a choice for future employment.

American Nurses' Association

The ANA first provided standards for geriatric care in 1973 and subsequently revised them in 1976 as standards of gerontological nursing practice (Figure 35.1). These standards provide special comments related to the ramifications of the aging process and the individuality of the older adult that are critical to the provision of excellent nursing care, and act as guidelines for professional practice. The ANA, through its Council on Gerontological Nursing, has also published subsequent documents that provide professional direction for nurses in gerontological care. The ANA *Statement on the Scope of Gerontological Nursing Practice* "contributes to the understanding of the scope and depth of nursing practice as well as raises questions about the character of the differences" (6). This statement also discusses societal changes that have affected care of the older adult, the nursing role, educational needs, and research needs that will advance the quality of care for the older adult. The document entitled "A Challenge for Change: The Role of Gerontological Nursing" goes beyond the former document, in that it describes the development of gerontological nursing and discusses essential components of a health care system for older adults (4). This discussion relates to the concepts of health promotion, health maintenance, disease prevention, self-help, and options in health care for the older adult. It also provides a nursing model for long-term care that delineates specific differentiations from medical care (Table 35.1). Issues in gerontological nursing are discussed with recommendations for change.

Such leadership at the national level is imperative if gerontological nursing is to develop and obtain the recognition it deserves as a specialty. Plans are currently being formulated to design a mechanism for national networking in gerontological nursing. Such a capability would enable gerontological nurses to communicate more effectively with one another regarding issues related to practice, education, and research. Individuals would have access to names of other nurses who share common research topics, or educational concerns, as well as disseminate exacting practice concepts to interested peers. Such activities promise to promote interest and enthusiasm in care of the older adult.

I. Data are systematically and continuously collected about the health status of the older adult. The data are accessible, communicated, and recorded.

II. Nursing diagnoses are derived from the identified normal responses of the individual to aging and the data collected about the health status of the older adult.

III. A plan of nursing care is developed in conjunction with the older adult and/or significant others that include goals derived from the nursing diagnoses.

IV. The plan of nursing care includes priorities and prescribed nursing approaches and measures to achieve the goals derived from the nursing diagnosis.

V. The plan of care is implemented using appropriate nursing actions.

VI. The older adult and/or significant others participate in determining the progress attained in the achievement of established goals.

VII. The older adult and/or significant others participate in the ongoing process of assessment, the setting of new goals, the reordering of priorities, the revision of plans for nursing care, and the initiation of new nursing actions.

Figure 35.1. Standards of Gerontological Nursing Practice

Source: American Nurses' Association. *Standards: Gerontological Nursing Practice.* Kansas City: American Nurses' Association, 1976. Reprinted with permission.

Development of Nurse Leaders in Gerontological Care

Although efforts to determine the pathogenesis of disease in aging are clearly medical, the health outcome of the older adult will be determined by a comprehensive nursing approach that addresses reasonable goals for the client and methods for attaining those goals. McClure and Nelson (19) summarize the primary nurse's role when they identify the two major role classifications as that of care giver and integrator. They state that the care giver role is one that "is best understood but at the same time, most underestimated." Care giver responsibilities described by them include the following:

- Dependency needs: bathing, grooming, toileting, feeding, safety
- Comfort needs: vigilance to signs and symptoms, including appropriate responses based on data obtained
- Therapeutic needs: medications, treatments, dressings
- Educational needs: including the fostering of coping mechanisms

McClure reminds us that nursing care is the main reason for inpatient facilities, and in relation to geriatric care it is likely that the nursing challenge will continue to be extensive, given the complexity and array of nursing care needs.

The second component, that of integration, speaks to the need for a coordinator of care and services in a way that enhances health and prevents exhaustion, confu-

sion, and client stress. The primary nurse integrates the various differentiated segments in the care of older adults. For example, in addition to the admitting diagnosis, an older adult may have hearing or vision impairment, decreased mental acuity, ambulation problems, loss of skin integrity, and lack of self-care skills such as feeding, toileting, and dressing, all of which may exacerbate the primary condition. Clearly, without an integrator, the older adult may receive fragmented care that may prove to be more injurious than therapeutic.

It is only through strong nursing leadership and nursing presence that we will be able to oversee and affect the clinical care of older adults in their respective health care settings. Ours is the domain of clinical care, and it is up to the profession of nursing to ensure that clinical interventions are influenced by nursing. In order to ensure that this happens, a "critical mass" of nurse clinicians, researchers, and educators focused on care of the older adult must develop. More educational programs with specialties in gerontological nursing, along with an active recruitment effort, may be an important step. On a positive note Thelma Wells, of the University of Michigan (30), has summarized progress in gerontological nursing and states that there has been a significant increase in the number of gerontological nursing textbooks as well as journals. She notes, however, that there are new problems emerging in the field: the graduate level student shortage, possible overexpansion beyond leadership capabilities, loss of focus in the field, and isolation from the mainstream of nursing. Issues of status and prestige continue to be a problem, with studies documenting geriatrics as the least preferred nursing specialty (27). Ours is a care-oriented health care system,

Table 35.1
Comparisons Between the Medical Model and the Nursing Model

	Medical Care	Nursing Care
Nursing and health needs	Secondary need	Major need
Setting for care delivery	Major need	Secondary need
Measurement of successful treatment	Number of diagnosed, appropriately treated, cured, or rehabilitated	Present level of physical, mental, social, and spiritual function compared with potential level of function
Treatment emphasis	Chief complaint: what's wrong, what's disabled; disability/illness orientation	Functional level: what's good, what's healthy; ability/health orientation
Focus of care	Individual organ—start with chief complaint	Holistic approach, total person—start where the person is
Duration of Care	Episodic	Continuing
Role of the patient, client, and family	Passivity, regressive-dependence	Active participation, progressive-independence

Source: Adapted from Philip G. Weiler. "Cost-effective Analysis: A Quandary for Geriatric Health Care Systems." *The Gerontologist,* October 1974, 415. Reprinted with permission from the American Nurses' Association, "A Challenge for Change: The Role of Gerontological Nursing," 1982.

and it may be that there is a sense of failure with older adults as clients because care may not be realistic. Value needs to be placed on the nurse's role in nurturing people through the dying process. Consideration of our own feelings regarding loss of function, beauty, autonomy, and health may provide some insight into the apparent lack of interest in this specialty.

National Organizations

Several key national organizations promote and enhance gerontological nursing. Membership in such organizations is one nursing action that enhances development and nursing presence in the field of gerontology/geriatrics.

The ANA *Council on Gerontological Nursing* is a key organization to be a part of. It provides a certification process that enables nurses to gain credentials in the field of gerontological nursing and provides an important network at the national level.

The Gerontological Society of America (GSA) provides valuable opportunities for gerontological nurses to communicate with a variety of gerontological professionals. During the past three years the nursing membership of the GSA has increased by more than 30 percent (13). Founded in 1945, the GSA serves more than 5,600 members, 11 percent of whom are nurses. This organization represents every state in the United States as well as more than thirty countries abroad. The interdisciplinary perspective that encompasses nursing, medicine, dentistry, social work, health policy professionals, and others reflects the diversity of people who are committed to the field of aging. Opportunities to serve in major leadership roles within the GSA are available to those prepared to do the work. The annual meeting, held each November, provides a forum for developing and presenting papers, round tables, and symposia on current aging issues.

The Association for Gerontology in Higher Education promotes the advancement and exchange of new knowledge in geriatrics and provides a forum for new teaching strategies and research findings in aging. Although more specific to educational issues, all professionals and students are invited to become members. Similarly almost all geographical areas of the country have state and local organizations that provide a way of communicating with others who share an interest in aging.

Although these organizations seem far removed from the day-to-day practice issues confronting nursing, they provide the impetus as well as information regarding funding for the development, recognition, and dissemination of ideas that enhance care of the older adult.

Issues Related to Care
of the Older Adult

Ethical Considerations

During the past decade issues that are ethical in nature have come to the forefront of American geriatric care. With an intensity that has never been demonstrated before, clinical care providers, lawyers, theologians, economists, and associations representing the elderly are providing documents, sponsoring forums, and developing policy that will shape the future of national policy related to ethical decision making as it affects the country's growing number of elderly.

Abrams and Buckner (1) state that "an essential component in enabling the young professional to develop a moral consciousness about his or her work is to have a considered and well-articulated concept of professional identity." Whether young or old, a professional identity is best understood by members of that profession. In order to maximize the benefits of such identities they must be clear to those who are not in the identified profession. Nurses, doctors, social workers, and lawyers need more opportunities to converse in an interdisciplinary fashion for the purpose of forming some common consensus about approaches to ethical decision making with the elderly. If not consensus, then at least the chance to better understand the thought development that goes into actions and decisions that affect the elderly, and thus affect our practices in a central way.

Gadow (14) states that contemporary views of aging are complex and varied. She provides the following examples as the spectrum of viewpoints commonly held in society today.

At the negative extreme, aging is viewed as the antithesis of health and vigor. This negativity is expressed in the clinical arena in a deceptively "objective" form in the designation of clinical changes as deterioration, disorganization, and disintegration. A less patently negative view is that aging is an unwelcome reminder of our mortality. The third is the charitable view that the elderly are underprivileged citizens and should be the recipients of our benevolence toward the oppressed—as atonement for past discrimination. A fourth view contends that aging as a clinical entity in its own right is a unique human phenomenon worthy of practitioners' and researchers' full attention. The elderly are, after all, biologically elite. The fifth view holds that the aged are a cultural treasure, a repository of wisdom and history.

Each of these value positions is in evidence today, and affects the clinical approach and decision making related to the elderly. Wetle states that "the first premise when considering ethical issues for the elderly is that there should be no special ethical issues unique to decision making with the elderly" (31). In order to provide older adults the same options in health care as their younger counterparts, their age should play no part in the decision-making process as to whether care should be offered or withheld. However, evidence suggests that this is not the case (7, 8). Primary nurses are in an optimal position to serve as advocates for older adults when difficult ethical issues arise over the opportunity for or extent of care that may be provided. As advocates, primary nurses may initiate dialogue in conjunction with or on behalf of the older adult that may improve communication and clarify expectations among all parties involved. Ostrovski states that "the erosion of caring as a component of health care has been attributed to specialization and the development of science and technology" (23). Professional nurses, as care givers and integrators, can and do make a difference but need to continue their vigilance to the special needs of older adults. Davis and Aroskar (10) outline the following six categories as bases for ethical decision making:

1. *Egoist:* Each should act and judge right and wrong in relation to his own advantage or his own greatest good.
2. *Deontologic:* Rightness or wrongness depends on certain invariant rules or principles. A moral judgment will be the same in any similar situation regardless of consequence.
3. *Utilitarian:* Rightness or wrongness is judged as related to the greatest good and the least amount of harm for the greatest number of people.
4. *Obligation:* This includes beneficence (the act of doing good, preventing harm, and removing evil) and distributive equal justice.
5. *Ideal Observer:* All related information in the dilemma is dispassionately reviewed and impartial action based on knowledge is taken.
6. *Justice or Fairness:* Each person is to have equal rights in negotiated statements of liberty for all.

Ebersole and Hess (11) believe that there are specific ethical considerations in the care of older adults (Figure 35.2), and comment that nurses are frequently victimized by a system that grants them great responsibility and little authority. They suggest that "perhaps making the client aware of dilemmas is a nursing function." In fact, although there is little research to document such activity, there is anecdotal evidence to suggest that pri-

- Political and economic considerations that guide the allocation of scarce resources
- Numerous demonstration projects that are not sustained and leave the aged stranded
- Finances of agencies limit number of visits (for instance, Visiting Nurses' Association limited to small number of visits; physicians limited to one visit per month to boarding care patients)
- The inappropriate extension of life
- The burdening expense of medical care and the need to deplete personal resources before assistance can be obtained
- Untrained, unqualified personnel caring for the ill aged in some settings
- Abuse of conservatorships and guardianships
- Inadequate care of the community aged

Figure 35.2. Major Ethical Dilemmas in the Care of the Aged

Source: P. Ebersole and P. Hess. *Toward Healthy Aging: Human Needs, Nursing Response.* St. Louis: C. V. Mosby, 1981, 626–27.

mary nurses play a powerful role in the awareness of older adults relative to health care options. This role needs to be promoted and supported for the benefit of older adults everywhere.

Research

The momentum and prestige of nursing research have been well described and illustrated in the nursing literature and nursing seminars at the local, state, and national levels. The ANA Council on Gerontological Nursing states:

The goal of research in gerontological nursing is to provide a scientific base for nursing practice for older adults and their families. . . . Research in gerontological nursing is focused on the interaction of the aging process, health status, and nursing practice in caring for older adults. (4)

This report goes on to enumerate the significant research issues and includes the following five needs:

1. Need for qualified nurse researchers interested in gerontology
2. Replication and review of existing findings
3. Recognition of high-priority research topics
4. Relationship of gerontological nursing research to education and practice
5. Multidisciplinary research

The Council summarizes by stating that gerontology cuts across numerous disciplines, and each discipline will gain by collaborating and building on previous work done by others.

Departments of nursing research are in evidence today more than ever before, and faculty in schools of nursing are increasingly expected to obtain research funds in order to advance the science of nursing, as well as to help fund their own teaching salaries. As each of us reads *Nursing Research* and similar journals, I would bet that occasionally the question "How did the author ever get started?" may occur to us. It is easy to feel overwhelmed and incompetent in the area of nursing research until one can bring it into a personal focus.

Nursing research that is interesting and of high quality develops from a personal interest and probably a clinical phenomenon that sparks a curiosity factor in the researcher. No matter how seemingly trivial, if it sustains researcher interest over time, it will probably sustain interest in others as well. Older adults can benefit greatly from nursing research projects on such topics as incontinence management, prevention of falls, elimination of iatrogenesis, and reorientation techniques, to name a few. The work has begun, but only the tip of the iceberg has been addressed, and the challenge for nursing is to identify and address research needs that will ultimately improve the health care of older adults.

Priorities in Nursing Assessment of the Older Adult

Older adults manifest specific normal age changes and health problems that are different from those of younger people. Crucial to the successful assessment of the health and well-being of elders is a holistic approach to the client with a sensitivity to the totality of the individual, as opposed to the collection of body system data. The loss of function in old age is generally linear and does not increase as one becomes older. It is the accumulation of age-related effects that causes the notable decline in old age. It is important for primary nurses to appreciate the variability of age-related changes within and among people as well as changes as they vary in groups and populations. The functions of cardiac output, glomerular filtration rate, and carbohydrate tolerance change markedly with age, whereas other functions, such as nerve conduction velocity and hematocrit, undergo no significant changes (21). Several excellent textbooks are now available that describe the various body system changes that constitute normal age changes as distinct from disease processes (1, 6, 8, 21, 25). Primary nurses who are caring for older adults should become familiar with these differences.

Assessment of the Older Person

There are several comprehensive texts that describe the elements of a thorough health assessment of the older adult (11, 21, 24, 32). However, a brief description of such an assessment is appropriate at this time.

Older people are known to exhibit specific normal age-related changes that are not normal in younger people. Examples of this phenomenon include gray hair and loss of subcutaneous fat. A successful health assessment will be predicated on the fact that the primary nurse is aware of what are normal age-related changes versus what are changes that are the result of a disease process. Fortunately more and more nursing education curricula are including content that describes physical assessment of the older adult so that it may soon be unnecessary to rely on clinical specialists to describe approaches and outcomes for the gerontological physical assessment.

Table 35.2, taken from Ebersole and Hess, summarizes normal physical findings in the elderly.

Biological changes in older adults are a continuation of decline that begins in middle adulthood. It is known that elders have a decreased ability to adapt to stressors and have more difficulty maintaining and regaining homeostasis. In clinical practice this means that usual evidence of disease may be slow to present itself and even slower in its resolution. The classic example in geriatrics relates to infection, and for older adults, body temperature does not rise characteristically as it does in younger people; nor does it return to normal in the usual period of time. *Psychological* changes in older people generally result from the major developmental tasks of maintaining independence, relinquishing power, coping with losses, initiating life review, and developing a philosophical perspective on life (21). Personality, however, remains relatively unchanged with age, except for some exaggeration of previous tendencies. The stubborn young man is more than likely to become a stubborn old man, and manifestations of marked differences implies the need for a workup to explore the possibility of a disease-related cause. There is, as yet, no definitive evidence that cognitive function declines in old age. Test measurements have come under close scrutiny in regard to this aspect, and age biases in testing instruments have been noted. Finally, *sociocultural* changes vary according to the societal context in which they are measured. Mezey and associates state

that "social age reflects performance of age-specific roles, and social age can be a state of development or a status confirmed by a social group" (21). Because everyone ages in his or her own unique way, it seems impossible to categorize an individual in any meaningful or truthful way. Professional nursing practice assumes that each older adult will be accorded an individualized assessment for the necessary health planning needs that will be successful for that person.

Clinical Management of Common Geriatric Disorders

Confusion

Confusion is a clinical phenomenon that is frequently mistaken as a diagnostic level. It is merely a symptom, and as such, confusion requires an in-depth review of systems for the purpose of identifying possible causative factors.

According to Kane and colleagues (18), in the community-dwelling population of elders over sixty-five, about 5 percent have some degree of cognitive impairment, while fully 20 percent of elders over seventy-five exhibit some cognitive dysfunction. Nursing homes have a 50 percent proportion of elders with cognitive impairment. This certainly presents a major nursing care challenge.

Wolanin and Phillips provide a comprehensive approach to care of the confused patient that has been widely recognized for its excellence (32). They state from the outset that the term confusion is used freely by health care professionals, yet it is unclearly defined and "is a label for the behaviors that caregivers recognize as being deviant from those expected from the client in a certain place and at a certain time." Geebie and Lavin have identified the following characteristics of confusion as data for the nursing diagnosis of confusion (15):

- Disorientation to place, person, time, object, and purpose after reality information is given
- Suspected impairment of attention span
- Restlessness
- Purposeless activity
- Anxiety
- Apprehension
- Fright
- Agitation
- Verbosity
- Confabulation

Table 35.2
Normal Physical Assessment Findings in the Elderly

System Assessed	Changes
Cardiovascular	
Cardiac output	Heart loses elasticity; therefore, decreased heart contractility in response to increased demands
Arterial circulation	Decreased vessel compliance with increased peripheral resistance to blood flow resulting from general or localized arteriosclerosis
Venous circulation	Does not exhibit change with aging in the absence of disease
Blood pressure	Significant increase in the systolic, slight increase in the diastolic, increase in peripheral resistance and pulse pressure
Heart	Dislocation of the apex because of kyphoscoliosis; therefore, diagnostic significance of location is lost
Murmurs	Diastolic murmurs in more than half the aged; the most common heard at the base of the heart because of sclerotic changes on the aortic valves
Peripheral pulses	Easily palpated because of increased arterial wall narrowing and loss of connective tissue; feeling of tortuous and rigid vessels
Heart rate	No changes with age at normal rest
Respiratory	
Pulmonary blood flow and diffusion	Decreased blood flow to the pulmonary circulation; decreased diffusion
Anatomical structure	Increased anteroposterior diameter
Respiratory accessory muscles	Degeneration and decreased strength; increased rigidity of chest wall
Internal pulmonic structure	Decreased pulmonary elasticity creates senile emphysema
	Shorter breaths taken with decreased maximum breathing capacity, vital capacity, residual volume, and functional capacity
	Airway resistance increases; less ventilation at the bases of the lung and more at the apex
Integumentary	
Texture	Skin loses elasticity; wrinkles, folding, sagging, dryness
Color	Spotty pigmentation in areas exposed to sun; face paler, even in the absence of anemia
Temperature	Extremities cooler; decreased perspiration
Fat distribution	Less on extremities; more on trunk
Hair color	Dull gray, white, yellow, or yellow-green
Hair distribution	Thins on scalp, axilla, pubic area, upper and lower extremities; decreased facial hair in men; women may develop chin and upper lip hair
Nails	Decreased growth rate
Genitourinary and Reproductive	
Renal blood flow	Because of decreased cardiac output, reduced filtration rate and renal efficiency; possibility of subsequent loss of protein from kidneys
Micturition	In men possibility of increased frequency as a result of prostatic enlargement
	In women decreased perineal muscle tone; therefore, urgency and stress incontinence
	Increased nocturia for both men and women
	Possibility that polyuria may be diabetes-related
	Decreased volume of urine may relate to decrease in intake, but evaluation needed
Incontinence	Increased occurrence with age, specifically in those with dementia
Male reproduction	
Testosterone production	Decreases; phases of intercourse slower, lengthened refractory time
Frequency of intercourse	No changes in libido and sexual satisfaction; decreased frequency to one or two times weekly
Testes	Decreased size; decreased sperm count, diminished viscosity of seminal fluid

(continued)

Table 35.2 (continued)

System Assessed	Changes
Genitourinary and Reproductive	
Female reproduction	
Estrogen	Decreased production with menopause
Breasts	Diminished breast tissue
Uterus	Decreased size; mucous secretions cease; possibility that uterine prolapse may occur as a result of muscle weakness
Vagina	Epithelial lining atrophies; narrow and shortened canal
Vaginal secretions	Become more alkaline as glycogen content increases and acidity declines
Gastrointestinal	
Mastication	Impaired because of partial or total loss of teeth, malocclusive bites, and ill-fitting dentures
Swallowing and carbohydrate digestion	Swallowing more difficult as salivary secretions diminish
	Reduced ptyalin production; therefore, impaired starch digestion
Esophagus	Decreased esophageal peristalsis
	Increased incidence of hiatus hernia with accompanying gaseous distension
Digestive enzymes	Decreased production of hydrochloric acid, pepsin, and pancreatic enzymes
Fat absorption	Delayed, affecting the rate of fat-soluble vitamins A, D, E, and K absorption
Intestinal peristalsis	Reduced gastrointestinal motility
	Constipation because of decreased mobility and roughage
Musculoskeletal	
Muscle strength and function	Decrease with loss of muscle mass; bony prominences normal in aged, since muscle mass decreased
Bone structure	Normal demineralization, more porous
	Shortening of the trunk as a result of intervertebral space narrowing
Joints	Become less mobile; tightening and fixation occur
	Activity may maintain function longer
	Normal posture changes; some kyphosis
	Range of motion limited
Anatomical size and height	Total decrease in size as loss of body protein and body water occur in proportion to decrease in basal metabolic rate
	Increased body fat; diminished in arms and legs, increased in trunk
	Decreased height from 2.5 to 10 cm from young adulthood
Nervous System	
Response to stimuli	All voluntary or automatic reflexes slower
	Decreased ability to respond to multiple stimuli
Sleep patterns	Stage IV sleep reduced in comparison to younger adulthood; increased frequency of spontaneous awakening
	Stay in bed longer but get less sleep; insomnia a problem that should be evaluated
Reflexes	Deep tendon reflexes responsive in the healthy aged
Ambulation	Kinesthetic sense less efficient; may demonstrate an extrapyramidal Parkinsonlike gait
	Basal ganglions of the nervous system influenced by the vascular changes and decreased oxygen supply
Voice	Decreased range, duration, and intensity of voice; may become higher pitched and monotonous
Sensory	
Vision	
Peripheral vision	Decreases
Lens accommodation	Decreases, requires corrective lenses
Ciliary body	Atrophy in accommodation of lens focus
Iris	Development of arcus senilis

(continued)

Table 35.2 (continued)

System Assessed	Changes
Sensory	
Choroid	Atrophy around disk
Lens	May develop opacity, cataract formation; more light necessary to see
Color	Fades or disappears
Macula	Degenerates
Conjunctiva	Thins and looks yellow
Tearing	Decreases; increased irritation and infection
Pupil	May be different in size
Cornea	Presence of arcus senilis
Retina	Observable vascular changes
Stimuli threshold	Increased threshold for light touch and pain; ischemic paresthesias common in the extremities
Hearing	Less perceptible high-frequency tones; hence greatly impaired language understanding; promotes confusion and seems to create increased rigidity in thought process
Gustatory	Decreased acuity as taste buds atrophy; may increase the amount of seasoning on food

Source: P. Ebersole and P. Hess. *Toward Healthy Aging: Human Needs, Nursing Response.* St. Louis: C. V. Mosby, 1985, 184–86. Reprinted with permission.

- Rambling speech
- Dependent and demanding attention-getting behavior
- Withdrawal
- Belligerence
- Combativeness
- Statements of confusion
- Facial expression specific to confusion

Each of these symptoms, or combinations of them, alerts the nurse to the possibility that the client is becoming, or in fact is, confused. Once a nursing diagnosis of confusion is made, the pathophysiology underlying the confusion is explored and usually can be attributed to the three general categories of *systemic problems,* such as hypoxia, hypoglycemia, or dehydration; *mechanical problems,* such as obstruction, or death of brain cells; and *presenile irreversible dementias,* such as Alzheimer's disease, Jakob–Creutzfeldt disease, and Pick's disease. The primary nurse's role in caring for the older adult with confusion primarily centers on the client's safety and comfort. It is important to differentiate between acute confusional states, chronic confusional states, and combinations of the two when planning care for the older adult. Client setting will mandate the inclusion of certain nursing interventions and incorporation of family, friends, and the older adult in deciding on approaches to confusion management that help ensure the success of the care plan. Guidelines

for providing a facilitative milieu for elderly with true dementia have been summarized by Wolanin and Phillips (32) and appear in Figure 35.3. Patience and understanding are probably the most therapeutic nursing skills available in the management of confusion. The nurse who finds her inner resources waning will do well to recognize her need for supports from colleagues to assure the continuity and success of the older adult's care.

Urinary Incontinence

Incontinence is a common and distressing condition in older adults, and its prevalence increases with age. The adverse effects of incontinence have been summarized by Kane and associates (18) and appear in Table 35.3. As in the case of confusion, successful management of incontinence requires an understanding of the underlying causative factors and the inclusion of the older adult in planning care for its control. Basic causes of incontinence include *urologic factors,* such as hyperactive bladder tone, increased outflow resistance, and sphincter weakness; *neurological factors,* such as central nervous system disease, peripheral neuropathy, and peripheral nerve damage; *locomotor* factors, such as immobility and inaccessible toilets; and *psychological factors,* such as depression, anger, and hostility (18).

Incontinence may be acute or chronic, and nursing

1. Make change slowly. The client must be well prepared for any physical, emotional, drug, nutritional, personnel, or geographical change.

2. Keep the client ambulatory as long as possible with daily exercise routine, including a walk in the sunshine.

3. Maintain a routine. A dependable world and a structured existence and environment are essential.

4. Provide social stimulation without overload. Maintain communication through every possible channel.

5. Avoid crowds or large spaces without boundaries. Avoid sensory overload.

6. Assist in organizing the personal aspects of the client's affairs—safekeeping of treasures, obtaining legal aid of attorney or ombudsman, and setting up file of personal papers.

7. Monitor use of health measures, including good nutrition, attention to mouth and teeth, and adequate shoes. Avoid the use of drugs.

8. Do not expect the client to understand or participate in complex activities or conversations.

9. Maintain positive input, such as reinforcement for any worthy act, to maintain the client's self-esteem and encourage self-participation in activities of daily living.

10. Ensure that information is available to the patient about the time and place: landmarks that provide reality—calendars with huge figures, clocks with all numbers for the hours, reality boards for institutions, and reminders of special events such as birthdays, anniversaries, and holidays.

11. Make bowel and bladder control consistent, using a routine. As the client's mind becomes hazier, use clothing with simple fasteners, or elastic wasitbands for pants.

12. Support the family, who in turn support the client, by simple reinforcement of their efforts with a special commendation. Respite care from the daily watching may enable them to care for the client in the home and visit him in the institution long after internal rewards have ceased to exist.

Figure 35.3.   Guidelines for Providing a Facilitative Environment for the Elderly Client with True Dementia

Source: M. O. Wolanin and L. R. F. Phillips. *Confusion: Prevention and Care.* St. Louis, C. V. Mosby, 1981, 332. Reprinted with permission.

Table 35.3
Effects of Urinary Incontinence

Physical health
  Skin breakdown
  Recurrent urinary tract infections
  Sepsis
  Death
Psychological health
  Withdrawal
  Isolation
  Depression
  Dependence
Socioeconomic factors
  Stress on family and friends
  Predisposition to institutionalization
  Costs of caring for incontinence
    Supplies (padding, catheters, etc.)
    Laundry
    Labor (nurses, housekeepers)

Source: R. L. Kane, J. Ouslander, and I. Abrass. *Essentials of Clinical Geriatrics.* New York: McGraw-Hill, 1984, 108. Reprinted with permission.

management will depend on evaluation of discernible patterns exhibited by the older adult over time. Supportive measures, such as bladder training programs, drug therapy, and corrective surgery, may be instituted to alleviate incontinence. However, nursing care that includes a positive attitude, excellent skin care, and regular scheduling will usually provide the most successful resolution of the problem.

Constipation

Constipation is common in older adults and may result from poor dietary habits, immobility, and chronic laxative abuse. Once the contributory factors have been identified, educational programming for the older adult regarding adequate fluid and bulk intake as well as regular toileting and exercise will help alleviate the problem. Miller conducted a clinical study that evaluated the effect of dietary fiber, fluid intake, and activity in a group of thirty-eight men with an average age of eighty-two (22). This study concluded that "a bowel regimen was significantly more effective than other medication regimens in reducing the incidence of constipation." Clearly the use of laxatives is a behavior that can be modified when primary nurses provide appropriate teaching strategies for the older adults they care for, with supportive follow-up and ongoing surveillance of the problem.

Falls

Falling is a geriatric syndrome that represents a serious source of morbidity and mortality. Although most falls are of little or no consequence, 6 percent of all falls result in fracture (24). Approximately 40 percent of falls in older adults are accidental and related to some environmental factor, such as a loose scatter rug or poor stairway lighting. Other causes include "drop-attacks," postural hypotension, central nervous system events, and cardiovascular events. Factors associated with falls among institutionalized elderly include recent admission, unsafe furniture, certain activities (such as toileting and transfers), wet floors, and low staff-patient ratios (14). Fife and co-workers conducted a study that assessed the degree of risk of falls for older adults at their acute care facility (12). Falls declined 61 percent with the implementation of their "Risk/Fall Program," and better documentation and care planning could also be noted. This is one example of how nursing interventions can make a difference in the care of the older adult.

When falls occur, careful evaluation of the older adult is necessary. Any premonitory or associated symptoms should be documented, as well as whether there was a loss of consciousness. Cardiac and seizure disorders must be ruled out. Bruising, areas of tenderness, and any alterations in neurological status should be noted and frequent vital signs instituted in cases where there is indication of need. Prevention of falls includes adaptation of the environment, such as bed rails, secure furniture, and proper lighting, as well as gait training and muscle-strengthening exercises when indicated.

Iatrogenic Disorders

Iatrogenesis can be thought of as unwanted outcomes secondary to therapeutic interventions in health care that result in health problems for the client. Examples of iatrogenic disorders include incontinence, polypharmacy, enforced dependency, and confusion. Older adults have a delicate balance between homeostasis and disability. They have a narrow therapeutic "window" that increases their susceptibility to toxic effects of therapies. The classic example of iatrogenesis usually involves a health problem that results from the treatment of some disorder by drug therapy. Because older adults have a reduced capability for metabolizing and excreting many drugs, they are at high risk for drug sensitivities. Steel reported that among 815 consecutive admissions to a hospital's general medical service, an overall rate of 497 iatrogenic events occurred (26). The nurse's role in the prevention of iatrogenic disorders among the older adults they care for cannot be overstated. Documentation of adverse side effects of prescribed therapies in the earliest stages can prevent the devastating effects that may develop over time. Sensitivity to "labeling" in older adults helps in the prevention of generalized nursing assessments that attribute symptoms to the aging process when, in fact, they are the result of improper therapy. In the words of Ron Cape, "The price of freedom from iatrogenic disease is external vigilance" (9).

Loneliness/Social Isolation

Loneliness and social isolation interfere with the older adult's sense of belonging and perceived self-worth. Examples of events that may trigger loneliness and social isolation include loss of familiar surroundings, perceived absence of loving family members, cognitive deterioration, and loss of health. Loneliness is usually a manifestation of some loss incurred by older adults. Ebersole and Hess describe four major sources of isolation that they believe result in interactional deprivations or exclusion (11):

1. attitudinal isolation—stems from an unacceptable appearance;
2. presentation isolation—stems from an unacceptable appearance;
3. behavioral isolation—involves unacceptable actions; and
4. geographical isolation—related to territorial restrictions.

These authors believe that these four factors are barriers to acceptance of older adults by others. Such a lack of acceptance inevitably leads to a loss of self-esteem and self-worth that is devastating.

Miller believes that self-esteem is "the evaluation component of self-concept; it is the individual's judgment about one's own worth" (22). Therefore, older adults who perceive themselves as valuable people have a confidence about life that enables them to interact meaningfully with their environment. On the other hand, for those older adults who have little sense of their own worth, these interactions are few and of little solace. Miller describes self-esteem as a "power source" in that it allows the following to occur:

- It enables the person to be an active participant in care.
- It helps the person develop confidence in interpersonal communication.
- It provides the person with accurate feedback, as opposed to inaccurate, derogatory feedback that occurs in people with low self-esteem.
- It enhances the potential for successful role performance.

Nursing care that is directed toward enhancing self-esteem of the older adult will do much to improve his or her sense of self-worth, which in turn is likely to decrease the loneliness or social isolation being felt. Nursing actions that are effective in breaking the cycle of social isolation and loneliness include a comprehensive assessment of the meaning of being alone for each older adult under consultation. Perhaps the older adult is satisfied with being alone. However, in cases where social isolation and loneliness exist the primary nurse may provide meaningful activities that enhance the older adult's sense of belonging. It is likely that a social history will be useful in order to discern previous coping patterns for the client in question. For some people, group activities may provide relief from loneliness and social isolation; others may do better with a one-to-one relationship. Successful interventions will depend on an evaluation of the activities and their perceived meaning to the older adult.

Finding Purpose in the Last Days of Life

Older adults who demonstrate indexes of life satisfaction later in life are often labeled "self-actualized." Self-actualization, as defined by Maslow, is the highest level of human function, and it implies that the person has inner convictions and beliefs that life has had value and continues to be of value. As the primary nurse plans care for the older adults, it is important for her to realize that a lifetime of behaviors and beliefs have come into making the person who he or she now is, and it is highly unlikely that any short-term intervention can make a demonstrable difference. It is more likely that nursing actions directed toward accepting the older adult for the person he or she is will provide the most comfort in the last days of life. Discussions with older adults that help elicit what, if any, activities provide personal enrichment can guide the primary nurse in health care planning. For some older adults, religion is important, while others prefer to focus on leisure activities. Personalized programs ensure that stereotypic senior citizen pro-

grams are avoided. A sensitivity to the differences inherent in all of us will be the best guide for planning nursing care.

DISCUSSION QUESTIONS

1. Given the increasing demand for gerontological nursing services in the United States, what organizations or institutions are available in your geographical area to enhance the well-being of the older adult as well as serve as a resource for gerontological nurses?
2. What ethical considerations are necessary for care of the confused older adult?
3. What research questions might be generated in relation to client education in later years?
4. What iatrogenic disorders are primarily the result of polypharmacy?
5. The prevention of falls is primarily a nursing consideration. What nursing actions are appropriate for such prevention?

REFERENCES

1. Abrams, N., and M. D. Buckner. *Medical Ethics.* Cambridge, Mass.: MIT Press, 1983.
2. Aiken, L. H., ed. *Nursing in the 1980's: Crises, Opportunities, Challenges.* Philadelphia: J. B. Lippincott, 1983.
3. American Nurses' Association. "Programs That Award a Master's Degree with Specialization in Gerontological Nursing." Kansas City: American Nurses' Association, 1980. Unpublished list.
4. American Nurses' Association. *A Challenge for Change: The Role of Gerontological Nursing.* Kansas City: American Nurses' Association, 1982.
5. American Nurses' Association. *Facts About Nursing: 1982–1983.* Kansas City: American Nurses' Association, 1983, 31.
6. American Nurses' Association. *A Statement on the Scope of Gerontological Nursing Practice.* Kansas City: American Nurses' Association, 1984.
7. Avorn, J., and E. L. Langer. "Induced Disability in Nursing Home Patients: A Controlled List." *Journal of the American Geriatrics Society* 30:6, 1982.
8. Besdine, R. W. "Decisions to Withhold Treatment from Nursing Home Residents." *Journal of the American Geriatrics Society* 31:602–6, 1983.
9. Cape, R. *Aging: Its Complex Management.* Hagerstown, Md.: Harper & Row, 1978.
10. Davis, A., and M. Aroskar. *Ethical Dilemmas and Nursing Practice.* New York: Appleton-Century-Crofts, 1978.

11. Ebersole, P., and P. Hess. *Toward Healthy Aging: Human Needs, Nursing Response.* 2d ed. St. Louis: C. V. Mosby, 1985.

12. Fife, D., P. Solomon, and M. Stanton. "A Risk/Fall Program: Code Orange for Success." *Nursing Management* 15:50–53, 1984.

13. Fulmer, T., and B. Hofland. "GSA: Your Communication Tool." *Journal of Gerontological Nursing* 11:22, February 1985.

14. Gadow, S. "Medicine, Ethics and the Elderly." In *Medical Ethics,* ed. N. Abrams and M. D. Buckner. Cambridge, Mass.: MIT Press, 1983.

15. Geebie, K. M., and M. A. Lavin, eds. *Classification of Nursing Diagnoses.* St. Louis: C. V. Mosby, 1975.

16. Gibson, R. M., and C. R. Fisher. "Age Differences in Health Care Spending, Fiscal Year 1977." *HCFA Health Note,* December 1978.

17. Health Care Financing Administration. Discussion Paper. *Long-term Care: Background and Future Directions.* U.S. Government Publication No. (HCFA) 81-200047.

18. Kane, R. L., J. Ouslander, and I. Abrass. *Essentials of Clinical Geriatrics.* New York: McGraw-Hill, 1984.

19. McClure, M., and J. Nelson. "Trends in Hospital Nursing." In *Nursing in the 1980's: Crises, Opportunities, Challenges,* ed. L. H. Aiken. Philadelphia: J. B. Lippincott, 1983.

20. Martinson, I. "Gerontological Nursing Comes of Age." *Journal of Gerontological Nursing* 10:8–11, 14–17, 1984.

21. Mezey, M. D., L. Rauckhorst, and S. Stokes. *Health Assessment of the Older Adult.* New York: Springer Publishing Co., 1980.

22. Miller, J. "Helping the Aged Manage Bowel Function." *Journal of Gerontological Nursing* 11:37–41, 1985.

23. Ostrovski, M. J. "Legalities and Ethics of Caring." In *Toward Healthy Aging: Human Needs and Nursing Response,* ed. P. Ebersole and P. Hess. St. Louis: C. V. Mosby, 1985.

24. Rowe, J. W., and R. W. Besdine. *Health and Disease in Old Age.* Boston: Little, Brown, 1983, 3.

25. Shields, E. M., and E. Kick. "Nursing Care in Nursing Homes." In *Nursing in the 1980's: Crises, Opportunities, Challenges,* ed. L. H. Aiken. Philadelphia: J. B. Lippincott, 1983.

26. Steel, K., P. M. Gertman, C. Crescenzi, and J. Anderson. "Iatrogenic Illness on a General Medical Service at a University Hospital." *New England Journal of Medicine* 304:638–42, 1981.

27. Tollett, S. M., and C. M. Adamson. "The Need for Gerontologic Content Within Nursing Curricula." *Journal of Gerontological Nursing* 8:21, 1982.

28. U.S. Census Bureau. *Reports and Projections Series,* 1982, 25.

29. U.S. Department of Health, Education, and Welfare, Public Health Service. *Selected Operating and Financial Characteristics of Nursing Homes, United States 1973–1974.* Washington, D.C.: National Nursing Home Printing Office, 1975, 10–11.

30. Wells, T. "What Does Commitment to Gerontological Nursing Really Mean?" *Journal of Gerontological Nursing* 8:434, 1982.

31. Wetle, T. "Ethical Issues in Long-term Care of the Aged." *Journal of Geriatric Psychiatry* 18:63–73, 1985.

32. Wolanin, M. O., and L. R. F. Phillips. *Confusion Prevention and Care.* St. Louis: C. V. Mosby, 1981.

CHAPTER 36

Chronic Obstructive Pulmonary Disease

GLORIA CALIANDRO

■

OBJECTIVES

After completing this chapter, the reader will be able to:

□ Define the term chronic obstructive pulmonary disease (COPD).

□ Identify the magnitude of COPD as a health problem in the United States.

□ Relate pathophysiology and complications of COPD to client problems that require nursing intervention.

□ Identify factors that contribute to the onset and progression of COPD.

□ State information specific to COPD that should be collected during a nursing assessment.

□ Relate common deviations from normal found during the assessment of the client with COPD to nursing diagnoses.

□ Discuss nursing intervention and evaluation related to selected nursing diagnoses for the client with COPD.

□ Identify ethical issues related to COPD.

Chronic obstructive pulmonary disease (COPD) is a clinical condition resulting from diseases that have the same basic problem: chronic obstruction of the smaller airways. Most commonly the term is applied to "those patients with chronic bronchitis, asthma, or anatomic emphysema who exhibit persistent obstruction of bronchial air flow" (8). Other terms that denote the same clinical syndrome are chronic obstructive lung disease (COLD) and chronic obstructive airway disease (COAD).

In the United States COPD is a major health problem. The following statistics give some indication of the magnitude of the problem. In 1981 more than 17 million Americans—one in every thirteen—reported having some form of COPD in the previous twelve months. More than 1,051,000 of them were hospitalized, the majority being elderly people with COPD. The cost of caring for elderly and disabled Medicare beneficiaries with COPD during the fiscal year 1979 was more than $535 million. The total care cost for persons with COPD is estimated to be in excess of $5 billion annually (19). This figure does not reflect earnings lost because of sick days.

Of the three diseases constituting COPD, chronic bronchitis is the most prevalent in the population between seventeen and sixty-four years of age, followed by asthma and emphysema, in that order (19). With the exception of asthma, which occurs more frequently among younger people, COPD is primarily a problem of those in late middle age and of older adults. Both chronic bronchitis and emphysema are more common in men than in women. Asthma, however, tends to occur more commonly in females. All forms of COPD are about five times as common in whites as in blacks (19).

From another perspective, COPD is a chronic problem that primarily occurs in a population with multiple health problems. An estimated 80 percent of older Americans have one or more chronic conditions. Of these people, approximately 12 million will be limited in their activities on the average of thirty-one to thirty-eight days per person per year (14). The vast majority of these people are not institutionalized, but are in their homes. Thus COPD is part of a much larger community health problem—the noninstitutionalized older adult with more than one chronic condition—that is particularly suited to primary nursing, where the emphasis is on assisting the client and the client's family to attain an acceptable level of self-care.

Although this chapter has been written for the health care professional, much of its contents can be adapted for teaching clients, their families, and the general public about COPD. It includes those subjects related to COPD that any person, professional or lay, needs to know in order to provide comprehensive care—the nature and scope of the problem, contributing factors, how COPD affects the person, and how to manage it effectively.

Overview of the Problem

Although chronic bronchitis, asthma, and emphysema pose a common problem—airway obstruction leading to hypoventilation—the diseases differ in their underlying pathology.

Chronic Bronchitis. Chronic bronchitis is characterized by a chronic, productive cough owing to prolonged exposure to respiratory irritants. It is said to exist when there is a cough with sputum production on most days for three or more months per year for two successive years in people for whom no other source of these symptoms can be found (7).

Both large and small airways are involved in chronic bronchitis. But the major site of airway resistance is in the smaller, peripheral airways (16). Common pathological findings of the airways are inflammation of the bronchial walls, hypertrophy and hyperplasia of mucus-secreting glands, increased mucus production, intraluminal mucus plugs, hypertrophy of smooth muscles, and fibrosis leading to narrowing and distortion of airways. The result is impaired ventilation, particularly exhalation.

Not all of the pathology of chronic bronchitis is irreversible. When the source of irritation is removed, the acute inflammation and mucus production and plugging may be reversed. But changes that occur with chronic inflammation, such as fibrosis, distortion, narrowing, and obliteration of smaller airways, are considered irreversible (16). Therefore, it behooves the person with chronic bronchitis to remove sources of bronchial irritation as quickly and permanently as possible to reduce the amount of irreversible lung damage.

Asthma.   Asthma is "characterized by intermittent attacks of dyspnea and wheezing caused by paroxysmal narrowing of the bronchial airways" (24). It occurs in people whose airways are hyperreactive to either extrinsic stimulants (extrinsic asthma) or intrinsic stimulants (intrinsic asthma). Examples of extrinsic stimulants that cause asthma are foods, medicines, pollens, and chemical dusts from industry. Intrinsic stimulants include such factors as exposure to cold, exercise, and emotions.

During an asthmatic attack there is generalized bronchoconstriction, edema of the mucosa of the bronchioles, and excessive mucus secretion, leading to trapping of air in the alveoli, hyperinflation of the lungs, and impaired ventilation. The person is in acute distress. With the administration of bronchodilators and the removal of the stimulus that precipitated the asthmatic attack, the pathology of asthma subsides. The person is then usually asymptomatic until the next acute asthmatic episode.

Emphysema.   Emphysema is characterized by a permanent change in the structure of the acinus, that portion of the airways distal to the terminal bronchioles. Destruction of the normal acinar structure leads to the most characteristic finding of emphysema—persistent reduction in the forced expiratory flow rate of air from the lungs. As the expiratory flow rate decreases and air is trapped in the distal air spaces, the lungs hyperinflate. This in turn leads to markedly increased residual lung volume, markedly reduced lung recoil, hyperresonant percussion sounds, depression of the diaphragm, and a barrel-shaped chest—all classic findings of emphysema.

Hypoventilation and ventilation-perfusion imbalance are characteristic of COPD, especially emphysema and chronic bronchitis. Oxygen and carbon dioxide normally pass freely across the respiratory membranes between the alveoli and the capillaries surrounding them. Because of trapping of air, the alveoli are not adequately ventilated, and gas exchange is impaired. Carbon dioxide is retained, oxygen intake into the alveoli is reduced, and exchange of these gases between the alveoli and the

surrounding capillaries is impaired. The degree of ventilation-perfusion imbalance varies between individuals, depending on how advanced the COPD is, whether or not the factors that contribute to the problem are removed, and the type of COPD the person has. People with chronic bronchitis tend to have a lower PaO_2 and a higher $PaCO_2$ more consistently than do people with emphysema.

The onset of symptoms of COPD, with the exception of asthma, is insidious. At first the person is unaware of a problem. He or she may notice breathlessness during physical exertion, such as running and climbing stairs, and attribute this to just being out of shape. There is usually a persistent cough, often labeled a smoker's cough and ignored. But as the problem progresses, the symptoms increase. If the person has chronic bronchitis, there is usually copious sputum and the chest is noisy on auscultation. Emphysematous clients have little sputum and their chests are quiet except for wheezing on expiration. Less exertion causes greater difficulty in breathing. Exhalation is normally effortless, but the person with advancing COPD must force air out of the lungs. The work of breathing is increased, exercise tolerance decreases, and fatigue increases (15).

Complications

Clients with COPD may develop a variety of complications, one of the most serious being acute respiratory failure. Acute respiratory failure occurs when there is a sudden elevation of the $PaCO_2$ above 50 mm Hg, accompanied by a PaO_2 below 50 mm Hg and a blood pH below 7.30. Because the client with COPD commonly has abnormal blood gas and pH values, it may not be easy to diagnose acute respiratory failure. A common cause of acute respiratory failure is respiratory tract infection. The lungs are unable to cope with the added burden of an infection, leading to increased retention of carbon dioxide, insufficient oxygen intake, and respiratory acidosis. The client is acutely ill and must be hospitalized. Treatment includes antibiotics, oxygen therapy, pulmonary toilet, bronchodilators, and measures to restore acid–base balance. If the client's respiration is severely depressed, he or she may be placed on a ventilator until respiration improves.

Another complication of COPD is pulmonary hypertension often associated with right ventricular hypertrophy. The client may or may not develop congestive heart failure as a result. Sudden weight gain, shortness of breath, and pedal edema are indicators of heart failure.

Spontaneous pneumothorax may occur in the client who has developed bullae—air-filled blebs—on the surface of the lungs. Rupture of these bullae causes the release of air into the normally negative pressure of the intrapleural space and can impair lung expansion. Symptoms of spontaneous pneumothorax include sudden sharp pain in the chest, followed by dyspnea, rapid respirations, and tachycardia. In some clients, air leakage stops after the initial rupture, ventilation is minimally impaired, and no treatment is necessary. For other clients, thoracentesis, closed chest drainage, or surgery may be necessary.

Owing to a compensatory increase in red blood cells resulting from chronic hypoxia and the subsequent thickening of blood, some clients with COPD develop intravascular clotting and pulmonary emboli. Symptoms of pulmonary embolism include sharp chest pain, hyperpnea, tachycardia, diaphoresis, hypotension, and cough with hemoptysis. Pulmonary embolism requires prompt treatment as the client may die. Treatment includes bed rest, anticoagulant therapy, oxygen therapy, and vasopressors to help maintain circulation if the client is hypotensive.

About 20 percent of the clients with COPD develop peptic ulcer (7, 27). The cause is unknown, but stress is thought to be a contributor. Symptoms of peptic ulcer include epigastric pain and loss of appetite and weight. Measures to reduce stress, such as counseling and relaxation exercises; medications to control acidity, such as antacids and cimetidine, a histamine H receptor inhibitor; and avoidance of food and drinks that irritate the gastric mucosa are used to relieve the problem.

Risk Factors

Smoking. Smoking contributes significantly to two forms of COPD, emphysema and chronic bronchitis. Not only is smoking irritating to the bronchial mucosa, but it also produces other effects that contribute to COPD. In one study, smokers, after only two cigarettes, had significantly more elastase, an enzyme that contributes to the destruction of the elastic fibers of the acini found in emphysema, than did nonsmokers (17). Smoking also impairs ciliary clearance of matter from the lungs, increases the leukocyte count, impairs the function of macrophages in the alveoli, and causes broncho-constriction (8). In another study a highly significant relationship was found between the number of cigarettes smoked per day and the number of years of smoking, and impairment of forced expiratory flow rate. The im-

pairment was even greater in older smokers who had respiratory problems as children (3).

Air Pollution. Although a less frequent cause of COPD than smoking, exposure to high concentrations of noxious gases, such as sulfur dioxide, and particulate matter as found in heavily industrialized and urbanized environments and some occupations, such as grain handlers, is associated with the onset and exacerbation of COPD (8). In a study of grain handlers in the northern United States, researchers concluded that these workers were more than four times as likely to have chronic bronchitis and wheezing than workers not exposed to grain dust (7).

Infection. Clients with COPD often give a history of more frequent or severe respiratory tract infections during childhood than do healthy people. Whether or not this contributes to the onset of COPD is questionable. There is little doubt that respiratory tract infections in clients with established COPD lead to an exacerbation of the problem (27).

Inheritance. Genetic inheritance is implicated in two types of COPD, extrinsic asthma and emphysema. Extrinsic asthma is a genetically determined hypersensitivity to certain substances or antigens. When initially exposed to the antigens, the asthmatic person develops immunoglobulin E (IgE), which attaches itself to mast cells of the bronchial tissues. Subsequent exposure causes chemical substances such as histamine and slow-reacting substance of anaphylaxis (SRS-A) to be liberated from the mast cells, producing the symptoms of asthma. A person with extrinsic asthma usually has a family history of allergies.

Studies have shown that people who inherit a protease inhibitor type Z (Pi Z) develop emphysema more often and earlier than do people with other genotypes for protease inhibitors (8, 27). People with Pi Z are deficient in alpha-antitrypsin, a substance that inhibits elastase and prevents damage to and alteration of the structure of the acini. Whereas most cases of emphysema occur in older people, clients with Pi Z develop emphysema between ages thirty and forty-five, especially when they smoke.

Age and Sex. Spirometric tests have shown that lung function decreases with age after early adulthood. How much of this decrease can be attributed to aging, as opposed to environmental and other factors, is questionable (27). Chronic bronchitis and emphysema primarily occur in older adults.

Generally more men than women have COPD, the exception being asthma, which is more prevalent in females. This may be related to the higher incidence of smoking among men.

Race and Socioeconomic Status. The incidence of COPD is almost five times greater in Caucasians than it is in blacks. The incidence is also higher in people living in poor socioeconomic conditions. Increased rates of respiratory infections, poor nutrition, inadequate medical care, and exposure to air pollution among poor people probably contribute to the increased incidence.

Prevention and Screening for Early Intervention

Smoking is considered the single most important factor that contributes to the onset and progression of chronic bronchitis and emphysema, as well as other important health problems. In recent years campaigns to educate the public about the hazards of smoking and to prohibit smoking in designated public places have made an impact on Americans.

In adults there has been a steady decline in smoking, and in 1983 the annual per capita consumption of cigarettes reached the lowest point in thirty-five years (11). Fewer teenagers than adults smoke, yet it is still a problem for them (29).

Other measures directed toward the reduction of COPD include air pollution control, particularly in industries where workers are exposed to high concentrations of noxious gases and organic and inorganic dusts. Miners, mill workers, grain handlers, and workers in plastics are only some of the workers who are exposed to high concentrations of air pollutants.

The role of the primary nurse in helping to improve the quality of air in industry includes identifying sources of air pollution and their actual and potential effects on clients, and recommending corrective action.

Most screening programs today combine a brief questionnaire with measures of forced expiratory flow rates and lung volumes to detect people with COPD. One limitation of these screening programs is that they are not sensitive enough to detect early airway obstruction in asymptomatic clients (9).

Overview of Management

Management of the client with COPD is a joint effort in which members of the health care team contribute according to their expertise to resolve acute and chronic problems. Areas in which the client usually will require assistance are nutrition, exercise, treatment of hypoventilation with such measures as bronchodilators and oxygen, treatment of respiratory tract infections, prevention and management of complications, and dealing with the impact of chronic illness.

The primary nurse's role as a member of the health team will encompass coordination of the therapeutic program, teaching, counseling, referral to appropriate health care resources, and implementing and evaluating a plan of comprehensive nursing care based on assessed client needs and problems.

Nursing Care

Assessment

Assessment of the person with COPD includes a nursing history, physical examination, and findings of laboratory tests to determine pulmonary function, blood gas levels, and acid–base balance. The latter two tests may be reserved for clients with advanced COPD in whom marked hypoventilation exists.

Information specific to COPD that is elicited during the nursing history includes the following:

- Onset, duration, and precipitating factors of such symptoms as shortness of breath, dyspnea, cough, sputum, wheezing, cyanosis, edema, decreased exercise tolerance, and fatigue
- History of smoking (how long, how much)
- Past history of respiratory tract infections and allergies
- Family history of COPD and allergies
- Occupation
- Home environment
- Activity–rest patterns
- Sleep patterns
- Nutrition
- Changes in body weight
- Client's knowledge of COPD and its management
- Impact of COPD on the client and family, emotionally, socially, and economically

- Client and family coping patterns
- Access to and use of health care resources

Information specific to COPD that is assessed during the physical examination is found in Table 36.1. In addition to the assessments listed, the nurse will also want to assess cardiovascular status in clients suspected of having cardiovascular complications of COPD.

Findings from tests of pulmonary function, blood gas levels, and acid–base balance complete the assessment. Those tests commonly done in COPD, together with the findings are found in Table 36.2.

Nursing Diagnoses

When caring for clients with COPD, the goal of nursing care is to help them become as self-sufficient as possible in managing their own health so that they can lead a satisfying, productive life. This goal is accomplished through teaching, counseling, caring, and supporting these clients, recognizing that their ability to care for themselves varies between individuals and within individuals at different points in time.

The following nursing diagnoses are common to clients with COPD and are discussed in detail in succeeding paragraphs:

- Potential noncompliance with no-smoking requirement related to such factors as insufficient knowledge of the detrimental effects of smoking and insufficient motivation
- Hypoventilation related to pathological changes within the lungs
- Activity intolerance related to fatigue
- Disturbance in sleep pattern related to such factors as transient nocturnal hypoxemia and coughing
- Nutritional deficits related to such factors as loss of appetite, fatigue, and general malaise
- Fear and anxiety related to the impact of COPD on the client and family
- Depression related to such factors as change in health status, the realities of chronic disease, and loss of self-esteem
- Social isolation related to such factors as loss of physical strength, impaired communication, and tension associated with chronic illness
- Impaired interpersonal relationships related to such factors as impaired communication and failure of others to appreciate the impact of COPD on the client

Planning and Implementation

Planning for nursing care is a mutual effort between the client, the client's family or care partner, and the primary nurse. Every effort should be made to help the client retain autonomy while recognizing the benefits of appropriate assistance from others. Planning begins at the point where the client is currently—physically, emo-

Table 36.1
Chest and Lungs Assessment in COPD

Assessment	Normal Finding	Finding in COPD
Thoracic configuration	Elliptical; ratio of anteroposterior diameter to transverse diameter 1:2	Barrel-shaped chest; increased anteroposterior diameter
Respiratory movements	Symmetrical expansion and contraction; no use of accessory muscle; no retraction	Retraction of supraclavicular fossa on inspiration. Expansion, especially of lower rib cage, may be decreased; use of accessory muscles as condition deteriorates.
Diaphragmatic excursion and level	Diaphragm located at level of T10; excursion 3–5 cm	Diaphragm depressed toward abdomen and relatively immobile as condition deteriorates.
Rate	16–20 breaths per minute	Increased
Percussion sounds	Resonant	Hyperresonant
Breath sounds	Peripheral lung—vesicular; apex—bronchovesicular; no adventitious sounds; inspiratory time > expiratory time over peripheral lung	Uneven sounds diminished at lung bases; scattered rales; rhonchi especially during expiration and clearing with cough; prolonged expiratory time

Table 36.2
Pulmonary Function, Blood Gas, and Acid–Base Tests in COPD

Test	Definition	Findings
Vital capacity	Maximum amount of air that can be exhaled after minimum inspiration	Normal or decreased
Forced vital capacity	Maximum amount of air that can be forcibly exhaled after maximum inspiration	Decreased
Residual volume	Volume of air remaining in the lungs after maximum expiration	Increased
Total lung capacity	Volume of air in fully expanded lungs	Normal or increased
Forced expiratory volume	Volume of air exhaled in a specified period of time—1 second in this instance—while exhaling forcibly	Decreased
Ratio of residual volume to total lung capacity		Markedly increased
Ratio of forced expiratory volume in 1 second to forced vital capacity		Decreased
Maximum midexpiratory flow rate	The maximum flow rate of expired air measured between 25% and 75% of the vital capacity maneuver	Decreased
Arterial O_2 Tension (P_aO_2)	Partial pressure of oxygen	Decreased
Arterial CO_2 Tension (P_aCO_2)	Partial pressure of carbon dioxide	Increased
Arterial pH	Measure of hydrogen ion concentration	Decreased
Serum bicarbonate	Measure of bicarbonate ion concentration	Increased with renal compensation for respiratory acidosis

tionally, and socially—and is directed toward building on the client's strengths as all work together toward nursing goals.

□ *Potential Noncompliance with No-Smoking Requirement.* All clients with COPD should be encouraged to stop smoking. Some of the positive effects observed in clients who stop smoking are diminished cough, fewer respiratory tract infections, improved timed forced expiratory volume, improved respiratory flow rates, and decreased mortality (20). Cessation of smoking can help to allay the progression of COPD.

Stopping smoking is a difficult task that requires a high degree of internal motivation, accompanied by external support and positive reinforcement. Advertising, peer pressure, self-image as a smoker, and being in the presence of smokers are only some of the factors that help to sustain the smoking habit. Strategies for breaking the smoking habit help the client to develop and sustain the motivation to stop smoking.

For some clients the fear of progressive illness, dis-

ability, and death is sufficient to cause them to stop smoking. This is particularly true when the client has known someone who died of COPD. Some clients, however, seem determined to follow a self-destructive course and are candidates for psychiatric help to understand and deal with their self-destructive behaviors.

Education about the hazards of smoking has contributed to the decline of cigarette smoking in the United States. Some of the most visible campaigns to decrease smoking have been waged by the federal government, through requirements for labeling cigarette packages and advertisements to alert the public about the hazards of smoking, the American Lung Association, the American Heart Association, and the American Cancer Society. Smoking has been banned in designated public places. Yet many people continue to smoke despite the knowledge of the hazards.

Other methods that have had limited success include using nonsmokers as role models (e.g., teachers, nurses, and other health care providers) for teenagers and adults, hypnosis, and increasing the taxes on tobacco.

For some clients the most effective way to stop smoking is to join a self-help group such as SmokEnders. Based on the principle of support by people who know firsthand what it is like to break the smoking habit, these self-help groups provide external support and motivation while the client develops his or her own internal motivation. If more than one person in the client's family smokes, stopping smoking should become a family project, with all members joining a self-help group.

□ *Hypoventilation.* Hypoventilation involves two separate problems: carbon dioxide retention and insufficient oxygen intake, leading to hypoxemia. In the client with COPD these problems are due to bronchoconstriction, mucus plugs in distal airways, trapping of air in the alveoli, and ventilation–perfusion imbalance. Nursing measures that aim to relieve hypoventilation are directed toward all of these causes.

The degree of hypoventilation that exists is determined by blood gas and acid–base values. Normal blood gas and acid–base values for arterial blood are found in Table 36.3. The client with COPD is frequently in respiratory acidosis, which means that the arterial pH is less than normal, and if the kidneys have compensated for this lowering of pH by retaining bicarbonate, the bicarbonate level will be increased. Oxygen levels are usually decreased and carbon dioxide levels are elevated. When hypoventilation is a chronic problem and the body has sufficient time to compensate, the client may tolerate a PaO_2 in the range of 35 to 40 mm Hg and a $PaCO_2$ of 80 mm Hg (8). The goal of nursing intervention, therefore, is not necessarily to return blood gas levels to normal, but to return them to a level at which the client can function without too much difficulty.

As soon as the diagnosis of COPD is established, the client is taught to breathe so that the best ventilation with the least effort is achieved. This can be accomplished by diaphragmatic breathing. The client assumes a comfortable position. For the client in acute distress the sitting position with forward leaning is best. The client is then instructed to relax the body, especially the muscles of the chest, shoulders, and arms, and to breathe deeply and slowly through the nose, imagining the air flowing deep into the lungs toward the center of the body. If done properly, the lower portion of the chest and the abdomen will expand. The client can feel this expansion with his or her hands. Then with the lips pursed and while using the abdominal muscles to help with exhalation, the client is instructed to breathe out slowly through the mouth. This exercise is repeated as often as necessary until it becomes habitual.

Chest percussion is an effective means of loosening mucus from the bronchial passageways so that it can be expelled. The client's family can be taught to do this, as well as to auscultate the client's lungs before percussing, to locate mucus, and afterward, to determine the effectiveness of the treatment.

Postural drainage aims to help relieve mucus drainage through the force of gravity. Chest percussion, deep breathing, administration of bronchodilators, and inhalation of moisture often precede postural drainage to increase mucus flow. Again, the client's family is taught to auscultate the client's chest, locate mucus, and then select a position that will promote drainage from the appropriate lung segments.

The best times for doing postural drainage are one hour before meals, late afternoon, and before retiring at night. The number of times it is done each day varies with the client's individual needs. It takes approximately thirty minutes to complete postural drainage, including time spent administering bronchodilators and other pretreatment measures and draining all lung segments. Because postural drainage is not effective for all clients, they are taught to evaluate its effects on themselves. If little mucus is expelled and there is little improvement in breathing and the client experiences excessive fatigue, the procedure is ineffective and should be discontinued.

There are two major groups of bronchial dilators used in the treatment of COPD. As shown in Table 36.4, one group consists of the methylxanthines, theophylline and its derivatives. These drugs produce bronchodilation by preventing the breakdown of cyclic AMP (adenosine monophosphate). In order to achieve best results, the client's serum levels are monitored periodically.

The second group of bronchodilators are the adrenergic (sympathomimetic) drugs. These produce bronchodilation by stimulating beta receptors in bronchial smooth muscles.

Table 36.3
Normal Blood Gas and Acid–Base Values
in Arterial Blood

Arterial O_2 Saturation (SaO_2)	93%–98%
Arterial O_2 Tension (PaO_2)	80–104 mm Hg
Arterial CO_2 Tension ($PaCO_2$)	36–42 mm Hg
pH	7.35–7.45
Bicarbonate	22–26 mEq/L

Table 36.4
Bronchodilator Drugs Used in COPD Treatment

Drug Type	Adverse Effects and Nursing Implications
Methylxanthine drugs Produce bronchodilation by inhibiting metabolism of cyclic AMP Examples: Theophylline (Bronkodyl, Elixophyllin, Slo-Phyllin, Theo-Bid, Theo-Dur), aminophylline (Aminodur, Amesec), oxtriphylline (Choledyl), dyphylline (Dilor)	Nervousness, insomnia, headache, dizziness, anxiety, confusion, tachycardia, rash, nausea, vomiting, and diarrhea Use cautiously in clients with history of cardiovascular disease, renal disease, gastritis, and peptic ulcer. Exert caution when using concurrently with other bronchodilators. Serum level of theophylline (includes all of the other theophylline derivatives listed under methylxanthine drugs) checked periodically.
Adrenergic drugs Produce bronchial smooth-muscle relaxation by activating $beta_2$-receptors and increasing cyclic AMP; may also activate $beta_1$-receptors, producing tachycardia, and $alpha_1$-receptors, producing vasoconstriction and increased blood pressure. Examples: Epinephrine, isoproterenol (Isuprel), metaproterenol (Allupent), terbutaline (Brethine, Bricanyl), isoetharine (Bronkosol, Bronchometer, Dilabron), albuterol (Proventil, Ventolin)	Restlessness, headache, palpitations, anxiety, tremors, weakness, pallor, elevated blood pressure, elevated serum glucose, increased angina, dizziness, nausea, and vomiting Use cautiously in clients with history of cardiovascular disease (including stroke), diabetes, and hyperthyroidism. Epinephrine is contraindicated in narrow-angle glaucoma. When more than one adrenergic drug is used concurrently, the effect is potentiated. Metaproterenol and isoetharine can produce paradoxical bronchial spasm. Frequent, repeated use of epinephrine can produce unresponsiveness to drug.

Both the methylxanthines and the adrenergic bronchodilators come in oral, parenteral, and aerosol preparations. Aerosol preparations are commonly used by the client to relieve acute distress. It is important to use the correct technique for administering aerosols. Either a hand nebulizer or a pressurized cartridge may be used to deliver the medication. The latter is preferred for weak clients who have difficulty squeezing a hand nebulizer. If a concentrated medication is to be used in a hand nebulizer, it is diluted with either sterile water or normal saline solution before administration. While holding the nebulizer between the lips, the client exhales as completely as possible. The client then inhales deeply, pressing either the pressurized cartridge or the hand nebulizer while doing so. The client holds his or her breath for about ten seconds to allow the medication to disperse throughout the lungs, and then exhales. The usual dose is one or two inhalations, but the client may repeat the medication until relief is obtained or tachycardia and shakiness occur (18, 28).

Corticosteroids may be used to relieve bronchospasm in asthmatics. Prednisone is usually given when other measures have proved ineffective.

Unless contraindicated (e.g., in clients with renal and cardiac problems causing fluid retention) clients with COPD are encouraged to drink at least one and one-half quarts of fluid daily. Room humidifiers may also be used, particularly during cold weather when the humidity is low. Both of these measures promote removal of mucus from the lungs. In asthmatic subjects the best response to humidified air comes when the air is breathed at room temperature. In one study investigators found that both heating and cooling the air before asthmatic subjects breathed it produced bronchospasm that lasted for up to ten minutes (the maximum time measured in the study) (1).

Low-flow oxygen therapy is usually indicated for clients with persistent resting hypoxemia (PaO_2 55 mm Hg), those suffering from significant sleep hypoxemia (25), those suffering from marked exertional hypoxemia, and those with cor pulmonale and pulmonary hypertension.

In some cases oxygen is administered intermittently during periods when clients are most susceptible to hypoxemia (e.g., during exercise and sleep). Research has shown, however, that continuous oxygen therapy is a better choice. In one study of 203 clients with hypoxemia owing to COPD who were followed for at least twelve months, those receiving continuous oxygen therapy had a significantly lower mortality rate than did those receiving intermittent oxygen for twelve hours daily, extending over the hours of sleep (8).

Either nasal prongs or Venturi masks that deliver a specified concentration of oxygen, regardless of flow rate, are most commonly used for clients with COPD. One advantage of nasal prongs is the client's ability to talk and eat while receiving oxygen. At a flow rate of 1 to 3 liters per minute, nasal prongs and Venturi masks deliver sufficient oxygen to relieve hypoxemia without depressing the client's respirations. In clients with severe COPD high concentrations of oxygen can depress the respiratory center, abolish the respiratory drive, and precipitate respiratory failure. Oxygen should be humidified to prevent drying of the respiratory tract and mucus plugging.

All clients who receive oxygen therapy are taught how to administer oxygen properly. Basic instruction includes when to use it, the proper flow rate, how to operate the equipment, safe use, storage and maintenance of equipment, and how to secure refills and help with equipment problems beyond their ability to handle. Because oxygen relieves acute distress, clients may be tempted to use it at a greater flow rate and more often than necessary. Such use is discouraged.

Two areas of concern related to oxygen therapy may necessitate client counseling. Some clients associate the use of oxygen with deterioration of their condition and death. They also may fear oxygen dependency. Such clients are encouraged to explore their fears and feelings and understand that oxygen therapy is not necessarily associated with deterioration, death, and dependency.

Other clients are so anxious when they have difficulty breathing that they automatically turn to oxygen if it is available before trying other measures to improve ventilation. Such clients may become dependent on oxygen. They are also encouraged to explore their feelings and try alternatives to oxygen therapy. Usually such clients require the supportive presence of a health care professional while they try alternative measures before they are willing to use them independently and alone. In the past, intermittent positive-pressure breathing therapy (IPPB) was used to improve ventilation and deliver aerosol medications to clients with COPD. The current view of IPPB is that other measures that are less expensive (e.g., hand nebulizers and bronchial hygiene) are as effective and do not have the hazards of IPPB. Therefore,

IPPB is used less frequently than in the past and only for selected clients who will benefit from it.

□ *Activity Intolerance.* Activity intolerance related to fatigue is a problem for many clients with COPD, appearing as an early symptom and increasing as the disease progresses. A number of factors may contribute to the fatigue, for example, hypoxemia, lack of sleep, poor nutrition, loss of muscle strength, and depression. As the aforementioned factors are discussed in other sections of this chapter, only nursing measures designed to help build muscle strength and cardiovascular fitness and to relax are discussed here.

Before instituting any program to build muscle strength and cardiovascular fitness in the client with COPD, the client's physical status must be assessed and exercise tolerance determined. This is ideally done by the client's physician in consultation with a physician whose expertise is in physical medicine and rehabilitation. Exercise programs should begin slowly and build gradually as the client's tolerance increases. The most successful programs in terms of long-term adherence to the program are those that are interesting, that are not beyond the client's physical abilities, and that do not require special equipment or places. Clients accept exercise programs better if the programs can be easily assimilated into their daily routines and life-styles.

Walking is an excellent means of improving cardiovascular/respiratory fitness and overcoming fatigue. It can be done almost any time and at any place and requires no special equipment except a good pair of shoes. Clients are taught to begin walking short distances on relatively flat terrain. As their strength improves, they may increase the distance and pace and go up grades. During inclement weather clients can continue their walking regimen in such places as enclosed shopping malls.

Becoming short of breath during exercise is not necessarily harmful for the client with COPD. Sustained moderate breathlessness resulting from exercise improves respiratory muscles and increases exercise capacity (10). Resting for a few minutes should relieve the shortness of breath. If it does not, the client is probably exercising too much and should proceed more slowly.

Another guide to determining whether or not the client is overexercising is the pulse rate. Clients can be taught to check their pulse rates before and after exercising. Generally the pulse rate should increase about twenty beats per minute more than the resting rate (15). Caution is necessary for clients with cardiac involvement.

The American Lung Association has developed an exercise program that aims to build muscle strength and increase joint flexibility in clients with COPD. (These exercises are contained in the booklet designed for client teaching entitled *Help Yourself to Better Breathing*. The booklet can be obtained from the American Lung Association.)

One of the most effective ways to relieve fatigue is to learn to relax. Clients with COPD have continuous stress, both emotionally and physically. As a result they are often tense, irritable, and tired. Numerous relaxation techniques are in vogue, many of them with audiotapes to help the client. Relaxation exercises should be done daily or more often, especially when the client feels tense.

The nurse can help clients prevent fatigue by assisting them to plan daily activities in a way that decreases energy expenditure while still doing those things that are important. Planning may include rearrangement of living and work space, clustering activities in one geographical area before moving to the next, and selecting activities that do not involve large energy expenditure. In Table 36.5 activities are categorized and listed by their approximate energy requirement.

□ *Disturbance in Sleep Pattern.* Research has shown that clients with COPD tend to sleep poorly. They have less rapid-eye-movement (REM) sleep, more changes in the stages of sleep, and less total sleep time than do normal subjects (12). These features are thought to be related to transient nocturnal hypoxemia, a phenomenon seen even in healthy adults and exaggerated in those with airway obstruction. As a result, clients with COPD are tired, irritable, and often have difficulty concentrating. They have the manifestations of sleep deprivation.

Measures that may facilitate sleep include having a quiet, well-ventilated, well-humidified dark room with a comfortable temperature. Postural drainage may be done at least one hour before retiring to assist ventilation. Immediately before or on retiring the client may do a relaxation exercise. Clients are encouraged to eat a smaller dinner at an earlier hour so that their stomachs are empty when they retire. Going to bed with a full stomach, particularly if the foods are heavy, places added stress on the cardiovascular and respiratory systems.

For some clients nocturnal oxygen therapy may be used. In one study it was shown that breathing oxygen while asleep reduced the number of hypoxemic episodes per night, increased the total sleep time, and increased

the amount of REM sleep, particularly in clients with elevated $PaCO_2$ and low PaO_2 (6).

Clients frequently remark that they are awakened at night by coughing and that this interferes with their sleep. In one study of nocturnal cough in patients with chronic bronchitis and emphysema, researchers confirmed that the vast majority of the patients coughed at night, but 85 percent of these coughing spells occurred while the clients were awake. Coughing during sleep was uncommon. Coughing spells were brief, lasting for less than four seconds (22).

□ *Nutritional Deficits.* If a client with COPD is overweight, it is important to lose weight to within the recommended levels for height and sex in order to reduce the workload on the heart and lungs. For many clients with COPD, however, the problem is not too much, but too little weight. Because of loss of appetite, fatigue, and not feeling well, they do not eat enough of the right foods to maintain an optimum nutritional status. At the same time they may be using excessive calories to supply the energy needed to breathe. In one study of clients with COPD, investigators found that the number of kilocalories consumed during a meal was less as the person's subjective experience of dyspnea increased (26). Both the overweight client and the underweight client require nutritional teaching and counseling.

□ *Fear and Anxiety.* Clients with COPD universally experience some degree of fear and anxiety during the course of illness. It may range from the mild anxiety associated with having to learn a new treatment procedure, to overwhelming panic experienced when the client is unable to breathe without struggle. Regardless of the degree of fear and anxiety, the client is uncomfortable and wants relief. If the anxiety is mild, such as that associated with learning a new procedure, the client may be motivated to learn, and thus achieve relief. But if the anxiety is severe, all of the client's efforts are directed toward obtaining immediate relief, either alone or with the aid of others, the latter being commonly demanded.

During anxiety the client is unable to identify what is causing the discomfort. There is an awareness that something is wrong and affecting him or her. But what this is, is unknown. With fear, the client is able to put a label on the problem and tell others why he or she feels uneasy. Some of the causes of fear and anxiety in the client with COPD are physical illness, mounting medical costs, inadequate income, loss of prestige and status, loss of position in the community, and hospital-

Table 36.5
Approximate Energy Expenditure in METs (Activities of 70-kg Person)

	Light (1–3 METs)		Moderate (3.5–6 METs)		Heavy (7+ METs)	
Personal care activities	Rest	1	Showering	3.5	Ambulation with braces or	
	Sitting	1	Using bedpan	4.0	crutches	6.5
	Standing (relaxed)	1	Walking downstairs	4.5	Walking upstairs	
	Eating	1	Conditioning exercises	4.5	with 17-lb load	7.5
	Conversation	1	Walking 3.5 mph	5.5		
	Dressing–undressing	2				
	Wash hands, face; shaving	2				
	Propelling wheelchair	2				
	Shaving	2.8				
	Bedside commode	3				
	Walking 2.5 mph	3				
Recreational activities	Walking level, slowly 1 mph	1.2	Walking level 3 mph	3.5	Tennis	6.0
	Painting, sitting	1.5	Bowling	3.5	Trotting horse	6.5
	Playing piano	2.0	Cycling 5.5 mph	3.5	Spading	7.0
	Driving	2.0	Badminton	3.5	Jogging level 5 mph	7.5
	Canoeing 2.5 mph	2.5	Canoeing, sailing	3.5	Skiing	8.0
	Horseback riding slowly	2.5	Golfing	4.0	Squash	8.5
	Volleyball	2.5	Swimming	4.0	Basketball	8.5
			Dancing	4.5	Tennis	8.5
			Gardening	4.5	Cycling 13 mph	9.0
					Gymnastics	10.0
					Football competition	10.0
Housework activities	Hand sewing	1.0	Ironing, standing	3.5	Mowing lawn by hand	6.5
	Sweeping floor	1.5	Scrubbing floors	3.5	Shoveling	7.0
	Machine sewing	1.5	Hanging wash	3.5	Ascending stairs	
	Polishing furniture	2.0	Cleaning windows	3.5	with 17-lb load	7.5
	Peeling potatoes	2.5	Beating carpets	4.0	Planting	7.5
	Washing small clothes	2.5	Plowing with tractor	4.5	Construction	
	Kneading dough	2.5	Lifting, carrying 20–44 lb	4.5	physical worker	6.5
	Cleaning windows	3.0	Carpentry	5.5	Pick and shovel work	8.0
	Making beds	3.0	Using pneumatic tools	6.0	Splitting wood by hand	10.0
	Desk work	1.2				
	Typing (electric)	1.2				
	Radio-TV repair	1.2				
	Draftsman	1.8				

Source: J. F. Miller. Coping with Chronic Illness. Philadelphia: F. A. Davis, 1983, 210.

ization. But the most overwhelming fear and anxiety are usually related to the fear of being unable to breathe and dying struggling for air. Regardless of what causes fear and anxiety, the client senses a certain powerlessness in being able to control what is happening to him or her. The health care system may be impinging on personal autonomy. There will be many things related to the illness that the client will not understand. And the client will be dependent, to some degree, on others for personal well-being.

How successfully a client copes with fear and anxiety depends on his or her understanding of what is causing personal discomfort, the adequacy of personal coping skills, and the support that the family gives. The kind of support the client receives from others is determined in part by the amount of anxiety the client generates in others. Anxious people create anxiety in others. It is also influenced by how close the person giving support is to the situation. Family members themselves may be suffering acute fear and anxiety as they watch a loved one suffer, and may be wondering what will become of both the loved one and themselves. When helping the anxious client, the nurse is often treating the family as well.

In order to help the client deal constructively with fear and anxiety, the nurse begins by helping the client to identify his or her perception of the problem and to separate reality from fantasy. The nurse helps the client to focus on and express feelings about what is happening and, when possible, to relate these feelings to everyday events that might have precipitated them. When specific events such as visiting a clinic or doing a procedure are identified as sources of fear and anxiety, the nurse and client can work together to find alternative ways of doing things to reduce the client's discomfort. It is important to encourage the client to weigh alternatives and make a decision so that he or she feels a recovery of control over the situation.

Clients are also encouraged to examine their coping mechanisms, identifying those that are constructive and those that are not. For instance, the client who denies that a problem exists and continues smoking is not coping effectively. But the client who admits a problem, expresses personal feelings, and begins to change his or her life-style is taking a positive approach toward the problem.

Telling a client what he or she can realistically expect, even when it is unpleasant, helps to reduce fear and anxiety. Many clients fear that they will die a terrible death, struggling and fighting for air to the last breath. Clients should be told that many people with COPD do not die of it. They may live many years and die of something else. But if they do die of COPD, most lapse into a coma near the end. Letting the client know that he or she may not be conscious and suffering to the end can be relieving (5).

Throughout the illness one of the most important things a nurse can do to relieve fear and anxiety is to be a caring presence for the client and family. Simply sitting beside the client while he or she talks or cries and holding the client's hand while giving oxygen to assist breathing can make the positive difference in how the client experiences the situation. For a more detailed discussion of caring, the reader is referred to chapter 2.

□ *Depression.*   All clients with COPD experience some degree of depression during the course of their illness. It may range from mild depression, in which the client experiences temporary feelings of sadness and discouragement, to more severe depression, in which the client begins to withdraw, feeling overwhelmed by life and unable to cope with problems.

A number of factors may contribute to depression, but for the client with COPD they usually stem from the change in health status and the reality of a chronic disease for which there is no cure, only palliative care. There may be loss of self-esteem associated with body changes, job changes, and inability to fulfill important role expectations. In one study of the effect of chronic pulmonary disease on the lives of women, the investigators concluded that women with COPD have a higher level of subjective stress and lower life satisfaction than do women who do not have COPD (26).

Often feeling helpless and ineffective in dealing with problems, the client turns increasingly inward and loses interest in other people and the environment. Feelings of tiredness, emptiness, and a lack of energy frequently ensue. Other people may view the client as antisocial and hostile. Family members may find it difficult to cope with the depressed client, especially when the client begins to act out depression through anger, dependency, and demanding behavior.

The nurse can help the client and family to cope with depression by helping them to recognize, first, that the client is depressed. It is easy to misinterpret behaviors that are associated with depression. Once the client and family gain insight into what is happening, more effective ways of handling feelings can be identified. For instance, if the client has a persistent pattern of acting out feelings of anger by blowing off steam at the nearest person, this behavior can be called to the client's attention and an alternative behavior discussed and tried. Instead of blowing off steam, the client can be helped to recognize anger and its cause and then talk out this anger with appropriate others.

Helping the client to develop a constructive philosophy of chronic illness can also be an antidote to depression. Two important aspects of such a philosophy are considered here.

When confronted with the diagnosis of chronic illness, some clients are almost overwhelmed by their perception of what lies ahead. They see problems stretching endlessly before them and getting worse. They see their life-styles changing in ways they do not want. They may even feel that their problems are taking charge of them instead of them being in charge of their problems. One strategy that I have used successfully with depressed persons to help them cope effectively with this situation is to help them live one day at a time. Briefly the strategy is as follows: Today is the only time I have to work with. Yesterday is past. I cannot retrieve it. Tomorrow has not come. What I do with today is up to me. I can make it a good day or a bad one. The choice is mine. There will be problems, but no one or no thing can make me have a bad day. Only I can decide how I will respond to what happens to me. Only I can determine what kind of day I will have. The quality of life I have depends on what I do with each day as it comes (4). Using this strategy consistently can help clients change their thought patterns and expectations and, consequently, what they experience.

The second aspect of philosophy to be considered is helping clients and their families to see chronic illness such as COPD as an opportunity for personal growth. Some clients seem to be overwhelmed by their problems and unable to move beyond them, but others, when threatened about the uncertainty of the future, are able to mobilize themselves toward positive change. Illness for them is a time when they can pause and reflect on their lives, searching for the meaning and direction for themselves. They examine what is important to them and begin to reorder their priorities so that they devote more of their time and energy to things most important to them. They recognize that illness poses limitations, but they view alternatives as opportunities. These clients grow because of their illness and often achieve a depth and richness they possibly might never have achieved if they did not have the problems of illness. For them the human experience is refined by facing and overcoming problems.

□ *Social Isolation and Impaired Interpersonal Relationships.* Two problems that tend to increase as the client's condition deteriorates are social isolation and difficulty maintaining harmonious interpersonal relationships. The client with COPD is often perceived as an irritable, demanding, self-centered, difficult person. In the hospital this may be the person the staff wants to avoid when possible because of the person's tendency to persistently demand something at the wrong time.

Many factors contribute to the client's behavior that causes others to label him or her as difficult. Loss of physical strength, difficulty communicating because of shortness of breath, chronic sleep deprivation, the tension of chronic problems that may be temporarily relieved but do not go away, loss of self-esteem, fear, anxiety, depression, and the narrowing of personal focus that occurs when a person's most basic need—the need for oxygen—is threatened are some of those factors.

The client with COPD can be challenging for those who are close to him or her and for health care providers.

In some hospitals clients with COPD are placed on nursing units where they are assigned to a primary nurse who has been prepared to deal with their problems and provide the care they need. But in other instances this arrangement is not possible, and tension arises as a staff that does not always understand clients with COPD attempts to cope with their demands. In these situations, having staff conferences in which staff members examine not only the client's behaviors that are causing problems, but also their own behaviors and how they impact on the client can be invaluable. Staff members are also encouraged to explore the human experience of chronic illness, what it does to a person, and how it affects behavior. If a psychiatric nurse consultant is available, he or she can be an excellent resource in helping the staff to understand the situation and identify alternative ways of coping.

Families of clients with COPD can also benefit from counseling. Although the primary nurse who is most familiar with the family can often provide this service, sometimes it may be best to have a psychiatric nurse consultant do it. In addition to exploring those same topics cited in the previous paragraph, the family is helped to examine feelings of guilt that often arise when they are overtaxed or do not think that they have given as much as they should to the client. Both family members and clients are encouraged to engage in activities outside the home. For family members it is particularly important to have some time each day to be alone and relax. At least once each week they should have an afternoon or evening out in which they can do something interesting and fun. Family members should never underestimate the value of time to themselves for strengthening their ability to cope with chronic illness.

Clients with COPD may consider moving to a warmer, drier climate. Generally this does not alter the progress of their condition unless they are allergic to environmental substances such as pollens. Clients should be encouraged to carefully weigh anticipated health benefits against the loss of friends and other social support systems. If the client considers moving to a mountainous area, the problems associated with low atmospheric oxygen found in high altitudes should be discussed. In one study it was found that emphysema deaths at altitudes over 7,000 feet occurred at a younger age, after a shorter duration of illness, and more commonly from cor pulmonale than at altitudes under 4,000 feet. Although the reasons for the increased mortality are not known, the investigators in the study suggested that it could stem from increased pulmonary hypertension owing to the hypoxia of lung disease, compounded by the hypoxia of high altitude (21).

Evaluation

Evaluation of nursing care is based on how well each of the client problems represented by nursing diagnoses were resolved. The following client behaviors and characteristics are representative of some that may be used to evaluate the nursing diagnoses included in this chapter.

Potential Noncompliance with No-Smoking Requirement. The client will engage in a program that supports smoking cessation and will stop smoking. The client will verbalize commitment to permanent abstinence from tobacco products. There should be some immediate evidence of efforts to stop smoking, although for some clients resolution of this problem may take months, during which there is gradual reduction of the number of cigarettes smoked per day.

Hypoventilation. The client's PaO_2 and $PaCO_2$ will remain within acceptable limits. The client will demonstrate competence in performing measures designed to aid ventilation (e.g., coughing and deep breathing). Although the client may give an acceptable return demonstration of measures, observing the client at home over a period of time better indicates continuing competence, which is important in managing chronic illness.

Disturbance in Sleep Pattern. The client will give evidence of using measures designed to promote sleep (e.g., relaxation exercises and environmental control). The client will sleep an optimum number of hours each night, based on sleeping patterns before the onset of the problem. Some improvement in sleep may be evident as early as one to two weeks after initiating nursing care.

Nutritional Deficits. The client and family will demonstrate knowledge of optimum nutrition and measures to improve food intake. The client's weight will move toward the optimum level for age, body build, and sex at a rate of approximately 1 pound per week.

Fear and Anxiety. The client will verbalize his or her perception of problems that can be associated with fear and anxiety, and feelings related to these problems. The client and family will identify coping mechanisms and recognize the effectiveness or ineffectiveness of these mechanisms. The client and family will begin to use more effective coping mechanisms. The client will have fewer manifestations of fear and anxiety (e.g., poor concentration, and reticence to engage in activities). Insight into more pressing problems may be manifest during the first few nursing contacts, but deeper problems often require months (sometimes years) of exploration before there is understanding.

Depression. The client will recognize depression and begin to use coping mechanisms to deal with it. The client will exhibit fewer manifestations of depression (e.g., withdrawal, feeling overwhelmed and unable to cope with life). Weeks to months may be required before significant change is evident.

Social Isolation. The client will exhibit less tendency toward social isolation by engaging in meaningful activities with others. The client will set appropriate priorities for expenditure of time and effort to promote socialization. Some evidence of the alleviation of this problem may be evident within a few weeks after initiating nursing care.

Impaired Interpersonal Relationships. The client and people with whom he or she relates will verbalize feelings of satisfaction with their relationships.

Ethical Issues

Two ethical principles often come into conflict when caring for the client with COPD. These are autonomy and a form of positive beneficence known as paternalism. Autonomy is defined as "a form of personal liberty of action where the individual determines his or her own course of action in accordance with a plan chosen by himself" (2). Paternalism, on the other hand, refers to acting as a father figure by making decisions for another person based on what you believe to be the best interests of that person. Health care providers, family, and friends may all act paternalistically, especially when they believe that the client has chosen the wrong course of action. The following illustrates the point.

A man has just been diagnosed as having emphysema. He has a history of smoking two packs of cigarettes per day for many years. As part of the initial plan of care, the physician advises the client not to smoke, and the primary nurse teaches him about the hazards of smoking and is quite direct in instructing him to stop smoking. When the man returns for a follow-up visit, the nurse learns that he is still smoking as much as always. The nurse becomes quite irritated with his seemingly irrational behavior and revises the plan for teaching self-care to include more graphic descriptions of what smoking does to the emphysematous person. But as the nurse is teaching, the client remarks that he is not sure he can give up smoking. After all, he has smoked most of his life. He is sure the nurse is right about what will happen to him, but to him, smoking is important. The nurse listens, thinking all the while how much more competent the nurse is to decide what is good for the client in this instance. After all, the nurse knows more about emphysema than this client does.

At this point the principles of autonomy and paternalism are in direct conflict. To a degree, both parties are right. The client does have the right to make a decision about smoking, and the nurse is right in wanting to help him and prevent him from doing further harm to himself. But the nurse is also committed to the concept of self-care, which solidly rests on the principle of autonomy.

The question is, what is best for the client? Is his right to exercise his freedom of choice and action more important than the nurse's desire to have him follow a course of action that, according to reliable professional literature, has proved most beneficial for a person with his diagnosis? How can they resolve the ethical conflict without sacrificing the client's right to autonomy and the nurse's moral commitment as a member of a helping profession to do what is best for the client? The issue of how to resolve conflicts between autonomy and paternalism is only one of the ethical issues the nurse will face in caring for the client with COPD. Another important issue is the allocation of resources.

Regarding the allocation of resources, such questions as the following are raised: What portion of governmental and private budgets should be allocated to prevention and treatment of chronic illness such as COPD? How should moneys be divided between prevention and treatment? Should the tobacco industry be taxed to pay for the health problems related to smoking? For long-term illnesses that have the potential for consuming all of a family's financial resources, who should pay for the treatment? Is it a responsibility of society, and if so, can society afford it? Although these are difficult questions to answer and relate to policy making, usually at the governmental level, the nurse has a responsibility as a citizen and health care professional to think about them and make his or her sentiments known to the appropriate people.

The ethical issues of caring for the chronically ill person are difficult. There are no easy answers, and there is no guarantee that the decision the nurse makes will be correct. The challenge is to thoroughly consider these issues before they are faced so that when the time arrives to decide, the nurse will be well grounded not only in his or her position, but also in that of the profession and society. For a more in-depth discussion of ethics the reader is referred to chapter 6.

CASE STUDY

Alton Clarke, a sixty-five-year-old self-employed shopkeeper, comes to the physician's office where he has been under continuing care for the past three years because of "increased shortness of breath and coughing with a lot of mucus." Three years ago he was diagnosed as having chronic bronchitis.

When you talk with Mr. Clarke you discover that he has been sleeping poorly for the past week, has not been eating well for the past two weeks, and has been more tired than usual for two weeks. Last week he felt as if he had caught a cold; it has not gone away. He has not taken his temperature, but he has felt warmer than usual. He has not taken any medication for his symptoms.

Physical examination yields the following findings: oral temperature of 99.6° F., respiratory rate 24 per minute, hyperresonant lung sounds with coarse rales and rhonchi in both lungs, and cough productive of thick, light yellow sputum.

While Mr. Clarke is dressing after the examination, you talk with Mrs. Clarke, who tells you that Mr. Clarke has seemed "blue" for the past month and has not gone out in the evening with his friends as he used to do. He has also been most reluctant to stay home from work, despite feeling bad, because their budget has been strained lately and they have no income unless he works. She is worried about her husband and does not know how to help him.

When Mr. Clarke was first diagnosed as having chronic bronchitis, you taught Mrs. Clarke how to percuss his chest to loosen mucus and assist him with postural drainage. Mrs. Clarke tells you she has discouraged him from doing this for the past week because he has felt so tired. She also tells you that Mr. Clarke has been smoking again, having stopped for the past two years.

1. Identify three problems in the situation that require nursing intervention. State them as nursing diagnoses.
2. Using your skills as teacher, counselor, and provider of direct physical care, describe the nursing intervention you could use to resolve the problems identified.
3. State expected outcomes of your nursing intervention.

REFERENCES

1. Aitken, M., and J. Marini. "Effect of Heat Delivery and Extraction on Airway Conductance in Normal and in Asthmatic Subjects." *American Review of Respiratory Disease* 131:357, 1985.

2. Beauchamp, T. L., and J. F. Childress. *Principles of Biomedical Ethics.* New York: Oxford University Press, 1979.

3. Burrows, B. "Quantitative Relationship Between Cigarette Smoking and Ventilatory Impairment." *American Review of Respiratory Disease* 115:195, 1977.

4. Caliandro, A. *You Can Make Your Life Count.* New York: Marble Arch, 1980.

5. Callahan, M. "COPD Makes a Bad First Impression but You'll Find Wonderful People Underneath." *Nursing* 12:72, 1982.

6. Calverly, P., et al. "The Effects of Oxygenation on Sleep Quality in Chronic Obstructive Bronchitis and Emphysema." *American Review of Respiratory Disease* 126:206, 1982.

7. *Chronic Obstructive Pulmonary Disease.* New York: American Lung Association, 1981.

8. "Continuous or Nocturnal Oxygen Therapy in Hypoxemic Chronic Obstructive Lung Disease." *Annals of Internal Medicine* 93:391, 1980.

9. Dopico, G. A., et al. "Epidemiologic Study of Clinical and Physiologic Parameters in Grain Handlers of Northern United States." *American Review of Respiratory Disease* 130:759, 1984.

10. "Exercise and the Breathless Bronchitic." *Lancet* 2:514, 1980.

11. Fielding, J. E. "Smoking: Health Effects and Control." *New England Journal of Medicine* 313:491, 1985.

12. Fleetham, J. A., and M. H. Kryger. "Sleep Disorders in Chronic Airflow Obstruction." *Medical Clinics of North America* 65:549, 1981.

13. Fleury, B., et al. "Work of Breathing in Patients with Chronic Obstructive Pulmonary Disease in Acute Respiratory Failure." *American Review of Respiratory Disease* 131:822, 1985.

14. *Healthy People—The Surgeon General's Report on Health Promotion and Disease Prevention.* Washington, D.C.: U.S. Department of Health, Education and Welfare, Public Health Service, 1979.

15. *Help Yourself to Better Breathing.* New York: American Lung Association, 1983.

16. Hogg, J., et al. Site and Nature of Airway Obstruction in Chronic Obstructive Lung Disease. *New England Journal of Medicine* 278:1355, 1968.

17. Janoff, A., L. Raju, and R. Dearing. "Levels of Elastase Activity in Bronchoalveolar Lavage Fluids of Healthy Smokers and Nonsmokers." *American Review of Respiratory Disease* 127:540, 1983.

18. Lertzman, M., and R. Cherniack. "Rehabilitation of Patients with Chronic Obstructive Pulmonary Disease." *American Review of Respiratory Disease* 114:1145, 1976.

19. *Magnitude of Lung Disease and Secular Trend over Past Decade: Chronic Obstructive Pulmonary Disease and Allied Conditions.* New York: American Lung Association, 1983.

20. Megaro, C. S. "The Natural History of Chronic Bronchitis in Tecumseh, Michigan." *American Review of Respiratory Disease* 127:158, 1983.

21. Moore, L. "Emphysema Mortality Is Increased in Colorado Residents at High Altitude." *American Review of Respiratory Disease* 126:225, 1982.

22. Power, J. T., et al. "Nocturnal Cough in Patients with Chronic Bronchitis and Emphysema." *American Review of Respiratory Disease* 130:999, 1984.

23. Rindfleisch, S., and C. W. Zwillich. "The Interaction Between Dyspnea and Caloric Consumption in C.O.P.D." *American Review of Respiratory Disease* 131:A164, 1985.

24. Robbins, S., M. Angell, and V. Kumar. *Basic Pathology.* 3d ed. Philadelphia: W. B. Saunders, 1981, ch. 13.

25. "Selection Criteria for Long-term Oxygen." *American Review of Respiratory Disease* 127:397, 1983.

26. Sexton, D. L. "The Effect of Chronic Obstructive Pulmonary Disease on the Lives of Women." *American Review of Respiratory Disease* 131:A164, 1985.

27. Task Force on Epidemiology of Respiratory Diseases. *Epidemiology of Respiratory Diseases.* Washington, D.C.: U.S. Department of Health and Human Services, Public Health Service, 1981.

28. "The Proper Use of Aerosol Bronchodilators." *Lancet* 1(8210):23, 1981.

29. U.S. Department of Health, Education and Welfare, *Health in the United States Chartbook.* Washington, D.C.: U.S. Department of Health, Education and Welfare, Public Health Service, 1980.

CHAPTER 37

Older Adults with Cerebral Vascular Disease

JOANNE DAMON

■

OBJECTIVES

After completing this chapter, the reader will be able to:

- Define the term *stroke* in terms of the etiology of each type.
- Describe the incidence of stroke in various populations.
- List the major risk factors in the development of stroke.
- Discuss the goals, objectives, and rationale for nursing intervention in stroke prevention.
- Describe the actions, complications, contraindications, and nursing implications of the most commonly used medications for stroke prevention and treatment.
- List the major nursing diagnoses in the physiological and sensory-perceptual domains.
- Identify the self-care responsibilities of clients, families, and communities in relation to residual neurological deficits and rehabilitation following a stroke.

Caring for the stroke client can be both challenging and rewarding. Few conditions affect as many aspects of clients' and their families' lives as stroke. Care that makes a positive difference requires a nurse who can appreciate both the impact stroke can have on the individual and family and the contribution rehabilitation can make to achieving a satisfactory quality of life. The focus of this chapter is on applying concepts of primary nursing to the care of the stroke client.

Overview

About 500,000 new strokes occur each year in the United States. Although no age-group is completely spared, the incidence of strokes reaches significant proportions only after age fifty-five. Strokes account for 250,000 deaths annually, and stroke is third among all causes of death, behind heart disease and cancer (25). Stroke also ranks high on the list of crippling diseases. Cerebrovascular disease is a major cause of hospitalization, accounting for half the clients hospitalized for neurologic disease. The residual disability after recovery from a stroke is substantial.

Although not as lethal as coronary heart disease, stroke is perhaps the most devastating manifestation of hypertension and atherosclerosis, incapacitating its victims and depriving them of their dignity and independence. Nonetheless, there is evidence that cerebrovascular disease need not accompany old age. All clients with a family history of or risk factors for stroke should see their physicians for an annual checkup in order to monitor a number of modifiable contributing factors that have been identified by prospective epidemiological studies. Such screening makes prevention possible by identifying potential candidates for corrective measures.

Incidence

Incidence rates reported for stroke vary somewhat, depending on the age composition of the sample, whether recurrent strokes are included, and whether the sample is based on the general population of hospitalizations. Incidence of stroke, nonfatal as well as fatal, is difficult to determine accurately. Few defined populations are available in which stroke has been studied over a sufficiently long time to draw conclusions about trends. Analysis of mortality data from several countries, including the United States, almost certainly indicates a decline in stroke mortality (14, 28). Morbidity statistics on the actual incidence of strokes are scarce and suffer from questionable comparability of cases over time (4, 13). However, studies of trends in stroke incidence and mortality in Framingham, Massachusetts, where uniform criteria and case ascertainment have been maintained over three decades, confirm a decline in stroke incidence.

Stroke is part of a larger problem of cardiovascular disease (CVD), and time trends must therefore be examined from the perspective of overall mortality. Age-adjusted CVD mortality rates have declined almost 32 percent over the past thirty years (14). This decrease has accelerated over the past decade. Life expectancy in the United States is now the longest in its history. The decline in CVD mortality has occurred in both sexes, in nonwhites as well as whites, and in all age-groups.

The sizable geographic differences in reported stroke death rates have narrowed, and stroke death rates from all regions have fallen over the past fifteen years (38, 44). The decline has been especially notable among nonwhites and among nonwhite women, who showed a 48.5 percent decrease in stroke mortality from 1960–75. These data represent a dramatic change in the racial patterns of stroke mortality.

It is currently not possible to determine whether the mortality is declining because of a fall in the incidence rate or because better treatment has lowered case fatality rates. It is not even clear if rates are declining for hospitalized or out-of-hospital clients. However, it is likely that the decline is real and that both primary prevention and better medical care have contributed to it.

Pathophysiology

The term cerebrovascular accident (or stroke) is used to label a sudden loss of cerebral function due to an ischemic or hemorrhagic event resulting in local neurologic deficits. Brain tissue that is deprived of an adequate supply of blood and oxygen undergoes ischemic changes that can result in necrosis or infarction. When hemorrhage occurs in the brain, increased intracranial pressure exerted by the extravasated blood can also lead to infarction. Infarction of brain tissue is irreversible (19). These deficits persist for more than twenty-four hours and may be reversible or permanent. The insult may be minimal, in which case the symptoms generally disappear, or it can result in coma and death. It is the nature of the precipitating cause that gives rise to the classification of the type of stroke.

The three most common causes of cerebrovascular accidents are thrombosis, embolism, and hemorrhage. Although cerebrovascular lesions may develop from a variety of underlying conditions, atherosclerosis is the principal condition leading to thrombosis and hemorrhage, whereas cerebral embolism is most commonly secondary to heart disease. In thrombosis, which is responsible for most strokes, a cerebral artery may be occluded or severely constricted by an atherosclerotic plaque or clot on its walls. Ischemia and infarction of brain tissue supplied by the occluded artery may follow, with congestion and edema of neighboring tissues. Hemorrhagic strokes are frequently secondary to rupture of a cerebral vessel whose wall has been weakened by the atherosclerotic process. Prolonged hypertension accelerates atherosclerosis and is a major cause of cerebral hemorrhage. The three main types of cerebrovascular lesions may occur in any of the cerebral arteries, the carotid arterial system, or the basilar-vertebral arterial system.

The specific neurologic abnormalities that follow a stroke depend primarily on the size and site of the vascular lesion. Since thrombosis is responsible for most strokes, and the middle cerebral artery and its branches are more frequently affected than any other cerebral vessel, the following discussion relates primarily to strokes due to thrombosis of the middle cerebral artery. Many of the specific focal signs associated with occlusion of a particular artery are present regardless of which cerebral artery is affected.

Thrombosis of a cerebral artery frequently occurs during sleep or shortly after the person arises in the morning. Often the individual has had some warning symptoms over a period of several days or months prior to the attack but has ignored them. There may be slight difficulty or slurring of speech, or numbness and weakness of the hands or legs, which may have lasted only a few minutes or about an hour. In contrast, the majority of people who develop cerebral hemorrhage are usually active at the time of onset and are indulging in fairly strenuous activities. Warning symptoms do not usually precede cerebral hemorrhage or embolism.

Involvement of the middle cerebral artery typically results in devastating effects—contralateral paralysis, contralateral sensory loss, visual field defect, and, if the lesion is in the dominant hemisphere, perhaps aphasia. The middle cerebral artery is the largest branch of the internal carotid artery, lying deep within the fissure of Sylvius. It branches out and supplies the lateral portions of the cerebral hemispheres. It also branches out to the basal ganglia, the internal capsule, and the thalamus; it is these branches, the lenticular and middle striate arteries, that are frequently affected. Unfortunately, the areas supplied by these branches of the middle cerebral artery are vital to effective functioning. The pyramidal tracts, controlling voluntary movement, originate in the cerebral cortex and pass as a bundle through the internal capsule. The majority of tracts cross in the medulla before arriving at the lower centers, where they initiate voluntary action. Damage to the blood supply of the internal capsule interferes with the passage of these impulses and results in contralateral hemiplegia. The extent and severity of the paralysis depend on the degree to which the cerebral vessels are involved. When impulses from the basal ganglia, which control complex involuntary movement, are unable to pass to the lower centers, rigidity and tremor are present.

If ascending fibers, carrying somesthetic sensations, pain, touch, temperature, and proprioception, are interrupted in the relay to the cortical sensory areas via the thalamus, then contralateral sensory loss results. It is also by way of the thalamus that visual impulses are projected to the visual cortex of the occipital lobe. A typical sign of involvement of the middle cerebral artery is homonymous hemianopsia, a loss in the right or left halves of the visual field in both eyes.

In vascular lesions of the middle cerebral artery, there is often some degree of motor and/or sensory aphasia if the dominant side of the hemisphere is involved. Most of the speech areas that have been identified are in and around areas of the dominant hemisphere supplied by branches of the middle cerebral artery.

The degree of permanence of any of the typical neurological abnormalities described cannot be predicted within the first few days or weeks after their onset. With recovery from the initial shock there is usually some improvement of the focal neurological signs, and they may continue to improve for several months. The healing process after a stroke takes six to twelve weeks. During this time edema around the damaged area may interfere with brain function; therefore, an accurate evaluation of the possible residual functioning of an individual is impossible.

Major Risk Factors

The major risk factors for stroke are those related to the development of atherosclerosis in general. Although hypertension is the most important predisposing factor, other important contributors are heart disease, diabetes, and the use of oral contraceptives. On the other hand, the impacts of some important risk factors of atherosclerotic cardiovascular disease, such as blood lipids, cigarette smoking, and obesity, are surprisingly modest. As the number of predisposing factors increases in a specific client, so, too, does the risk of stroke.

Hypertension. This is the preeminent predisposing factor for stroke. Although the mechanism of action has not yet been clearly identified, it is presumed that hypertension accelerates the development of atherosclerosis. The risk increases as blood pressure increases, and a high systolic pressure has been found to be as significant as a high diastolic pressure (22). While it has been consistently demonstrated that the incidence of stroke among native Americans and Orientals does not differ significantly from that of whites, no such consistent data have emerged regarding the black community. Some epidemiological studies support the belief that the black population has a predisposition to stroke, while other studies negate this finding (50).

Cardiac Impairment. Evidence of cardiac impairment, such as an electrocardiogram (ECG) exhibiting left ventricular hypertrophy (LVH), or even a rapid heart rate, is associated with an increased risk of stroke in general and brain infarctions in particular. Even after adjustment for blood pressure and other associated cardiovascular factors, there is still a significant residual impact of LVH on stroke incidence.

A rapid heart rate is also associated with increased risk, but this is significant only in men. Adjustment for other concomitant risk factors results in a loss of statistical significance, indicating that much of the increased risk is attributable to the higher blood pressures in those with rapid heart rates.

Transient Ischemic Attack (TIA). The contribution of transient ischemic attack or previous stroke to present stroke risk has been clearly demonstrated. Episodes of TIA are widely accepted as the precursor of thrombotic stroke. Clients experiencing TIA have a ten times greater probability of stroke than the non-TIA population of comparable age and gender (50).

Diabetes Mellitus. The relative and attributable risks associated with diabetes mellitus are substantial. Brain infarctions occur at about two and a half times the expected rate in diabetic men and are almost four times more common in diabetic women (compared with nondiabetics of the same age and sex). The triggering mechanism is unclear, but it has been suggested that diabetics have a low glucose tolerance and that this may potentiate stroke (50). It has been demonstrated that the use of hormonal contraceptives also reduces glucose tolerance. Diabetes has also been found to hasten the atherosclerotic process in both large and small arteries.

Minor Risk Factors

Blood Lipids. Although the relationship of serum lipids to the development of coronary heart disease is well established, their association with stroke has been equivocal. This is puzzling in view of the consistent relationship of blood lipids to coronary heart disease, a process with the same underlying pathology as atherothrombotic brain infarction (23).

Hematocrit. Although pathologically elevated hematocrit values have long been recognized as a stroke hazard, it was not appreciated until reported by the Framingham study (22). The increased risk of brain infarction with hematocrits above 45 percent may be due to greater blood viscosity, which increases sharply when hematocrits exceed this value. The risk of cerebral infarction with high hematocrit values may be greatest when there is severe atherosclerosis in the smaller vessels of the deep structures of the brain rather than in the cortical areas (46).

Family History. Since there is a strong familial component in essential hypertension, it seems likely that there is also a genetic influence in stroke (50). Familial susceptibility to stroke could derive from an innate reduced capacity to tolerate the various stroke risk factors.

Environmental Factors

A number of environmental factors involving life-style may play a role in the evolution of stroke.

Cigarette Smoking. Cigarette smoking, which is a powerful contributor to the incidence of coronary heart disease and occlusive peripheral arterial disease, does not rank high among the risk factors for stroke.

Oral Contraceptives. Between 1950 and 1970 neurologists began reporting vascular brain syndromes in young women using birth control pills. Subsequent studies have supported the view that there is increased risk of transient cerebral and retinal ischemic attacks and of bland and hemorrhagic infarcts of the brain in patients taking oral estrogen preparations.

The risk is augmented in certain identifiable subgroups of the female population, including those with coexisting hypertension, those with a history of migraine, those who are over thirty-five years of age, those who have taken the pill for a prolonged period, and those having diabetes or hyperlipidemia. The risk of cardiovascular complications in general is increased by cigarette smoking. High-estrogen-content pills have been implicated as the greatest offenders.

Prevention and Screening for Early Intervention

Stroke or TIA should be regarded as a failure of prevention. Measures to diagnose and treat the already afflicted stroke patient are for the most part too little and too late. In the case of cerebral infarction and cerebral hemorrhage, physicians need to shift their attention from applying high-technology instrumentation to the client with advanced cerebrovascular disease to the more mundane business of modifying risk factors for disease prevention in the presymptomatic stroke candidate (7).

Nurses should continually assess their clients for even modest elevations in blood pressure and early signs of cardiac impairment and should encourage preventive health measures with respect to obesity, cigarette smoking, and physical inactivity. Each physician and primary nurse can identify prime candidates for stroke among asymptomatic clients. Control of severe and moderately severe hypertension will definitely prevent stroke; however, these clients will require vigorous and sustained therapy to maintain normotension. Medical treatment of the adult population of the United States known to have mild hypertension (diastolic pressure between 98 and 105 mm Hg) requires significant therapeutic effort by the physician and the nurse and considerable expense

for the client. In addition, antihypertensive drugs have adverse effects that limit their acceptance by clients and reduce clients' compliance with the medical regimen.

Effective means of reducing the risk of cardiovascular disease include losing weight, reducing salt intake, and giving up cigarette smoking. By considering a client's history of cigarette smoking, ECG, blood glucose level, systolic blood pressure, and serum cholesterol, the doctor or nurse can formulate a cardiovascular risk profile, and the risk of stroke, cardiovascular heart disease, or peripheral arterial disease can be determined. It is to those persons most at risk that vigorous antihypertensive therapy should be applied. The nurse must estimate the degree of compliance to expect from each client, by reviewing medications currently used by the client as well as the client's history of compliance.

Overview of Management

In this chapter, management of the stroke client is divided into three components: (a) management of major associated problems (hypertension, diabetes mellitus, and cardiac impairment), (b) drug therapy, and (c) rehabilitation. As this section indicates, the primary nurse has a role in management, but the unique role of the nurse emerges in relation to management of nursing diagnoses, which are discussed in a subsequent section.

Associated Problems

Hypertension. Edema and ischemia may result in an increase in intracranial pressure, requiring a somewhat elevated blood pressure to maintain cerebral blood flow. A too-rapid reduction in blood pressure may result in increased infarct size or a new stroke. Medical treatment is conservative and includes bed rest and a low-sodium diet. Antihypertensive drugs may be introduced cautiously when the neurological condition is stabilized. Nursing management includes rigorous monitoring of blood pressure; provision of a restful, low-stress environment; and avoidance of Valsalva maneuver.

Diabetes Mellitus. Immobility, hospitalization, and change in life-style alter metabolic needs at the same time that dietary intake may be limited by swallowing and chewing difficulties and decreased appetite. Medical management requires frequent monitoring of blood glucose levels and frequent adjustments of diet and insulin.

Nursing management includes monitoring of intake and output. Consultation with the family and dietitian may assist in providing acceptable foods that the client can eat. Clients may need assistance with eating to prevent fatigue and to ensure that the prescribed diet is maintained. Small meals with between-meal supplements may be necessary. For additional information about care of the diabetic client, the reader is referred to chapter 33.

Cardiac Impairment. Medical treatment may vary with the specific cardiac disease. Diagnostic workup is required, and the client must be on a cardiac monitor until stable. The nurse must observe the client closely for changes in neurological status indicating further embolization. Arrhythmias, venous distention, and heart and lung sounds should be monitored. Clients' energy should be conserved, and they should be assisted with care and allowed frequent rest periods.

Drug Therapy

Hyperosmotic Agents. When the cerebral edema accompanying a stroke threatens to cause herniation, intravenous mannitol is the drug of choice. The hyperosmotic agent reduces the intracranial pressure due to edema. It must be used with caution in clients with renal dysfunction, as the increased circulatory volume may compromise damaged kidneys. Side effects of mannitol include fever, angina, pulmonary congestion, headache, and blurred vision. The nurse must carefully monitor intake and output, body weight, and electrolytes because clients may quickly become dehydrated.

Antihypertensives. Thiazide diuretics are considered the cornerstone of antihypertensive therapy by the majority of physicians and are usually the first drugs prescribed. If the client's hypertension cannot be controlled by thiazides alone, moderately potent antihypertensive drugs (propanolol, methyldopa, reserpine) are prescribed in the second step. If the client's blood pressure remains high, then hydralazine, an even more potent drug, is added. If, at this point, the client's blood pressure still fails to respond to medication, the nurse and physician must reassess the compliance of the client with the regimen.

Clients receiving antihypertensive drug therapy may develop acute hypotensive reactions characterized by faintness, weakness, and nausea; clients therefore must be taught how to prevent acute hypotensive reactions as well as what to do should a reaction occur. For additional information about care of the hypertensive client, the reader is referred to chapter 30.

Corticosteroids. Dexamethasone (Decadron) is used to treat the stroke client. When this drug is used, the initial dose is tapered over a period of seven to ten days. Decadron helps break the cycle of increasing intracranial pressure by reducing the inflammatory reaction. Although commonly used, its benefit in the treatment of stroke is questionable, and additional research in this area is needed.

Anticoagulants. Anticoagulants are used to prevent stroke resulting from infarction (thrombus, embolus). These are given to slow the blood's coagulation time, with the goal of preventing further clot formation. Anticoagulants are prescribed only if hemorrhage has been ruled out.

Heparin is used as the first step in anticoagulation. It is most effective when administered by continuous intravenous infusion of 1000 units/hour or until the partial prothrombin time (PTT) is two to three times normal. Treatment usually lasts seven to ten days. Complications include bleeding and easy bruising.

Long-term anticoagulation is accomplished through the oral administration of warfarin (Coumadin, Panwarfarin), which inhibits prothrombin synthesis and decreases the vitamin K–dependent clotting factors. The usual dosage is 5–10 mg/day. A prothrombin time (PT) of two to two and a half times normal is desirable. Treatment in stroke syndromes lasts three to six months. Excessive bleeding is the primary complication. A client taking warfarin on a long-term basis must know the following: the signs and symptoms of anticoagulant overdosage; the drugs with which warfarin interacts; the rationale for avoiding modifications in diet; the importance of avoiding trauma; the importance of a Medic-Alert bracelet; and the need for routine blood testing.

Antiplatelet Vasodilators. Several vasodilators have been reported to have an antiplatelet aggregate effect, which has spurred interest in conducting trials with aspirin and with oral anticoagulants for clients with thromboembolic disorders.

Acetylsalicylic acid (aspirin, ASA) is used to prevent platelet aggregation at the site of an atherosclerotic plaque. The dosage of 320 mg four times a day or 640 mg twice a day is administered orally. The complication of gastrointestinal bleeding may be reduced by administering aspirin with meals. It is contraindicated in clients with peptic ulcer and must be used with caution when anticoagulants are also being taken. The duration of treatment is indefinite.

Dipyridamole (Persantine) also inhibits platelet aggregation. It is used alone or with aspirin in treating TIAs and is administered orally in doses of 50 mg to 75 mg three or four times a day with aspirin. Complications include nausea and vomiting. The duration of treatment is indefinite.

Anticonvulsants.   Clients who have suffered cerebral vascular hemorrhages are the most likely candidates for anticonvulsants.

Dilantin, the drug of choice, acts on the motor cortex by promoting efflux of sodium from neurons, which stabilizes the threshold against hyperexcitability and reduces the membrane sodium gradient, preventing cortical seizure foci from stimulating adjacent cortical areas. The usual maintenance dose is 400–600 mg orally every day. Dilantin should be administered with at least one-half glass of water immediately before, with, or immediately after meals, to minimize gastric irritation. The nurse should inform the client that the drug may impart a harmless pink or red to red-brown coloration to the urine. Clients over sixty years of age are more likely to show evidence of toxicity than younger clients. These clients should be monitored closely, especially during dosage adjustment. Liver-function tests, blood counts, and urinalyses are recommended prior to therapy and at monthly intervals. Hydantoin derivatives may interfere with folic acid metabolism, with resulting megaloplastic anemia. Folic acid therapy may be prescribed. Clients should be instructed not to alter the prescribed regimen. Status epilepticus and seizure may be precipitated when an anticonvulsant is abruptly withdrawn (12).

Rehabilitation

Rehabilitation is the process that enables a disabled or ill client to achieve maximum physical, mental, and social well-being. The three goals of rehabilitative management are to prevent deformity, to maintain function, and to restore or retrain the remaining functions to maximum effectiveness.

Some of the deficits observed during the initial phase of stroke are not permanent but are due to cerebral edema. Therefore, the plan of care for the stroke client during this early phase must be fluid and must reflect the gradual changes and return of function. Generally speaking, rehabilitation should begin twelve to twenty-four hours after stabilization of neurological findings.

Although it is difficult to predict how much functional improvement can be expected for any given client, a number of factors have been identified to assist in establishing rehabilitation potential. The following factors are associated with a good prognosis for functional recovery: (a) positive acceptance of the disability on the part of the client, (b) presence in the home of a spouse or other family member to assist the client, (c) good bladder control, (d) good visual-motor coordination, (e) early return of muscle tone, (f) early return of tendon reflexes, (g) early return of voluntary motion, (h) good strength in muscles of hands and trunk, and (i) skill in feeding (8). Work toward the first two goals begins when the client enters the health care system. For example, upon admission of the hemiplegic client, the nurse attempts to prevent deformity in the client by passive exercises, ROM exercises, and proper positioning. In addition, measures to maintain the function of the respiratory and gastrointestinal system are implemented. With the physiological stabilization of the client, the focus shifts to restoration of function. During this stage the client begins to relearn and regain control over bodily actions and functions that are deficient or lost because of the stroke. Activities might focus on speech, walking, bowel and bladder control, and activities of daily living.

Paralysis affecting the extremities, trunk, and face in various combinations is the hallmark of the stroke victim. The involved extremities may be completely paralyzed (hemiplegia), or there may be mild weakness. The degree of paralysis is usually greater early in the illness; recovery from paralysis is most rapid in the first eight to twelve weeks. This is because edema and pressure from other sources may temporarily impair brain function in some areas.

Hemiplegic clients do better if they are able to realize early in their illness that doing certain things for themselves, although difficult, is beneficial. Activity is an important part of treatment. Encouragement is frequently needed to get a client to use the paretic limb to its maximum potential; there is a tendency to do everything with the unaffected limb. Special care must be taken when implementing the rehabilitation plan. Rehabilitation should begin slowly and increase within the client's capabilities, to avoid frustrating the client and thus causing a setback.

As soon as they can sit up in bed, hemiplegic clients are encouraged to perform all the self-care activities they can, using the unaffected hand (e.g., brushing teeth, eating, combing hair, shaving, and bathing). This helps preserve the adult pattern of independent self-care. Gait training can begin when the client can stand comfortably without fatigue for fifteen to twenty minutes.

Clients with a cerebrovascular accident are often as much victims of professional discouragement as they are of the stroke itself. The rate of recovery is usually rapid at the beginning and then gradually slows down; ultimately, clients are usually left with some permanent residual effects. The fullest possible recovery for most clients is achieved by utilizing a learning method of setting short-range, short-term goals and focusing upon these, short step by short step (37).

Continuity of Care. Continuity of care is essential if the goals of the original rehabilitation program are to be fulfilled. The primary nurse must assume responsibility for providing referrals for follow-up care. Primary nursing supports this accountability for client care outcomes.

Client discharge referrals must be done prior to discharge from an acute care facility, not as an afterthought while the client is preparing to leave. Evidence continues to mount that clients regress physically, emotionally, and socially when follow-up care is not available.

Nursing Care

Caring for the stroke client can be challenging because of the potential social, emotional, and physical impact of disability on the client and family. Emphasis throughout the acute and rehabilitative phases is on comprehensive, individualized nursing care that aims to restore the client and family to an optimum level of functioning. The client's and family's quality of life often depends on the quality of care the primary nurse gives, and this in turn depends on an accurate assessment of the needs and problems of the client and family.

Assessment

A thorough history and physical examination of the stroke client is a vital addition to the data gathered in special diagnostic tests. When complete, this data provides a comprehensive picture of the client's problems and needs and an adequate basis for comprehensive care. An assessment profile specific to the stroke client is found in Figure 37.1.

Health History. The initial interview with the client or the client's family should answer two basic questions:

Where is the lesion? and What caused it? This helps the health care team predict some of the deficits that may occur. But equally important is assessment of actual deficits, particularly as they relate to communication and self-care. This is explored in depth with the client and family.

Valuable information can be obtained from the client's past history and may give the physician and nurse insight into the cause of the stroke. The presence of hypertension, diabetes, and heart disease poses complications in the management of stroke. Each of these conditions will significantly affect the client's response to the stroke and must be considered when planning both the medical and nursing regimens.

The risk factors that are correlated with stroke may be divided into three categories: nonreversible; partially reversible; and reversible. The nonreversible risk factors include sex, age, race, and heredity. The partially reversible risk factors are hypertension, diabetes mellitus, cardiac impairments, and blood lipid abnormalities. Any one of these diseases doubles the risk of stroke. When they occur in combination, the risk is further compounded. The incidence of stroke may be reduced by improved detection and management of these specific conditions. The reversible risk factors include smoking and obesity.

Because stroke can have such a great impact on the client and family, assessment of their life-style, coping mechanisms, interpersonal relationships, and resources is vital. Planning for a life with a disability—if there is one following stroke—appropriately begins with an accurate understanding of the client as a person living with a family in a community that has resources that may or may not be used. This is the point of departure in establishing rehabilitation goals.

Physical Examination. A thorough general physical examination should always be performed. This includes evaluation of all peripheral pulses that may suggest the presence of other occlusive diseases. A complete detailed neurological examination is important because it may detect an unsuspected primary disorder. In addition, it is vital to identify any persistent neurological deficit, which separates a client with a cerebral infarction from one with a TIA. The examination also provides a baseline for any postoperative neurological changes.

The blood pressure of both upper extremities should be recorded to identify the presence of hypertension and a difference between the blood pressure of the two upper extremities, which may suggest occlusive disease of

ASSESSMENT PROFILE

Subjective Data
Current problem/complaint: _____
_____
_____

Onset of Difficulty

Yes	No	
		I. Sudden loss of speech or change in speech _____
		attack sudden _____
		attack gradual _____
		precipitating event _____
		event cleared completely _____
		how many attacks in the last 12 months? _____
		when was most recent event? _____

Yes	No	
		about how long do the attacks usually last? _____
		—just a second or two
		—several seconds to a few minutes
		—a few minutes to 1 hour
		—about 1 hour to 6 hours
		—about 6 hours to 24 hours
		—more than 24 hours

Yes	No	
		Symptoms occurring at the same time as the speech difficulty:
		visual disturbance
		numbness or tingling of face, fingers, extremities
		blackouts or fainting
		headache
		paralysis or weakness of arm or leg
		light-headedness or dizzy spell
		convulsions or seizures
		generalized weakness
		other: _____

The same protocol applies for the following areas of data collection:
  II. Numbness, tingling, or loss of feeling in arms, legs, or face
  III. Weakness or paralysis of extremities
  IV. Loss or change in vision (monocular blindness)
  V. Episodes of dizziness, light-headedness, or loss of balance

(continued)

Figure 37.1. Assessment Screening Tool: *Stroke Risk Profile*

History of Illness

	Client				*Family*	
	Yes	No			Yes	No
	___	___	hypertension		___	___
	___	___	hypotension		___	___
	___	___	diabetes		___	___
	___	___	heart disease		___	___
	___	___	stroke		___	___
	___	___	transient ischemic attacks		___	___
	___	___	smoking		___	___
	___	___	estrogen therapy		___	___
	___	___	obesity		___	___
	___	___	immobility (decreased mobility)		___	___

Medications:

_____

_____

_____

_____

Dietary History
Special Diet: _____

Dietary Restriction: _____

Objective Data

Weight _____   Age _____   Gender _____

Blood pressure _____   Right arm _____   Left arm _____

Apical pulse rate _____   Radial pulse rate _____

Carotid pulses (palpate one side at a time)

Right _____   Left _____

Superficial temporal artery pulse (palpate both sides simultaneously)

Right _____   Left _____

Bruits may be heard over the thoracic, cervical, and cranial arteries.
1. Systolic bruit may be heard at the carotid bifurcation at the angle of the jaw.

   Right _____   Left _____

2. Augmentation murmur may be heard over the orbit of the eye.

   Right _____   Left _____

Figure 37.1.   (*continued*)

Precordium
1. Diastolic apical rumble may be heard over the mitral valve. _____

2. Diastolic gallop may be heard during ventricular filling. _____

Laboratory Data

Hemoglobin _____

Hematocrit _____

Blood glucose _____

Urine glucose _____

Platelets _____

Prothrombin time _____ (if client is on anticoagulant therapy)
(Prothrombin time is usually checked once a day for ten days, then three times a week, and then once every 1 to 2 weeks. Client should generally remain at a level of 15 to 17 seconds with the normal value of 12 seconds.)

Figure 37.1. (*continued*)

the arteries of the aortic arch. Palpation and auscultation of carotid arteries and vertebral arteries in the neck may reveal diminished or absent pulsation, suggesting occlusive disease. Bruits are produced by turbulence from the flow of blood in a vessel and usually are transmitted distally from the side of an atherosclerotic lesion.

Diagnostic Tests. All clients with stroke or recent TIA should be admitted to the hospital. After a careful physical and neurological examination, the client should undergo bed rest, and an evaluation should be initiated not only to confirm the diagnosis of stroke but also to identify the specific cause. It is most important to direct the diagnostic workup in such a way as to differentiate between ischemic and hemorrhage stroke. The diagnostic workup is dictated by the urgency of the situation.

Some of the neurodiagnostic tests are simple and painless; others, complex and painful. Some of these tests are potentially life-threatening (for example, cerebral angiogram); nurses must be prepared to detect and correct complications promptly. The nurse should be cognizant of the fact that many stroke clients in the acute phase are unable to communicate (aphasia) and will therefore not be able to ask questions about the tests. The supportive care by the nurse is very important during this phase; it will enhance the client's sense of well-being and promote confidence in unfamiliar people and procedures. The nurse will also facilitate the expression of fears and other concerns and will answer requests for information by clients and significant others.

An electrocardiogram should be performed at the time of admission to exclude the possibility of myocardial infarction or arrhythmia. Continuous cardiac monitoring by the use of a Holter monitor is particularly effective in detecting intermittent cardiac arrhythmias. If embolic stroke is a possibility, echocardiogram is particularly useful in the diagnosis of valvular heart disease.

X-ray studies of the neck may reveal calcification in the carotid artery or severe osteophytes that may compress the vertebral arteries. A skull roentgenogram may suggest a neoplasm or other mass by a pineal shift or by evidence of increased intracranial pressure. Cranial calcification may suggest an aneurysm, an arteriovenous malformation, an atherosclerotic vessel, or a brain tumor.

An electroencephalogram is particularly useful in showing possible seizure activity, which is encountered especially in hemorrhage or superficial embolic infarctions.

Computed tomography (CT scan) is particularly useful during the early phase in distinguishing hemorrhage from infarction.

Lumbar puncture enables a sample of cerebral spinal fluid to be taken. The presence of blood in an atraumatic lumbar puncture confirms the presence of a hemorrhagic stroke. Xanthochromia is another abnormal finding indicating that old blood is present, evidence of past bleeding.

Following a lumbar puncture, the nurse should carefully monitor any reactions to the procedure, including nausea, vomiting, urinary retention, and headache. When it is necessary to perform a lumbar puncture, the client with known or possible increased intracranial pressure should be observed closely for herniation syndrome (change in level of consciousness, rising blood pressure, headache) (1).

Recently, several noninvasive tests, such as ophthalmodynamometry, oculoplethysmography, cerebral blood flow measurements, and various types of ultrasound imaging of the carotid artery, have been developed for carotid disease. Such noninvasive procedures may be particularly helpful in defining the indications for angiography in clients with probable TIA who have medical or other contraindications to angiography. The advantages of noninvasive procedures are that they are relatively inexpensive, are performed in outpatient settings, take only thirty minutes to one hour; are painless, and pose no risk to health. The main disadvantage is that they are not definitive, with high reportings of false negatives and false positives. When these studies are performed in proper clinical settings, such information may be helpful in deciding whether to proceed with cerebral angiography.

The most definitive test in the evaluation of cerebrovascular disease is an aortic arch study and cerebral angiography. The indications for such a study in stroke clients are as follows: (a) when diagnosis is in doubt, particularly if the client is deteriorating; (b) when neck vessel surgery is considered in clients with carotid transient ischemic attacks; (c) in all clients with bloody spinal taps and evidence of intracranial hemorrhage on CT scan, to confirm presence of aneurysm or arteriovenous malformation.

The cerebral angiogram should be performed when the client is considered in optimal condition for surgery (when blood pressure and vital signs are stable). Although cerebral angiography is a relatively safe procedure, with morbidity and mortality less than 1 percent, it should be reserved for clients in whom the findings will significantly influence management. As with any invasive procedure, the potential hazards must be carefully weighed against the expected benefits.

During testing, the nurse concentrates on reducing the anxiety of the client and family by clarifying and reinforcing information about the diagnostic tests and examination. The nurse should make every effort to assist the physician in performing the diagnostic tests, noting the client's responses as well as providing the physical and emotional support needed. The nurse must share information about untoward reactions after cerebral angiography, which include local and/or systemic allergic reactions to the contrast material, spasm or occlusion of the vessel by the clot, hemorrhage, and obstructive clot about the femoral injection site.

Nursing Diagnoses

Based on the findings of the assessment, the nurse caring for a stroke client might expect to encounter the following nursing diagnoses:

1. Ineffective airway clearance, impaired gas exchange, or altered respiratory function related to immobility.
2. Altered physical mobility related to alterations in lower and upper limbs (hemiplegia, hemiparesis).
3. Altered skin integrity related to immobility.
4. Altered nutrition: reduced food intake related to hypovigilance, indifference, impaired communication.
5. Self-care deficits related to neuromuscular impairment—paresis, apraxia, visual/sensory defects, unilateral neglect.
6. Altered bowel elimination: diarrhea related to improper feeding.
7. Altered bowel elimination: constipation related to impaired bowel tone, weak abdominal musculature, inadequate dietary bulk, immobility, inadequate fluid intake.
8. Altered bladder elimination: urinary incontinence related to impaired central control of micturation, impaired communication, hypovigilance.
9. Sensory-perceptual alterations (hemianopsia, central blindness, diplopia, nystagmus, and loss of touch, proprioception, pain, and temperature sensation.
10. Impaired communication related to damage to the left-hemisphere brain structures.
11. Ineffective coping of the individual and family related to the sudden onset of a potentially devastating illness with long-term effects.
12. Altered thought processes (hypovigilance, indifference, decreased attention span, impaired ability to solve problems) related to impaired cerebral circulation, damage to brain structures.
13. Knowledge deficits of the individual and family related to lack of information about stroke, cognitive deficits.

Planning and Implementation

Emphasis during the early or acute phase of stroke is on good nursing care, with the goals being to prevent secondary disability and deformity and to preserve residual function. Rehabilitation begins as soon as possible, even while life-saving medical management is the predominant concern. Attention is given to nursing diagnoses as they relate to the total plan of care.

☐ *Ineffective Airway Clearance, Impaired Gas Exchange, or Altered Respiratory Function.* The nurse assesses the client for signs of hypoxia (e.g., restlessness, confusion, and cyanosis). Respiration is facilitated by (a) keeping the tongue from obstructing the airway, (b) frequent suctioning as necessary, (c) oxygen administration as prescribed, (d) turning the client every two hours, and (e) monitoring blood gases if ordered. Some clients may be on respirators and/or have tracheostomies.

☐ *Altered Physical Mobility.* Paralysis affecting the extremities, trunk, and face in various combinations is the hallmark of the stroke victim. There may be paralysis and sensory impairment of the contralateral side of the body. Most common is paralysis of half of the body (hemiplegia), with weakness of the lower half of the face (central facial palsy). Depending on the level of the lesion, varying combinations of ipsilateral and contralateral motor and sensory loss may be present. Initially, paralysis is usually flaccid, and the deep tendon reflexes are decreased. In twenty-four to forty-eight hours, the reflexes may become more active, commonly hyperactive (7).

Recovery from paralysis is most rapid in the first eight to twelve weeks, although improvement is seen months after the stroke. Generally the more severe the initial paralysis, the less the functional recovery of the involved extremity. Many factors affect recovery, including the general medical condition, disability from previous strokes, secondary disabilities, and client cooperation. Frequent changes of body position, active and passive range of motion exercises, adequate support of body parts, maintenance of proper body alignment, and early ambulation help preserve body functioning and facilitate mobility.

☐ *Altered Skin Integrity.* During the acute stage of stroke, clients are completely dependent upon nurses for protecting their skin from injury. The stroke client who is not able to change position independently should have a program of scheduled position changes to prevent sustained pressure. Improper positioning can lead to the development of pressure sores just as readily as failure to change positions at all. Clients who use wheelchairs must also be positioned and repositioned properly, since sustained pressure can be just as hazardous in the sitting position. With loss of sensation and motor function from stroke, the mechanisms that usually protect against mechanical injury to the skin are absent. The client may be unaware that any trauma has occurred to affected extremities during transfer from one place to another. Clients should be instructed to guide and protect paralyzed limbs.

Mobilizing the client is important in preventing pressure sore formation, because it promotes circulation to all areas and involves shifting of the body.

Dependence of the limbs may contribute to an increase of interstitial fluid. This can progress to edema and tissue breakdown. Elastic hose that are too tight, wrinkled, or left in place too long only serve as tourniquets and hide the color, temperature, and condition of the skin of the feet and legs. It is recommended that elastic hose be removed frequently to observe the condition of the feet and legs. The nurse as well as the client and family should make daily observations of the skin, to check for evidence of breaks in the skin and reddened or ischemic areas. Special attention should be given to the skin over bony prominences and under splints, braces, restraints, and other equipment that can exert pressure and irritate the skin. Any areas of redness or impaired circulation should be considered the beginning of a pressure sore. Massage and range-of-motion exercises to promote circulation should be an integral part of the program for prevention of tissue breakdown.

☐ *Altered Nutrition: Reduced Food Intake.* In the acute phase of stroke, the nutritional needs of the client are a secondary concern. The client may be maintained for up to ten days on intravenous fluids. Facial weakness on the affected side and dysphagia (difficulty in swallowing) present special problems. If the client is conscious and able to swallow without aspirating, oral feeding is encouraged.

The first oral feeding should be approached with caution, as the gag reflex may not be intact. In order to check this before initiating a feeding, the back of the throat may be gently stimulated with a tongue blade. If the gag reflex is absent, the feeding should be deferred and exercises to stimulate swallowing begun. The speech therapist, occupational therapist, or physical therapist is usually responsible for designing this program. However, the primary nurse may be called upon to develop this program in certain clinical settings.

If the gag reflex is present, the nurse may proceed with the feeding. The client should be placed in a high-Fowler's position for the feeding as well as for fifteen minutes before and after the feeding. For the first feeding, foods should be selected that are easy to swallow (e.g., puréed foods). Liquids often promote coughing. Milk products should be avoided because they tend to increase the viscosity of mucus and increase salivation. Foods should be placed on the unaffected side of the mouth. Stroking the neck or pressing down on the top of the head decreases laryngeal tension and promotes swallowing. The nurse should ensure that the atmosphere is unrushed and nonstressful. Each feeding must be followed by scrupulous oral hygiene, as food tends to collect on the affected side.

□ *Self-Care Deficits.* Personal self-care activities involve three major areas. The first area includes personal hygiene activities (bathing, oral hygiene, grooming) and ability to attend to one's own bowel and bladder needs. The second area of activity is dressing; the third, eating.

There are innumerable assistive devices for dressing, eating, and personal hygiene. Further resources are suggested in the list of references at the end of the chapter.

Most hemiplegic clients can achieve independence in the essential activities of daily living. Routines should be established for each client that can be followed at home and that will enable him or her to care for his or her own needs.

With activities of daily living, the physical therapist, the occupational therapist, and the primary nurse work closely together in order to coordinate and reinforce each other's teaching. Cooperation from the family, friends, and health care personnel in giving the encouragement and time necessary for self-care may require skillful explanation and persuasion.

At mealtime, stroke clients' food should be prepared and arranged so that they can feed themselves with assistance only when necessary. Special eating utensils and other self-help devices may be needed. Sometimes the nurse or family may be able to make some of these self-help items. Devices also may be available from an occupational therapist.

Whether clients feed themselves or are assisted by the nurse, food should be placed in the uninvolved side of the mouth (a mirror helps clients do this). The nurse should check frequently to prevent the accumulation of food in the weakened side of the mouth.

Independence in dressing should be achieved early. Relearning how to dress and undress is almost always a struggle for the client. However, after mastering even a small part of dressing, clients begin to regain dignity and self-respect. The nurse and the occupational therapist work together in this area, reinforcing each other's instructions.

The hemiplegic client should also be instructed in transferring out of bed and onto a wheelchair, in using the toilet and shower, and in one-handed manipulative skills for other needs.

Most hemiplegics can be taught one-handed home-making and kitchen activities, and they should be instructed in energy-saving principles similar to those used by clients with heart disease. Some aspects of homemaking can be practiced in the hospital, such as folding linen, rinsing out clothes, bedmaking, and cleaning. A number of assistive devices can be useful in promoting independent functioning.

Emphasis should be placed on activities that are either useful or interesting to the client. Assistive devices should be provided specifically for each client's needs and should be withdrawn when no longer necessary.

□ *Altered Bowel Elimination: Diarrhea.* If the stroke client is unable to take food orally, tube feedings may be initiated, usually by the nasogastric route. While the most common side effect of tube feeding is constipation, diarrhea is also noted. Diarrhea in tube-fed clients is caused by feeding too fast, too high a concentration of formula, and lactose intolerance. Nursing interventions include reducing the rate of infusion and introducing formula gradually, from a quarter to a half to full strength as tolerated, and notifying the physician for changes in formula.

□ *Altered Bowel Elimination: Constipation.* During the acute stage following a stroke, constipation and fecal impaction are common. They are compounded by bed rest and inactivity and the absence of an adequate diet. As soon as the client can be mobilized and can tolerate a diet, the nurse begins bowel retraining. Information about the premorbid bowel pattern helps the nurse give individualized management. The client's fluid intake must be maintained at a level of 1,500–2,000 cc/day unless contraindicated for medical reasons. Roughage should be included in the diet as tolerated. The client should be allowed adequate time on the toilet at the time of day consistent with previous patterns of defecation. As clients resume more normal activity, bowel medications, such as suppositories, stool softeners, and laxatives, may be discontinued.

□ *Altered Bladder Elimination: Urinary Incontinence.* In the acute stage of stroke, the primary genitourinary problem is poor bladder control resulting in incontinence. Initially, an indwelling catheter is helpful. However, chronic use of a catheter prolongs bladder retraining and promotes the development of urinary tract infections. Indwelling catheters should be avoided. An adequate fluid intake is critical for bladder retraining. A bedpan or urinal should be offered every two hours. Disposable diapers for adults are easy to change and keep the client dry. The nurse *must* explain to the client that the diapers are for short-term use only and may prevent long-term problems. For male clients, condom catheters may be used. Long-term fluid restriction to reduce urinary soiling can lead to dehydration and skin problems. Intermittent catheterization or external devices may be used for short periods of time, until bladder retraining can be attempted.

If the client is unable to regain bladder control, a serious care problem develops. A coordinated training program by all members of the nursing staff is a major primary nursing responsibility. Until bladder and bowel control are attained, further rehabilitation efforts will be hampered.

□ *Sensory/Perceptual Alterations.* Lesions in any of the three major cerebral arterial systems that supply the parietal lobe may result in perceptual alterations, such as disturbance of body image, spatial judgment, and sensory interpretation. To recognize and assess perceptual alterations, the nurse should determine whether the client ignores input from one side of the body or environment even when vision is intact. Evidence of neglect includes failure to wash or dress one side of the body, "forgetting" the affected limbs (which may be seen dangling over the edge of the bed or entangled in wheelchair spokes), or failure to perceive persons or objects in the left visual space that are recognized normally from the right. The nurse should also determine whether the client judges spatial relations correctly. Can the client reach for an article, follow routine directions or commands to use the right or left extremity, or determine when the body is in an upright position?

Another category of problems might be described as sensory rather than perceptual. When damage to the brain affects the sensory cortex of the parietal lobe, sensation on the contralateral side will be lost or diminished. As the client loses tactile sensation from one side of the body, one source of information to the brain is eliminated. The client may need to watch rather than feel as a guide to activity.

Damage to the visual pathways anywhere along their route from the optic chiasm to the occipital lobe will result in visual field deficits, loss of vision, and, therefore, loss of input from part of external space.

Hemianopsia and homonymous hemianopsia refer to blindness in one-half of each visual field. Testing for visual field defects in the brain-damaged client should be performed during the acute phase of illness as well as during the rehabilitation period. Persistent disregard of objects in part of the visual field should alert the nurse to this possibility. The client needs to be trained to compensate for these deficits. After the initial stress of the illness, the nurse may begin placing items necessary for activities of daily living on the unaffected side.

Initially, the nurse compensates for the perceptual problem by arranging the environment within the client's perceptual field. Later, the client is instructed to consciously attend to the neglected side. The position of the affected arm or leg in space must be checked by the client to prevent unfelt trauma. Other visual problems may include diplopia, loss of the corneal reflex, and ptosis.

□ *Impaired Communication.* Evaluation of the ability to communicate and the presence of visual impairment should also be an integral part of early rehabilitation. Loss of function in these areas is not only quite disturbing to the client, but it seriously affects his or her ability to cooperate in rehabilitation efforts.

It is important that nurses possess skills that will enable them to make a basic assessment of the speech problem. The nurse's assessment should consist of neurological and psychological data and an assessment of speech status.

If the client is unable to respond, the nurse should collect data from the family that will give clues to the client's interests, hobbies, and occupation, as well as general social information. It is helpful to know the client's level of education and to have some idea of his or her intelligence.

The services of a speech therapist are desirable if the stroke has caused receptive or expressive aphasia, but the nurse can also assist in this area. If the person has difficulty following verbal directions, a demonstration of the action desired may help. Persons who have suffered strokes may not be able to express themselves clearly, but it should not be assumed that they cannot hear. Encourage clients' attempts to communicate. Make every effort to include them in planning care by asking simple questions to allow them to express preferences. Remember that in spite of limitations, the person who has suffered a stroke is still an intelligent, sensitive human being with awareness of the attitudes of those caring for him or her.

Several investigators believe that therapy for aphasia should begin as quickly as possible following the stroke to provide the aphasic client as much language stimulation as possible (30).

It is important for nurses to differentiate aphasic from dysarthric speech. Dysarthria results from weakness or paralysis of the muscles of the lips, tongue, and larynx or loss of sensation. With dysarthria the client understands and comprehends language but has difficulty pronouncing words and may slur them. The dysarthric client can understand verbal speech, read, and write, unless the dominant hand is paralyzed. Recovery from aphasia depends on a number of factors, including age, etiology of aphasia, severity of initial aphasia, and personality prior to the stroke.

□ *Ineffective Coping of the Individual and Family.* Both the client and family are challenged by an illness that varies in degree of physical disability and in some clients may include impaired thought processes. Destructive behaviors toward self, anger, excessive fatigue, and anxiety are some of the behavioral changes that may be observed in the client. Although individual problems exist for varying lengths of time, living with a stroke is a long-term situation for both client and family.

Family members must cope with three important aspects of the client's behavior. First, they must recognize those changes that are caused by neurological deficits and cannot be changed. Second, they must cope with the client's response to the loss at the same time that they are dealing with their own response. Third, they must deal with behavior that they have reinforced in the early stages of the illness. For example, the client may be reluctant to resume dressing independently, and the family unconsciously reinforces the behavior by continuing to assist with dressing. This may be due both to lack of knowledge and to guilt. Consequently, family members may be hesitant to assert themselves because they are afraid of a recurrence.

Family therapy is a helpful adjunct to a rehabilitation program. Family needs include support and reassurance, accurate and complete information about the disease and treatment, and assistance during this crisis period.

□ *Altered Thought Processes.* It is difficult, if not impossible, for nurses to create conditions for effective learning unless their teaching methodologies are adapted to the alterations in cognitive function that accompany

brain damage. Impaired memory, a short attention span, and poor judgment can prevent generalizing from one activity to another (26).

Teaching methods and the environment must be modified to facilitate learning in the client with alterations in sensation and perception. Learning requires concentration. The environment should be quiet and free of distractions, and the client should be taught when he or she is most alert (usually early in the day). Sessions should be short enough to correspond to the attention span. To combat difficulties in generalizing, tasks should be learned in the environment in which they will be needed.

Perceptual alterations may affect learning in various ways. Neglect of paralyzed limbs affects the ability of clients to learn to dress, since they repeatedly forget to dress the affected side. The nurse can call attention to the affected side by saying, "What about your weak arm?" The nurse can also attach brightly colored labels to a shirt sleeve or pant leg, which will attract the attention of stroke clients.

Individual clients may be unable to simplify problems and may become overwhelmed and immobilized as a result, or their attempts at solution may be haphazard and therefore futile. Nurses must break down problems into component parts, subsequently designing measures to deal with each. For clients who continue to have difficulty with problem solving, simple written lists of the steps used in performing common activities promote both safety and independence. Clients should be encouraged to assume responsibility for themselves, if their abilities seem to be marginal (14).

Anticipatory guidance in problem solving should be included as soon as possible. In this way, many problems can be prevented. Clients should be asked about the problems they anticipate and should be allowed to work them out in this supportive environment.

□ *Knowledge Deficits of the Individual and Family.* Families and clients are usually eager for information and the opportunity to discuss the impact of stroke on their lives. Client and family counseling should be instituted at the time of initial evaluation and continued throughout treatment. The patient's ability to learn is affected by the damage to his or her brain. Patients should not be labeled slow, stubborn, or unmotivated or dismissed as "lost causes" (33).

Sometimes families and clients develop patterns of interaction that are detrimental to the long-term health of the client. Families that overreact to the stroke may respond by keeping the client in a dependent position.

Patients and families should be counseled throughout the client's illness on the best ways of supporting the client.

Evaluation

Determining how stroke will affect each client is difficult. It is often impossible to predict how the client will be two days, seven days, or three weeks later, or how much recovery of function there is likely to be. It is important to keep in mind that virtually all clients who survive do improve to some degree. Thus, assessment and intervention for the stroke client does not remain static but must continually be updated as the client progresses. An understanding of the usual progress of recovery will help the primary nurse to plan realistically for care.

Timetables of goal attainment by the stroke client are beneficial in projecting the outcomes of nursing actions. These timetables assist nurses not only in planning nursing care but also in projecting costs. The nurse can play a vital role in seeing that the client has every opportunity for maximum recovery. This requires astute observation, and experience will enable the nurse to design care that will meet both immediate and long-term needs. Most clients who survive do improve functionally, and expert nursing care can significantly improve the likelihood that the patient will successfully adapt to permanent disabilities (2).

In the context of the nursing diagnoses discussed in this chapter, sample behaviors that indicate movement toward resolution of problems are illustrated below.

Ineffective Airway Clearance, Impaired Gas Exchange, or Altered Respiratory Function. The client will not exhibit any manifestations of hypoxia (e.g., restlessness, confusion, cyanosis, or abnormal blood-gas values).

Altered Physical Mobility. The client will perform activities within the limitations of neuromuscular disability.

Altered Skin Integrity. The client will not exhibit any manifestations of skin breakdown (e.g., redness and ulceration).

Altered Nutrition: Reduced Food Intake. The client will ingest sufficient calories and nutrients to meet the body's demands.

Self-Care Deficits. The client and family will verbalize a realistic perception of the client's ability to perform self-care activities. The client will perform self-care activities regularly, considering personal limitations.

Altered Bowel Elimination: Diarrhea, Constipation. The client will have normal bowel elimination, according to a pattern optimal for the individual.

Altered Bladder Elimination: Urinary Incontinence. The client (if possible) and family will verbalize an understanding of the relationship between stroke and urinary incontinence. The client will participate in bladder training.

Sensory/Perceptual Alterations. The client and family will recognize sensory/perceptual deficits (e.g., loss of tactile sensation and spatial judgment).

Impaired Communication. The client will consistently use modes of communication appropriate to the type and level of deficit.

Ineffective Coping of the Individual and Family. The client and family will identify past coping mechanisms that were successful in dealing with stressors similar to the ones currently encountered. The client and family will identify the impact of stressors on them.

Altered Thought Processes. When teaching methods are adapted to the client's needs, the client will demonstrate the ability to perform tasks (e.g., activities of daily living).

Knowledge Deficits of the Individual and Family. The client and family will demonstrate an understanding of the impact of stroke on their lives. The client and family will be able to differentiate between deficits that can be changed and those that cannot.

Ethical and Legal Issues

Because stroke can affect every aspect of the individual—physical, intellectual, emotional, and social—the nurse caring for the stroke client is frequently faced with ethical and legal dilemmas. How can the client's need for self-determination be reconciled with physical, intellectual, emotional, and social deficits? How far can the nurse go in making decisions for the client when the client seems either unwilling or unable to make a decision? When should legal consultation be sought to determine the client's ability to make decisions, especially as they relate to finances?

When caring for the client who is emotionally unstable, physically impaired, and uncommunicative, how can the nurse protect the client's right to respect as an individual? How can the nurse best serve the client as an advocate?

CASE STUDY

Dr. Norton, a seventy-year-old, internationally known physicist, is being discharged from an acute-care facility to his home in one week. You are the primary nurse and are working with the nursing staff to provide continuity of care when he goes home.

During your assessment of Dr. Norton you find that he has left-sided weakness and is unable to stand without assistance. He is able to feed himself and perform personal hygiene with some assistance. His speech is unaffected, but he is depressed because he feels that he will be a burden to his wife when he returns home. As you talk about his feelings, he begins to cry and then tells you that he sees no purpose to his life now.

When you talk with his wife, you discover that she has no relatives living in the region and has no friends who can help her on a sustained basis, even a friend with whom she can talk. She feels overwhelmed by her impending role as primary care giver, although she knows you will make frequent visits and manage Dr. Norton's care.

1. Identify three actual and potential problems that require nursing intervention and state them as nursing diagnoses.
2. Specify interventions needed for each of these nursing diagnoses.
3. Discuss your role as teacher and counselor in helping the Norton family to cope with their situation.
4. What information may you share with Mrs. Norton to help her understand her husband's partial paralysis, particularly as it relates to functional recovery?

REFERENCES

1. Ball, P. "Preventing Stroke Through Non-Invasive Carotid Artery Assessment." *Journal of Neurosurgical Nursing* 14:182, 1982.
2. Blanco, K. "The Aphasic Patient." *Journal of Neurosurgical Nursing* 14:34, 1982.
3. Carpenito, L. J. *Nursing Diagnosis: Application to Clinical Practice.* Philadelphia: J. B. Lippincott, 1983.
4. Christie, I. "Stroke in Melbourne: A Study of the Relationship Between a Teaching Hospital and the Community." *Medical Journal of Australia* 1:565, 1976.
5. Coakley, C. A., et al. "Technical Aspects of Real-Time Ultrasound Arteriography." *Bruit* 4:40, 1980.
6. Darley, F. L. "Threat or Neglect." *ASAA* 21:628.
7. Feldman, J. L., and M. E. Schultz. "Rehabilitation After a Stroke." *Nursing Digest* 4:63, 1976.
8. Gersten, J. "Rehabilitation Potential." In *Stroke and Its Rehabilitation,* ed. S. Licht. Baltimore: Williams & Wilkins, 1975, 435–71.
9. Grabois, M. "Rehabilitation of Patients with Completed Strokes." In *Diagnosis and Management of Strokes and TIA's,* ed. J. S. Meyer and T. Shaw. Menlo Park, Calif.: Addison-Wesley, 1982.
10. Graham, L. "Stroke Rehabilitation—A Creative Process." *Canadian Nurse* 72:22, 1976.
11. Granger, C. V., et al. "Measurements of Outcome for Stroke Patients." *Stroke* 6:34, 1975.
12. Govoni, L. E., and J. E. Hayes. *Drugs and Nursing Implications.* 3d ed. New York: Appleton-Century-Crofts, 1978.
13. Hansen, B. S., and J. Marquardson. "Incidence of Stroke in Frederiksberg, Denmark." *Stroke* 8:663, 1977.
14. Harborman, S., R. Capildeo, and F. C. Rose. "The Changing Mortality from Cerebrovascular Disease." *Quarterly Journal of Medicine* 47:71, 1978.
15. Harmsen, P., and G. Tibblin. "A Stroke Register in Goteborg, Sweden." *Acta Medica Scandinavica* 191:463, 1972.
16. Hecaen, H., and M. L. Albert. *Human Neuropsychology.* New York: John Wiley & Sons, 1978.
17. Henderson, V. A. "Preserving the Essence of Nursing in a Technological Age." *Journal of Advanced Nursing* 5:245, 1980.
18. Hickey, J. *Quick Reference to Neurological Nursing.* Philadelphia: J. B. Lippincott, 1984.
19. Hurwitz, L. J., and G. F. Adams. "Rehabilitation of Hemiplegia: Indices of Assessment and Prognosis." *British Medical Journal* 1:94, 1972.
20. Joseph, L. S. "Self-care and the Nursing Process." *Nursing Clinics of North America* 15:131, 1980.
21. Kannel, W. B., et al. "Components of Blood Pressure and Risk of Atherothrombotic Brain Infarction: The Framingham Study." *Stroke* 7:327, 1976.
22. Kannel, W. B., et al. "Hemoglobin and the Risk of Cerebral Infarction: The Framingham Study." *Stroke* 3:409, 1972.
23. Kannel, W. B., P. A. Wolf, and T. R. Dawber. "Hypertension and Cardiac Impairments Increase Stroke Risk." *Geriatrics* 33:71, 1978.
24. Kartchner, M. M., and L. P. McRae. "Non-Invasive Evaluation and Management of the Asymptomatic Carotid Bruit." *Surgery* 82:841, 1977.
25. Kurtzke, J. F. "An Introduction to the Epidemiology of

Cerebrovascular Diseases." In *Cerebrovascular Diseases*, ed. P. Scheinburg. New York: Raven Press, 1976.

26. Laughlin, H. P. *The Fatigue Reactions, the Neuröses*. Eastington: Butterworth, 1967.

27. Levine, M. E. "The Four Conservation Principles of Nursing." *Nursing Forum* 6:45, 1967.

28. Levy, R. I. "Stroke Decline: Implications and Prospects." *New England Journal of Medicine* 300:490, 1979.

29. Licht, S., ed. *Stroke and Its Rehabilitation*. Baltimore: Waverly Press, 1975.

30. Louis, M. C., and S. M. Povse. "Aphasia and Endurance: Considerations in the Assessment and Care of the Stroke Patient." *Nursing Clinics of North America* 15:265, 1980.

31. Luckman, J., and K. Sorensen, eds. *Medical Surgical Nursing: A Physiologic Approach*. 2d ed. Philadelphia: W. B. Saunders, 1980.

32. McCartney, V. C. "Rehabilitation and Dignity for the Stroke Patient." *Nursing Clinics of North America* 19:693, 1974.

33. Mahoney, E. K. "Alterations in Cognitive Functioning in the Brain Damaged Patient." *Nursing Clinics of North America* 15:283, 1980.

34. Maida, M. J. "Regional Cerebral Blood Flow: Patient Correlations." *Journal of Neurosurgical Nursing* 14:309, 1982.

35. Marquardson, J. "The Natural History of Acute Cerebrovascular Disease: A Retrospective of 769 Patients." *Acta Neurologica Scandinavica* 45:11, 1969.

36. Masi, A. T., and M. Dagdale. "Cerebrovascular Diseases Associated with Use of Oral Contraceptives: A Review of the English Language Literature." *Annals of Internal Medicine* 72:111, 1970.

37. Matheney, R. "Cerebrovascular Accident and Personality Organization." *Nursing Clinics of North America* 1:443, 1966.

38. Moriyama, I. M., D. E. Drueger, and F. Stamer. *Cerebrovascular Diseases in the United States*. Cambridge, Mass.: Harvard University Press, 1971.

39. Mullin, V. I. "Implementing the Self-care Concept in the Acute Care Setting." *Nursing Clinics of North America* 15:177, 1980.

40. Myco, G. "Stroke and Its Rehabilitation: The Perceived Role of the Nurse in Medical and Nursing Literature." *Journal of Advanced Nursing* 9:429, 1984.

41. O'Brien, M. T., and P. J. Pallett. *Total Care of the Stroke Patient*. Boston: Little, Brown, 1978.

42. Report of the Joint Committee for Stroke Facilities. "IV. Guidelines for the Nursing Care of Stroke Patients." *Stroke* 3:637, 1972.

43. Russell, J. B., and D. S. Sumner. Ultrasonic Arteriography. Southern Illinois University School of Medicine Vascular Research Lab—St. Johns Hospital, Springfield, Ill., 1980.

44. Soltero, I., et al. "Trends in Mortality for Cerebrovascular Disease in the USA." *Stroke* 9:349, 1960.

45. Stryker, R. *Rehabilitation Aspects of Acute and Chronic Nursing Care*. Philadelphia: W. B. Saunders, 1977, 127–45.

46. Tohgi, H., et al. "Importance of the Hematocrit as a Risk Factor in Cerebral Infarction." *Stroke* 9:369, 1978.

47. Waterman, J. W. "Nursing Management of Stroke: Acute Care. Part I." *Cardiovascular Nursing*. American Heart Association, January–February 1985.

48. Waterman, J. W. "Nursing Management of Stroke: Acute Care. Part II." *Cardiovascular Nursing*. American Heart Association, March–April 1985.

49. Whisnant, J. "Concepts of Cerebrovascular Disease." *Stroke* 9:1, 1978.

50. Wolf, P. A., et al. "The Declining Incidence of Stroke: The Framingham Study." *Stroke* 9:97, 1978.

CHAPTER 38

Caring for the Person with Arthritis

MILA AMORIN-NODELMAN

DAISY CRUZ-RICHMAN

■

OBJECTIVES

After completing this chapter, the reader will be able to:

- Differentiate the pathophysiological alterations in rheumatoid arthritis (RA) from those in osteoarthritis (OA).
- Describe at least three manifestations of RA.
- Describe at least three manifestations of OA.
- List five questions that should be included in the physical assessment of the client with arthritis.
- List five questions that should be included in the psychosocial assessment of the client with arthritis.
- Describe at least two diagnostic tests that may be used to differentiate RA from OA.
- Explain the actions and side effects of at least three drugs used in treating RA and OA.
- Formulate at least three nursing diagnoses for clients with RA and OA.
- Design a plan of nursing interventions for clients with RA and OA.
- Identify at least five expected outcomes of the proposed nursing interventions.

Arthritis, a chronic and potentially disabling disease, is a health problem of considerable magnitude. The term *arthritis,* which denotes inflammation of a joint, embraces a variety of more than one hundred related rheumatic diseases. In the United States today, arthritis in some form affects more than 36 million people, and based on prevalence statistics, about a million people will develop arthritis each year (3).

Arthritis can affect every aspect of the client's life, requiring major adaptations for many. Research studies have indicated that in addition to the physical consequences of the disease, concomitant psychological disturbances also exist (11, 27). The psychosocial areas are of significance, both because they are affected by and because they in turn affect the client's response to illness. Thus, the nurse should be cognizant of the interrelationship between the physical and psychosocial factors as they affect the client's overall functioning in the face of a potentially disabling disease.

Because of the chronic nature of the disease, arthritis also produces a financial burden on clients and their families. However, the extent of disease costs from the perspective of an individual client is difficult to ascertain. In addition to direct medical costs, there are also the indirect costs of the client's lost income and productivity. A research study reported that indirect costs due to lost income were at least three times the direct medical costs (39).

Moreover, many people spend much money on quack treatments, despite numerous proven methods of treatment. Hopes of obtaining miracle cures, combined with limited knowledge of the disease, lead millions of people to try unproven and quack remedies totaling an estimated $1 billion each year (3). Quackery may prevent clients from seeking appropriate care or may even cause them serious harm.

Unfortunately, arthritis is often viewed by many as either a minor problem or a crippling disease. Although there is currently no known cure for this serious health problem, much can be done to prevent or reduce its disabling effects. With teaching and counseling, the nurse can play a vital role in preventing or decreasing the potential impact of arthritis.

In this chapter, discussion will focus on rheumatoid arthritis (RA) and osteoarthritis (OA), the two most prevalent types of arthritis. Using the nursing process framework, this chapter will also describe the care of arthritic clients with the ultimate goals of helping them to develop successful adaptive skills and to function fully in spite of illness.

Overview of Rheumatoid Arthritis

Rheumatoid arthritis (RA) is a chronic systemic inflammatory disease of the synovium that leads eventually to destruction of the joints. The inflammatory process may involve the tendons, ligaments, fascia, and muscle and may extend into the bone. Normally, the synovium consists of cells called synoviocytes, which are known for their phagocytic and excretory functions as well as for lubricating the articular cartilage (6, 9, 12).

There are almost seven million people afflicted with RA in the United States. Prevalence among women is three times that among men. Although RA can occur at any age, the peak incidence of onset occurs in the forty to sixty age-group, and there is an increasing prevalence among elderly people up to age seventy (3, 8).

Etiology

The cause of RA remains unknown. Researchers have focused on several factors, such as autoimmunity, infection, genetics, nutrition, endocrine problems, environment, and psychosocial stress. In spite of numerous and intensive studies, there is no conclusive evidence that these factors are related to the cause of RA. However, more and more researchers believe that an autoimmune response precipitates the inflammation, because of the presence of rheumatoid factors in the synovial fluid and plasma of clients with RA. Rheumatoid factors are antibodies against immunoglobulin G (IgG) (6).

Another factor that is gaining more attention as a possible cause of RA is infection. It has been suggested that there is a "specific initiating external factor" that precipitates autoimmunity. Some researchers believe that the infection is caused by bacteria or virus. Because some viral infections have incited inflammatory rheumatic disorders, the virus is seen as the possible initiator of the immunologic and subsequent inflammatory process in RA (8). It has also been suggested that a decreased function of T-suppressor cells may produce autoimmunity reaction (6).

Other studies have proposed that RA may be a genetic disorder because familial tendencies have been noted. It has been discovered that 54 percent of clients with RA have a certain genetic marker called HLA-DR4 antigen. However, a genetic cause of RA has yet to be identified, since HLA-DR4 has also been found in healthy persons (5, 6).

Pathophysiology

RA can affect a single joint or every joint in the body. The most commonly involved joints are the smaller peripheral joints, such as the proximal interphalangeal, metacarpophalangeal, metatarsophalangeal, wrists, elbows, and ankles, although larger bones like the hips, knees, cervical spine, and temporomandibular joints are frequently involved. There is bilateral or symmetrical involvement of peripheral joints (9).

In RA the affected joint goes through four pathologic stages: (a) synovitis, (b) pannus formation, (c) fibrous ankylosis, and (d) bony ankylosis.

In the first stage, synovitis, the synovium is inflamed, causing pain, warmth, and swelling. Eventually leukocytes, lymphocytes, and plasma cells infiltrate the joints, and fibrin forms. As inflammation continues, synovial joints thicken. The inflamed synovial villi adhere to the surface of the articular cartilage and spread progressively over the cartilage. This inflammatory granulation tissue, called pannus, eventually destroys and erodes the articular cartilage, extending to the joint capsule, surrounding ligaments and subchondral bone. (See Figure 38.1.) If the disease continues to progress, fibrous ankylosis develops, and joint mobility is restricted because of partial or total obliteration of the joint space. Calcification of the fibrous tissue causes bony ankylosis, a firm fusion of the affected joints (6).

Clinical Manifestations

RA occurs insidiously and rapidly, with unexplainable remissions and exacerbations. Severe pain and disability may develop within a number of days. Prodromal symptoms may include fatigue, malaise, anorexia, weight loss, and low-grade fever. The client may indicate the presence of generalized joint pain and stiffness, which lasts for about thirty minutes or so upon waking up in the morning and begins to subside during the day. This morning joint stiffness is typical of inflammatory joint disease and diagnostically important. Other complaints may include cold hands and feet, numbness, and a tingling sensation. This paresthesia may indicate median nerve compression, the cause of carpal tunnel syndrome (7).

Early joint involvement in RA usually begins in the proximal interphalangeal and metacarpophalangeal joints of the hand and the metatarsophalangeal joints of the feet, followed, in a symmetrical pattern, by other joints such as the wrist, elbows, knees, shoulders, and hips. The affected joints are swollen, warm to the touch, tender, and painful. Because of the swelling caused by synovial hypertrophy and effusion, the fingers appear fusiform or spindle-shaped (6).

Pain, an outstanding symptom of RA, may be due to swelling, excessive strain on the capsule and ligaments from effusion within the joint cavity, and inflammation of synovial tissues. The pain is intensified through use of the affected joint and alleviated through rest. Pain leads to limitation of movement of the affected joint and extremity. As the disease progresses, limitation of movement is worsened by the eventual muscle atrophy and tendon involvement, until the joints are completely locked and immobile because of fibrous ankylosis (6, 9).

Joint instability and subluxation (partial dislocation) may occur during the latter part of the disease because of the destructive effects of chronic inflammation on the joints, stretched ligaments and joint capsule, atrophied muscle, and fixed tendons (6). Osteoporosis may also occur as a result of the inflammation within the joint and subsequent joint erosion.

Other deformities seen in RA include subcutaneous nodules (commonly over the elbow), ulnar deviation, hyperextension of the proximal interphalangeal joints ("swan neck" deformity), and flexion of the distal interphalangeal joints (boutonniere deformity). Flexion deformities may affect the hips, the elbows, and the small

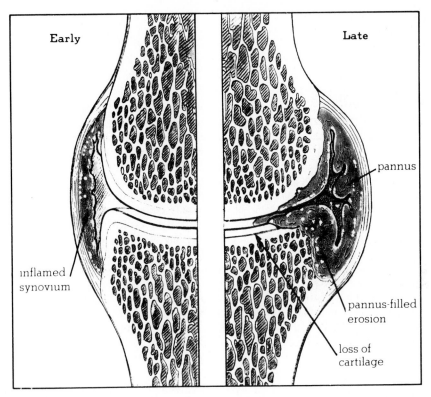

Figure 38.1.   Rheumatoid Arthritis
Source: From M. E. Koerner, "Adult Arthritis: A Look at Some of Its Forms." Reprinted with permission from *American Journal of Nursing,* Vol. 83, No. 2, February 1983, © American Journal of Nursing Company.

joints of the toes and hands; valgus deformities are seen at the knees (6).

Because RA is a systemic inflammatory disorder, it may affect many organs other than the joints. The presence of abnormal immunoglobulin and lymphocytes in the blood may cause inflammation in other parts of the body. When the lungs are involved, there may be pleuritis, pleural effusion, fibrosing alveolitis, and pneumoconiosis (Caplan's syndrome). Pulmonary nodules also may occur and rupture, causing pneumothorax. This involvement causes high morbidity in clients with RA. Myocarditis, pericarditis, and the presence of rheumatoid nodules in the myocardium and in the valves may occur. Ocular manifestations include scleritis, keratoconjunctivitis sicca, and conjunctivitis. Decreased lubrication in the eyes may precipitate corneal ulceration. Carpal tunnel syndrome (paresthesia in the fingers) is a common neuromuscular manifestation of RA. Rheuma-

toid vasculitis may occur and, depending on the size of the vessel involved, may cause either minimal ischemia or total occlusion of the blood vessel and gangrene. Felty's syndrome—which is characterized by splenomegaly, leukopenia, thrombocytopenia, severe anemia, leg ulceration, and lymphadenopathy—is another systemic manifestation of RA. Sjogren's syndrome mainly affects women over fifty years old; it is characterized by decreased salivary and lacrimal secretions due to the presence of lymphocytes in the salivary and lacrimal glands. It occurs also in the trachea, bronchi, vagina, rectum, and nose (6, 8, 9).

Risk Factors

Based on statistics provided by the Arthritis Foundation, RA affects females more than males, by a 3:1 ratio

(3). Age seems to be another risk factor. Although RA affects all age-groups, there is an increasing prevalence among older adults, beginning in middle life.

Prevention and Screening for Early Intervention

In spite of research efforts, the etiology of RA remains unknown. Therefore, prevention is not possible at present. The nurse can, however, play a significant role in screening clients for early intervention.

The nurse's knowledge of the etiological theories, risk factors, incidence rates, and major clinical manifestations of the disease is essential for effective screening of clients for RA. For example, because genetic studies suggest a hereditary influence, special attention should be directed to clients with family histories of RA. There should also be a careful screening of women between the ages of thirty-five and fifty-five because of RA's tendency to afflict women in this age-group. Because RA may be detected early in the course of the disease, in instances of suspected rheumatic disease the nurse should focus on questioning clients regarding the physical manifestations of RA.

Recognizing that education is a significant tool in early detection, the nurse should participate actively in informing the public about the disease, integrating client education into everyday nursing practice. In addition to programs geared to understanding the disease and its treatments, the public should be informed of existing agencies in their communities, such as chapters of the Arthritis Foundation. These provide an array of services, including educational programs, support groups, home living–assistance programs, and research and treatment centers across the country.

Nursing Care

The problems facing anyone with arthritis are multidimensional, and care requires the cooperation and collaboration of all health care professionals. The impact of arthritis on clients and their families is considerable and poses a challenge for the professional nurse. Comprehensive, client-centered nursing care begins with assessment.

Assessment

The emphasis in assessment should be on the client's functional abilities, not the disease condition. The following should serve as a guide to assessment with specific attention to the client as an individual.

Health History. In general, the health history should include major areas such as the present illness, important physical manifestations, past health, family health, and a review of systems.

The history of the present illness in an RA client focuses on the involvement of the musculoskeletal system. In particular, attention should be directed to the clinical manifestations associated with RA. As with other rheumatic diseases, RA's significant manifestations are pain, swelling, limitation of motion, stiffness, weakness, and fatigue. These specific features should encompass details of the manifestations in five dimensions—namely, bodily location, quality and quantity, sequence, aggravating and alleviating factors, and other associated manifestations.

After the history of the present illness is elicited, the client's past health, including information concerning all previous major illnesses, should be discussed. The past history can reveal previous conditions related to the present illness that were not treated or manifestations that were treated differently in the past.

A family tree is an essential tool for recording pertinent data regarding illnesses that might be related to the client's present illness. A number of disorders, such as RA, have suspected genetic influences.

Since RA is a systemic disease, it is important to include a review of systems. This is a final, systematic evaluation of other symptoms or illnesses that the client has or may have had.

Because arthritis affects the client's psychosocial life, the nurse should also focus on the client's psychosocial adaptation to the stress of illness, assessing factors in the client's psychosocial functioning before and during the illness.

The nurse should focus on the client's perceptions and responses to illness, coping skills, and support systems during a stressful event. Special attention should be directed to specific arthritis-related stressors and to the client's adaptive or maladaptive abilities. Other psychosocial areas that are affected by the disease—and should therefore be included—are the client's self-concept, sexuality, and family relationships. In addition, the nurse should elicit information about the client's financial and work situations, activities of daily living (ADL), and social activities.

Physical Assessment. Physical assessment of the client with RA concentrates on the musculoskeletal system. Assessments of joints and skeletal muscles are performed simultaneously. The joint assessment consists of four basic techniques: inspection, palpation, range of motion (ROM), and muscle strength testing. Inspection and palpation are performed first, followed by ROM and muscle strength testing.

Before the physical assessment begins, the client should be told what to expect. The findings can be shared with the client as the assessment is being performed. To ensure accuracy, findings should be recorded immediately. Relaxation and active participation by the client can make the physical assessment more accurate and productive.

The assessment of the musculoskeletal system should proceed in an orderly, logical manner, beginning with observation of the client's posture and gait. The joints are then examined sequentially, starting with the upper extremities and proceeding to the trunk and lower extremities.

The nurse begins by inspecting and palpating simultaneously the joints and extremities of both sides of the body for position and symmetry. Each joint is then assessed for shape, size, skin color, warmth, swelling, tenderness, pain, and deformities. In RA, there are signs of joint inflammation (redness, swelling, warmth, and pain) and tenderness. The most commonly involved joints are the proximal interphalangeal, metacarpophalangeal, and metatarsophalangeal joints. Deformities of the hands and feet are common in RA. Rheumatoid nodules may be present. During palpation, the client may complain of pain or experience tenderness. Handling joints gently helps reduce discomfort.

Muscles are inspected bilaterally for symmetry in size and shape and palpated for tone, tenderness, and pain. Any muscle atrophy or hypertrophy should be noted.

Following inspection and palpation, the nurse assesses the joints for active and passive range of motion. In RA, joint movement is limited; in severe cases, range of motion is diminished markedly. The nurse should note the presence of crepitus. During ROM assessment, complaints of pain and tenderness are elicited from the client. To prevent increased pain and inflammation, a swollen or painful joint should not be ranged fully.

There are a variety of methods to test the client's muscle strength. One method is the grip test, in which the client grasps and squeezes a partially inflated (20 mm Hg) sphygmomanometer cuff. The client performs this procedure three times, and the mean pressure achieved is recorded. Otherwise, the client's muscle strength may

be graded on a 5 through 0 scale (9). Grade 5 indicates that the client has normal strength with complete range of motion against gravity with full resistance. Grade 4 indicates good muscle strength with complete range of motion against gravity with some resistance. Grade 3 indicates fair strength with complete range of motion against gravity. Grade 2 indicates poor strength without complete range of motion against gravity. Grade 1 indicates trace of slight muscle contraction without joint motion. Grade 0 indicates no muscle strength and no indication of muscle contraction (paralysis). Muscle strength and ROM are usually decreased in RA (9).

Diagnostic Tests. In addition to the client's history and the results of the physical assessment, several tests are used to confirm the diagnosis of RA.

Although a nonspecific test, the erythrocyte sedimentation rate (ESR) is a useful index of inflammatory activity. It is usually elevated in RA, though a normal ESR does not necessarily exclude RA (6, 7).

A normocytic anemia that does not respond to iron therapy is common in RA. Usually there is leukocytosis.

Roentgenographic examinations are useful for confirming the diagnosis of RA and following its progress. Soft-tissue swelling is present during the early phase of the disease. Later in the disease process, there are osteoporotic changes around the affected joints, erosions in the cartilage, and narrowed space between joints. Much later, x-rays show obvious destruction of bone ends, with subluxation and other deformities (7).

Synovial fluid aspiration helps determine the presence or absence of infection in the involved joint and the degree of joint inflammation. Normally, the synovial fluid is clear to light yellow in color, is viscous, and contains less that 200 cells per cubic millimeter of leukocytes. Clients with RA have abnormal synovial fluid because of the inflammatory process. Their synovial fluid becomes cloudy and less viscous, and the leukocyte count is increased, usually above 5,000 to 50,000 per cubic millimeter. It is very important that strict asepsis be observed during synovial fluid aspiration. After the test, a small pressure dressing is applied to the involved joint (23).

Eighty-five percent of the clients with RA have rheumatoid factor (RF) antibody against IgG bodies. It should be noted, however, that RF is increased in other conditions, such as tuberculosis, liver disease, bacterial endocarditis, acute viral infections, and syphilis. RFs are found in 3 percent to 5 percent of normal individuals, the incidence increasing with age (7, 23).

Nursing Diagnoses

Based on the clinical manifestations, the health history, the objective and subjective assessment data, and the diagnostic findings, the client's major problems may include:

1. Alteration in comfort related to joint pain and stiffness.
2. Impaired physical mobility related to pain and deformity.
3. Ineffective individual and family coping related to the stress of illness.
4. Disturbance in self-concept related to decrease in body image, self-esteem, identity, and role performance.
5. Sexual dysfunction related to decrease in body image and pain, stiffness, limited ROM.

In addition to the aforementioned nursing diagnoses, there may be alteration in nutrition, sleep pattern disturbance, and dysfunctional grieving.

Planning and Implementation

Once the diagnosis of RA has been established, it is the primary nurse's responsibility to educate the client regarding the disease process, to encourage self-care, and to emphasize the significance of commitment to the therapeutic regimen.

Based on the preceding nursing diagnoses, goals of nursing intervention include relief of pain and discomfort, maintenance of mobility, prevention of deformity, development of effective coping skills, development of positive self-concept, and positive sexual expression and response.

□ *Alteration in Comfort.* Pain is a paramount problem for the client with RA. Although it may vary in intensity, it is often severe and increases with movement. The client may be unable to perform even the simplest activities of daily living. Contractures may develop, leading to total disability.

It is of the utmost importance that the nurse anticipate, assess, and evaluate the type and severity of the client's pain. Everyone perceives pain differently, and it is therefore most reliable to ask the client to describe the pain (perhaps using a pain rating scale) and to express the degree of satisfaction with the present comfort level. The nurse should also assume a primary role in educating the client and family about possible comfort measures.

Measures to relieve pain include rest and proper positioning, application of heat and cold, pharmacologic agents, relaxation techniques, and surgery. Rest helps alleviate pain and inflammation, and is indicated during the acute phase of RA until there is objective and subjective improvement of acute inflammation. Because of differences in opinion regarding the amount of rest required during the acute stage, ten to twelve hours a day of rest has been recommended for some clients, and hospitalization may be necessary. A balanced program of rest and activity is important to prevent muscle atrophy and ankylosis as well as to control fatigue and joint inflammation (7, 21).

Nurses can help clients rest by organizing other activities and therapies around the time the client is not sleeping or resting. While activity is restricted, it is essential that the nurse help prevent contractures and deformities and minimize pain by proper positioning, which is changed at least once every two hours. A firm mattress with footboard, trochanter rolls, and splints to support and maintain proper body alignment should be provided. Measures to prevent flexion deformity and other complications such as thrombophlebitis should be taken while the client is in a supine position. Pillows should not be placed under the knees. A small, thin pillow under the head is preferred to prevent cervical flexion. Splints may be used on the involved joints to help maintain alignment to prevent pain and trauma during moving. Splints should be checked periodically because ill-fitted ones can cause skin damage. The client should be encouraged to lie prone at least twice daily. This helps relax the lower back, hips, and knees and helps maintain functional alignment and prevent hip flexion (43). Skin assessment and care is necessary to prevent breakdown and infection, especially if the client is on steroid therapy.

The nurse should also assess and evaluate the client's psychological status. Psychological rest is just as important as physical rest. The nurse plays an important role in identifying the client's emotions and perceptions regarding pain. Helping the client cope with the severity and chronicity of illness and to develop self-help skills can decrease suffering and enhance self-esteem.

Heat and cold therapy may be used to relieve pain and inflammation. Heat, which helps decrease swelling and relax muscle spasms, may be applied in various ways—locally or to the entire body, moist or dry. Examples are warm moist compresses, warm baths or showers, whirlpool baths, heating pads, ultrasound, and paraffin baths. Cold application may be advised to some clients to decrease pain during acute inflammation.

Clients are taught about the use of heat and cold. Cost and availability should be considered. Hot baths, showers, or soaks are simple and already available at home. The use of baths allows the client to do range-of-motion exercises because of the floating effect of water. Heat reaches its maximal effect in twenty to thirty minutes; more prolonged use of heat is not recommended. Safety precautions, such as protecting the skin during the treatment, should be discussed. Heat and cold applications are contraindicated for clients with poor circulation, decreased sensation, and heat hypersensitivity. Elderly clients should be especially careful when using this treatment (14, 38).

Medications are used to alleviate pain and inflammation. The nurse has a primary role in teaching the client and family about medications. Clients must understand the importance of strict adherence to times and dosage of medications even if pain and inflammation have subsided or they begin to feel better. Because the client has to take multiple medications, a schedule may be helpful. Table 38.1 lists medications used in treating arthritis.

Among the salicylates, acetylsalicylic acid (ASA), commonly known as aspirin, is the most widely used drug during initial treatment. It has analgesic as well as anti-inflammatory effects. The dosage may range from twelve to twenty-four tablets per day in divided doses every three or four hours, depending on the need and response of the client. The serum salicylate level should be tested in order to monitor the treatment's effectiveness. ASA commonly causes gastric irritation and should therefore be taken with food or antacids. Salicylate preparations are available that help decrease gastric irritation; these include enteric coated aspirin (Ecotrin), buffered aspirin (Bufferin), choline salicylate, and magnesium salicylate (28, 31).

Nonsteroidal anti-inflammatory drugs (NSAIDs) are used if clients cannot tolerate salicylates or if their conditions are not adequately controlled by salicylates. Currently available NSAIDs are listed in Table 38.1. Like aspirin, these drugs also have analgesic and anti-inflammatory effects, but they do not change the disease process. Because pain is decreased, function and mobility are maintained; however, manifestations of inflammation recur rather rapidly after they are discontinued (16).

Sometimes, analgesic drugs such as codeine, pentazocine, Darvon, or Tylenol may be prescribed in addition to salicylates or NSAIDs to provide additional pain relief. The client should be informed that these drugs do not decrease the inflammation, and he or she should therefore continue to take the anti-inflammatory medications. Narcotics should be given only when absolutely necessary. The client may easily become addicted because of the chronicity of pain.

Remissive drugs such as gold, d-penicillamine, and hydrochloroquine sulfate may be given in RA when ASA and other NSAIDs fail to control inflammation, pain, or development of bony erosions. These drugs seem to be more effective in causing remission, but it takes several months before the full beneficial effects become evident. They are also more difficult to administer, and close monitoring is needed because of serious adverse effects.

The mechanism of the action of gold is unknown, but it induces remission in many clients and can prevent future structural damage to joints. Myochrysine and Solganol are the most commonly given gold compounds; they are administered intramuscularly. A newer oral preparation, Auranofin, is being made available (31).

Hydrochloroquine sulfate (Plaquenil) is an antimalarial drug that may be used as an alternative to gold or d-penicillamine. It may be given to clients with an early onset of progressive synovitis. Its use requires an eye examination because it can cause severe retinal damage that may lead to irreversible blindness (25).

D-penicillamine has effects similar to those of gold. Its exact mechanism of action is not known, either. It is used to treat clients with severe rheumatoid vasculitis and those who have developed toxic effects from gold (25).

Corticosteroids, the most potent anti-inflammatory agents, are used when there is persistent synovitis and progressive destruction. Because of the potentially serious side effects of long-term use of steroids, small doses are recommended. High doses of intravenous corticosteroids (pulse therapy) may be given at specific intervals during an acute and severe exacerbation of the disease process (31).

Intra-articular corticosteroid injections are sometimes used to suppress inflammation in specific joints and to relieve pain. The effect, though almost immediate, lasts for only a few hours to several weeks. Since a foreign object is being introduced inside the joint, it is imperative that strict aseptic precautions be observed.

Immunosuppressive drugs are also used to treat RA. They are given to clients who develop chronic, aggressive disease that has failed to respond to other types of drug therapy. Because they depress the immune system, immunosuppressive drugs increase the risk of cancer.

Experimental treatment modalities, including plas-

Table 38.1

Drugs Used in Rheumatoid Arthritis and Osteoarthritis

Drug	Action	Side/Toxic Effects	Nursing Implications
Anti-inflammatory Agents Salicylates Aspirin (ASA), sodium salicylate Choline salicylate	Analgesic, anti-inflammatory and antipyretic. Decrease inflammatory process and fever by inhibiting prostaglandins production.	Gastric irritations, bleeding, tinnitus, hearing loss, skin eruptions urticaria, Asthma.	Client should take medication after meals, with food, milk or an antacid, or large amounts of water. Client should take medication regularly to maintain effective levels at 20–30%. Observe bleeding precautions. Client should avoid cuts and bruises. Client should avoid alcohol. Enteric coated and buffered salicylates are available if ASA is not tolerated. Client should avoid other medications containing aspirin.
Nonsteroidal Agents (NSAIDS) Naproxen (Naprosyn) Sulindec (Clinoril) Indomethacin (Indocin) Fenoprofen (Nalfon) Phenylbutazone (Butazolidin) Ibuprofen (Motrin)	Analgesic and anti-inflammatory. Also inhibits the production of prostaglandins.	Nausea and vomitng, gastric irritation, and ulcer, but less frequently than ASA. Headache dizziness, blurred vision, urticaria, and bleeding.	Recommended if client cannot tolerate ASA. Client should take medication with meals, milk, or an antacid. Observe for toxic effects on GIT, blood, renal and CNS. Indocin is not recommended for long-term use. Interferes with diuretics. ASA decreases therapeutic effects when given with indomethacin.
Remittive Drugs Gold compounds Aurothioglucose (Solganal) Gold sodium thiomalate (Myochrysine) Auranofin P.O. is being tested	Anti-inflammatory. Mechanism of action is unknown, but seems to inhibit the activity of lyosomal enzyme, decrease lymphocyte proliferation.	Bone marrow depression, skin rash, mouth ulceration, stomatitis, dermatitis, nephropathy, corneal deposits, liver damage.	Administered intramuscularly. Used when inflammation is not relieved by NSAIDs and salicylates. Slow-acting drugs take 3–6 months to work. Assess for skin rash, dermatitis, mouth lesion, metallic taste in mouth, CBC. Urinalysis before each injection. Discontinue medication if toxic effects occur. Contraindicated in renal and hepatic disorders. Client should avoid exposure to sunlight. Good oral hy-

Drug	Action/Use	Side Effects	Nursing Considerations
			giene to decrease risk of stomatitis. Dimercaprol (BAL) is an antidote to gold overdosage.
Antimalarial Drugs Hydroxychloroquine sulfate (Plaquenil sulfate) Chloroquine hydrochloride & phosphate (Aralen hydrochloride & phosphate) Quinacrine hydrochloride (Atabrine)	Mechanism of action is unknown, but has anti-inflammatory effect. Induces remissions.	Skin rash, hyperpigmentation, headache, dizziness, nausea, retinopathy, blood dyscrasia, bone marrow depression.	Slow-acting drugs, take 3–6 months to take effect. Client should have regular eye examination every 3–4 months because drugs cause retinal damage and blindness. Client should take medication with meals or milk. Contraindicated in hepatic and renal disorder and alcoholism.
3 D-Penicillamine (Cuprimine)	Mechanism of action is unknown, but is presumed to act on immune system and decrease immune complexes in the blood and synovial fluid.	Skin rash, pruritis, blood dyscrasia, "lupuslike" syndrome, myasthenia gravis, loss of sense of taste, nephrotic syndrome.	Onset of action is 3–6 months. Monitor CBC. Urinalysis monthly. Pyrodoxine P.O. is given, since vitamin B_6 absorption is affected by penicillamine. Client should take medication on empty stomach or 2 hours after food or iron intake. Penicillin allergy is not a contraindication.
Corticosteroids Prednisone Prednisolone	Potent anti-inflammatory drugs used to relieve acute exacerbation. Drugs are reserved for clients with intolerable pain and stiffness.	Gastrointestinal tract ulceration, hypertension, edema, hypocalcemia, osteoporosis, prone to infection. Cushingoid features, diabetes, insomnia, decreased healing, adrenal crisis if abruptly withdrawn, cataracts, glaucoma, skin atrophy, and bruising.	Client should take medication with food, antacid, or milk. Client should not increase or decrease or discontinue medication without notifying physician. Monitor side effects such as electrolyte imbalance, edema. Client should carry identification card that states name of drug and dosage. Long-term use of medication should be avoided. Stress will require increase of dosage.
Immunosuppressive Drugs Cyclophosphamide (Cytoxan) Azathioprine (Imuran) Chlorambucil (Leukeran)	Mechanism of action is unknown, but they suppress the immune system	Alopecia, bone marrow suppression, gastrointestinal ulceration, decreased resistance to infection, hemorrhage, cystitis. Carcinogenic.	Monitor blood. Urinalysis weekly. Obtain client's consent before therapy. Client should increase fluid intake. Should not be used in children or women of childbearing age.

mapheresis or lymphoplasmapheresis, thoracic duct drainage, and lymph node irradiation, are being investigated in an effort to find a cure for RA. The immune system, which some investigators believe may be responsible for the inflammatory process in RA, seems to be the main focus for these experimental treatments. Although favorable results have been obtained, more studies examining the therapeutic efficacy of these treatments are needed (16, 40).

Relaxation techniques, such as breathing exercises, meditation, imagery, yoga, and therapeutic touch, can be used in conjunction with other pain-relief measures. Relaxation can help alleviate pain through distraction, decreased fatigue, separating the self from the pain sensation, and increased self-control.

Surgery is indicated when medical management fails. A variety of surgical procedures, such as synovectomy, osteotomy, arthrodesis, and replacement arthroplasty, may be performed to relieve pain caused by the diseased joints, to increase function, and to correct deformities. Surgery for arthritis is no longer performed during the advanced stage of the disease process, though early and aggressive surgery may effectively prevent deformities related to RA (19).

In spite of the successful results of some joint surgeries, it is important that the client be carefully selected and given an adequate preoperative preparation. Factors to evaluate before surgery are the client's present state of joint disease, medical health, age, weight, and attitude toward surgery. Infection and poor skin integrity are contraindications to surgery, as are lack of motivation, inappropriate expectations, and severe psychological problems. The client must be informed and must comprehend fully the surgical procedure and its expected benefits as well as possible complications.

Thorough discharge teaching of the client and family includes activity limitations, exercises, safety precautions, medications, follow-up care, and physical therapy as prescribed.

It is crucial that the client and family understand the importance of following the necessary rehabilitation measures after surgery. The nurse should allay the client's fear and anxiety before discharge. Discharge planning and teaching are initiated early. Referral to community agencies for follow-up care and assistance may facilitate adjustment of the client to the home environment.

Because of the debilitating and crippling effects of RA and OA and persistent pain, clients often resort to "miraculous" treatments and "quack" cures and remedies for pain relief. Even cost is often not a deterrent. Clients

and their families should therefore be warned about the dangers of quack remedies such as herbs, metabolic therapy, special diets, hormones, vaccines, devices, and special clinics; these remedies may delay or interfere with the course of treatment. A better understanding of the disease process helps the client and family avoid such quack remedies.

□ *Impaired Physical Mobility.* Chronic pain and joint swelling in arthritis often limit joint use. Joint inactivity contributes to decreased joint range, diminished muscle strength, and eventually loss of function. Joints may also lose their normal ROM because of deformity and atrophy of muscles. In an effort to avoid pain, clients tend to immobilize the involved joints, even when they know that they need some activity.

The major nursing interventions in helping a client maintain mobility and prevent deformity are a regular schedule of exercise (with balance between rest and activity) and knowledge of body mechanics. The nurse should emphasize to the client that exercise must be carried out on a daily basis because usual activities of daily living (ADL) do not move joints their full range. If the exercises produce pain, the nurse (through assisted exercises) helps the client perform the required motions.

When the client has swollen and painfully inflamed or damaged joints, isometric exercises contract the muscles, and joints are not moved. Isometric contractions must last at least five seconds and be repeated five to six times per day for maximum effectiveness (5). To develop muscle strength, resistive exercises are performed, mainly on non-weight-bearing positions (to prevent additional stress to the joint). Isotonic exercises, which require repetitive joint motion, should be used with caution.

Clients must be supervised until they can perform the aforementioned exercises correctly, without causing additional trauma to affected joints. The nurse observes and evaluates the client's tolerance of the exercise program. During exercises it is not uncommon for clients to complain of pain that persists for a short time. However, pain that lasts for more than a half-hour after exercises may indicate that the exercises are excessive and that modifications are needed. To help decrease pain and to facilitate movement, the nurse reinforces the use of heat and cold applications, analgesics, stress reduction, and relaxation techniques before exercise.

When physical therapy is prescribed, the nurse collaborates with the therapist on the client's program of exercises. Physical therapy is significant because it prevents and corrects deformities, strengthens weakened muscles, and improves functioning. Deformities are prevented and corrected by a program of vigorous positioning and an active exercise program.

There should be a balance between therapeutic exercise and rest. Too much of either can be harmful. When clients complain of fatigue, their exercise tolerance must be evaluated. Overactivity can aggravate rather than reduce joint symptoms. When acute inflammation occurs, rest may be more important than exercise. Joint rest is essential for protecting inflamed or damaged joints.

Resting affected joints involves the use of splints, traction, assistive devices, and other mechanical devices. Simple splints support the joints in optimal position to relieve pain and help prevent deformity. Traction may help relieve compression on nerve roots. Canes, crutches, and other mechanical devices are helpful for local support when weight-bearing joints are involved.

Self-care, with special attention to the individual client's limitations, is encouraged. Because clients may experience pain and stiffness when they move, they should not be rushed during activities. Correct posture and body mechanics should be emphasized at all times. Clients should be informed about the variety of self-care appliances designed to help them maintain their maximum level of independence. These include such things as eating utensils with special handles, long-handled combs, and specially elevated toilet seats and chairs.

There is no specific dietary regimen in the treatment of arthritis, although a well-balanced diet is recommended. If a client is obese, a weight-reducing diet may help to relieve joints of the stress of supporting excessive amounts of weight.

☐ *Ineffective Individual and Family Coping.* Stress threatens one's equilibrium and challenges one's adaptive abilities. Because it affects every aspect of the client's life, arthritis imposes various physical and psychosocial stressors on the client and family, placing a burden on their repertoire of coping mechanisms. Moreover, since these stressors threaten the client's physical integrity and self-system simultaneously, the potential for taxing the client's and family's coping abilities is greater. Faced with this stressful event, both the client and family are vulnerable to situational crisis.

The chronic, unpredictable nature of arthritis engenders an array of emotional responses. As the client perceives that his or her self-system is threatened, feelings of anxiety, anger, hostility, depression, and alienation may emerge. Anxiety, in all its expressions and with all its concomitant somatic manifestations, becomes the predominant emotional reaction.

The nurse plans care directed toward helping the client and family identify anxiety-producing stressors and use effective coping skills. Adapting successfully to the stress of arthritis can reduce the potential occurrence of situational crisis.

Through an atmosphere of unconditional acceptance, the nurse encourages the client and family to acknowledge and verbalize their feelings of anxiety. Such emotional reactions, it should be stressed, are normal. In accepting the client's and family's feelings of anxiety, the nurse must continually clarify personal feelings without reciprocal anxiety, which can have detrimental effects on the therapeutic process.

After acknowledging the presence of anxiety, it is important to discuss its possible causes. By active listening, the nurse can help the client and family identify specific stressors. Often it is the nurse, as the most constant provider of care, to whom the client and family express their problems. The nurse must therefore use every opportunity to respond in a manner that helps them build their coping skills.

The nurse should determine the client's and family's past experiences and ways of coping with stressful situations. If coping mechanisms have been adaptive, the nurse encourages their use. For example, denial may be used as an effective mechanism for allaying anxiety immediately after a stressful event. If denial is gradually eliminated as the stress begins to subside, the individual may better adapt to the situation (15). When coping mechanisms are ineffective, the nurse can share perceptions regarding their ineffectiveness and assist the client and family in exploring new and effective coping mechanisms.

One way of helping the client and family to cope is to reexamine the nature of the stressors. Is the appraisal of the situation realistic? Do the client and family have accurate information about the disease? For example, if they have anxieties and fears about the crippling effects of arthritis, emphasize that such effects can be prevented. Educating the client and family about the disease process is vital. Information helps to defuse anxieties and to identify realities with which they must deal.

Self-help groups such as those conducted by local chapters of the Arthritis Foundation can provide excellent support for the client and family. Community resources, social networks, relationships with family and friends, and spiritual strength may all be drawn upon. Physical activity and relaxation techniques may be helpful in reducing anxiety.

Because stress is fundamental to the human condition and life is not totally anxiety-free, the nurse encourages the client and family to tolerate mild anxiety and use its constructive aspects. During mild anxiety, when the perceptual field is increased, learning tends to peak.

When the usual repertoire of coping skills proves ineffective in dealing with stress, the level of anxiety rises and a crisis emerges. Through anticipatory guidance, the nurse can help the client and family to resolve a crisis. Using Aguilera's framework on crisis intervention, the nurse focuses on balancing factors such as perception of the event, situational supports, and coping mechanisms (1). The nurse aids the client and family in understanding the impact of crisis and resolving accompanying issues. Clarification of issues facilitates perception of cause-and-effect relationships. Efforts by the nurse are directed first toward support and recognition of effective coping skills. The nurse then encourages the appropriate use of support systems. For additional information about stress and crisis, the reader is referred to chapters 15 and 16.

Successful crisis resolution is more likely to occur if one's perception of the event is realistic, if there are available support systems, and if coping mechanisms alleviate anxiety. When the client's and family's coping skills are weakened, the nurse can provide extra support until they regain equilibrium.

□ *Disturbance in Self-Concept.*   Because of the chronicity of the disease, combined with the resultant alterations in physical and psychosocial functions, arthritis can present a continuing threat to the client's self-concept. Self-concept can be altered by arthritis-related stressors affecting one's body image, self-esteem, role performance, and identity. Disturbances in self-concept create a stressful situation for the client and family. Often, clients experience a change in feelings and perceptions about themselves, with a concomitant decrease in self-worth. Because of long-standing illness, the client may constantly be faced with feelings of worthlessness.

Changes in physical appearance obviously affect body image. The significance of a change in body image is influenced by one's perception of the alteration. The greater the significance of body image within one's self-concept, the greater the threat that an altered body image may be to one's perception of self.

The deformities caused by arthritis may also affect the client's self-esteem and identity. Side effects from long-term corticosteroids therapy, such as obesity, buffalo hump, moon face, and ecchymosis, can lead to perceived loss of physical attractiveness. Moreover, chronic pain, stiffness, and limited ROM may reduce the client's efforts to attend to physical appearance.

The client with physical disabilities may feel unattractive and may withdraw from social activities, resulting in the inability to maintain relationships or meet members of the opposite sex. Relationships between spouses may be threatened. Because of the spouse's fears and concerns about the client's condition, patterns of sexual expression may change.

Manifestations of role strain are reflected in one's role performance. Role strain, which may be expressed by the client as feelings of frustration or inadequacy, can lead to altered role performance. This is characterized by changes in the client's self-perception of role and the ability to maintain family roles. Furthermore, arthritis can interfere with the client's capacity to assume roles in work and other social situations.

With regard to role performance, the client is especially threatened during exacerbations of the disease. As the client becomes aware of limitations in role performance, conflicts between reality and personal expectations of productivity and independence may arise. Independence is threatened when clients must ask for assistance with self-care activities from their families; concerns about becoming a burden are intensified. As clients lose independence, social withdrawal may occur. Loss of independence can be devastating to one's ego. The client's altered role performance may also affect self-esteem and identity.

In helping the client achieve a positive self-concept, interventions focus on the client's adaptation to changes affecting body image, roles, self-esteem, and identity.

Because the client's self-worth is reduced, it is important that the nurses analyze their own feelings of worthlessness. Through this introspective analysis, nurses can establish an empathic relationship with the client. Equally significant is the nurse's ability to identify the signs of disturbed self-concept. Through an accepting attitude, the nurse encourages clients to discuss feelings regarding specific stressors that affect self-concept. By encouraging discussion, the nurse can correct misconceptions and can communicate that emotional reactions to the changes produced by arthritis are acceptable.

To effectively provide care, nurses should be aware of their potential negative and positive impact on the client's self-concept. Accepting clients as worthy human beings despite physical alterations can stimulate positive self-perceptions.

The nurse should be sensitive to and support behaviors indicating that clients are starting to adapt to physical alterations. For example, clients may begin to discuss real or imagined changes in themselves or express anger, rage, or grief while discussing physical alterations. While nurses accept the clients' negative feelings or negative perceptions about themselves, they also assist clients in recognizing the positive aspects of their personalities. It is critical that nurses reinforce realistic perceptions. Clients need time to adapt to the changes affecting their self-concepts. Through a supportive environment, the nurse can help them proceed through recognized stages of adaptation—shock, panic, defensive retreat, acknowledgment, and adaptation (42).

To foster clients' sense of control, the nurse enlists their participation in decisions affecting care and promotes client independence and self-management. Encouraging self-care activities and providing positive reinforcement will also enhance clients' self-esteem. Bearing in mind clients' limitations and strengths, the nurse includes activities in which they will achieve some success.

Because changes in client roles affect families, the nurse should likewise involve the family when planning care. During exacerbations of the disease, the family may need to assist the client in ADL and fulfill the client's usual roles in the family. As a result, the family may need to reorganize their life-style, often changing family dynamics. Thus, it is essential to encourage the client and family to maintain effective communication. Moreover, the client should be encouraged to maintain social activities and relationships with friends and peers. The nurse should also provide information about community support groups.

Stuart and Sundeen propose a step-by-step approach to help a client achieve a positive self-concept (41). This approach begins with the client's self-awareness, self-exploration, and self-evaluation of all aspects of personality, particularly in relation to the present stressful situation. Once insight into problems is developed, the client formulates realistic goals, which consist of possible solutions, including adaptive behaviors. Finally, the client must be committed to achieving these goals. It is important for the nurse to support clients while they proceed through this step-by-step approach.

Continuing support and understanding from the nurse and family can provide a sense of stability until the client achieves a positive self-concept.

□ *Sexual Dysfunction.* Broadly defined, sexuality encompasses the physical, emotional, and social aspects of the client's sexual being and behavior. It includes a desire for warmth, intimacy, contact, tenderness, and love. Sexual concerns and problems are common in arthritis because the disease can interfere with many physical and psychosocial aspects of normal sexuality.

Numerous factors can contribute to sexual dysfunction. Arthritis superimposes on the normal concerns and problems of sexual adjustments the compounding factor of chronic disease and potential disability. In a client with arthritis, sexual concerns and problems may arise from mechanical problems due to pain, stiffness, and limited ROM. These problems can present obstacles to the client's capacity for sexual expression and response. Arthritic involvement of the hip, knees, and lumbar spine may also cause mechanical problems that interfere with sexual performance. Because of restrictions in joint mobility, some clients may have difficulty assuming a comfortable position during sexual intercourse.

Sexual identity is a major part of self-concept. Therefore, changes in self-concept will lead to changes in sexuality, and vice versa.

Disturbed self-concept engenders various emotional reactions. Depression, for example, slows all body functions and decreases libido. It must be recognized that physical and psychosocial alterations produced by arthritis can lead to a generalized state of ill health, which in turn can lead to diminished libido. Additionally, drug therapy—particularly corticosteroids—can reduce sexual drive.

When caring for a client with sexual dysfunction, it is of the utmost importance for the nurse to involve the client's sexual partner in all aspects of care. In general, clients should be encouraged to maintain a closer relationship and open communication with their sexual partners and to have a positive attitude toward sexuality.

In the initial phase of the nurse-client relationship, the nurse communicates to the client that topics related to sexuality are acceptable. An atmosphere of acceptance and a nonjudgmental attitude help the client to discuss freely any sexual concerns or problems. Because of the personal and sensitive nature of the subject, some clients may be embarrassed to ask direct questions related to sexuality. Being sensitive to clues helps the nurse recognize when the client has a concern in this area.

Sexual counseling is an integral part of the nurse's role. To counsel clients effectively, nurses must examine their own values and belief systems related to sexual behaviors. A critical factor is the level of self-awareness, which has a direct impact on the ability to counsel effectively. It is vital for nurses to respect the client's sexual attitudes and clarify their own to prevent conflicts during counseling.

To help make sexual activity possible and comfortable for the client, nurses can reinforce certain measures to relieve some of the physical and psychological manifestations of the disease. These measures include the use of warm baths or showers, stress reduction and relaxation techniques, and analgesics before sexual intercourse. Consideration must be given to alternative positions during sexual intercourse. For clients with back pain, a lateral position may be preferable. With increased disability in women, intercourse may be possible if a posterior approach is used by the man. A sidelying position may alleviate problems in the joints of the hands and arms. Problems in these joints may interfere with foreplay. Arthritis can also force a client to find alternative ways of sexual expression. In this instance, it is imperative that the nurse explore with the client alternative methods of meeting sexual needs.

Evaluation

Specific criteria for evaluating the outcome of nursing interventions are directed toward nursing diagnoses.

Alteration in Comfort

1. The client will use measures to prevent or manage pain (e.g., rest, heat and cold treatment, anti-inflammatory agents, and relaxation techniques).
2. The client will perform measures to increase stability and mobility after surgery (e.g., exercises to strengthen muscles) and will ambulate progressively better until no assistive device is needed.

Impaired Physical Mobility

1. The client will demonstrate competence in performing a program of exercise to maintain joint movement and muscle strength and to prevent deformity. Also, the client will evaluate his or her need for rest when the exercises result in fatigue. With a regular program of exercise, improved mobility without any manifestations of deformity should be expected.
2. The client will use correct body mechanics to maintain optimal mobility.

Ineffective Individual and Family Coping

1. The client and family will use effective adaptive strategies in dealing with specific arthritis-related stressors.
2. The client and family will utilize available resources. The client will maintain relationships with friends and peers and will participate in social activities or use community resources such as those provided by the Arthritis Foundation.

Disturbance in Self-Concept

1. The client will verbalize feelings regarding specific arthritis-related changes that affect body image, self-esteem, roles, and identity. The client will share feelings with the nurse and family.
2. The client will use effective strategies to cope with altered roles, which directly affect self-concept. For example, the client will accept assistance from his or her family during exacerbations of the disease and will perform self-care when able.

Sexual Dysfunction

1. The client will discuss with the nurse or sexual partner his or her feelings regarding sexual concerns and problems associated with arthritis.
2. The client will demonstrate competence in performing measures designed to facilitate comfortable sexual activity. These measures include use of heat applications, relaxation techniques, and analgesics prior to sexual activity or use of alternative positions or methods of sexual expression.

Overview of Osteoarthritis

Osteoarthritis (OA), also known as degenerative or senescent arthritis, is the most common form of arthritis. Unlike RA, it is a nonsystemic disease and is characterized primarily by degeneration of articular cartilage.

There are about 16 million people with OA in the United States (3). The disease affects both men and women, with prevalence being greater in men under age forty-five and in women over age fifty-five. However, the disease has universal prevalence by age eighty, as evidenced by radiographic examination (44). It is known to be the leading cause of joint pain and subsequent disablement in middle-aged and elderly individuals (7).

Etiology

The exact cause of OA is not yet known. However, certain factors may contribute to its development. Although there is a higher incidence of the disease among the elderly, specialists now believe that OA is not an inevitable part of aging, claiming that it is more likely the result of sustained exposure to pathophysiological processes during early years in life. It is not clear how aging relates to the onset of OA because of the difference in the biochemical alterations seen in OA and aging (29).

Risk Factors

Several groups are at risk for OA. Age is a high-risk factor: the elderly are more prone to develop OA because of physiological changes in the joints from repeated mechanical stresses to the joints over time (29).

Occupation is another risk factor. Studies indicate that OA is prevalent among individuals exposed to prolonged and/or excessive stresses, which may create inordinate wear and hypertrophic remodeling reactions in some joints (20, 29). Examples of these individuals are miners, athletes, farmers, and dock workers.

Sex is also considered a risk factor. Females, especially those over fifty-five years of age, have not only a higher incidence of OA but also more severe, multiple-joint involvement. Experimental studies have suggested that estrogens may have a protective effect against OA, although there is no conclusive evidence (29). However, males under age forty-five are also predisposed to OA.

There is a possible familial predisposition to OA; studies have shown that Heberden's nodes are three times as common in sisters of women with OA as in others (29).

Research has shown that obesity is a predisposing factor in OA because it causes increased stress on weight-bearing joints (29).

Other risk factors include injury, joint surgery, fracture, previous joint disorder, prolonged immobility, and developmental defects such as bowleg deformity.

Pathophysiology

Unlike rheumatoid arthritis, in which the alterations are seen in the synovium, in OA pathologic changes (specifically, progressive degeneration and destruction) take place in the articular cartilage. Normally, the articular cartilage is a white, translucent material that covers the end of the bone and acts as a shock absorber by providing a smooth surface between the bones.

OA affects primarily the weight-bearing joints (hips and knees), the terminal interphalangeal joints of the fingers, and the lumbar and cervical spines. However, other joints can be involved.

As a result of the joint's repeated exposure to mechanical stresses, there is an altered balance between the mechanical demands and joint durability. The articular cartilage loses its elasticity and eventually its ability to absorb shock.

OA occurs in three stages: first, there is degeneration of the articular cartilage; second, remodeling of bone; and third, formation of new bone. The degeneration of the articular cartilage is related to the breakdown of its essential component (called chondrocyte), resulting in the destruction of the cartilage and, indirectly, in the stiffening of the subchondral bone (13, 20, 36). Once this occurs, the protective function of the cartilage is impaired. Continued stress on the joint is likely to cause further damage and breakdown of the collagen network that holds the articular cartilage together. As the cartilage wears away, the surface of the bone is exposed, new bone forms, and bony spurs form at the joint margins (36). (See Figure 38.2.) Eventually, mechanical interference of joint function ensues.

Clinical Manifestations

OA has an insidious onset, with manifestations usually not appearing before age forty. Unlike RA, OA does not have systemic effects and does not cause severe debilitation and crippling.

Pain is its primary symptom. The client usually describes having an obscure, aching pain during and after activity. It is relieved by rest. As the disease progresses, the pain may persist even during rest. Pain at night may also occur, especially when the disease process becomes severe (29).

The articular cartilage is insensitive to pain, but the joint capsule and associated tendons, periosteum, and ligaments are highly sensitive. The alterations that take place in the articular cartilage during the disease process stimulate the nerve endings of the joint capsule, thus causing the pain of OA (13).

The pain in OA may be associated with stiffness. The joint stiffness of OA differs from that of RA in that it is localized to involved joints and lasts for shorter durations (less than thirty minutes). It is more pronounced upon awakening and after periods of rest during the day. The pain may also be related to weather, although

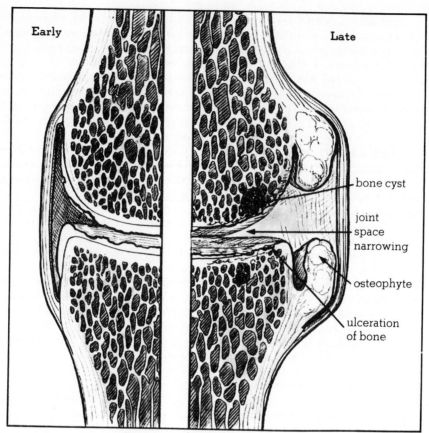

Figure 38.2. Osteoarthritis

Source: From M. E. Koerner, "Adult Arthritis: A Look at Some of Its Forms." Reprinted with permission from *American Journal of Nursing,* Vol. 83, No. 2, February 1983, © American Journal of Nursing Company.

the nature of the relationship is unclear. The stiffness of OA is not as severe as that of RA, but limitation of joint movement may occur as the disease progresses. Pain, muscle spasms, and contracture compound this problem (29).

Crepitus or crunching of the involved joint may be heard or palpated. This is related to coarsened or roughened joint surface and loss of cartilage.

OA is also characterized by the presence of joint enlargement. This may occur because of the proliferation of bone spurs or the development of secondary synovitis, which occurs particularly in the knees.

OA is accompanied by characteristic hand deformities. Heberden's nodes are bony enlargements in the distal interphalangeal joints of the fingers. Bouchard's nodes are bony swellings occurring at the proximal interphalangeal joints. These hand deformities may cause pain, numbness, and decreased hand dexterity (29).

Prevention and Screening for Early Intervention

The exact cause of OA is still unknown. Since prevention is not yet possible, efforts should be directed toward screening clients for early intervention.

A number of factors predisposing individuals to OA have been identified. Attention to these factors is valuable during the screening process. The factors include aging, obesity, family history of the disease, previous joint trauma, athletics, and abuse or strenuous physical labor in any age-group. In addition to the predisposing factors, questions regarding the physical manifestations of OA should be asked of the client when the disease is suspected.

Finally, the significance of the nurse's involvement in educating the public regarding the disease cannot be overemphasized. Educational programs should include community resources for the client and family.

Nursing Care

Assessment of the client with OA follows the same plan described earlier for the client with RA.

A review of the client's history, laboratory data, diagnostic findings, and x-ray results are all essential in collecting objective data.

Health History. The health history of a client with OA consists of data regarding the client's present illness, past health, and family history, with emphasis on the development of the disease, including details of its physical manifestations. These include pain, swelling, limitation of motion, stiffness, and weakness.

Pain, the most common manifestation of OA, is more pronounced with activity and is relieved by rest. The OA client usually complains of stiffness after periods of rest, and morning stiffness, which is more pronounced after rising, usually lasts for less than thirty minutes.

Psychosocial assessment of OA clients is found in the discussion of RA clients.

The focus of the physical assessment in OA, like RA, is the musculoskeletal system, using the techniques of inspection, palpation, ROM, and muscle-strength testing. Descriptions of the techniques for joint assessment are found in the discussion of RA.

In addition to the general aspects of joint assessment, the nurse should be knowledgeable about the major characteristics of OA. The nurse inspects the joints for swelling that may indicate effusion or synovitis. The finger joints are frequently involved, although OA usually occurs in weight-bearing joints. In OA, the distal interphalangeal and the proximal interphalangeal joints are characteristically involved. Bony nodules may be present, and on inspection and palpation, these may prove inflamed or painful. Crepitus may be heard or palpated, if present.

With OA, ROM is usually limited, and when the disease is severe, ROM is greatly reduced. Assessment of the vertebral column should be included because it is usually involved in clients with OA.

Diagnostic Tests. Roentgenographic examination is the most useful diagnostic tool in confirming the diagnosis of OA. It shows the characteristic alterations and/or changes in the involved joint(s). It also helps in assessing the severity of joint damage. X-ray findings may reveal narrowing of joint space, appearance of osteophytes or spurs at the marginal aspects of the joints, bone sclerosis, and subluxation (which is a late finding) (13).

Serologic results in OA are normal, unless the client has other health problems. The rheumatoid-factor test is negative, although it may be positive among older clients. False positive rheumatoid factor increases with age among normal individuals (36).

Examination of the synovial fluid, which is viscous, clear, and "noninflammatory" in OA clients, will not help in the diagnosis of OA, though it may rule out synovitis, infection, and hemiarthrosis (13).

Bone and joint scanning are useful in assessing the extent and severity of OA (29).

Nursing Diagnoses

Based on the clinical manifestations, health history, objective and subjective assessment data, and diagnostic findings, the client's major problems may include:

1. Alteration in comfort related to joint pain and stiffness.
2. Impaired physical mobility related to pain and deformity.
3. Ineffective individual and family coping related to the stress of illness.
4. Disturbance in self-concept related to decrease in body image, self-esteem, identity, and role performance.
5. Sexual dysfunction related to decrease in body image and to pain, stiffness, and limited ROM.

These major problems may be accompanied by alteration in nutrition, sleep pattern disturbance, and dysfunctional grieving.

Planning and Implementation

General goals related to the aforementioned nursing diagnoses are relief of discomfort and pain, maintenance of mobility and prevention of deformity, effective individual and family coping skills, positive self-concept, and positive sexual expression and response.

Alteration in Comfort. The measures for pain relief for the OA client are basically the same as those for the RA client. However, some variations do exist.

Bed rest is not necessary, although rest of the affected joints is helpful in alleviating the pain and may help delay the progression of the disease process (28). The client and family should be taught how to differentiate pain from stiffness. Stiffness in OA occurs after prolonged periods of rest. Therefore, the client should be instructed to avoid sitting for long periods of time. It should be stressed that pain can be relieved by preventing undue stress or movement of the affected joints through rest and alteration of activities of daily living. A balance of rest and activity is essential for the client's health.

Heat application is an integral part of the treatment program. Moist heat is preferred to dry heat because of its better conductive properties. Therapeutic exercises should be encouraged during and after the treatment.

Pharmacologic agents used to treat OA are not as extensive as those used with RA. There is no known drug to prevent the degenerative process that takes place in OA, although drugs are available that relieve pain. Salicylates seem to be the drugs of choice for this. NSAIDs may be prescribed primarily for their analgesic effect, not for their anti-inflammatory effect. Systemic steroid treatment is not recommended. However, intra-articular injections of steroids may temporarily relieve the pain. (See Table 38.1.)

The use of appropriate assistive devices, such as canes, crutches, or walkers, will help decrease stress on weight-bearing joints, thus minimizing pain. Splints and other supportive appliances (e.g., cervical collar) can be helpful and effective in relieving pain as well.

Although the client is taught by the physical therapist, reinforcement is an important nursing responsibility. The cane should be used on the opposite side of the involved joint. Attention to good posture and body mechanics should also be emphasized. Since a large majority of clients with OA are elderly, safety precautions should be reiterated to both client and family.

It may be necessary to allay the client's fear of assistive devices. Some clients refuse to use these devices because they believe they will be labeled "crippled" or will become dependent on them.

Weight reduction is recommended for obese clients. Excess weight puts added strain on involved joints, notably the hips and knees.

Surgery may be performed to relieve pain and correct deformity. Procedures include osteotomy, arthrodesis, arthroplasty, and total joint replacement. These surgical interventions were discussed previously under rheumatoid arthritis.

Although gross deformities are not seen in osteoarthritis, the intervention for nursing diagnoses 2–5 is essentially the same as that described for the client with rheumatoid arthritis.

Evaluation

Expected outcomes for the evaluation of nursing interventions for the OA client are similar to those for the RA client.

Ethical Issues

Ethical issues in the treatment of arthritis relate primarily to the person's right to self-determination and respect as an individual. Arthritic clients vary in the degree of their disability and, consequently, in their ability for self-management. A major goal of care for arthritic clients is self-management. The nurse and family must both decide when to intervene in assisting the client. How much independence is possible, given the client's level of disability, and when and how should others intervene? Allowing clients to struggle with self-care that is painful and beyond their capabilities sometimes leads to frustration and a sense of defeat and failure. Yet too much intervention too soon can lead to a feeling of being deprived of the right to try. Clients may feel they are being treated like children and may become resentful. Getting to know the client well and being sensitive to cues about feelings and attitudes toward care can help the nurse deal constructively with these issues.

CASE STUDY

Ms. Beatrice Josephs is a forty-five-year-old mother of two sons, aged twelve and ten. She works part time in a delicatessen managed by her husband. She describes herself to the nurse as an "outgoing person," saying, "I like to keep myself busy all the time."

Ms. Josephs has been diagnosed as having RA for a year now. At present, she reports to the nurse that she experiences pain, morning stiffness, and joint swelling, which became severe in the past two months. Because of these manifestations, she has had to curtail some of her social activities with friends.

Further, she says that her daily chores at home, such as cooking, cleaning the house, and doing the laundry, tire her easily.

She also states that her family understands her condition. She says that although her husband is supportive, they have limited time together because of her husband's busy schedule.

1. Identify further data to collect regarding Ms. Josephs's physical manifestations.
2. Differentiate her physical manifestations from those seen in clients with OA.
3. Describe specific nursing measures to assist Ms. Josephs in relieving her pain, morning stiffness, and joint swelling.
4. Identify Ms. Josephs's potential psychosocial disturbances.
5. Describe specific nursing measures to assist Ms. Josephs in dealing with her potential psychosocial disturbances.

REFERENCES

1. Aguilera, D. C., and J. M. Messick. *Crisis Intervention: Theory and Methodology.* 4th ed. St. Louis: C. V. Mosby Co., 1982.
2. Amstutz, H., and W. Kim. "Osteoarthritis of the Hip." In *Osteoarthritis: Diagnosis and Management,* ed. R. Moskowitz et al. Philadelphia: W. B. Saunders Co., 1984.
3. Arthritis Foundation. *Arthritis: A Serious Look at the Facts.* Atlanta: Arthritis Foundation, 1984.
4. Arthritis Medical Information Service. *Rheumatoid Arthritis.* Atlanta: Arthritis Foundation, 1984.
5. Banwell, B. F. "Exercise and Mobility." *Nursing Clinics of North America,* 1984, 19:605.
6. Barnes, C. G. "Rheumatoid Arthritis." In *Mason and Currey's Clinical Rheumatology,* ed. H. L. Currey. United Kingdom: Pitman Press, 1980, 30–60.
7. Beeson, P., and W. McDermott. *Cecil-Loeb Textbook of Medicine.* Philadelphia: W. B. Saunders Co., 1971.
8. Bennett, C. J. "Rheumatoid Arthritis." In *Cecil Textbook of Medicine,* ed. J. B. Wyngaarden and L. H. Smith. Philadelphia: W. B. Saunders Co., 1985, 1911–17.
9. Bluestone, R. "Rheumatoid Arthritis." In *Rheumatology,* ed. R. Bluestone. Boston: Houghton Mifflin Professional Publishers, 1980, 129–41.
10. Brassell, M. P. "Rehabilitation Nursing and the Surgical Patient." In *Rheumatology,* ed. R. Bluestone. Boston: Houghton Mifflin Professional Publishers, 1980.
11. Burckhardt, C. S. "The Impact of Arthritis on Quality of Life." *Nursing Research,* 1985, 34:11.
12. Cracchiolo, A. "The Surgical Approach to Degenerative Joint Disease." In *Rheumatology,* ed. R. Bluestone. Boston: Houghton Mifflin Professional Publishers, 1980, 77–90.
13. Currey, H. L. "Osteoarthritis." In *Mason and Currey's Clinical Rheumatology.* United Kingdom: Pitman Press, 1980, 96–105.
14. Downey, J. "The Psychiatrist in Arthritic Management." In *Rehabilitation Management of Rheumatic Conditions.* ed. G. E. Ehrlich. Baltimore: Williams and Wilkins, 1980, 29–35.
15. Elliot, S. "Denial as an Effective Mechanism to Allay Anxiety Following a Stressful Event." *Journal of Psychiatric Nursing,* 1980, 18:11.
16. Furst, D. E. "Nonsteroidal Anti-inflammatory Drugs." In *Rheumatology,* ed. R. Bluestone. Boston: Houghton Mifflin Professional Publishers, 1980, 235–45.
17. Groer, M. E., and M. E. Shekleton. *Basic Pathophysiology: A Conceptual Approach.* St. Louis: C. V. Mosby Co., 1979.
18. Hawley, D. J. "Nontraditional Treatments of Arthritis." *Nursing Clinics North America,* 1984, 19:663.
19. Hedley, A., and A. Cracchiolo. "The Role of Surgery." In *Rheumatology,* ed. R. Bluestone. Boston: Houghton Mifflin Professional Publishers, 1980.
20. Howell, D. F. "Osteoarthritis." In *Cecil Textbook of Medicine,* ed. J. B. Wyngaarden and L. H. Smith. Philadelphia: W. B. Saunders Co., 1985, 1951–54.
21. Johnson, J. A., and E. C. Repp. "Nonpharmacologic Pain Management in Arthritis." *Nursing Clinics of North America,* 1984, 19:583.
22. Kaufman, M. "Complications from Arthritic Surgery." In *Rehabilitation Management of Rheumatic Conditions,* ed. G. E. Ehrlich. Baltimore: Williams and Wilkins, 1980.
23. Kee, J. L. *Laboratory and Diagnostic Tests with Nursing Implications.* East Norwalk, Conn.: Appleton-Century-Crofts, 1983.
24. Koerner, M. E., and G. R. Dickinson. "Adult Arthritis: A Look at Some of Its Forms." *American Journal of Nursing,* 1983, 83:255.
25. Louis, J. S. "Additional Drugs for Rheumatoid Arthritis." In *Rheumatology,* ed. R. Bluestone. Boston: Houghton Mifflin Professional Publishers, 1980, 246–51.
26. Meenan, R. F., et al. "The Costs of Rheumatoid Arthritis." *Arthritis and Rheumatism,* 1978, 21:827.
27. Meenan, R. F., et al. "The Impact of Chronic Disease: A Sociomedical Profile of Rheumatoid Arthritis." *Arthritis and Rheumatism,* 1981, 24:544.
28. Moskowitz, R. W. *Clinical Rheumatology.* 2d ed. Philadelphia: Lea & Febiger, 1982.
29. Moskowitz, R. W., et al. *Osteoarthritis: Diagnosis and Management.* Philadelphia: W. B. Saunders Co., 1984.
30. Moskowitz, R. W. "Osteoarthritis: Signs and Symptoms." In *Osteoarthritis: Diagnosis and Management,* ed. R. W. Moskowitz et al. Philadelphia: W. B. Saunders Co., 1984, 149–54.
31. Neuberger, G. B. "The Role of the Nurse with Patients on Drug Therapy." *Nursing Clinics of North America,* 1984, 19:593.
32. Pigg, J. S. "Nursing Care of the Hospitalized Patient with Rheumatoid Arthritis." In *Rehabilitation Management of*

Rheumatic Conditions, ed. G. E. Ehrlich. Baltimore: Williams and Wilkins, 1980, 76–103.

33. Pigg, J. S., and P. M. Schroeder. "Frequently Occurring Problems of Patients with Rheumatic Diseases." *Nursing Clinics of North America,* 1984, 19:697.

34. Polley, H. F., and G. G. Hunder, *Physical Examination of the Joints.* 2d ed. Philadelphia: W. B. Saunders Co., 1978, 1–44.

35. Porth, C. *Pathophysiology: Concepts of Altered Health Status.* Philadelphia: J. B. Lippincott, 1982.

36. Price, S., and L. M. Wilson. *Pathophysiology: Clinical Concepts of Disease Processes.* 2d ed. New York: Mc-Graw-Hill Book Co., 1982.

37. Reza, M. "Extraarticular Manifestations of Rheumatoid Arthritis." In *Rheumatology,* ed. R. Bluestone. Boston: Houghton Mifflin Professional Publishers, 1980, 142–60.

38. Simpson, C. "Heat, Cold or Both." *American Journal of Nursing,* 1983, 83:270.

39. Spitz, P. W. "The Medical, Personal, and Social Costs of Rheumatoid Arthritis." *Nursing Clinics of North America,* 1984, 19:575.

40. Strands, C., and S. Clark. "Adult Arthritis: Drugs and Remedies." *American Journal of Nursing,* 1983, 83:266.

41. Stuart, G. W., and S. J. Sundeen. *Principles and Practice of Psychiatric Nursing.* St. Louis: C. V. Mosby Co., 1983.

42. Sultenfuss, S. R. "Psychosocial Issues and Therapeutic Interview." In *Principles of Ostomy Care,* ed. D. C. Broadwell and B. S. Jackson. St. Louis: C. V. Mosby Co., 1982.

43. Sutton, J. D. "The Hospitalized Patient with Arthritis." *Nursing Clinics of North America,* 1984, 19:617.

44. Valkenburg, H. A. "Osteoarthritis in Some Developing Countries." *Journal of Rheumatology,* 1983, 10:20.

CHAPTER 39

Older Adults with Degenerative Neuromuscular Disease

JOANNA HOFFMAN

■

OBJECTIVES

After completing this chapter, the reader will be able to:

- Identify the magnitude of multiple sclerosis, Parkinson's disease, and Alzheimer's disease in the United States.
- Relate the pathophysiology of multiple sclerosis, Parkinson's disease, and Alzheimer's disease to client problems requiring nursing intervention.
- Identify factors associated with the onset and progression of multiple sclerosis, Parkinson's disease, and Alzheimer's disease.
- Identify measures that can be used to screen clients for early intervention and to prevent Parkinson's disease.
- Relate the nursing assessment of the client with multiple sclerosis, Parkinson's disease, and Alzheimer's disease to nursing diagnoses.
- Discuss nursing intervention and evaluation related to selected nursing diagnoses for clients with multiple sclerosis, Parkinson's disease, and Alzheimer's disease.
- Recall research needs related to clients with progressive neurological dysfunction.
- Recall ethical issues related to clients with progressive neurological dysfunction.

Management of progressive neurological dysfunction is a challenge for all health care workers, especially the primary nurse. Clients with a degenerative disease experience depression, fear, and anger. They may withdraw from society. Families are in a dilemma, torn by feelings of guilt and grief, the need to care for the ill member, and the need to lead their own lives. Nurses can help clients by alleviating their physical symptoms when possible, preventing complications, assisting in maximizing activities of daily living (ADL), and helping them adjust to their disease. Nurses can assist families by offering understanding, counseling, and referrals.

Three of the frequently seen neuromuscular diseases—multiple sclerosis, Parkinson's disease, and Alzheimer's disease—have been selected to demonstrate the application of concepts of primary nursing to people with neurological dysfunction. This chapter discusses the nature of the neurological dysfunction characteristic of each of these disorders and their management and nursing care.

Overview of Multiple Sclerosis

Multiple sclerosis (MS) was first described over a hundred years ago by the French neurologist Charcot. It is a progressive disease of the neurological system characterized by exacerbations and remissions of symptoms related to diverse body functions.

Multiple sclerosis clients can expect to live 90 percent or more of their expected life span. The cause of death in most MS clients is the same as in the population as a whole, heart disease being the primary factor. It is rare for a case to follow a rapidly progressive course. Only 10 percent of the clients will continue to deteriorate after the initial onset of symptoms (25).

Causes of an exacerbation (worsening of all symptoms with the appearance of new symptoms) are still primarily speculative. It is known that infections or exposure to increased temperatures will exaggerate symptoms. This type of exacerbation usually subsides when the precipitating cause is removed. Families tend to report emotional stress as a cause of exacerbation, but it is difficult to prove or disprove the role of emotions in MS, especially since the sudden appearance of new symptoms is a cause of emotional stress.

A remission is either a partial or total clearing of symptoms that lasts more than twenty-four hours. To be significant, a remission should last at least a month. About 20 percent of MS clients have remissions lasting for months or years with complete freedom from all symptoms of the disease (17). For most clients the disease remains chronic and progressive.

Incidence and Risk Factors

Epidemiologists use prevalence rates (the proportion of the population that has MS at any given time) rather than the incidence rate (the proportion of people newly diagnosed) when discussing MS. Prevalence studies show a correlation between MS and latitude. The disease increases in incidence as the distance from the equator increases. The disease is almost nonexistent in the tropics and has a relatively high rate of incidence in the temperate zones. This environmental and latitudinal effect was markedly evident in a recent study of veterans of World War II and the Korean War (11). Veterans who grew up in temperate zones and moved to subtropical regions had the same rate of MS as those still living in temperate zones. Veterans who grew up in southern areas and later moved to northern latitudes retained a lower rate of MS. These findings imply that there may be an environmental cause of MS, with the actual disease process being initiated years before the onset of symptoms.

In temperate climates, MS has been found to attack women at a higher rate than men—almost two to one in the United States (27). The onset in women seems to be just before age thirty. It is somewhat later in men. Worldwide, the difference in rates by sex is not as pronounced, although the rate in women remains slightly higher than in men. Black and Asian populations have a lower rate.

In actual numbers the prevalence of the disease in the northern United States today is fifty cases per 100,000 persons of all ages (23). Onset occurs between ages fifteen and fifty-five. The first symptoms usually appear around age thirty. Because of the remissions and exacerbations seen in the majority of clients with MS, many years may pass between the onset of symptoms and the actual diagnosis of the disease.

Other geographical areas with a prevalence rate similar to the northern United States are Canada, Iceland, the United Kingdom, Northern Europe, and southern New Zealand. Exceptionally high rates (300 per 100,000 population) are seen in the Orkney Islands, north of Scotland. Researchers have attempted to explain this high incidence as a result of canine distemper epidemics (3). Canine distemper is caused by a virus that attacks the central nervous system of dogs. This virus is very similar to the human measles virus. In the past fifty years, there have been frequent distemper epidemics in the Orkney Islands, especially during World War II, when many soldiers were stationed there before being sent to European battlefields. Since 1959 canine distemper has been controlled and epidemics of it have been less severe. There has been a corresponding reduction in the number of newly diagnosed cases of MS on the islands. This reduction in cases has prompted some researchers to propose that canine distemper vaccines in dogs and measles vaccines in humans might be effective in preventing MS. This theory is still highly controversial, but it does support a possible viral cause of MS.

Viruses have long been thought to be a possible cause of MS, with the measles virus being the most extensively researched. The measles (rubella) virus can cause a chronic nervous system disease in childhood called subacute sclerosing panencephalitis. As early as 1962, persons with MS were found to have increased measles antibodies in their bloodstreams. Recent evidence has shown that most MS clients have more antiviral antibodies in the cerebral spinal fluid (CSF) than control groups (12).

Other research describes a reactivation of latent brain viruses that cause exacerbations in MS (4). This finding supports the possibility that an immune system response, initiated by a virus, may be involved in MS. The virus is believed to be defective in some way, thus causing autoimmunity in the central nervous system (CNS). Immunoglobulin G (IgG) increases in the spinal fluid of MS clients. IgG is associated with long-term immunity after two or more episodes of viral infection, thus supporting the theory that latent brain viruses are a cause of MS.

Whether or not antibodies in the CSF are a cause of the myelin destruction or are a result of the inflammatory process of demyelination remains controversial. All that is known for certain is that T cells are elevated during periods of remission and suppressed during exacerbations (8).

Pathophysiology

Multiple sclerosis is characterized by progressive destruction of the myelin sheath covering the axons in the CNS. The primary neuropathology is degeneration of oligodendrocytes (myelin-forming cells of the CNS) and proliferation of astrocytes (star-shaped nerve cells). Astrocyte proliferation causes plaques or sclerotic tissue formation. These sclerotic lesions occur in numerous sites throughout the CNS, brain, spinal cord, and optic nerve and give the disease its name—multiple sclerosis or disseminated sclerosis.

The degree of disability depends on the areas in the CNS that are involved. When the brain stem or cerebellum is affected, the symptoms are more severe, and the prognosis is serious. These clients eventually require total care. With spinal cord involvement, the symptoms appear slowly, with longer periods of remission. With cerebral involvement, dementia may become a primary concern (9). Most clients exhibit symptoms from more than one primary lesion, since the disease is characterized by multiple lesions. Symptoms of MS associated with sites of lesions in the CNS are presented in Table 39.1.

The cause of the myelin destruction is as yet unknown. Current research focuses primarily on three areas—environmental, immunological, and biological causes.

Overveiw of Management

Management is primarily aimed at control of symptoms and prevention of exacerbations. Adrenocorticotrophic hormone (ACTH) and prednisone have been found useful in treating acute inflammations and exacerbations. These steroids are given only for brief periods—usually no more than a month at a time—to prevent the common serious complications of long-term steroid therapy.

Spasticity is usually treated with antispasmodic drugs, such as baclofen (Lioresal) and diazepam (Valium). Sensory disorders such as paresthesias are usually not

Table 39.1
Symptoms of Multiple Sclerosis
According to Site of Lesion

Site of Lesion	Symptoms
Spinal cord	Paraparesia
	Sensory changes in limbs
	Spasticity
	Bladder dysfunction
Brain stem	Tremors
	Dysphagia
	Scanning speech
	Nystagmus
Cerebral	Memory alterations
	Impaired coordination
	Dementia

Note: Most patients exhibit a combination of symptoms. Cranial nerve involvement will cause symptoms specific to area affected.

treated unless pain is severe. If severe pain is apparent, carbamazepine (Tegretol) is the current drug of choice.

The urinary incontinence, frequency, and urgency experienced by a majority of MS clients are sometimes controlled with anticholinergics, the most common being propantheline bromide (Pro-Banthine). Examples of drugs used in the treatment of MS may be found in Table 39.2.

Immunosuppressive treatment is a relatively new therapy for MS and is still in the experimental stage. Plasma exchange (plasmaphoresis) has been used for some clients with MS with no long-term beneficial or nonbeneficial effects. ACTH, in combination with Cytoxan, is the usual drug protocol for immunosuppressive treatment. With this therapy, the client has increased risk of infection, hemorrhagic cystitis, bladder cancer, and leukemia (9). It is used only when all other remedies have proved incapable of stabilizing a rapidly progressive course of the disease.

Various dietary treatments for MS have been tried, with no noticeable alterations in the course of the disease. Allergen-free diets, gluten-free diets, low-fat diets, and high-vitamin diets have all been investigated. Fad diets continue to appear. Clients should be encouraged to make certain that any diet used is nutritionally sound. Whatever diet the client selects should be nutritious and well balanced and should contain adequate vitamins. Roughage should be included to help counteract any constipation. If tremors occur, extra calories should be

provided. If urinary tract infections occur, diets high in protein and cranberries should be used to increase urinary acidity.

The National Multiple Sclerosis Society is the only voluntary health organization in the United States supporting worldwide research into the cause of and cure for the disease. Some of the exciting new research projects supported by this organization are treatment with 4-aminopyridine and treatment with cyclosporin. Injections of 4-aminopyridine restore conduction in blocked nerve fibers for up to four hours by slowing down nerve impulses, strengthening them, and enabling them to cross demyelinated zones. The effect on the nerves of this drug is similar to the effect of cold temperatures. Within ten minutes of receiving the drug, clients experience mild to marked improvement in vision and gait, lasting about four hours. The drug does not halt the progression of the disease, but works by controlling the symptoms, the same way L-dopa works in Parkinson's disease.

Cyclosporin, a drug currently used to prevent rejection of organ transplants, is also being tested in MS clients. Since T-lymphocytes are elevated during exacerbations, the cyclosporin, by inhibiting the immune response, may reduce or reverse the autoimmune response in MS. Cyclophosphamide, classified as an alkylating agent, is also currently under investigation in treating MS. Its usefulness may be in preventing exacerbations.

Along with new drug treatments, research is under way to identify the genes in the body that control immune responses. In other studies, researchers are comparing the normal amino acid peptides in the myelin sheath with those of viral proteins that are almost identical (15).

Nursing Care

Nursing care, either in a hospital or at home, is aimed at maintaining optimal function. The client should remain independent for as long as possible. Physical abilities should be assessed in a realistic manner. As function decreases, the nurse must help the client and family set realistic and attainable goals for self-care.

Assessment

Nursing care of the client with MS derives from a comprehensive data base that includes the nursing history, physical examination, and findings of diagnostic tests.

Table 39.2
Drugs Used in the Management of Multiple Sclerosis

Category and Drug	Indications for Use	Nursing Considerations
Corticosteroids Prednisone Dexamethasone Hydrocortisone	Short-term use for control of exacerbations; immunosuppression.	Should use for one month or less; restrict salt intake when taking drugs; do not stop abruptly; numerous side effects when used longer than one month.
Cholinergics Urecholine Prostigmin	Urinary retention; flaccid bladder (failure to empty).	Causes hypotension; may increase muscle weakness.
Anticholinergic Pro-Banthine (propantheline bromide)	Urinary frequency and urgency; spastic bladder (failure to store).	Do not use if glaucoma present; can potentiate sleeping aids.
Antispasmodics Valium (diazepam)	Spasticity and muscle weakness.	Avoid activities that require alertness; addictive; do not mix with alcohol.
Baclofen (Lioresal)	Spasticity and unstable bladder.	Do not stop abruptly; can cause hallucinations; do not use with other CNS depressants; may increase fatigue; do not mix with alcohol.

Nursing History.   The nursing history is usually the first major source of data collected. The areas normally covered in a comprehensive nursing history include: demographic data, major complaints, history of present illness, past health history, family health history, social and personal history, a review of systems, learning needs, self-care ability, access to and use of health resources, and ability to cope with chronic illness.

A close family member should be included in the interview if there is any evidence of the client's inability to convey information in a coherent manner. If the client is unreliable, the nursing history may have to be obtained entirely from family members. The family interview should include questions regarding personality or behavior changes and bizarre physical complaints, such as sudden blindness or deafness lasting only a few seconds.

Tact is required when obtaining the history either from the family or client. Extra time should be allowed for a full discussion of what a symptom might include. The onset of neurological disease may be so gradual that it is only through a careful interview that changes in behavior may be seen. Paradoxically, those who may see the client infrequently may notice unusual facial expressions, voice or speech alterations, or posture changes before close family members do. Close family or friends may fail to notice any insidious changes.

During the nursing history, the nurse must be alert to any signs of depression. Clients become frustrated over gradually increasing memory loss, tremors, or malaise and may become genuinely depressed by their increasing incapacities. It is often difficult to determine whether depression is a result of the symptoms or a cause of the symptoms. A careful history can sometimes bring out the very early symptoms overlooked by the client and the family—symptoms that may have begun to cause the stress and depression.

Physical Examination.   When dealing with long-term degenerative diseases, the nurse may be responsible for conducting an independent, ongoing neurological assessment of the client and assisting with any special neurodiagnostic procedures requested by the physician. Regardless of the setting (home, clinic, hospital, or emergency room), the neurological assessment should have similar components. Examination of cranial nerves, mental status, sensory status, language and speech status, and motor status should be included. The sequence of the assessment is of no importance, but the individual nurse-examiner should develop a system that encourages completeness and thoroughness without overtaxing the energy of a weakened or easily exhausted client. A comprehensive procedure for examining the twelve cranial nerves is outlined in Table 39.3.

Table 39.3
Cranial Nerve Assessment

Cranial Nerve	Assessment Procedure
I. Olfactory	Clear nasal passages; ask client to identify familiar odors such as oil, perfume, or clove; check both nostrils.
II. Optic	Determine visual field; view fundus with ophthalmoscope.
III. Oculomotor IV. Trochlear V. Abducens	Examine all together; pupil reaction to light; ability to follow objects.
V. Trigeminal	Assess sensations of pain, touch, temperature on face and cheek; ability to bite and open mouth.
VII. Facial	Test tongue for taste of sweet, sour, bitter substances; observe symmetry of face; raise eyebrows, close eyes; smile.
VIII. Acoustic	Check hearing by bone and air conduction.
IX. Glossopharyngeal X. Vagus	Assess gag reflex; swallowing; ability to speak and cough on command.
XI. Spinal Accessory	Ability to shrug shoulders and rotate head against resistance.
XII. Hypoglossal	Ability to protrude tongue on demand.

The sensory status of the trunk and extremities is tested for superficial and deep sensations. The examiner determines the extent of sensory response by touching the client. Cotton balls, a sharp object, or hot or cold water can be used as stimuli for light touch, pain, or temperature sensations, respectively. Suspected areas of sensory loss should be mapped out on a body diagram to facilitate identification of possible CNS lesion sites. Areas of increased or intensified sensations (hyperesthesia) should also be noted. Paresthesia, or abnormal sensations such as burning, itching, numbness, or prickly feelings, may be evident. All abnormal or unusual sensations should be noted.

Testing for sensations in deep-lying structures is done by vibration. Placing a tuning fork over joints in the legs and asking the client to describe the feeling will identify the presence of deep sensations. Pain perception is best noted by compression of the Achilles tendon.

Language and speech problems are evaluated during the interview. If gross abnormalities are noticed, the cli-

ent should be referred to a speech pathologist for a definite diagnosis and possible treatment.

When evaluating motor function, muscles are inspected for contractures, atrophy, tremor, tone, and abnormal movements. All joints are put through range-of-motion tests, and muscle groups are tested for strength. Coordination is assessed by asking the client to do two simple movements concurrently, such as touching the nose and tapping one foot. Usually, close observation of gait and balance while the client is walking or climbing stairs provides clues regarding weakness or spasticity of legs. The Romberg test may be used to evaluate balance.

Inspection and documentation of basic body build and posture is necessary on initial evaluation so that comparisons can be made during future examinations. Palpation of a muscle mass is done to determine turgor, firmness, or tenderness. Muscle tone can best be evaluated through resistance of muscles to passive manipulation. Extremity muscles are also evaluated in this manner. Tone is a reflex phenomenon with both afferent and efferent nerve components. Muscles become flaccid when there is loss of motor and sensory nerve supply. With degenerative diseases, it is important to measure muscle mass and watch for signs of hypertrophy.

Abnormal movements usually noted are tremors and spasms. Ataxic gaits should be differentiated from simple difficulties in walking that occur as a result of serious illness or chronic inactivity.

Mental Status Examination.   The mental status examination begins with an assessment of the client's ability to pay attention to the examiner. Always check if eyeglasses or hearing aids are normally used by the client before beginning the examination. Ask questions in a tactful manner and explain that this is a routine procedure. Some clients become very offended when nurses ask seemingly ridiculous questions like "Do you know what year this is?" Always provide for privacy, even if the examination is to be primarily verbal.

Included in the mental status examination is orientation to person, place, and time. This is usually done with direct questioning by asking, "What is your name?" or "Do you know the name of this hospital?" Disorientation to person or place indicates a profound disorder. It is common to forget temporarily the day of the week or the date of the month.

Affect and mood are both evaluated during the procedure. Important behaviors to note are the client's emotional lability, body posture, facial expression, and appropriateness of affect. A description of the general appearance, behavior, and attitude should be included in a mental status examination.

If degenerative brain disease is suspected, perception and comprehension must be evaluated. Changes may be very subtle and go unnoticed on initial interviews. Types of agnosias are presented in Table 39.4.

Memory and thought processes, along with knowledge of simple arithmetic calculations, should be evaluated. Recent memory may be evaluated by asking the client to repeat a series of five or ten numbers or words. Normally a person can repeat five to eight words or numbers.

When evaluating thought processes, be alert for coherent and logical sentences. Perseveration, neologisms, word salads, and confabulations will become apparent during questioning.

Judgment is best evaluated by situational questioning, asking the client to respond to a specific situation such as "What should you do when you see smoke coming from a neighbor's window?" Many times, observing behavior will provide data about a person's judgment. A tremulous client who insists on climbing stairs alone when told to request assistance is demonstrating poor judgment.

Abstract thinking can be assessed by asking the client to explain simple proverbs such as Haste makes waste or A stitch in time saves nine.

Diagnostic Tests. Although examination of cerebral spinal fluid shows an increase in IgG and viral antibodies, a diagnosis of MS is still based on clinical evidence after ruling out all other possible causes of symptoms.

Initially, symptoms of MS are transient, brief in duration, and ignored by the client. The most common early symptom is sensory impairment. The client may complain of numbness or a tingling sensation (paresthesia) in any or all limbs. Muscle weakness is usually noted, and after repeated exacerbations, the weakness may progress to paralysis.

Visual problems may be an initial sign of sclerosis of the optic nerve. An ophthalmic examination may reveal that the optic nerve is pale. The client may complain of blurred vision, double vision, or sudden color blindness.

Temporary gait changes and lack of coordination are often early transient symptoms. Many MS-afflicted women with coordination problems are accused falsely of overindulging in alcohol. Transient muscle weakness gives rise to accusations of laziness. Thus, many women experience a gradual loss of self-esteem, which is reinforced by later symptoms, such as urinary bladder incontinence.

Not all symptoms occur simultaneously, and occasionally a thorough history will not elicit all the symptoms the client might have experienced. If a symptom was short-lasting, it may have been overlooked or forgotten by the client.

A final diagnosis is sometimes not made until late in the disease when Charcot's triad of symptoms is seen. This triad includes nystagmus (oscillating movement of the eyes), scanning speech (staccatolike speech with pauses between syllables), and intention tremor (tremor when voluntary motion is attempted).

Diagnosis in the early stage is rare. Physicians prefer to observe the client over a period of time, perhaps months or years, before making a diagnosis of MS. One simple diagnostic procedure is observation of the client when exposed to increased temperatures. This precipitates symptoms that otherwise are concealed. Nerves may be able to conduct impulses, even when damaged, under normal body conditions. But when the body temperature rises, the damaged nerve is no longer able to function because of the loss of myelin. For this reason, clients are very susceptible to increases in symptoms with only a slight increase in body temperature—0.1°F or 0.06°C. Sitting in a hot bath—104°F to 108°F—can evoke previous symptoms as well as those not yet experienced. Symptoms abate when the client gets out of the tub.

Visually and auditorially evoked potential studies are useful in identifying multiple lesions not yet apparent (7). In these noninvasive procedures, the electroencephalograph (EEG) records changes in brain waves as a result of specific stimuli, either visual or auditory. The

Table 39.4
Types of Agnosias

Agnosia	Deficit
Auditory agnosia	Inability to interpret sounds
Finger agnosia	Inability to identify fingers of one's own hands or of others
Optic agnosia	Inability to interpret visual images
Prosopagnosia	Inability to recognize familiar faces
Tactile agnosia	Inability to distinguish objects by sense of touch

resulting changes in the EEG are evaluated with computer assistance and can pinpoint lesions in the brain.

Somatosensorially evoked potential studies are done by stimulating nerves in the arms and legs and recording resulting electrical impulses from appropriate areas of the brain with an EEG. To be of value in diagnosing MS, EEG must be combined with other evaluation methods.

Intracranial computed tomography (CT scan) is useful in evaluating the extent of the disease by examining various layers of the brain and producing a detailed image. Newer procedures, such as magnetic resonance imaging (MRI) and positron emission tomography, also are being used to produce detailed, cross-sectional images of the brain. They are, however, costly and not available in many hospitals.

There is a tendency to do exhaustive testing (including myelography, an invasive procedure) in an effort to rule out tumors or other CNS disorders before making a diagnosis of MS. Many clients willingly submit to potentially harmful invasive procedures in order to discover the underlying cause of symptoms they have had for years. Medical and nursing personnel are both responsible for providing clients with enough information to make an informed decision and to give informed consent for invasive procedures.

Nursing Diagnoses

Although nursing diagnoses are individualized for each client, based upon the findings of the nursing assessment, the diagnoses in this section related to MS represent those typical of many clients. These diagnoses are:

1. Self-care deficit related to such factors as muscle spasticity and lack of adequate environmental supports.
2. Disturbance in self-esteem related to such factors as altered body image, perceived inadequacy, and role changes.
3. Altered patterns of urinary elimination related to such factors as urinary retention and incontinence.
4. Ineffectual family coping related to such factors as inadequate understanding of the client's abilities in terms of the disease process and the chronicity of problems.
5. Social isolation related to such factors as impaired physical mobility and impaired cognitive ability.
6. Sleep disturbances related to such factors as fatigue and anxiety.

Planning and Implementation

Nursing care plans based on nursing diagnoses in MS clients should be developed on an individual basis after a thorough collection of data. Numerous motor and sensory changes may occur, depending on the site of lesions in the CNS. Physical, social, and psychological problems occur simultaneously and interact.

☐ *Self-Care Deficit.* Self-care deficits are not apparent in the early stages of the disease. Even with marked muscle spasticity and weakness, clients may be able to care for themselves with environmental alterations designed to compensate for their limitations. For example, even though clients living at home may report that they can no longer bathe themselves, in reality they often can with an appropriate environment. Support bars in the bathroom or shower may overcome this deficit.

During the early stages of the disease, the client is generally able to be up and about with little or no assistance. As the disease progresses, it is important to assist clients in coping with a gradual loss of independent functioning. If there is mental deterioration affecting judgment, supervision may need to be increased.

The "slapping and staggering" gait may be minimized by having the client lean to the less affected side and place the heel of the foot on the floor first. Physical exertion must be avoided, and daily planning should include periods of rest. Providing periods of rest during self-care activities can help reduce fatigue.

As the disease progresses, the physical nursing care must continue to be aggressive in order to prevent complications of immobility. As clients gradually become unable to function without assistance in their activities of daily living, their needs should be anticipated and satisfied in a matter-of-fact way. This helps decrease discouragement and depression.

☐ *Disturbance in Self-Esteem.* Self-esteem disturbances may be a result of altered body image, the client's perceived inadequacy, or a loss of the parenting role. MS has been called the crippler of young adults. For many, the symptoms appear in their most productive years, when they are working and raising a family. Feelings of failure and grief for loss of function are usually present. These negative feelings are apparent through the client's verbalizations (e.g., "I can't even cook for my children any more"). Some MS clients are accused of being lazy or hysterical early in the course of the disease. The weakness and staggering walk may have caused the patient to be ridiculed or accused of being drunk. Urinary dysfunction and incontinence may have caused embarrassment. Rebuilding the client's feelings of self-worth are an important part of nursing care.

□ *Urinary Elimination.* Urinary dysfunction is a frequently encountered problem for clients and their families. It is usually not an initial symptom, but during the course of the disease 90 percent of the clients will experience this problem (9). Bladder symptoms and their associated urinary tract infections shorten the life span of the MS client. Common complaints are retention, frequency, urgency, nocturia, and incontinence. Educational and vocational pursuits may need to be curtailed, and social and sexual activities may become strained.

A diagnosis of the specific problem must be made. It cannot be based on symptoms alone, since identical symptoms may be evident with both retention (failure to empty) and a hyperactive bladder (failure to store). Because lesions may be anywhere in the spinal cord, bladder dysfunction can be as varied as the course of the disease. The most common cause is upper motor neuron lesions. Both client and family need a careful explanation of why an insidious disease of the brain and spinal cord can affect urinary output.

Once there is an understanding of the genitourinary system and how it is affected, learning to manage the dysfunction can begin. Education includes a discussion of the signs and symptoms of autonomic hyperreflexia, since this can become a life-threatening crisis situation.

Pharmacological agents often either help to alleviate or eliminate some symptoms. Intermittent self-catheterization may be considered. Women can be taught clean, intermittent self-catheterization with the aid of a mirror and may eventually be able to do it by touch alone in the privacy of their bathroom.

It is important to set reasonable goals for improving bladder function. Goals may include decreasing voiding frequency to permit short periods of time for shopping or attending church, decreasing the number of urinary tract infections, and preventing incontinence at night.

Infections can be reduced by eliminating residual urine. Baclofen (Lioresal) is useful for controlling bladder spasms that impede urinary flow. Mechanical means for eliminating residual urine, such as self-catheterization and suprapubic tapping, may also be helpful. The nurse may have to assist the client through a trial-and-error period before the most appropriate medications and techniques are determined.

Client and family teaching is an important nursing measure in bladder dysfunction. Restoration of function may be possible through consistent compliance with prescribed treatment, but like many other problems associated with MS, urinary dysfunction may recur. Periodic urodynamic studies, urine cultures, and residual urine determinations are needed to monitor the effects of interventions and to detect early signs of increased dysfunction and complications. Sexual counseling can eliminate embarrassment and help clients adjust to decreased sensations in the genital areas.

□ *Ineffectual Family Coping.* Ineffectual family coping is a common long-term problem associated with MS. The primary care giver may be a client's spouse, parent, or child. Care givers are observed for signs of exhaustion and verbalizations of guilt and discouragement. With MS, the care giver may not fully understand the nature of the disease and may expect the client to be able to do more than he or she is capable of. Feelings of animosity between them may be apparent.

Family health considerations are a part of the nursing care plan. The physical and emotional strains of caring for long-term chronically ill individuals at home places a tremendous financial and social burden on family care givers and all other family members. If dementia is present, the strain is intensified. Family members and care givers must be alert to the client's physical needs and wandering attention. They must communicate affection and provide reassurance that all is well even when the client may not recognize them.

Currently, most disabled clients living in the family setting are cared for by women—wives, daughters, or daughters-in-law—who may also be aging (22). Changing patterns in the sex roles in general and the increased number of working women have not significantly altered the role of the female as care giver within the family structure.

Planning and providing for holistic home care for both the client and family is a nursing challenge. Families may have scheduled contact with health care providers, but most seek assistance only in a crisis or when there has been a breakdown in the internal family support system. Providing and assisting families in locating community health services and support groups is a nursing responsibility.

Information about the disease and its progression and possible ramifications is necessary before family members can make any decisions regarding long-term care of the client. Nurses must remain nonjudgmental and supportive as the family makes decisions. The primary concern must be the safety and well-being of the client. Primary care givers often must cope for sustained periods of time with difficult problems such as incontinence, combativeness, and abrupt mood swings, all of which can increase family stress. If the client is totally bedridden and no longer aware of the environment, the nurse may initiate discussions about alternatives to home care by the family.

The decision to seek placement in a nursing home should be based on judgments about what will best serve the client and family. Each family has unique capacities and tolerances, and families are therefore best evaluated on an individual basis. The kinds (e.g., respite care centers and day care centers) and amount of support services available to the family may make the difference between success and failure in home care.

☐ *Social Isolation.*   Social isolation may result from impaired physical mobility and/or impaired cognitive ability. Statements such as "I have few visitors" or "My daughter hasn't been to see me in a month" indicate probable feelings of isolation. MS clients may make excuses for the family's lack of attention, yet it is important to remember that social isolation can affect self-esteem, cause depression, and increase stress—all of which may increase psychological distance between the client and family.

Helping the client adjust to a changing social situation is a difficult task. Encouraging hobbies appropriate to the client's motor abilities and referral to occupational therapy may be helpful.

Reading may be suggested for clients whose sight is sufficient. If double vision causes difficulty, an eye patch worn over one eye may help. Book holders may be used by clients whose arms are too weak to support a book.

Social isolation of homebound and/or institutionalized elderly and disabled clients, a growing problem in the United States, is difficult to prevent entirely. Nurses may be able to decrease it by identifying clients, contacting community groups and agencies that provide either telephone or home visiting services, and arranging transportation to day care centers.

☐ *Sleep Disturbances.*   Too much or too little sleep are common complaints in clients with degenerative neuromuscular disease. Common causes include increased fatigue, anxiety, short-term memory loss, and anticipatory grieving.

Preventing exhaustion and planning daily activities with a regular routine may encourage restful sleep. Going to bed at the same time every night may also be helpful. Medications are used only when other sleep-inducing measures fail.

During remission, sufficient rest is important, since fatigue can cause relapse. Eating a well-balanced diet, exercising regularly, and avoiding infections that may increase body temperature also help prevent relapses.

Evaluation

The following behaviors may be used to measure the outcomes of nursing interventions.

Self-Care Deficits.   The client and family will verbalize understanding of the client's self-care ability. The client will perform self-care activities at optimum level, considering personal limitations.

Disturbances in Self-Esteem.   The client will verbalize a positive self-image and will engage in meaningful activities with others and derive satisfaction from them.

Ineffectual Family Coping.   The client and family will verbalize realistic perceptions of their coping skills and will demonstrate increased ability to handle difficult situations.

Social Isolation.   The client will engage in meaningful activities with others, both within the home (or institution) and outside, when feasible.

Sleep Disturbances.   The client will have adequate periods of restful sleep.

Overview of Parkinson's Disease

In 1817 James Parkinson, an English physician, wrote a short essay entitled "Essay on the Shaking Palsy," which described clients with a slowly progressive physical disease characterized by tremors, weakness, and gait changes (2). This illness is now called Parkinson's disease or primary Parkinsonism. Its origin is unknown, a factor that differentiates it from secondary Parkinsonism, which can be related to causes such as exposure to certain drugs. Distinguishing clinical manifestations include involuntary shaking movements of the limbs (tremors), muscle rigidity, bradykinesia (slowness of movement), and loss of postural reflexes.

Incidence

Parkinson's disease begins slowly and insidiously and is not confined to the elderly. Recent surveys show that it is more widespread than previously thought (19). It has been diagnosed in adults as young as thirty, but the incidence increases significantly with advancing age. Approximately 1 percent of the population over fifty in the United States has Parkinson's disease (21). One in seven clients first show signs of it before age fifty. Approximately 75 percent of those who develop it do so between the ages of fifty and sixty-five. It affects men slightly more than women.

With the exception of black populations in the United States and South Africa, where the incidence is lower, the worldwide incidence of Parkinson's disease is similar to that found in the United States (21).

Pathophysiology

Parkinson's disease (PD) is associated with a dopamine deficiency in the nigrostriatal complex of the midbrain. Dopamine is necessary for the transmission of neurological impulses from the nigrostriatal (substantia nigra) to cells in the corpus striatum. (See Figure 39.1.) In PD, the black-pigmented dopaminergic neurons in the substantia nigra degenerate, resulting in decreased manufacture and storage of dopamine in the upper midbrain.

In addition to being a neurotransmitter, dopamine is an important modulator of movement and a chemical messenger in the regulation of pituitary hormones. It affects mood and behavior.

The body normally makes dopamine from tyrosine, an essential amino acid found in protein-rich foods, such as red meats and legumes. Tyrosine is changed by liver enzymes into tyrosine hydroxylase and then into levodopa (L-dopa). Most of the L-dopa in the body is excreted by the kidneys. Only a small amount crosses the blood-brain barrier, where it is converted to dopamine, the active neurotransmitter. Dopamine is then stored in the cells of the substantia nigra and released into the corpus striatum when neurons are stimulated. The inability to store and release dopamine results in parkinsonian symptoms.

The fundamental cause of dopamine deficiency remains unknown, but the effects can be identified. In addition to tremors, rigidity, and bradykinesia, clients walk with a shuffling gait, small steps, and increased propulsion. The arms are flexed and unswinging, the posture stooped and flexed.

There are changes in the autonomic nervous system manifested by increased perspiration, seborrhea, oily skin, orthostatic hypotension, and urinary retention. In more advanced cases of Parkinson's disease, there are affect changes, with decreased facial expressions and vital lung capacity causing a low speaking voice.

Two subgroups of Parkinson's disease have been identified. One group has primarily postural instability and gait difficulty. Muscle rigidity interferes with voluntary movements and can lead to severe incapacitation and disability. The head, hips, and knees flex in a fetallike position, causing postural instability and gait changes, especially the short steps called "marche à petits pas." Clients are often confined to a wheelchair.

Gait changes can occur early in the disease and are the primary cause of falls and secondary injuries. The client is unable to maintain balance because of the absence of a normal reflex righting response. Cogwheeling (rigidity with rhythmical fluctuations in intensity) can often be felt in muscles by the examiner. In a very thin client, the cogwheeling may be seen in large muscles.

In the second subgroup, in which tremors are the dominant feature, the prognosis is more favorable. The parkinsonian tremor is slow and rhythmical. It occurs when voluntary muscles are relaxed and is reduced during voluntary motion, sleep, and anesthesia. Tremors are not normally present in large muscles affected by rigidity, but rather in the smaller muscles of the arms. Tremors can migrate to other muscle groups. Stress and anxiety increase tremors, yet with determination, some clients are able to control them for several minutes. A sudden emotional shock can stop a tremor for several minutes, although it resumes with increased intensity. It was once thought that stress caused Parkinson's symptoms because of their prominence after an emotional upset. In clients exhibiting a sudden onset of symptoms, a careful history will usually reveal unrecognized symptoms that existed prior to the stressful event.

Risk Factors

Although the incidence of Parkinson's disease is about 1 percent in the general population and may reach 10 percent in the population over age sixty-five, there are still no apparent risk factors. The cause remains idiopathic, with no evidence of hereditary or genetic predispositions. Exposure to carbon monoxide and manganese and long-term use of tricyclic antidepressants may increase one's risk for secondary Parkinsonism. Drug-induced symptoms are more common in persons over age sixty and are usually reversible if the drugs are discontinued.

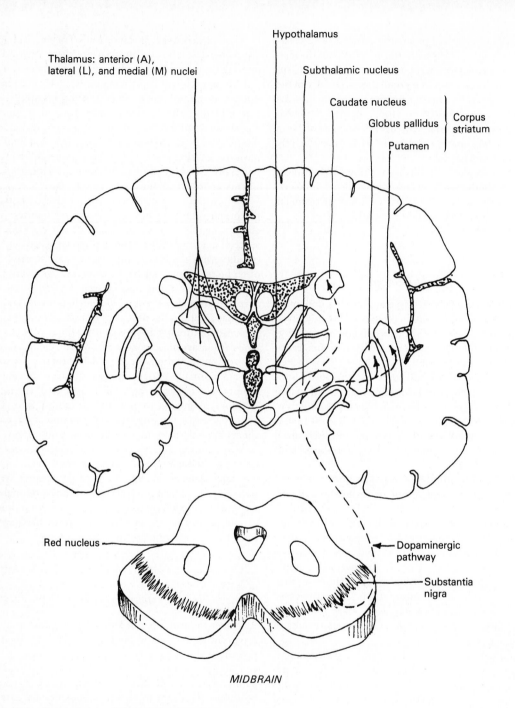

Figure 39.1. Transmission of Neurological Impulses
Source: Courtesy of Eugene Canava, Nurse/Artist

Prevention and Screening for Early Intervention

Prevention of secondary Parkinsonism includes educating the public about exposure to substances associated with parkinsonian symptoms. For example, exposure to carbon monoxide should be minimized. Proper ventilation of areas such as closed garages and tunnels is essential. Employees who are constantly exposed to high concentrations of carbon monoxide should be rotated to areas with low concentrations. Carbon monoxide levels in the environment should be monitored continuously.

Occupational health nurses should be aware of situations in which manganese is used, such as the production of nonmagnetic steel products. Manganese levels of employees in these situations should be monitored bimonthly. The normal serum level for this trace element is 4–20 mcg/100 ml.

Clients on tricyclic antidepressants should have their blood levels of these drugs checked every three months. Dosage should not exceed the therapeutic range.

Since Parkinson's disease has an insidious and highly variable onset, the primary screening measure is a good health history. Early symptoms are vague and nonspecific and are frequently missed or assumed to have other causes. Clients may complain of anxiety, depression, restlessness, aching in muscles, and changes in handwriting. In the early stages, muscle rigidity is more common than tremors. Functional changes may include fatigue, constipation, and unilateral difficulty when moving. Differentiating the onset of PD from psychological causes and stroke (especially when there is unilateral muscle involvement) is difficult unless a thorough and accurate history is available.

Overview of Management

The treatment of choice for Parkinson's disease is drug therapy. Drugs that are currently used are listed in Table 39.5. Prior to the development of oral dopamine precursors and agonists, the drug of choice was an anticholinergic such as trihexyphenidyl HCl (Artane) or benztropine mesylate (Cogentin). Anticholinergics work by blocking the neurotransmitter acetylcholine, which has an action opposite that of dopamine. Anticholinergics help to reestablish the equilibrium between acetylcholine and today are used as an adjunct to levodopa.

Anticholinergics are useful when muscle rigidity and stiffness are the primary signs of Parkinson's disease. In many instances, they are the initial treatment. They are also used for clients having drug-induced Parkinsonism when it is necessary to continue potent tranquilizers or antidepressants causing extrapyramidal symptoms (e.g., tremors).

Levodopa is the most effective drug available for the control of Parkinson's disease. Dopamine itself is not useful, since it does not cross the blood-brain barrier and is destroyed in the gastrointestinal tract. Instead, levodopa (L-dopa), the metabolic precursor of dopamine, is used. When used alone, large doses of levodopa are necessary to counteract the effect of an enzyme that occurs abundantly outside the brain, dopa-decarboxylase. This enzyme converts most of the levodopa to dopamine before it enters the brain, causing excessive waste.

Carboxylase inhibitors are now used in conjunction with levodopa, thus reducing the levodopa dosage by as much as 75 percent. Sinemet, a commonly used drug, contains the decarboxylase inhibitor carbidopa and levodopa in combination. Even with combination drugs, one or two weeks of treatment may be needed before any improvement in symptoms is noted. Hospitalization is generally necessary when initiating levodopa therapy because of the high incidence of adverse reactions. Obviously, clients may be monitored more closely, and safe and effective dosage levels may be determined more easily, in the hospital. Initially, clients experience relief of symptoms, such as improvement in bradykinesia and less rigidity for four to five hours, when levodopa is given three times a day. Tremors and instability contributing to falls are least changed by levodopa. Individual reactions vary greatly, and for those with a good response to the medication, the effects can be startling, enabling the person to resume normal activities. Life expectancy also increases.

After a few years of treatment, however, the duration of relief following each dose is shorter. Some clients alter their own dose schedule, taking smaller doses at more frequent intervals in order to maintain mobility. But not all clients experience this waning effect of the medication. Levodopa does not stop the underlying disease process. Instead it can be an effective replacement therapy. Levodopa has not been found to be effective in treating drug-induced Parkinsonism.

Gradually building up therapeutic levels of levodopa can help to reduce common side effects, such as nausea, vomiting, and loss of appetite. Psychological manifestations include delirium, hallucinations, hostility, and

Table 39.5
Drugs for Parkinson's Disease

Category and Drug	Indications for Use	Nursing Considerations
Dopaminergic Levodopa (L-Dopa) Levodopa + carbidopa (Sinemet)	Bradykinesia, tremors, rigidity.	Frequent side effects when L-dopa used alone; causes orthostatic hypotension, nightmares, hallucinations. Do not use vitamin pills if L-dopa used alone. Combinations reduce side effects; dosage needs careful regulation.
Anticholinergics Artane (Trihexyphenidyl HCl) Cogentin (benztropine mesylate)	Tremors and control of extrapyramidal disorders.	Can increase difficulty swallowing.
Antihistamines Benadryl (diphenhydramine)	Rigidity and akinesia.	Tolerance may develop; do not mix with alcohol; sedative effect may be very strong.
Antiviral agents Symmetral (Amantadine HCl)	Reduces drug-induced extra-pyramidal reactions; rigidity.	Do not stop suddenly, since this can initiate Parkinsonism crisis; orthostatic hypotension, especially in early morning.
Parlodel (bromocriptine mesylate)	Prevention of peak-dose dyskinesia from L-dopa.	Can cause hypotension, dizziness, and headache; incidence of side effects is 68%; nausea is most common.

paranoia. Before the availability of decarboxylase inhibitors, one in five clients had to stop levodopa because of severe side effects (6). Dosage is usually reduced when side effects are seen, then slowly increased to a therapeutic level.

The progressive nature of Parkinson's disease requires lifelong drug therapy accompanied by the increased risk of side effects. Abnormal induced movements, sometimes referred to as dyskinesias, commonly occur. These include nodding of the head, protrusion of the tongue, and increased respiratory movement (16). Other effects of long-term therapy include painful cramping of the feet early in the morning before taking the initial dose for the day, postural instability, and dementia. These effects possibly result from the progressive nature of the disease and not from levodopa, but some authors believe the drug does aggravate symptoms after long-term use.

Currently, some physicians prefer to withhold levodopa until the client has problems with activities of daily living. Others prefer to start clients on low doses, thus reserving some of the benefits for later years. The decision to begin levodopa therapy is individualized for each client.

Bromocriptine mesylate (Parlodel), a derivative of ergot and a medication originally developed to prevent milk formation in postpartum women, mimics the effect of dopamine in the brain (16). When used in large doses, it produces a strong antiparkinsonian effect, but side effects are frequent and severe. A therapeutic response with fewer fluctuations and dyskinesias is produced when it is given in smaller doses combined with levodopa. The long-term side effects of levodopa are also decreased.

New innovations in drug therapies and increased understanding of the role of dopamine in the body are changing health care workers' perceptions of Parkinson's disease. Much is still unknown about the disease, but knowing that a previously untreatable illness can now be explained in terms of a chemical disorder of the brain continues to stimulate researchers and give hope to sufferers. An exciting treatment under investigation in other countries is autotransplantation of adrenal medullary tissue into the caudate nucleus of the brain, causing a revitalization of the nigrostriatal system and relief of symptoms.

Nursing Care

All clients with Parkinson's disease need individual care based on their nursing diagnoses and the stage of the disease process. Long-term care of progressive diseases requires comprehensive care by a primary nurse.

Assessment

Assessment of the client with Parkinson's disease follows the same guidelines for nursing history and physical examination described in the section related to multiple sclerosis.

Nursing Diagnoses

Nursing diagnoses in clients with Parkinson's disease are made on an individual basis after a thorough neurological assessment. As with all progressive neuromuscular diseases, there are two primary desired client outcomes: the client functions at the highest level of ability in all aspects of ADL, and the client is free of severe complications.

Selected nursing diagnoses covered in this section of the chapter are:

1. Activity intolerance related to such factors as tremors and muscle rigidity.
2. Safety deficits related to such factors as lack of motor control.
3. Nutritional deficits related to such factors as dysphagia and bradykinesia.
4. Altered bowel elimination (constipation) related to such factors as reduced physical activity and medications.
5. Impaired communication related to such factors as impaired motor control.
6. Ineffectual family coping related to such factors as the demands of the treatment program and the chronicity of problems.

Planning and Implementation

☐ **Activity Intolerance.** Promotion of physical exercise is an important aspect of care. Medical treatment and drug therapy may delay severe disability for several years, but the potential for contractures is increased if physical exercise decreases. A program of physical therapy is essential for every client with Parkinson's disease regardless of age. Goals of treatment are to keep muscles healthy and efficient and to prevent deformities and depression.

Exercise can help the client maintain physical abilities, prevent muscle atrophy, and decrease hazards of immobility. Maintaining independence through activities also helps decrease depression. Clients and their families can be taught how to do exercises and establish a program that is appropriate for the client's needs and abilities.

For some clients, initiating quick movements and sustaining regular actions over a period of time are especially difficult. Techniques that can help the client include using visual, audio, or tactile stimuli to initiate movement. Seeing a shoe before the foot helps some clients step forward. Listening to or humming marching tunes may help the client maintain a steady walking pace.

Freezing, the sudden inability to move when walking, can be overcome in some instances by making a deliberate effort to stand straight and consciously put one foot before the other. Sometimes taking a step backward helps. Pulling the client increases freezing and may cause falls.

☐ **Safety Deficits.** Safety measures are necessary, particularly in the home. Scatter rugs are removed because they can cause falls. Handrails in the bathroom and hallways facilitate ambulation. Cutlery handles may be enlarged with rubber tubing or padding to help prevent cuts. If tremors are severe, plastic drinking cups or straws may be used instead of glass. Care is taken when serving and eating hot foods to prevent burns.

☐ **Nutritional Deficits.** Nutritional deficits can have serious consequences for clients with Parkinson's disease. Clients with dysphagia need appetizing foods that are easily eaten. Bradykinesia makes eating slow; use of warming trays helps keep food warm and appetizing during extended meals. If the client becomes fatigued, six small meals a day may be offered instead of three large ones.

☐ **Altered Bowel Elimination—Constipation.** Constipation can be a problem because of reduced physical activity and the use of medications. Fluids and roughage must be included in the daily diet. Stool softeners and rectal suppositories may be used and are preferable to enemas. Many clients become overly concerned about their bowels and need to be reassured that daily bowel movements are not necessary for good health.

☐ *Impaired Communication.* Communication skills are often impaired by Parkinson's disease. Speech can sometimes be improved by having clients read aloud and use the lips in an exaggerated manner. The microphagia characteristic of Parkinson's disease sometimes improves with levodopa and with writing on wide-lined paper.

☐ *Ineffectual Family Coping.* Since more than 90 percent of all clients are cared for at home, careful evaluation of the home situation is necessary. The economic, physical, social, and psychological burdens on the family can be overwhelming. Serious problems may be averted by identifying them and intervening before problems become significant and by educating the family about the disease.

Treatment programs are planned cooperatively with the family care givers. Family schedules can be used to plan for the sharing of responsibilities and to allow clients ample time for activities of daily living. It is important to remember that each family has individual cultural, social, emotional, and religious needs that must be considered when planning home care.

As the disease progresses, clients may have personality changes characterized by irritability, querulousness, and stubbornness. They may make excessive demands on family members. In the later stages, insomnia is common and may be alleviated with sedatives. In general, care is directed toward making both the client and family as comfortable as possible.

Evaluation

Behaviors that exemplify the client's and family's ability to meet expected outcomes of nursing intervention include the following.

Activity Intolerance. The client will achieve an optimum level of activity, considering physical limitations.

Safety Deficits. The client and family will identify potential environmental hazards to safety, and measures will be taken to correct them.

Nutritional Deficits. The client and family will adopt eating practices that accommodate the needs of the client (e.g., allowing sufficient time for meals).

Altered Bowel Elimination—Constipation. Clients will engage in measures known to facilitate bowel elimination (e.g., eating sufficient roughage).

Impaired Communication. The client will recognize communication difficulties and will use measures that aim to improve communication.

Ineffectual Family Coping. The family will verbalize a more positive attitude toward care of the client and will demonstrate effective coping skills when dealing with problems.

Overview of Alzheimer's Disease

The term Alzheimer's disease was coined in 1906 after Alois Alzheimer, a German physician, presented a case report of dementia in a middle-aged woman (5). At the time, Alzheimer's disease was considered to be a distinct problem affecting persons under sixty-five years of age. Persons over sixty-five were diagnosed as having senile dementia, believed to be a normal part of the aging process.

Today researchers no longer consider Alzheimer's disease a distinct problem based on age. Regardless of the age of onset, the disease symptomatology and pathology are the same, although the progression of Alzheimer's disease is more rapid in younger persons. The term senile dementia of the Alzheimer's type is still sometimes used to identify the disease in older clients.

Incidence

About 10 percent of the population over sixty-five in the United States has Alzheimer's disease. By age eighty, about 20 percent of the population has it. Overall, about 1.5 to 2 million Americans suffer from Alzheimer's disease. When one considers the rapidly growing number of elderly persons in the United States, the disease's future impact could be enormous. It is projected that by 2025, 25 percent of the population in the United States will be over sixty-five, and one-third of the population will reach at least eighty years of age (22). Because of the potential incidence by the year 2000, Alzheimer's disease has been called the disease of the century. It currently accounts for almost half of all admissions to nursing homes (1).

Pathophysiology

Alzheimer's disease is characterized by gross brain atrophy in the frontal and temporal lobes. Postmortem examinations of the brain reveal destruction of neurons in the nucleus basalis in the base of the forebrain. These neurons are responsible for the production of the neurotransmitter acetylcholine. In addition, there are neurofibrillary tangles and neuritic plaques, sometimes referred to as Alzheimer's lesions. Plaque formation causes the progressive loss of intellectual function.

Symptoms of Alzheimer's disease normally develop slowly and follow similar patterns of progressive intellectual decline. Four phases of the disease have been identified (13). Phase I is insidious, with the person having less energy and drive. In phase II, the client is able to function, but evidence of impairment is apparent. Difficulty in handling financial matters surfaces. In phase III, the client exhibits markedly altered behaviors and has little warmth or affection for family members. Severe mental disability requires continuous supervision. In phase IV, clients can no longer recognize the major care giver or family members. Incontinence and mutism occur, although they may be evident earlier in some clients.

It may take up to fifteen years for a client to progress from phase I to phase IV. When the onset occurs at an early age, progression to the later phases is rapid. Some older clients stabilize at phase II or III, with minimal progression beyond that point. Considering the variability among clients, it is important to individualize treatment.

Risk Factors

Although various theories about the cause of Alzheimer's disease are being considered, no risk factors except advanced age have been found. Clusters of individuals with Alzheimer's disease have been identified in some families, but there is no consistent pattern of incidence. Persons with Down's syndrome, a genetic disorder, have a much higher rate after age forty (26).

Prior head injury with loss of consciousness may be a precipitating factor, but evidence remains inconclusive. In one study, 26 percent of the clients with Alzheimer's disease had a history of severe head injury, a rate much higher than the control group (14).

Theories of viral causation abound. Two rare dementias occurring in humans—Creutzfeldt-Jacob disease and Kuru—are believed to be caused by submicroscopic agents and are characterized by neurotic plaque formation similar to Alzheimer's disease. Both of these diseases are transmissible. There is no evidence that Alzheimer's disease is transmitted between human beings.

A high concentration of aluminum has been found in the neurofibrillary tangles of Alzheimer's disease, thus leading researchers to suspect that exposure to toxins and trace metals may be a precipitating factor. Aluminum is neurotoxic to man, yet it is mildly elevated in normal elderly persons (24). It has no known function in the human body.

Other factors associated with Alzheimer's disease that are currently under investigation include immunological causes, chromosomal abnormalities, alterations in brain glucose metabolism, and alterations in brain chemistry. To date, neither these nor any other factors have been proved to be associated with Alzheimer's disease. Arteriosclerosis and lack of oxygen to the brain have been ruled out as causes, however.

Screening for Early Intervention

A clinical diagnosis of Alzheimer's disease is made in progressively dementing individuals after other illnesses that may cause memory loss have been excluded. A complete history is needed to rule out other conditions that may resemble Alzheimer's disease, such as past multiple cerebral infarctions leading to a condition currently termed multiple-infarct dementia. Pernicious anemia, drug reactions, and hydrocephalus can also cause cognitive impairment similar to Alzheimer's disease. These problems are treatable, and an early diagnosis may prevent further mental decline. A definitive diagnosis of Alzheimer's disease is made on the basis of findings from brain biopsy, which is not practical because of its invasiveness, and autopsy.

When Alzheimer's disease is suspected, a thorough physical, neurological, and psychiatric evaluation is imperative. Mental-status examinations and psychometric tests are used in conjunction with computerized axial tomography (CT). Measuring cognitive decline is possible after an initial assessment of mental function has been established. Areas of investigation that may yield clinically useful methods of early diagnosis and monitoring of the disease process include longitudinal electroencephalograph studies, magnetic resonance imaging (MRI), and positron emission tomography (PET).

Overview of Management

Current treatment of Alzheimer's disease is supportive and symptomatic. Psychotropic drugs such as chlorpromazine hydrochloride (Thorazine) and diazepam (Valium) help control agitation. Sleeping medications may reduce nocturnal wandering, but dosages must be monitored carefully in the elderly because of the long half-life of some medications. Acetylcholinesterase inhibitors such as physostigmine salicylate (Antilirium) may be used to manage diminished cholinergic function, yet the modest increase in cognitive ability resulting from them may make their use impractical. Better results have been obtained through the use of a combination of cholinergic precursors and cholinesterase inhibitors (20).

Nootropics, a new class of psychotropic agents used primarily in postoperative neurosurgery clients, are being studied extensively in the treatment of Alzheimer's disease. When they are given to elderly individuals in controlled situations, memory, alertness, and socialization improve. When used in combination with cholinergic precursors, they may prove useful in treating Alzheimer's disease (18). Neuropeptides, vasodilators, and psychostimulants are also being investigated. Studies using tetrahydroaminoacridine (THA) are currently planned on a national level. The limited research for review on THA appears promising. However, the fact remains that currently there is no specific treatment for Alzheimer's disease.

Nursing Care

Alzheimer's disease has a poor prognosis, eventual deterioration and death being due to a variety of complications resulting from progressive immobility and mental deterioration. Physical illness or any other stressful situation can accelerate progression. Promoting physical and mental health through supportive care is a priority. Nursing care aims to prolong cognitive and self-care abilities in the client and to support the family.

Assessment

Assessment of the client with Alzheimer's disease follows the guidelines for the nursing history and physical examination found earlier in this chapter. When collect-

ing data, the nurse should remember that Alzheimer's disease develops slowly, and evidence of dysfunction changes with time.

Nursing Diagnoses

Nursing diagnoses presented and discussed for clients with multiple sclerosis and Parkinson's disease may be applicable to the client with Alzheimer's disease. For example, the client with Alzheimer's disease may have nutritional deficits, self-care deficits, activity intolerance, sleep disturbances, and social isolation. To minimize redundancy, only three of the possible nursing diagnoses are considered here. These are:

1. Cognitive impairment with memory loss related to neurological deterioration.
2. Alteration in communication patterns related to such factors as neurological deterioration and panic.
3. Ineffectual family coping related to such factors as personality changes, loss of memory, and unpredictable behavior in the client.

Planning and Implementation

☐ *Cognitive Impairment with Memory Loss.* In the early stages of the disease, memory loss sometimes can be compensated for through use of the logic and judgment that remain intact. Lists, calendars, and clocks kept in all rooms may increase orientation. A consistent daily routine minimizes confusion and allows family members to plan activities around the client's daily routine. Drawers and cabinets can be labeled to help the client find things, and updated family snapshots can be kept in sight to help the client remember who family members are.

☐ *Alteration in Communication Patterns.* Communication impairment in the early stages of Alzheimer's disease is usually evidenced by difficulty finding words to express thoughts. As the disease progresses, loss of language skills, particularly agnosia (the inability to comprehend auditory, visual, and tactile stimuli), increases. Eventually, the client may be unable to recognize himself or herself and others. This may be most disturbing to the client; panic sometimes ensues. Holding the client and gently telling him or her that all is well and safe and providing a calm, safe environment can be therapeutic.

☐ *Ineffectual Family Coping.* Personality changes are a major cause of stress for families. Clients may be quite hostile and combative, creating a situation almost impossible to cope with in the home. Clients also may wander from their homes and may be unable to remember names and addresses, thus posing safety problems. It is helpful for these clients to wear identification at all times.

Alzheimer's disease is probably the most disruptive of the neurological diseases because of the symptoms and behaviors associated with it—loss of memory, poor judgment, lack of communication skills, unpredictability, embarrassing and dangerous behavior, incontinence, and wandering. These symptoms and behaviors require constant supervision. Because clients are unable to give gratifying feedback to care givers, and because there are few services available to many families, these clients are prime candidates for admission to nursing homes. Care givers, especially when they are alone and elderly, need substantial support systems to enable them to meet their own needs as well as those of the client.

Many times nursing-home placement is requested only after families have endured unrelenting, prolonged strain and social isolation. For care givers who choose to continue care at home, the nurse can help by obtaining assistance. Day care programs for impaired elderly are available in larger communities throughout the United States.

When placement in a long-term facility is probable, the family can be assisted in making a decision by asking such questions as "Does the client know where he or she is?" "Is constant care required?" "Is the client safe from inadvertent harm at home?" and "Is wandering increasing?" The answers to these questions may indicate that constant care in a protected environment with twenty-four-hour supervision is needed. Such care is beyond the ability of most families, yet relinquishing the role of care giver is often difficult. Being supportive, understanding, and nonjudgmental and simply letting families know they are not alone can help them through this difficult experience.

Finances should be discussed early in Alzheimer's disease, before the client becomes so mentally impaired that he or she cannot make a decision competently. If the client is able to make decisions, trust funds may be established to protect assets and income. It is most important for someone to be legally empowered to assume responsibility for the client's finances when mental deterioration makes this impossible for the client. Since the disease is seldom diagnosed in the early stages, many families must depend on court-appointed conservatorships (usually a family member) to handle the client's finances.

Promoting community awareness of Alzheimer's disease can increase community support and legislation to provide assistance to families. Respite services are another kind of assistance that helps relieve family stress and may delay client institutionalization; they include day care centers, short-term hospitalization, and visitors who relieve family members.

Evaluation

Client and family behaviors that indicate the degree to which nursing intervention is effective include the following.

Cognitive Impairment with Memory Loss. The client will use appropriate aids to help compensate for memory deficits.

Alteration in Communication Patterns. Family members will verbalize their understanding of communication deficits inherent in the disease. Family members will use appropriate comfort measures for the client experiencing fear about communication deficits.

Ineffectual Family Coping. Family members will verbalize an understanding of the personality and behavioral changes that can occur in Alzheimer's disease. Family members will discuss alternative forms of care (e.g., long-term placement) with the primary nurse. Family members together with the client will plan for financial management, unless the client has deteriorated to the point of legal incompetence.

Research Needs in Alzheimer's Disease

President Ronald Reagan, in proclaiming November 1983 as National Alzheimer's Disease Month, stated:

> The emotional, financial, and social consequences of Alzheimer's disease are so devastating that it deserves special attention. Science and clinical medicine are striving to improve understanding of what causes Alzheimer's disease and how to treat it successfully. Right now, research is the only hope for victims and families. (22)

Research on all progressive neuromuscular diseases is vital. Nursing can make a contribution with research into family care, coping abilities, and benefits of support services. More specifically, research into how families can be assisted in identifying problems early in the course of the disease, how families can help care givers to cope, the effects of day care and respite services on families, and nursing interventions needed in long-term situations can make a substantial contribution to the quality of life and care for clients and their families. Nursing interventions now assumed to be effective—for example, those used to deal with thought impairment, memory loss, and disorientation—require research validation.

Ethical Questions

The biblical proclamation to honor thy father and mother seems to conflict with the contemporary belief that children and parents should be independent of each other. Ethical questions such as the following arise from this change in expectations about parent-child relationships.

1. What is the moral obligation of children toward their elderly parents?
2. Do the changes in health, longevity, and social circumstances of elderly and neurologically impaired people justify a shift in traditional moral obligations?
3. Is it legitimate for society to demand that government assume much of the burden for direct care of the neurologically impaired?
4. What constitutes neglect and abuse of the impaired adult? It is important to remember that abuse and neglect are not limited to the physical, but may include emotional and financial abuse and neglect. What is the nurse's responsibility in identifying and reporting neglect and/or abuse?

Summary

Three of the more common progressive neurological diseases are discussed in terms of incidence, pathophysiology, and nursing and medical management. Nursing care is developed in the context of the nursing process.

Before planning nursing care, a complete health history and nursing assessment is necessary. Comprehensive nursing care is, in most instances, directed toward the following nursing diagnoses: impaired mobility, self-care deficits, impaired communication, altered sleep patterns, knowledge deficits, altered nutrition, and impaired family coping.

Progressive neurological diseases such as multiple sclerosis, Parkinson's disease, and Alzheimer's disease involve long-term problems that are highly stressful to both client and family. Many clients will require placement in long-term care facilities when the family or other care givers are unable to meet the demands of the client's care. Hospitalization or other institutionalization is best determined on an individual basis after a thorough assessment of the client's status and the family's resources and ability to provide care.

As the life span of the American population increases, nurses can expect to see more clients with progressive neurological diseases, especially among persons over eighty years old. Nurses have much to offer these clients and their families and can make the difference between their being able to maintain an acceptable quality of life and delay institutionalization and their being overwhelmed by chronic problems.

CASE STUDY 1

Mary Smith, a thirty-four-year-old female engineer, is admitted to the hospital with a diagnosis of rule out multiple sclerosis. She is scheduled for neurological testing and examination. Over the past year, Ms. Smith noticed occasional visual problems. She also complained of feeling tired and weak by midday. After work she rests, often not getting up for meals. She is planning to marry in three months and is concerned about how her physical condition will affect her fiancé. At the present time, he is very concerned and supportive, offering reassurance and love.

1. Discuss the major problems in the clinical diagnosis of multiple sclerosis. What laboratory and neurological testing will probably be done?
2. How can a warm bath be used to evaluate Ms. Smith's condition?
3. What are other motor and sensory symptoms that may indicate multiple sclerosis?
4. Urinary bladder dysfunction is a major long-term complication of multiple sclerosis. Describe medical and nursing management of bladder dysfunction.
5. If Ms. Smith has an exacerbating-remitting form of the disease, what information regarding prognosis and long-term care is needed? How can the nurse offer support and guidance during the diagnostic phase of the disease?

CASE STUDY 2

Mr. Brown, age seventy-two, was admitted to the hospital with a broken arm, which he sustained in a fall down a short flight of stairs. During the health history, his wife told the nurse that he has been having difficulty getting out of bed in the morning. His walking has been slower than normal, and recently he has had difficulty with his balance. She noticed a slight tremor in his hands while he was eating but attributed this to his age. The onset of symptoms was gradual. Mrs. Brown first noticed a change in her husband two or three years ago. Medical intervention was not considered by the family, who believed that aging caused the changes in his behavior.

1. What classic symptoms of Parkinson's disease does Mr. Brown have? Describe the typical onset of Parkinson's disease.
2. Describe the knowledge deficits in this family. How can the nurse approach the family effectively and plan health teaching?
3. What complication of Parkinson's disease does Mr. Brown have? What are other complications, and how can they be prevented?
4. If drug therapy with L-dopa is used, what must the family be taught about the medication and the course of treatment?
5. What tips can be given to Mrs. Brown to enable her to care for her husband and help him maintain his independence?

CASE STUDY 3

Mr. Jones, age sixty-eight, has been caring for his sixty-seven-year-old wife, Sara, for six years with only occasional assistance from a married daughter, who works full time and has four children. Mr. Jones recently joined a support group for spouses of individuals with Alzheimer's disease.

Mrs. Jones has periods of complete forgetfulness during which she does not recognize her husband. Sometimes she reacts violently toward him and calls him stupid. His voice reveals anger when he discusses his wife's behavior. At present, Mr. Jones is quite depressed, especially because his plans for his retirement years are not being met.

1. What can the nurse do to help Mr. Jones cope with his feelings about his wife's behavior?
2. What type of agnosia does Mrs. Jones have? What other types of agnosia may she develop?
3. How can the nurse help Mr. Jones to consider institutionalization for his wife?
4. Discuss the long-term financial, social, and emotional effects of Alzheimer's disease on the family.

REFERENCES

1. Brody, E. M., M. P. Lawton, and B. Liebowitz. "Senile Dementia: Public Policy and Adequate Institutional Care." *American Journal of Public Health,* 1984, 74:1381.
2. Calne, S. "Parkinson's Disease—Helping the Patient With a Movement Disorder." *Canadian Nurse,* 1984, 80:35.
3. Cook, S., et al. "Declining Incidence of Multiple Sclerosis in the Orkney Islands." *Neurology,* 1985, 35:545.
4. Coyle, P. K. "CSF Immune Complexes in Multiple Sclerosis." *Neurology,* 1985, 35:398.
5. Dodson, J. "The Slow Death: Alzheimer's Disease." *Journal of Neurosurgical Nursing,* 1984, 16:270.
6. Garrett, E. "Parkinsonism: Forgotten Considerations in Medical Treatment and Nursing Care." *Journal of Neurosurgical Nursing,* 1982, 14:13.
7. Guibilato, T., and J. Metcalf. "Evoked Potentials: Nursing Perspective." *Journal of Neurosurgical Nursing,* 1984, 16:241.
8. Hartshorn, J. C. "Immunosuppressive Treatment of MS." *Journal of Neurosurgical Nursing,* 1984, 16:275.
9. Holland, N. J., P. Wiesel-Levison, and M. G. Madonna. "Community Care of the Patient with Multiple Sclerosis." *Rehabilitation Nursing,* 1984, 9:18.
10. Jankovic, J., J. Orman, and J. Berger. "Placebo-Controlled Study of Mesulergine in Parkinson's Disease." *Neurology,* 1985, 35:161.
11. Kurtzke, J., G. Beebe, and J. Norman. "Epidemiology of Multiple Sclerosis in United States Veterans: Migration and Risk of MS." *Neurology,* 1985, 35:672.
12. Lewis, S. M. "Viral and Immunopathology in Multiple Sclerosis." *Journal of Neurosurgical Nursing,* 1983, 15:346.
13. Mayeux, R., Y. Stern, and S. Spanton. "Heterogeneity in Dementia of the Alzheimer's Type: Evidence of Subgroups." *Neurology,* 1985, 35:453.
14. Mortimer, J., et al. "Head Injury as a Risk Factor in Alzheimer's Disease." *Neurology,* 1985, 35:264.
15. National Multiple Sclerosis Society. *News Release* (Research nos. 091285, 0702485, 062984, 041385). New York: National Multiple Sclerosis Society, 1985.
16. Rinne, U. K. "Combined Bromocriptine-Levodopa Therapy Early in Parkinson's Disease." *Neurology,* 1985, 35:1196.
17. Scheinberg, L. C. *Multiple Sclerosis: A Guide for Patients and Their Families.* New York: Raven Press, 1983, 41.
18. Schneck, M. K. "Nootropics." In *Alzheimer's Disease: The Standard Reference,* ed. B. Reisberg. New York: Free Press, 1983, 362–68.
19. Schoenberg, B. S., D. W. Anderson, and A. G. Haerer. "Prevalence of PD in the Biracial Population of Copial County, Mississippi." *Neurology,* 1985, 35:841.
20. Sitaram, N., et al. "Combination Treatment of Alzheimer's Dementia." In *Alzheimer's Disease: The Standard Reference,* ed. B. Reisberg. New York: Free Press, 1983, 355–61.

21. Stern, G., and A. Lees. *Parkinson's Disease: The Facts.* New York: Oxford University Press, 1982, 3.

22. U.S. Department of Health and Human Services. *Report of the Secretary's Task Force on Alzheimer's Disease.* DHHS Publication no. ADM 84-1323, September 1984, 49.

23. Waksman, B. H., and W. E. Reynolds. *Research on Multiple Sclerosis.* Rev. ed. New York: National Multiple Sclerosis Society, 1982, 25–27.

24. Wells, C. "Chronic Brain Disease: An Update on Alcoholism, Parkinson's Disease and Dementia." *Hospital and Community Psychiatry,* 1982, 33:111.

25. Whittington, L. "Multiple Sclerosis: Dealing with Reality." *Canadian Nursing,* 1983, 79:34.

26. Wisniewski, K. E., "Alzheimer's Disease in Down's Syndrome." *Neurology,* 1985, 35:957.

27. World Health Organization. *World Health Statistics Annual.* Geneva, Switzerland: WHO, 1984, 180.

28. Zetusky, W., J. Jankovic, and F. J. Perozzola. "The Heterogeneity of Parkinson's Disease." *Neurology,* 1985, 35:522.

INDEX

.

Abandonment, parental, 263
Abdominal system, substance abuse and, 243
Abortion, spontaneous, maternal age and, 365
Abruptio placenta, 365
Abusive families, 250–264
  abused spouse in, 256
  adolescents in, 254–256
  assessment of members in, 254, 255
  characteristics of, 251–253
  children in, 254–256
  elderly abuse in, 256
  establishing relationship with, 253–254
  interventions for, 257, 259–262
    primary prevention in, 257, 259
    secondary prevention in, 259–260
    tertiary prevention in, 260–262
  legal aspects of, 263–264
  nursing diagnosis and, 256–257, 258–259
  outcome evaluation and, 262–263
  problem of, 250–251
Accidents
  falling, older adults and, 555
  school environment and, 162–163
Accountability, 51. *See also* Quality assurance
  occupational health nursing and, 180
  sexually transmitted disease and, 427
Accreditation, home care and, 186–187
Acetylsalicylic acid
  antiplatelet effect of, 580–581
  arthritis treatment with, 601, 602
Achondroplasia, paternal age and, 366
Acid-base values
  COPD, 564
  normal, 565
Acidosis
  metabolic, renal failure and, 480
  respiratory, COPD and, 565
Acquired immunodeficiency syndrome (AIDS), 522–537
  assessment in, 530–531
  chest x-ray in, 436
  complications of, 525
  ethical and legal issues in, 536–537
  evaluation in, 535–536
  immunosuppression and, 523–524
  implementation in, 531–535
  intravenous drug abuse and, 246–247
  management of, 528–530
  natural history of, 525, 526

  nervous system effects of, 524
  nursing diagnoses in, 531
  planning in, 531–535
  prevention of, 525, 527–528
  screening for, 528
  transmission of, 524–525
  tuberculosis and, 430
    chemotherapy for, 437
Activity(ies). *See also* Exercise
  AIDS and, 535
  energy requirements of, 569
  intolerance of
    COPD and, 567–568
    Parkinson's disease and, 629
    renal failure and, 482
Acute respiratory failure, COPD and, 560
Adaptation, stages of, 510, 514
Addiction. *See* Substance abuse
Administrator(s). *See also* Nurse administrators
  resistance to self-care of, 32–33
  school health, 152–153
Adolescence
  abuse in, 254–256
  AIDS information and, 528
  chronic illness in, 383–384
  grief and, 231–232
  nutrition in, 146–147
Adoption, 378
  breast-feeding and, 338–339
  infertility and, 370
Adrenergic drugs, COPD and, 565–566
Adrenergic inhibitors, side effects of, 464–465
Advocacy
  nutrition and, 140–141
  older parents and, 372
AFP (alpha-fetoprotein), 368
Age. *See also* Adolescence; Child(ren); Elderly; Infancy
  Alzheimer's disease and, 630
  COPD and, 561–562
  coronary artery disease and, 490
  ESRD incidence and, 474
  nutritional needs and, 142–148. *See also* Life cycle, nutrition and
  osteoarthritis and, 609
  parenting and, 363–372. *See also* Parent(s), older
  rheumatoid arthritis and, 598
Agency policy
  ethics and, 86–87
  written, 67–68

Agency standards. *See also* Standards of nursing practice
  tice
  home care and, 186–187
Aging, demographics of, 544
Agnosias, types of, 621
AIDS. *See* Acquired immunodeficiency syndrome
"AIDS anxiety," 530
AIDS dementia, 535
AIDS-related complex (ARC), 525
AIDS-related retrovirus. *See* Human immunodeficiency virus
  ciency virus
Air pollution, COPD and, 561
Alcohol abuse, 237. *See also* Substance abuse
  physiology of, 238–240
  withdrawal from, 247
Alcohol intake, 141
  hypertension and, 454
Aldosteronism, hypertension and, 451
Allergy
  asthma and, 387–391
  breast-feeding and, 331
Alpha$_1$-adrenergic blocker, side effects of, 465
Alpha-fetoprotein, 368
Aluminum encephalopathy, 474
Aluminum hydroxide, renal failure and, 481
Alzheimer's disease, 553, 630–634
  assessment of, 632
  cognitive impairment in, 632
  communication pattern alterations in, 632
  early intervention in, 631
  evaluation and, 633
  family coping with, 632–633
  implementation and, 632–633
  incidence of, 630
  management of, 632
  memory loss in, 632
  nursing diagnoses and, 632
  pathophysiology of, 631
  planning and, 632–633
  research needs in, 633–634
  risk factors for, 631
Ambulatory status, home care and, 190
Amebiasis, 415
  treatment of, 420
Amenorrhea, oral contraceptives and, 314–315
American Association of Occupational Health Nurses, 169, 178
American Heart Association, smoking cessation recommendations of, 491
  ommendations of, 491
American Nurses' Association
  Council on Gerontological Nursing of, 547
  geriatric care standards of, 545–546
  home care standards of, 187
  quality assurance definition of, 51
  standards of nursing practice of, 53–54, 57–60
    research and, 92

Amniocentesis, 366–368
  risks and concerns of, 368–369
Amniography, 368
Analgesic drugs, arthritis treatment with, 601
Androgenic agents, chronic renal failure and, 477
Anemia
  chemotherapy and, 288
  renal failure and, 473
Angina pectoris, 488, 497. *See also* Coronary artery disease
  disease
  treatment of, 497, 498
Angiography, cerebrovascular disease diagnosis and, 586
  586
Angiotensin-converting enzyme inhibitors, side effects of, 465
  of, 465
Ankylosis, 596
Anorexia
  chemotherapy and, 289
  renal failure and, 481
Antenatal testing, 366–369
Anthropometric measurements, 136–137
Anticancer treatment, 274, 275
Anticholinergics, Parkinson's disease treatment with, 627, 628
  627, 628
Anticipatory guidance
  older parents and, 372
  stress management and, 211
Anticoagulants, stroke and, 580
Anticonvulsants, cerebrovascular disease treatment and, 581
  and, 581
Antidepressants, Parkinson's disease and, 625, 627
Antihistamines
  chronic renal failure and, 477
  Parkinson's disease treatment with, 628
Antihypertensive drugs, 462–463, 464–465, 580
  chronic renal failure and, 477
Anti-inflammatory drugs, 601, 602
Antimalarial drugs, arthritis treatment with, 601, 603
Antiplatelet vasodilators, 580–581
Antipruritics, chronic renal failure and, 477
Antituberculosis chemotherapy, 437–439
  adverse effects of, 442–443
Antiviral drugs, Parkinson's disease treatment with, 628
  628
Anxiety. *See also* Stress
  AIDS and, 531–532
  chemotherapy and, 291
  COPD and, 568–570
  coronary artery disease and, 499–500
  definition of, 500
  renal failure and, 483
  rheumatoid arthritis and, 605
  tuberculosis and, 441, 444
Aphasia, dysarthria versus, 590
Apnea, sleep
  home monitoring of, 401
  SIDS and, 399

Areola, 332
Arrhythmias, 489
Arterial pressure. *See* Blood pressure; Hypertension
Arterial wall, changes in, hypertension and, 452
Arthritis, 595–613
  ethical issues in, 612
  osteoarthritis, 608
    assessment of, 611
    clinical manifestations of, 609–610
    early intervention in, 610–611
    etiology of, 608–609
    evaluation and, 612
    nursing diagnoses and, 611
    pathophysiology of, 609, 610
    planning and, 611–612
    risk factors for, 609
  rheumatoid, 595
    assessment of, 598–599
    clinical manifestations of, 596–597
    early intervention in, 598
    etiology of, 595–596
    evaluation and, 608
    implementation and, 600–608
    nursing diagnoses and, 600
    pathophysiology of, 596, 597
    planning and, 600–608
    risk factors for, 597–598
Aspirin
  antiplatelet effect of, 580–581
  arthritis treatment with, 601, 602
Assault. *See* Abusive families
Assessment, 7. *See also* Self-assessment
  abusive families and, 254–256
  Alzheimer's disease, 632
  cancer nursing and, 284–293
    Cancer Nursing Assessment Tool for, 284–287
    Prechemotherapy Nursing Assessment Model for, 288–293
  cerebral palsy, 392
  chronic renal failure, 476, 478, 479
  communication in, 37–38
  community, 112–118. *See also* Community, assessment of
  COPD, 562–563, 564
  coronary artery disease, 493–494, 495, 496
  crisis and, 219–220
  diabetes, 512–514
  grief, 233
  HIV infection, 530–531
  hypertension, 457–458
  multiple sclerosis, 618–622
  nutrition, 134–138
  older adults and, 549–550, 551–553
  rheumatoid arthritis, 598–599
  school nurse and, 158–161
  self-care and, 30–31

sexually transmitted disease, 422–423, 424
SIDS, 402–403
stress, 207–208
stroke, 582–586
substance abuse and, 242–243
tuberculosis, 434–437
Association for Gerontology in Higher Education, 547
Asthma, 387–391, 560
  allergy proofing of home and, 389
  child with, nursing care of, 387–388
  self-care responsibilities and, 388–391
Atherosclerosis, 488. *See also* Coronary artery disease
  diabetes and, 509
  hypertension and, 451
Attachment(s)
  loss and, 226
  stressors and, 205–206
Attitudes, communication and, 40
Attitudinal barriers, cancer nursing care and, 278–281, 282
Audit, 49
Autonomic gastroparesis, diabetes and, 508
Autonomy
  COPD and, 572–573
  principle of, 8
Avoidance behaviors, cancer nursing care and, 277
Azidothymidine (AZT), AIDS and, 529

Bacillus of Calmette and Guérin, vaccination with, tuberculosis and, 434
Bacteriologic examination, tuberculosis and, 436–437
Barbiturates
  abuse of, 240–241
  overdose of, 246
Barclay v. Campbell, 76
Bass v. Barksdale, 74
Battered child syndrome, 250. *See also* Child(ren), abused
Battered spouse, 256, 261
  law and, 263–264
Bayer v. Smith, 76
Bayley Scales of Infant Development, abuse and, 254
BCG vaccine, tuberculosis and, 434
Belmon v. St. Francis Cabrini Hospital, 71–72
Bereavement. *See* Grief
Beta-adrenergic blockers
  angina pectoris treatment with, 498
  side effects of, 464
Bibliographic data bases, 93, 94
Biochemical disorders, antenatal testing for, 367–368
Birth. *See* Childbirth
Birth control. *See* Family planning; Oral contraceptives
Birth defects. *See also* Chronically ill child(ren)
  maternal age and, 366
Black Lung Association, 178

Bladder. *See also* Genitourinary system; Urinary *entries*
    neurogenic, diabetes and, 508
Bleiler v. Bodnar, 69–70
Blood alcohol concentration, 238
Blood gas values
    COPD, 564
    normal, 565
Blood glucose monitoring, 510–511
Blood pressure
    high. *See* Hypertension
    measurement of
        factors affecting, 455
        interpretation to client of, 456–457
        technique of, 455–456
    self-monitoring of, 461–462
Blood screening, HIV antibody, 528
Blood transfusion, AIDS transmission by, 524
Body image
    loss of, 232, 233
    rheumatoid arthritis and, 606
Body weight, 136–137, 141. *See also* Obesity
    reduction in, hypertension and, 461
Bonding, maternal-infant, breast-feeding and, 331
Bone, renal failure and, 480–481
Bony ankylosis, 596
Booster effect, tuberculosis and, 435
Bottle-feeding, supplemental, 336–337. *See also* Breast-feeding
Bouchard's nodes, 610
Bowel disturbances
    abused children and, 254
    AIDS and, 535
    chemotherapy and, 289
    older adults and, 554–555
    Parkinson's disease and, 629–630
    renal failure and, 472, 482
    stroke and, 588
Bra, nursing, 339–340
Brain
    alcohol abuse and, 238–239
    degenerative diseases of, 616–635. *See also* Alzheimer's disease; Multiple sclerosis; Parkinson's disease
Breakthrough bleeding, oral contraceptives and, 314–315
Breast cancer, early detection of, 268
Breast-feeding, 328–346
    adequacy of intake and, 337–338
    adopted children and, 338–339
    advantages of, 328–331
    anatomy and physiology of, 331–332
    assuring breathing during, 334
    breast care and, 335
    breast pumps and, 336
    breast size and, 336

cesarean birth and, 337
    contraception and, 339
    contraindications to, 342
    diet and, 335
    factors encouraging, 343–344
    father's role and, 339
    frequency and duration of, 334–335
    infant breast swelling and, 338
    infant stools and, 338
    intervention in, 345–346
    inverted nipples and, 336
    leaking breasts and, 338
    low-birth-weight infant and, 342, 343
    manual expression of milk and, 341–342
    mastitis and, 335
    medication aftereffects and, 340–341
    milk delivery in, 332–333
    multiple births and, 342–343
    pollution and, 340
    positioning for, 333–334
    premature infant and, 342, 343
    public, 339–340
    reasons to stop, 344–345
    rest and, 335–336
    siblings' role and, 339
    solid foods and, 338
    storage of milk and, 341–342
    sucking techniques and, 337
    supplements and, 336–337
    techniques of, 333
    teething and, 337
    timing of, 340
    weaning from, 341
    work/social schedule and, 341
Breast pumps, 336
Breathing, diaphragmatic, 565
Bromocriptine mesylate (Parlodel), 628
Bronchitis, chronic, 559–560. *See also* Chronic obstructive pulmonary disease
Bronchodilators, 565–566
Brown Lung Association, 178
Burnout, 211–212
    cancer nursing and, 280
    working mothers and, 357

Caffeine
    breast-feeding and, 340
    hypertension and, 454
Calcium, recommended daily allowances of, 143
    pregnancy and, 144
Calcium antagonists, angina pectoris treatment with, 498
Calcium level, renal failure and, 480–481
Cancer, 266–305
    coping ability and, 274, 276
    diagnostic stage of, 273

early detection of, 267–269, 270–272
end stage of, 273–274
extent of, 274, 275
intermediate stage of, 273
Kaposi's sarcoma, AIDS and, 525
patient-need dynamics and, 269, 272
prevention of, 267–269, 270–271
primary nursing role and, 276, 277
stages of, 272–274
treatment for, 274, 275
type of, 274, 275
warning signals of, 268
Cancer nursing
barriers to care in, 277–283, 294–296, 300–305
attitudinal, 278–281, 282
cognitive, 281, 283, 294–296
interpersonal, 296, 300–305
"cure-versus-care" dilemma and, 279, 280
development of, 276, 277
outcome standards for, 296, 297–299
Cancer Nursing Assessment Tool, 284–287
Candidiasis, treatment of, 420
CAPD (continuous ambulatory peritoneal dialysis), 476
Capillary blood glucose monitoring, 511
Capreomycin, tuberculosis treatment with, 439
Carbohydrate intake, 141
Carbon monoxide, Parkinson's disease and, 625, 627
Carboxylase inhibitors, levodopa with, 627
Cardiac function
hypertension and, 453
stroke and, 578, 580
Cardiac neuropathy, diabetes and, 508
Cardiomyopathy, alcohol abuse and, 239
Cardiovascular disease, 486. *See also* Coronary artery disease
Cardiovascular system
chemotherapy and, 290
elderly and, 551
renal failure effects on, 472
substance abuse and, 243
Care giver, responsibilities of, gerontological nursing and, 546–547
Caring. *See also* Self-care
beneficial results of, 25–26
capacity for, 22–25
components of, 20
essential ingredients of, 19–20
meaning of, 18–19
process of, 21
and relationship to nursing, 20–22
Carpal tunnel syndrome, 597
Carter v. St. Vincent Infirmary, 72
Catecholamines, hypertension and, 452
Central adrenergic inhibitors, side effects of, 464

Central nervous system
alcohol abuse and, 238–239
HIV effect on, 524
Cerebral palsy, 391–396
child with, assessment of, 392
legal and ethical issues in, 395–396
prevention of, nurse's role in, 391–392
universal self-care needs and, 392–395
Cerebrovascular disease, 576–592
assessment in, 582–586
cardiac impairment and, 578, 580
diabetes and, 509, 578, 579–580
drug therapy for, 580–581
ethical and legal issues in, 591–592
evaluation in, 591
hypertension and, 453, 578, 579
implementation in, 587–591
incidence of, 576
management of, 579–582
nursing diagnoses in, 586
pathophysiology of, 576–578
planning in, 587–591
prevention of, 579
rehabilitation after, 581–582
risk factors for, 578–579
Certification
home care agency, 187
school nurse, 153
Cervical cancer, early detection of, 268
Cervical cap, 323, 324
Cesarean birth, breast-feeding after, 337
Chancroid, treatment of, 421
Change strategies, barriers to, 61
Chemotherapy, 275
assessment before, 288–293
tuberculosis and, 430, 437–439
adverse effects of, 442–443
Chest pain. *See* Angina pectoris
Chest percussion, COPD and, 565
Chest x-ray examination, tuberculosis and, 436
Child(ren). *See also* School health
abused, 250
characteristics of, 254–256
law and, 263
sexually, 252–253, 261
chronically ill, 381–396. *See also* Chronically ill child(ren)
coronary heart disease prevention for, 492, 493
death of, leading causes of, 158
divorce impact on, 375–376
home care for, 186
loss and, 230–231
role of, breast-feeding and, 339
welfare of, maternal employment effects on, 351–352

Child Abuse and Treatment Act of 1974, 250. *See also*
    Child(ren), abused
Child care, maternal employment and, 352–354
Childbirth. *See also* Pregnancy
    abusive families and, 251
    cesarean, breast-feeding after, 337
    drug aftereffects from, breast-feeding and, 340–341
    sociocultural context of, 126–128
Chlamydia, 415
    treatment of, 420
Cholesterol
    coronary artery disease and, 489–490
    hypertension and, 454
    reduction of, dietary changes for, 491–492
Cholesterol intake, 141
Christopher v. Dow Chemical Company, 74
Chromosomal abnormalities
    maternal age and, 366
    paternal age and, 366
Chromosomal examination, antenatal, 367
Chronic illness. *See also* Chronically ill child; *specific
        illness*
    adaptation to, 507, 510. *See also* Coping ability
Chronic obstructive pulmonary disease (COPD), 559–
        573
    activity intolerance and, 567–568
    assessment in, 562–563, 564
    asthma, 560
    bronchitis, 559–560
    climate and, 571–572
    complications of, 560–561
    depression and, 570–571
    emphysema, 560
    ethical issues in, 572–573
    evaluation in, 572
    fear and anxiety and, 568–570
    hypoventilation and, 565–567
    implementation in, 563–572
    management of, 562
    nursing diagnoses in, 563
    nutritional deficits and, 568
    planning in, 563–572
    prevention of, 562
    risk factors for, 561–562
    sleep disturbances and, 568
    smoking cessation and, 564–565
    social isolation and, 571–572
Chronic renal failure (CRF), 471
    assessment of, 476, 478, 479
    causes of, 475
    complications of, 473–474
    early intervention in, 474–475
    evaluation and, 483–484
    management of, 475–476, 477–478
    nursing diagnoses and, 478–483
    stages of, 472

Chronic sorrow, 384
Chronically ill child(ren), 381–396
    asthma in, 387–391
    cerebral palsy in, 391–396
    legal and ethical issues with, 395–396
    nurse's role and, 381–387
        community and, 386–387
        family and, 384–386
        growth and development and, 382–384
        research recommendations for, 396
Cigarette smoking
    angina and, 497
    COPD and, 561, 562, 564–565
    coronary artery disease and, 489, 491
    stroke and, 579
Cignetti v. Camel, 75
Cirrhosis, alcohol abuse and, 239
Client(s)
    assignment of, 13
    caring for. *See* Caring
    knowledge level of, 39–40. *See also* Knowledge defi-
        cit(s)
    needs of, cancer and, 269, 272, 274, 276
    nurse's relationship with. *See* Nurse-client relation-
        ship
    and resistance to self-care, 31
    rights of, 8
        home care and, 195
    self-concept of, 39
Client behavior, ethical decision making and, 85
Client classification system, home care and, 191–192
Client teaching
    cancer nursing and, 294
    condoms and, 321
    coronary artery disease and, diet and, 492
    diabetes and, 511, 515, 516, 517, 519
    diaphragm use and, 323
    HIV infection and, 535
    inadequate, 73–74
    IUD and, 318–319
    nutrition and, 139
    older parents and, 371
    oral contraceptives and, 316–317
    spermicides and, 322
    stroke and, 590–591
Clotting, intravascular, COPD and, 561
CMV (cytomegalovirus), AIDS and, 525
Cocaine, 240
Code for Nurses, 85–86
Cognitive barriers, cancer nursing care and, 281, 283,
        294–296
Cognitive functioning
    AIDS and, 535
    Alzheimer's disease and, 632
    chemotherapy and, 291–293
Coitus interruptus, 324

Cold application, rheumatoid arthritis and, 600–601
Collaboration
    cancer nursing and, 295
    nurse-client, 7, 43–44
    occupational health nursing and, 175, 180–181
    of team members, 45
Collegial relationship, 14
Colostrum, 330
Coma, hyperosmolar hyperglycemic nonketotic, 508
Committee for Occupational Safety and Health
        (COSH), 177
Communication, 37–45
    attitudes and, 40
    cancer nursing and, 300–305
    collaborating in, 43–44
    feelings and, 40–41
    impaired
        Alzheimer's disease and, 632
        Parkinson's disease and, 630
        stroke and, 589–590
    knowledge and, 39–40
    listening and, 43
    model of, 37–39
    needs and, 41–42
    negligence and, 74–75
    negotiating in, 44. *See also* Negotiation
    personality type and, 41
    self-concept and, 39
    sociocultural factors in, 42–43
    with team members, 45
    therapeutic skills in, 304
    values and, 40
Community
    assessment of, 112–118
        data base analysis in, 116–117
        data base establishment in, 113–115
        high-level wellness and, 118
        nursing process after, 117–118
        nursing process application in, 112
        purpose of, 113
    chronically ill child and, 386–387
    definition of, 112–113
    health needs of, 117
    school health and, 153
    self-care concept and, 30–31
    sexually transmitted disease and, 426–427
Community education, AIDS and, 527–528
"Community of solution" approach, 113
Community resources
    occupational health nursing and, 177–178
    SIDS and, 407
Community services, referral to, home care and, 196–197
Community standards, 68–69
Compliance. *See* Noncompliance

Condom, 321
    AIDS and, 525, 527
Condylomata acuminata, treatment of, 421
Confidentiality
    AIDS and, 536–537
    occupational health nursing and, 180
Conflict, negotiation and, 44
Confusion, older adults and, 550, 553, 554. *See also*
        Alzheimer's disease
Congestive heart failure, 489
Constipation
    AIDS and, 535
    older adults and, 554–555
    Parkinson's disease and, 629–630
    renal failure and, 473, 482
    stroke and, 588
Consumer, home health service selection by, 188, 189
Consumerism, 12
Continuous ambulatory peritoneal dialysis (CAPD),
        476
Contraception, 312–325. *See also* Family planning;
        Oral contraceptives
    breast-feeding and, 339
Contract, standard of care and, 70–71
Control, negotiation versus, 99
Cooper v. National Motor Bearing Company, Inc., 75
Cooperative model, 44
COPD. *See* Chronic obstructive pulmonary disease
Coping ability. *See also* Stress
    AIDS and, 533–534
    Alzheimer's disease and, 632–633
    cancer and, 274, 276
        chemotherapy and, 292
    multiple sclerosis and, 623–624
    Parkinson's disease and, 630
    rheumatoid arthritis and, 605–606
    stroke and, 590
Coronary artery disease, 487–501
    complications of, 488–489
    diabetes and, 509
    ethical and legal issues in, 501
    hypertension and, 452
    incidence of, 487–488
    management of, 492–493
    nursing care for, 493–501
        assessment in, 493–494, 495, 496
        evaluation in, 500–501
        implementation in, 494–500
        nursing diagnoses in, 494
        planning in, 494–500
    pathophysiology of, 488
    prevention of, 490–492
    risk factors in, 489–490
Corticosteroids
    arthritis treatment with, 601, 603
    stroke therapy and, 580

COSH (Committee for Occupational Safety and Health), 177
Costs, 11
  breast-feeding, 331
  cerebral palsy and, 395
  diabetes and, 518–519
  prospective payment and, 61–62
  substance abuse, 237
  third-party payers and, ethical decision making and, 87–88
Coughing, COPD and, sleep disturbance and, 568
Coumadin (warfarin), 580
Council on Gerontological Nursing, 547
Counseling
  family, COPD and, 571
  genetic, 369
  grief and, 233–234
  marital, SIDS and, 405–406
  nutrition, 138–139
  school nurse and, 162
  sexual, rheumatoid arthritis and, 607
  sibling, SIDS and, 404–405
Court decisions, 66–67
"Crabs," treatment of, 420
Cranial nerve assessment, 620
CRF. *See* Chronic renal failure
Crisis
  classification of, 216–217
  divorce as, 376
  stress and, 216
Crisis intervention, 217–224
  assessment and, 219–220
  older parents and, 372
  primary nurse in, 224
  principles of, 220–222
  self-care and, 223–224
  SIDS and, 403–404
  stages of, 222–223
  suicidal client and, 217–219
Cromolyn sodium, 391
Culture
  capacity for caring and, 24
  communication and, 42–43
  food and, 123–124, 136
  health beliefs and, 120–131. *See also* Health beliefs
  occupational health nursing and, 178–179
Cushing's syndrome, hypertension and, 451
Cycloserine, tuberculosis treatment with, 439
Cytomegalovirus (CMV), AIDS and, 525

Data base(s), 93, 94
  analysis of, community assessment and, 116–117
  establishment of, community assessment and, 113–115
  information sources for, 115
Day care, 353

Death. *See also* Grief
  in children and young adults, leading causes of, 158
  coronary heart disease and, 487, 488
  in infancy. *See also* Sudden infant death syndrome
    maternal age and, 365
  maternal, age and, 364
Decadron (dexamethasone), stroke therapy and, 580
Decision making, 13
  ethical, 84, 548
  legal, 65–69
Defense mechanisms, chronically ill adolescent and, 384
Defensive medicine, 369
Deficiency diseases, 123
Deficit Reduction Act of 1984, home care accreditation and, 187
Degenerative arthritis, 608–612
Degenerative neuromuscular disease, 616–635. *See also* Alzheimer's disease; Multiple sclerosis; Parkinson's disease
Dementia. *See also* Alzheimer's disease
  AIDS and, 535
  elderly and, 553, 554
Demographics
  aging and, 544
  home care and, 189
  hypertension and, 449
  occupational health nursing and, 170–171
Denial/protection syndrome, 301
  AIDS and, 532
Denver Developmental Screening Test, abuse and, 254
Depo-Provera, 318
Depression
  COPD and, 570–571
  coronary artery disease and, 499–500
  renal failure and, 482–483
Development, growth and, chronically ill child and, 382–384
Developmental assessment, abusive families and, 254
Developmental crises, 217
Developmental loss, 227
Developmental-nutritional needs, 142–148. *See also* Life cycle, nutrition and
Developmental self-care requisites, 29
Developmental tasks, family, 258–259
Dexamethasone (Decadron), stroke therapy and, 580
Diabetes, 505–520
  assessment in, 512–514
  classification of, 505
  complications of, 507, 508–509
  coronary artery disease and, 490
  diagnosis of, 505–507
  ethical and legal issues in, 518–519
  evaluation in, 517–518
  implementation in, 514–517
  management of, 507–511

nursing diagnoses in, 514
planning in, 514–517
pregnancy and, maternal age and, 364–365
prevention of, 511–512
psychosocial aspects of, 507
renal failure and, 475
screening for, 512
stroke and, 509, 578, 579–580
Diagnostic and Statistical Manual of Mental Disor-
   ders, anxiety definition of, 500
Diagnostic-related groups (DRGs), 11, 62
   home care and, 184, 194–195
Diagnostic tests
   cerebrovascular disease and, 585–586
   coronary artery disease and, 496
   diabetes and, 513–514
   multiple sclerosis and, 621–622
   osteoarthritis and, 611
   rheumatoid arthritis and, 599
   substance abuse and, 243–244
   tuberculosis and, 434–437
Dialysis, 476
   electrolyte balance and, 480
   nutrition and, 481
Diaper rash, cerebral palsy and, 393
Diaphragm, contraception with, 322–323
Diaphragmatic breathing, 565
Diarrhea
   AIDS and, 535
   diabetes and, 508
   stroke and, 588
Diet. *See also* Nutrition
   asthma and, 388
   breast-feeding and, 335
   cholesterol reduction and, 491–492
   diabetes and, 508–509
   hypertension and, 454, 460–461
   multiple sclerosis and, 618
Diet recall, 135
Dilantin, cerebrovascular disease treatment and, 581
Dilemmas, ethical, 82
Dipyridamole (Persantine), antiplatelet effect of, 581
Discomfort. *See also* Pain
   AIDS and, 532–533
   osteoarthritis and, 612
   rheumatoid arthritis and, 600–601, 604
Disease
   illness and. *See also* Illness; *specific disease*
      sociocultural context of, 128–129
   sexually transmitted, 414–428. *See also* Sexually
      transmitted diseases
Disfigurement, loss and, 232, 233
Disinfection, AIDS and, 527–528
Dispositional crises, 217
Distress, 204
Diuretics, side effects of, 464

Divorce, 375–377
   grief and, 232–233
"Divorce Myth, The," 377
Documentation, 72–73
   client teaching and, 74
   ethics and, 87
   home care service, 191–192
Dopamine deficiency, 625. *See also* Parkinson's disease
Down's syndrome, maternal age and, 366
DRGs. *See* Diagnostic-related groups
Drugs
   abuse of. *See* Substance abuse
   aftereffects of, breast-feeding and, 340–341
   Alzheimer's disease management and, 632
   antihypertensive, 462–463, 464–465
   arthritis treatment with, 601, 602–603
   chronic renal failure and, 477–478
   diabetes management with, 509–510, 511
   multiple sclerosis management with, 617–618, 619
   Parkinson's disease treatment with, 627–629
   prescribing, 66
   stroke management and, 580–581
   tuberculosis, 437–439
      adverse effects of, 442–443
Dysarthria, aphasia versus, 590
Dysrhythmias, 489

Ectopic pregnancy, maternal age and, 365
Education. *See also* Client teaching; Community education; Nursing education
   level of, abusive families and, 252
   school nurse and, 163–165
Education for All Handicapped Children Act of 1975,
   153
Educational neglect, 263
EEG. *See* Electroencephalogram
Elderly, 544–556
   abuse of, 256
      law and, 264
   assessment of, 549–550, 551–553
   cerebrovascular disease in, 576–592. *See also* Cere-
      brovascular disease
   confusion in, 550, 553, 554. *See also* Alzheimer's
      disease
   constipation in, 554–555
   demographics of aging and, 544
   ethical considerations and, 548–549
   falling in, 555
   health care resource utilization by, 544
   iatrogenic disorders in, 555
   life satisfaction of, 556
   loneliness in, 555–556
   long-term care of, 544
   nursing resources for, 544–547
   nutrition programs for, 140
   nutritional needs of, 147–148

Elderly (*continued*)
  research on, 549
  urinary incontinence in, 553–554
Electrocardiogram, cerebrovascular disease and, 585
Electroencephalogram
  cerebrovascular disease and, 585
  multiple sclerosis and, 621–622
Electrolyte balance, renal failure and, 480–481
Embolism, cerebral, 577
Emergency alert system, 196
Emergency care, school, 161–162
Emotional factors. *See also specific emotion*
  AIDS and, 531–534
  communication and, 40–41
  COPD and, 568–572
  coronary artery disease and, 499–500
  diabetes and, 507, 510
  hypertension and, 454
  nutrition and, 136
    old age and, 148
  renal failure and, 482–483
  rheumatoid arthritis and, 600, 605–607
  sexually transmitted disease and, 425
  stroke and, 590
Emotional support
  caring and, 25–26
  older parents and, 371–372
Empathy, abusive families and, 253
Emphysema, 560. *See also* Chronic obstructive pulmo-
    nary disease
Employers, resistance to self-care of, 32–33
Employment. *See* Occupational health; Working
    mothers
Encephalopathy
  AIDS and, 535
  aluminum, 474
Endocrine system, renal failure effects on, 472
End-stage renal disease (ESRD), 471, 472
  ethical issues in, 484
  management of, 475–476, 477–478
  nursing diagnoses and, 478–483
  risk factors for, 474
Enuresis, abused children and, 254
Environment
  asthma and, 389–390
  climate and, COPD and, 571–572
  disease ecology of agriculture and, 121–126. *See*
    also Health beliefs, environment and
  ethical decision making and, 85–88
  home care and, 190
  interpersonal, 104
  occupational, 175–179
    working mothers and, 355
  pollution in
    breast-feeding and, 340
    COPD and, 561

school, 162–163
  stroke and, 578–579
  system, 102
Enzyme deficiency, antenatal testing for, 367–368
Esophagus, alcohol abuse and, 239
ESRD. *See* End-stage renal disease
Essential hypertension, 450–453. *See also* Hyperten-
    sion
Estrogens, oral. *See also* Oral contraceptives
  postcoital contraception with, 318
Ethambutol, tuberculosis treatment with, 438
  adverse effects of, 443
Ethanol. *See also* Alcohol abuse; Alcohol intake
  chemical reaction of, 238–240
Ethical issues, 81–88
  agency policy and, 86–87
  AIDS and, 536–537
  arthritis and, 612
  cerebral palsy and, 395–396
  client behaviors and, 85
  COPD and, 572–573
  coronary artery disease and, 501
  decision making and, 84, 548
  degenerative neuromuscular diseases and, 634
  diabetes and, 518–519
  dilemmas in, 82
  end-stage renal disease and, 484
  external environments and, 85
  hypertension and, 466–467
  individualism and, 81
  internal environments and, 84–85
  legal issues versus, 81
  older adults and, 548–549
  professional standards and, 85–86
  public health and, 82
  resource allocation, 83
  respect and, 83–84
  self-determination and, 82–83
  sexually transmitted disease and, 427–428
  stroke and, 591–592
  substance abuse and, 247
  third-party payers and, 87–88
  tuberculosis and, 444–445
Ethionamide, tuberculosis treatment with, 439
Ethnonursing, 42
Eustress, 204
Evaluation, 7–8. *See also* Peer review
  AIDS and, 535–536
  Alzheimer's disease and, 633
  communication in, 39
  COPD and, 572
  coronary artery disease and, 500–501
  diabetes and, 517–518
  hypertension and, 466
  multiple sclerosis and, 624
  nutrition and, 137

Parkinson's disease and, 630
renal failure and, 483–484
research versus, 55
rheumatoid arthritis and, 608
sexually transmitted disease and, 427
stroke and, 591
substance abuse and, 245–246
tuberculosis and, 444
Exercise. *See also* Activity(ies)
COPD and, 567–568
coronary artery disease and, 490, 492, 497–499
diabetes management and, 510
hypertension and, 461
rheumatoid arthritis and, 604–605
stress and, 358
Expanded Food and Nutrition Education Program, 140
Eye(s)
diabetes and, 509, 513–514
hypertension and, 453
Eye tests, 160

Fallopian tubes
blockage of, 370
ligation of, 325
Falls, older adults and, 555
Family(ies)
abuse in, 250–264. *See also* Abusive families
adoption and, 378. *See also* Adoption
chronically ill child(ren) and, 381–396. *See also* Chronically ill child(ren)
coping of
AIDS and, 533–534
Alzheimer's disease and, 632–633
chemotherapy and, 292
multiple sclerosis and, 623–624
Parkinson's disease and, 630
rheumatoid arthritis and, 605–606, 607
stroke and, 590
counseling of, COPD and, 571
divorce and, 375–377. *See also* Divorce
education of, cancer nursing and, 294
grieving, SIDS and, 401–402. *See also* Sudden infant death syndrome
home care and, 190, 195, 197
older parents in, 363–372. *See also* Parent(s), older
remarriage and, 377–378
self-care concept and, 30–31
sexually transmitted disease and, 426
stepparenting and, 377–378
working mothers in, 350–360. *See also* Working mothers
Family day care, 353
Family development, phases of, 258–259
Family planning, 312–325
barrier methods in, 321–323

breast-feeding and, 339
failure rates of, 315
intrauterine devices in, 318–321
natural methods of, 323–324
older parents and, 363–372. *See also* Parent(s), older
oral contraceptives in, 312–317. *See also* Oral contraceptives
postcoital contraceptives in, 317–318
progestin injections in, 318
spermicides in, 322
sterilization in, 324–325
unreliable methods of, 324
Fat, hypertension and, 454
Fat intake, 141
coronary artery disease and, 490
Father. *See also* Parent(s)
age of, 366
role of, breast-feeding and, 339
Father-daughter incest, 252
Fatigue
breast-feeding and, 335–336, 344
COPD and, 567
Fear
AIDS and, 531–532
COPD and, 568–570
coronary artery disease and, 499–500
grief and, 227–228
renal failure and, 483
Federal laws, school health and, 153
Federal nutrition programs, 140–141
Feedback loop, 103
Feet, diabetes and, 513
Fein v. Permanente Medical Group, 69
Female infertility, 370
Ferrous sulfate, renal failure and, 473
Fertility, age and, 369–370
Fertility awareness, 323–324, 325
Fertilization, in vitro, 370
Fetal alcohol syndrome, 237, 239–240
Fetoscopy, 368
Fibrous ankylosis, 596
Fluid intake, stroke and, 588
Fluid volume, renal failure and, 479–480
Folacin, recommended daily allowances of, 143
Folate deficiency, alcohol abuse and, 239
Folic acid, renal failure and, 481
Food. *See also* Diet; Nutrition
cultural meanings of, 123–124
solid, when to start, 338
Food diary, 135
Food frequencies, 135
Food Stamp Program, 140
Formula, infant, supplemental, 336–337
Foster care, abusive families and, 262

Gag reflex, stroke and, 587–588
Gastrointestinal system. *See also* Bowel disturbances
chemotherapy and, 289
elderly and, 552
Gastroparesis, autonomic, diabetes and, 508
Gay men, AIDS and, 524, 534
Gender
antenatal identification of, 367
COPD and, 562
coronary artery disease and, 490
divorce impact on children and, 376
osteoarthritis and, 609
rheumatoid arthritis and, 597
Gene mutations, parental age and, 366
General adaptation syndrome, 206
Genetic counseling, 369
Genetics
capacity for caring and, 23
COPD and, 561
coronary artery disease and, 490, 492, 493
diabetes and, 506
stroke and, 578
Genital herpes, 415–416
diagnosis of, 424
treatment of, 420
Genital warts, treatment of, 421
Genitourinary system. *See also* Urinary *entries*
chemotherapy and, 290
elderly and, 551
stroke and, 588–589
substance abuse and, 243
Genitourinary tuberculosis, 434
Gerontological nursing, 544–547. *See also* Elderly
Gerontological Society of America (GSA), 547
Giardiasis, 415
treatment of, 420
Glucose intolerance. *See also* Diabetes
classification of, 505
Glucose tolerance test, oral, 505–506
Glycosylated hemoglobin, 513
Goal(s)
crisis intervention, 220
hypertension and, 460
reestablishment of, abusive families and, 262–263
system, 102
Goal-directed care, 6
Gold compounds, arthritis treatment with, 601, 602–603
Gonorrhea, 416–417
diagnosis of, 424
treatment of, 419
Granuloma inguinale, treatment of, 420–421
Grief, 226–234
abnormal, 229–230
adolescence and, 231–232
AIDS and, 534

assessment of, 233
body image loss and, 232
children and, 230–231
chronic, 230
chronically ill child and, 381, 384–385. *See also* Chronically ill child(ren)
delayed, 229
divorce and, 232–233
inhibited, 229–230
intervention in, 233–234
loss and, 227–228
normal phases of, 228–229, 230
ripple effect and, 228
self-understanding and, 234
SIDS and, 401–402
GSA (Gerontological Society of America), 547
Guidelines for the Investigative Functions of Nurses, 91
Gynecological system, substance abuse and, 243

Hallucinogens, 241
Handicapped child(ren). *See* Chronically ill child(ren)
Hazards, occupational, 175
Headache, hypertension and, 452
Health agencies, 177. *See also* Agency *entries; specific type*
Health belief model, 460
Health beliefs, 120–131
environment and, 121–126
Chinese, 124
cultural meanings of food and, 123–124
deficiency diseases and, 123
hunger and, 123
malaria and, 122
native Americans and, 124–125
nutrition and, 122–123
schistosomiasis and, 122
smallpox and, 125
maternity and, 126–128
sociocultural context and, 128–131
Health care costs, 11
Health care delivery, changes in, 12
Health care settings, 8–9. *See also specific setting, e.g.,* Home care
capacity for caring and, 24–25
self-care feasibility and, 33–34
Health care system, 101–104
Health deviation self-care requisites, 29
Health education. *See also* Client teaching; Nursing education
school nurse and, 163–165
Health maintenance, home care and, 196
Health PAC, 178
Health practices, stress management and, 209
Health professionals. *See* Professional *entries; specific type*

Health team
    communication within, 45
    nutrition, 137–138
Hearing testing, 160–161
Heart. *See also* Cardiac function; Cardiovascular system; Coronary artery disease
    alcohol abuse and, 239
    inflammation surrounding, renal failure and, 473–474
Heart failure, congestive, 489
Heat therapy, rheumatoid arthritis and, 600, 601
Heberden's nodes, 610
Hematinics, chronic renal failure and, 477
Hematocrit, stroke and, 578
Hematologic system, renal failure effects on, 472
Hematopoietic system, chemotherapy and, 288
Hemianopsia, 589
Hemiplegia, stroke and, 581–582, 587
    self-care and, 588
Hemodialysis, 476
    activity intolerance and, 482
    electrolyte balance and, 480
Hemoglobin, glycosylated, 513
Hemorrhage, pregnancy and, maternal age and, 365
Hemorrhagic stroke, 577
Henderson, Virginia, self-care concept of, 27–28
Heparin, stroke and, 580
Hepatotoxicity, chemotherapy and, 289
Heredity
    capacity for caring and, 23
    COPD and, 561
    coronary artery disease and, 490, 492, 493
    diabetes and, 506
    stroke and, 578
Heroin, 240
Herpes simplex, 415–416
    diagnosis of, 424
    treatment of, 420
Hexosaminidase A, deficiency of, antenatal testing for, 367–368
High-density lipoprotein, coronary artery disease and, 489
High-level wellness, community, 112, 118
HIV. *See* Human immunodeficiency virus
Holistic care, 6
Holistic Nursing, 22
Home apnea monitoring, SIDS prevention and, 401
Home blood glucose monitoring, 510–511
Home care, 184–197
    abusive families and, 261
    client rights in, 195
    components of, 185–186
    definition of, 185–186
    documentation in, 191–192
    future of, 194–195
    levels of, 186

    nurse's role in, 195–197
    past and present of, 184–185
    quality assurance in, 194
    reimbursement issues in, 192–194
    standards of, 186–191
        agency, 186–187
        agency selection and, 187, 188
        external changes and, 187, 189
        individual, 187
        internal changes and, 189–191
Home health agencies, number of, 185
Home Health Agency Survey Report, 187
Home health aides, 185
Homemaker/attendant care, 186
Homemakers, stresses of, 356–357
Homonymous hemianopsia, 589
Homosexual men, AIDS and, 524, 534
Hospice, 185–186
Hospitals. *See also* Institutions
    nursing care in, abuse victims and, 260–261
    nursing education development in, 10
Human immunodeficiency virus (HIV), 523–524. *See also* Acquired immunodeficiency syndrome
    antibody to, screening for, 528
    natural history of, 525, 526
    nervous system effects of, 524
    nonsexual exposure to, 527
    transmission of, 524–525
Humanistic values, 24
Humoral control, hypertension and, 449, 450
Hunger, 123
Hydantoin derivatives, cerebrovascular disease treatment and, 581
Hydrochloroquine sulfate (Plaquenil), arthritis treatment with, 601, 603
Hypercalcemia, renal failure and, 480–481
Hyperglycemia. *See* Diabetes
Hyperkalemia, renal failure and, 480
Hyperosmolar hyperglycemic nonketotic coma, 508
Hyperosmotic agents, stroke and, 580
Hypersensitivity. *See* Allergy
Hypertension, 448–467
    classification of, 448
    clinical manifestations of, 452–453
    complications of, 453
    coronary artery disease and, 489
    determinants of, 449, 450
    early intervention in, prevention and screening for, 454–457
    essential, 450–453
    ethical and legal issues in, 466–467
    food and drugs implicated in, 451
    humoral control and, 449, 450
    intravascular volume autoregulation and, 449
    nursing care and, 457–466
        assessment in, 457–458

Hypertension (*continued*)
    diet and, 460–461
    drug therapy and, 462–463, 464–465
    evaluation in, 466
    implementation in, 459–466
    noncompliance and, 463, 465–466
    nursing diagnoses in, 458–459
    planning in, 459–466
    self-care and, 459–460
    self-monitoring and, 461–462
    stress management and, 461, 462
    weight reduction methods and, 461
  prevalence of, 448–449
  pulmonary, COPD and, 560
  renal failure and, 474
  risk factors for, 453–454
  secondary, 449–450, 451
  stroke and, 453, 578, 579
  sympathetic nervous system and, 449
Hypervolemia, renal failure and, 479
Hypoglycemia, 508
Hypoglycemic agents, oral, 509–510
Hypokalemia, renal failure and, 480
Hypomenorrhea, oral contraceptives and, 314–315
Hypoventilation, COPD and, 565–567
Hypovolemia, renal failure and, 479, 480

Iatrogenic disorders, older adults and, 555
IDDM (insulin-dependent diabetes mellitus), 506. *See also* Diabetes
Illness. *See also specific illness*
  chronic. *See also* Chronically ill child(ren)
    adaptation to, 507, 510
  crisis intervention and, 222
  disease and, sociocultural context of, 128–129
  nutrition and, 148–149
  occupational, 173
  social, 129–130
  terminal, adolescence and, 232
  therapy for, home care and, 196
Immunization. *See* Vaccine(s)
Immunodeficiency, acquired. *See* Acquired immunodeficiency syndrome (AIDS)
Immunological properties, breast-feeding and, 330–331
Immunosuppressive drugs
  arthritis treatment with, 601, 603
  multiple sclerosis treatment with, 618
Implementation, 7
  abusive families and, 257, 259–262
  AIDS and, 531–535
  Alzheimer's disease and, 632–633
  communication in, 38–39
  COPD and, 563–572
  coronary artery disease and, 494–500
  diabetes and, 514–517

hypertension and, 459–466
multiple sclerosis and, 622–624
nutrition and, 137
osteoarthritis and, 611–612
Parkinson's disease and, 629–630
rheumatoid arthritis and, 600–608
sexually transmitted disease and, 423–427
stroke and, 587–591
substance abuse and, 244–245
tuberculosis and, 441–443
Impotence. *See* Sexual dysfunction
In vitro fertilization, 370
Inborn errors of metabolism, antenatal testing for, 367–368
Incest, 252–253
Incontinence, urinary
  older adults and, 553–554
  stroke and, 588–589
Individualistic ethics, 81–82
Individualized care, 6
Industrial hygienists, 175. *See also* Occupational health
Infancy. *See also* Child(ren)
  cerebral palsy prevention in, 391
  gonorrhea in, 416
  home care and, 186
  nutrition in, 145–146. *See also* Breast-feeding
  risks in, maternal age and, 365–366
  sudden death in, 399–407. *See also* Sudden infant death syndrome
Infertility
  age and, 369–370
  gonorrhea and, 416
Information systems, quality assurance and, 60
Informed consent, 75–78
INH (isoniazid), 438, 440, 442
Institutions
  capacity for caring and, 24–25
  nursing research support by, 92
  primary nursing impact on, 14–15
  resistance to self-care of, 32–33
  systems approach to, 101–104
Insulin deficiency, 506
Insulin-dependent diabetes mellitus (IDDM), 506. *See also* Diabetes
Insulin reaction, 508
Insulin resistance, 506–507
Insulin therapy, 510, 511
Insurance. *See also* Third-party payers
  negligence and, 75
Integrator, responsibilities of, gerontological nursing and, 547
Integumentary system
  chemotherapy and, 288
  diabetes and, 513
  elderly and, 551

renal failure and, 473, 482
stroke and, 587
substance abuse and, 243
Intensive level of care, 186
Intermediate level of care, 186
Intermittent positive-pressure breathing (IPPB), 567
Interpersonal climate, 104
Interpersonal relationship(s)
AIDS and, 533
cancer nursing and, 296, 300–305
COPD and, 571–572
male-female, maternal employment and, 351
nursing as, 21. *See also* Nurse-client relationship
stress management and, 209
Interpersonal resolution strategy, self-assessment of,
cancer nursing and, 303
Intervention. *See* Implementation; *specific intervention; specific problem*
Intrauterine devices, 318–321
Intravascular clotting, COPD and, 561
Intravascular volume, autoregulation of, hypertension
and, 449
Intravenous drug abuse, AIDS and, 246–247, 524,
527
Inverted nipples, breast-feeding and, 336
Iodine, recommended daily allowances of, 143
IPPB (intermittent positive-pressure breathing), 567
Iron, recommended daily allowances of, 143
pregnancy and, 144
Iron supplements, renal failure and, 473
Isoniazid
adverse effects of, 442
tuberculosis prophylaxis with, 440
tuberculosis treatment with, 438
IUDs, 318–321

Joint Commission on Accreditation of Healthcare Organizations (JCAHO), 48–49
home care standards and, 187
standards for nursing services of, 54
Joints, arthritis and. *See* Arthritis
Journals, nursing research, 93

Kanamycin, tuberculosis treatment with, 439
Kaposi's sarcoma, AIDS and, 525
Keith-Wagner-Barker scale, 453
Ketoacidosis, diabetic, 508
Kidney. *See* Renal *entries*
Kirk v. Michael Reese Hospital, 76
Knowledge, communication and, 39–40
Knowledge deficit(s)
chemotherapy and, 293
diabetes and, 515
HIV and, 535
hypertension and, 459–463

sexually transmitted disease and, 425
stroke and, 590–591
Kohlberg's moral reasoning stages, 84–85
Korotkoff sounds, 456
Korsakoff's syndrome, 238
Kwashiorkor, 123

Labor. *See also* Childbirth
prolonged, older woman and, 365
Laboratory studies, home care and, 186
Lact-Aid, 342, 343
Lactation, 332. *See also* Breast-feeding
diet during, 335
Lateral thinking, 8
Law, 65–67
abusive families and, 263–264
AIDS and, 536–537
school health and, 153
Laxatives, chronic renal failure and, 477–478
Learning, barriers to, 515
Legal responsibilities, 65–78
cerebral palsy and, 395–396
coronary artery disease and, 501
decision-making model and, 65–69
diabetes and, 518–519
ethical issues versus, 81
hypertension and, 466–467
informed consent and, 75–78
malpractice and, 69–73
professional negligence and, 73–75
sexually transmitted disease and, 427
stroke and, 591–592
substance abuse and, 247
tuberculosis and, 444–445
Legislation, 65–66
occupational health and, 176–177
Leininger's caring constructs, 19
Let-down reflex, 332–333
Levodopa, Parkinson's disease treatment with, 627–628
LGV (lymphogranuloma venereum), treatment of, 420
Licensure
home care agency, 187
regulations and, 67
Life cycle, nutrition and, 142–148
adolescence and, 146–147
infancy and, 145–146
old age and, 147–148
pregnancy and, 143–145
Life processes, wellness and, 22
Life satisfaction, older adults and, 556
Life transitions, anticipated, crises of, 217
Lipid level
coronary artery disease and, 489–490
hypertension and, 454

Lipid level (*continued*)
  reduction of, 491–492
  stroke and, 578
Listening, communication and, 43
Litigation, 66–67
Liver, alcohol abuse and, 239, 243–244
Living will, 76–78
Loneliness. *See also* Social isolation
  older adults and, 555–556
Long-term care
  Alzheimer's disease and, 633
  older adults and, 544, 545
Loop diuretics, side effects of, 464
Loss. *See also* Grief
  of body image, 232, 233
  children and, 230–231
  implications of, 226–227
  ripple effect in, 228
  types of, 227
Low-birth-weight babies
  breast-feeding of, 342, 343
  maternal age and, 365–366
Low-density lipoprotein, coronary artery disease and,
  489–490
Lower extremities, diabetes and, 513
Lumbar puncture, cerebrovascular disease and, 585–
  586
Lungs. *See* Pulmonary *entries*; Respiratory system
Lymphadenopathy, AIDS and, 525
Lymphogranuloma venereum, treatment of, 420

Magnesium, recommended daily allowances of, 143
Maintenance level of care, 186
Malaria, 122
Male-female relationships, maternal employment and,
  351
Male infertility, 370
Mallory-Weiss syndrome, 239
Malpractice, 69–73
Maltreatment, 263. *See also* Abusive families
Manganese, Parkinson's disease and, 627
Mannitol, stroke and, 580
Mantoux test, 434–435
Marasmus, 123
Marfan's syndrome, paternal age and, 366
Marihuana, 241
Marital counseling, SIDS and, 405–406
Marital relationship, maternal employment and, 351
Marital strife
  abusive families and, 251
  chronically ill child(ren) and, 385
Marker Model, 52
Maslow's hierarchy of needs, 514
Mastitis, breast-feeding and, 335

Maternal age, 363–364
  infant risks and, 365–366
  pregnancy risks and, 364–365
Maternal fatigue, breast-feeding and, 335–336, 344
Maternal-infant bonding, breast-feeding and, 331
Maternal mortality, age and, 364
Maternal nutrition, breast-feeding and, 335
Maternity, sociocultural context of, 126
Mayerhoff's major ingredients of caring, 19
Meals-on-Wheels, 186
Mediation, 99
  divorce, 376
Medic Alert ID, 518
Medicaid, 11
  home care and, 193
Medical diagnosis, home care and, 190
Medical equipment, home care and, 186
Medical model
  nursing model versus, gerontological nursing and,
    546
  occupational health nursing and, 172–173
  self-care model versus, 31, 32
Medical social service, home care and, 185
Medicare, 11
  home care and, 184, 192–193
Medications. *See* Drugs
Meditation, stress management and, 211
Medroxyprogesterone acetate, 318
Memory loss, Alzheimer's disease and, 632
Menstrual cycle, oral contraceptives and, 314–315
Mental status
  home care and, 190
  multiple sclerosis and, 620–621
  substance abuse and, 243
Metabolic acidosis, renal failure and, 480
Metabolic system, renal failure effects on, 472
Metabolism, inborn errors of, antenatal testing for,
  367–368
Methylxanthines, 390, 565–566
Mifepristone (RU 486), postcoital contraception with,
  318
Miliary tuberculosis, 434
Milk, lack of, breast-feeding and, 344
Milk-ejection reflex, 332–333
Minerals, recommended daily allowances of, 142–143
Miscarriage, maternal age and, 365
Mobility
  rheumatoid arthritis and, 604–605
  stroke and, 587
Molluscum contagiosum, treatment of, 421
Moniliasis, treatment of, 420
Moral reasoning, 84–85. *See also* Ethical issues
Moralizing, abusive families and, 251
"Morning-after" pill, 317–318
Mortality. *See* Death
Motherhood. *See also* Maternal *entries*; Parent(s)

sociocultural context of, 126
work/social schedule and, breast-feeding and, 341
Motherhood mandate, 354–355
Mourning. *See* Grief
Mouth, diabetes and, 513
Mucositis rating scale, 283
Multiple births
  breast-feeding and, 342–343
  maternal age and, 369
Multiple sclerosis, 616–624
  assessment of, 618–622
  evaluation and, 624
  family coping with, 623–624
  implementation and, 622–624
  incidence of, 616–617
  management of, 617–618, 619
  nursing diagnoses and, 622
  pathophysiology of, 617, 618
  planning and, 622–624
  risk factors for, 617
  self-care and, 622
  self-esteem and, 622–623
  sleep disturbances and, 624
  social isolation and, 624
  urinary elimination and, 623
Musculoskeletal system. *See also* Arthritis
  cerebral palsy and, 395
  elderly and, 552
  multiple sclerosis and, 620
  renal failure effects on, 473
  substance abuse and, 243
Mycobacteria, 432–433
Myocardial infarction, 488–489
  sexual dysfunction after, 499

Naloxone, 246
Narcotic antagonists, 246
Nasal prongs, 567
National Association for Home Care (NAHC), 185
National Center on Child Abuse and Neglect, 250
National Diabetes Data Group, 505
National gerontological nursing organizations, 547
National Institute of Occupational Safety and Health (NIOSH), 173, 176
National League for Nursing (NLN), home care standards of, 186–187
National Multiple Sclerosis Society, 618
National Organization for Women (NOW), 12
National School Health Project, 154
National School Lunch and Breakfast programs, 140
Native Americans, disease ecology and, 124–125
"Nature versus nurture" debate, 23
Nausea, chemotherapy and, 289
Needs
  cancer patient, 269, 272
  communication and, 41–42

community, 117
  hierarchy of, 514
Neglect, 263. *See also* Abusive families
Negligence, 73–77
  malpractice versus, 69–70
  standard of care and, 70–72
Negotiation, 98–101
  communication and, 44
  control versus, 99
  hypertension control and, 467
  primary nursing role and, 104–106
  suggestions for, 99–101
Neisseria gonorrhoeae. See Gonorrhea
Nephropathy, diabetic, 509
Nerve conduction velocity studies, 513
Nervous system
  alcohol abuse and, 238–239
  chemotherapy and, 290
  elderly and, 552
  HIV effect on, 524
  renal failure effects on, 473
  substance abuse and, 238–239, 243
  sympathetic, hypertension and, 449
Neurogenic bladder, diabetes and, 508
Neurological impulses, transmission of, 626
Neuromuscular disease, 616–635
  Alzheimer's disease, 630–634. *See also* Alzheimer's disease
  ethical issues in, 634
  multiple sclerosis, 616–624. *See also* Multiple sclerosis
  Parkinson's disease, 624–630. *See also* Parkinson's disease
Neuropathy
  chronic renal failure and, 474
  diabetic, 508
  isoniazid and, 442
Niacin, recommended daily allowances of, 143
NIDDM (non-insulin-dependent diabetes mellitus), 506–507. *See also* Diabetes
Nightingale, Florence, 9–10, 27
  quality assurance and, 48
NIOSH (National Institute of Occupational Safety and Health), 173, 176
Nipple(s)
  anatomy of, 332
  complications of, breast-feeding and, 344
  inverted, breast-feeding and, 336
Nipple shields, 336
Nitrates, angina pectoris and, 498
Noncompliance
  antihypertensive therapy and, 463, 465–466
  antituberculosis chemotherapy and, 443–444
  coronary artery disease and, 494–497, 499
  diabetes and, 515–517, 519

Noncompliance (*continued*)
  to no-smoking requirement and COPD, 564–565
  sociocultural context of, 129–130
Nongonococcal urethritis, treatment of, 421
Non-insulin-dependent diabetes mellitus (NIDDM),
    506–507. *See also* Diabetes
Nonsteroidal anti-inflammatory drugs (NSAIDs), 601,
    602
Nontherapeutic Interpersonal Nurse Behavior Cycle,
    300
Nootropics, Alzheimer's disease and, 632
Norepinephrine, hypertension and, 452
Norethindrone enanthate, 318
Noristerat, 318
Notes on Nursing, 27
NSAIDs (nonsteroidal anti-inflammatory drugs), 601,
    602
Nurse(s), 11
  stresses of, 357. *See also* Professional stress
Nurse administrators, nursing research support by, 92
Nurse practice acts, 65–67
Nurse-client collaboration, 7, 43–44
Nurse-client relationship
  abusive families and, 253–254
  cancer and, 296, 300–305. *See also* Cancer nursing
  caring and, 20–21
  communication in, 37. *See also* Communication
  crisis intervention and, 220
  home care and, 197
  STD care and, 422
Nurses Environmental Health Watch, 178
Nursing
  as commitment to action, 21
  core versus trim of, 20
  as interpersonal relationship, 21
  as process, 20–21
  purpose of, 21–22
Nursing audit, 49
Nursing care subsystems, 104, 105
Nursing diagnosis, 7
  abusive families and, 256–257
  AIDS and, 531
  Alzheimer's disease and, 632
  cancer stages and, 274
  cancer therapy methods and, 275
  cancer types and extent and, 275
  COPD and, 563
  coronary artery disease and, 494
  diabetes and, 514
  home care and, 190, 192
  hypertension and, 458–459
  multiple sclerosis and, 622
  osteoarthritis and, 611
  Parkinson's disease and, 629
  renal failure and, 478–483
  rheumatoid arthritis and, 600

  sexually transmitted disease and, 423
  stroke and, 586
  substance abuse and, 244
  tuberculosis and, 440–441
Nursing education
  development of, 10
  gerontological nursing in, 544–545
  school health preparation in, 155–156
  socialization process in, 14
Nursing homes, 544, 545
  Alzheimer's disease and, 633
Nursing leaders, gerontological, development of, 546–
    547
Nursing model(s)
  differences in, 32
  medical model versus, gerontological nursing and,
    546
  occupational health nursing and, 171–172
Nursing practice. *See* Practice models
  standards of. *See* Standards of nursing practice
Nursing process. *See also specific step*
  abusive families and, 253–263. *See also* Abusive
    families
  community assessment and, 112
  steps in, 7–8
  thinking and, 8
Nursing systems
  self-care and, 29–30
  SIDS families and, 406–407
Nutrient intake, calculation of, 135
Nutrition, 134–149. *See also* Diet
  abused child and, 254
  AIDS and, 529–530, 534
  COPD and, 568
  coronary artery disease and, 491–492
  developmental needs for, 142–148
    adolescence and, 146–147
    infancy and, 145–146. *See also* Breast-feeding
    old age and, 147–148
    pregnancy and, 143–145
  environment and, impact of agriculture on, 122–
    124
  intervention in, 138–141
  maternal, breast-feeding and, 335
  Parkinson's disease and, 629
  renal failure and, 481–482
  status of, determination of, 134–138
  stroke and, 587–588
  therapeutic needs for, health deviation and, 148–
    149
  universal needs for, 141–143
Nutrition health team, 137–138
Nutritional support services, home care and, 186
Nutritionist, role of, 138

Obesity
  adult, breast-fed infants and, 330

coronary artery disease and, 490
hypertension and, 454, 461
Occupational health, 169–181
  business versus health conflict and, 169–170
  common programs for, 180
  environment and, 175–179
    community resources in, 177–178
    legal and political factors in, 176–177
    management-labor relationship in, 175–176
    physical, 175
    sociocultural, 178–179
  future directions of, 181
  knowledge versus skills and, 170, 171
  medical model and, 172–173
  need for nursing services in, 169
  nursing in, 179–181
    accountability and, 180
    collaboration and, 180–181
    confidentiality and, 180
    informal and formal authority and, 179–180
  nursing model and, 171–172
  osteoarthritis and, 609
  Parkinson's disease and, 627
  worker as person and, 170–171
  worker model and, 173–175
Occupational history form, 174
Occupational Safety and Health Act of 1970, 176–177
Occupational therapy, home care and, 185
"Office hypertension," 453
Old tuberculin (OT), 434
Older adults, 544–556. *See also* Elderly
Older Americans Act, nutrition programs in, 140
Ophthalmology. *See* Eye *entries*
Opiates, overdose of, 246
Oral contraceptives, 312–317
  breast-feeding and, 339
  contraindications to, 315–316
  effectiveness of, 312, 314, 315
  health benefits of, 314
  mode of action of, 312
  patient teaching and, 316–317
  postcoital use of, 317–318
  side effects of, 314–315
  stroke and, 579
Oral glucose tolerance test (OGTT), 505–506
Oral hypoglycemic agents, 509–510
Orem's self-care concept, 28–30
  assessment and, 30
  SIDS families and, 406–407
Organ donation, 475
OSHA, 176–177
Osteoarthritis, 608–612
  alteration in comfort and, 612
  assessment of, 611
  clinical manifestations of, 609–610
  drugs used in, 602–603

early intervention in, 610–611
  etiology of, 608–609
  implementation and, 611–612
  nursing diagnosis and, 611
  pathophysiology of, 609, 610
  planning and, 611–612
  risk factors for, 609
Outcome criteria, evaluation of, 7
  abusive families and, 262–263
Outcome standards, 53
Outcome Standards for Cancer Nursing Practice, 296, 297–299
Outreach, abusive families and, 253–254
Overdose, 246
Overweight
  adult, breast-fed infants and, 330
  coronary artery disease and, 490
  hypertension and, 454, 461
Ovulation, failure of, 370
Oxygen therapy, COPD and, 566–567
Oxytocin, lactation and, 332

Pain. *See also* Discomfort
  chest. *See* Angina pectoris
  loss and, 226–227
  osteoarthritis and, 609–610
  rheumatoid arthritis and, 596, 600–601, 604
Pancreatitis, alcohol abuse and, 239
Panwarfarin (warfarin), 580
Para-aminosalicylic acid, tuberculosis treatment with, 439
Paralysis, stroke and, 581–582, 587
  self-care and, 588
Parent(s). *See also* Family(ies); Father; Maternal *entries*; Motherhood
  adoptive, 378
  child-care sharing and, 353
  of chronically ill child(ren), 385
  grieving, SIDS and, 401–402. *See also* Sudden infant death syndrome
  older, 363–372
    adoption and, 370
    antenatal testing and, 366–369
    definition of, 363–364
    developmental implications of, 371
    father as, 366
    genetic counseling and, 369
    infant risks and, 365–366
    infertility and, 369–370
    multiple births and, 369
    nursing care for, 371–372
    pregnancy risks and, 364–365
Parenthood. *See also* Stepparenting
  as crisis state, 372
Parkinson's disease, 624–630
  activity intolerance in, 629

Parkinson's disease (*continued*)
    assessment of, 629
    constipation in, 629–630
    evaluation and, 630
    family coping with, 630
    impaired communication in, 630
    implementation and, 629–630
    incidence of, 624–625
    management of, 627–629
    nursing diagnoses and, 629
    nutritional deficits in, 629
    pathophysiology of, 625
    planning and, 629–630
    prevention of, 627
    risk factors for, 625
    safety deficits in, 629
Parlodel (bromocriptine mesylate), 628
Paternalism, COPD and, 572–573
Patient(s). *See* Client(s)
Payment. *See* Costs; Reimbursement; *specific type*
Pediatric home care, 186
Pediatrics. *See* Child(ren); Infancy
Pediculosis, treatment of, 420
Peer pressure, school health education and, 164–165
Peer review, 51
Peer-support group
    divorced parents and, 377
    hypertension and, 459–460
    professional stress management and, 212
    smoking cessation, 565
    stress management and, 462
    weight reduction and, 461
Pelvic inflammatory disease (PID)
    gonorrhea and, 416
    IUDs and, 318
Penkava v. Kasbohn, 70
Pentobarbital, abuse of, 240
Peptic ulcer, COPD and, 561
Perception
    AIDS and altered, 535
    stroke and altered, 589
    styles of, 41
Pericarditis, renal failure and, 473–474
Peripheral adrenergic antagonists, side effects of, 465
Peripheral neuropathy
    chronic renal failure and, 474
    diabetes and, 508
    isoniazid and, 442
Peripheral vascular disease, diabetes and, 509
Peritoneal dialysis, 476
    electrolyte balance and, 480
Persantine (dipyridamole), antiplatelet effect of, 581
Persistent generalized lymphadenopathy (PGL), AIDS and, 525
Personal philosophy, capacity for caring and, 22–23

Personality
    communication and, 41
    hypertension and, 454
Phosphate binding agents, chronic renal failure and, 478
Phosphate level, renal failure and, 481
Phosphorus, recommended daily allowances of, 143
Physical examination
    cerebrovascular disease and, 582, 585
    coronary artery disease and, 494, 495
    HIV infection and, 530–531
    hypertension and, 458
    multiple sclerosis and, 619–620
    rheumatoid arthritis and, 599
    school, 159–160
    substance abuse and, 243
    workplace, 172–173
Physical mobility
    rheumatoid arthritis and, 604–605
    stroke and, 587
Physical therapy
    home care and, 185
    rheumatoid arthritis and, 604–605
Pick's disease, 553
PID. *See* Pelvic inflammatory disease
Placebo response, 130–131
Placenta previa, 365
Planning, 7
    AIDS and, 531–535
    Alzheimer's disease and, 632–633
    COPD and, 563–572
    coronary artery disease and, 494–500
    diabetes and, 514–517
    hypertension and, 459–466
    multiple sclerosis and, 622–624
    nutrition and, 137
    osteoarthritis and, 611–612
    Parkinson's disease and, 629–630
    rheumatoid arthritis and, 600–608
    sexually transmitted disease and, 423–427
    stroke and, 587–591
    substance abuse and, 244–245
    tuberculosis and, 441–443
Plaquenil (hydrochloroquine sulfate), arthritis treatment with, 601, 603
Pneumocystis pneumonia, AIDS and, 525
Pneumothorax
    rheumatoid arthritis and, 597
    spontaneous, COPD and, 561
Policy
    ethics and, 86–87
    written, 67–68
Pollution
    breast-feeding and, 340
    COPD and, 561
Positive attitudes, caring and, 26

Postcoital contraception, 317–318
    IUD and, 321
Postpartum hemorrhage, 365
Postural drainage, COPD and, 565
Potassium level, renal failure and, 480
Potassium-sparing agents, side effects of, 464
Poverty levels, occupational health nursing and, 178–179
Power, information and, 12
PPD (purified protein derivative of tuberculin), 434, 435
Practice models, 10–11, 13–14
Prechemotherapy Nursing Assessment Model, 288–293
Prednisone, asthma and, 391
Pregnancy
    age and. *See* Parent(s), older
    AIDS and, 528
    alcohol consumption during, 237, 239–240
    herpes simplex and, 415–416
    nutrition and, 143–145
    occupational stresses and, 355, 356
    prevention of. *See* Family planning
    risks of, older woman and, 364–365
    taboos surrounding, 127–128
Premature babies
    breast-feeding of, 342, 343
    maternal age and, 365–366
Prenatal testing, 366–369
Prescribing drugs, 66
Primary Health/Preventing Disease: Objectives for the Nation, 164
Primary nursing
    characteristics of, 6–7
    institutional impact of, 14–15
    philosophy of, 6
    practice models for, 10–11, 13–14
    settings for, 8–9
Private insurance. *See* Third-party payers
Problem solving
    American Nurses' Association quality assurance model and, 57–58
    crisis intervention and, 221
Process, nursing as, 20–21. *See also* Nursing process
Process standards, 53
Professional development, stages of, 14
Professional groups, occupational health and, 178
Professional negligence. *See* Negligence
Professional resistance, self-care framework and, 31–32
Professional standards. *See* Ethical issues; Standard of care; Standards of nursing practice
Professional stress, 211–212, 357
    cancer nursing and, 280
Professionals, quality care and, 50–51
Progestasert-T, 318, 319

Progestins. *See also* Oral contraceptives
    high dose, postcoital contraception with, 318
    injections of, long-acting, 318
Project Health PACT, 164
Prospective payment, 61–62. *See also* Diagnostic-related groups
    home care and, 194
Protein, recommended daily allowances of, 142
    AIDS and, 534
    pregnancy and, 144
    renal failure and, 481
Psychiatric emergencies, 217
Psychological factors. *See also* Grief; Stress
    aging and, 550
    AIDS and, 531–534
    COPD and, 568–572
    coronary artery disease and, 499–500
    diabetes and, 507, 510
    hypertension and, 454
    nutrition and, 136
        old age and, 148
    renal failure and, 482–483
    rheumatoid arthritis and, 600, 605–607
    sexually transmitted disease and, 425
    stroke and, 590
Psychological support
    caring and, 25–26
    older parents and, 371–372
Psychopathology, crises reflecting, 217
Psychosocial assessment
    chemotherapy and, 291–293
    hypertension and, 458
Psychotropic drugs, Alzheimer's disease and, 632
Public health ethic, 82
Public health nursing, self-care and, 27
Public Law 93-247, 250
Public Law 94-142, 153
Pulmonary disease, chronic obstructive. *See* Chronic obstructive pulmonary disease
Pulmonary emboli, COPD and, 561
Pulmonary fibrosis, chemotherapy and, 289
Pulmonary hypertension, COPD and, 560
Pulmonary system. *See also* Respiratory system
    renal failure effects on, 472
Pulmonary tuberculosis. *See also* Tuberculosis
    signs and symptoms of, 434
Pulse rate, activity and, COPD and, 567
Purified protein derivative of tuberculin (PPD), 434, 435
Pyrazinamide, tuberculosis treatment with, 438
    adverse effects of, 443

Quality appraisal process, 56–57
Quality assurance, 48–62
    accountability and, 51. *See also* Accountability
    ANA model of, 57–60

Quality assurance (*continued*)
    change and, 60–61
    definitions of, 51–52
    development of, 48–50
    establishing programs for, 58–60
    historical perspective on, 48
    home care and, 194
    improvement and, 60–61
    information systems and, 60
    peer review and, 51
    professionals and, 50–51
    prospective payment plans and, 61–62
    quality care indicators and, 54–55
    review and evaluation in, 55
    standards of nursing practice and, 52–60. *See also*
        Standards of nursing practice

Race
    COPD and, 562
    coronary artery disease and, 490
Radiation therapy, 275
Rapport, establishment of, crisis intervention and,
        220
Rauwolfia alkaloids, side effects of, 465
Recommended daily dietary allowances, 142–143
    AIDS and, 534
Referral
    cancer nursing and, 294–295
    divorced parents and, 377
    home care and, 190, 196–197
    older parents and, 372
Regulations, 67
Rehabilitation
    of SIDS families, 407
    stroke, 581–582
Rehabilitative Potential Patient Classification System,
        191–192
Reimbursement, home care and, 189, 192–194
Relationships. *See* Interpersonal relationship(s);
        Nurse-client relationship
Relaxation, stress management and, 209–211
Religiosity, abusive families and, 251
Remarriage, 377–378
Renal disease, end-stage, 471, 472
    ethical issues in, 484
    management of, 475–476
    nursing diagnoses and, 478–483
    risk factors for, 474
Renal failure
    chronic, 471
        assessment of, 476, 478, 479
        causes of, 475
        complications of, 473–474
        early intervention in, 474–475
        evaluation and, 483–484

        management of, 475–476, 477–478
        nursing diagnoses and, 478–483
        stages of, 472
    frank, 472
    systemic effects of, 472–473
Renal function, 471
    chemotherapy and, 290
    hypertension and, 453
Renal hypertension, clinical manifestations of, 452
Renal insufficiency, 472
Renal reserve, diminished, 472
Renal transplantation, 475
Renin, plasma, hypertension and, 451–452
Renin-angiotensin-aldosterone system, 450
Reproductive system. *See also* Family planning; Preg-
        nancy
    elderly and, 551–552
    occupational stress effects on, 355, 356
Research, 91–96
    access to, 92–94
    conducting, 94–95
    critiquing, 95
    educational level and, 91
    evaluation versus, 55
    gerontological nursing, 549
    journals reporting, 93
    neuromuscular diseases and, 633–634
    process of
        commitment to, 92
        elements of, 94
    school nursing issues for, 165
    support of, 92
    use of, facilitating the, 95–96
    value of, 92
Research Appraisal Checklist, 95
Resources
    allocation of, 83
        COPD and, 573
    cancer nursing and, 294
    community
        occupational health nursing and, 177–178
        SIDS and, 407
    supply of, 103
    utilization of, older adults and, 544
Respect, ethics and, 83–84
Respiratory acidosis, COPD and, 565
Respiratory failure, COPD and acute, 560
Respiratory system. *See also* Pulmonary *entries*
    chemotherapy and, 289
    elderly and, 551
    infections of, COPD and, 561
    stroke and, 587
    substance abuse and, 243
Rest
    AIDS and, 535
    asthma and, 388–389

breast-feeding and, 335–336
rheumatoid arthritis and, 605
Retina, hypertension and, 453
Retinopathy, diabetic, 509
Retrovir (zidovudine), AIDS and, 529
Rheumatoid arthritis, 595–608
    alteration in comfort and, 600–601, 604
    clinical manifestations of, 596–597
    coping with, 605–606
    drugs used in, 601, 602–603
    etiology of, 595–596
    mobility impairment in, 604–605
    pathophysiology of, 596, 597
    risk factors for, 597–598
    sexual dysfunction and, 607–608
Riboflavin, recommended daily allowances of, 143
Rifampin, tuberculosis treatment with, 438
    adverse effects of, 442–443
Risk management, 49
Role alterations
    AIDS and, 533
    rheumatoid arthritis and, 606
Role conflict, working mothers and, 355–356
Rooting reflex, 334
RU 486 (mifepristone), postcoital contraception with, 318
Rules, regulations and, 67

Safe sex, 525, 527
Safety
    Parkinson's disease and, 629
    school environment and, 162–163
Safety engineers, occupational health nursing and, 175
Salicylates, arthritis treatment with, 601
Salt intake, 141
    hypertension and, 460–461
Scabies, treatment of, 421
Schistosomiasis, 122
School health, 152–165
    definition of, 152
    factors affecting, 152–153
    nurse's role in
        children's health needs and, 157
        counseling and, 162
        current status of, 155–157
        emergency care and, 161–162
        environment and, 162–163
        health appraisal and, 158–161
        health education and, 163–165
        historical perspective on, 154–155
        primary health care provision and, 162
        special services and, 162
    program components of, 152

research issues in, 165
role of, 154
School health program, 152
School nursing, 152
Scoliosis, screening for, 161
Scratch test, 387–388
Screening programs, school, 160–161
Secobarbital, abuse of, 240
Seizures, cerebral palsy and, 395
Self-actualization, older adults and, 556
Self-assessment, cancer nursing and, 302, 303
Self-care, 26–34
    assessment and, 30–31
    child(ren) with asthma and, 388–391
    child(ren) with cerebral palsy and, 392–395
    client resistance and, 31
    communication model for, 38. *See also* Communication
    concept within nursing of, 27–28
    crisis intervention and, 223–224
    Henderson's concept of, 27–28
    hypertension and, 459–460
    multiple sclerosis and, 622
    nutrition and, 134–149. *See also* Nutrition
    Orem's concept of, 28–30
        SIDS families and, 406–407
    professional resistance and, 31–32
    promotion of, 31, 33
    rheumatoid arthritis and, 605
    sexually transmitted disease and, 425–427
    stroke and, 588
Self-care deficit, 29
Self-care model, traditional model versus, 31, 32
Self-care philosophy, beliefs compatible with, 23
Self-concept
    communication and, 39
    rheumatoid arthritis and, 606–607
Self-determination, 82–83
Self-esteem
    multiple sclerosis and, 622–623
    older adults and, 555–556
Self-examination, cancer detection and, 268
Self-growth, capacity for caring and, 23
Self-help groups. *See* Support groups
Self-help movement, 12
Self-image
    AIDS and, 532
    crisis and, 221–222
Self-monitoring
    blood glucose, 510–511
    blood pressure, 461–462
Self-pay, home care and, 193–194
Self-reliance, crisis and, 222
Self-understanding, grief and, 234
Senescent arthritis, 608–612

Sensory-perceptual alterations
  AIDS and, 535
  stroke and, 589
Sensory status
  elderly and, 552–553
  multiple sclerosis and, 620
Sermcheif v. Gonzales, 66
Settings. *See also* Health care settings; *specific setting,*
      e.g., Home care
  capacity for caring and, 24–25
  self-care feasibility and, 33–34
Sex
  antenatal identification of, 367
  COPD and, 562
  coronary artery disease and, 490
  divorce impact on children and, 376
  osteoarthritis and, 609
  rheumatoid arthritis and, 597
Sexual abuse, 252–253
  nursing care after, 261
Sexual activity, safe, AIDS and, 525, 527
Sexual dysfunction
  coronary artery disease and, 499
  diabetes and, 508
  rheumatoid arthritis and, 607–608
Sexually transmitted diseases, 414–428. *See also* Ac-
      quired immunodeficiency syndrome (AIDS)
  amebiasis, 415
  assessment of, 422–423, 424
  early intervention in, 417
  emotional responses to, 425
  ethical and legal issues in, 427–428
  evaluation and, 427
  giardiasis, 415
  gonorrhea, 416–417
  herpes simplex, 415–416
  knowledge deficit and, 425
  management of, 417–418, 419–421
  nursing care for, 418, 422
  nursing diagnosis and, 423
  potential transmission of, 423–425
  self-care deficits and, 425–427
  statistics on, 414
  syphilis, 416
  trichomoniasis, 415
Shift rotation, stress and, 357
Siblings
  of chronically ill child(ren), 385–386
  counseling of, SIDS and, 404–405
SIDS. *See* Sudden infant death syndrome
Single working mothers, 356
Skeletal system. *See* Musculoskeletal system
Skin. *See* Integumentary system
Skin fold thickness, 137
Sleep apnea
  home monitoring of, 401
  SIDS and, 399

Sleep disorders
  abused children and, 254
  AIDS and, 535
  alcohol abuse and, 239
  COPD and, 568
  multiple sclerosis and, 624
  renal failure and, 482
Smallpox, 125
Smoking
  angina and, 497
  COPD and, 561, 562, 564–565
  coronary artery disease and, 489, 491
  stroke and, 579
Snellen test, 160
Social illness, 129–130
Social interaction, cerebral palsy and, 393
Social isolation
  AIDS and, 532–533
  COPD and, 571–572
  multiple sclerosis and, 624
  older adults and, 555–556
Social Security Act, 12
Socialization process, 14
Sociocultural factors
  aging and, 550
  communication and, 42–43
  health beliefs and, 120–131. *See also* Health beliefs
  motherhood and, 126
  occupational health and, 178–179
Socioeconomic factors
  COPD and, 562
  hypertension and, 449
  nutrition and, 136
    old age and, 148
Sodium intake, 141
  hypertension and, 460–461
Solid foods, when to start, 338
Sorrow. *See also* Grief
  chronic, 384
Spatial perception, stroke and, 589
Speech pathology
  home care and, 185
  stroke and, 589–590
Sperm count, 370
Spermicides, 322
Sphygmomanometer, 455–456
Spontaneous abortion, maternal age and, 365
Spousal relationship, maternal employment and, 351
Spouse abuse, 256, 261
  law and, 263–264
Sputum specimens, tuberculosis and, 436
Standard of care. *See also* Ethical issues
  breach in, 71–72
  existence of, 70–71
Standards of nursing practice, 52, 69
  ANA, 53–54, 57–60

gerontological nursing and, 545–546
    research and, 92
compliance with, measurement of, 55–60
criteria and, 55–56
data source selection and, 56
home care and, 186–187
JCAHO, 54
purpose of, 52
quality appraisal process and, 56–57
time frame and, 56
types of, 52–53
State laws, school health and, 153
State licensure, home care agency, 187
STDs. *See* Sexually transmitted diseases
Stepparenting, 377–378
Sterilization, 324–325
Stool softeners, chronic renal failure and, 477
Stools, breast-fed baby and, 338
Streptomycin, tuberculosis treatment with, 438
    adverse effects of, 443
Stress, 204–213. *See also* Anxiety
    adoption and, 378
    assessment of, 207–208
    cancer patients and, 269, 272
    coronary artery disease and, 490, 492
    crisis and, 216, 217
    definitions of, 204
    exercise and, 358
    homemakers and, 356–357
    hypertension and, 454, 461
    intervention in, 208–211
    professional, 211–212, 357
        cancer nursing and, 280
    renal failure and, 482–483
    response to, 206–207
        determinants of, 207
    rheumatoid arthritis and, 605
    sources of, 205–206
    working mothers and, 354–357
Stroke, 576–592. *See also* Cerebrovascular disease
Structural approach, community assessment and, 113
Structural-organizational routines, 103–104
Structure standards, 52–53
Substance abuse, 237–248
    abusive families and, 252
    assessment of, 242–243
    barbiturates and, 240–241
    cocaine and, 240
    complications of, 246–247
    diagnostic tests for, 243–244
    early intervention in, 241–242
    ethanol and, 238–240
    ethical issues in, 247
    etiology of, 238
    evaluation in, 245–246
    hallucinogens and, 241

heroin and, 240
    implementation and, 244–245
    intravenous, AIDS and, 246–247, 524, 527
    legal issues in, 247
    marihuana and, 241
    nursing diagnoses and, 244
    planning and, 244–245
    prevention of, 241–242
    risk factors for, 241
Sudden infant death syndrome, 399–407
    community resources for, 407
    etiological theories of, 399
    family rehabilitation after, 407
    incidence of, 399
    prevention of
        primary, 400–401
        secondary, 401–402
        tertiary, 402
    risk factors for, 400
    sleep apnea and, 399
    treatment and, 402–407
Suicidal client, crisis intervention and, 217–219
Sulfonylureas, oral, 509–510
Supervisory neglect, 263
Superwoman syndrome, 356
Supplemental Food Program for Women, Infants, and
        Children (WIC), 140
Support groups
    divorced parents and, 377
    hypertension and, 459–460
    professional stress and, 212
    smoking cessation, 565
    stress management and, 462
    weight reduction and, 461
Support system
    abusive families and, 251
    crisis intervention and, 221
    older parents and, 371–372
    SIDS and, 407
Surgery
    arthritis treatment with, 604
    cancer and, 275
    crisis intervention and, 222
    grief and, 233
Sympathetic nervous system, hypertension and, 449
Sympathomimetics
    COPD and, 565–566
    hypertension and, 451
Synovial fluid, rheumatoid arthritis diagnosis and, 599
Synovitis, 596
Syphilis, 416
    diagnosis of, 424
    treatment of, 419
Systems approach, 101–104
    community assessment and, 112–113

Taboos, pregnancy and, 127–128
Tax Equity and Fiscal Responsibility Act of 1981, home care and, 184
Taxonomy, 128
Tay-Sachs disease, 367–368
Teaching. *See* Client teaching; Nursing education
Team members
  communication with, 45
  nutrition and, 137–138
Team nursing, 10
  model for, 13
Technologies, home care and, 189
Teenagers. *See* Adolescence
Teething, breast-feeding and, 337
Telephone reassurance services, 186
Temper tantrums, abused children and, 254
Terminal illness. *See also specific illness, e.g.,* Cancer
  adolescence and, 232
Testicular cancer, early detection of, 268
Tetrahydrocannabinol (THC), 241
Theophylline, 390, 565–566
Thiamine, recommended daily allowances of, 143
Thiazides, side effects of, 464
Third-party payers
  ethical decision making and, 87–88
  home care and, 193
Thrombocytopenia, chemotherapy and, 288
Thrombosis
  cerebrovascular accident and, 577
  myocardial infarction and, 488–489
Thumb-sucking, abused children and, 254
TIA, 578. *See also* Cerebrovascular disease
Tinea cruris, treatment of, 421
Tobacco
  angina and, 497
  COPD and, 561, 562, 564–565
  coronary artery disease and, 489, 491
  stroke and, 579
Toilet training, cerebral palsy and, 393
Toxemia, maternal age and, 365
Transfusion, AIDS transmission by, 524
Transient ischemic attack (TIA), 578. *See also* Cerebrovascular disease
Transplantation, renal, 475
Transportation, home care and, 186
Traumatic stress, crises resulting from, 217
Tremors, Parkinson's disease and, 625
Treponema pallidum, 416
Trichomoniasis, 415
  treatment of, 420
Tricyclic antidepressants, Parkinson's disease and, 625, 627
Triglycerides, coronary artery disease and, 490
Triplets, breast-feeding of, 342–343
Trisomy 13, 367

Trisomy 21, 367
  maternal age and, 366
Trust, establishment of, crisis intervention and, 220
Tubal ligation, 325
Tuberculin skin test, 434–435
Tuberculosis, 430–445
  adverse medication effects and, 442–443, 444
  anxiety and, 441, 444
  diagnosis of, 434–437
  ethical and legal issues in, 444–445
  etiology of, 432–433
  evaluation and, 444
  management of, 437–439
    noncompliance and, 443–444
  new infection potential and, 441–442, 444
  nursing diagnoses and, 440–441
  pathophysiology of, 433–434
  prevention of, 439–440
  transmission of, 433
Tumors, AIDS and, 525
Twins
  breast-feeding of, 342–343
  incidence of, maternal age and, 369
Type A Behavior and Your Heart, 490
Tyramine-containing foods, 451

Ulcer, peptic, COPD and, 561
Unemployment rates, occupational health nursing and, 178
Universal self-care requisites, 28–29
  cerebral palsy and, 392–395
Universality, in ethics, 83
Uremia, 471. *See also* Renal failure
  skin integrity and, 482
Urethritis, nongonococcal, treatment of, 421
Urinary dysfunction, multiple sclerosis and, 623
Urinary incontinence
  older adults and, 553–554
  stroke and, 588–589
Urinary tract infections, renal failure and, 475
Utter v. United Hospital Center, 67–68

Vaccine(s)
  AIDS, 528
  BCG, tuberculosis and, 434
Vaginal spermicides, 322
Vaginal sponge, 323
Vaginitis, nonspecific, treatment of, 421
Variola major, 125
Vascular system
  diabetes and, 509
  hypertension and, 453
Vasectomy, 325
Vasodilators
  antiplatelet, 580–581
  side effects of, 465

Vasomotor control, hypertension and, 451
Vegetarians, breast-feeding and, 335
Venereal diseases. *See* Sexually transmitted diseases
Venturi masks, 567
Verbal negativism, cancer and, 277
Vertical thinking, 8
Very low density lipoprotein, 489–490
Vial of Life Program, 196
Villers v. Puritan-Bennett Corporation, 73
Violence. *See* Abusive families
Vision screening, school, 160
Visiting nurses, 10, 184. *See also* Home care
Vitamin D, 481
Vitamins, recommended daily allowances of, 142–143
Volume alterations, renal failure and, 479–480
Volunteers, home care and, 186
Vomiting, chemotherapy and, 289

Wald, Lillian, 10, 184
Warfarin (Coumadin, Panwarfarin), 580
Warts, genital, treatment of, 421
Watson's carative factors, 19–20
Weaning, 341
Weight, 136–137, 141. *See also* Obesity
Weight reduction, hypertension and, 461
Wellness. *See also* High-level wellness
   life processes and, 22
   occupational health programs for, 180
Wernicke's syndrome, 238
Western cultures. *See also* Sociocultural factors
   childbirth imagery in, 126–127
White Lung Association, 178
Wholeness concept, community assessment and, 113
WIC program, 140
Witch's milk, 338
Withdrawal
   alcohol, 247
   heroin, 240

Women
   abused, 256, 261
   law and, 263–264
   infertility of, 370
   working, motherhood and, 352. *See also* Working mothers
Women's movement, 12–13
   abusive families and, 252
Women's Occupational Health Resource Center, 178
Worker model, occupational health nursing and, 173–175
Working mothers, 350–360
   child care and, 352–354
   child welfare and, 351–352
   family life and, 350–351
   homemakers, 356–357
   issues affecting, 352
   male-female relationships and, 351
   nurses as, 357
   nursing care planning for, 357–359
   schedule of, breast-feeding and, 341
   single, 356
   stress and, 354–357
Workplace. *See* Occupational health
Written policies, 67–68

Xanthochromia, 585
X-ray examination
   cerebrovascular disease and, 585
   chest, tuberculosis and, 436

Yasko's symptom management model, 294
Young adults, death in, leading causes of, 158

Zidovudine (Retrovir), AIDS and, 529
Zinc, recommended daily allowances of, 143
Zubrod scale, modified, 291